pediatric NURSING

caring for children

pediatric NURSING
caring for children

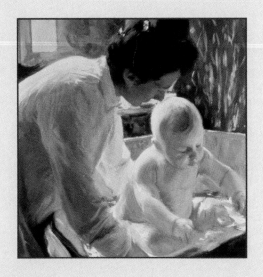

Jane Ball, RN, CPNP, DrPH
Director
Emergency Medical Services for Children National Resource Center
Children's National Medical Center
Washington, DC

Ruth Bindler, RNC, MS
Associate Professor
Intercollegiate Center for Nursing Education
Washington State University
Spokane, Washington

Appleton & Lange
Stamford, Connecticut

Notice: The authors and the publisher of this volume have taken care to make certain that the doses of drugs and schedules of treatment are correct and compatible with the standards generally accepted at the time of publication. Nevertheless, as new information becomes available, changes in treatment and in the use of drugs become necessary. The reader is advised to carefully consult the instruction and information material included in the package insert of each drug, therapeutic agent, or equipment before carrying out interventions. This advice is especially important when using new or infrequently used drugs or performing techniques or skills that are not routine. The authors and publisher disclaim any liability, loss, injury, or damage incurred as a consequence, directly or indirectly, or the use and application of any of the contents of this volume.

www.appletonlange.com

99 00 01 02 03 / 10 9 8 7 6 5 4 3 2 1

Prentice Hall International (UK) Limited, *London*
Prentice Hall of Australia Pty. Limited, *Sydney*
Prentice Hall Canada, Inc., *Toronto*
Prentice Hall Hispanoamericana, S.A., *Mexico*
Prentice Hall of India Private Limited, *New Delhi*
Prentice Hall of Japan, Inc., *Tokyo*
Simon & Schuster Asia Pte. Ltd., *Singapore*
Editora Prentice Hall do Brasil Ltda., *Rio de Janeiro*
Prentice Hall, *Upper Saddle River, New Jersey*
ISBN: 0-8385-8123-4

Cover art: *In the Morning* by Boris Mihajlovic Kustodiev (1878–1927) Russian State Museum, St. Petersburg, Russia

Library of Congress Cataloging-in-Publication Data

Pediatric nursing : caring for children / Jane Ball, Ruth Bindler, — 2nd ed.
    p. cm.
  Includes bibliographical references and index.
  ISBN 0-8385-8123-4 (case : alk. paper)
  1. Pediatric nursing.   I. Ball, Jane.   II. Bindler, Ruth McGillis.
    [DNLM: 1. Pediatric Nursing—methods. 2. Nursing Care—in infancy & childhood. 3. Nursing Assessment—methods.   WY 159P3733 1999]
RJ245.P4414   1999
610.73′62—dc21
DNLM/DLC
for Library of Congress   98-25825
                                       CIP

Acquisitions Editor: David P. Carroll
Development Editor: Donna Frassetto
Production Editors: Karen Davis, Angela Dion
Art Coordinator: Eve Siegel
Designer: Libby Schmitz

ISBN 0-8385-8123-4

9 780838 581230

90000

PRINTED IN THE UNITED STATES OF AMERICA

BRIEF CONTENTS

DETAILED CONTENTS

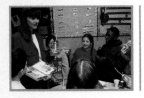

1. NURSE'S ROLE IN CARE OF THE ILL AND INJURED CHILD / 2
Hospital, Community Settings, and Home

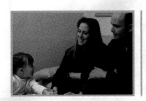

2. GROWTH AND DEVELOPMENT / 26

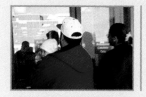

3. PEDIATRIC ASSESSMENT / 92

4. NURSING CONSIDERATIONS FOR THE HOSPITALIZED CHILD / 176

5. NURSING CONSIDERATIONS FOR THE CHILD IN THE COMMUNITY / 208

6. THE CHILD WITH A LIFE-THREATENING ILLNESS OR INJURY / 238

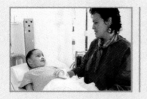

7. PAIN ASSESSMENT AND MANAGEMENT / 264

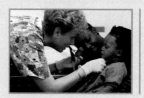

8. ALTERATIONS IN FLUID, ELECTROLYTE, AND ACID–BASE BALANCE / 288

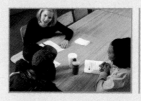

9. ALTERATIONS IN IMMUNE FUNCTION / 338

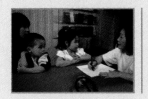

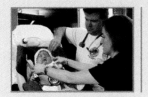

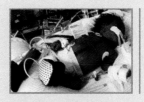

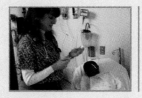

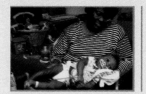

14. ALTERATIONS IN CELLULAR
   GROWTH / 540

15. ALTERATIONS IN GASTROINTESTINAL
FUNCTION / 590

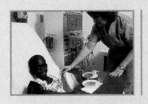

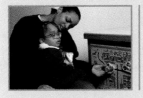

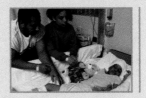

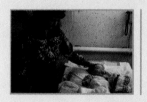

19. ALTERATIONS IN MUSCULOSKELETAL FUNCTION / 816

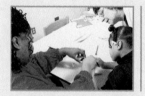

20. ALTERATIONS IN ENDOCRINE FUNCTION / 862

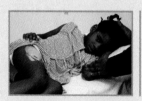

21. ALTERATIONS IN SKIN INTEGRITY / 906

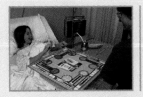

22. ALTERATIONS IN PSYCHOSOCIAL FUNCTION / 952

CONTRIBUTORS TO THE FIRST EDITION

Jan Dalby, RNC, MS
Maternal Clinical Nurse Specialist
St. Mary's Hospital
Richmond, Virginia
(Alterations in Genitourinary Function)

Linda Felver, RN, PhD
Associate Professor
School of Nursing
Oregon Health Sciences University
Portland, Oregon
(Alterations in Fluid & Electrolyte and Acid–Base
Balance)

Darla Gowan, RN, FNPC, MN
Nurse Practitioner
Kosair Children's Hospital
Louisville, Kentucky
(Alterations in Skin Integrity)

Joyce Griffin, RN, OCN, PhD
Associate Professor
Nursing Department
Fairleigh Dickinson University
Teaneck, New Jersey
(Alterations in Immune Function, Alterations in
Hematologic Function)

Sandra Jo Hammer, RN, MPH, MSN
Nursing Supervisor
Children's Hospital, Oakland
Oakland, California
(Infectious and Communicable Diseases)

Linda Kinrade, RN, PNP, MN
Professor
Department of Nursing
California State University
Hayward, California
(Alterations in Cellular Growth)

Katherine Morris, RN, CPNP
Nurse Clinician
Department of Pediatrics
Endocrinology & Metabolic Division
Medical College of Virginia
Richmond, Virginia
(Alterations in Endocrine Function)

Jean Moss, ARNP, CPNP, PhD
Pediatric Nurse Practitioner
Planned Parenthood
Child Health Clinic
Claremont, New Hampshire
(Alterations in Eye, Ear, Nose, and Throat Function)

Ruth Novitt-Schumacher, RN, MSN
Pediatric Nursing Instructor
Maternal Child Department
University of Illinois at Chicago
Chicago, Illinois
(Alterations in Gastrointestinal Function)

Nan Peterson, RN, MS
Clinical Nurse Manager
Pediatric Intensive Care Program
University of Wisconsin Children's Hospital
Madison, Wisconsin
(The Child with a Life-Threatening Illness or Injury)

Deborah Thomas, RNC, MSN
Pediatric Psychiatric Clinical Nurse Specialist
Kosair Children's Hospital
Louisville, Kentucky
(Alterations in Psychosocial Function)

Robert Wayner, MD
Neurosurgeon
The Neurological Clinic
Laguna Hills, California
(Alterations in Neurologic Function)

Amy Weigelt-Leinweber, RN, BSN
Staff Nurse
Shriners Hospital for Crippled Children
Spokane, Washington
(Alterations in Musculoskeletal Function)

Marcia Wellington, RN, MS
Education Coordinator
Emergency Trauma Services
Children's National Medical Center
Washington, D.C.
(Alterations in Neurologic Function, Atlas of Pediatric
Procedures)

Rosemarie C. Westberg, RN, MSN
Associate Professor, Nursing
Northern Virginia Community College
Annandale, Virginia
(Alterations in Respiratory Function)

REVIEWERS

Ann Bello, RN, MA
Norwalk Community Technical College
Norwalk, Connecticut

Linda Connolly, RN, MS
Department of Nursing
Orange County Community College
Middletown, New York

Sherry Cyza
Nursing Instructor
Department of Nursing
Normandale Community College
Bloomington, Minnesota

Neysa Dobson, RN
Laboratory Preceptor Director
Intercollegiate Center for Nursing Education
Spokane, Washington

Mary Ann Dono, RN, MA, CPN
St. Vincent's Hospital
School of Nursing
New York, New York

Karen Frank, RNC, MS
Pediatric Clinical Specialist
Johns Hopkins Hospital
Baltimore, Maryland

Robert Greenburg, OD
Pediatric Vision System Specialist
Reston, Virginia

Cathleen M. Homrighaus, RN, MSN
Faculty, Pediatric Nursing
St. Joseph's Hospital Health Center
School of Nursing
Syracuse, New York

Jane Jech, RN
Inver Hills Community College
Inver Hills, Minnesota

Tracy Kelly, MSN, CPNP
Pediatric Nursing Practitioner
Pediatric Bone Marrow Program
Duke University
Durham, North Carolina

Sue Khanna, MEd, EdD, RNC
Assistant Professor
School of Nursing
Pace University
Pleasantville, New York

Susan Millet, PhD, CSNP
Certified Family Nurse Practitioner
Presbyterian Medical Group
Albuquerque, New Mexico

Debra Ann Mills, MSN, RN
Salt Lake Community College
Salt Lake City, Utah

R. Stanley Robinson, MD
Ophthalmologist
Rockwood Clinic
Spokane, Washington

Marilyn M. Rowe, RN, BSN, MA
Nursing Faculty
South Suburban College
South Holland, Illinois

Vicki Sandin, RN, MS
Pediatric Oncology Nurse
Deaconess Hospital
Spokane, Washington

Karen Sullivan, RN, MSN
Community Health Nurse
The Montgomery County, Maryland School Health
   Services
Rockville, Maryland

PREFACE

Practicing nurses must make tough choices every day in caring for children. Faculty members must make similar choices in preparing students to practice safely and effectively in the clinical setting. What information must students have to provide care? What is the best way to prepare students to practice in the acute care clinical setting? What is the best way for students to learn how to help families care for their children in the home and community?

The goal of the second edition of this book is to provide a core of pediatric nursing content that will prepare students for practice and provide them with the tools for continued self-learning. Students who learn which questions to ask, when to ask them, how to evaluate the answers, and how to think from a multidisciplinary perspective in any clinical setting will be able to learn and adapt to a changing health care system.

This book reflects how students learn and apply information and is structured to reflect clinical and academic realities.

- The first reality is that faculty have only 4 to 9 weeks to prepare students to become clinically safe pediatric nurses.
- The second reality is that pediatric health care and clinical experiences for students occur in a wide range of settings.
- The third reality is that there are defined, acceptable standards of care for specific problems.
- The fourth reality is that if students learn how to make decisions about what is important, they will be able to adapt to future changes in clinical practice.

▶ THIS BOOK REFLECTS THE REALITIES OF PEDIATRIC NURSING TODAY

The first edition of this book focused on the nursing care of children and their families in an acute care environment. In the second edition, the focus has been expanded to reflect the realities of the dramatic shift of pediatric health care out of the hospital and into ambulatory, home, and community settings. Advances in technology and practice along with efforts to control health care costs have resulted in major changes in the way in which pediatric nursing care is provided. Much acute care is now managed by families in the home after a brief hospitalization or same-day procedure. More families are providing long-term home care for children who previously would have been hospitalized for a complex health condition.

Because many graduating nurses go on to practice in acute care facilities, this edition continues to emphasize the information necessary to prepare students to work in that setting. Students who understand how to effectively care for and communicate with children and families in an acute care setting where children are extremely ill can readily transfer these skills to other nursing situations and environments.

A unique characteristic of this book continues to be the emphasis throughout of the impact that injury has on childhood mortality, hospitalizations, disability, and the general care of children. In this book, an effort is made to describe common pediatric injuries and related nursing care by body system. Injury prevention has been emphasized whereever possible.

In this edition, there is a much greater emphasis on helping parents and families care for children following discharge from the hospital, as well as in community settings—including day care, school, and managed care environments. The nurse's role in preparing a family for their child's discharge from an acute care facility is the transitional step to nursing care in the home and community. There is solid coverage of long-term management of complex health conditions as these problems are especially challenging to manage in community settings. Selected ambulatory pediatric conditions are also included because students will see these conditions in everyday life and in the hospital where these conditions are secondary to the presenting problem. Nursing actions to enhance health promotion among children are emphasized throughout the text and in the scenarios that begin each chapter.

THE BOOK IS ORGANIZED BY BODY SYSTEM, WITH THE NURSING PROCESS AS THE FRAMEWORK FOR CARE

The book is organized by body system rather than age group for several reasons: this approach makes it easier for students to find information, study, prepare for clinical experiences, and review for the National Council of State Boards of Nursing Licensure Examination (NCLEX). The key to this book is integration. No child is treated in isolation, so the emphasis throughout is on the child and family. The nursing process provides the underlying structure for the book.

SEVERAL THEMES ARE INTEGRATED THROUGHOUT THE BOOK IN THE NARRATIVE, ART, LEGENDS, LABELS, AND MARGIN NOTES

Critical thinking and problem solving, communication, cultural diversity, growth and development, assessment, and legal and ethical concerns are themes fundamental to daily nursing practice. As in the first edition, these themes continue to be interwoven through narrative, margin notes, and art, resulting in a unique, integrated presentation that engages students and makes them active participants in the material, rather than passive recipients of information. Students and faculty can therefore make use of important applied information where and when it is most appropriate.

- **Critical thinking** principles are integrated in the organization, pedagogy, writing style, and art. Students practice critical thinking and problem-solving skills in their everyday lives. Many students have not, however, learned to apply these skills to the practice of nursing. This book will help students understand how their normal curiosity and problem-solving skills can be applied to pediatric nursing. They will learn, by example, which questions to ask, when, and why.

- **Communication** is one of the most important skills that students need to learn. Effective communication is the very fiber of nursing practice. This book integrates communication skills in an applied manner where students can most benefit.

- Current demographic trends demand that nurses be culturally sensitive. **Cultural considerations,** like the other five themes, are integrated throughout the book where appropriate. Students deal with cultural diversity as part of everyday practice and need to know when and why these differences are important in the care of children. Cultural information appears in the body of the text and in the art and is highlighted in margin notes.

- Knowledge of **growth and development** and **assessment** are central to the effective practice of pediatric nursing. A separate chapter is devoted to each area. In addition, both topics are integrated where appropriate in the narrative, art, labels, and legend copy and are highlighted in the margin as applied information where necessary. This supports students' need to know relevant information associated with a specific topic or concept to help them apply theoretical information to clinical nursing practice.

- Throughout the book, **legal and ethical concerns** are provided in margin notes. This material is designed to sensitize students to thinking about the implications of what they do on a daily basis and to consider whether or not there are legal and ethical repercussions to their actions.

New to this edition are an emphasis on **research considerations** and **home and community considerations.** The relevance of nursing research to many facets of pediatric nursing care is emphasized throughout the text and in margin notes that highlight the results of specific studies. Important home or community concerns are also highlighted in the margin as applied information, supplementing the expanded focus on these settings throughout the book.

THE FOUR-COLOR TEXT AND ART PROGRAM ENHANCE LEARNING AND ENGAGE THE INSTRUCTOR AND STUDENT

The first edition of this text pioneered a unique handling of narrative, art, figure labels, and legend copy that prevented duplication of information in text and art unless there was a reason to provide additional reinforcement. Many photographs were included to prepare students for the realities of the clinical setting. We have continued this approach in the second edition. Photography continues to reinforce the focus on a child and family with a health problem or health promotion need, rather than on a problem or need that happens to be associated with a child. In this edition, many new four-color illustrations have been added to reinforce students' understanding of anatomy and physiology, and pathophysiologic processes. Line drawings superimposed over photographs enable students to learn the relationship of internal structures to surface anatomy.

The art, labeling, and legend copy continue to play an active and untraditional teaching role by engaging the student directly with strong visual images. For this reason, you will notice that sometimes labels contain descriptive and applied information. This approach ties explanations directly to the art rather than forcing the student to move back and forth between text and art. Some of the labels ask a question of the student that is then answered either in the legend or in the body of the text. This encourages students to think about what they are seeing and to test their knowledge, rather than passively absorbing information.

CHANGES TO THE SECOND EDITION

Each chapter has undergone a significant revision to update clinical information and expand related home and community care. Six new care plans are included to reflect this new focus. Several other changes will be readily apparent as you use this edition. First, each chapter has a new opening scenario to set the stage for content to be learned. A chapter on caring for the child in the community was added to address key nursing concepts for pediatric nursing care outside of the hospital setting. Home and community nursing care guidelines have been integrated throughout all elements of the book. The chapters on fluid and electrolyte balance and acid–base balance were combined into one, more focused chapter. Infectious and communicable diseases are now covered in a chapter rather than the atlas format of the first edition. In response to requests from faculty and students, the first edition's atlas of pediatric procedures has been pulled out to appear as a separate book accompanying this textbook. The *Quick Reference to Pediatric Clinical Skills* has been reformatted and expanded, enabling it to be used more easily in the clinical setting.

STUDENT AND FACULTY MATERIAL

The student resource guide has been coordinated closely with this text. It will help students improve their communication skills and will assist them in reviewing the material covered in both the text and lectures. The resource guide includes a combination of exercises that will reinforce students' critical thinking skills while helping them to learn pediatric nursing.

Faculty material includes an instructor's manual, containing additional critical thinking exercises and learning resources; a testbank of NCLEX-format questions; and a transparency package.

* * * * * * *

In this second edition, we continue to make difficult choices about what to include and how extensively to cover each topic. Our decisions in this edition continue to reflect the extensive research conducted among faculty and students prior to the writing of the first edition. At the same time, we recognize the significant changes than have taken place in pediatric health care over the past 3 to 4 years. Our emphasis is clearly on the most common problems and needs that students will see in the acute care, home, and community settings. The information presented in the book is applied and designed to make students think in the same way that they will need to think in clinical practice. The interplay between the art and text is unique, interesting, and designed to engage students and make them active participants in learning.

We are confident that this edition represents a solid core of essential information that will continue to prepare students for the changing realities of clinical practice in pediatrics.

Jane Ball
Ruth Bindler

ACKNOWLEDGMENTS

The production of any textbook is the result of a dedicated team of professionals who support the authors. This has been especially true for this second edition, which was nearly as significant an undertaking as the original creation. Appleton & Lange Senior Editor Dave Carroll and Nursing Editor-in-Chief Sally Barhydt were generous in their support, enabling us to build on the tremendous response to the first edition. It was our great fortune to have Donna Frassetto return as our developmental editor. Her editing gives the book a uniform voice. She assured consistency from chapter to chapter by tracking the content organization, illustrations, care plans, and the major themes, focusing on the total book when we could only focus on an individual chapter. Words do not come close to describing how valuable her contribution was to this edition.

Several other individuals made major contributions to the textbook. Our primary photographer, George Dodson, continues to amaze us with his ability to make children comfortable and to capture their images in all types of settings. Roy Ramsey also contributed many new photographs, which reflect his commitment to quality. The production team at Appleton & Lange worked tirelessly to build on and expand the visual appeal of the first edition. Our thanks go to Libby Schmitz, who created the new design for this edition, and to Eve Siegel, who managed the complex and multifaceted art program. Our production editor, Karen Davis, capably addressed all of the book's editing and production details with assistance from Angela Dion.

Several hospitals and other sites allowed us to photograph children in the actual settings in which they receive care. In Washington, DC, children were photographed at Lafayette Elementary School, and in several units of the Children's National Medical Center and of the Hospital for Sick Children. Special thanks to Wayne Neal, Janice LePlatte, Michael Ciarrocchi, Joan Confer, Jenny Rohrer, and Cathy Raischer for their assistance in coordinating these photo sessions. In Spokane, Washington, children were photographed in Shriners Hospital, Sacred Heart Medical Center, and Deaconess Medical Center. Our thanks to Diane Hoffman and Vicki Sandin for arranging some of these photo shoots. We are again grateful for the opportunity to use the skills laboratory at the Intercollegiate Center for Nursing Education in Spokane, Washington, and for the assistance of Neysa Dobson in providing needed equipment and verifying the appropriateness of techniques demonstrated in many photographs. Darina Green of the Head Start Center in Spokane and day care provider Linda Berna also facilitated our photographing of children. Hope Thommes of New Hope Home Care graciously arranged for us to photograph children in their homes.

We sincerely thank all the parents and children who allowed us to illustrate development, pediatric health care conditions, and nursing care with their pictures in the hospital, home, and community settings.

Finally, we must acknowledge the enduring support and sacrifices of our families. They made it possible to dedicate endless hours to writing, reviewing, and editing the chapters of this book.

GUIDE TO KEY FEATURES

CHAPTER OPENING VIGNETTES

Chapter opening scenarios provide realistic case studies that are often followed throughout the chapter. Vignettes assist in turning clinical cases into real-life depictions of children, their families, and nurses

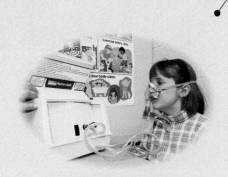

Jessica, 8 years old, is anxious because her asthma attack is getting worse. Her teacher sees that she is having trouble breathing, so she sends her to the school health office for treatment. Jessica has such severe asthma that a nebulizer is kept at school for her to use. This treatment will often relieve Jessica's symptoms and permit her to return to classes. However, in this case, the asthma attack does not respond to the treatment, and the school contacts her mother to come pick her up from school. This means another visit to the emergency department for treatment.

Jessica has had asthma since she was 2 years old and has needed to stay in the hospital for severe asthma attacks twice over the past 2 years. Fortunately, her asthma attack improves with the medications provided in the emergency department, and she can go home after a couple of hours. Jessica does not like to miss school or to worry her mother. Her mother wishes there were some way to reduce the number and severity of her asthma attacks.

What are some possible triggers of Jessica's asthma attacks at school? What measures can be taken to control her asthma on a daily basis and reduce the number of attacks? What special arrangements are needed to permit a child to receive care for asthma or another chronic situation while at school?

NURSING CONSIDERATIONS FOR THE CHILD IN THE COMMUNITY 5

"Sometimes Jessica's asthma attacks really frighten me because she struggles so hard to breathe. I don't like to send her out of class too soon, but I don't want to make her condition worse. I wish I knew what to do!"

TERMINOLOGY

- **chronic condition** A health condition that lasts or is expected to last 3 months or more
- **developmental surveillance** A continuous process of skilled observations of a child's fine and gross motor, language, and psychosocial behavior milestones through encounters during child health visits
- **disability** Impairment in one or more of five categories of function—cognition, communication, motor abilities, social abilities, or patterns of interactions
- **health supervision** The process of health promotion services, growth and development monitoring, and disease and injury prevention throughout the child's life
- **medical home** A primary care provider or regular source of health care.
- **medically fragile** Children who need skilled nursing care with or without medical equipment to support vital functions
- **screening tests** Procedures used to detect the presence of a health condition before symptoms are apparent
- **sensitivity** Screening test value stated as the percentage of children testing positive for a condition who truly have that condition.
- **specificity** Screening test value stated as the percentage of children testing negative for a condition who do not have that condition.

TERMINOLOGY

Important vocabulary terms are identified and defined at the beginning of each chapter. New terms are printed in boldface type as they are introduced within the chapter.

PARENT TEACHING GUIDELINES

Important instructions for parent teaching are included in convenient tables.

10-6 Parent Teaching: Guidelines for Evaluating Fever in Children

Call your health care provider immediately if:
- The child is under 2 months old or has a fever over 40.1°C (104.2°F).
- The child is crying inconsolably or whimpering.
- The child cries when moved or otherwise touched by the parent or other family members.
- The child is difficult to awaken.
- The child's neck is stiff.
- There are any purple spots present on the skin.
- Breathing is difficult and no better after the nose is cleared.
- The child is drooling saliva and is unable to swallow anything.
- The child has a convulsion.
- The child acts or looks very sick.

Call your health care provider within 24 hours if:
- The child is 2–4 months old (unless fever occurs within 48 hours of a DTP shot and the infant has no other serious symptoms).
- The fever is higher than 40.1°C (104.2°F) (especially if the child is under 3 years old).
- The child complains of burning or pain with urination.
- The fever has been present more than 24 hours without an obvious cause or location of infection.
- The fever went away for more than 24 hours and then returned.
- The fever has been present for more than 72 hours.

Modified from Hay, W.W., Jr., Groothuis, J.R., Hayward, A.R., & Levin, M.J. (Eds.). (1997). Current pediatric diagnosis and treatment (13th ed.). Stamford, CT: Appleton & Lange.

Care of the Child in the Health Care Setting

Nursing care of children with infectious diseases in health care settings focuses on preventing the spread of infection. Children with suspicious rashes should be isolated from other children. When possible, hard surfaces in the examining room where the child was seen should be wiped down with antiseptic solution before another child uses the room. Linens are disposed of in appropriately marked linen bags.

Nursing care for treatment of fever includes administering antipyretics, removing unnecessary clothing, and encouraging increased fluid intake. Tepid baths or sponging may be ordered when the child's temperature is greater than 40°C (104°F) while waiting for the antipyretic to work. Use water that is about 26.6°C (80°F).

Children are often admitted to the hospital for treatment of severe infections. In addition, countless numbers of **nosocomial** (hospital-acquired) **infections** occur each year. The fecal–oral and respiratory routes are the most common sources of infections in children. All items with which the infected child comes into contact are considered contaminated (linens, toys, medical equipment, etc.) Transmission-based precautions, including isolation, must be implemented to reduce exposure of other children and staff to the infectious agent. Follow your facility's standard precautions and transmission-based precautions to reduce the spread of infectious diseases to staff and other patients. Bring any questions and concerns to your hospital's infection control [?]. (Refer to the *Quick Reference to Pediatric Clinical Skills* accompanying [?]xt for more detailed information.)

RESEARCH CONSIDERATIONS

A recent study compared fever reduction in febrile children with temperatures of more than 38.9°C (102°F) when given acetaminophen alone or with a 15-minute tepid sponge bath. No significant differences were found in temperature between the two study groups over a 2-hour period. However, the children who were given sponge baths had significantly higher discomfort scores.[19]

INTEGRATION OF ART, LABELS, AND FIGURE LEGENDS

Difficult concepts are simplified by using figure labels and legends to highlight important points being illustrated.

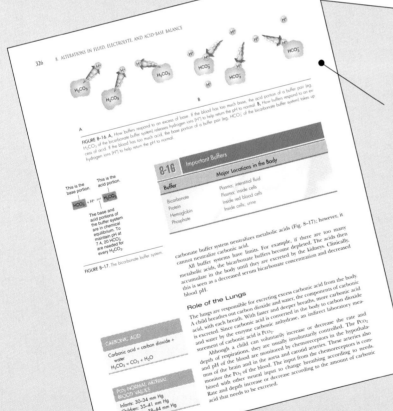

8. ALTERATIONS IN FLUID, ELECTROLYTE, AND ACID-BASE BALANCE   326

A

B

FIGURE 8-16. **A,** How buffers respond to an excess of base. If the blood has too much base, the acid portion of a buffer pair (eg, H_2CO_3) of the bicarbonate buffer system) releases hydrogen ions (H^+) to help return the pH to normal. **B,** How buffers respond to an excess of acid. If the blood has too much acid, the base portion of a buffer pair (eg, HCO_3^-) of the bicarbonate buffer system) takes up hydrogen ions (H^+) to help return the pH to normal.

This is the base portion.   This is the acid portion.

$$HCO_3^- + H^+ \rightleftharpoons H_2CO_3$$

The base and acid portions of the buffer system are in chemical equilibrium. To maintain pH at 7.4, 20 HCO_3 are needed for every H_2CO_3.

FIGURE 8-17. The bicarbonate buffer system.

8-16 Important Buffers

Buffer	Major Locations in the Body
Bicarbonate	Plasma; interstitial fluid
Protein	Plasma; inside cells
Hemoglobin	Inside red blood cells
Phosphate	Inside cells, urine

carbonate buffer system neutralizes metabolic acids (Fig. 8-17); however, it cannot neutralize carbonic acid.

All buffer systems have limits. For example, if there are too many metabolic acids, the bicarbonate buffers become depleted. The acids then accumulate in the body until they are excreted by the kidneys. Clinically, this is seen as a decreased serum bicarbonate concentration and decreased blood pH.

Role of the Lungs

The lungs are responsible for excreting excess carbonic acid from the body. A child breathes out carbon dioxide and water, the components of carbonic acid, with each breath. With faster and deeper breaths, more carbonic acid is excreted. Since carbonic acid is converted in the body to carbon dioxide and water by the enzyme carbonic anhydrase, an indirect laboratory measurement of carbonic acid is P_{CO_2}.

Although a child can voluntarily increase or decrease the rate and depth of respirations, they are usually involuntarily controlled. The P_{CO_2} and pH of the blood are monitored by chemoreceptors in the hypothalamus of the brain and in the aorta and carotid arteries. These arteries also monitor the P_{O_2} of the blood. The input from the chemoreceptors is combined with other neural input to change breathing according to needs. Rate and depth increase or decrease according to the amount of carbonic acid that needs to be excreted.

CARBONIC ACID

Carbonic acid = carbon dioxide + water
$$H_2CO_3 = CO_2 + H_2O$$

P_{CO_2} NORMAL ARTERIAL BLOOD VALUES

Infants: 30–34 mm Hg
Children: 35–41 mm Hg
Adolescents: 38–44 mm Hg

FIGURE 3–21. Cross section of the ear. The tympanic membrane normally has a triangular light reflex with the base on the nasal side pointing toward the center. The bony landmarks, the umbo and handle of malleus, are seen through the tympanic membrane.

SAFETY PRECAUTIONS

Never irrigate the ear canal if any discharge is present. Cold water should never be used for irrigation.

GROWTH & DEVELOPMENT CONSIDERATIONS

Indicators of hearing loss in an infant:
- No startle reaction to loud noises
- Does not turn toward sounds by 4 months of age
- Babbles as a young infant but does not keep babbling or develop speech sounds after 6 months of age

Indicators of hearing loss in a young child:
- No speech by 2 years of age
- Speech sounds are not distinct at appropriate ages

obstructed by cerumen or a foreign body, irrigation can be used to clean the canal.

The tympanic membrane, which separates the outer ear from the middle ear, is usually pearly gray and translucent. It reflects light, and the bones (ossicles) in the middle ear are normally visible. When the pneumatic attachment is squeezed, the tympanic membrane normally moves in and out in response to the positive and negative pressure applied (Fig. 3–21). Table 3–10 lists the abnormal findings of a tympanic membrane examination and their associated conditions.

HEARING ASSESSMENT

Hearing evaluation is important in children of all ages because hearing is essential for normal speech development and learning. Often hearing must be evaluated by inspection of the child's responses to various auditory stimuli. Hearing loss may occur at any time during early childhood as the result of birth trauma, frequent otitis media, meningitis, or antibiotics that damage cranial nerve VIII.

Use hearing and speech articulation milestones as an initial hearing screen. Select an age-appropriate method to screen hearing. When a hearing deficiency is suspected as a result of screening, the child is referred for audiometry, tympanometry, or evoked response to obtain the most accurate evaluation of hearing.

Infants and Toddlers

Select noisemakers with different frequencies, such as a rattle, bell, and tissue paper, that will attract the young child's attention. Ask the parent or an assistant to entertain the infant with a quiet toy, such as a teddy bear. Stand behind the infant, about 2 feet (60 cm) away from the infant's ear but outside the infant's field of vision, and make a soft sound

---

GROWTH AND EVALUATING DIETARY INTAKE   171

CLINICAL TIP

...e best response to deep tendon re... testing is achieved when the child ...laxed or distracted. Children often ...ipate the knee jerk and either ...m up or exaggerate the re... Making the child focus on an... ...et of muscles may provide a ...accurate response. When testing ...exes on the lower legs, have ...d press his or her hands to... ...r try to pull them apart when ...together.

NEEDED

...gth measuring device ...ate standardized ...es ...collection tools

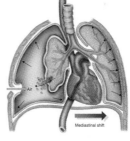

CULTURAL CONSIDERATIONS

Although growth curves have been standardized on the U.S. population, they can be used on children of different ethnic groups. Children of first- or second-generation immigrants to the United States follow patterns of growth similar to those of the children whose families have ... United States ... lower percentile.

...tes for infants, children, and adolescents by sex. Identify which percentile for weight, length or height, weight for length, and head circumference for age the child falls in. Children normally fall between the 10th and 90th percentiles for weight, length or height, and weight for length. A measurement below the 10th percentile of weight for length may indicate undernutrition, whereas a measurement over the 90th percentile for length may indicate overnutrition. Measurements of weight, length, or height below the 10th percentile may be normal in some cultural groups.

...ength intersect, mark an X on the spot where the ...the child's length or height, ...e child's age and sex. For ... Appendix A gives standardized growth

---

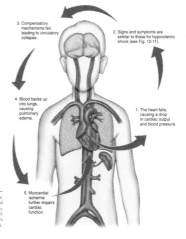

FIGURE 12-13. Obstructive shock can occur when a tension pneumothorax obstructs blood flow to and from the heart. Here, the great vessels are compressed during the mediastinal shift.

Mediastinal shift

3. Compensatory mechanisms fail, leading to circulatory collapse.

2. Signs and symptoms are similar to those for hypovolemic shock (see Fig. 12-11).

4. Blood backs up into lungs, causing pulmonary edema.

1. The heart fails, causing a drop in cardiac output and blood pressure.

5. Myocardial ischemia further impairs cardiac function.

FIGURE 12-14. When the heart fails, cardiac output and blood pressure decrease. Blood backs up into the lungs, causing pulmonary edema. Inadequate amounts of oxygen reach the myocardium, further impairing the heart's pumping action. The result is cardiogenic shock.

CARE PLANS FOR HOME AND COMMUNITY CARE

Care plans for home, school, or community care are included to demonstrate that care is provided in a variety of settings.

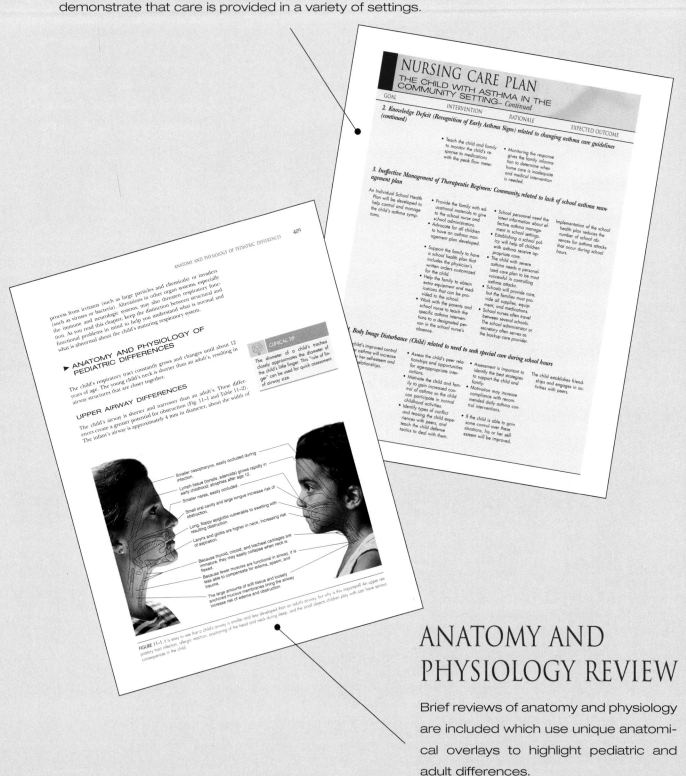

process from irritants (such as large particles and chemicals) or invaders (such as viruses or bacteria). Alterations in other organ systems, especially the immune and neurologic systems, may also threaten respiratory function. As you read this chapter, keep the distinction between structural and functional problems in mind to help you understand what is normal and what is abnormal about the child's maturing respiratory system.

▶ ANATOMY AND PHYSIOLOGY OF PEDIATRIC DIFFERENCES

The child's respiratory tract constantly grows and changes until about 12 years of age. The young child's neck is shorter than an adult's, resulting in airway structures that are closer together.

UPPER AIRWAY DIFFERENCES

The child's airway is shorter and narrower than an adult's. These differences create a greater potential for obstruction (Fig. 11–1 and Table 11–2). The infant's airway is approximately 4 mm in diameter, about the width of

CLINICAL TIP

The diameter of a child's trachea closely approximates the diameter of the child's little finger. This "rule of finger" can be used for quick assessment of airway size.

Smaller nasopharynx, easily occluded during infection.

Lymph tissue (tonsils, adenoids) grows rapidly in early childhood, atrophies after age 12.

Smaller nares, easily occluded.

Small oral cavity and large tongue increase risk of obstruction.

Long, floppy epiglottis vulnerable to swelling with resulting obstruction.

Larynx and glottis are higher in neck, increasing risk of aspiration.

Because thyroid, cricoid, and tracheal cartilages are immature, they may easily collapse when neck is flexed.

Because fewer muscles are functional in airway, it is less able to compensate for edema, spasm, and trauma.

The large amounts of soft tissue and loosely anchored mucous membranes lining the airway increase risk of edema and obstruction.

FIGURE 11–1. It is easy to see that a child's airway is smaller and less developed than an adult's airway, but why is this important? An upper respiratory tract infection, allergic reaction, positioning of the head and neck during sleep, and the small objects children play with can have serious consequences in the child.

NURSING CARE PLAN
THE CHILD WITH ASTHMA IN THE COMMUNITY SETTING— *Continued*

GOAL	INTERVENTION	RATIONALE	EXPECTED OUTCOME

2 Knowledge Deficit (Recognition of Early Asthma Signs) related to changing asthma care guidelines
(continued)

- Teach the child and family to monitor the child's response to medications with the peak flow meter.

- Monitoring the response gives the family information to determine when home care is inadequate and medical intervention is needed.

3. Ineffective Management of Therapeutic Regimen: Community, related to lack of school asthma management plan

An Individual School Health Plan will be developed to help control and manage the child's asthma symptoms.

- Provide the family with educational materials to give to the school nurse and school administrators.
- Advocate for all children to have an asthma management plan developed.
- Support the family to have a school health plan that includes the physician's written orders customized for the child.
- Help the family to obtain extra equipment and medications that can be provided to the school.
- Work with the parents and school nurse to teach the specific asthma interventions to a designated person in the school nurse's absence.

- School personnel need the latest information about effective asthma management in school settings.
- Establishing a school policy will help all children with asthma receive appropriate care.
- The child with severe asthma needs a personalized care plan to be most successful in controlling asthma attacks.
- Schools will provide care, but the families must provide all supplies, equipment, and medications.
- School nurses often travel between several schools. The school administrator or secretary often serves as the backup care provider.

Implementation of the school health plan reduces the number of school absences for asthma attacks that occur during school hours.

4. Body Image Disturbance (Child) related to need to seek special care during school hours

child's improved control ... asthma will increase ... her self-esteem and ... relationships.

- Assess the child's peer relationships and opportunities for age-appropriate interactions.
- Motivate the child and family to gain increased control of asthma so the child can participate in normal childhood activities.
- Identify types of conflict and teasing the child experiences with peers, and teach the child defense tactics to deal with them.

- Assessment is important to identify the best strategies to support the child and family.
- Motivation may increase compliance with recommended daily asthma control interventions.
- If the child is able to gain some control over these situations, his or her self-esteem will be improved.

The child establishes friendships and engages in activities with peers.

ANATOMY AND PHYSIOLOGY REVIEW

Brief reviews of anatomy and physiology are included which use unique anatomical overlays to highlight pediatric and adult differences.

NURSING CARE PLANS

pediatric
NURSING

caring for children

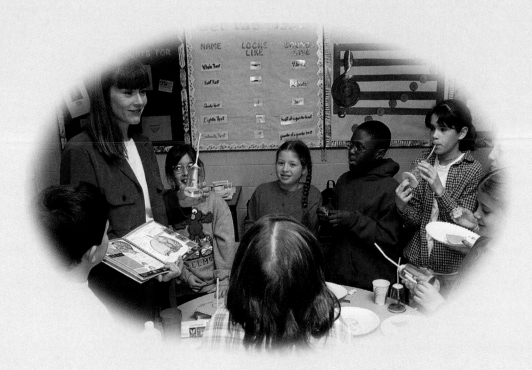

Bethany and several of her classmates have asthma. If her asthma is not kept under control, Bethany has a difficult time concentrating in school because her attention is focused on breathing. Several times over the past 2 years, she had to go to the doctor or the emergency department to obtain treatment for severe asthma attacks. These attacks caused her to miss a lot of school. Although Bethany has medications to help control her asthma, she did not always use them because she was afraid the other children would view her as "different."

The number of children with asthma in the elementary school prompted the school nurse to start an asthma club. Her purpose in starting this club was to help the children with asthma learn more about their illness and ways to control the condition. She had discovered that very few children understand how to recognize the early signs of an asthma attack. As a result, treatment often is not begun as soon as symptoms occur. Teaching the children about the condition has also enabled them to explain to peers why they sometimes have difficulty breathing and need to take medications.

Over the past few months, Bethany has learned to recognize signs of an asthma attack and when to use her inhaler. She has had to seek emergency treatment less often. She also enjoys knowing she has friends who are like her, working hard to "breathe easier."

NURSE'S ROLE IN CARE OF THE ILL AND INJURED CHILD
Hospital, Community Settings, and Home

1

"The asthma club has really helped these children become more confident in managing their asthma. It helps them to know that they have other friends with this condition."

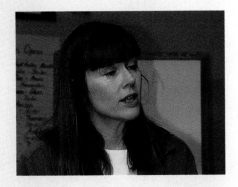

TERMINOLOGY

- **advance directives** A patient's living will or appointed durable power of attorney for health care decisions.
- **assent** Voluntary agreement to participate in a research project or to accept treatment.
- **continuity of care** An interdisciplinary process of facilitating a patient's transition between and among settings based on changing needs and available resources.
- **continuum of care** A system of care that includes each of the following elements: primary care, illness or injury prevention, acute care in the hospital, and restorative care in either the home or a rehabilitation center until patient is reintegrated into family and community.
- **critical pathways** Comprehensive interdisciplinary care plans for a specific condition that describe the sequence and timing of interventions that should result in desired patient outcomes.
- **emancipated minors** Self-supporting adolescents under 18 years of age not subject to parental control.
- **family-centered care** A philosophy of care that integrates the family's values and potential contributions in the plans for and provision of care to the child.

- **informed consent** A formal preauthorization for an invasive procedure or participation in research.
- **mature minors** Adolescents of 14 and 15 years of age who are able to understand treatment risks and who in some states can consent to or refuse treatment.
- **moral dilemma** A conflict of social values and ethical principles that support different courses of action.
- **morbidity** An illness or injury that limits activity, requires medical attention or hospitalization, or results in a chronic condition.
- **quality assurance** A process for monitoring the procedures and outcomes of care that uses indicators to measure compliance with standards of care.
- **quality improvement** The continuous study and improvement of the processes and outcomes of providing health care services to meet the needs of patients by examining the system and processes of care and service delivery.
- **risk management** A process established by a health care institution to identify, evaluate, and reduce the risk of injury to patients, staff, and visitors and thereby reduce the institution's liability.

Nurses in many settings come into contact with children who have asthma. Nurses are important members of the health care team during all phases of the **continuum of care** (a system of care that includes each of the following elements: illness or injury prevention, acute care in the hospital, and restorative care in either the home or rehabilitation center until the child is reintegrated into the family and community). In which of these roles did the school nurse help Bethany and her friends? In what other settings is pediatric nursing care provided? How many different roles for nurses can you identify for children with a health care problem throughout the continuum of care? This chapter reviews concepts important to pediatric nursing: the role of the nurse in pediatrics, the contemporary climate of pediatric health care, and legal and ethical issues.

What is the role of the nurse in working with children who have asthma? In how many different settings could you find nurses providing care to children with asthma? Does the type of nursing care provided to children by nurses differ among these settings? Regardless of the setting in which nurses work, assessment, nursing care interventions, and patient education are universal roles for nurses. This chapter defines the various roles and settings for the nursing care of children and the important challenges in providing that care.

▶ ROLE OF THE NURSE IN PEDIATRICS

CLINICAL PRACTICE

Pediatric nursing focuses on protecting children from illness and injury, assisting them to attain optimal levels of health, regardless of health problems, and rehabilitation. This focus fits with the American Nurses Association definition of the scope of nursing practice: "the nursing diagnosis and treatment of human responses to health and to illness."[1] The nursing roles in caring for children and their families include direct care, patient education, advocacy, and case management.

Direct Nursing Care

The primary role of pediatric nurses is to provide direct nursing care to children and their families. The nursing process provides the framework for delivery of direct pediatric nursing care. The nurse assesses the child, identifies the nursing diagnoses that describe the responses of the child and family to the illness or injury, and implements and evaluates nursing care. This care is designed to meet the child's physical and emotional needs. It is tailored to the child's developmental stage, giving the child additional responsibility for self-care with increasing age.

Nurses play an important role in minimizing the psychologic and physical distress experienced by children and their families. Providing support to children and their families is one component of direct nursing care. This often involves listening to the concerns of children and parents and simply being present during stressful or emotional experiences. Nurses can help families by suggesting ways to support their children in the hospital, in out-of-hospital settings, and in the home.

Patient Education

Patient education improves treatment results. In pediatric nursing, patient education is especially difficult because nurses must be prepared to work

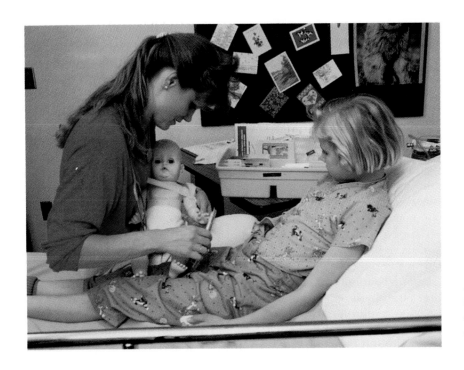

FIGURE 1–1. Explaining procedures can reduce the patient's and family's fears and anxieties about what to expect as well as teach procedures and proper home care.

with children at various levels of understanding and change the behavior of family members.

As patient educators, nurses help children adapt to the hospital setting and prepare them for procedures (Fig. 1–1). Most hospitals encourage a parent to stay with the child and to provide much of the direct and the supportive care. Nurses teach parents to watch for important signs, to increase the child's comfort, and even to provide advanced care. Taking an active role prepares the parent to assume total responsibility for care after the child leaves the hospital.

Counseling is another form of patient education. Counseling may involve guidance, such as injury-prevention strategies and anticipatory guidance to promote development. Nurse specialists or other experienced nurses are often responsible for counseling that is directed toward helping the child or family solve a problem.

Patient Advocacy

Advocacy—acting to safeguard and advance the interests of another—is directed at enabling the child and family to adjust to the changes in the child's health in their own way. To be an effective advocate, the nurse must be aware of the child's and the family's needs, the family's resources, and the health care services available in the hospital and the community. The nurse can then assist the family and the child to make informed choices about these services and to act in the child's best interests.

As advocates, nurses also ensure that the policies and resources of health care agencies meet the psychosocial needs of children and their families. The nurse must also protect the child and family by taking appropriate actions related to any incidents of incompetent, unethical, or illegal practices by any member of the health care team.

Case Management

What happens when a child has significant health problems? Can you handle it all?

When a child has a significant health problem or handicapping condition, health care professionals (physicians, nurses, social workers, physical and occupational therapists, and other specialists) create an interdisciplinary plan to meet the child's medical, nursing, developmental, educational, and psychosocial needs. Because nurses spend large amounts of time providing nursing care for the child and family, they often know more than other health care professionals about the family's wishes and resources. As a member of the interdisciplinary care plan team, the nurse serves as an advocate to ensure that the care plan considers the family's wishes and contains appropriate services. The nurse often becomes the child's case manager, coordinating the implementation of the interdisciplinary care plan. Sometimes the parent or a social worker becomes the case manager.

Case management is a process of coordinating the delivery of health care services in a manner that focuses on both quality and cost outcomes. This is often a collaborative practice with other health care providers that promotes **continuity of care** (an interdisciplinary process of facilitating a patient's transition between and among settings based on changing needs and available resources). The nurse case manager has control over the use of health care resources that are considered appropriate for the patient's condition and links the child and family to these services. The goal is to help the child and family have the best health care outcome, while controlling the cost of health care services. Case management may be used for care of the patient when hospitalized as well as for long-term care of chronic conditions.

Discharge planning is a form of case management. Good discharge planning promotes a smooth, rapid, and safe transition into the community and improves the results of treatment begun in the hospital. To be a discharge planner, the nurse needs to know about community medical resources, home care agencies qualified to care for children, educational interventions, and services reimbursed by the child's health plan or other financial resources.

NURSING PROCESS IN PEDIATRIC CARE

Can you describe how the five steps of the nursing process relate to children? Pediatric nurses use the nursing process to identify and solve problems and to plan patient care. The systematic framework for practice that the nursing process provides is the same for pediatric patients as for other patients.

- *Assessment* involves collecting patient and family data and performing physical examinations during community-based health services, at admission, periodically during the child's hospitalization, and when home care services are provided. The nurse analyzes and synthesizes data to make a judgment about the patient's problems.

- *Nursing diagnoses* describe the health promotion and health patterns that nurses can manage. Once health patterns have been identified, specific nursing actions can be planned.

- *Nursing care plans* are based on goals that will improve the child's or family's dysfunctional health patterns. Specific planned outcomes should be realistic. The family and the nurse (and the child, when old enough) should agree with the care plan goals.

Standard care plans for specific diagnoses are often used in the pediatric unit of the hospital and by home health agencies. The nurse is responsible for individualizing standard care plans based on data collected from the child's assessment and from evaluation of the child's response to care. Individualized nursing action plans provide directions for nursing care.

- *Implementation* is the carrying out of interventions outlined in the nursing care plan. Interventions may be modified if the child's responses are undesirable.

- *Evaluation* is the use of specific objective and subjective measures (often called outcome measures or criteria) to assess the child's and family's progress in reaching the goals defined in the nursing care plan. Following the evaluation of the child's and family's progress toward the goals, the nursing care plan may be modified. For example, as the child's condition improves and goals are attained, new goals and nursing action plans must be defined. Data from ongoing assessments are collected to guide the revision of the care plan.

Critical pathways are comprehensive interdisciplinary care plans for a specific condition that describe the sequence and timing of interventions that should result in expected patient outcomes. The care plans are based on a synthesis of research and past medical decision making to identify the most effective practices for a patient's condition. They address nursing care, nutrition, diagnostic tests, medications and other treatments, mobility and activity, patient teaching, and discharge planning. Critical pathways are adopted within a health care setting to reduce variation in patient management and to limit costs of care.[2,3] Many nurses are engaged in research to identify cost-effective plans for care.

SETTINGS FOR PEDIATRIC NURSING CARE

Pediatric nurses function in many different settings. Within the hospital, acute care may be provided in the emergency department, observation or short-stay unit, postanesthesia unit, intensive care unit, general pediatric inpatient unit, and various outpatient clinics. Pediatric nurses working with children and families on a general pediatric hospital unit promote health improvement in several ways:

- By gathering data and assessing the health of children and their families
- By providing ordered medical therapies
- By providing nursing care in a manner that preserves as many of the child's and family's normal routines as possible while maintaining the family unit
- By working with the family and health care team to develop an individualized health care plan and a discharge plan, or to implement a critical pathway plan

The hospital stay is now integrated into a continuum that allows children to complete therapy at home, at school, or in other community settings. Pediatric nurses assist families in making the transition from the acute hospital setting to:

- The home, for a short recuperation or long-term management
- A rehabilitation center or long-term care hospital
- A nurse-managed home care or hospice program

Managing the child's transition from acute care to another setting involves planning the discharge, implementing interdisciplinary plans, helping the family to develop an emergency care plan in the event their child has an unexpected health care crisis, and collaborating with a broad range of health care professionals.

Pediatric nurses also work in several other health care settings.

- In *pediatricians' offices* and *health maintenance organizations,* nurses assess children, provide telephone counseling, and support and counsel families about growth and development and nutrition.

- In *hospital clinic settings,* nurses assess children, assist with medical procedures, and educate families to ensure the continuous management of the child's health care problem.

- In *home health agencies,* nurses provide home care to children with acute and chronic conditions. Children need medical treatment and nursing care for acute, self-limited, chronic, and terminal conditions. Care may involve visits for specific interventions such as medication administration or "private duty" care (one-to-one nursing care).

- In *rehabilitation centers,* nurses provide inpatient care to help restore children to an optimal state and plan for discharge management of chronic conditions.

- In *schools,* nurses assess children, monitor their health status, and provide health education to teachers and children. Many children who are assisted by technology or have chronic conditions attend school. Individual School Health Plans are developed, implemented, and evaluated by the school nurse. In the case of Bethany and her friends from the asthma club, patient education helps them become more independent in managing their asthma.

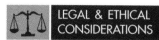

LEGAL & ETHICAL CONSIDERATIONS

The Education for All Handicapped Children Act, P.L. 94-142, provides free appropriate education to all handicapped children between 2 and 21 years of age. Provisions for needed medical care must be available in the school setting. Education for the Handicapped Act Amendments of 1986, P.L. 99-457, provides federal funding to states for multidisciplinary programs of early intervention services for handicapped infants and toddlers.

► CONTEMPORARY CLIMATE FOR PEDIATRIC NURSING CARE

More than 82 million children under the age of 21 live in the United States. They account for 31.6% of the population.[4] (See Fig. 1–2 for a dis-

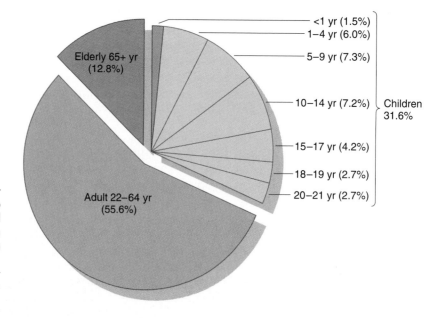

FIGURE 1–2. In 1995, children from birth to 21 years of age accounted for about one third of the population in the United States, with slightly over one fourth of the total population being under 17 years of age.
From US Bureau of the Census. (1996). Statistical abstract of the United States (116th ed.). Washington, DC: US Department of Commerce.

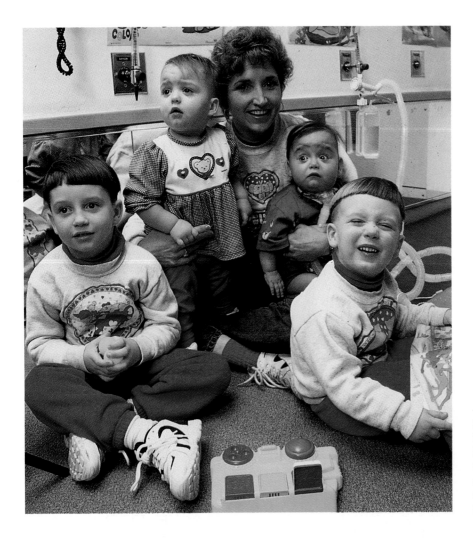

FIGURE 1–3. Many facilities now encourage family visitation for children with health problems that require long-term hospitalization. Extended family visits enable parents to learn about the child's care, and provide siblings with opportunities to interact with the hospitalized child.

tribution of the population by age group.) At one time children were valued primarily as laborers. Over the past century, however, the unique needs and qualities of children have been recognized. In today's society, children are considered to have special value; they are vulnerable and need protection.

FAMILY-CENTERED CARE

Efforts to address and meet the emotional, social, and developmental needs of children and families seeking health care in all settings is a concept known as **family-centered care.** The importance of the family in helping the child recover from illnesses and injuries is recognized by integrating them into the health care plan (Fig. 1–3). Families are often considered partners in the child's care, learning about the child's condition and participating in decisions regarding the child's care. Thus, families gain greater confidence and competence in caring for their children, which has become even more important as families play an ever-increasing role in providing care for children's health care problems. The key elements of family-centered care are provided in Table 1–1.

1-1	Key Elements of Family-Centered Care

- Incorporating into policy and practice the recognition that the *family is the constant* in a child's life, while the service systems and support personnel within those systems fluctuate.
- Facilitating family/professional collaboration at all levels of hospital, home, and community care:
  - care of an individual child
  - program development, implementation, evaluation, and evolution
  - policy formation
- Exchanging complete and unbiased information between family members and professionals in a supportive manner at all times.
- Incorporating into policy and practice the recognition and honoring of cultural diversity, strengths, and individuality within and across all families, including ethnic, racial, spiritual, social, economic, educational, and geographic diversity.
- Recognizing and respecting different methods of coping and implementing comprehensive policies and programs that provide developmental, educational, emotional, environmental, and financial supports to meet the diverse needs of families.
- Encouraging and facilitating family-to-family support and networking.
- Ensuring that home, hospital, and community service and support systems for children needing specialized health and developmental care and their families are flexible, accessible, and comprehensive in responding to diverse family-identified needs.
- Appreciating families as families and children as children, and recognizing that they possess a wide range of strengths, concerns, emotions, and aspirations beyond their need for specialized health and developmental services and support.

From Shelton, T.L., & Stepanek, J.S. (1994). Family-centered care for children needing specialized health and developmental services. Bethesda, MD: Association for the Care of Children's Health.

CULTURALLY SENSITIVE CARE

The U.S. population has a varied mix of cultural groups, with ever-increasing diversity. More than 25% of all children under 5 years of age are from families of minority populations.[5] Culture develops from socially learned beliefs, lifestyles, values, and integrated patterns of behavior that are characteristic of the family and community. The cultural background and values of children and their parents are often quite different from those of the nurse.

Specific elements that contribute to a family's value system include the following:

- Religion and social beliefs
- Presence and influence of the extended family, as well as socialization within the ethnic group
- Communication patterns
- Beliefs and understanding about the concepts of health and illness
- Permissible physical contact with strangers
- Education

Specific differences in beliefs between families and health care providers are common in the following areas:

- Help-seeking behaviors
- Causes of diseases or illnesses
- Death and dying

CULTURAL CONSIDERATIONS

Conflicts can occur within a family when traditional rituals and practices of the family's elders do not conform with current health care practices. Nurses need to be sensitive to the potential implications for the child's health care, especially after the child is discharged from the hospital. When cultural values are not part of the nursing care plan, parents may be forced to decide whether the family's beliefs should take priority over the health care professional's guidance.

- Caretaking and caregiving
- Child-rearing practices

These elements in differing degrees influence the cultural beliefs and values of an ethnic group, making the group unique. Misunderstandings may occur when the health care professional and the family come from different cultural groups. In addition, past experiences with care may have made the family angry or suspicious of providers. Nurses must be able to recognize, respect, and respond to ethnic diversity in a way that leads to a mutually desirable outcome.

When the family's cultural values are incorporated into the care plan, the family is more likely to accept and comply with the needed care, especially in the home care setting. Avoid imposing your personal cultural values on the children and families in your care. By learning about the values of the different ethnic groups in the community—their religious beliefs that have an impact on health care practices, their beliefs about common illnesses, and their specific healing practices—you can develop an individualized nursing care plan for each child and family.

PEDIATRIC HEALTH STATISTICS

Children have different health care problems than adults, and the problems may depend on age and development. For example, the leading causes of infant mortality (death occurring during the first year of life) vary according to the age of the infant (Fig. 1–4).

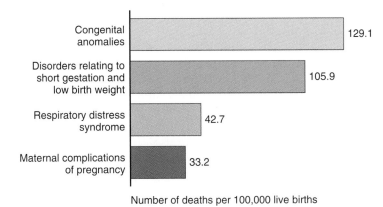

A

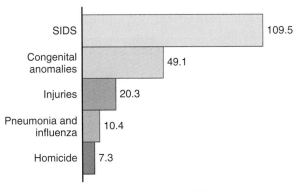

B

FIGURE 1–4. Leading causes of death in the United States in 1993 **(A)** in infants up to 28 days old and **(B)** in infants 1 to 12 months old. *From National Center for Health Statistics. (1996). Vital statistics of the United States: Vol. 2. Mortality. Part A. Washington, DC: Public Health Service.*

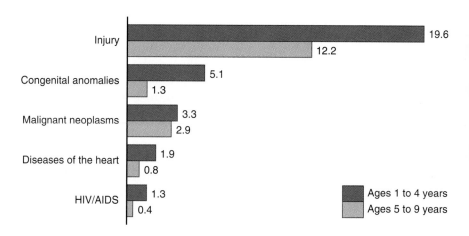

FIGURE 1–5. Age-specific death rate per 100,000 children in the United States in 1992. The leading cause of death in children between the ages of 1 and 9 years was injury. Why do you think that is? Do you think these data still apply today? Which type of injury has the highest rate of death? Firearms? Fires? Motor vehicle accidents? Falls? See Figure 1–6 for the answer.
From National Center for Health Statistics. (1995). National Vital Statistics System. Unpublished data.

The leading causes of death in neonates (birth to 28 days of age) are congenital anomalies, low birth weight, respiratory distress syndrome, and maternal complications of pregnancy. Sudden infant death syndrome accounts for nearly 67% of deaths to infants in the postneonatal period (between 1 and 12 months of age). Figure 1–4 shows the relative frequency of other major causes of death in the postneonatal period.[6] What could account for homicide as the fifth leading cause of death in infants?

The most common cause of death for children between 1 and 9 years of age is injury. Congenital anomalies, cancer, diseases of the heart, and infection with the human immunodeficiency virus (HIV)/acquired immunodeficiency syndrome (AIDS) are the other major causes. Figure 1–5 shows the distribution of these causes by age group. The major causes of death from unintentional injury in childhood include motor vehicle crashes (passengers and pedestrians), drowning, fires and burns, firearms, and falls (Fig. 1–6).[7]

Unintentional injury continues to be the leading cause of death in adolescents. Homicide, suicide, cancer, and congenital anomalies are other major causes of death (Fig. 1–7). Of all deaths from unintentional injury, motor vehicle crashes are the leading cause, followed by drowning, fires and burns, firearms, and falls (Fig. 1–8).

The U.S. government set objectives to improve the health of children and young adults in the 1990s in the report entitled *Healthy People 2000.*

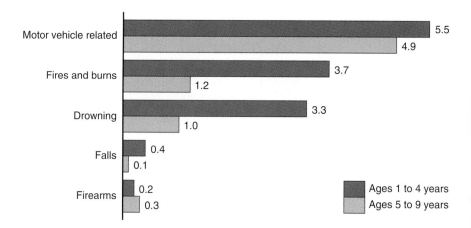

FIGURE 1–6. Death rates from unintentional injuries per 100,000 children ages 1 to 9 years in the United States in 1992. Which type of unintentional injury is the most common?
From National Center for Health Statistics. (1995). National Vital Statistics System. Unpublished data.

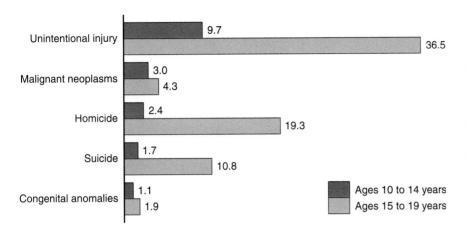

FIGURE 1–7. Death rates per 100,000 adolescents in the United States in 1992. Do you notice any difference in the rates of homicide as the child gets older? Do you think that these numbers would vary between socioeconomic and cultural groups? Why do you think there are differences? Are your conclusions supported by fact or are they influenced by your personal bias?
From National Center for Health Statistics. (1994). National Vital Statistic System. Unpublished data.

These objectives have focused on reducing the incidence of death and disability from the major causes of death shown in Figure 1–7. Federal funding is available to health care institutions for the development of programs aimed at reducing the number of deaths from these factors in specific high-risk groups.

Morbidity (an illness or injury that limits activity, requires medical attention or hospitalization, or results in a chronic condition) also varies according to the age of the child. In 1993, there were 3.4 million hospital discharges for children between 1 and 21 years of age, an average of 4 discharges per 100 children.[6] Figure 1–9 compares the leading causes of hospitalization of children by age group in 1989 and 1993. Respiratory diseases are the leading cause of hospitalization in children between 1 and 9 years of age, accounting for 35% of hospital discharges in this age group. Injury is among the top three causes of hospitalization in all age groups between 1 and 21 years of age. Another important cause of hospitalization is diseases of the digestive system. Pregnancy, childbirth, and mental disorders are among the leading causes of hospitalization in adolescents between 15 and 21 years of age.[6]

In 1993, chronic illnesses and impairments limited the activities of more than 4.7 million children between 1 and 19 years of age. More boys than girls had activity limitations between 1 and 19 years of age.[7]

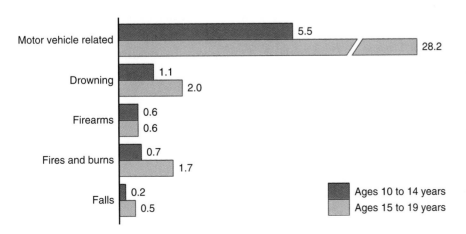

FIGURE 1–8. Death rates from unintentional injuries per 100,000 adolescents in the United States in 1992. Why do you think that motor vehicle–related accidents jump so significantly in the 15- to 19-year-old age group? Can you see ways to use these data with patients and families during patient teaching and when talking with them while providing care?
From National Center for Health Statistics. (1994). Division of Vital Statistics. Public Health Service. Unpublished data.

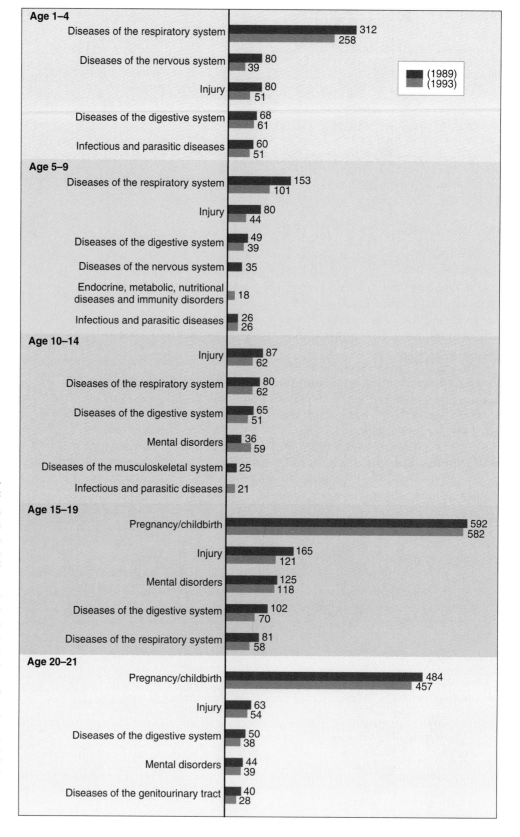

FIGURE 1-9. The leading causes of hospitalization in the United States in 1993 are much the same as those in 1989 in those 21 years and under, but the rates have changed substantially (number of hospital discharges [in 1000s]). What does this tell you about the change in the health care system between 1989 and 1993? What do you think the current hospitalization numbers are today? How can you apply this information when providing care and patient education?
From National Center for Health Statistics. (1990). Hospital discharge survey, 1989. In Maternal and Child Health Bureau. (1991). Child health USA '91. (DHHS Publication No. HRS-M-CH 91-1). Washington, DC: National Center for Education in Maternal and Child Health. Child health USA '95. (DHHS Publication No. HRSA-M-DSEA-96-5). Washington, DC: Government Printing Office.

HEALTH CARE ISSUES

Health Care Technology

Research and technology have enabled many children with congenital anomalies and low birth weights to survive, with and without chronic conditions. Lifesaving technology has also created such burdens as high costs of health care and stresses on the functioning of the child's family. Many children with chronic conditions or complications of acute illnesses and injuries are managed in long-term care hospitals, rehabilitation centers, or home care programs (Fig. 1–10). Approximately 400,000 children in the United States are unable to engage in normal childhood activities or depend on some form of medical technology[8] (Fig. 1–11).

Health Care Financing

Not all children in the United States have access to health care. In 1994, 10 million children, nearly 15% of those below 18 years of age, had no health insurance and 25.2% were covered by public insurance programs such as Medicaid. Of all children who lived in poverty in 1994, 22.3% had no health insurance and 64.9% were covered by public insurance.[6] Most of these children had difficulty obtaining the most basic preventive health care, including immunizations (Fig. 1–12).

Efforts to provide universal access to health care for children continue to grow. Congress recently passed legislation to enable more children to obtain access to essential health care services. Managed care is an effort to coordinate and provide quality care while preventing unnecessary care and controlling costs. Significant changes in health care practices are occurring in response to these health insurance programs. Most state Medicaid programs are converting to a managed-care process.

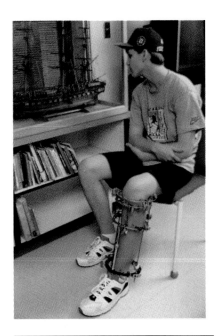

FIGURE 1–10. At the time of this photograph, Joey had been at Shriner's Hospital for over 8 months undergoing external fixation (lengthening the leg), which is a long and painful process. It is important that children undergoing long-term care continue their schooling, develop friendships with other children in the hospital, maintain contact with their friends at home, and learn self-care.

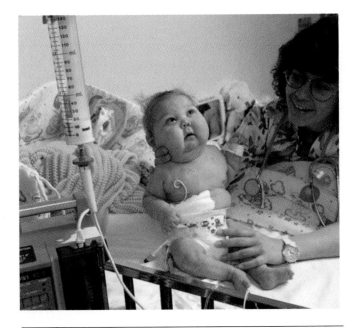

FIGURE 1–11. This child is dependent on the latest technology for necessary nutrients.

LEGAL & ETHICAL CONSIDERATIONS

The Child Health Insurance Program, P.L. 105-33, provides health coverage to low-income, uninsured children. Covered services must match benefits comparable to the Blue Cross Blue Shield plan for federal employees, a state employee health plan, or the plan of the largest health maintenance organization in the state. Medicaid can be expanded or the state may create a new program for children's health. Children at 200% of the poverty level are targeted by this program.[9]

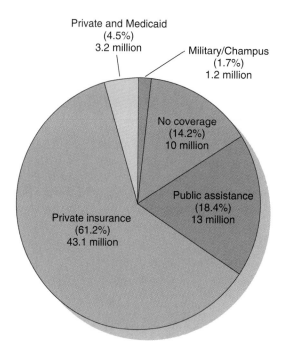

FIGURE 1–12. In the United States, how is health care of children paid for? These data from 1994 shows that our taxes support nearly 38% of the costs. What can you do to help? Something as simple as counseling parents about injury prevention and providing immunizations while a child is under care for other problems can prevent potential health problems. Part of good nursing care is supporting the well-being of the child in addition to caring for the presenting problem.
From US General Accounting Office. (1996). Health insurance for children: Private insurance continues to deteriorate. (HEHS-96-129). Washington, DC: Author.

Many children with severe chronic illnesses can be treated at home rather than by continued hospitalization. A 1989 study reported that more than 1 million children had a severe chronic illness that required ongoing home care.[10] After studies found that home health care was substantially less expensive than hospital care,[10] Congress amended laws to permit payment of home care services with federal funds. Technologic advances have resulted in the design of portable medical and infusion therapy equipment for home care. Some families have regained control over their lives by cre-

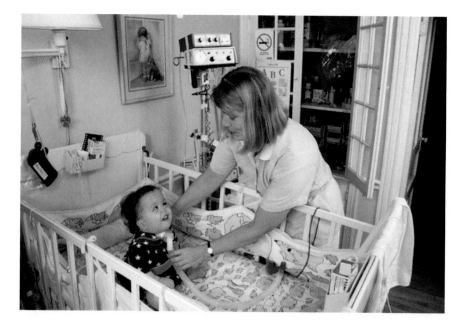

FIGURE 1–13. It is often desirable from a family and cost perspective to provide health care in the home, and technologic advances have made this possible. But is it really less costly to provide care in the home for a child with technology assistance? How does one factor in parents' out-of-pocket expenses for medical supplies that are not reimbursed? Lost time from work or the need for a parent to discontinue employment to care for the child? The emotional strain on families who care for their child 24 hours a day, 7 days a week? What support is needed by these families to continue providing this level of care at home?

ating intensive care units in their homes (Fig. 1–13). Children who 10 years ago would have died of respiratory, neurologic, or other medical conditions are thriving with home care and are participating in family, community, and school life.

▶ LEGAL CONCEPTS AND RESPONSIBILITIES

REGULATION OF NURSING PRACTICE

Because nurses are accountable for their professional actions, each state regulates nursing practice with a Nurse Practice Act. In many states, nursing is defined as "the nursing diagnosis and treatment of human responses to health and to illness."[1] A state's Nurse Practice Act defines the legal roles and responsibilities of nurses. Become familiar with the Nurse Practice Act in your state.

As professionals, nurses set standards for education and practice that conform to state regulations. Professional nursing organizations and state agencies that accredit nursing programs modify the standards for nursing education as the science of nursing progresses. Nurses in professional organizations develop Standards of Nursing Practice. These standards describe the public and patient responsibilities for which nurses are accountable.

Standards of clinical nursing practice developed by the American Nurses Association define standards for both nursing care and performance.[1] Standards of care describe the competent level of nursing care using the nursing process and form the foundation of clinical decision making. Standards of performance describe the nurse's behavior in the professional role and include such criteria as quality of care, performance appraisal, collegiality, resource utilization, ethics, research, education, and collaboration. Specific standards have also been developed for pediatric clinical nursing practice (Table 1–2).

ACCOUNTABILITY AND RISK MANAGEMENT

Accountability

The family entrusts the child's care to the health care team. Family members expect this team to provide good medical and nursing care and to avoid mistakes that cause harm. Nurses are personally accountable for expanding their knowledge base, for recognizing important changes in the child's condition that require intervention, and for taking action as necessary to protect the child.

Risk Management

Health care institutions make every effort to promote optimal patient care and reduce liability by various activities:

- **Risk management** is a process established by a health care institution to identify, evaluate, and reduce the risk of injury to patients, staff, and visitors, and thereby reduce the institution's liability.

1-2	Professional Practice Standards for Pediatric Clinical Nursing Practice

Standards of Care for the Pediatric Nurse Include
- Collecting health data.
- Analyzing the assessment data in determining diagnoses.
- Developing a plan of care that prescribes interventions to attain expected outcomes.
- Implementing the interventions identified in the plan of care.
- Evaluating the child's and family's progress toward attainment of outcomes.

Standards of Performance for the Pediatric Nurse Include
- Systematically evaluating the quality and effectiveness of pediatric nursing practice.
- Evaluating his or her own nursing practice in relation to professional practice standards and relevant statutes and regulations.
- Acquiring and maintaining current knowledge in pediatric nursing practice.
- Contributing to the professional development of peers, colleagues, and others.
- Making decisions and taking action on behalf of children and their families that are determined in an ethical manner.
- Collaborating with the child, family, and health care providers in providing patient care.
- Using research findings in practice.
- Considering factors related to safety, effectiveness, and cost in planning and delivering care.

From American Nurses Association & the Society of Pediatric Nurses. (1996). Statement on the scope and standards of pediatric clinical nursing practice. (MCH-17). Washington, DC: American Nurses Publishing. © 1996 American Nurses Publishing, American Nurses Foundation/ American Nurses Association, 600 Maryland Ave SW, Suite 100W, Washington, DC 20024–2571.

CLINICAL TIP

Policy and procedure manuals should be current and provide guidance on patient care and the use of technology, specifically related to potentially serious situations.

LEGAL & ETHICAL CONSIDERATIONS

The patient's record is a legal document that is admissible evidence in court. Information in the patient's record must be legibly written in objective terms. When recording a patient's response to therapy, the nurse needs to include physiologic responses and exact quotes. The date, time, and nurse's signature and title are required.

- **Quality assurance** is a process used to monitor the procedures and outcomes of care using indicators to measure compliance with standards of care.

- **Quality improvement** is the continuous study and improvement of the processes and outcomes of providing health care services to meet the needs of patients, by examining the systems and processes of how care and services are delivered.

Nurses participate in the development of institutional policies and standards of nursing practice. Hospitals and home health agencies encourage the development of diagnosis-specific nursing care plans or interdisciplinary critical pathways that serve as minimal institutional standards of care.

During the development of institutional standards of care, indicators of effective care by nurses and other providers are identified. These indicators may measure either the process of care, the institution's systems, or the expected outcome of care for a specific patient condition. Patient records are regularly reviewed to identify deviations from the institutional standards or critical pathways. When deviations from expected processes and outcomes are identified, opportunities to improve the system or processes of care provision are explored with all care providers. Recommendations for the revision of institutional standards to further improve care by nurses and other health providers in the institution often result.

Documentation of nursing care is an essential part of risk management and quality assurance. If a patient record is subpoenaed, documented care is considered the only care provided, regardless of the quality of undocumented care. The patient assessment, the nursing care plan, and the child's responses to medical therapies and nursing care, including the regularly scheduled evaluation of the patient's progress toward nursing goals, must all be documented accurately and sequentially. Nurses must also report any untoward incidents that could inhibit the patient's recovery.

► LEGAL AND ETHICAL ISSUES IN PEDIATRIC CARE

Shanti, a 15-year-old girl with acute myelocytic leukemia, has come out of her second remission with an acute onset of fever, joint pain, and petechiae. A bone marrow transplant is one of the few remaining therapeutic options. While Shanti has agreed to a transplant if a suitable donor is found, she does not want to be resuscitated and placed on life support equipment should she have a cardiac arrest. She has talked extensively with the hospital chaplain and social worker and feels comfortable with her decision. Her parents want an all-out effort to sustain her life until a donor is located.

Shanti's case illustrates the legal and ethical dilemmas in caring for children. At what age can children make an informed decision about whether to accept or refuse treatment? What happens when the parents and child have conflicting opinions about treatment? How are ethical decisions resolved?

INFORMED CONSENT

Informed consent is a formal preauthorization for an invasive procedure or participation in research. Consent must be given voluntarily. Parents, as the legal custodians of minor children, are customarily requested to give informed consent on behalf of a child. When parents are divorced, either may give informed consent. Both children and parents must understand that they have the right to refuse treatment at any time. In an emergency, consent for treatment to preserve life or limb is not required.

Children under 18 or 21 years of age, depending on state law, can legally give informed consent in the following circumstances:[11]

- When they are minor parents of the child patient
- When they are **emancipated minors** (self-supporting adolescents under 18 years of age, not subject to parental control)
- When they are adolescents between 16 and 18 years of age seeking birth control, mental health counseling, or substance abuse treatment

Mature minors (14- and 15-year-old adolescents who are able to understand treatment risks) can give consent for treatment or refuse treatment in some states.

Children should become more actively involved in decision making about treatment procedures as their reasoning skills develop. Children too young to give informed consent can be given age-appropriate information about their condition and asked about their care preferences. Their parents, however, make ultimate decisions regarding their care (Fig. 1–14).

With regard to participation in research, federal guidelines state that children 7 years of age and older must receive information about a research

LEGAL & ETHICAL CONSIDERATIONS

Information that the physician must provide to obtain informed consent includes a detailed description of the treatment, possible benefits and significant risks associated with the proposed treatments, possible alternative treatments, and notification of a parent's or guardian's right to refuse treatment on behalf of the child.

CLINICAL TIP

The physician is legally responsible for obtaining informed consent. The nurse's role in obtaining informed consent includes the following:
- Alerting physicians to the need for informed consent
- Responding to questions asked by parents and children
- Serving as a witness when parents sign consent forms or give verbal consent by telephone

GROWTH & DEVELOPMENT CONSIDERATIONS

By 7 or 8 years of age, a child is able to understand concrete explanations about informed consent for research participation. By age 11, a child's abstract reasoning and logic are advanced. By age 14, an adolescent can weigh options and make decisions regarding consent as capably as an adult.

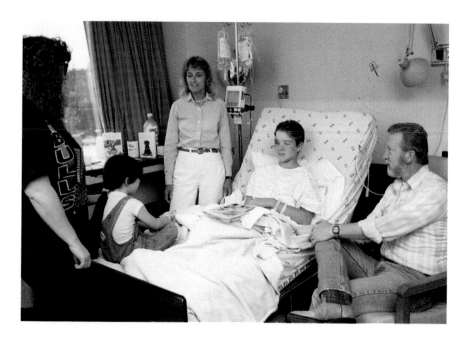

FIGURE 1–14. Children need to be actively involved in decisions regarding their care when appropriate. The nurse (behind bed) has brought the entire family together to discuss the child's care in a positive and honest manner.

project and give **assent** (the voluntary agreement to participate in a research project or to accept treatment) before they are enrolled. Children should be given adequate time to ask questions and be told that they have the right to refuse to participate in the study.[12,13]

CHILD'S RIGHTS VERSUS PARENTS' RIGHTS

Parents or guardians have absolute authority to make choices about their child's health care except in specific cases:[11]

- When the child and parents do not agree on major treatment options
- When the parents' choice of treatment does not permit lifesaving treatment for the child
- When there is a potential conflict of interest between the child and parents, such as with suspected child abuse or neglect
- When the parents are incapacitated and cannot make a decision (eg, critically injured in the same motor vehicle crash)

In some cases, the court may be requested to appoint a proxy decision maker for the child or to determine that the child is capable of making a major treatment decision.

CONFIDENTIALITY

When the child is an emancipated or mature minor, the physician may provide birth control and treatment for sexually transmitted diseases including HIV/AIDS, pregnancy, and substance abuse without informing the child's parents.[11] If the child has a reportable disease, confidentiality may create a public health hazard. In such cases, the health care professional is obligated to report the presence of the disease to the appropriate state or county agency.[14,15] Suspected cases of child abuse must be reported to the appropriate agency specified by state law. In the current

LEGAL & ETHICAL CONSIDERATIONS

Obtain legal advice for complex family issues related to guardianship, divorced parents disagreeing over care, or a caregiver who is not the legal guardian.

LEGAL & ETHICAL CONSIDERATIONS

Jehovah's Witnesses oppose blood transfusions for themselves and their children because they believe transfusions are equivalent to the oral intake of blood, which is morally and spiritually wrong according to their interpretation of the Bible (Leviticus 17:13–14). A Jehovah's Witness who receives a transfusion believes he or she has committed a sin and may have forfeited everlasting life. Transfusions of any blood products, including plasma and the patient's own blood, are forbidden.

health care system, the complexities of treatment and the numbers of health care providers involved make it more difficult to maintain confidentiality.

PATIENT SELF-DETERMINATION ACT

The federal Patient Self-Determination Act directs health care institutions to inform hospitalized patients about their rights, which include expressing a preference for treatment options and making **advance directives** (writing a living will or authorizing a durable power of attorney for health care decisions on the patient's behalf). Nurses often discuss these issues with patients and their families.[16] Minor children and their parents should also be informed of their rights.

Do Not Resuscitate orders have become more common for children with terminal illnesses in which no further treatments are possible or desired. In many cases, these children are cared for at home or in a hospice program, but some still attend school. Implementation of Do Not Resuscitate orders for such children then becomes a community issue, to assure that no resuscitation measures are initiated by any emergency care provider when the child has a life-threatening event. State health policies must be developed so children with these signed orders are easily identified and appropriate documentation of the orders is on file.

ETHICAL ISSUES

Ethics is the philosophic study of morality, moral judgments, and moral problems. Ethical issues may arise from a **moral dilemma** (a conflict of social values and ethical principles that support different courses of action). Technology makes it possible to sustain the lives of children who previously would have died, thus creating many ethical issues. Problems may develop because physicians, nurses, and parents have differing opinions about treatments for an infant or child with a serious or fatal condition. Nurses often face ethical dilemmas when providing care to such a child. They witness parents struggling to decide among treatment options. Ethical issues in pediatrics are often more complex because most children lack the capacity to make or to participate in medical decisions that directly affect them.

Ethical decision making is based on respect for persons and their ability to make decisions independently. All individuals must be treated without prejudice, regardless of race, gender, religious preference, cultural or educational background, financial status, or sexual orientation.[17] Health care professionals may have different values from patients, based on culture and life experiences.

Certain principles guide decision making about treatment when moral dilemmas exist. A major principle is to avoid harm and provide beneficial care to the child. When making treatment decisions in pediatrics, health care professionals must determine whether their responsibility is limited to the child or includes the interests of the parents. The health care institution's ethics committee should make treatment decisions using the process of data collection and evaluation outlined in Table 1–3. Often this ethics committee develops guidelines to help health care providers with ethical decision making for common issues. Courts should make ethical decisions only when health care professionals and parents are unable to agree about providing or withholding treatment.

 CLINICAL TIP

Breeching confidentiality is a potential problem for adolescents, who are just learning whom they can trust in the health care system. Make sure you openly discuss the limits of confidentiality for such things as mandatory reporting requirements with the patient and family. Inadvertent disclosure of personal information may lead to psychologic, social, or physical harm in some patients.

1-3   Steps in Making Ethical Decisions

Collect Information
What decisions are needed?
Who are the key persons involved?
What information will help make the situation more clear?
Are there any legal constraints?

Identify the Ethical Issues or Concerns of the Situation
What are their historical roots, the religious and philosophical positions?
What are the current societal views of each issue?

Define the Personal and Professional Moral Positions on the Issues
What personal constraints are raised by the issues?
What is the professional code for guidance?
Are there any conflicting loyalties or obligations?
What are the moral positions of the key individuals involved?

Identify Any Value Conflicts
What is the basis for the conflict?
What is the possible resolution?

Decision Making
Who should make the decision?
What are the possible actions and their anticipated outcome?
What is the moral justification for each action?
Which action fits the criteria for this situation?
Decide on a course of action and carry it out.

Evaluate the Results of the Decision Action
Did the expected outcome occur?
Is a new decision needed?
Is the decision process complete?

Adapted from Thompson, J.B., & Thompson, H.O. (1981). Ethics in nursing. New York: Macmillan Publishing.

Terminating Life-Sustaining Treatment

Baby Tim at 1 day of age has severe myelomeningocele with hydrocephalus. His physicians are seeking his parents' consent for surgical placement of a shunt to control the progression of hydrocephalus. Regardless of medical care and surgical intervention, the infant is expected to have a severe handicap. The parents, after much consideration and discussions with their family and pastor, have requested that life-sustaining treatment be withheld.

What happens when the parents' request differs from the opinion of physicians? How do federal regulations for care of infants with severe defects affect current health care practice?

Federal "Baby Doe" regulations were developed to protect the rights of infants with severe defects. Parents of such infants are usually the ultimate decision makers about the child's care. They may want to terminate treatment because of the tremendous social, emotional, and financial burden.[18] Physicians may believe treatment will help the child and improve the quality of life (sometimes defined as a meaningful existence or an ability to develop human relationships). Federal regulations require a formalized ethical decision-making process before physicians accept or reject a parent's wishes. The most common question brought before ethics committees is whether to terminate life-sustaining treatment.

Justifications for withholding, withdrawing, or limiting therapy include the following:[17]

- The treatment in question will not work.
- The burdens of the treatment outweigh the benefits, or the quality of life is poor after treatment.
- The burdens of the disease outweigh the benefits of continued survival, or the quality of life is poor before the treatment.

Each of these conditions is considered according to the individual beliefs of the members of the ethics committee and their perceptions of the value of specific interventions for an individual child. Treatment to save the infant's life is elected if it has the potential for improving the quality of life as well. Physicians are not obligated to offer interventions that cause extreme pain and suffering when there is no or limited potential benefit. Treatments that only prolong life represent a misuse of expensive health care resources.

Organ Transplantation Issues

The death of a child can benefit another child through organ transplantation. The National Organ Transplant Act (PL98-507) generated laws, regulations, and guidelines for organ collection and transplantation.[11] For example, the transplant team cannot provide care to the potential donor. The institution has specific requirements to approach family members when brain death is suspected or confirmed to request organ donation.

Regulations are important because too few organs are available for patients needing transplantation. The limited supply of organs has created numerous ethical issues. Which patients on the waiting list should receive the organs available? Should families be permitted to pay donor families for organs? Should the family's ability to pay for an organ transplant give a child higher priority for an organ? What are the brain death and nonheartbeating criteria for children that enable organ collection to proceed?

► SUMMARY

Many topics discussed in this chapter reflect the current challenges children and their families face in the health care system—access to health care, specific disease and injury risks, and ethical and legal concerns. Fortunately, pediatric nursing often involves caring for children who have episodes of acute illness or injury and who recover quickly without serious consequences. The challenge and gratification of pediatric nursing are to provide appropriate care in a supportive environment that promotes the family unit and the child's development.

REFERENCES

1. American Nurses Association. (1991). *Standards of clinical nursing practice*. (NP-79). Kansas City, MO: Author.
2. Merritt, T.A., Palmer, D., Bergman, D.A., & Shiono, P.H. (1997). Clinical practice guidelines in pediatric and newborn medicine. Implications for their use in practice. *Pediatrics, 99*(1), 100–114.
3. Turley, K.M., Higgins, S.S., Archer-Duste, H., & Cafferty, P. (1995). Role of the clinical nurse coordinator in successful implementation of critical pathways in

pediatric cardiovascular surgery patients. *Progress in Cardiovascular Nursing, 10*(1), 22–26.

4. U.S. Bureau of the Census. (1996). *Statistical abstract of the United States, 1996.* (116th ed.). Washington, DC: U.S. Department of Commerce.

5. MacKune-Karrer, B., & Taylor, E.H. (1995). Toward multiculturality: Implications for the pediatrician. *Pediatric Clinics of North America, 42*(1), 21–30.

6. Maternal and Child Health Bureau. (1996). *Child health USA '95.* (DHHS Publication No. HRSA-M-DSEA-96-5). Washington, DC: Government Printing Office.

7. Maternal and Child Health Bureau. (1995). *Child health USA '94.* (DHHS Publication No. HRSA-MCH-95-1). Washington, DC: Government Printing Office.

8. Klug, R.M. (1992). Selecting a home care agency. *Pediatric Nursing, 8,* 504–506.

9. Association of Maternal and Child Health Professionals. (1997). *AMCHP Updates, 6*(4), 10–11, Washington, DC: Author.

10. U.S. General Accounting Office. (1989). *Home care experiences of families with chronically ill children.* Washington, DC: Author.

11. Frader, J., & Thompson, A. (1994). Ethical issues in the pediatric intensive care unit. *Pediatric Clinics of North America, 41*(6), 1405–1421.

12. U.S. Department of Health and Human Services. (1983). *Protection of human subjects: Code of federal regulations, 45 CFR #46, Subpart D.*

13. Thurber, F.W., Deatrick, J.A., & Grey, M. (1992). Children's participation in research: Their right to consent. *Journal of Pediatric Nursing, 7,* 165–170.

14. King, N.M.P., & Cross, A.W. (1989). Children as decision makers: Guidelines for pediatricians. *Journal of Pediatrics, 115,* 10–16.

15. Fiesta, J. (1992). Protecting children: A public duty to report. *Nursing Management, 23,* 14–15.

16. Badzek, L.A. (1992). What you need to know about advance directives. *Nursing '92, 22,* 58–59.

17. Cassidy, R.C., & Fleischman, A.R. (1996). *Pediatric ethics—From principles to practice.* Amsterdam, The Netherlands: Harwood Academic Publishers.

18. Schlomann, P. (1992). Ethical considerations of aggressive care of the very low birth weight infant. *Neonatal Network, 11,* 31–36.

ADDITIONAL RESOURCES

Cohen, E.L., & Cesta, T.G. (1993). *Nursing case management: From concept to evaluation.* St. Louis: Mosby.

Crummette, B.D., & Boatwright, D.N. (1991). Case management in inpatient pediatric nursing. *Pediatric Nursing, 17,* 469–473.

Davis, B.D., & Steele, S. (1991). Case management for young children with special health care needs. *Pediatric Nursing, 17,* 15–19.

Davis, F.D. (1989). Organ procurement and transplantation. *Nursing Clinics of North America, 24,* 823–826.

Erlen, J.A., & Holzman, I.R. (1988). Anencephalic infants: Should they be organ donors? *Pediatric Nursing, 14,* 60–63.

Everson-Bates, S. (1988). Research involving children: Ethical concerns and dilemmas. *Journal of Pediatric Nursing, 2,* 234–239.

Joint Commission for the Accreditation of Health Care Organizations. (1996). *1996 Accreditation manual for health care network* (Vol. 1). Oakbrook Terrace, IL: Author.

Johnson, B.H., Jeppson, E.S., & Redburn, L. (1992). *Caring for children and families: Guidelines for hospitals.* Bethesda, MD: Association for the Care of Children's Health.

Jones, N.E. (1992). Childhood injuries: An epidemiologic approach. *Pediatric Nursing, 18,* 235–239.

Malloy, C. (1992). Children and poverty: America's future at risk. *Pediatric Nursing, 18,* 553–557.

McClowry, S.G. (1993). Pediatric nursing psychosocial care: A vision beyond hospitalization. *Pediatric Nursing, 19,* 146–148.

McCubbin, H.I., Thompson, E.A., Thompson, A.I., et al. (1993). Culture, ethnicity, and the family: Critical factors in childhood chronic illnesses and disabilities. *Pediatrics, 91*(5), 1063–1070.

Rushton, C.H. (1995). The Baby K case: Ethical challenges of preserving professional integrity. *Pediatric Nursing, 21,* 367–372.

Rushton, C.H., & Hogue, E.E. (1993). When parents demand "everything." *Pediatric Nursing, 19,* 180–183.

Rushton, C.H., & Infante, M.C. (1995). Keeping secrets: The ethical and legal challenges. *Pediatric Nursing, 21,* 479–482.

Schuman, A.J. (1997). Home sweet home: The best place for pediatric care. *Contemporary Pediatrics, 14*(3), 91–104.

Selekman, J. (1991). Pediatric rehabilitation: From concepts to practice. *Pediatric Nursing, 17,* 11–14.

Solnit, A.J., Schowalter, J.E., & Nordhaus, B.F. (1995). Best interests of the child in the family and community. *Pediatric Clinics of North America, 42*(1), 181–191.

Spector, R.E. (1996). *Cultural diversity in health and illness* (4th ed.). Stamford, CT: Appleton & Lange.

Thurber, F., Berry, B., & Cameron, M.E. (1991). The role of school nursing in the United States. *Journal of Pediatric Nursing, 5,* 135–140.

U.S. General Accounting Office. (1996). *Health maintenance for children—Private insurance continues to deteriorate.* (HEHS-96-129). Washington, DC: Author.

Vikell, J.H. (1991). The process of quality management. *Pediatric Nursing, 17,* 618–619.

Zagorsky, E.S. (1993). Caring for families who follow alternative health care practices. *Pediatric Nursing, 19,* 71–75.

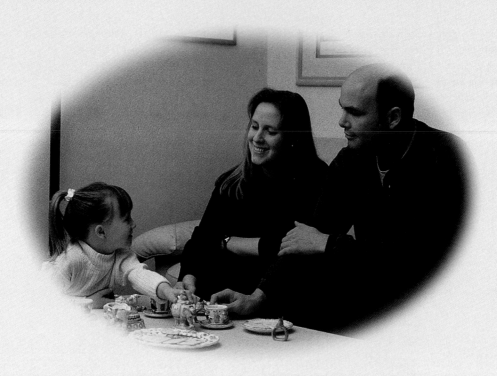

Four-and-a-half-year-old Sara returns home from preschool and gets out her favorite tea set. When her father arrives home from work, she asks her parents to sit down with her and have a "tea party." Although her parents have been busy and are eager to get on with the tasks of the evening, they know that the tea party is an important time to connect with Sara. She pours "tea" for them and snacks on some crackers and bananas herself. This special time for her is even more important now that she has a new baby sister and has had to give up her place as the only child in the family.

Once the tea party is over, Sara holds her new sister and cuddles briefly, then plays with her Barbie doll. Although she enjoys this independent play, she comes to her parents for comfort when she scrapes her hand and when she needs help changing Barbie's clothes. After dinner, Sara draws pictures, listens to the story her father reads, and goes to sleep.

Sara's play today has been inside the house, but she often plays outside with the other children in her neighborhood and at preschool. She enjoys playing on the swing set and riding her bicycle with training wheels. Sara is small for her age in comparison with her friends, but her motor abilities are average for her age group.

GROWTH AND DEVELOPMENT 2

"Watching Sara grow is fascinating and scary. She is changing so fast, learning new things. It is hard to keep up with her. It is an exciting time."

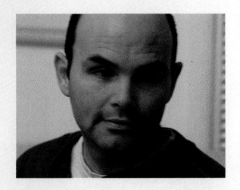

TERMINOLOGY

- **accommodation** The process of changing one's cognitive structures to include data from recent experiences.
- **anticipatory guidance** The process of understanding upcoming developmental needs and then teaching caretakers to meet those needs.
- **assimilation** The process of incorporating new experiences into one's cognitive awareness
- **associative play** A type of play that emerges in preschool years when children interact with one another, engaging in similar activities and participating in groups.
- **cephalocaudal development** The process by which development proceeds from the head downward through the body and toward the feet.
- **conservation** The knowledge that matter is not changed when its form is altered.
- **cooperative play** A type of play that emerges in school years when children join into groups to achieve a goal or play a game.
- **defense mechanisms** Techniques used by the ego to unconsciously change reality, thereby protecting itself from excessive anxiety.
- **development** An increase in capability or function.
- **dramatic play** A type of play in which a child acts out the drama of daily life.

- **expressive jargon** Use of unintelligible words with normal speech intonations as if truly communicating in words; common in toddlerhood.
- **growth** An increase in physical size.
- **nature** The genetic or hereditary capability of an individual.
- **nurture** The effects of environment on an individual's performance.
- **object permanence** The knowledge that an object or person continues to exist when not seen, heard, or felt.
- **parallel play** A type of play that emerges in toddlerhood when children play side by side with similar or different toys, demonstrating little or no social interaction.
- **proximodistal development** The process by which development proceeds from the center of the body outward to the extremities.
- **puberty** Period of life when the ability to reproduce sexually begins; characterized by maturation of the genital organs, development of the secondary sex characteristics, and (in females) the onset of menstruation.
- **sensitive periods** Times when an individual is especially responsive to certain environmental effects; sometimes called critical periods.

Children develop as they interact with their surroundings. They learn skills at different ages, but the order in which they learn them is universal. In the preceding scenario, Sara's activities provide examples of her level of development, which is characteristic of most preschoolers. We also see examples of factors, such as nutrition and culture, that influence children's development. Although an observer might describe Sara as a "typical preschooler," every child is unique, bringing different life experiences and personality to his or her individual circumstances.

To highlight the important facets of development that are explored in this chapter, let us begin by examining what was accomplished during Sara's afternoon and evening activities (Fig. 2–1).

Physical Growth and Development

Sara is smaller than many of her peers. However, her gross motor skills of running and jumping are well developed. Fine motor skills are evident in her ability to feed herself, manipulate toy dishes, and draw pictures.

Cognitive Development

Sara's evening activity demonstrates and enhances her cognitive learning. She learns new words and grammar by speaking with others. Her atten-

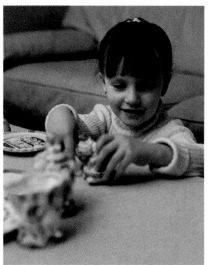

A

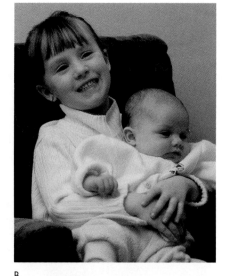

B

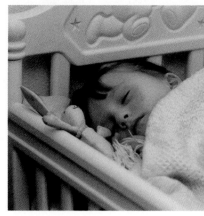

C

D

FIGURE 2–1. Carefully observing all of a child's activities helps determine what stage of growth and development the child has reached. **A,** Sara's play with her parents demonstrates physical and social skills. **B,** The birth of a new sibling offers challenges and rewards for the preschooler. **C,** Children need to be nurtured and to develop trust. **D,** Adequate sleep is needed to promote growth and development.

dance at preschool offers experiences that assist her in learning letters, colors, and other concepts. The variety of toys her parents provide ensure that her cognitive development will be maximized at home.

Play

Sara's play is typical of preschoolers in that she enjoys a mixture of solitary play and associative play with other young children (see Fig. 2–3).

Nutrition

Sara eats foods from all the food groups similar to those enjoyed by the rest of her family. Smaller servings and more frequent meals are the norm for preschoolers. Sara needs to eat a snack when she returns home from preschool so she will have energy to engage in activities until dinnertime. At this age, children can be given some choices in the foods they eat. Meal manners typical of her family's culture are being taught, as when Sara serves her parents during the tea party.

Injury Prevention

Cognitive and physical development mirror the changing hazards to the health and well-being of children. Sara might be injured in a car accident, particularly if not secured by a seatbelt. The playground and her bicycle are some other potential sources of injury. Although Sara's physical skills are well developed, she does not yet understand all of the hazards around her; therefore, she needs close supervision. Nurses use **anticipatory guidance** to discuss safety hazards and injury prevention for children of various ages with their parents.

Personality and Temperament

Sara has always had what experts term an "easy" temperament; that is, she readily adopts a regular schedule for eating and sleeping, her mood is generally pleasant, and she is easily comforted when upset. These temperamental characteristics form a critical link to communication with family, teachers, and friends.

Communication

Sara has learned words from her parents, preschool friends, and others. She understands most speech and uses complete, short sentences. She has refined her social skills and is able to cooperate with others. Feedback from others has helped to form her self-image and promote learning.

In this chapter, you will learn general principles of growth and development and will explore several theories related to childhood development, as well as their nursing applications. Each age group, from infancy through adolescence, is described in detail. Developmental milestones, physical and cognitive characteristics, health and safety concerns, and communication strategies are presented. This basic information will help you provide developmentally appropriate care for children in each age group.

▶ PRINCIPLES OF GROWTH AND DEVELOPMENT

It is essential to understand the concepts of growth and development when learning to care for children. **Growth** refers to an increase in physical size. **Development** refers to an increase in capability or function. The quantitative changes in body organ functioning, ability to communicate, and performance of motor skills unfold over time.

Each child displays a unique maturational pattern during the process of development. Although the exact age at which skills emerge differs, the sequence or order of skill performance is uniform among children. Skill development proceeds according to two processes: from the head down and from the center of the body out to the extremities. Development that proceeds from the head downward through the body and toward the feet is called **cephalocaudal development** (Fig. 2–2). For example, at birth, an infant's head is much larger proportionately than the trunk or extremities. Similarly, infants learn to hold up their heads before sitting, and to sit before standing. Skills such as walking that involve the legs and feet develop last in infancy. Development that proceeds from the center of the body outward to the extremities is called **proximodistal development** (see Fig. 2–2). For example, infants are first able to control the trunk, then the arms; only later are fine motor movements of the fingers possible.

During the childhood years, extraordinary changes occur in all aspects of development. Physical size, motor skills, cognitive ability, language, sensory ability, and psychosocial patterns all undergo major transformations. Nurses study normal patterns of development so they can perform thorough pediatric assessments and identify children who demonstrate slow or abnormal development. These assessments can guide the nurse in planning interventions for the child and family, such as referring the child for a diagnostic evaluation or rehabilitation, or teaching the parents how to provide adequate stimulation for the child. When development is proceeding normally, the nurse uses his or her knowledge of these normal patterns to plan teaching approaches based on the child's cognitive and language ability, to offer appropriate toys and activ-

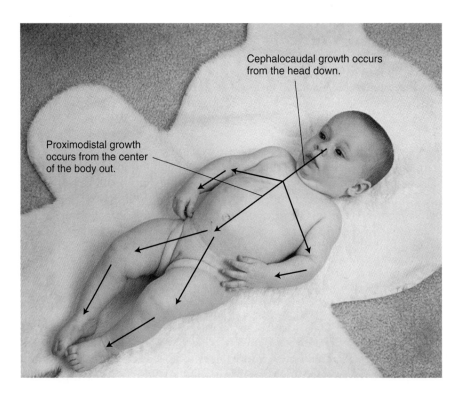

FIGURE 2–2. In normal *cephalocaudal* growth, the child gains control of the head and neck before the trunk and the limbs. In normal *proximodistal* growth, the child controls arm movements before hand movements. For example, the child reaches for objects before being able to grasp them. Children gain control of their hands before their fingers; that is, they can hold things with the entire hand before they can pick something up with just their fingers.

ities during illness, and to respond therapeutically during interactions with the child.

▶ MAJOR THEORIES OF DEVELOPMENT

Child development is a complex process. Many theorists have attempted to organize their observations of behavior into a description of principles or a set of stages. Each theory focuses on a particular facet of development. Most developmental theorists separate children into age groups by common characteristics (Table 2–1).

FREUD'S THEORY OF PSYCHOSEXUAL DEVELOPMENT

Theoretical Framework

The psychoanalytic techniques used by Freud led him to believe that early childhood experiences form the unconscious motivation for actions in later life. He developed a theory that sexual energy is centered in specific parts of the body at certain ages. Unresolved conflict and unmet needs at a certain stage lead to a fixation of development at that stage.

Freud viewed the personality as a structure with three parts: the *id* is the basic sexual energy that is present at birth and drives the individual to seek pleasure; the *ego* is the realistic part of the person, which develops during infancy and searches for acceptable methods of meeting sexual needs; and the *superego* is the moral system, which develops in childhood and contains a set of values and conscience.[1] The ego protects itself from excess anxiety by use of **defense mechanisms,** including regression to earlier stages and repression or forgetting of painful experiences such as child abuse (Table 2–2).

Stages

Oral (Birth to 1 Year)
The infant derives pleasure largely from the mouth, with sucking and eating as primary desires.

SIGMUND FREUD (1856–1939)

Freud was a physician in Vienna, Austria. His work with adults who were experiencing a variety of nervous disorders led Freud to develop the approach called psychoanalysis, which explored the driving forces of the unconscious mind.[1]

2-1 Developmental Age Groups

infancy—Birth to 12 months. Includes infants or babies up to 1 year of age who require a high level of care in daily activities.

toddlerhood—1–3 years. Characterized by increased motor ability and independent behavior.

preschool—3–6 years. The preschooler refines gross and fine motor ability and language skills and often participates in a preschool learning program.

school age—6–12 years. Begins with entry into a school system and is characterized by growing intellectual skills, physical ability, and independence.

adolescence—12–18 years. Begins with entry into the teen years. Mature cognitive thought, formation of identity, and influence of peers are important characteristics of adolescence.

2-2	Common Defense Mechanisms Used by Children	
Defense Mechanism	Definition	Example
Regression	Return to an earlier behavior	A previously toilet-trained child becomes incontinent when separated from parents during a hospitalization.
Repression	Involuntary forgetting of uncomfortable situations	An abused child cannot consciously recall episodes of abuse.
Rationalization	An attempt to make unacceptable feelings acceptable	A child explains hitting another because "he took my toy."
Fantasy	A creation of the mind to help deal with unacceptable fear	A hospitalized child who is weak pretends to be Superman.

Anal (1–3 Years)
The young child's pleasure is centered in the anal area, with control over body secretions as a prime force in behavior.

Phallic (3–6 Years)
Sexual energy becomes centered in the genitalia as the child works out relationships with parents of the same and opposite sexes (Oedipus and Electra complexes).

Latency (6–12 Years)
Sexual energy is at rest in the passage between earlier stages and adolescence.

Genital (12 Years to Adulthood)
Mature sexuality is achieved as physical growth is completed and relationships with others occur.

Nursing Application

Freud emphasized the importance of meeting the needs of each stage in order to move successfully into future developmental stages. The crisis of illness can interfere with normal developmental processes and add challenges for the nurse striving to meet an ill child's needs. For example, the importance of sucking in infancy guides the nurse to provide a pacifier for the infant who cannot have oral fluids. The preschool child's concern about sexuality guides the nurse to provide privacy and clear explanations during any procedures involving the genital area. It may be necessary to teach parents that masturbation by the young child is normal and to help parents deal with it. The adolescent's focus on relationships suggests that the nurse should include questions about significant friends during history taking. Table 2–3 summarizes ways in which the nurse can apply these theoretical concepts to the care of children.

2-3   Nursing Applications of Theories of Freud, Erikson, Piaget

Age Group	Developmental Stages	Nursing Applications
Infant (birth to 1 year)	Oral stage (Freud): The baby obtains pleasure and comfort through the mouth. Trust versus mistrust stage (Erikson): The baby establishes a sense of trust when basic needs are met. Sensorimotor stage (Piaget): The baby learns from movement and sensory input.	When a baby is NPO, offer a pacifier if not contraindicated. After painful procedures, offer a baby a bottle or pacifier or have the mother breast-feed. Hold the hospitalized baby often. **(1)** Offer comfort after painful procedures. Meet the baby's needs for food and hygiene. Encourage parents to room in. Manage pain effectively with use of pain medications and other measures. Use crib mobiles, manipulative toys, wall murals, and bright colors to provide interesting stimuli and comfort. Use toys to distract the baby during procedures and assessments.
Toddler (1–3 years)	Anal stage (Freud): The child derives gratification from control over bodily excretions. Autonomy versus shame and doubt stage (Erikson): The child is increasingly independent in many spheres of life. Sensorimotor stage (end); preoperational stage (beginning) (Piaget): The child shows increasing curiosity and explorative behavior. Language skills improve.	Ask about toilet training and the child's rituals and words for elimination during admission history. Continue child's normal patterns of elimination in the hospital. Do not begin toilet training during illness or hospitalization. Accept regression in toileting during illness or hospitalization. Have potty chairs available in hospital. Allow self-feeding opportunities. Encourage child to remove and put on own clothes, brush teeth, or assist with hygiene. **(2)** If restraint for a procedure is necessary, proceed quickly, providing explanations and comfort. Ensure safe surroundings to allow opportunities to manipulate objects. Name objects and give simple explanations.

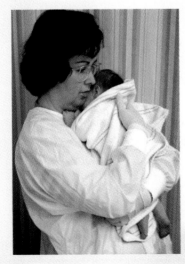

(1)

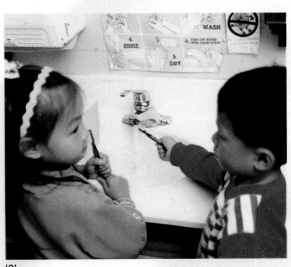

(2)

Continued . . .

2-3   Nursing Applications of Theories of Freud, Erikson, Piaget (continued)

Age Group	Developmental Stages	Nursing Applications
Preschooler (3–6 years)	Phallic stage (Freud): The child initially identifies with the parent of the opposite sex but by the end of this stage has identified with the same-sex parent. Initiative versus guilt stage (Erikson): The child likes to initiate play activities. Preoperational stage (Piaget): The child is increasingly verbal but has some limitations in thought processes. Causality is often confused, so the child may feel responsible for causing an illness.	Be alert for children who appear more comfortable with male or female nurses, and attempt to accommodate them. Encourage parental involvement in care. Plan for playtime and offer a variety of materials from which to choose. Offer medical equipment for play to lessen anxiety about strange objects. **(3)** Assess children's concerns as expressed through their drawings. Accept the child's choices and expressions of feelings. Offer explanations about all procedures and treatments. Clearly explain that the child is not responsible for causing the illness.
School age (6–12 years)	Latency stage (Freud): The child places importance on privacy and understanding the body. Industry versus inferiority stage (Erikson): The child gains a sense of self-worth from involvement in activities. Concrete operational stage (Piaget): The child is capable of mature thought when allowed to manipulate and see objects.	Provide gowns, covers, and underwear. Knock on door before entering. Explain treatments and procedures. Encourage the child to continue school work while hospitalized. Encourage child to bring favorite pasttimes to the hospital. **(4)** Help child adjust to limitations on favorite activities. Give clear instructions about details of treatment. Show the child equipment that will be used in treatment.

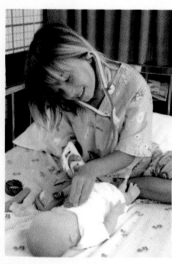

(3)

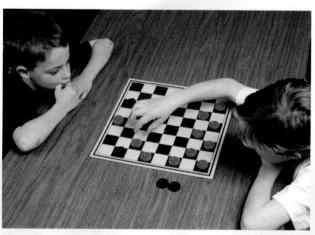

(4)

2-3	Nursing Applications of Theories of Freud, Erikson, Piaget (continued)	
Age Group	**Developmental Stages**	**Nursing Applications**
Adolescent (12–18 years)	Genital stage (Freud): The adolescent's focus is on genital function and relationships.	Ensure access to gynecologic care for adolescent girls. Provide information on sexuality. Ensure privacy during health care. Have brochures and videos available for teaching about sexuality.
	Identity versus role confusion stage (Erikson): The adolescent's search for self-identity leads to independence from parents and reliance on peers.	Provide a separate recreation room for teens who are hospitalized. **(5)** Take health history and perform examinations without parents present. Introduce adolescent to other teens with same health problem.
	Formal operational stage (Piaget): The adolescent is capable of mature, abstract thought.	Give clear and complete information about health care and treatments. Offer both written and verbal instructions. Continue to provide education about the disease to the adolescent with a chronic illness, as mature thought now leads to greater understanding.

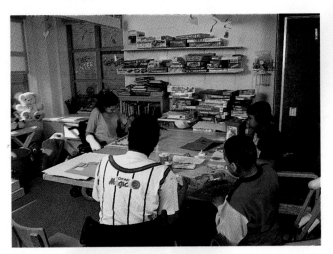

(5)

AUTONOMY VERSUS SHAME AND DOUBT

The toddler likes to show autonomy by exerting control over toys and activities.

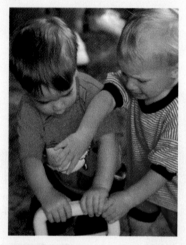

INDUSTRY VERSUS INFERIORITY

A child takes pride in accomplishments in sports.

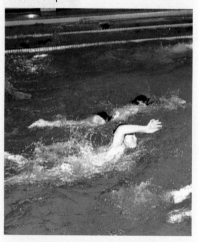

ERIKSON'S THEORY OF PSYCHOSOCIAL DEVELOPMENT

Theoretical Framework

Erikson's theory establishes psychosocial stages during eight periods of human life. For each stage Erikson identifies a *crisis*, that is, a particular challenge that exists for healthy personality development to occur.[2,3] The word "crisis" in this context refers to normal maturational social needs rather than to a single critical event. Each developmental crisis has two possible outcomes. When needs are met, the consequence is healthy and the individual moves on to future stages with particular strengths. When needs are not met, an unhealthy outcome occurs that will influence future social relationships.

Stages

Trust versus Mistrust (Birth to 1 Year)
The task of the first year of life is to establish trust in the people providing care. Trust is fostered by provision of food, clean clothing, touch, and comfort. If basic needs are not met, the infant will eventually learn to mistrust others.

Autonomy versus Shame and Doubt (1–3 Years)
The toddler's sense of autonomy or independence is shown by controlling body excretions, saying no when asked to do something, and directing motor activity. Children who are consistently criticized for expressions of autonomy or for lack of control—for example, during toilet training—will develop a sense of shame about themselves and doubt in their abilities.

Initiative versus Guilt (3–6 Years)
The young child initiates new activities and considers new ideas. This interest in exploring the world creates a child who is involved and busy. Constant criticism, on the other hand, leads to feelings of guilt and a lack of purpose.

Industry versus Inferiority (6–12 Years)
The middle years of childhood are characterized by development of new interests and by involvement in activities. The child takes pride in accomplishments in sports, school, home, and community. If the child cannot accomplish what is expected, however, the result will be a sense of inferiority.

Identity versus Role Confusion (12–18 Years)
In adolescence, as the body matures and thought processes become more complex, a new sense of identity or self is established. The self, family, peer group, and community are all examined and redefined. The adolescent who is unable to establish a meaningful definition of self will experience confusion in one or more roles of life.

Nursing Application

Erikson's theory is directly applicable to the nursing care of children. The social situations created by health care provide opportunities for meeting children's needs. The child's usual support from family, peers, and others is interrupted by hospitalization. The challenge of hospitalization also adds a situational crisis to the normal developmental crisis a child is experiencing.

Although the nurse may meet many of the hospitalized child's needs, continued parental involvement is necessary to ensure progression through expected developmental stages (see Table 2–3).

PIAGET'S THEORY OF COGNITIVE DEVELOPMENT

Theoretical Framework

Based on his observations and work with children, Piaget formulated a theory of cognitive (or intellectual) development. He believed that the child's view of the world is influenced largely by age and maturational ability. Given nurturing experiences, the child's ability to think matures naturally.[4] The child incorporates new experiences via **assimilation** and changes to deal with these experiences by the process of **accommodation.**

Stages

Sensorimotor (Birth to 2 Years)
Infants learn about the world by input obtained through the senses and by their motor activity. Six substages are characteristic of this stage.

Use of Reflexes (Birth to 1 Month). The infant begins life with a set of reflexes such as sucking, rooting, and grasping. By using these reflexes, the infant receives stimulation via touch, sound, smell, and vision. The reflexes thus pave the way for the first learning to occur.

Primary Circular Reactions (1–4 Months). Once the infant responds reflexively, the pleasure gained from that response causes repetition of the behavior. For example, if a toy grasped reflexively makes noise and is interesting to look at, the infant will grasp it again.

Secondary Circular Reactions (4–8 Months). Awareness of the environment grows as the infant begins to connect cause and effect. The sounds of bottle preparation will lead to excited behavior. If an object is partially hidden, the infant will attempt to uncover and retrieve it.

Coordination of Secondary Schemes (8–12 Months). Intentional behavior is observed as the infant uses learned behavior to obtain objects, create sounds, or engage in other pleasurable activity. **Object permanence** (the knowledge that something continues to exist even when out of sight) begins when the infant remembers where a hidden object is likely to be found; it is no longer "out of sight, out of mind."

Tertiary Circular Reactions (12–18 Months). Curiosity, experimentation, and exploration predominate as the toddler tries out actions to learn results. Objects are turned in every direction, placed in the mouth, used for banging, and inserted in containers as their qualities and uses are explored.

Mental Combinations (18–24 Months). Language provides a new tool for the toddler to use in understanding the world. Language enables the child to think about events and objects before or after they occur. Object permanence is now fully developed as the child actively searches for objects in various locations and out of view.

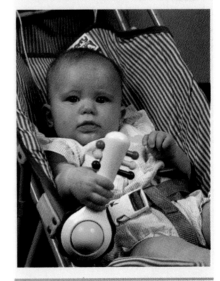

Preoperational (2–7 Years)

The young child thinks by using words as symbols, but logic is not well developed. During the preconceptual substage (2–4 years), vocabulary and comprehension increase greatly but the child is egocentric (that is, unable to see things from the perspective of another). In the intuitive substage (4–7 years), the child relies on transductive reasoning (that is, drawing conclusions from one general fact to another). For example, when a child disobeys a parent and then falls and breaks an arm that day, the child may ascribe the broken arm to bad behavior. Cause-and-effect relationships are often unrealistic or a result of "magical thinking" (the belief that events occur because of thoughts or wishing).

Concrete Operational (7–11 Years)

Transductive reasoning has given way to a more accurate understanding of cause and effect. The child can reason quite well if concrete objects are used in teaching or experimentation. The concept of conservation (that matter does not change when its form is altered) is learned at this age.

Formal Operational (11 Years to Adulthood)

Fully mature intellectual thought has now been attained. The adolescent can think abstractly about objects or concepts and consider different alternatives or outcomes.

Nursing Application

Piaget's theory is essential to pediatric nursing. The nurse must understand a child's thought processes in order to design stimulating activities and meaningful, appropriate teaching plans. Understanding a child's concept of time suggests to the nurse how far in advance to prepare that child for procedures. Similarly, the nurse's decision to offer manipulative toys, read stories, draw pictures, or give the child reading matter to explain health care measures depends on the child's cognitive stage of development (see Table 2–3).

KOHLBERG'S THEORY OF MORAL DEVELOPMENT

Theoretical Framework

LAWRENCE KOHLBERG
(B. 1927)

Kohlberg used Piaget's cognitive stage theory as the basis for his theory of moral development. He worked with children in his native Germany and in many other countries, including Kenya, Taiwan, and Mexico.[5]

Kohlberg's focus is on a particular type of cognitive development, that concerned with moral decisions. He presented stories involving moral dilemmas to children and adults and asked them to solve the dilemmas. Kohlberg then analyzed the motives they expressed when making decisions about the best course to take. Based on the explanations given, Kohlberg established three levels of moral reasoning. Although he provided age guidelines, he stated that they are approximate and that many people never reach the highest (postconventional) stage of development.[5]

Stages

Preconventional (4–7 Years)
Decisions are based on the desire to please others and to avoid punishment.

Conventional (7–11 Years)
Conscience or an internal set of standards becomes important. Rules are important and must be followed to please other people and "be good."

Postconventional (12 Years and Older)

The individual has internalized ethical standards on which to base decisions. Social responsibility is recognized. The value in each of two differing moral approaches can be considered and a decision made.

Nursing Application

Decision making is required in many areas of health care. Children can be assisted to make decisions about health care and to consider alternatives when available. The nurse should keep in mind that young children may agree to participate in research simply because they want to comply with adults and appear cooperative.

SOCIAL LEARNING THEORY

Theoretical Framework

Bandura, a contemporary psychologist, believes that children learn through their social contacts with adults and other children. Children imitate (or model) the behavior they see; if the behavior is positively reinforced, they tend to repeat it. The external environment and the child's internal processes are key elements in social learning theory.[6]

Nursing Application

The importance of modeling behavior can readily be applied in health care. Children are more likely to cooperate if they see adults or other children performing a task willingly. A frightened child may watch another child perform vision screening or have blood drawn and then decide to allow the procedure to take place. Contact with positive role models is useful when teaching children and adolescents self-care for chronic diseases such as diabetes. Positive reinforcement should be given for desired performance.

BEHAVIORISM

Theoretical Framework

Watson studied the research of Pavlov and Skinner, who demonstrated that actions are determined by responses from the environment. Pavlov and, later, Skinner worked with animals, presenting a stimulus such as food and pairing it with another stimulus such as a ringing bell. Eventually the animal being fed began to salivate when the bell rang. As Skinner and then Watson began to apply these concepts to children, they showed that behaviors can be elicited by positive reinforcement, such as a food treat, or extinguished by negative reinforcement, such as by scolding or withdrawal of attention. Watson believed that he could make of a child anyone he desired—from a professional to a thief or beggar—simply by reinforcing behavior in certain ways.[7]

Nursing Application

Behaviorism has been criticized for its simplicity and its denial of the inherent capability of persons to respond willfully to events in the environment. This theory does, however, have some use in health care. When particular behaviors are desired, positive reinforcement can be established to

ALBERT BANDURA (B. 1925)

Bandura is a Canadian who has conducted psychologic research at Stanford University for many years. He believes that children learn from their social environment, particularly by modeling the observed behaviors of others.[6]

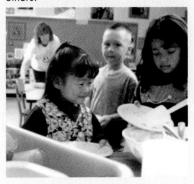

JOHN WATSON (1878–1958)

Watson was an American scientist who applied the work of animal behaviorists, such as Ivan Pavlov and B.F. Skinner, to children.[7]

encourage these behaviors. Behavioral techniques are also used to alter behavior of misbehaving children or to teach skills to handicapped children. Parents often use reinforcement in toilet training and other skills learned in childhood.

ECOLOGIC THEORY

Theoretical Framework

You may have noticed that there is controversy among theorists concerning the relative importance of heredity versus environment—or nature versus nurture—in human development. **Nature** refers to the genetic or hereditary capability of an individual. **Nurture** refers to the effects of the environment on a person's performance (Fig. 2–3). Piaget believed in the importance of internal cognitive structures that unfold at their appointed times, given any environment that provides basic opportunities. He emphasized the strength of nature. The behaviorist John Watson, on the other hand, believed that behaviors are primarily shaped by environmental responses; he thus stressed the predominance of nurture. Contemporary developmental theories increasingly recognize the interaction of nature and nurture in determining the child's development.

The ecologic theory of development was formulated by Urie Bronfenbrenner to explain the unique relationship of the child in all of life's settings, from close to remote.[8] Ecologic theory emphasizes the presence of mutual interactions between the child and these various settings. Neither

---

NATURE VERSUS NURTURE

Does nature or nurture have primary importance in the theories of Erikson, Kohlberg, Freud, and social learning? Think about whether each of the theories emphasizes the role of heredity (nature) or the role of the environment (nurture) in influencing the development of children.

URIE BRONFENBRENNER (B. 1917)

Bronfenbrenner, a professor at Cornell University, has established the ecologic theory of development. He views the child as interacting with the environment at different levels, or systems.[8]

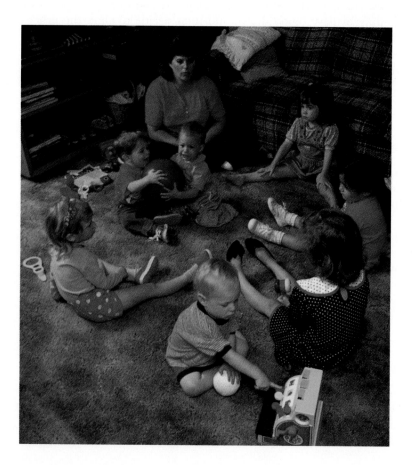

FIGURE 2–3. Children exposed to pleasant stimulation and who are supported by an adult will develop and refine their skills faster. Group play such as this provides an environment for both motor skill and psychosocial development. Can you identify which skills are being developed?

nature nor nurture is considered of more importance. Bronfenbrenner believes each child brings a unique set of genes—as well as specific attributes such as age, gender, health, and other characteristics—to his or her interactions with the environment. The child then interacts in many settings at different levels or systems (Fig. 2–4).

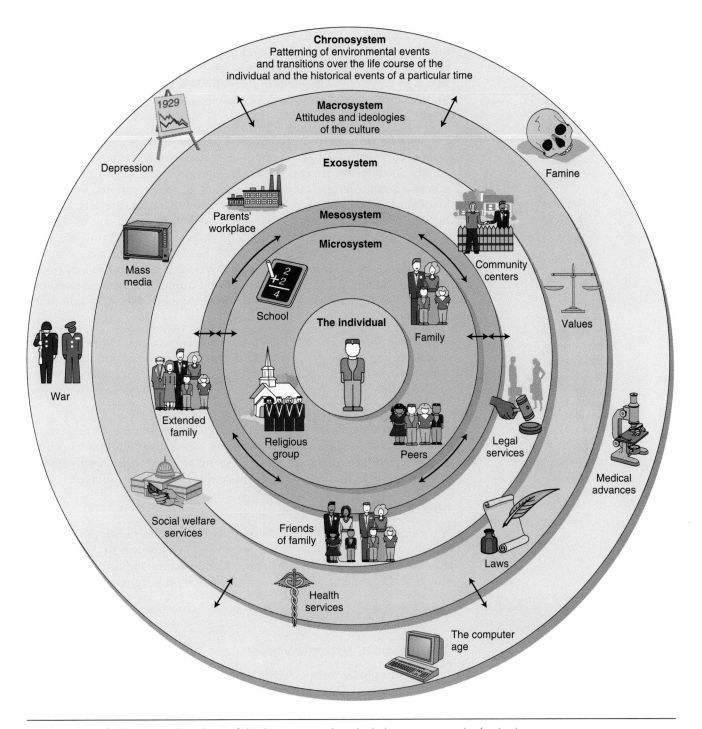

FIGURE 2–4. Bronfenbrenner's ecologic theory of development views the individual as interacting within five levels or systems.
Redrawn from Santrock, J.W. (1997). Life span development. Madison, WI: Brown & Benchmark. Based on Bronfenbrenner's work in Contexts of child rearing: Problems and prospects. (1979). American Psychologist, 34, 844–850, and Ecology of the family as a context for human development: Research perspectives. (1986). Developmental Psychology, 22, 723–742.

Levels/Systems

Microsystem. This level is defined as the daily, consistent, close relationships such as home, child care, school, friends, and neighbors. For the child with a chronic illness requiring regular care, the health care providers may even be part of the microsystem. In the ecologic model, the child influences each of these settings in addition to being influenced by them, with reciprocal interactions.

Mesosystem. This level includes relationships of microsystems with one another. For example, two microsystems for most children are the home and the school. The relationships between these microsystems are shown by parents' involvement in their children's school. This involvement, in turn, influences the effects of the home and school settings on the children.

Exosystem. This level is composed of those settings that influence the child even though the child is not in close daily contact with the system. Examples include the parents' jobs and the governing board of the local school district. Although the child may not go to the parents' workplaces, he or she can be influenced by policies related to health care, sick leave, inflexible work hours, overtime, or travel or even by the mood of the boss (through its impact on the parent). The child's needs may influence a parent to give up a certain job, or to work harder to obtain money for the child's education. Likewise, when a local school board votes to ban certain books or to finance a field trip, the child is influenced by these decisions; the child, in turn, can help establish an atmosphere that will guide future school board decisions.

Macrosystem. This level includes the beliefs, values, and behaviors expressed in the child's environment. Culture is a powerful influence in the macrosystem, as is the political system. For instance, a democratic system creates different beliefs, values, and even eating practices than an anarchic system.

Chronosystem. This final level brings the perspective of time to the previous settings. The time period during which the child grows up influences views of health and illness. For example, the experiences of children with influenza in the 19th versus 20th centuries are quite different.

Nursing Application

Nurses use ecologic theory when they assess the child's settings to identify influences on development. Table 2–4 provides an assessment tool based on this theory. Interventions are planned to enhance the strengths of the child's settings and to improve on areas that are not supportive.

TEMPERAMENT THEORY

Theoretical Framework

In contrast to behaviorists such as Watson or maturational theorists such as Piaget, Chess and Thomas recognize the innate qualities of personality that each individual brings to the events of daily life. They, like Bronfenbrenner, believe the child is an individual who both influences and is influenced by the environment. However, Chess and Thomas focus on one specific aspect of development—the wide spectrum of behaviors possible in children, identifying nine parameters of response to daily events (Table 2–5). Infants generally display clusters of responses, which Chess and Thomas have classified

2-4   Assessment of Ecologic Systems in Childhood

Microsystem
Parents
Significant others in close contact
Child care arrangements
School
Neighborhood contacts
Clubs
Friends, peers
Religious community (eg, churches, synagogues)

Mesosytems
Parents' involvement in child care or school
Parents' involvement in community
Parents' relationship with significant others (eg, grandparents, care providers)
Influences of religious community (eg, church, synagogue) on parents and school

Exosystems
Community centers
Local political influences
Parents' work
Parents' friends and activities
Social services
Health care
Libraries

Macrosystems
Cultural group membership
Beliefs and values of group
Political structure

Chronosystem
Child's age
Parents' ages

Ask yourself:
- How does the child influence each system?
- How is the child influenced by each system?
- Where does this lead you in planning interventions for the child?

---

into three major personality types (Table 2–6). Although most children do not demonstrate all behaviors described for a particular type, they usually show a grouping indicative of one personality type.[10]

Recent research demonstrates that personality characteristics displayed during infancy are often consistent with those seen later in life. The ability to predict future characteristics is not possible, however, because of the complex and dynamic interaction of personality traits and environmental reactions.

Many other researchers have expanded the work of Chess and Thomas, developing assessment tools for temperament types. The concept of "goodness of fit" is an outgrowth of this theory. Goodness of fit refers to whether parents' expectations of their child's behavior are consistent with the child's temperament type. For example, an infant who is very active and reacts strongly to verbal stimuli may be unable to sleep well when placed in a room with older siblings. A child who is slow to warm up may not perform well in the first few months at a new school, much to parents' disappoint-

2-5   Nine Parameters of Personality

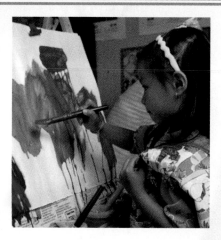

1. **Activity level.** The degree of motion during eating, playing, sleeping, bathing. Scored as high, medium, or low.
2. **Rhythmicity.** The regularity of schedule maintained for sleep, hunger, elimination. Scored as regular, variable, or irregular.
3. **Approach or withdrawal.** The response to a new stimulus such as a food, activity, or person. Scored as approachable, variable, or withdrawn.
4. **Adaptability.** The degree of adaptation to new situations. Scored as adaptive, variable, or nonadaptive.
5. **Threshold of responsiveness.** The intensity of stimulation needed to elicit a response to sensory input, objects in the environment, or people. Scored as high, medium, or low.
6. **Intensity of reaction.** The degree of response to situations. Scored as positive, variable, or negative.
7. **Quality of mood.** The predominant mood during daily activity and in response to stimuli. Scored as positive, variable, or negative.
8. **Distractibility.** The ability of environmental stimuli to interfere with the child's activity. Scored as distractible, variable, or nondistractible.
9. **Attention span and persistence.** The amount of time devoted to activities (compared with other children of the same age) and the degree of ability to stick with an activity in spite of obstacles. Scored as persistent, variable, or nonpersistent.[10]

ment. When parents understand a child's temperament characteristics, they are better able to shape the environment to meet the child's needs.

Nursing Application

The concept of personality type or temperament is a useful one for nurses.[11] Nurses can assess the temperament of young children and alter the environment to meet their needs. This may involve moving a hospitalized child to a single room to ensure adequate rest if the child is easily stimulated, or allowing a shy child time to become accustomed to new surroundings and equipment before beginning new procedures or treatments.

Parents are often relieved to learn about temperament characteristics. They learn to appreciate their children's qualities and to adapt the envi-

2-6   Patterns of Temperament

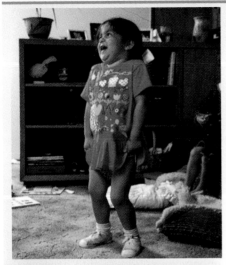

The **"easy" child** is generally moderate in activity; shows regularity in patterns of eating, sleeping, and elimination; and is usually positive in mood and when subjected to new stimuli. The easy child adapts to new situations and is able to accept rules and work well with others. About 40% of children in the New York Longitudinal Study displayed this personality type.

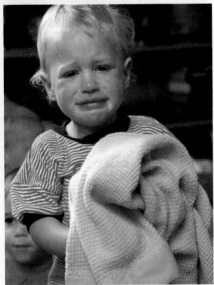

The **"difficult" child** displays irregular schedules for eating, sleeping, and elimination; adapts slowly to new situations and persons; and displays a predominantly negative mood. Intense reactions to the environment are common. About 10% of children in the New York Longitudinal Study displayed this personality type.

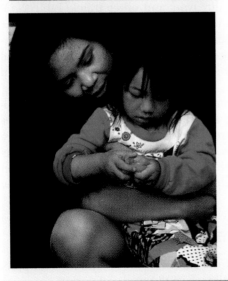

The **"slow-to-warm-up" child** has reactions of mild intensity and slow adaptability to new situations. The child displays initial withdrawal followed by gradual, quiet, and slow interaction with the environment. About 15% of children in the New York Longitudinal Study displayed this personality type.

The remaining 35% of children studied showed some characteristics of each personality type.[10]

2-7	Ways to Improve Goodness of Fit Between Parents and Child	
Child's Behavior	**Parent's Activity**	
Extremely active	Plan periods of active play several times in day. Have restful periods before bedtime to foster sleep.	
Shy	Allow time to adapt at own pace to new people and situations.	
Easily stimulated	Have quiet room for sleeping as an infant. Have quiet room for homework as a school-age child.	
Short attention span	Provide projects that can be completed in a short period. Gradually encourage longer periods at activities.	

ronment to meet the children's needs. A burden of guilt can also be lifted from parents who feel that they are responsible for their child's actions. The nurse can teach parents ways of enhancing goodness of fit between the child's personality and the environment (Table 2–7).

► INFLUENCES ON DEVELOPMENT

As we have seen, both nature and nurture are important in determining individual patterns of development. The interaction of these two forces can explain differences in time frames for skills acquisition, personality variations between identical twins, and other unique characteristics of individuals. Several of the factors that contribute to individual differences are explored in more detail next.

GENETICS

THE HUMAN GENOME PROJECT

This project was begun in 1988 by the United States Congress to fund research that would lead to mapping of all human genes by the year 2005. The United States has joined with other nations in seeking to understand the basic unit of heredity.

Each child inherits 23 chromosomes from the mother's egg and 23 from the father's sperm, resulting in a unique individual with 46 chromosomes. Every chromosome carries many genes that determine physical characteristics, intellectual potential, personality type, and other traits (Table 2–8). Children are born with the potential for certain features; however, their interaction with the environment influences how and to what extent particular traits are manifested. For example, a child may have the potential for a high level of intellectual performance, but because he or she lives in an unstimulating environment, that potential is never reached.

Chromosomal abnormalities that lead to such conditions as Down syndrome may result from factors such as radiation exposure, parental age, or parental disease states. Some children also inherit genes that lead to diseases such as cystic fibrosis. A family history of these diseases is usually present, although they may appear without an identifiable history. This is because genes sometimes mutate, leading to an initial incidence of a genetic disorder.

PRENATAL INFLUENCES

Some Asian cultures calculate age from the time of conception. This practice acknowledges the profound influence of the prenatal period.

2-8   Laws of Mendelian Inheritance

Dominant inheritance   A gene that produces a trait whenever it is present. Achondroplasia dwarfism is one example.

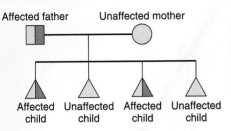

In each pregnancy there is a 50% chance that the child will have the characteristic.

Recessive inheritance   A gene that produces a trait only when paired with another like gene. Examples include cystic fibrosis, Tay-Sachs disease, and phenylketonuria.

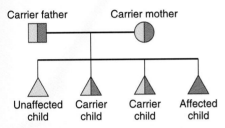

In each pregnancy, there is a 25% chance that the child will have the characteristic, a 25% chance that the child will be unaffected, and a 50% chance that the child will be a carrier of the characteristic.

X-linked inheritance   A disease carried in either a dominant or recessive fashion on the X chromosome. Hemophilia is a common example of an X-linked disorder.

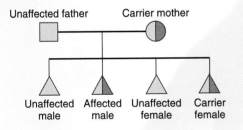

In each pregnancy with a male birth, there is a 50% chance that the child will have the characteristic and a 50% chance that the child will be unaffected. In each pregnancy with a female birth, there is a 50% chance that the child will be a carrier and a 50% chance that the child will be unaffected.

Chromosome defect   Disorders caused by nondisjunction or translocation of chromosomes. Down syndrome is usually caused by a trisomy of chromosome 21.

The mother's nutrition and general state of health play a part in pregnancy outcome. Poor nutrition can lead to small infants, compromised neurologic performance, or low maternal stores of iron and resultant anemia in the newborn.[12] Maternal smoking is associated with low-birth-weight infants. Ingestion of alcoholic beverages, including beer and wine, during pregnancy may lead to fetal alcohol syndrome (Fig. 2–5). Illicit drug use by the mother may result in neonatal addiction, convulsions, hyperirritability, poor social responsiveness, and other neurologic disturbances.

Even prescription drugs may adversely affect the fetus. An example is the drug thalidomide, which was commonly used in Europe to treat nausea

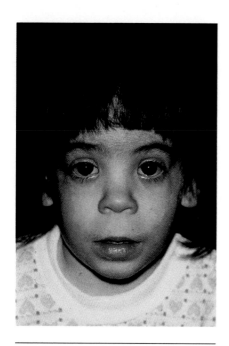

FIGURE 2–5. Fetal alcohol syndrome.
Courtesy of Dr. Sterling Clarren, Seattle, WA. Clarren, S.K. & Smith, D.W. (1978). The fetal alcohol syndrome. New England Journal of Medicine 298, *1063–1067. Copyright © 1978 Massassuchets Medical Society. All rights reserved.*

2-9	Effects of Divorce	
Age (years)	**Behavior**	
3–5	Fear, anxiety, and dread in daily life events Regression Searching and questioning Self-blame Increased aggression	
6–8	Extreme sadness Fantasies and panic Worries about lack of food, money, caretaking	
9–12	Intense anger Somatic complaints Confused self-identity	
13–18	Withdrawal from family Concern about sex and marriage Sense of loss Anger	

Adapted from Wallerstein, J., & Kelly, J. (1996). Surviving the breakup. New York: Harper Collins.

during the 1950s. This drug resulted in the birth of infants with limb abnormalities to women who used the drug during pregnancy. Other drugs can cause bleeding, stained teeth, impaired hearing, or other defects in the infant.[13]

Some maternal illnesses are harmful to the developing fetus. An example is rubella (German measles), which is rarely a serious disease for adults but which can cause deafness, vision defects, heart defects, and mental retardation in the fetus if it is acquired by a pregnant woman. A fetus can also acquire diseases, such as acquired immunodeficiency syndrome (AIDS)/human immunodeficiency virus (HIV) infection or hepatitis B from the mother.

Radiation, chemicals, and other environmental hazards may adversely affect a fetus when the mother is exposed to these influences during her pregnancy. The best outcomes for infants occur when mothers eat well; exercise regularly; seek early prenatal care; refrain from use of drugs, alcohol, tobacco, and excessive caffeine; and follow general principles of good health.

OTHER INFLUENCES

Family Structure

The families into which children are born influence them profoundly. Children are supported in different ways and acquire different world views depending on such factors as whether one or both parents work, how many siblings are present, and whether an extended family is close by. Note should be made of variations in family structure such as single parent, homosexual parents, extended family, and step-parents.

First-born children tend to be concerned with achievement and grades, often become leaders, and more commonly obtain advanced degrees. Last-born children more often demonstrate a relaxed approach to school and achievements.[14]

Nearly half of all marriages in the United States end in divorce. Divorce has a profound effect on children, varying with the child's age and cognitive stage. Young children who have limited ability to understand divorce may show such behavioral manifestations as crying, sleep disturbance, regression, and aggressive behavior[15] (see Table 2–9). Remarriage, single parenting, and joint custody arrangements all create special challenges for families.

School

Once a child is 5 or 6 years of age, several hours daily are spent in a school setting. Physical skills are developed through participation in education and sports. Psychosocial stages are met as the child interacts with children and adults and achieves social interaction patterns and pride in accomplishments. The presentation of concepts that challenge thought processes enhance cognitive development.

Although the primary role of schools is educational, they also perform several health-related functions. School health screening programs play an important role in identifying children with such health problems as hearing loss, visual impairment, and scoliosis.

Many schools teach good nutrition, healthful living, safe sexual practices, and other health-related subjects. A school nurse may be present, at least part time, to plan these classes or to work with teachers, as well as to provide emergency health care when needed. With the increase in mainstreaming, school staff now have the responsibility for administering medications, maintaining urinary catheters, and providing respiratory care and other treatments to ensure the child's proper growth and development.

Stress

The adverse effect of stress on adults is well documented. More recently the impact of stress on children has been recognized. Children manifest stress in a variety of ways, including regressive behavior, interrupted sleep, hyperactive behavior, gastrointestinal symptoms, crying, and withdrawal from normal events. Common stressful events for children include moving to a new home or school, marital difficulties in the family, abuse, and being expected to achieve at an extremely high level in school or sports[16] (Fig. 2–6).

The child experiencing stress has more frequent respiratory and gastrointestinal illnesses and is more likely to be the victim of an accident. The negative long-term effects of stress on body organs and systems suggest that children under stress are more likely to develop illnesses such as strokes, hypertension, and heart attacks later in life.

Socioeconomic Influences

Basic financial stability contributes much to the general health and well-being of children. The United States has the world's largest gross national product but does not meet the needs of many of its children. One quarter of all women in the United States receive no prenatal care in the first trimester of pregnancy, which contributes to a high infant mortality rate. One in four children in the United States is born into poverty, increasing the child's risk of prematurity, health problems, and abuse.[17]

Low socioeconomic status and unemployment are associated with a number of risk factors for children's development, such as poor nutrition,

RESEARCH CONSIDERATIONS

In one study of inner-city poor minority families with young children, the most commonly reported stressors for families related to food, shelter, transportation, medical care, information, and personal-time needs. The researchers identified important supports for these families—including family members, friends, and professionals—and suggested that health care professionals can help families gain access to these supports.[19]

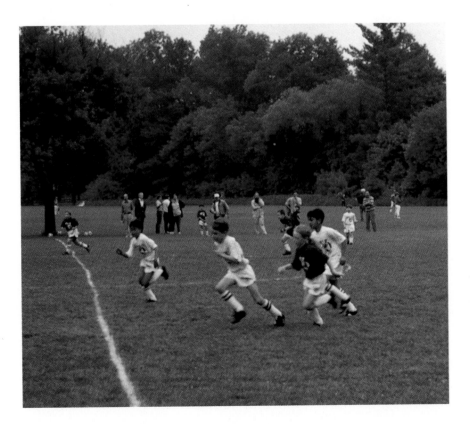

FIGURE 2–6. Sports can be an excellent way for children to develop their psychosocial, cognitive, and motor skills. However, when coaches and parents make demands of children beyond their developmental capabilities, the resultant stress can be manifested in gastrointestinal disorders, sleep disturbance, or other physical and psychosocial symptoms. *Courtesy Rebecca Scheirer, Kensington, Maryland.*

lack of immunization, increased injuries, and a high rate of teenage pregnancy.[18] Homelessness is one example of an economic problem that places children at risk. Families are the fastest growing group of homeless people. Homeless children do not usually have health insurance. They are more likely to lack immunizations, proper nutrition, a safe environment, and stable school and family situations.[20]

Community

The community in which a child lives may support the child's development or, conversely, expose the child to hazards. Social programs such as Head Start preschools, sports activities, after-school programs, and child abuse treatment centers offer valuable services that improve the experiences of growing children. On the other hand, an economically depressed community with scant services and a high homicide rate is unsupportive and hazardous for growing children.

The physical environment is supportive when the child is provided with sidewalks on which to walk to school, open spaces in which to learn and play, and clean air to breathe. Children who must walk to school on unsafe roads, have access to contaminated water supplies, or live near polluting manufacturing companies or in crowded housing or old structures are at risk for injuries and health problems such as lead poisoning.

Culture

The traditional customs of the many cultural groups represented in North American society influence the development of the children in these

2-10	Traditional Foods of Various Cultures	
Culture	**Traditional Foods**	**Special Notes**
African-American	Okra, kale, collard, and other greens; red and lima beans; black-eyed peas; corn bread; grits; pork products; tongue; chitterlings	Foods are similar to those common to all Southerners.
Orthodox Jewish	Kosher foods	Pork products and shellfish are prohibited. Milk and meat are not mixed or eaten at the same meal.
Native American	Blue corn meal, meats, fish, fruits, berries, greens	Practices vary among tribes. Milk products may not be widely used.
Mexican American	Beans, rice, cheese, corn, tortillas, enchiladas, burritos, avocados, chilies, melons, tomatoes	All meats and foods are labeled as "hot" or "cold," which does not relate to temperature. "Hot" foods such as cheese, eggs, onions, peppers, and beef are used to treat "cold" diseases such as cancer, teething, colds, and stomach cramps. "Cold" foods such as fruits and vegetables, dairy products, or chicken are used to treat "hot" diseases such as fever, rashes, or constipation.
Chinese American	Rice, tofu, bok choy, bean sprouts, water chestnuts, bamboo shoots, snow peas, melons, pineapple, duck, shellfish, thinly sliced beef, pork, or chicken	Special seasonings such as soy sauce and oyster sauce are used. Monosodium glutamate (MSG) used for cooking can increase salt intake. Lactose intolerance is frequent.
East Indian American	Wheat, rice, barley, chick peas, leafy green vegetables, potatoes, melons, berries	East Indian Hindus are vegetarians. Special spices are used for flavoring.

groups. Foods commonly eaten vary among people with different cultural backgrounds (Table 2–10) and influence the incidence of health problems such as cardiovascular disease in these groups. The Native American practice of carrying infants on boards often delays walking when it is measured against the norm for walking on some developmental tests. Children who are carried by straddling the mother's hips or back for extended periods have a low incidence of developmental dysplasia of the hip since this keeps their hips in an abducted position.

All cultural groups have rules regarding patterns of social interaction. Schedules of language acquisition are determined by the number of languages spoken and the amount of speech in the home. The particular social roles assumed by men and women in the culture affect school activities and ultimately career choices. Attitudes toward touching and other methods of encouraging developmental skills vary among cultures.

Media

The violence on television and in video games has been associated with aggressive behavior in children[22] (Fig. 2–7). A rating system for television shows has recently been adopted to indicate whether a show contains violence, sexual content, or language that might not be appropriate for children. Parents now have more information to assist them in guiding children's television viewing. They also can use lockout mechanisms that will turn the television off either after a certain period of viewing time or when violent shows are on. An increased amount of television viewing time is associated with above-normal weight, lower reading and intellectual test scores, and poorer sports performance.[23,24] Parents at home and nurses in the hospital should be aware of the shows children are watching, make decisions about their suitability, and be available to discuss the content with children.

 CULTURAL CONSIDERATIONS

Cultural differences in childrearing influence personality. For example, Japanese children are taught to respect parents and elders. Gender distinctions are the basis for social behaviors. Girls are praised for maintaining poise, grace, and control; boys for showing determination and strength of will in overcoming obstacles.

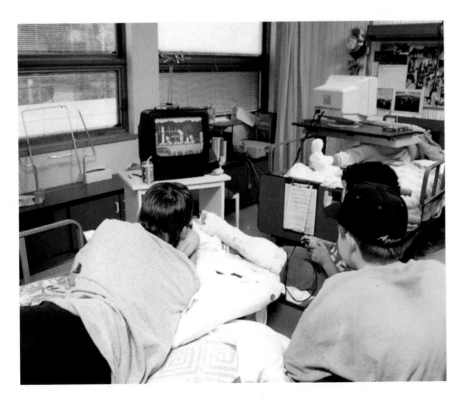

FIGURE 2–7. Some research suggests a correlation between violence on TV, in the movies, and in video games and aggressive behavior in children. Nurses should determine the parents' preference for what the child should watch when they are not with the child.

► INFANT (BIRTH TO 1 YEAR)

Can you imagine tripling your present weight in one year? Or becoming proficient in understanding fundamental words in a new language and even speaking a few? These and many more accomplishments take place in the first year of life. Starting the year as a mainly reflexive creature, the infant can walk and communicate by the year's end. Never again in life is development so swift (Fig. 2–8).

PHYSICAL GROWTH AND DEVELOPMENT

The first year of life is one of rapid change for the infant. The birth weight usually doubles by about 5 months and triples by the end of the first year (Fig. 2–9). Height increases by about a foot during this year. Teeth begin to erupt at about 6 months, and by the end of the first year the infant has six to eight deciduous teeth (see Chap. 3).

Body organs and systems, although not fully mature at 1 year, function differently than they did at birth. Kidney and liver maturation helps the 1-year-old excrete drugs or other toxic substances more readily than in the first weeks of life. The changing body proportions mirror changes in developing internal organs. Maturation of the nervous system is demonstrated by increased control over body movements, enabling the infant to sit, stand, and walk. Sensory function also increases as the infant begins to discriminate visual images, sounds, and tastes (Table 2–11).

CULTURAL CONSIDERATIONS

Health care providers in the United States use one set of growth charts for all children, but these charts do not take into account variations related to hereditary differences. African-American infants generally weigh less at birth than white infants but grow faster during childhood, thereby attaining a larger size. Some Asian groups have a hereditary predisposition to short stature. A review of parental and sibling size provides important data about the effects of cultural heritage. When height and weight are assessed, it is most important that growth follows the same percentile curve.

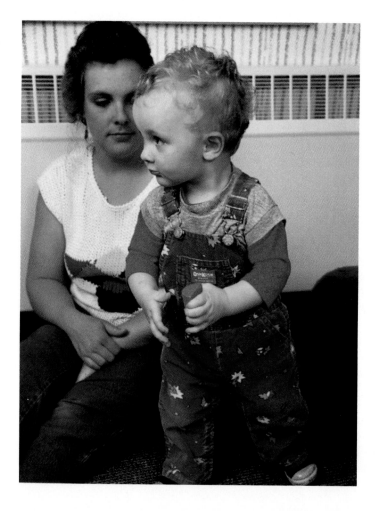

FIGURE 2–8. A 12-month-old child will have tripled his birth weight, learned to walk, and will be beginning to talk.

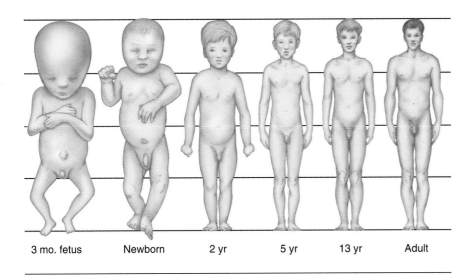

| 3 mo. fetus | Newborn | 2 yr | 5 yr | 13 yr | Adult |

FIGURE 2–9. Body proportions at various ages.

COGNITIVE DEVELOPMENT

The brain continues to increase in complexity during the first year. Most of the growth involves maturation of cells, with only a small increase in number of cells. This growth of the brain is accompanied by development of its functions. One has only to compare the behavior of an infant shortly after birth with that of a 1-year-old to understand the incredible maturation of brain function. The newborn's eyes widen in response to sound; the 1-year-old turns to the sound and recognizes its significance. The 2-month-old cries and coos; the 1-year-old says a few words and understands many more. The 6-week-old grasps a rattle for the first time; the 1-year-old reaches for toys and feeds himself or herself.

The infant's behaviors provide clues about thought processes. Piaget's work outlines the infant's actions in a set of rapidly progressing changes in the first year of life. The infant receives stimulation through sight, sound, and feeling, which the maturing brain interprets. This input from the environment interacts with internal cognitive abilities to enhance cognitive functioning.

PLAY

An 8-month-old infant is sitting on the floor, grasping blocks and banging them on the floor. When a parent walks by, the infant laughs and waves hands and feet wildly (Fig. 2–10). Physical capabilities enable the infant to move toward and reach out for objects of interest. Cognitive ability is reflected in manipulation of the blocks to create different sounds. Social interaction enhances play. The presence of a parent or other person increases interest in surroundings and teaches the infant different ways to play.

The play of infants begins in a reflexive manner. When an infant moves extremities or grasps objects, the foundations of play are established. Pleasure is gained from the feel and sound of these activities, and they gradually are performed purposefully. For example, when a parent places a rattle in the hand of a 6-week-old infant, the infant grasps it reflexively. As the hands move randomly, the rattle makes an enjoyable sound. The infant learns to move the rattle to create the sound and then finally to grasp the rattle at will to play with it.

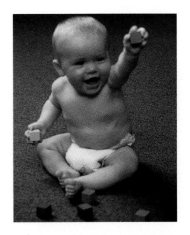

FIGURE 2–10. Garrett shows us that an 8-month-old child can play with blocks, demonstrating physical, cognitive, and social capabilities.

Age	Physical Growth	Fine Motor Ability	Gross Motor Ability	Sensory Ability	Nutrition
Birth to 1 month	Gains 5–7 oz (140–200 g)/week Grows 1.5 cm (½ in.) in first month Head circumference increases 1.5 cm (½ in.)/month	Holds hand in fist (1) Draws arms and legs to body when crying	Inborn reflexes such as startle and rooting are predominant activity May lift head briefly if prone (2) Alerts to high-pitched voices Comforts with touch (3)	Prefers to look at faces and black-and-white geometric designs Follows objects in line of vision (4)	Eats every 2–3 hours, breast or bottle, 2–3 oz (60–90 mL) per feeding

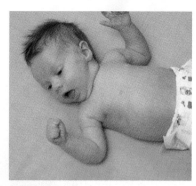

(1) Holds hand in fist

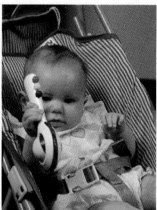

(2) May lift head

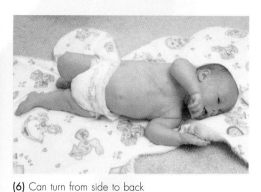

(3) Comforts with touch

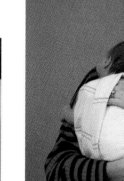

(4) Follows objects

| 2–4 months | Gains 5–7 oz (140–200 g)/week Grows 1.5 cm (½ in.)/month Head circumference increases 1.5 cm (½ in.)/month Posterior fontanel closes Eats 120 mL/kg/24 hr (2 oz/lb/24 hr) | Holds rattle when placed in hand (5) Looks at and plays with own fingers Readily brings objects from hand to mouth | Moro reflex fading in strength Can turn from side to back and then return (6) Decrease in head lag when pulled to sitting; sits with head held in midline with some bobbing When prone, holds head and supports weight on forearms (7) | Follows objects 180° Turns head to look for voices and sounds | Has coordinated suck-swallow Establishes regular eating pattern of 3–4 oz (90–120 mL) every 3–4 hours |

(5) Holds rattle

(6) Can turn from side to back

(7) Holds head up and supports weight with arms

2-11	Growth and Development Milestones During Infancy (continued)

Age	Physical Growth	Fine Motor Ability	Gross Motor Ability	Sensory Ability	Nutrition
4–6 months	Gains 5–7 oz (140–200 g)/week Doubles birth weight 5–6 months Grows 1.5 cm (½ in.)/month Head circumference increases 1.5 cm (½ in.)/month Teeth may begin erupting by 6 months Eats 100 mL/kg/24 hr (1½ oz/lb/24 hr)	Grasps rattles and other objects at will; drops them to pick up another offered object (8) Mouths objects Holds feet and pulls to mouth Holds bottle Grasps with whole hand (palmar grasp) Manipulates objects (9)	Head held steady when sitting No head lag when pulled to sitting Turns from abdomen to back by 4 months and then back to abdomen by 6 months When held standing supports much of own weight (10)	Examines complex visual images Watches the course of a falling object Responds readily to sounds	Eats 4–5 oz (100–150 g) four or more times/day Begins baby food, usually rice cereal

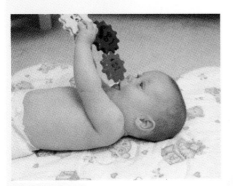

(8) Grasps objects at will

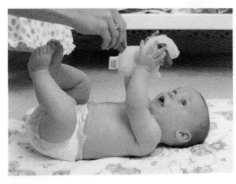

(9) Manipulates objects

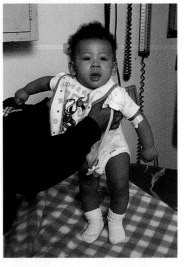

(10) Supports most of weight when held standing

Age	Physical Growth	Fine Motor Ability	Gross Motor Ability	Sensory Ability	Nutrition
6–8 months	Gains 3–5 oz (85–140 g)/week Grows 1 cm (⅜ in.)/month Growth rate slower than first 6 months	Bangs two objects held in hands Transfers objects from one hand to the other Beginning pincer grasp at times	Most inborn reflexes extinguished Sits alone steadily without support by 8 months (11) Likes to bounce on legs when held in standing position	Recognizes own name and responds by looking and smiling Enjoys small and complex objects at play	Eats 6–8 oz (160–225 g) four times/day Eats baby food such as rice cereal, fruits, and vegetables

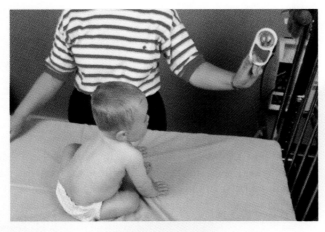

(11) Sits alone without support

Continued . . .

2-11	Growth and Development Milestones During Infancy (continued)				
Age	Physical Growth	Fine Motor Ability	Gross Motor Ability	Sensory Ability	Nutrition
8–10 months	Gains 3–5 oz (85–140 g)/week Grows 1 cm (⅜ in.)/month	Picks up small objects **(12)** Uses pincer grasp well **(14)**	Crawls or pulls whole body along floor by arms **(13)** Creeps by using hands and knees to keep trunk off floor Pulls self to standing and sitting by 10 months Recovers balance when sitting	Understands words such as "no" and "cracker" May say one word in addition to "mama" and "dada" Recognizes sound without difficulty	Eats 6 oz (160 g) four times/day Enjoys soft finger foods **(15)**

(12) Picks up small objects

(13) Crawls or pulls body by arms

(14) Uses pincer grab well

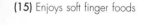
(15) Enjoys soft finger foods

The next phase of infant play focuses on manipulative behavior. The infant examines toys closely, looking at them, touching them, and placing them in the mouth. The infant learns a great deal about texture, qualities of objects, and all aspects of the surroundings. At the same time, interaction with others becomes an important part of play. The social nature of play is obvious as the infant plays with other children and adults.

Toward the end of the first year the infant's ability to move in space enlarges the sphere of play (Fig. 2–11). Once the infant is crawling or walking, he or she can get to new places, find new toys, discover forgotten objects, or

2-11	Growth and Development Milestones During Infancy (continued)				
Age	Physical Growth	Fine Motor Ability	Gross Motor Ability	Sensory Ability	Nutrition
10–12 months	Gains 3–5 oz (85–140 g)/week Grows 1 cm (³⁄₈ in.)/month Head circumference equals chest circumference Triples birth weight by 1 year	May hold crayon or pencil and make mark on paper Places objects into containers through holes (16)	Stands alone (17) Walks holding onto furniture Sits down from standing (18)	Plays peek-a-boo and patty cake	6–8 oz (160–225 g) four times/day Uses cup with lid and attempts to feed self with spoon though spills often (19) Eating most soft table foods with family

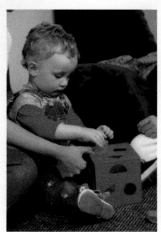
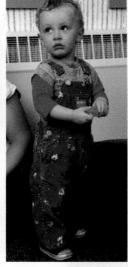
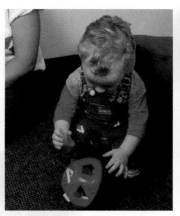
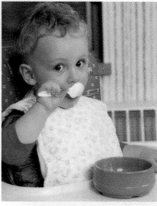

(16) Places objects in container through holes

(17) Stands alone

(18) Sits down from standing

(19) Feeds self with spoon

seek out other people for interaction. Play is a reflection of every aspect of development, as well as a method for enhancing learning and maturation (Table 2–12).

NUTRITION

From the first feeding of a few ounces of breast milk or formula to a meal of soft table foods with the family at 1 year of age, the infant demonstrates an amazing growth in ability to ingest and digest a wide variety of foods. Never again will the individual have such a high metabolic rate or high intake requirements in relation to size, or such a change in the types of food eaten. Meeting these needs is made difficult by the small size of the infant's stomach and the immaturity of the digestive system. The great physical activity necessitates a high caloric intake. Nutrient demands for protein and vitamins must be met for the cells of the nervous system and body organs to develop properly.

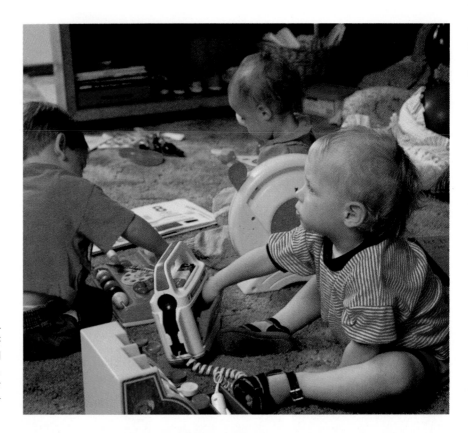

FIGURE 2–11. Mobility enlarges the sphere of play, allowing the child to seek new toys and spaces and to seek out people for interaction. Which psychosocial, cognitive, and motor skills do you see taking place in this photograph?

2-12   Favorite Toys and Activities in Infancy

Birth to 2 months
Mobiles, black-and-white patterns, mirrors
Music boxes, singing, tape players, soft voices
Rocking and cuddling
Moving legs and arms while singing and talking
Varying stimuli—different rooms, sounds, visual images

3–6 months
Rattles
Stuffed animals
Soft toys with contrasting colors
Noise-making objects that are easily grasped

6–12 months
Large blocks
Teething toys
Toys that pop apart and back together
Nesting cups and other objects that fit into one another or stack
Surprise toys such as jack-in-the-box
Social interaction with adults and other children
Games such as peek-a-boo
Soft balls
Push and pull toys

Early Breast- or Bottle-Feeding

The first decision parents have to make about their infant's food intake is whether to breast-feed or bottle-feed. Citing the nutritional, immunologic, and psychosocial benefits of breast-feeding, the American Academy of Pediatrics encourages mothers to breast-feed for the first few months of life. Breast milk naturally provides all necessary nutrients for the infant, as well as immunity against several diseases.[12]

Providing breast-feeding information and instruction positively influences the number of women who decide to breast-feed and increases the number of months mothers choose to breast-feed. Some hospitals have lactation specialists who assist breast-feeding mothers; in others, the staff nurses provide this service. Home visits or phone calls from the hospital nursing staff and telephone numbers for support organizations such as LaLeche League can provide mothers with needed breast-feeding information or problem-solving suggestions. Support programs are especially helpful to mothers who have difficulty breast-feeding, feel unsure how it will fit into family and work life, or have an infant with problems related to feeding, such as prematurity. The mother of a hospitalized child will need special support to continue breast-feeding. The mother should be encouraged to come to the hospital to feed her baby on the same schedule as at home. If the infant cannot breast-feed, many hospitals have electric pumps so the mother can maintain lactation. Often hospitals provide some meals for the mother to help maintain quality nutrition for the baby.

 SAFETY PRECAUTIONS

Formula can be mixed with tap water but must be refrigerated once mixed. Formula that the baby does not drink should be discarded after use and not kept for future feedings. This minimizes the chance for bacteria to grow and to cause illness in the baby.

2-13 Advantages and Disadvantages of Formula Preparations

Formula Preparation	How Packaged	Advantages	Disadvantages
Ready to feed	Bottles or cans	No preparation needed	Most expensive type of formula
Concentrate	Cans of concentrated liquid	Easy to add equal amounts of formula concentrate and water directly into bottle and shake	Can be incorrectly measured, leading to inadequate or unsafe nutrition for infant; requires access to clean water supply such as city tap water or bottled water; well water may have too high a mineral concentration
Powder	Cans	Least expensive type of formula	Can be incorrectly measured, leading to inadequate or unsafe nutrition for infant; requires shaking to mix thoroughly; requires access to clean water supply such as city tap water or bottled water; well water may have too high a mineral concentration

COMMON BABY FORMULAS

Milk-based Formulas
Enfamil
Good Nature
Similac
SMA
Soy-based Formulas
Isomil
Nursoy
ProSobee
Soyalac
Specialized Formulas
Lofenalac (low phenylketonuria)
Nutramigen (casein hydrolysate)
Portagen (sodium caseinate)

CLINICAL TIP

Nursing bottle mouth syndrome occurs when an infant is allowed to nurse or drink from a bottle for long periods, especially when sleeping. The milk, juice, or other fluid pools around the upper anterior teeth, salivary flow decreases, and acid buffering is decreased, resulting in tooth decay.

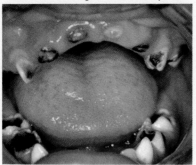

Teach parents to avoid putting the child to bed with a bottle. Encourage pacifier use or a bottle of water instead. Mothers who breast-feed should also be cautioned to limit nursing to specific feeding times so that milk will not pool in the mouth during sleep.[25]

Courtesy Dr. Lezley McIlveen, Department of Dentistry, Children's National Medical Center, Washington, D.C.

FOODS THAT COMMONLY CAUSE CHOKING

Hot dogs
Nuts
Popcorn
Hard candy
Ice cubes
Grapes
Uncooked vegetable chunks
Lumps of peanut butter

Some women decide against breast-feeding or are unable to breast-feed. Nurses can provide these mothers with information about formula feeding. Three types of infant formula are available—ready to feed, concentrate, and powder. All are nutritionally adequate for infants. The nurse can help the parents decide which preparation of formula is best suited for their infant (Table 2–13). Some infants, such as those with phenylketonuria, other metabolic disorders, or disorders affecting dietary intake, will require specialized formulas. Breast- or bottle-feeding is assessed at each contact with health professionals to identify potential teaching needs.

Introduction of Other Foods

When should other foods be added to the infant's diet? Although some parents add other foods when the infant is only days or weeks old, it is best to take cues from the infant's developmental milestones. The American Academy of Pediatrics recommends introducing semisolid food at 4–6 months. At this age the protrusion reflex (or tongue thrust) decreases and the infant can sit well with support.[26]

The first food added to the infant's diet is usually rice cereal. The advantage of introducing cereal first is that it provides iron at an age when the infant's prenatal iron stores begin to decrease, seldom causes allergy, and is easy to digest. A tablespoon or two is fed to the infant once or twice daily, just before formula or breast-feeding. The infant may appear to spit out the food at first because of the normal tongue thrust. Parents should not interpret this early feeding behavior as indicating dislike for the food. With a little practice the infant becomes adept at spoon feeding.

Once the infant eats $\frac{1}{4}$ cup of cereal twice a day, usually at 6–8 months of age, vegetables or fruits can be introduced (Table 2–14). By 8–10 months of age, most fruits and vegetables have been introduced and strained meats can be added to the infant's diet. Finger foods are introduced during the second half of the first year as the infant's palmar and then finger grasp develops and as teeth begin to erupt. Infants enjoy toast, O-shaped cereal, finely sliced meats, and small pieces of cooked, softened vegetables. Advise parents to use caution in providing finger foods to the infant. Hard foods slip easily into the throat and may cause choking. As food and juice intake increases, formula or breast-feedings decrease in amount and frequency (Table 2–15).

INJURY PREVENTION

Injuries are a major cause of death in childhood. The infant is particularly vulnerable to injuries when not adequately supervised. Increasing mobility during the second half of the first year challenges parents to childproof the home and environment. The nurse can provide anticipatory guidance to help prevent unintentional injuries (Table 2–16).

PERSONALITY AND TEMPERAMENT

Why does one infant frequently awaken at night crying while another sleeps for 8–10 hours undisturbed? Why does one infant smile much of the time and react positively to interactions while another is withdrawn with unfamiliar people and frequently frowns and cries? Such differences in responses to the environment are believed to be inborn characteristics of temperament. Infants are born with a tendency to react in certain ways to noise

2-14   Introduction of Solid Foods in Infancy

Recommendation	Rationale
Introduce rice cereal at 4–6 months.	Rice cereal is easy to digest, has low allergenic potential, and contains iron.
Introduce fruits or vegetables at 6–8 months.	Fruits and vegetables provide needed vitamins.
Introduce meats at 8–10 months.	Meats are harder to digest, have high protein load, and should not be fed until close to 1 year of age.
Use single-food prepared baby foods rather than combination meals.	Combination meals usually contain more sugar, salt, and fillers.
Introduce one new food at a time, waiting at least 3 days to introduce another.	If a food allergy develops, it will be easy to identify.
Avoid carrots, beets, and spinach before 4 months of age.	Their nitrates can be converted to nitrite by young infants, causing methemoglobinemia.
Infants can be fed mashed portions of table foods such as carrots, rice, and potatoes.	This is a less expensive alternative to jars of commercially prepared baby food; it allows parents of various cultural groups to feed ethnic foods to infants.
Avoid adding sugar, salt, spices when mixing own baby foods.	Infants need not become accustomed to these flavors; they may get too much sodium from salt or develop gastric distress from some spices.
Avoid honey until at least 1 year of age.	Infants cannot detoxify *Clostridium botulinum* spores sometimes present in honey and can develop botulism.

and to interact differently with people. They may display varying degrees of regularity in activities of eating and sleeping, and manifest a capacity for concentrating on tasks for different amounts of time.

Nursing assessment identifies personality characteristics of the infant that the nurse can share with the parents. With this information, the parents can appreciate more fully the uniqueness of their infant and design experiences to meet the infant's needs. Parents can learn to modify the environment to promote adaptation. For example, an infant who does not adapt easily to new situations may cry, withdraw, or develop another way of coping when adjusting to new people or places. Parents might be advised to use one or two baby-sitters rather than engaging new sitters frequently. If the infant is easily distracted when eating, parents can feed the infant in a quiet setting to encourage a focus on eating. Although the infant's temperament is unchanged, the ability to fit with the environment is enhanced.

COMMUNICATION

Even at a few weeks of age, infants communicate and engage in two-way interaction. Comfort is expressed by soft sounds, cuddling, and eye contact.

COMMUNICATION STRATEGIES: INFANT

Hold for feedings.
Hold, rock, and talk to infant often.
Talk and sing frequently during care.
Tell names of objects.
Use high-pitched voice with newborns.
When the infant is upset, swaddle and hold securely.

2-15	Typical Daily Intake at Various Ages					
	Breakfast	**Snack**	**Lunch**	**Snack**	**Dinner**	**Snack**
Infant 6 months	2 T rice cereal with 2 oz (60 mL) formula	4 oz (120 mL) formula or breast milk	6 oz (180 mL) formula or breast milk	6 oz (180 mL) formula or breast milk	2 T rice cereal with 2 oz (60 mL) formula, then 6 oz (180 mL) formula or breast milk	4 oz (120 mL) formula or breast milk
12 months	6 oz (180 mL) apple juice 4 T rice cereal with 4 oz (120 mL) milk	3 crackers ½ cup (120 mL) milk	1 thin slice (½ oz [14 g]) of turkey ½ cup soft cooked carrots 1 cup (240 mL) milk	½ slice of cheese ½ cup (120 mL) juice	¼ cup plain pasta ¼ cup thin sliced apple chunks ½ cup (120 mL) milk	½ cup yogurt
Toddler	¼ cup (60 mL) orange juice ¼ cup cereal with ½ cup (120 mL) milk ¼ banana	5 crackers ½ cup (120 mL) milk	2 thin slices (1 oz [28 g]) of turkey with ½ slice of bread ½ cup cooked carrots 1 cup (240 mL) milk	1 slice cheese ½ cup (120 mL) juice	¼ cup plain pasta ¼–½ cup thin sliced apple chunks ½ cup (120 mL) milk	½ cup yogurt
Preschooler	½ cup (120 mL) orange juice ⅓ cup cereal with 3/4 cup (180 mL) milk ½ banana	5 crackers ½ orange ½ cup (120 mL) milk	3 thin slices (1½ oz [42 g]) of turkey with ½ slice bread ¼ cup cooked carrots ¾ cup (180 mL) milk	1 slice cheese ½ cup (120 mL) juice	¼ cup plain pasta with meat sauce ½ cup thin sliced apple chunks ½ cup (120 mL) milk	½ cup yogurt
School-age child	½ cup (120 mL) orange juice ¾ cup cereal with 1 cup (240 mL) milk ½ bagel with jam		4 thin slices (2 oz [56 g]) of turkey with 1 slice bread and condiments Apple 1 cup (240 mL) milk 1 oatmeal cookie	1½ cups popcorn 1 cup (240 mL) lemonade	½ cup pasta with meat sauce Dinner salad 1 slice garlic bread 1 cup (240 mL) milk	1 cup pudding or yogurt
Adolescent	½ cup (120 mL) orange juice 1 cup cereal 1 cup (240 mL) milk 1 bagel with 1 T peanut butter and jam		3 oz (84 g) meat with 2 slices of bread plus condiments Apple 1 cup (240 mL) milk 1 oatmeal cookie	3 cups popcorn 1 cup (240 mL) lemonade	1½ cup pasta with meat sauce 1 slice garlic bread Salad with dressing 1 cup (240 mL) milk	1 cup pudding Fruit

2-16   Injury Prevention in Infancy

Hazard	Developmental Characteristics	Preventive Measures
Falls	Mobility increases in first year of life, progressing from squirming movements to crawling, rolling, and standing	Do not leave infant unsecured in infant seat, even in newborn period. Do not place on high surfaces such as tables or beds unless holding child. **(1)** Once mobile by crawling, keep doors to stairways closed or use gates. Standing walkers have led to many injuries and are not recommended.
Burns	Infant is dependent on caretakers for environmental control. The second half of the first year is marked by crawling and increased mobility. Objects are explored by touching and placing in mouth.	Check temperature of bath water and food/liquids for drinking. Cover electrical outlets. Supervise infant so that play with electrical cords cannot occur.
Motor vehicle crashes	Infant is dependent on caretakers for placement in car. On impact with another motor vehicle, an infant held on a lap acts as a torpedo.	Use only approved restraint systems (according to Federal Motor Vehicle Safety Standards) (see Table 2–22). The seat must be used for every trip, even if very short. The seat must be properly buckled to the car's lap belt system. **(2)**
Drowning	Infant cannot swim and is unable to lift head.	Never leave infant alone in a bath of even 2.5 (1 in.) of water. Supervise when in water even when a life preserver is worn. Flotation devices such as arm inflatables are not certified life preservers.

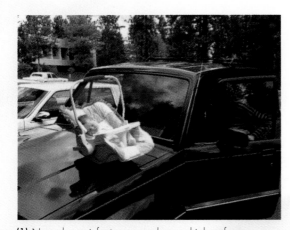

(1) Never leave infant unsecured or on high surface.

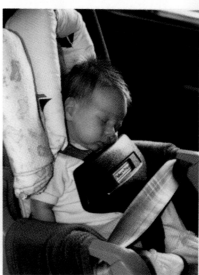

(2) Always use approved restraint system. Place infant in rear-facing seat in backseat of car

Continued . . .

The infant displays discomfort by thrashing the extremities, arching the back, and crying vigorously. From these rudimentary skills, communication ability continues to develop until the infant speaks several words at the end of the first year of life (Table 2–17).

Nurses assess communication to identify possible abnormalities or developmental delays. Language ability may be assessed with the Denver II De-

2-16   Injury Prevention in Infancy (continued)

Hazard	Developmental Characteristics	Preventive Measures
Poisoning	Infant is dependent on caretakers to keep harmful substances out of reach. The second half of infancy is marked by exploratory reaching and mouthing objects.	Keep medicines out of reach. Teach proper dosage and administration of medicines to parents. Cleaning products and other harmful substances should not be stored where the infant can reach them. Remove plants from play areas. Have poison control center number by telephone.
Choking	Infant explores objects by placing them in the mouth. **(3)**	Avoid foods that commonly cause choking. Keep small toys away from infants, especially toys labeled "not intended for use in those under 3 years."
Suffocation	Young infant has minimal head control and may be unable to move if vomiting or having difficulty breathing.	Position infant on side for sleep, particularly after feeding. Do not place pillows, stuffed toys, or other objects near head. Do not use plastic in crib. Avoid latex balloons. **(4)**
Strangulation	Infant is able to get head into railings or crib slats but cannot remove it.	Be sure older cribs have slats spaced 6 cm (2⅜ in.) or less apart. The mattress must fit tightly against the crib rails.

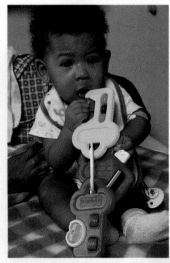

(3) Explores objects with mouth.

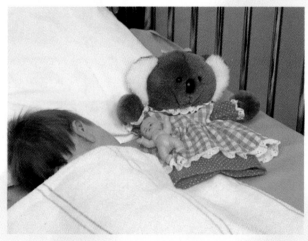

(4) Place infant on side after eating, keep toys clear. The nurse should remove the unsafe toys and pillow from this infant's crib.

velopmental Test and other specialized language screening tools (see Chap. 5). Normal infants understand (receptive speech) more words than they can speak (expressive speech). Abnormalities may be caused by a hearing deficit, developmental delay, or lack of verbal stimulation from caretakers. Further assessment may be required to pinpoint the cause of the abnormality.

Nursing interventions focus on providing a stimulating environment. Parents are encouraged to speak to infants and teach words. Hospital nurses should include the infant's known words when providing care.

2-17	Patterns of Infant Communication
Age	**Behavior**
Birth to 2 months	Coos Babbles Comfort sounds Cries
3–6 months	Vocalizations with play and favorite people Laughs Cries less Squeals and makes pleasure sounds Multisyllabic babbling
6–9 months	Increasing vowel and consonant sounds Links syllables together Speech-like rhythm when "talking" with adult
9–12 months	Understands "no" and other simple commands Says "dada" and "mama" to identify parents Learns one or two other words Receptive speech surpasses expressive speech

► TODDLER (1–3 YEARS)

Toddlerhood is sometimes called the first adolescence. An infant only months before, the child from 1 to 3 years is now displaying independence and negativism. Pride in newfound accomplishments emerges.

PHYSICAL GROWTH AND DEVELOPMENT

The rate of growth slows during the second year of life. By age 2, the birth weight has usually quadrupled and the child is about one half of the adult height. Body proportions begin to change, with legs longer and head smaller in proportion to body size than during infancy (see Fig. 2–9). The toddler has a pot-bellied appearance and stands with feet apart to provide a wide base of support. By approximately 33 months, eruption of deciduous teeth is complete, with 20 teeth present.

Gross motor activity develops rapidly (Table 2–18), as the toddler progresses from walking to running, kicking, and riding a Big Wheel tricycle (Fig. 2–12). As physical maturation occurs, the toddler develops the ability to control elimination patterns (Table 2–19).

COGNITIVE DEVELOPMENT

During the toddler years the child moves from the sensorimotor to the preoperational stage of development. The early use of language awakens in the 1-year-old the ability to think about objects or people when they are absent. Object permanence is well developed.

At about 2 years of age, the increasing use of words as symbols enables the toddler to use preoperational thought. Rudimentary problem solving, creative thought, and an understanding of cause-and-effect relationships are now possible.

CULTURAL CONSIDERATIONS

In traditional Native American families, children are allowed to unfold and develop naturally at their own pace. Children thus wean and toilet-train themselves at their own pace with little interference or pressure from parents.

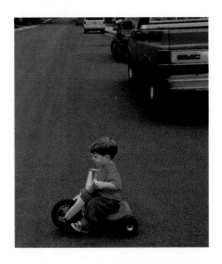

FIGURE 2–12. This toddler has learned to ride a Big Wheel, which he is doing right into the street. Toddlers must be closely watched to prevent injury.

2-18   Growth and Development Milestones During Toddlerhood

Age	Physical Growth	Fine Motor Ability	Gross Motor Ability	Sensory Ability	Nutrition
1–2 years	Gains 227 g (8 oz) or more per month Grows 9–12 cm (3.5–5 in.) during this year Anterior fontanel closes	By end of 2nd year, builds a tower of four blocks (1) Scribbles on paper (2) Can undress self (3) Throws a ball	Runs Walks up and down stairs (5) Likes push and pull toys (6)	Visual acuity 20/50	Eats three meals per day with snacks Drinks regular milk or follow-up formula Uses cup and spoon but often prefers finger foods
2–3 years	Gains 1.4–2.3 kg (3–5 lb)/year Grows 5–6.5 cm (2–2.5 in.)/year	Draws a circle and other rudimentary forms Learns to pour Learning to dress self (4)	Jumps Kicks ball (7) Throws ball overhand		May begin to use fork but still needs food cut into bite-size pieces

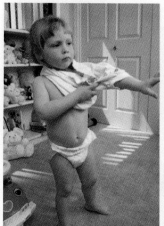
(1) Second year tower of four blocks

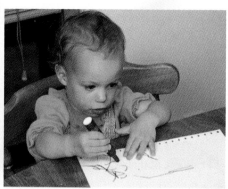
(2) Scribbles on paper

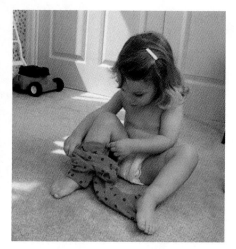
(3) Can undress self

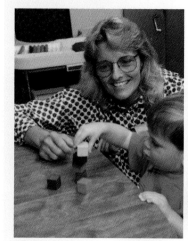
(4) Learning to dress self

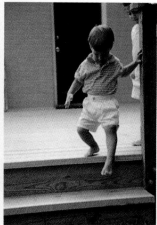
(5) Walks up and down stairs

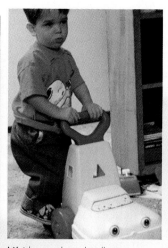
(6) Likes push and pull toys

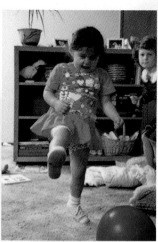
(7) Jumps and kicks ball

2-19 Toilet Training

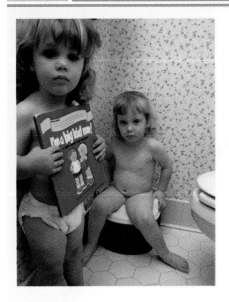

When are children ready to learn toileting? Are parents responsible for the differences in ages at which toilet training is accomplished? Does toilet training provide clues to a child's intellectual ability?

We know that children are not ready for toilet training until several developmental capabilities exist: to stand and walk well, to pull pants up and down, to recognize the need to eliminate and then to be able to wait until in the bathroom. Once this readiness is apparent, the child can be given a small potty chair and the procedure explained.

Children often prefer their own chair on the floor to using the large toilet. The child should be placed on the chair at regular intervals for a few moments and can be given reward or praise for successes. If the child seems not to understand or does not wish to cooperate, it is best to wait a few weeks and then try again. Just as all of development is subject to individual timetables, toilet training occurs with considerable variability from one child to another. Identify for parents the developmental characteristics of their child and encourage them to appreciate without anxiety the unfolding of skills. These timetables are not predictive of future development.

The child who is ill or hospitalized or has other stress often regresses in toilet training activities. It is best to quietly reinstitute attempts at training after the trauma. Potty chairs should be available on pediatric units and toileting habits identified during initial assessment so that regular routines can be followed and the child's usual words for elimination can be used.

PLAY

Many changes in play patterns occur between infancy and toddlerhood. The toddler's motor skills enable him or her to bang pegs into a pounding board with a hammer. The social nature of toddler play is also readily seen. Toddlers find the company of other children pleasurable, even though socially interactive play may not occur. Two toddlers tend to play with similar objects side by side, occasionally trading toys and words. This is called **parallel play.** This playtime with other children assists toddlers to develop social skills. Toddlers engage in play activities they have seen at home, such as pounding with a hammer and talking on the phone. This imitative behavior teaches them new actions and skills (Fig. 2–13).

Physical skills are manifested in play as toddlers push and pull objects, climb in and out and up and down, run, ride a Big Wheel, turn the pages of books, and scribble with a pen. Both gross motor and fine motor abilities are enhanced during this age period.

Cognitive understanding enables the toddler to manipulate objects and learn about their qualities. Stacking blocks and placing rings on a building tower teach spatial relationships and other lessons that provide a foundation for future learning. Various kinds of play objects should be provided for the toddler to meet play needs. These play needs can easily be met whether the child is hospitalized or at home (Table 2–20).

NUTRITION

Why do parents of toddlers frequently become concerned about the small amount of food their children eat? Why do toddlers seem to survive and even thrive with minimal food intake? The toddler often displays the phenomenon of **physiologic anorexia,** caused when the extremely high metabolic demands of infancy slow to keep pace with the more moderate growth rate of toddlerhood. Although it can appear that the toddler eats nothing

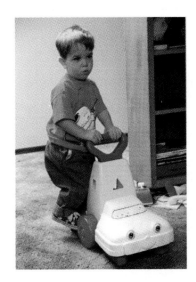

FIGURE 2–13. Imitative play such as pushing and pulling allows the toddler to develop gross and fine motor skills.

2-20   Favorite Toys and Activities in Toddlerhood

Play Need	Types of Toys and Activities
Facilitate imitative behavior	Play kitchen Grocery carts Pounding board Toy phone
Encourage gross motor activity and provide an outlet for stress	Big Wheel tricycle Soft ball and bat Water and sand Bean bag toss
Foster fine motor skills	Cloth books Large pencil and paper Wooden puzzles
Facilitate cognitive growth	Educational television shows Music Stories and books

at times, intake over days or a week is generally sufficient and balanced enough to meet the body's demands for nutrients and energy.

Advise parents to offer a variety of nutritious foods several times daily (three meals and two snacks) and let the toddler make choices from the foods offered. Small portions are also more appealing to the toddler. A general rule of thumb for food quantity at a meal is one tablespoon of each food per year of age (see Table 2–15). The toddler should drink 16–24 oz (½–¾ L) of milk daily. Caution parents against giving the toddler more than a quart (a liter) of milk daily, since this interferes with the desire to eat other foods, leading to an unbalanced diet.

The toddler displays characteristic autonomy (independence) during mealtime. Advise parents to provide opportunities for self-feeding of food with fingers and utensils, and to allow some simple choices, such as type of juice. Because social skills are developing, the hospitalized toddler may eat better if allowed to have meals with parents or other hospitalized children.

INJURY PREVENTION

By 1 year of age, unintentional injuries are by far the leading cause of death in children.[27] Injuries also cause disfigurement and other ongoing health problems. Nurses intervene to care for injured children in the hospital and are responsible for making sure that the hospital environment is free of safety hazards. Nurses are also instrumental in teaching parents how to make the toddler's environment safe (Tables 2–21 and 2–22).

PERSONALITY AND TEMPERAMENT

The toddler retains most of the temperamental characteristics identified during infancy but may demonstrate some changes. The normal developmental progression of toddlerhood also plays a part in responses. For example, the infant who previously responded positively to stimuli, such as a new baby-sitter, may appear more negative in toddlerhood. The increasing independence characteristic of this age is shown by the toddler's use of

2-21   Injury Prevention in Toddlerhood

	Hazard	Developmental Characteristics	Preventive Measures
	Falls	Gross motor skills improve. Toddler is able to move chairs to counters and can climb up ladders.	Supervise toddler closely. Provide safe climbing toys. Begin to teach acceptable places for climbing.
	Poisoning	Gross motor skills enable toddler to climb onto chairs and then cabinets. Medicines, cosmetics, and other poisonous substances are easily reached.	Keep medicines and other poisonous materials locked away. Use child-resistant containers and cupboard closures. Have poison control center number by telephone. Keep syrup of ipecac in home.
	Burns	Toddler is tall enough to reach stove top. Toddler can walk to fireplace and may reach into fire.	Keep pot handles turned inward on stove. Do not burn fires without close supervision. Use a fire screen.
	Motor vehicle crashes	Toddler may be able to undo seat belt, may resist using car seat, demonstrating characteristic negativism and autonomy.	Insist on safety seat use for all trips (see Table 2–22). Use approved safety seats only, such as forward-facing convertible seat. Toddler is not large enough to use car seat belts.

Continued . . .

the word *no.* The parent and child constantly adapt their responses to each other and learn anew how to communicate with each other.

COMMUNICATION

Because of the phenomenal growth of language skills during the toddler period, adults should communicate frequently with children in this age

2-21   Injury Prevention in Toddlerhood (continued)

	Hazard	Developmental Characteristics	Preventive Measures
	Drowning	Toddler can walk onto docks or pool decks. Toddler may stand on or climb seats on boat. Toddler may fall into buckets, toilets, and fish tanks and be unable to get top of body out.	Supervise any child near water. Swimming classes do not protect a toddler from drowning. Use child-resistant pool covers. Use approved child life jackets near water and on boats. Empty buckets when not in use.

2-22   Parent Teaching: Use of Infant and Child Car Seats

Weight below 9 kg (20 lb)
Use infant or convertible seat in back seat of car in backward-facing position.
Keep infant reclined at 45 degrees.
Never place the infant in the front passenger seat.
Fasten seat securely to car using car seat belt and following manufacturer instructions.
Adjust harnesses to fit snugly at shoulders and legs.
When using an infant seat, move to a larger seat before the infant's head reaches the top of shell.
When using a convertible seat from birth, use one with a 5-point harness.

Birth–18 kg (40 lb)
When using a convertible seat, use reclined for rear-facing and upright for forward-facing position.
Follow manufacturer instructions for proper positions at specified child weights for that product.
When using a convertible seat, move to a high-backed child seat or booster when child's ears are above the seat.
Always place the seat in rear seat of the vehicle.

Above 13.6 or 18 kg–27 or 36.3 kg (30 or 40 lb–60 or 80 lb)
Use booster seat for children who have outgrown convertible/toddler seats.
Follow manufacturer instructions for use and for specified child weights for the product.
Use booster seat until the vehicle lap and shoulder belts fit correctly.
Have all children 12 years and under ride in the rear seat, whether or not in a car seat.
Note: Air bags can cause serious injury and death when a child is in a car seat in the front passenger seat. Even when not in a car seat, and when the vehicle is not equipped with a passenger side air bag, the back seat is the safest for all children.

From National Safety Council (1998). Child Passenger Safety. Washington DC: Author.

2-23   Communicating With a Toddler

Procedures such as drawing blood can be frightening for a toddler. Effective communication minimizes the trauma caused by such procedures:

- Avoid telling toddlers about the procedure too far in advance. They do not have an understanding of time and can become quite anxious.
- Use simple terminology. "We need to get a little blood from your arm. It will help us to find out if you are getting better." If the parent is willing, say, "Your Mom will hold your arm still so we can do it quickly."
- Allow the toddler to cry. Acknowledge that it must be frightening and that you understand.
- Perform the procedure in a treatment room so that the toddler's bed and room are a safe haven.
- Be sure the toddler is restrained, with the joints above and below the procedure immobilized.
- Use a Band-Aid to cover up the site. This can reassure the toddler that the body is still intact.
- Allow the toddler to choose a reward such as a sticker after the procedure.
- Praise the toddler for cooperation and acknowledge that you know this was difficult.
- Comfort the toddler by rocking, offering a favorite drink, playing music, and holding. If parents are present, they can offer the comfort needed.

---

group. Toddlers imitate words and speech intonations, as well as the social interactions they observe.

At the beginning of toddlerhood, the child may use four to six words in addition to "mama" and "dada." Receptive speech (the ability to understand words) far outpaces expressive speech. By the end of toddlerhood, however, the 3-year-old has a vocabulary of almost 1000 words and uses short sentences.

Communication occurs in many ways, some of which are nonverbal. Toddler communication includes pointing, pulling an adult over to a room or object, and speaking in expressive jargon. **Expressive jargon** is using unintelligible words with normal speech intonations as if truly communicating in words. Another communication method occurs when the toddler cries, pounds feet, displays a temper tantrum, or uses other means to illustrate dismay. These powerful communication methods can upset parents, who often need suggestions for handling them. It is best to verbalize the feelings shown by the toddler, for example, by saying, "You must be very upset that you cannot have that candy. When you stop crying you can come out of your room," and then to ignore further negative behavior. The toddler's search for autonomy and independence creates a need for such behavior. Sometimes an upset toddler responds well to holding, rocking, and stroking.

Parents and nurses can promote a toddler's communication by speaking frequently, naming objects, explaining procedures in simple terms, expressing feelings that the toddler seems to be displaying, and encouraging speech. The toddler from a bilingual home is at an optimal age to learn two languages. If the parents do not speak English, the toddler will benefit from a day-care experience so that both languages can be learned.

The nurse who understands the communication skills of toddlers is able to assess expressive and receptive language and communicate effectively, thereby promoting positive health care experiences for these children (Table 2–23).

COMMUNICATION STRATEGIES: TODDLER

Give short, clear instructions.
Do not give choices if none exist.
Offer a choice of two alternatives when possible.
Approach positively.
Tell toddler what you are doing, names of objects.

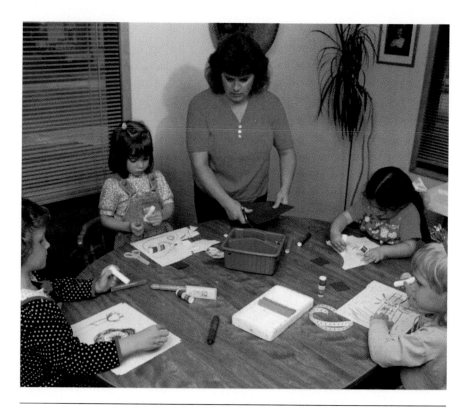

FIGURE 2–14. Preschoolers have well-developed language, motor, and social skills, and they can work creatively together on an art project, as this group is doing at a day-care center in Spokane.

▶ PRESCHOOL CHILD (3–6 YEARS)

The preschool years are a time of new initiative and independence. Most children are in a day-care center or school for part of the day and learn a great deal from this social contact. Language skills are well developed, and the child is able to understand and speak clearly. Endless projects characterize the world of busy preschoolers. They may work with play dough to form animals, then cut out and paste paper, then draw and color (Fig. 2–14).

PHYSICAL GROWTH AND DEVELOPMENT

Preschoolers grow slowly and steadily, with most growth taking place in long bones of the arms and legs. The short, chubby toddler gradually gives way to a slender, long-legged preschooler (Table 2–24).

Physical skills continue to develop (Fig. 2–15). The preschooler runs with ease, holds a bat, and throws balls of various types. Writing ability increases, and the preschooler enjoys drawing and learning to write a few letters.

COGNITIVE DEVELOPMENT

The preschooler exhibits characteristics of preoperational thought. Symbols or words are used to represent objects and people, enabling the young child to think about them. This is a milestone in intellectual development; however, the preschooler still has some limitations in thought (Table 2–25).

Physical Growth

Gains 1.5–2/5 kg (3–5 lb)/year Grows 4–6 cm (1½–2½ in.)/year

Fine Motor Ability

Uses scissors **(1)**
Draws circle, square, cross **(2)**
Draws at least a six-part person
Enjoys art projects such as pasting, string-
  ing beads, using clay
Learns to tie shoes at end of preschool
  years **(3)**
Buttons **(4)**
Brushes teeth **(5)**

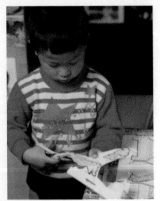

(1) Uses scissors

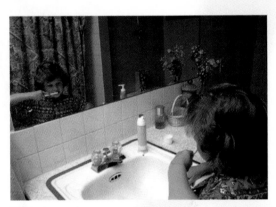

(2) Draws circle, square, cross

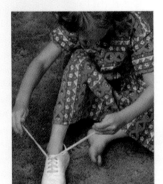

(3) Ties shoes

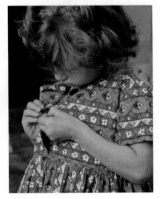

(4) Buttons clothes

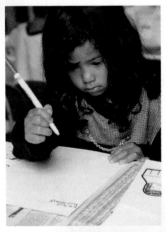

(5) Brushes teeth

Gross Motor Ability

Throws a ball overhand
Climbs well **(6)**
Ride tricycle **(7)**

Sensory Ability

Visual acuity continues to improve
Can focus on and learn letters and
  numbers **(8)**

Fine Motor Ability

Eats three meals with snacks
Uses spoon, fork, and knife

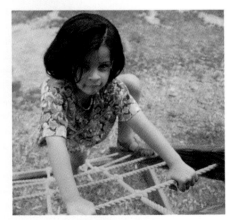

(6) Climbs well

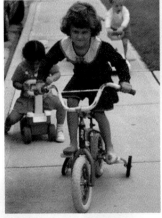

(7) Rides bicycle or bicycle with
training wheels

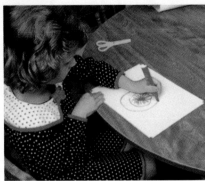

(8) Learns letters and numbers

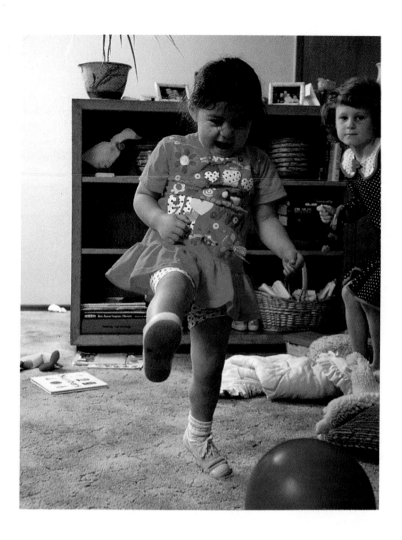

FIGURE 2–15. Preschoolers continue to develop more advanced skills, such as kicking a ball without falling down.

2-25	Characteristics of Preoperational Thought[28]		
Characteristic	**Definition**	**Example**	
Egocentrism	Ability to see things only from one's own point of view	The child who cannot understand why parents may need to leave the hospital for work when the child wishes them to be present	
Transductive reasoning	Connecting two events in a cause–effect relationship simply because they occur together in time	A child who, awakening after surgery and feeling pain, notices the intravenous infusion and believes that it is causing the pain	
Centration	Focusing on only one particular aspect of a situation	The child who is concerned about breathing through an anesthesia mask and will not listen to any other aspects of preoperative teaching	
Animism	Giving lifelike qualities to nonliving things	The child who views a monitoring machine as alive because it beeps	

PLAY

The preschooler has begun playing in a new way. Toddlers simply play side by side with friends, each engaging in his or her own activities, but preschoolers interact with others during play. One child cuts out colored paper while her friend glues it on paper in a design. This new type of interaction is called **associative play** (Fig. 2–16).

In addition to this social dimension of play, other aspects of play also differ. The preschooler enjoys large motor activities such as swinging, riding a tricycle, and throwing a ball. Increasing manual dexterity is demonstrated in greater complexity of drawings and manipulation of blocks and modeling. These changes necessitate planning of playtime to include appropriate activities. Preschool programs and child life departments in hospitals help meet this important need.

Materials provided for play can be simple but should guide activities in which the child engages. Since fine motor activities are popular, paper, pens, scissors, glue, and a variety of other such objects should be available. The child can use them to create important images such as pictures of people, hospital beds, or friends. A collection of dolls, furniture, and clothing can be manipulated to represent parents and children, nurses and physicians, teachers, or other significant people. Because fantasy life is so powerful at this age, the preschooler readily uses props to engage in **dramatic play,** that is, the living out of the drama of human life (Fig. 2–17).

The nurse can use playtime to assess the preschool child's developmental level, knowledge about health care, and emotions related to health care experiences. Observations about objects chosen for play, content of dramatic play, and pictures drawn can provide important assessment data. The nurse can also use play periods to teach the child about health care procedures and offer an outlet for expression of emotions (Table 2–26).

NUTRITION

The diet of the preschooler is similar to that of the toddler, but mealtime is now a more social event. Preschoolers like the company of others while they eat, and they enjoy helping with food preparation and table setting. Involving them in these tasks can provide a forum for teaching about nutritious foods and principle' of preparation such as the need for refrigeration, safety around stoves, and cleanliness.

Although the rate of growth is slow and steady during the preschool years, the child has periods of food jags (eating only a few foods for several days or weeks) and greater or lesser intake. Advise parents to assess food intake over a 1- or 2-week period rather than at each meal to obtain a more accurate impression of total intake. Food jags can be handled by providing the desired food along with other foods to foster choice. The child who chooses not to eat at snacktime or mealtime should not be given other foods in between. Three meals and two or three snacks daily are the norm (see Table 2–15).

The preschool period is a good time to encourage good dental habits. Children can begin to brush their own teeth with parental supervision and help to reach all tooth surfaces. Parents should floss their children's teeth, give fluoride as ordered if the water supply is not fluoridated (Table 2–27), and schedule the first dental visit so the child can become accustomed to the routine of periodic dental care.[29]

INJURY PREVENTION

The increasing independence of preschool children puts them at risk of injury. The 3–7-year-old group is at high risk of injury from fire, drowning,

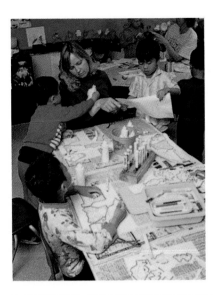

FIGURE 2–16. These preschoolers are participating in associative play, which means they can interact. One child is cutting out shapes, and the other is gluing them in place. Of course, every job needs a supervisor, who can be seen on the right.

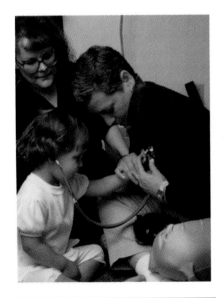

FIGURE 2–17. Jasmine is participating in dramatic play with a nurse while her mother looks on. In dramatic play the child uses props to play out the drama of human life. It can be an excellent way for a nurse to assess the developmental level of children while talking to them. Notice that the child and the nurse are on the floor at the same level and the atmosphere is informal. Why is it important to be at the same level as the child?

2-26	Favorite Toys and Activities in the Preschool Years
Play Need	**Types of Toys and Activities**
Facilitate associative play	Simple games Puzzles Nursery rhymes, songs
Promote dramatic play	Dolls and doll clothes Play houses and hospitals Dress-up clothes Puppets
Encourage outlet for stress	Pens, paper Glue, scissors
Facilitate cognitive growth	Educational television shows Music Stories and books

and motor vehicle and pedestrian accidents.[27] Nurses can teach parents preventive measures and can also begin to include preschoolers in safety teaching (Table 2–28).

PERSONALITY AND TEMPERAMENT

Characteristics of personality observed in infancy tend to persist over time. The preschooler may need assistance as these characteristics are expressed in the new situations of preschool or nursery school. An excessively active child, for example, will need gentle, consistent handling to adjust to the structure of a classroom. Encourage parents to visit preschool programs to choose the one that would best foster growth in their child. Some preschoolers enjoy the structured learning of a program that focuses on cognitive skills, whereas others are happier and more open to learning in a small group that provides much time for free play. Nurses can help parents to identify their child's personality or temperament characteristics and to find the best environment for growth.

2-27	Recommended Daily Fluoride Dosages		
	Amount of Fluoride in Water Supply		
Age	Under 0.3 ppm	0.3–0.6 ppm	Above 0.6 ppm
6 months to 3 years	0.25 mg	0	0
3–6 years	0.50 mg	0.25 mg	0
6–16 years	1.00 mg	0.50 mg	0

ppm, parts per million.
Note: Fluoride is available as a liquid to be mixed in a small amount of food or fluid for the infant and toddler and as a chewable tablet for the older child. It acts both systemically to promote strong teeth before they erupt and topically to strengthen tooth surfaces with which it comes in contact.
From Bindler, R.M., & Howry, L.B. (1997). Pediatric drugs and nursing implications (2nd ed.). Stamford, CT: Appleton & Lange, pp. 253–255.

2-28   Injury Prevention in the Preschool Years

	Hazards	Developmental Characteristics	Preventive Measures
	Motor vehicle crashes	Older preschooler independently gets into car and puts on seat belt. Child may forget to belt up or may do so incorrectly.	Verify that child is belted in properly before starting car. Child restraint systems must be used until child weighs 18 kg (40 lb) and is 100 cm (40 in.) tall.
	Motor vehicle and pedestrian accidents	Preschooler increasingly plays outside alone or with friends. Preschooler is unable to judge speed of moving car and assumes driver knows that he or she is present.	Teach child never to go into road. A safe, preferably enclosed, play yard is recommended.
	Drowning	Preschooler who has had swimming lessons may choose to go into a lake or pool.	Teach child never to go into water without an adult. Provide supervision whenever child is near water.
	Burns	Preschooler can understand the hazards of fire.	Teach child to stop, drop, and roll if clothes are on fire. Practice escapes from home are useful. A visit to a fire station can reinforce learning. Teach child how to call 911.
	Needle sticks in hospital	Preschooler can ambulate and is interested in new objects.	Keep needles out of reach. Remove from unit immediately after use.
	Electrical injury in hospital	Preschooler is mobile and may trip over cords and equipment or may choose to examine them.	Avoid use of electrical cords if possible. Keep equipment out of major traffic areas. Keep beds away from electrical outlets. Monitor child closely.

COMMUNICATION

Language skills blossom during the preschool years. The vocabulary grows to over 2000 words, and children speak in complete sentences of several words and use all parts of speech. They practice these newfound language skills by endlessly talking and asking questions.

The sophisticated speech of preschoolers mirrors the development occurring in their minds and helps them to learn about the world around them. However, this speech can be quite deceptive. Although preschoolers use many words, their grasp of meaning is usually literal and may not match that of adults. These literal interpretations have important implications for health care providers. For example, the preschooler who is told she will be "put to sleep" for surgery may think of a pet recently euthanised; the child who is told that a dye will be injected for a diagnostic test may think he is going to die; mention of "a little stick" in the arm can cause images of tree branches rather than of a simple immunization.

The child may also have difficulty focusing on the content of a conversation. The preschooler is egocentric and may be unable to move from individual thoughts to those the nurse is proposing, as the following conversation illustrates:

Nurse: I'd like to tell you about the operation that you will have tomorrow.
Sharisse: OK. Did you know my brother just got a new squirt gun?
Nurse: That's nice. Now, first thing in the morning you will wake up early and your foot will be scrubbed with a special soap.
Sharisse: The gun can spurt for about 40 feet—you have to pump it up.
Nurse: We'll talk about that later. Let me tell you about your operation now. After your foot is scrubbed, the nurse will measure your blood pressure and temperature and feel the pulse in your arm. Do you remember my doing those things today?
Sharisse: Yes. And I got a sticker when I came into the hospital today, too. Do you know that my Mom is going to stay here tonight?

In this interchange Sharisse is engaging in **collective monologue,** in which separate conversations occur even though each person waits for the other to speak. Though waiting for the nurse to speak, Sharisse is not generally responding to the nurse's content but is instead focusing on content from her own mind. The nurse needs to respond to Sharisse's content and then reinsert more facts about the preparations for surgery.

Concrete visual aids such as pictures of a child undergoing the same procedure or a book to read together enhance teaching by meeting the child's developmental needs. Handling medical equipment such as intravenous bags and stethoscopes increases interest and helps the child to focus. Teaching may have to be done in several short sessions rather than one long session.

COMMUNICATION STRATEGIES: PRESCHOOLER

Allow time for child to integrate explanations.
Verbalize frequently to the child.
Use drawings and stories to explain care.
Use accurate names for bodily functions.
Allow choices.

► SCHOOL-AGE CHILD (6–12 YEARS)

Errol, 10 years old, arrives home from school shortly after 3 PM each day. He immediately calls his friends and goes to visit one of them. They are building models of cars and collecting baseball cards. Endless hours are spent on these projects and on discussions of events at school that day (Fig. 2–18).

Nine-year-old Karen practices soccer two afternoons a week and plays in games each weekend. She also is learning to play the flute and spends her free time at home practicing. Although practice time is not her favorite part of music, Karen enjoys the performances and wants to play well in

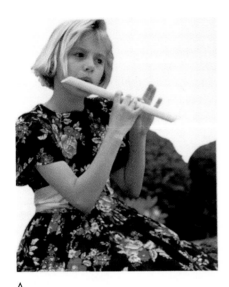

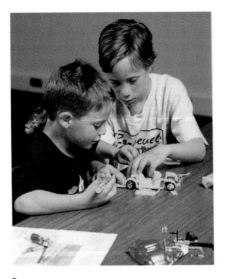

A

B

FIGURE 2-18. A, School-age children may take part in activities that require practice. This is a consideration when children are hospitalized and unable to practice or perform. Why? B, School-age children enjoy spending time with others the same age on projects and discussing the activities of the day. This is an important consideration when they are in an acute-care setting. When you are in the clinical setting, look for facilities where this type of interaction is taking place.

front of her friends and teacher. Her parents now allow her to ride her bike unaccompanied to the store or to a friend's house.

These two school-age children demonstrate common characteristics of their age group. They are in a stage of industry in which it is important to the child to perform useful work. Meaningful activities take on great importance and are usually carried out in the company of peers. A sense of achievement in these activities is important to develop self-esteem and to prevent a sense of inferiority or poor self-worth.

PHYSICAL GROWTH AND DEVELOPMENT

School age is the last period in which girls and boys are close in size and body proportions. As the long bones continue to grow, leg length increases (see Fig. 2-9). Fat gives way to muscle, and the child appears leaner. Jaw proportions change as the first deciduous tooth is lost at 6 years and permanent teeth begin to erupt. Body organs and the immune system mature, resulting in fewer illnesses among school-age children. Medications are less likely to cause serious side effects, since they can be metabolized more easily. The urinary system can adjust to changes in fluid status. Physical skills are also refined as children begin to play sports, and fine motor skills are well developed through school activities (Table 2-29 and Fig. 2-19).

COGNITIVE DEVELOPMENT

The child enters the stage of concrete operational thought at about 7 years. This stage enables school-age children to consider alternative solutions and solve problems. However, school-age children continue to rely on concrete experiences and materials to form their thought content.

During the school-age years the child learns the concept of **conservation** (that matter is not changed when its form is altered). At earlier ages, a child believes that when water is poured from a short, wide glass into a tall, thin glass, there is more water in the taller glass. The school-age child recognizes that although it may look like the taller glass holds more water, the quantity is the same. The concept of conservation is helpful when the nurse

2-29 Growth and Development Milestones During the School-Age Years

Physical Growth	Fine Motor Ability	Gross Motor Ability	Sensory Ability	Nutrition
Gains 1.4–2.2 kg (3–5 lb)/year Grows 4–6 cm (1½–2½ in.)/year	Enjoys craft projects Plays card and board games	Rides two-wheeler **(1)** Jumps rope **(2)** Roller skates or ice skates	Can read Able to concentrate for longer periods on activities by filtering out surrounding sounds **(3)**	Eats three meals per day Enjoys preparing own food

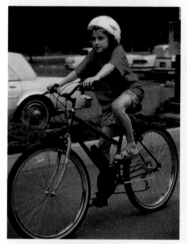

(1) Rides two-wheeler

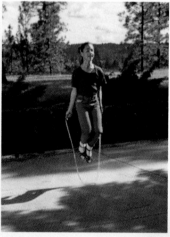

(2) Jumps rope

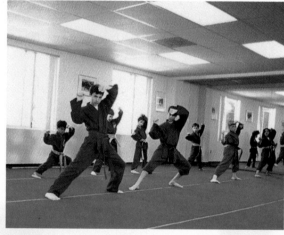

(3) Concentrates on activities for longer periods

explains medical treatments. The school-age child understands that an incision will heal, that a cast will be removed, and that an arm will look the same as before once the intravenous infusion is removed.

PLAY

When the preschool teacher tries to organize a game of baseball, both the teacher and the children become frustrated. Not only are the children physically unable to hold a bat and hit a ball, but they seem to have no understanding of the rules of the game and do not want to wait for their turn at bat. By 6 years of age, however, children have acquired the physical ability to hold the bat properly and may occasionally hit the ball. School-age children also understand that everyone has a role—the pitcher, the catcher, the batter, the outfielders. They cooperate with one another to form a team, are eager to learn the rules of the game, and want to ensure that these rules are followed exactly (Table 2–30).

The characteristics of play exhibited by the school-age child are cooperation with others and the ability to play a part in order to contribute to a unified whole. This type of play is called **cooperative play.** The concrete nature of cognitive thought leads to a reliance on rules to provide structure and security. Children have an increasing desire to spend much of playtime with friends, which demonstrates the social component of play. Play is an extremely important method of learning and living for the school-age child.

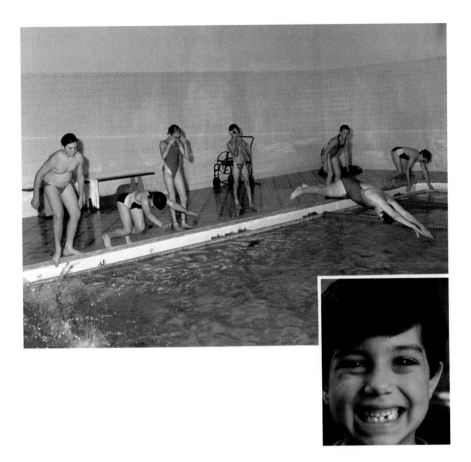

FIGURE 2–19. School-age girls and boys enjoy participating in sports. They begin to lose fat while developing their muscles, so they appear leaner than at earlier ages. *Inset,* Front teeth are lost around age 6. The family may have rituals associated with the loss of teeth that could affect the child's behavior if he loses a tooth while in the hospital.

When a child is hospitalized, the separation from playmates can lead to feelings of sadness and purposelessness. School-age children often feel better when placed in multibed units with other children. Games can be devised even when children are wheelchair bound (Fig. 2–20). Normal, rewarding parts of play should be integrated into care. Friends should be

2-30	Favorite Play Activities of School-Age Children
Play Need	**Types of Activities**
Foster gross motor activity	Ball sports Skating Dance lessons Water and snow skiing Biking
Promote sense of industry	Musical instrument Collections (eg, stamps, miniatures) Hobbies Board and video games
Facilitate cognitive growth	Reading Crafts Word puzzles

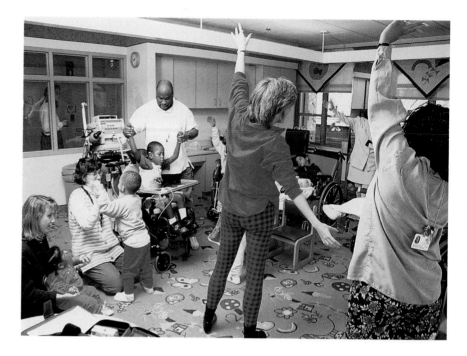

FIGURE 2–20. The nurse can help the child and family accept and adjust to new circumstances. Encouraging the child in a wheelchair to participate in group activities can help build confidence in physical skills. Good self-esteem, goal attainment, personal satisfaction, and general health are the continued benefits.

encouraged to visit or call a hospitalized child. Discharge planning for the child who has had a cast or brace applied should address the activities the child can engage in and those the child must avoid. Reinforce the importance of playing games with friends.

NUTRITION

The school-age years are a period of gradual growth when energy requirements remain at a steady level. The child is increasingly responsible for preparing snacks and even some parts of the meal. This makes the school-age years an appropriate time to teach children how to choose nutritious foods and how to plan a well-balanced meal (see Table 2–15). Because school-age children still operate at the concrete level of cognitive thought, nutrition teaching is best presented by using pictures, samples of foods, videotapes, handouts, and hands-on experience.

School-age children often prefer the types of food eaten at home and may be resistant to new food items. A hospitalized child may refuse to eat, slowing the recuperative process. Encourage family members to bring favorite foods from home that meet nutritional requirements. This can be especially helpful for children from nondominant cultural groups. A child accustomed to a diet of rice, tofu, marinated chicken, and vegetables may not enjoy a hamburger and fries. Many hospitals allow children to plan a pizza night or sponsor other events to encourage eating. By school age, food has become strongly associated with social interaction, so it is beneficial to have children eat together or to encourage family members to take the child off the unit to eat or to bring in food from home and eat with their child.

The start of adolescence (age 12) generally begins a rapid increase in growth (the so-called adolescent growth spurt). However, growth spurts sometimes occur before that time. Girls may begin a growth spurt by 9 or 10 years and boys a year or so later (see Fig. 2–21). Nutritional needs increase dramatically with this spurt, as discussed in the following section on the adolescent.

The loss of the first deciduous teeth and the eruption of permanent teeth usually occur at about age 6, or at the beginning of the school-age pe-

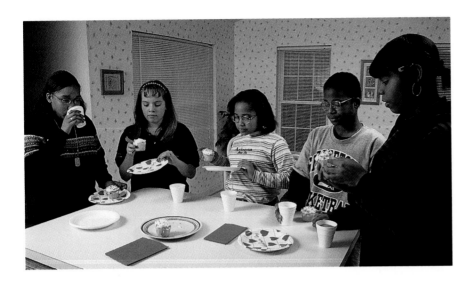

FIGURE 2–21. Because girls have a growth spurt earlier than boys, girls often are taller than boys of the same age. Remember what it was like at your first dance?

riod. Of the 30 permanent teeth, 22–26 erupt by age 12 and the remaining molars follow during the teenage years. The school-age child should be closely monitored to ensure that brushing and flossing are adequate, that fluoride is taken if the water supply is unfluoridated, that dental care is obtained to provide for examination of teeth and alignment, and that loose teeth are identified before surgery or other events that may lead to loss of a tooth.

INJURY PREVENTION

Because school-age children play in unsupervised settings for longer periods, they are at risk for different types of injuries than younger children (Table 2–31). Motor vehicle crashes are still common, but firearm and burn injuries increase in incidence.[27] Safety teaching should be an integral part of each school's curriculum.

PERSONALITY AND TEMPERAMENT

The enduring aspects of temperament continue to be manifested during the school years. The child classified as "difficult" at an earlier age may now have trouble in the classroom. Advise parents to provide a quiet setting for homework and to reward the child for concentration. For example, after homework is completed, a television show can be watched. Creative efforts and alternative methods of learning should be valued. Encourage parents to see their children as individuals who may not all learn in the same way. The "slow-to-warm-up" child may need encouragement to try new activities and to share experiences with others, while the "easy" child will readily adapt to new schools, people, and experiences.

COMMUNICATION

During the school-age years, the child should learn how to correct any lingering pronunciation or grammatical errors. Vocabulary increases, and the child is taught about parts of speech in school. School-age children enjoy writing and can be encouraged to keep a journal of their experiences while in the hospital as a method of dealing with anxiety. The literal translation of words characteristic of preschoolers is uncommon among school-age children.

COMMUNICATION STRATEGIES: SCHOOL-AGE CHILD

Provide concrete examples of pictures or materials to accompany verbal descriptions.

Assess knowledge before planning teaching.

Allow child to select rewards following procedures.

Teach techniques such as counting or visualization to manage difficult situations.

Include child in discussions and history with parent.

2-31   Injury Prevention in the School-Age Years

	Hazard	Developmental Characteristics	Preventive Measures
	Motor vehicle/ pedestrian/ biking crashes	Child plays outside; may follow ball into road; rides two-wheeler.	Teach child safe outside play, especially near streets. Reinforce use of bike helmet. Teach biking safety rules and provide safe places for riding.
	Firearms	Child may have been shown location of guns; is interested in showing them to friends.	Teach child never to touch guns without parent present. Guns should be kept unloaded and locked away. Guns and ammunition should be stored in different locations. Be sure guns have trigger locks.
	Burns	Child may perform experiments with flames or toxic substances.	Teach child what to do in case of fire or if toxic substances touch skin or eyes. Reinforce teaching about 911.
	Assault	Child may be left alone after school and may walk, bike, or take public transportation alone.	Provide telephone numbers of people to contact in case of an emergency or if child feels lonely. Leave child alone for brief periods initially, and evaluate child's success in managing time. Teach child not to accept rides from or talk to or open doors to strangers. Teach child how to answer the phone.

▶ ADOLESCENT (12–18 YEARS)

Adolescence is a time of passage signaling the end of childhood and the beginning of adulthood. Although adolescents differ in behaviors and accomplishments, they are in a period of identity formation. If a healthy identity and sense of self-worth are not developed in this period, role confusion and purposeless struggling will ensue. The adolescents in your care will represent various degrees of identity formation, and each will offer unique challenges.

PHYSICAL GROWTH AND DEVELOPMENT

The physical changes ending in **puberty,** or sexual maturity, begin near the end of the school-age period. The prepubescent period is marked by a growth spurt at an average age of 10 years for girls and 13 years for boys (Fig. 2–21). The increase in height and weight is generally remarkable and is completed in 2–3 years (Table 2–32). The growth spurt in girls is accompanied by an increase in breast size and growth of pubic hair. Menstruation occurs last and signals achievement of puberty. In boys the growth spurt is accompanied by growth in size of the penis and testes and by growth of pubic hair. Deepening of the voice and growth of facial hair occur later, at the time of puberty. See Chapter 3 for a description of the pubertal stages.

During adolescence children grow stronger and more muscular and establish characteristic male and female patterns of fat distribution. The apocrine and eccrine glands mature, leading to increased sweating and a distinct odor to perspiration. All body organs are now fully mature, enabling the adolescent to take adult doses of medications.

The adolescent must adapt to a rapidly changing body for several years. These physical changes and hormonal variations offer challenges to identity formation.

COGNITIVE DEVELOPMENT

Adolescence marks the beginning of Piaget's last stage of cognitive development, the stage of formal operational thought. The adolescent no longer depends on concrete experiences as the basis of thought but develops the ability to reason abstractly. Such concepts as justice, truth, beauty, and power can be understood. The adolescent revels in this newfound ability and spends a great deal of time thinking, reading, and talking about abstract concepts.

The ability to think and act independently leads many adolescents to rebel against parental authority. Through these actions, adolescents seek to establish their own identity and values.

ACTIVITIES

Maturity leads to new activities. Adolescents may drive, ride buses, or bike independently. They are less dependent on parents for transportation and spend more time with friends. Activities include participation in sports and extracurricular school activities, as well as "hanging out" and attending movies or concerts with friends (Table 2–33). The peer group becomes the focus of activities (Fig. 2–22), regardless of the teen's interests. Peers are important in establishing identity and providing meaning. Although same-sex interactions predominate, boy–girl relationships are more common than at earlier stages. Adolescents thus participate in and learn from social interactions fundamental to adult relationships.

NUTRITION

Most adolescents need well over 2000 calories daily to support the growth spurt, and some adolescent boys require nearly 3000 calories daily. When teenagers are active in a variety of sports, these requirements increase fur-

2-32 Growth and Development Milestones During Adolescence

Physical Growth	Fine Motor Ability	Gross Motor Ability	Sensory Ability	Nutrition
Variation in age of growth spurt During growth spurt, girls gain 7–25 kg (15–55 lb) and grow 2.5–20 cm (2–8 in.); boys gain approximately 7–29.5 kg (15–65 lb) and grow 11–30 cm (4½–12 in.)	Skills are well developed (1)	New sports activities attempted and muscle development continues (2) Some lack of coordination common during growth spurt	Fully developed	Large appetite, which increases during growth spurt Eats many meals with friends; food choices influenced by peers (3)

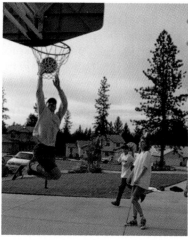

(2) New sports activites attempted

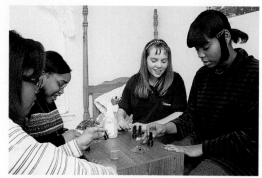

(1) Skills are well developed

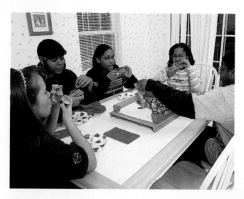

(3) Eats many meals with friends

ther. Because adolescents prepare much of their own food and often eat with friends, they need to be taught about good nutrition. Developing a diet that includes a large number of calories, meets vitamin and mineral requirements, and is acceptable to the teen may be a challenge (see Table 2–15). An adolescent who does not like the hospital lunch and reaches into a bag for a soft drink and chips may be receptive to juice and pizza, a more nutritious meal. Small improvements should be viewed positively as they may lead to further changes.

Some common deficits in diets of adolescents are iron, calcium, and zinc. Iron and calcium deficiencies are often greater problems for girls due to low intake of meat and dairy products. Loss of blood through menstruation further contributes to their low iron levels. Nutritional teaching and offering snacks high in these minerals can help to provide for these needs. The adolescent who restricts food intake because of a disease process such as anorexia nervosa or bulimia is at high risk for nutritional deficits. Health care visits for any purpose should incorporate assessment of height and weight and patterns of food intake. Because the peer group influence is important, group sessions in which adolescents eat lunch together while nutritional information is presented provide a forum for influencing food habits.

INJURY PREVENTION

Motor vehicle crashes, suicide, and homicide cause 75% of adolescent deaths.[27] Teenagers have access to potentially harmful objects, such as firearms, motor vehicles, and boats. They often think that no harm can come to them. This encourages adolescents to put themselves at high risk from dangerous behaviors (Table 2–34).

Suicide among adolescents has increased by 300% over the past two decades.[30] The high rate of stress experienced by today's teenagers coupled with easy access to harmful substances and firearms promotes death by suicide.

Nurses can be instrumental in assessing the potential for injury of adolescents seen in practice. Teaching about prevention is most successful when young people who have been injured share their experiences with other adolescents. A national health objective for the year 2000 is to reduce the teen suicide rate by more than 25%.

Violence is an increasingly important factor in adolescent injury. Homicide is the number one cause of death for young black males. The environment should be assessed for factors contributing to violence and adolescents at risk referred to special programs for violence prevention. Abuse in homes and schools must be reported to law enforcement agencies when nurses are aware that it may have occurred.

2-33   Favorite Activities in Adolescence

Sports
Ball sports
Gymnastics
Water and snow skiing
Swimming
School team sports

School Activities
Drama
Yearbook
Class officer
Committee participation

Peer Group Activities
Movies
Dances
Driving
Eating out

Quiet Activities
Reading
School work
Television and video games
Music

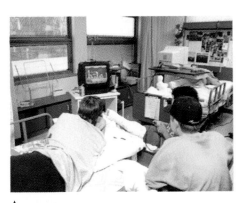

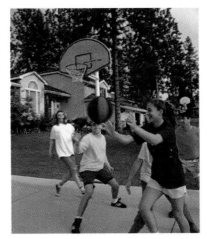

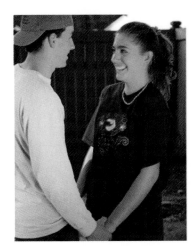

A   B   C

FIGURE 2–22. Social interaction between children of same and opposite sex is as important inside the acute care setting as it is outside. **A,** Teenage interaction inside hospital. **B,** Teenagers enjoy playing together. **C,** Emotional relationships form during adolescence.

2-34	Injury Prevention in Adolescence		
	Hazard	**Developmental Characteristics**	**Preventive Measures**
	Motor vehicle crashes	Adolescents learn to drive, enjoy new independence, and often feel invulnerable.	Insist on driver's education classes. Enforce rules about safe driving. Seat belts should be used for every trip. Discourage drug and alcohol use. Get treatment for teenagers who are known substance abusers.
	Sporting injuries	Adolescents may participate in physically challenging sports such as soccer, gymnastics, or football. They may be allowed to drive motorboats.	Encourage use of protective sporting gear. Teach safe boating practices. Perform teaching related to hazards of drug and alcohol use, especially when using motorized equipment.
	Drowning	Adolescents overestimate endurance when swimming. They take risks diving.	Encourage swimming only with friends. Reinforce rules and teach them about risks.

PERSONALITY AND TEMPERAMENT

Characteristics of temperament manifested during childhood usually remain stable in the teenage years. For instance, the adolescent who was a calm, scheduled infant and child often demonstrates initiative to regulate study times and other routines. Similarly, the adolescent who was an easily stimulated infant may now have a messy room, a harried schedule with assignments always completed late, and an interest in many activities. It is also common for an adolescent who was an easy child to become more difficult because of the psychologic changes of adolescence and the need to assert independence.

As during the child's earlier ages, the nurse's role may be to inform parents of different personality types and to help them support the teen's uniqueness while providing necessary structure and feedback. Nurses can help parents to understand their teen's personality type and to work with the adolescent to meet expectations of teachers and others in authority.

COMMUNICATION

All parts of speech are used and understood by the adolescent. Colloquialisms and slang are commonly used with the peer group. The adolescent often studies a foreign language in school, having the ability to understand and analyze grammar and sentence structure.

The adolescent increasingly leaves the home base and establishes close ties with peers. These relationships become the basis for identity formation. There is generally a period of stress or crisis before a strong identity can emerge. The adolescent may try out new roles by learning a new sport or other skills, experimenting with drugs or alcohol, wearing different styles of clothing, or trying other activities. It is important to provide positive role models and a variety of experiences to help the adolescent make wise choices.

The adolescent also has a need to leave the past, to be different, and to change from former patterns to establish his or her own identity. Rules that are repeated constantly and dogmatically will probably be broken in the adolescent's quest for self-identity. This poses difficulties when the adolescent has a health problem, such as diabetes or a heart problem, that requires ongoing care. Introducing the adolescent to other teens who manage the same problem appropriately is usually more successful than telling the adolescent what to do.

Privacy should be ensured during the taking of health histories or interventions with teens. Even if a parent is present for part of a history or examination, the adolescent should be given the opportunity to relay information or ask questions alone with the health care provider. The adolescent should be given a choice of whether to have a parent present during an examination or while care is provided. Most information shared by an adolescent is confidential. Some states mandate disclosure of certain information to parents such as an adolescent's desire for an abortion. In these cases, the adolescent should be informed of what will be disclosed to the parent.

Setting up teen rooms (recreation rooms for use only by adolescents) or separate adolescent units in hospitals can provide necessary peer support during hospitalization. Most adolescents are not pleased when placed on a unit or in a room with young children. Choices should be allowed whenever possible. These might include preference for evening or morning bathing, the type of clothes to wear while hospitalized, timing of treatments, and who should be allowed to visit and for how long. Use of contracts with adolescents may increase compliance. Firmness, gentleness, choices, and respect must all be balanced during care of adolescent patients.

COMMUNICATION STRATEGIES: ADOLESCENT
Provide written as well as verbal explanations.
Direct history and explanations to teen alone; then include parent.
Allow for safe exploration of topics by suggesting that teen is similar to other teens. ("Many teens with diabetes have questions about. . . . How about you?")
Arrange meetings for discussions with other teens.

SEXUALITY

With maturation of the body and increased secretion of hormones the adolescent achieves sexual maturity. This is a complex process involving growing interactions with members of the opposite sex, an interplay of the forces of society and family, and identity formation. The early adolescent progresses from dances and other social events with members of the opposite sex to the late adolescent who is mature sexually and may have regular sexual encounters. About half of all male teens in the United States have had intercourse by the age of 16 years, and about half of female teens by 17 years.[32]

Teenagers need information about their bodies and emerging sexuality. They should understand the interests and forces they experience. Including sex education in school classes and health care encounters is important. Information on methods to prevent sexually transmitted diseases is given, with most school districts now providing some teaching on AIDS. Far more common risks to teens, however, are diseases such as gonorrhea and herpes. Health histories should include questions on sexual activity, sexually transmitted diseases, and birth control use and understanding. Most hospitals routinely perform pregnancy screening on adolescent girls before elective procedures.

Adolescents will benefit from clear information about sexuality, an opportunity to develop relationships with adolescents in various settings, an open atmosphere at home and school where problems and issues can be discussed, and previous experience in problem solving and self–decision making. Sexual issues should be among topics that adolescents can discuss openly in a variety of settings. Alternatives and support for their decisions should be available.

 REFERENCES

1. Gemelli, R. (1996). *Normal child and adolescent development* (pp. 101–104). Washington, DC: American Psychiatric Press.
2. Erikson, E. (1963). *Childhood and society* (pp. 247–273). New York: W.W. Norton.
3. Erikson, E. (1968). *Identity: Youth and crisis* (pp. 91–96). New York: W.W. Norton.
4. Ginsburg, H., & Opper, S. (1969). *Piaget's theory of intellectual development* (pp. 1–25). Englewood Cliffs, NJ: Prentice-Hall.
5. Santrock, J. (1997). *Life-span development.* (pp. 344–347). Madison, WI: Brown & Benchmark.
6. Bandura, A. (1986). *Social foundations of thought and action: A social cognitive theory.* Englewood Cliffs, NJ: Prentice-Hall.
7. Santrock, J. (1997). *Life-span development.* (pp. 43–44). Madison, WI: Brown & Benchmark.
8. Bronfenbrenner, U. (1986). Ecology of the family as a context for human development: Research perspectives. *Developmental Psychology, 22,* 723–742.
9. Klaus, M.S., & Kennell, H. (1983). *Bonding: The beginnings of parent–infant attachment.* New York: New American Library.
10. Chess, S., & Thomas, A. (1995). *Temperament in clinical practice.* New York: Guilford Press.
11. Melvin, N. (1995). Children's temperament: Intervention for parents. *Journal of Pediatric Nursing, 10*(3), 152–159.
12. Worthington-Roberts, B., & Williams, S. (1993). *Nutrition in pregnancy and lactation* (5th ed., pp. 87–165). St. Louis: Mosby.
13. Briggs, G., Freeman, R., & Yaffe, S. (1994). *Drugs in pregnancy and lactation* (3rd ed.). Baltimore: Williams & Wilkins.
14. Santrock, J. (1997). *Life-span development* (pp. 249–252). Madison, WI: Brown & Benchmark.
15. Wallerstein, J.S. , Corbin, S.B., & Lewis, J.M. (1988). Children of divorce: A ten year study. In E.M. Hetherinton & J.B. Arasteh (Eds.), *Impact of divorce, single parenting, and stepparenting on children* (pp. 197–214). Hillsdale, NJ: Erlbaum Publishers.
16. Elkind, D. (1981). *The hurried child* (pp. 3–22). Menlo Park, CA: Addison-Wesley.
17. Children's Defense Fund. (1997). Key facts about children. *CDF Reports, 17*(2), 6.
18. Johnson, C., Miranda, L., Sherman, A., & Weill, J. (1991). *Child poverty in America.* Washington, DC: Children's Defense Fund.
19. Baxter, A., & Kahn, J.V. (1996). Effective early intervention for inner-city infants and toddlers: Assessing social supports, needs, and stress. *Infant-Toddler Intervention Transdisciplinary Journal, 6*(3), 197–211.
20. Murata, J., Mace, J.P., & Strehlow, A., et al. (1992). Disease patterns in homeless children: A comparison with national data. *Journal of Pediatric Nursing, 7*(3), 196–204.
21. Wagner, J.D., Menke, E.M., & Ciccone, J.K. (1995). What is known about the health of rural homeless families? *Public Health Nursing, 12*(6), 400–408.
22. Groer, M., & Howell, M. (1990). Autonomic and cardiovascular responses of preschool children to television programs. *Journal of Child and Adolescent Psychiatric Mental Health Nursing, 3*(3), 134–138.
23. Dietz, W.H., & Gortmaker, S.L. (1985). Do we fatten our children at the television set? Obesity and television viewing in children and adolescents. *Pediatrics, 75,* 807–812.

24. Dietz, W.H., Bandini, L.G., Morelli, J.A., Peers, K.F., & Ching, P.L. (1994). Effect of sedentary activities on resting metabolic rate. *American Journal of Clinical Nutrition, 59*(3), 556–559.

25. Barnes, G.P., Parker, W.A., Lyon, T.C., Drum, M.A., & Coleman, G.C. (1992). Ethnicity, locations, age and fluoridation factors in baby bottle tooth decay and caries prevalence of Head Start children. *Public Health Report, 10*(2), 167–173.

26. Trahms, C.M., & Pipes, P. (1997). *Nutrition in infancy and childhood* (6th ed., pp. 101–102). St. Louis: WCB/McGraw Hill.

27. Overby, K.J. (1996). Pediatric health supervision. In A.M. Rudolph, J.I.E. Hoffman, & C.D. Rudolph, (Eds.), *Rudolph's pediatrics* (20th ed., p. 27). Stamford, CT: Appleton & Lange.

28. Piaget, J. (1972). *The child's conception of the world.* Totowa, NJ: Littlefield, Adams Co.

29. Overby, K.J. (1996). Pediatric health supervision. In A.M. Rudolph, J.I.E. Hoffman, & C.D. Rudolph, (Eds.), *Rudolph's pediatrics.* (20th ed., p. 21). Stamford, CT: Appleton & Lange.

30. Troiano, R.P., Flegel, K.M., Kuczmarski, R.J., Campbell, S.M., & Johnson C.L. (1995). Overweight prevalence and trends for children and adolescents. *Archives of Pediatric and Adolescent Medicine, 149,* 1085–1091.

31. MMWR. (1995). Suicide among children, adolescents, and young adults—United States, 1980–1992. *MMWR, 44*(15), 289–291.

32. Neinstein, L.S. (1991). *Adolescent health care—A practical guide* (2nd ed., pp. 537–545). Baltimore: Urban & Schwarzenberg.

 ## ADDITIONAL RESOURCES

Brenner, A. (1984). *Helping children cope with stress.* Lexington, MA: Lexington Books.

Children's Defense Fund. (1997). *The state of America's children.* Washington, DC: Author.

Centers for Disease Control. (1992). *Youth suicide prevention programs: A resource guide.* Atlanta: U.S. Department of Health and Human Services.

Chess, S., & Thomas, A. (1996). *Temperament: Theory and practice.* New York: Brunner/Mazel.

Cross cultural medicine. (1992). *Western Journal of Medicine, 157*(3), 248–373.

Edelman, M. (1991). *The measure of our success.* Boston: Beacon Press.

Elkind, D. (1987). *Miseducation.* New York: Alfred Knopf.

Flavell, J. (1963). *The developmental psychology of Jean Piaget.* New York: D. Van Nostrand Co.

Heatherington, E.M., & Blechman, E.A. (1996). *Stress, coping and resiliency in children.* Mahwah, NJ: L. Erlbaum Associates.

Institute of Medicine. (1992). *Nutrition during pregnancy and lactation.* Washington, DC: National Academy Press.

Lazarus, R.S. (1993). Coping theory and research: Past, present, and future. *Psychosomatic Medicine, 55,* 234–247.

Medoff-Cooper, B. (1995). Infant temperament: Implications for parenting from birth through 1 year. *Journal of Pediatric Nursing, 10*(3), 141–145.

Mohrbacher, N., & Stock, J. (1991). *The breastfeeding answer book.* Franklin Park, IL: LaLeche League International.

Nelms, B.C. (1996). Suicide—Can we help prevent it? *Journal of Pediatric Health Care, 10*(3), 97–98.

Piaget, J. (1969). *The child's conception of physical causality.* Totowa, NJ: Littlefield, Adams & Co.

Piaget, J. (1973). *The psychology of intelligence.* Totowa, NJ: Littlefield, Adams & Co.

Rennie, J. (1994). Grading the gene tests. *Scientific American, 270*(6), 88–97.

Spector, R. (1996). *Cultural diversity in health and illness* (4th ed.). Stamford, CT: Appleton & Lange.

Tomlinson, P.S., Harbaugh, B.L., & Anderson, K.H. (1996). Children's temperament at 3 months and 6 years old: Stability, reliability, and measurement issues. *Issues in Comprehensive Pediatric Nursing, 19*(1), 33–47.

Wallace, M.R. (1995). Temperament and the hospitalized child. *Journal of Pediatric Nursing, 10*(3), 173–180.

Williams, J.K., & Lea, D.H. (1995). Applying new genetic technologies: Assessment and ethical considerations. *The Nurse Practitioner, 20*(7), 16–26.

Williams, J.K., & Lessick, M. (1996). Genome research: Implications for children. *Pediatric Nursing, 22*(1), 40–46.

Yoos, H.L., Kitzman, H., Olds, D.L., & Overacker, I. (1995). Child rearing beliefs in the African-American community: Implications for culturally competent pediatric care. *Journal of Pediatric Nursing, 10*(6), 343–353.

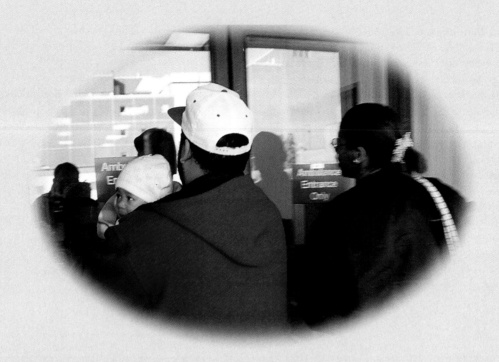

L atoya, 6 months old, is brought by her mother and father to the emergency room. She is an emergency admission from the local pediatrician's office with a diagnosis of bronchiolitis. As Latoya's nurse, you are responsible for assessing her condition after she arrives on the pediatric nursing unit.

What information do you look for, and in what order do you gather this information? What techniques can you use to obtain information about Latoya's condition? How do you organize your findings to make sense of them?

The patient history and physical examination provide a structure and a sequence for collecting and analyzing relevant *assessment* data. The initial physical examination findings provide the baseline for monitoring Latoya's response to treatment. Analysis of the assessment data also enables you to form nursing diagnoses and to develop a nursing care plan to direct the nursing care that Latoya will receive.

PEDIATRIC ASSESSMENT 3

"I was scared when we brought Latoya to the hospital. She looked helpless, afraid, and sick. The nurses and doctors took over when we got to the hospital, and I felt better because they seemed to know what to do."

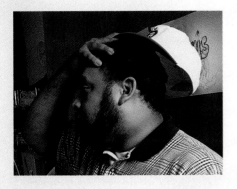

TERMINOLOGY

- **assessment** The process of collecting information about a child and family to develop the nursing diagnoses. The assessment process includes the patient history, physical examination, and analysis of the collected data to identify relevant information.
- **auscultation** The technique of listening to sounds produced by the airway, lungs, stomach, heart, and blood vessels to identify their characteristics. Auscultation is usually performed with the stethoscope to enhance the sounds heard.
- **clinical judgment** Analyzing and synthesizing data from the patient history, physical examination, screening tests, and laboratory studies to make decisions about the child's health problems. This is also called diagnostic reasoning.
- **effective communication** Information exchanged among the nurse, parent, and child that is clearly understood by all persons involved in the conversation.
- **inspection** The technique of purposeful observation by carefully looking at the characteristics of the child's physical features and be-

haviors. Physical feature characteristics include size, shape, color, movement, position, and location.
- **nonverbal behavior** The use of facial expression, eye contact, touch, posture, gestures, and body movements that communicate feelings during a conversation.
- **palpation** The technique of touch to identify characteristics of the skin, internal organs, and masses. Characteristics include texture, moistness, tenderness, temperature, position, shape, consistency, and mobility of masses and organs.
- **percussion** The technique of striking the surface of the body, either directly or indirectly, to set up vibrations that reveal the density of underlying tissues and borders of internal organs.
- **range of motion** The direction and extent to which a particular joint is capable of moving, either independently or with assistance.
- **review of systems** A comprehensive interview to identify and record the parent's or child's health concerns and health problems by body system; provides an overview of the child's health status.

Do examination techniques need to vary for children of different ages? How does the nurse gain cooperation for the examination from infants and toddlers? This chapter answers these questions and provides an overview of pediatric assessment, including history taking and examination techniques geared to the unique needs of pediatric patients. Strategies for obtaining the child's history are presented first. The remainder of the chapter then outlines a systematic process for physical examination of the child and guidelines for nutritional assessment.

► ANATOMIC AND PHYSIOLOGIC CHARACTERISTICS OF CHILDREN

It is readily apparent that infants and children are smaller than adults. Significant differences in physiology also normally exist between children and adults. Knowledge of pediatric anatomic and physiologic differences will aid in recognizing normal variations found during the physical examination. It also assists with understanding the different physiologic responses children have to illness and injury. Figure 3–1 provides an

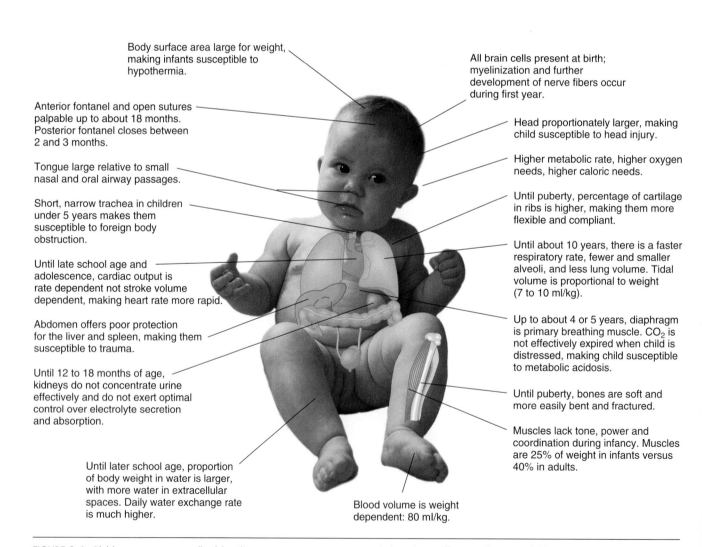

Body surface area large for weight, making infants susceptible to hypothermia.

Anterior fontanel and open sutures palpable up to about 18 months. Posterior fontanel closes between 2 and 3 months.

Tongue large relative to small nasal and oral airway passages.

Short, narrow trachea in children under 5 years makes them susceptible to foreign body obstruction.

Until late school age and adolescence, cardiac output is rate dependent not stroke volume dependent, making heart rate more rapid.

Abdomen offers poor protection for the liver and spleen, making them susceptible to trauma.

Until 12 to 18 months of age, kidneys do not concentrate urine effectively and do not exert optimal control over electrolyte secretion and absorption.

Until later school age, proportion of body weight in water is larger, with more water in extracellular spaces. Daily water exchange rate is much higher.

All brain cells present at birth; myelinization and further development of nerve fibers occur during first year.

Head proportionately larger, making child susceptible to head injury.

Higher metabolic rate, higher oxygen needs, higher caloric needs.

Until puberty, percentage of cartilage in ribs is higher, making them more flexible and compliant.

Until about 10 years, there is a faster respiratory rate, fewer and smaller alveoli, and less lung volume. Tidal volume is proportional to weight (7 to 10 ml/kg).

Up to about 4 or 5 years, diaphragm is primary breathing muscle. CO_2 is not effectively expired when child is distressed, making child susceptible to metabolic acidosis.

Until puberty, bones are soft and more easily bent and fractured.

Muscles lack tone, power and coordination during infancy. Muscles are 25% of weight in infants versus 40% in adults.

Blood volume is weight dependent: 80 ml/kg.

FIGURE 3–1. Children are not just small adults. There are important anatomic and physiologic differences between children and adults that will change based on a child's growth and development. Can you identify which of these differences are of greatest concern for the hospitalized child and why?

overview of important anatomic and physiologic differences between children and adults.

► OBTAINING THE CHILD'S HISTORY

COMMUNICATION STRATEGIES

What makes communication effective? What does it mean when a parent or caretaker will not look you in the eye when speaking with you? What types of cues indicate that a parent may be withholding historical information?

The health history interview is a very personal conversation with a parent, caretaker, or adolescent during which private concerns and feelings are shared. Try to ensure that this exchange of information with the parent or the child is clearly understood by both parties, that it is an **effective communication.** Effective communication is difficult to accomplish because parents and children often do not correctly interpret what the nurse says, just as you may not understand completely what the parent or child says. People's interpretation of information is based on their life experiences, culture, and education.

Strategies to Build a Rapport With the Family

As you begin the history, make sure the parents understand the purpose of the interview and that the information will be used appropriately. To develop rapport, demonstrate your interest in and concern for the child and family during the interview. This rapport forms the foundation for the collaborative relationship between the nurse and parent that will provide the best nursing care for the child. The following strategies help to establish rapport with the child's family during the nursing history:

- *Introduce yourself* (your name, title or position, and your role in caring for the child). To demonstrate respect, ask all family members present what name they prefer you to use when talking with them.

- *Explain the purpose of the interview* and why the nursing history is different from the information collected from other health professionals. For example, "The nurses will use this information to plan nursing care best suited for your child."

- *Provide privacy* and remove as many distractions as possible during the interview. If the patient's room does not offer privacy, attempt to find a vacant patient room or lounge.

- *Direct the focus of the interview* with open-ended questions. Use close-ended questions or directing statements to clarify information. Open-ended questions are useful to initiate the interview, develop a rapport, and understand the parent's perceptions of the child's problem; for example, "Tell me what problems led to Roberto's admission to the hospital." Close-ended questions are used to obtain detailed information; for example, "How high was Tommy's fever this morning?"

- *Ask one question at a time* so that the parent or child understands what piece of information you want and so that you know which question the parent is answering. "Does any member of your family have diabetes, heart disease, or sickle cell anemia?" is a multiple question. Ask about each disease separately to ensure the most accurate response.

- *Involve the child in the interview* by asking age-appropriate questions. Young children can be asked "What is your doll's name?" or "Where does it hurt?" Demonstrating an interest in the child initiates develop-

CULTURAL CONSIDERATIONS

Some cultural groups, particularly Asians, try to anticipate the answers you want to hear or say yes even if they do not understand the question. This is done in an effort to please you or as an expression of politeness. Remember to phrase your questions in a neutral manner.

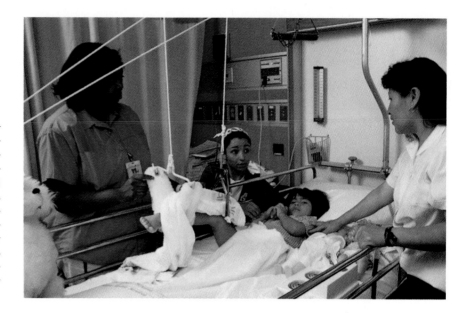

FIGURE 3–2. Selecting and using an interpreter. Most hospitals have designated interpreters that you should use. If not, find a professional interpreter whom you have identified beforehand and who knows medical terms and the typical cultural norms of the family. The interpreter *(center)* should be positioned to improve communication. Maintain eye contact with the parent or patient, not the interpreter. To ensure confidentiality of information for parents, avoid using a family member for history taking.

ment of rapport with both child and parents. Ask older children and teens questions about their illness or injury. Offer them an opportunity to privately discuss their major concerns when their parents are not present.

- *Be honest* with the child when answering questions or when giving information about what will happen. Children need to learn that they can trust you.

- *Choose the language style* best understood by the parent and child. Commonly used phrases can have different meanings to persons in various regions of the country or to different ethnic groups. To improve communication, request frequent feedback from the parents or child to ensure that their interpretation of phrases is accurate.

- *Use an interpreter to improve communication* when you are not fluent in the family's primary language (Fig. 3–2).

Careful Listening

Complete attention is necessary to "hear" and accurately interpret information the parents and child give during the nursing history. Carefully *listen* to the information provided by the parent, as well as how it is expressed, and *observe behavior* during the interaction.

- Does the parent hesitate or avoid answering certain questions?

- Pay attention to the parent's attitude or tone of voice when the child's problems are discussed. Determine if it is consistent with the seriousness of the child's problem. The tone of voice can reveal anxiety, anger, or lack of concern.

- Be alert to any underlying themes. For example, the parent who talks about the child's diagnosis, but repeatedly refers to the impact of the illness on the family's finances or on meeting the needs of other family members, is requesting that these issues be addressed.

- Observe the parent's **nonverbal behavior** (posture, gestures, body movements, eye contact, and facial expression) for consistency with the words and tone of voice used. Is the parent interested in and appropriately concerned about the child's condition? Behaviors such as sitting up straight, making eye contact, and appearing apprehensive reflect appropriate concern for the child. Physical withdrawal, failure to make eye contact, or a happy expression could be inconsistent with the child's serious condition.

Subtle nonverbal and verbal cues often indicate that the parent has not provided complete information about the child's problem. Observe for behaviors such as avoiding eye contact, change in voice pitch, or hesitation when responding to a question. Being supportive and asking clarifying questions encourage further description or the expression of information that is difficult for the parent or child to share; for example, "It sounds like that was a very difficult experience. How did Latasha react?"

Encourage parents to share information, even if it is private or sensitive, especially when it influences nursing care planning. Often parents avoid sharing some information because they want to make a good impression, or they do not understand the value of the missing information. If a hesitation to share information is detected, briefly explain why the question was asked, for example, to make their child's hospital experience more pleasant or to begin planning for the child's discharge and home care.

In some cases the parent becomes too agitated, upset, or angry to continue responding to questions. When the information is not needed immediately, move on to another portion of the history to determine whether the parent is able to respond to other questions. Depending on the emotional status of the parent, it may be more appropriate to collect the remaining historical data at a later time.

DATA TO BE COLLECTED

The child's health, medical, and personal-social history is collected and organized to plan the child's nursing care. A modification of the Burns Classification System is the data-collection framework selected for this text.[2,3] Physiologic, psychosocial, and developmental data are organized to help develop the nursing diagnoses and the nursing care plan. Be alert for nonverbal cues (Fig. 3–3).

> **CULTURAL CONSIDERATIONS**
>
> Eye contact with the interviewer may be avoided by many cultural groups (Asian, Native American, and Middle Eastern patients) because it is considered impolite, aggressive, or a sign of disrespect.[1]

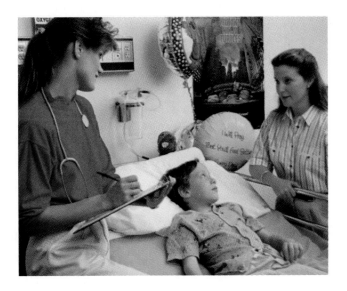

FIGURE 3–3. While you are collecting physiologic data you should be observing patient behavior.

Patient Information

Obtain the child's name and nickname, age, sex, and ethnic origin. The child's birth date, race, religion, address, and phone number can be obtained from the admission form. Ask the parent for an emergency contact address and phone number, as well as a work phone number. The person providing the patient history and that person's relationship to the patient are recorded.

Physiologic Data

Information about the child's health problems and diseases is collected chronologically in a format similar to the traditional medical history.

- The *chief complaint* is the child's primary problem or reason for hospital admission or visit to a health care setting, stated in the parent's or child's exact words.

- The *history of the present illness or injury* is a detailed description of the current health problem. This includes the onset and sequence of events, characteristics of and changes in symptoms over time, influencing factors, and the current status of the problem. Each problem is described separately. Table 3–1 lists the specific data to be collected about each illness and injury.

- The *past history* is a more detailed description of the child's prior health problems. It includes the birth history and all major past illnesses and injuries. A detailed and complete birth history is obtained when the child's present problem may be related to the birth history (Table 3–2). Record the child's age at the time of each illness, injury, related surgery, or hospitalization. Obtain information about each specific diagnosis, treatment, outcomes, complications or residual problems, and the child's reaction to the event (Table 3–3).

3-1	History of Present Illness or Injury

Characteristic	Defining Variables
Onset	Sudden or gradual, previous episodes, date and time began
Type of symptom	Pain, itching, cough, vomiting, runny nose, diarrhea, rash, etc
Location	Generalized or localized—anatomically precise
Duration	Continuous or episodic, length of episodes
Severity	Effect on daily activities, eg, interrupted sleep, decreased appetite, incapacitation
Influencing factors	What relieves or aggravates symptoms, what precipitated the problem, recent exposure to infection or allergen
Past evaluation for the problem	Laboratory studies, physician's office or hospital where done, results of past examinations
Previous and current treatment	Prescribed and over-the-counter drugs used, other measures tried (heat, ice, rest), response to treatments

3-2 **Birth History**

Prenatal
Mother's age, health during pregnancy, prenatal care, weight gained, special diet, expected date of delivery
Details of illnesses, x-ray findings, hospitalizations, medications, complications, and timing during pregnancy
Prior obstetric history

Antenatal—Description of Delivery
Site of delivery (hospital, home, birthing center)
Labor induced or spontaneous
Vaginal or cesarean section, forceps or suction used, vertex or breech position
Single or multiple birth

Condition of Baby at Birth
Weight, Apgar score, cried immediately
Need for incubator, oxygen, suctioning, ventilator
Any abnormalities detected, meconium staining

Postnatal
Difficulties in the nursery—feeding, respiratory difficulties, jaundice, cyanosis, rashes
Length of hospital stay, special nursery, home with mother
Breast or bottle fed, weight gained in hospital
Medical care needed in first week—admission to hospital

- The *current health status* is a detailed description of the child's typical health status. Obtain information about allergies, current medications, immunization status, activities and exercise, sleep patterns, nutrition, safety measures used, and health maintenance care (Table 3–4).

- The **review of systems** provides a comprehensive overview of the child's health. This is an opportunity to identify additional signs and symptoms associated with the child's admission problem or to identify other problems that have no direct relationship to the child's significant health problem but could be factors complicating nursing care or home care. For example, asking about any urinary problems may reveal that a child still wets the bed at 7 years of age, although the admission is for a femur fracture. The nurse would then need to consider how bedwetting might cause problems with the spica cast. For each problem, obtain the treatment, outcomes, residual prob-

3-3 **Past Illnesses and Injuries**

Illnesses	Major illnesses including common communicable diseases
Injuries	Major injuries, their mechanism (cause) and severity
Surgery	Specific type, day surgery or hospitalized
Hospitalizations	Reason and length of hospitalization
Transfusions	Circumstances, reactions

3-4	Current Health Status

Health Maintenance
Name of primary health care provider; last visit
Name of dentist; last visit
Other health care providers

Allergies
To food, medication, animals, insect bites, environment, etc
Type of reaction

Immunizations
Types, dates received, unexpected reactions

Safety Measures Used
Car restraint system
Window guards
Medication storage
Sports protective gear
Smoke detectors
Bicycle helmet
Firearm storage
Other

Activities and Exercise
Physical mobility
Play and/or sports activities
Limitations and adaptive equipment

Nutrition
Formula fed or breast-fed
When solid foods introduced
Eating and snacking habits
Variety of foods consumed, junk foods eaten
Appetite

Sleep
Length and timing of naps and nighttime sleep
Nightmares or night terrors
Other sleep disturbances
Where the child sleeps
Bedtime rituals

lems, and age at time of onset. Data-collection guidelines are given in Table 3–5.

- The *familial and hereditary diseases* summarize the major familial and hereditary diseases in family members, including the parents, grandparents, aunts, uncles, and siblings. Collect information about the health status of each parent. Record information in either a pedigree or a narrative format. Specific diseases the nurse inquires about are listed in Table 3–6.

Psychosocial Data

Obtain information about family composition to establish a socioeconomic and sociologic context within which to plan the child's care in the hospital and at home.

3-5 Review of Systems

Body Systems	Examples of Problems to Identify
General	General growth pattern, overall health status, ability to keep up with other children or tires easily with feeding or activity, fever, sleep patterns
	Allergies, type of reaction (hives, rash, respiratory difficulty, swelling, nausea), seasonal or with each exposure
Skin and lymph	Rashes, dry skin, itching, changes in skin color or texture, tendency for bruising, swollen or tender lymph glands
Hair and nails	Hair loss, changes in color or texture, use of dye or chemicals on hair
	Abnormalities of nail growth or color
Head	Headaches, head injuries
Eyes	Vision problems, squinting, crossed eyes, lazy eye, wears glasses, eye infections, redness, tearing, burning, rubbing, swelling eyelids
Ears	Ear infections, frequent discharge from ears, or tubes in ears
	Hearing loss (no response to loud noises or questions, inattentiveness, was hearing test ever done?)
Nose and sinuses	Nosebleeds, nasal congestion, colds with runny nose, sinus pain or infections
	Nasal obstruction, difficulty breathing, snoring at night
Mouth and throat	Mouth breathing, difficulty swallowing, sore throats, strep infections
	Tooth eruption, cavities, braces
	Voice change, hoarseness, speech problems
Cardiac and hematologic	Heart murmur, anemia, hypertension, cyanosis, edema, rheumatic fever, chest pain
Chest and respiratory	Trouble breathing, choking episodes, cough, wheezing, cyanosis, exposure to tuberculosis, other infections
Gastrointestinal	Bowel movements, frequency, color, regularity, consistency, discomfort, constipation or diarrhea, abdominal pain, bleeding from rectum, flatulence
	Nausea or vomiting, appetite
Urinary	Frequency, urgency, dysuria, dribbling, enuresis, strength of urinary stream
	Toilet trained—age when day and night dryness attained
Reproductive	For pubescent children
Female	Menses onset, amount, duration, frequency, discomfort, problems; vaginal discharge, breast development
Male	Puberty onset, emissions, erections, pain or discharge from penis, swelling or pain in testicles
Both	Sexual activity, use of contraception, sexually transmitted diseases
Musculoskeletal	Weakness, clumsiness, poor coordination, balance, tremors, abnormal gait, painful muscles or joints, swelling or redness of joints, fractures
Neurologic	Seizures, fainting spells, dizziness, numbness, learning problems, attention span, hyperactivity, memory problems

3-6 Familial or Hereditary Diseases

Infectious diseases	Tuberculosis, HIV, or hepatitis
Heart disease	Heart defects, myocardial infarctions, hypertension, hyperlipidemia
Allergic disorders	Eczema, hay fever, or asthma
Eye disorders	Glaucoma or cataracts
Hematologic disorders	Sickle cell anemia, thalassemia, G6PD deficiency, leukemia
Lung disorders	Cystic fibrosis
Cancer	Type
Endocrine disorders	Diabetes mellitus
Mental disorders	Mental retardation, epilepsy, Huntington chorea, psychiatric disorders
Musculoskeletal disorders	Arthritis, muscular dystrophy
Gastrointestinal disorders	Ulcers, colitis, kidney disease

- Family composition, including family members in the home, their relationship to the child, marital status of parents or other family structure, and persons participating in the care of the child
- Household members employed, family income, and financial resources or agencies used such as health insurance, food stamps, or Temporary Assistance for Needy Families
- Description of the housing and home environment (atmosphere, emotional stresses, family activities); safe play area; use of city or well water; and availability of electricity, heat, and refrigeration
- School or day-care arrangements; description of the neighborhood, including playgrounds, transportation, and proximity to stores

Information about daily routines, psychosocial data, and other living patterns forms the basis for many nursing diagnoses and development of an individualized nursing care plan. Collection of information should focus on issues that have an impact on the quality of daily living, even if some data seem to overlap with disease data (Table 3–7). The psychosocial history for adolescents should focus on critical areas in their lives (home environment, employment and education, activities, drugs, sexual activity/sexuality, suicide and depression, and safety) that may contribute to a less than optimal environment for normal growth and development.[4] Screening questions that can be used are found in Table 3–8.

3-7	Daily Living Patterns

Role Relationships
Family relationships/alterations in family process
Peer relationships
Social interactions: eg, day care, preschool, school
Communication

Self-Perception/Self-Concept
Personal identity and role identity
Self-esteem
Body image/nonvisible disorder

Coping/Stress Tolerance
Temperament
Coping behaviors
Discipline
Any substance abuse

Values and Beliefs
Religion
Personal values/beliefs

Home Care Provided for Child's Condition
Resources needed/available
Knowledge and skills of parents, other family members
Respite care available

Sensory/Perceptual Problems
Adaptations to daily living for any sensory loss (vision, hearing, cognitive, or motor)

Adapted from Burns, C. (1992). A new assessment model and tool for pediatric nurse practitioners. Journal of Pediatric Health Care, 6, 73–81.

3-8 Adolescent Psychosocial Assessment Using the HEADSSS Screening Tool

Home Environment
- With whom do you live?
- Have there been any recent changes in your living situation?
- How are things between your parents (or parent and significant other adult) at home?
- Are your parents employed?

Employment and Education
- Are you currently in school?
- What are your favorite subjects?
- How are your school grades?
- Have you ever been expelled from school or missed a lot of time?
- Do your friends attend school?
- What are your future education or employment plans?

Activities
- What do you do in your spare time?
- What do you do for fun?
- Whom do you spend time with?

Drugs
- Have you ever tried street drugs? Alcohol? Steroids? Have you ever smoked or chewed tobacco?
- Are you still using these drugs? Are any of your friends using or selling any drugs?

Sexual Activity/Sexuality
- What is your sexual orientation?
- Are you sexually active?
  At what age did you start having sex?
  How many sexual partners do you have?
  Do you (or your partner) use condoms?
  Do you (or your partner) use contraceptives?
- Have you ever been abused, either physically or sexually?

Suicide/Depression
- Are you ever sad or tearful? Tired or unmotivated?
- Have you ever felt that life is not worth living? Have you ever thought about or tried to hurt yourself? Do you have a suicide plan?

Safety
- Do you use a seat belt or bicycle helmet?
- Do you ever get into dangerous situations where you could be hurt?
- Is there a gun in your home? Have you ever learned about gun safety?

Modified from Goldenring, J.M., & Cohen, E. (1988). Getting into adolescent heads. Contemporary Pediatrics, 5, 75–90.

Developmental Data

Information about the child's motor, cognitive, language, and social development is recorded. Ask the parent about the child's milestones and current fine and gross motor skills. Obtain the age at which the child first used words appropriately and the current words used or language ability. For children in school, ask about academic performance to assess cognitive development. Ask the parent about the child's manner of interaction with other children, family members, and strangers.

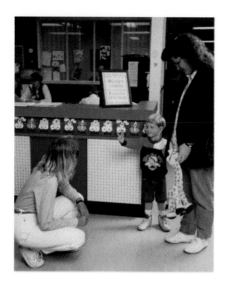

FIGURE 3–4. Examination of the child begins from the first contact. You should be observing the behavior of the child and parent by using visual cues to make a proper assessment. Does the child appear well nourished? Does the child appear secure with the parent?

The developmental data will help the nurse plan nursing care appropriate for the child. Guidelines for a nursing assessment of development can be found in Chapter 5.

▶ GENERAL APPRAISAL

The examination begins when you first meet the child, either when admitting the child to the nursing unit or in the patient's room (Fig. 3–4). Measure the infant's weight, length, and head circumference. If the child can stand, a standing height measurement is substituted for length (Fig. 3–5). Take the child's temperature, heart rate, respiratory rate, and blood pressure. Refer to the *Quick Reference to Pediatric Clinical Skills* accompanying this text for technique.

Observe the child's general appearance and behavior. The child should appear well nourished and well developed. Infants and young children are often fearful and seek reassurance from their parents. The child may resist interacting with you until rapport is established.

Observe the behavior and tone of voice used by the parent when he or she is talking to the child. Is the child encouraged to speak? Is the child appropriately reassured or supported by the parent? The child should feel secure with the parent and perceive permission to interact with the nurse.

▶ ASSESSING SKIN AND HAIR CHARACTERISTICS AND INTEGRITY

What is indicated when the child's skin is not uniform in color or when it feels spongy to the touch? What are each of the primary skin lesions called,

EXAMINATION TECHNIQUES

- **inspection** Purposeful observation of the child's physical features and behaviors. Physical feature characteristics include size, shape, color, movement, position, and location.
- **palpation** Use of touch to identify characteristics of the skin, internal organs, and masses. Characteristics include texture, moistness, tenderness, temperature, position, shape, consistency, and mobility of masses and organs.
- **auscultation** Listening to sounds produced by the airway, lungs, stomach, heart, and blood vessels to identify their characteristics. Auscultation is usually performed with a stethoscope to enhance the sounds heard.
- **percussion** Striking the surface of the body, either directly or indirectly, to set up vibrations that reveal the density of underlying tissues and borders of internal organs.

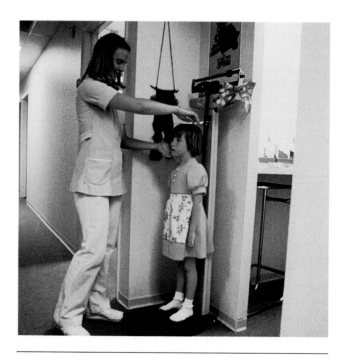

FIGURE 3–5. Standing height measurements are taken routinely at each well-child visit to assess the child's rate of growth.

and what characteristics are used to describe each of them? How can cyanosis and jaundice be detected in dark-skinned children? Why is skin turgor assessed? How is the presence of head lice identified in a child?

Examination of the skin requires good lighting to detect variations in skin color and to identify lesions. Daylight is preferred, but it is not always available. Rather than inspecting the entire skin surface of the child at one time, the nurse examines the child's skin simultaneously with other body systems as each region of the body is exposed.

INSPECTION OF THE SKIN

The child's skin is inspected for color and the presence of imperfections, elevations, or other lesions.

Skin Color

The color of the child's skin usually has an even distribution. The skin is inspected for color variations—such as increased or decreased pigmentation, pallor, mottling, bruises, erythema, cyanosis, or jaundice—that may be associated with local or generalized conditions. Some variations in skin color are common and normal, such as freckles found in the white population and Mongolian spots found on dark-skinned infants (Fig. 3–6). Bruises are common on the knees, shins, and lower arms as children stumble and fall. Bruises on other parts of the body, especially in various stages of healing, should raise a suspicion of child abuse.

When a skin color abnormality is suspected, the buccal mucosa and tongue should be inspected to confirm the color change. This is especially important in darker skinned children because the mucous membranes are usually pink, regardless of skin color. The gums are pressed lightly for 1–2 seconds. Any residual color, such as jaundice or cyanosis, is more easily detected in blanched skin. Jaundice may also be noticed in the sclerae of the eyes. Generalized cyanosis is associated with respiratory and cardiac disorders. Jaundice is associated with liver disorders.

CLINICAL TIP

The palms of the hands and soles of the feet are often lighter than the rest of the skin surface in darker skinned children. In addition, their lips may appear slightly bluish.

EQUIPMENT NEEDED

Gloves

CLINICAL TIP

The color of the bruise provides clues to its age.[5]

Color	Age of Bruise
Reddish blue	Up to 48 hours
Brownish blue	2–3 days
Brownish green	4–7 days
Greenish yellow	7–10 days
Yellow-brown	More than 8 days
Normal skin color	2–4 weeks

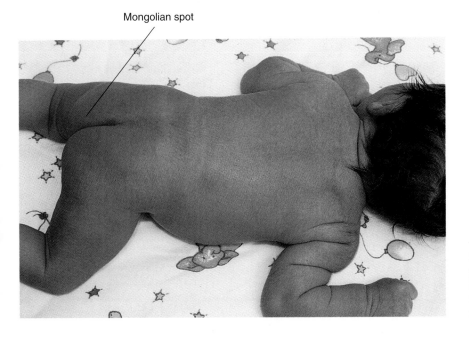

Mongolian spot

FIGURE 3–6. *Mongolian spots* are large patches of bluish-colored skin often seen on the buttocks. They are a normal occurrence in dark-skinned infants, but are sometimes incorrectly thought to be bruises.

PALPATION OF THE SKIN

Palpation of the skin provides a sense of its characteristics: temperature, texture, moistness, and resilience or turgor. To evaluate these characteristics, the nurse lightly touches or strokes the skin surface. The nurse follows standard precautions by wearing gloves when palpating mucous membranes, open wounds, and lesions.

Temperature

The child's skin normally feels cool to the touch. A general evaluation of skin temperature can be obtained by placing the wrist or dorsum of the hand against the child's skin. Excessively warm skin may indicate the presence of fever or inflammation, whereas abnormally cool skin may be a sign of shock or cold exposure.

Texture

Children have soft, smooth skin over the entire body. Any areas of roughness, thickening, or induration (area of extra firmness with a distinct border) should be identified. Abnormalities in texture are associated with endocrine disorders, chronic irritation, and inflammation.

Moistness

The child's skin is normally dry to the touch. The skin may feel slightly damp when the child has been exercising or crying. Excessive sweating without exertion is associated with a fever or with an uncorrected congenital heart defect.

Resilience (Turgor)

The child's skin is taut, elastic, and mobile because of the balanced distribution of intracellular and extracellular fluids. To evaluate skin turgor, the examiner pinches a small amount of skin on the abdomen between the thumb and forefinger, releases the skin, and watches the speed of recoil (Fig. 3–7). If the skin rapidly returns to its previous contour, good skin turgor is indicated. When poor skin turgor is present, the skin tents or stands up rather than resuming its previous contour. Poor skin turgor is commonly associated with dehydration.

CLINICAL TIP

The degree of dehydration, or weight loss caused by dehydration, can be estimated from the time it takes tented skin to return to its natural configuration.[6]

Weight Loss from Dehydration	Time to Return to Normal
<5%	<2 sec
5–8%	2–3 sec
9–10%	3–4 sec
>10%	>4 sec

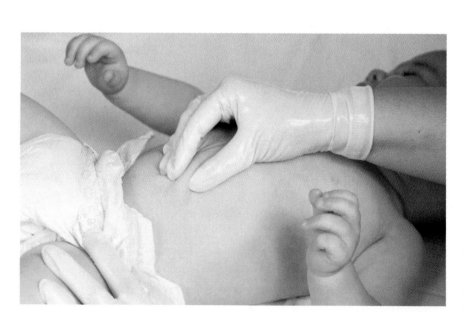

FIGURE 3–7. Tenting of the skin associated with poor skin turgor. Skin with normal turgor will return to a flat position quickly.

If *edema,* an accumulation of excess fluid in the interstitial spaces, is present, the skin feels doughy or boggy. To test for the degree of edema present, the examiner presses for 5 seconds against a bone beneath the area of puffy skin, releases the pressure, and observes how rapidly the indentation disappears. If the indentation disappears rapidly, the edema is "nonpitting." Slow disappearance of the indentation indicates "pitting" edema, which is commonly associated with kidney or heart disorders.

Capillary Refill and Small-Vein Filling Times

Two techniques are used to determine the adequacy of tissue perfusion (oxygen circulating to the tissues). When tissue perfusion is inadequate, immediately assess the child for shock or a physical constriction such as a cast or bandage that is too tight. The capillary refill time is normally less than 2 seconds (Fig. 3–8A and B). The small-vein filling time is normally less than 4 seconds (Fig. 3–8C and D).

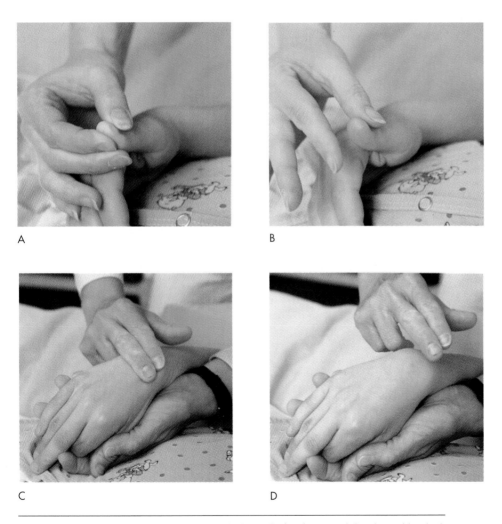

A B

C D

FIGURE 3–8. Capillary refill technique: **A,** Pinch the end of a finger until the skin is blanched. **B,** Quickly release the finger and watch the blood return to the veins. Count the seconds it takes for the color to return or veins to fill. Slow color return or vein filling time could be related to shock or constriction due to a tight bandage or cast. Small vein filling time technique: **C,** Using the index finger, milk a vein on the dorsum of the hand or foot from proximal to distal. **D,** Release your pressure and color should return promptly. Technique for small-vein filling time.

3-9   Common Primary Skin Lesions and Associated Condition

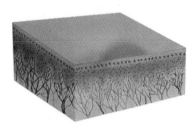

Lesion Name: Macule
Description:
Flat, nonpalpable, diameter <1 cm (1/2 in.)
Example: Freckle, rubella, rubeola, petechiae

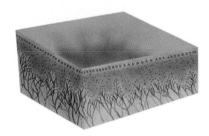

Lesion Name: Patch
Description:
Macule, diameter >1 cm (1/2 in.)
Example: Vitiligo, Mongolian spot

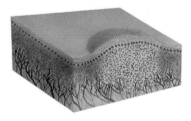

Lesion Name: Papule
Description:
Elevated, firm, diameter <1 cm (1/2 in.)
Example: Warts, pigmented nevi

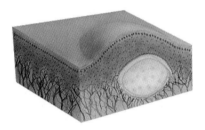

Lesion Name: Nodule
Description:
Elevated, firm, deeper in dermis than papule, diameter 1–2 cm (1/2 in.–1 in.)
Example: Erythema nodosum

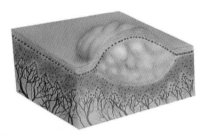

Lesion Name: Tumor
Description:
Elevated, solid, diameter >2 cm (1 in.)
Example: Neoplasm, hemangioma

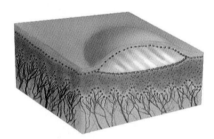

Lesion Name: Vesicle
Description:
Elevated, filled with fluid, diameter <1 cm (1/2 in.)
Example: Early chicken pox, herpes simplex

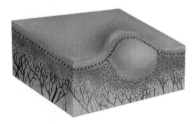

Lesion Name: Pustule
Description:
Vesicle filled with purulent fluid
Example: Impetigo, acne

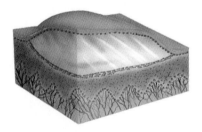

Lesion Name: Bulla
Description:
Vesicle diameter >1 cm (1/2 in.)
Example: Burn blister

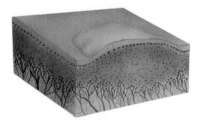

Lesion Name: Wheal
Description:
Irregular elevated solid area of edematous skin
Example: Urticaria, insect bite

SKIN LESIONS

Skin lesions are usually an indication of an abnormal skin condition. Characteristics of these lesions—location, size, type of lesion, pattern, and discharge, if present—provide clues about the cause of the condition. Inspect and palpate the isolated or generalized skin color abnormalities, elevations, lesions, or injuries to describe all characteristics present.

Primary lesions (such as macules, papules, and vesicles) are often the skin's initial response to injury or infection. Mongolian spots and freckles are normal findings also classified as primary lesions. Secondary lesions (such as scars, ulcers, fissures) are the result of irritation, infection, and delayed healing of primary lesions. Table 3–9 describes common primary lesions.

INSPECTION OF THE HAIR

Inspect the scalp hair for color, distribution, and cleanliness. The hair shafts should be evenly colored, shiny, and either curly or straight. Variation in hair color not caused by bleaching can be associated with a nutritional deficiency. Normally, hair is distributed evenly over the scalp. Investigate areas of hair loss. Hair loss in a child may result from tight braids or skin lesions such as ringworm (see Table 21–6). Notice any unusual hair growth patterns. An unusually low hairline on the neck or forehead may be associated with a congenital disorder such as hypothyroidism.

Children are frequently exposed to head lice. Inspect the individual hair shafts for small nits (lice eggs) that adhere to the hair (Fig. 3–9). None should be present.

Observe the distribution of body hair as other skin surfaces are exposed during examination. Fine hair covers most areas of the body. The presence of body hair in unexpected places should be noted. For example, a tuft of hair at the base of the spine often indicates a spinal defect.

It is important to note the age at which pubic and axillary hair develops in the child. Development at an unusually young age is associated with precocious puberty.

COMMON PATTERNS OF SKIN LESIONS

Annular: Circular, begins in center and spreads to periphery
Polycyclic: Annular lesions running together
Linear: In a row or stripe
Groups: Clustered
Gyrate: Twisted, spiral, coiled

GROWTH & DEVELOPMENT CONSIDERATIONS

Pubic hair begins to develop in children between 8 and 12 years of age, and axillary hair develops about 6 months later. Facial hair is noted in boys shortly after axillary hair develops.

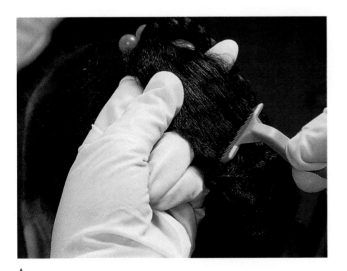

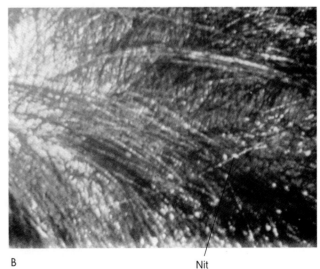

Nit

A
B

FIGURE 3–9. **A,** Inspecting for head lice with a fine-tooth comb. **B,** Nits on hair.
B, courtesy of Reed and Carnich Pharmaceuticals.

PALPATION OF THE HAIR

Palpate the hair shafts for texture. Hair should feel soft or silky with fine or thick shafts. Endocrine conditions such as hypothyroidism may result in coarse, brittle hair. Part the hair in various spots over the head to inspect and palpate the scalp for crusting or other lesions. If lesions are present, describe them using the characteristics in Table 3–9.

▶ ASSESSING THE HEAD FOR SKULL CHARACTERISTICS AND FACIAL FEATURES

What can cause a child's head or face to be asymmetric? How does a normal fontanel feel? What does an unusually large or small head suggest in an infant? What is the ping-pong phenomenon and what does it indicate?

INSPECTION OF THE HEAD AND FACE

Head

During early childhood the skull's sutures permit expansion for brain growth. Infants and young children normally have a rounded skull with a prominent occipital area. The shape of the head changes during childhood, and the occipital area becomes less prominent. An abnormal skull shape can result from premature closure of the sutures.

The head circumference of infants and young children is routinely measured until 5 years of age to ensure that adequate growth for brain development has occurred. The *Quick Reference to Pediatric Clinical Skills* accompanying this text describes the proper technique. A larger than normal head is associated with hydrocephalus, and a smaller than normal head suggests microcephaly.

EQUIPMENT NEEDED

Tape measure

CLINICAL TIP

Children who were low-birth-weight infants often have a flat, elongated skull because the soft skull bones were flattened by the weight of the head early in infancy.

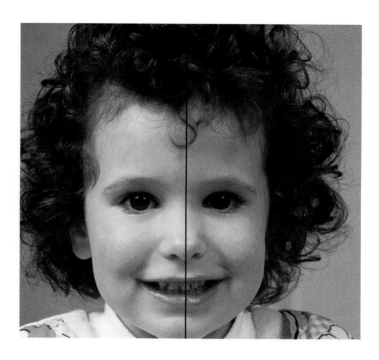

FIGURE 3–10. Draw an imaginary line down the middle of the face over the nose and compare the features on each side. Significant asymmetry may be caused by paralysis of cranial nerve V or VII, in utero positioning, and swelling from infection, allergy, or trauma.

Face

Inspect the child's face for symmetry during several facial expressions such as resting, smiling, talking, and crying (Fig. 3–10). Significant asymmetry may result from paralysis of trigeminal or facial nerves (cranial nerves V or VII), in utero positioning, and swelling from infection, allergy, or trauma.

Next inspect the face for unusual facial features such as coarseness, wide eye spacing, or disproportionate size. Tremors, tics, and twitching of facial muscles are often associated with seizures.

PALPATION OF THE SKULL

Palpate the skull in infants and young children to assess the sutures and fontanels and to detect soft bones (Fig. 3–11).

Sutures

Use your fingerpads to palpate each suture line. The edge of each bone in the suture line is felt, but normally there is no separation of the two bones. If additional bone edges are felt, it may indicate a skull fracture.

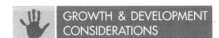

GROWTH & DEVELOPMENT CONSIDERATIONS

The suture lines of the skull are seldom palpated after 2 years of age. After that time the sutures rarely split.

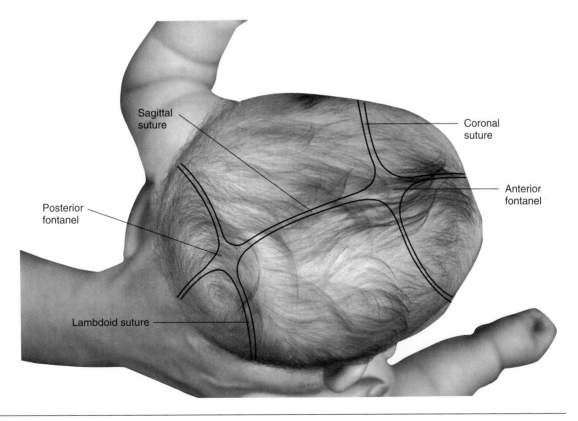

FIGURE 3–11. The sutures are separations between the bones of the skull that have not yet joined. The fontanels are formed at the intersection of these sutures where bone has not yet formed. Fontanels are covered by tough membranous tissue that protects the brain. The posterior fontanel closes between 2 and 3 months. The anterior fontanel and sutures are palpable up to the age of 18 months.

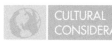

CULTURAL CONSIDERATIONS

The head is a sacred part of the body to Southeast Asians. Ask for permission before touching the infant's head to palpate the sutures and fontanels.[1] When a Hispanic child is examined, however, not touching the head is considered bad luck.

Fontanels

At the intersection of the sutures, palpate the anterior and posterior fontanels. The fontanel should feel flat and firm inside the bony edges. The anterior fontanel is normally smaller than 5 cm (2 in.) in diameter at 6 months of age and then becomes progressively smaller. It closes between 12 and 18 months of age. The posterior fontanel closes between 2 and 3 months of age.

A tense fontanel, bulging above the margin of the skull, is an indication of increased intracranial pressure. A soft fontanel, sunken below the margin of the skull, is associated with dehydration.

Craniotabes

Craniotabes is a snapping, ping-pong sensation associated with soft bones. Press firmly above and behind the ears. If craniotabes is present, a small section of bone suddenly sinks and then snaps back up when compression is lifted. Craniotabes is an abnormal finding associated with hydrocephalus and rickets.

▶ ASSESSING EYE STRUCTURES, FUNCTION, AND VISION

What is one of the most common eye problems that occurs during childhood? What do bulging or sunken eyeballs look like? What is the red reflex and what does it indicate? How is eye muscle balance tested? Is it normal for a child's visual acuity to be different at certain ages?

INSPECTION OF THE EXTERNAL EYE STRUCTURES

The function of the external and internal eye structures and related cranial nerves makes vision possible. The external eye structures, including the eyeballs, eyelids, and eye muscles, are inspected. The function of cranial nerves II, III, IV, and VI, which innervate the eye structures, is also tested (Fig. 3–12).

Eye Size and Spacing

Inspect the eyes and surrounding tissues simultaneously when examining facial features. The eyes should be the same size but not unusually large or small. Observe for eye bulging, which can be identified by retracted eyelids or a sunken appearance. Bulging may be associated with a tumor, and a sunken appearance may reflect dehydration.

Next inspect the eyes to see if they are appropriately distanced from each other. *Hypertelorism,* or widely spaced eyes, can be a normal variation in children.

Eyelids

Inspect the eyelids for color, size, position, mobility, and condition of the eyelashes. Eyelids should be the same color as surrounding facial skin and free of swelling or inflammation along the edges. Sebaceous glands that look like yellow striations are often present near the hair follicles. Eyelashes curl away from the eye to prevent irritation of the conjunctivae.

EQUIPMENT NEEDED

Ophthalmoscope
Vision chart
Penlight
Small toy
Index card or paper cup

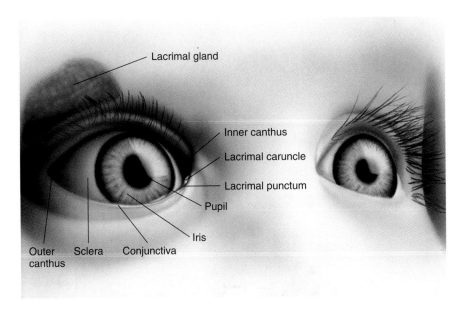

Inspect the conjunctivae lining the eyelids by pulling down the lower lid and then everting the upper lid. The conjunctivae should be pink and glossy. The lacrimal punctum, the opening for the lacrimal gland on each lid, is located near the medial canthus. No redness or excess tearing should be present.

When the eyes are open, inspect the level at which the upper and lower lids cross the eye. Each lid normally covers part of the iris but not any portion of the pupil. The lids should also close completely over the iris and cornea. Ptosis, drooping of the lid over the pupil, is often associated with injury to the oculomotor nerve, cranial nerve III. Sunset sign, in which the sclera is seen between the upper lid and the iris, may indicate retracted eyelids or hydrocephalus.

Inspect the eyes for the palpebral slant (Fig. 3–13). The eyelids of most people open horizontally. An upward or Mongolian slant is a normal finding in Asian children; however, children with Down syndrome also often have a Mongolian slant (Fig. 3–14). A downward or anti-Mongolian slant is seen in some children as a normal variation.

Eye Color

Inspect the color of each sclera, iris, and bulbar conjunctiva. The sclera is normally white or ivory in darker skinned children. Sclerae of another color suggest the presence of an underlying disease. For example, yellow sclerae indicate jaundice. Typically the iris is blue or light colored at birth and becomes pigmented within 6 months. Inspect the iris for the presence of Brushfield spots, white specks in a linear pattern around the iris circumference, which are often associated with Down syndrome. The bulbar conjunctivae, which cover the sclera to the edge of the cornea, are normally clear. Redness can indicate eyestrain, allergies, or irritation.

Pupils

Inspect the pupils for size and shape. Normally the pupils are round, clear, and equal in size. Some children have a coloboma, a keyhole-shaped pupil

 CLINICAL TIP

The eyelids of newborns are often swollen and difficult to open after antibiotics are instilled at birth to prevent infection.

 CLINICAL TIP

Children of Asian descent often have an extra fold of skin, known as the epicanthal fold, covering all or part of the medial canthus of the eye.

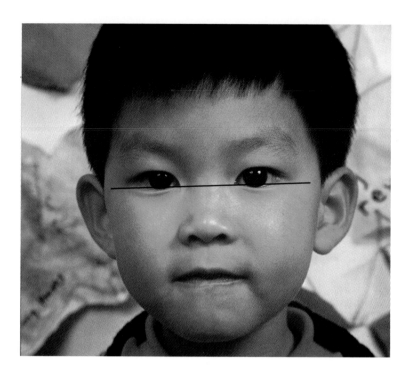

FIGURE 3–13. Draw an imaginary line across the medial canthi and extend it to each side of the face to identify the slant of the palpebral fissures. When the line crosses the lateral canthi, the palpebral fissures are horizontal and no slant is present. When the lateral canthi fall above the imaginary line, the eyes have an upward or Mongolian slant. A downward or anti-Mongolian slant is present when the lateral canthi fall below the imaginary line. Epicanthal folds are present when an extra fold of skin partially or completely covers the caruncles in the medial canthi. Which type of slant does this child have?

caused by a notch in the iris. The presence of this sign can indicate that the child has other congenital anomalies.

To test the pupillary response to light, shine a bright light into one eye. A brisk constriction of both the pupil exposed to direct light and the other pupil is a normal finding.

To test pupillary response to accommodation, ask the child to look first at a near object (for example, a toy) and then at a distant object (for example, a picture on the wall). The expected response is pupil constriction with near objects and pupil dilation with distant objects. This procedure tests the optic nerve, cranial nerve II.

INSPECTION OF THE EYE MUSCLES

One of the most common pediatric eye disorders is strabismus, or crossed eyes. This condition is important to detect because, if uncorrected, it can cause vision impairment. Several tests are used to detect the presence of a muscle imbalance that can result in strabismus. These tests include the evaluation of extraocular movements, the corneal light reflex, and the cover–uncover test.

Extraocular Movements

Seat the child at your eye level to evaluate the extraocular movements. Hold a toy or penlight 30 cm (12 in.) from the child's eyes and move it through the six cardinal fields of gaze. The child's head may need to be held still until fine motor eye movement develops. Both eyes should move together, tracking the object. This procedure tests the oculomotor, trochlear, and abducens nerves (cranial nerves III, IV, and VI) (Fig. 3–15).

Corneal Light Reflex

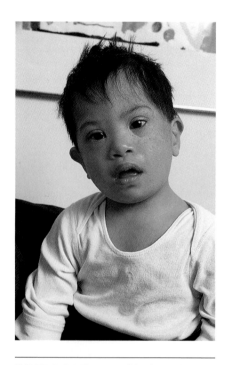

FIGURE 3–14. The eyes of this boy with Down syndrome show a Mongolian slant.

To test the corneal light reflex, shine a light on the child's nose, midway between the eyes. Identify the location where the light is reflected on each

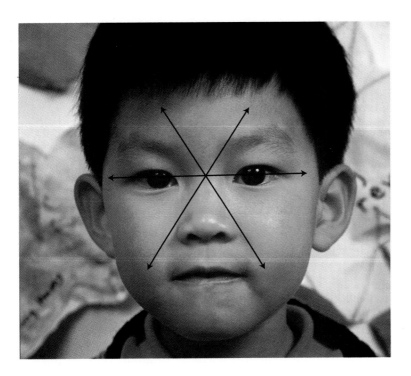

FIGURE 3–15. Begin the eye muscle examination with inspection of the extraocular movements. Have the child sit at your eye level. Hold a toy or penlight about 30 cm (12 in.) from the child's eyes and move it through the six cardinal fields of gaze. Both eyes should move together, tracking the object. This procedure tests cranial nerves III, IV, and VI.

eye. The light reflection is normally symmetric, at the same spot on each cornea. An asymmetric corneal light reflex indicates strabismus (see Fig. 3–12).

Cover–Uncover Test

The cover–uncover test can be used only for older, cooperative children. While standing slightly to one side but in a position from which you are still able to see the child's eyes, ask the child to look at a picture on the wall. Cover one of the child's eyes with an index card and simultaneously inspect the uncovered eye for movement as it focuses on the picture. Then remove the card from the covered eye and inspect it for movement as it focuses on the picture. Repeat the procedure with the child's other eye covered. Because the eyes work together, no obvious movement of either eye is expected. Eye movement indicates a muscle imbalance.

VISION ASSESSMENT

Because vision is such an important sense for learning, assessment is essential to detect any serious problems. Vision is evaluated using an age-appropriate vision test, but no simple method exists. It is possible to assess the presence of vision in infants and children by observing their behavior in response to certain maneuvers and during play.

Infants and Toddlers

When the infant's eyes are open, test the blink reflex by moving your hand quickly toward the infant's eyes. A quick blink is the normal response. Absence of the blink reflex can indicate that the infant is blind.

To test an infant's ability to visually track an object, hold a light or toy about 15 cm (6 in.) from the infant's eyes. When the infant has fixated on or is staring at the object, move it slowly to each side. The infant should follow the object with the eyes and by moving the head.

GROWTH & DEVELOPMENT CONSIDERATIONS

Research has discovered that newborns have vision good enough at birth to prefer faces to other patterns and to follow a moving object. The child's visual acuity develops during early childhood.[6]

Age	Visual Acuity
3 years	20/50
4 years	20/40
5 years	20/30
6 years	20/20

Once an infant has developed skills to reach for and then pick up objects, observe play behavior to evaluate vision. The ability to easily find and pick up small toys is a good indicator of vision in children under 3 years of age.

Standardized Vision Charts

Standardized vision charts cannot be used to test vision until the child can understand directions and cooperate, usually at about 3 or 4 years of age. The Snellen E chart or Picture chart can be used to test visual acuity of preschool-age children just as the Snellen Letter chart is used for school-age children and adolescents. The *Quick Reference to Pediatric Clinical Skills* accompanying this text describes the use of these charts.

INSPECTION OF THE INTERNAL EYE STRUCTURES

The funduscopic examination allows you to inspect the structures of the internal eye—the retina, optic disc, arteries and veins, and macula (Fig. 3–16). This examination takes extensive practice because the ophthalmoscope is a complex instrument to master and because the examination is difficult to perform on uncooperative children. Most often it is performed by experienced examiners.

Darkening the room will cause the child's pupils to dilate. Explain the procedure to the child to gain his or her cooperation. Have a picture on the wall or have the parent or assistant hold a toy for the child to stare at so that the child's eye will not have to be held open forcibly.

Using the Ophthalmoscope

The ophthalmoscope has a lens-and-mirror system and a bright light for inspecting the structures of the internal eye (Fig. 3–17). Different lens powers are arranged on the rotating disk of the ophthalmic head. This system permits compensation for vision difference between the child and the examiner. The black-numbered plus lenses magnify images, and the red-

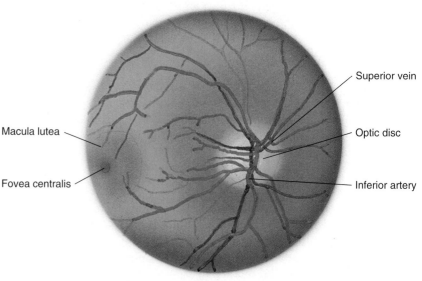

Macula lutea

Fovea centralis

Superior vein

Optic disc

Inferior artery

Retina

FIGURE 3–16. Normal fundus.

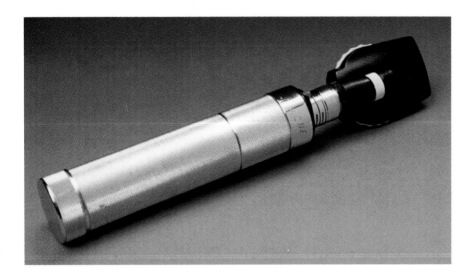

FIGURE 3–17. Ophthalmoscope.

numbered minus lenses reduce them in a range of powers. The lenses can be changed by turning the disk with the forefinger.

Turn the ophthalmoscope on and set the lens power at 0. Keep your forefinger on the disk to change the lens power as needed. Hold the ophthalmoscope so you can see through the lens. Rest the top against your eyebrow and the handle against your cheek to keep the instrument stabilized. The right eye is used to examine the child's right eye and the left eye to examine the child's left eye. This position is best for visualizing the eye, and it reduces direct exposure to infection. Place a hand on the child's head for stabilization.

Red Reflex

Shine the ophthalmoscope light at the child's eye from a distance of 30 cm (12 in.). The first image seen is the red reflex, the red glow of the vascular retina. When the red reflex is seen, the ophthalmoscope is being used correctly and the child's lens is clear. Black spots or opacities within the red reflex are abnormal and may indicate congenital cataracts. If a white reflex is seen rather than a red reflex, a retinoblastoma may be present. The red reflex can also be tested by shining a small flashlight into the eye.

Visualizing the Internal Eye Structures

Slowly move closer to the child. Deeper levels of the vitreous humor are inspected before the pink retina comes into view. The retina is a deeper pink in dark-skinned children. A blood vessel is the first retinal structure usually seen. Continue moving closer to the child's eye and adjust the plus or minus lenses to focus on this blood vessel. Retinal arteries appear smaller and brighter red than veins. The blood vessels branch to spread and cover the retina.

Inspect and follow the branching of the blood vessels toward the nose until they merge into the optic disc. Dark areas along the blood vessels may indicate retinal hemorrhages. Carefully inspect sites where arteries and veins cross. Notches and indentations at these sites are associated with hypertension.

The optic disc margin is normally sharply defined, round, and yellow to creamy pink. Blurring of the disc margins or bulging of the optic disc is a sign of increased intracranial pressure. The diameter of the optic disc is used to identify the location of other landmarks on the retina.

CLINICAL TIP

Keep the red reflex in view to make sure your head and the ophthalmoscope move as one unit. If you lose the red reflex when moving closer to the child, move back, find the red reflex, and start again.

The macula is located approximately 2 disc diameters lateral to the optic disc. To see the macula, ask the child to look at the light. It appears as a yellow dot surrounded by deep pink. The macula is inspected last because the bright light causes the child to blink and look away.

► ASSESSING THE EAR STRUCTURES AND HEARING

How do you identify proper ear placement on the head? What is the significance of low-set ears? Why is otitis media the most common ear problem during early childhood? What play activities can be used to test hearing in young children? How do you evaluate the hearing of an older child?

INSPECTION OF THE EXTERNAL EAR STRUCTURES

The position and characteristics of the pinna, the external ear, are inspected as a continuation of the head and eye examination. The pinna is considered "low set" when the top lies completely below an imaginary line drawn through the medial and lateral canthi of the eye toward the ear. Low-set ears are often associated with congenital renal disorders (Fig. 3–18).

Inspect the pinna for any malformation. The pinna should be completely formed, with an open auditory canal. Next, inspect the tissue around the pinna for abnormalities. A pit or hole in front of the auditory canal may indicate the presence of a sinus. If the pinna protrudes outward, there may be swelling behind the ear, a sign of mastoiditis.

Inspect the external auditory canal for any discharge. A foul-smelling, purulent discharge may indicate the presence of a foreign body or an infection in the external canal. Clear fluid or a blood-tinged discharge may indicate a cerebrospinal fluid leak caused by a basilar skull fracture.

EQUIPMENT NEEDED

Otoscope
Noisemakers (bell, rattle, tissue paper)
Tuning fork, 500–1000 Hz

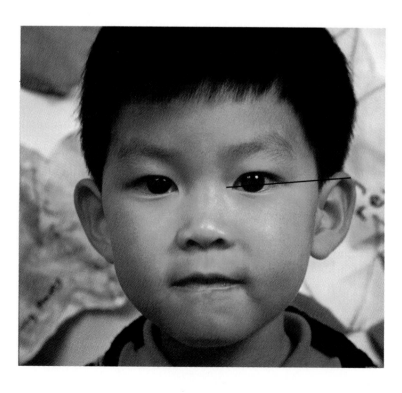

FIGURE 3–18. To detect the correct placement of the external ears, draw an imaginary line through the medial and lateral canthi of the eye toward the ear. This line normally passes through the upper portion of the pinna. The pinna is considered "low set" when the top lies completely below the imaginary line. Low-set ears are often associated with renal disorders. Is this a normal ear placement? Yes, it is.

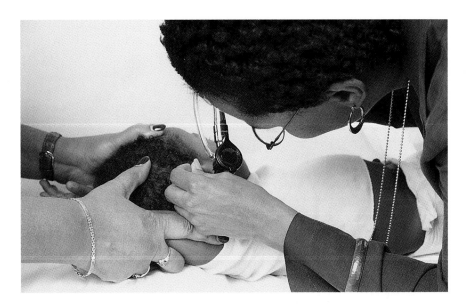

FIGURE 3-19. To restrain an uncooperative child, place the child prone on the examining table. Have an assistant hold the child's arms next to the head to restrain the child's head movements. Restrain the child's body movements by lying across the child's body. Keep your hands free to hold the otoscope and position the external ear.

INSPECTION OF THE TYMPANIC MEMBRANE

Examination of the tympanic membrane is important in infants and young children because they are prone to otitis media, a middle ear infection. The eustachian tubes are shorter, wider, and more horizontally positioned in infants and young children than in older children and adults. This positioning enables bacteria to move up the eustachian tube from the pharynx, causing an infection.

The otoscope, an instrument with a magnifying lens, bright light, and speculum, is used to examine the internal auditory canal and tympanic membrane.

Infants and young children often resist having their ears inspected with the otoscope because of past painful experiences. The otoscopic examination is often delayed until portions of the assessment requiring cooperation are completed. Use simple explanations to prepare the child. Let the child play with the otoscope or demonstrate how it is used on the parent or a doll. Figure 3–19 illustrates one method that can be used to restrain an uncooperative child.

Using the Otoscope

To begin the otoscopic examination, hold the handle of the otoscope in the palm of your hand with your thumb pointed toward the base of the handle. If a pneumatic squeeze bulb is used, hold it between the index finger and the handle. Choose the largest ear speculum that fits into the auditory canal to form a seal for testing the movement of the tympanic membrane. A large speculum is also less likely to injure the auditory canal if the child moves suddenly.

Hold the otoscope in the hand closest to the child's face and when the child is cooperative rest the back of your hand against the child's head to stabilize it. Use your other hand to pull the pinna toward the back of the head and either up or down. Pulling the pinna straightens the auditory canal and improves inspection of the tympanic membrane (Fig. 3–20).

Slowly insert the speculum into the auditory canal, inspecting the walls for signs of irritation, discharge, or a foreign body. The walls of the auditory canal are normally pink, and some cerumen is present. Children often put beads, peas, or other small objects into their ears. If the auditory canal is

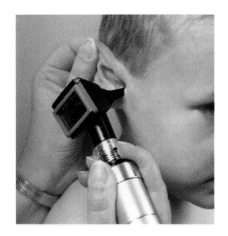

FIGURE 3-20. To straighten the auditory canal: pull the pinna back and up for children over 3 years of age; pull the pinna down and back for children under 3 years of age.

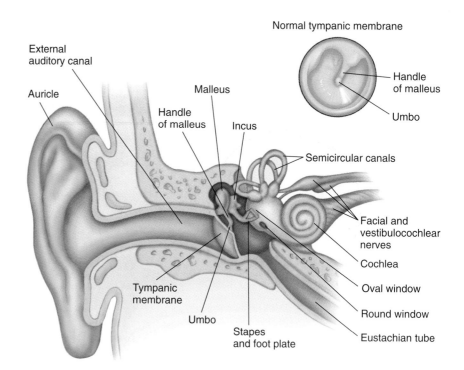

FIGURE 3–21. Cross section of the ear. The tympanic membrane normally has a triangular light reflex with the base on the nasal side pointing toward the center. The bony landmarks, the umbo and handle of malleus, are seen through the tympanic membrane.

SAFETY PRECAUTIONS

Never irrigate the ear canal if any discharge is present. Cold water should never be used for irrigation.

GROWTH & DEVELOPMENT CONSIDERATIONS

Indicators of hearing loss in an infant:
- No startle reaction to loud noises
- Does not turn toward sounds by 4 months of age
- Babbles as a young infant but does not keep babbling or develop speech sounds after 6 months of age

Indicators of hearing loss in a young child:
- No speech by 2 years of age
- Speech sounds are not distinct at appropriate ages

obstructed by cerumen or a foreign body, irrigation can be used to clean the canal.

The tympanic membrane, which separates the outer ear from the middle ear, is usually pearly gray and translucent. It reflects light, and the bones (ossicles) in the middle ear are normally visible. When the pneumatic attachment is squeezed, the tympanic membrane normally moves in and out in response to the positive and negative pressure applied (Fig. 3–21). Table 3–10 lists the abnormal findings of a tympanic membrane examination and their associated conditions.

HEARING ASSESSMENT

Hearing evaluation is important in children of all ages because hearing is essential for normal speech development and learning. Often hearing must be evaluated by inspection of the child's responses to various auditory stimuli. Hearing loss may occur at any time during early childhood as the result of birth trauma, frequent otitis media, meningitis, or antibiotics that damage cranial nerve VIII.

Use hearing and speech articulation milestones as an initial hearing screen. Select an age-appropriate method to screen hearing. When a hearing deficiency is suspected as a result of screening, the child is referred for audiometry, tympanometry, or evoked response to obtain the most accurate evaluation of hearing.

Infants and Toddlers

Select noisemakers with different frequencies, such as a rattle, bell, and tissue paper, that will attract the young child's attention. Ask the parent or an assistant to entertain the infant with a quiet toy, such as a teddy bear. Stand behind the infant, about 2 feet (60 cm) away from the infant's ear but outside the infant's field of vision, and make a soft sound

3-10	Unexpected Findings on Examination of the Tympanic Membrane and Their Associated Conditions	
Characteristics of Tympanic Membrane	**Unexpected Findings**	**Associated Conditions**
Color	Redness	Infection in middle ear
	Slight redness	Prolonged crying
	Amber	Serous fluid in middle ear
	Deep red or blue	Blood in middle ear
Light reflex	Absent	Bulging tympanic membrane, infection in middle ear
	Distorted, loss of triangular shape	Retracted tympanic membrane, serous fluid in middle ear
Bony landmarks	Extra prominent	Retracted tympanic membrane, serous fluid in middle ear
Movement	No motility	Infection or fluid in middle ear
	Excess motility	Healed perforation

with the noisemaker. Have the parent or your assistant observe the child for any of the following responses when the noisemaker is used: widening the eyes, briefly stopping all activity to listen, or turning the head toward the sound. Repeat the test in the other ear and with the other noisemakers.

Preschool and Older Children

Whispered words are used to evaluate the hearing of children over 3 years of age. Position your head about 12 inches (30 cm) away from the child's ear, but out of the range of vision so the child cannot read your lips. Use words easily recognized by the child, such as Mickey Mouse, hot dog, and Popsicle, and ask the child to repeat the words. Repeat the test with different words in the opposite ear. The child should correctly repeat the whispered words.

An alternative procedure is used to assess hearing when the child will not cooperate by repeating the whispered words. In a whisper, direct the child to point to different parts of the body or objects, for example, "Show me your eyes" and "Point to your mouth." Children should point to the correct body part each time.

Bone and Air Conduction of Sound

A tuning fork is used to evaluate the hearing of school-age children who can follow directions. Stroke the tines of the tuning fork to begin the vibration. Avoid touching the vibrating tines, which will dampen the sound. Bone conduction is tested when the handle of the tuning fork is placed on the child's skull. Air conduction is tested when the vibrating tines are held close to the child's ear (Fig. 3–22).

To perform the *Weber test*, place the vibrating tuning fork on top of the child's skull in the midline. Ask the child to tell you where the sound is heard the best, either in both ears equally or in one ear. The sound should be heard equally in both ears.

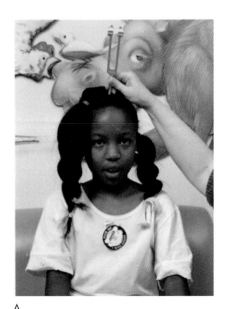

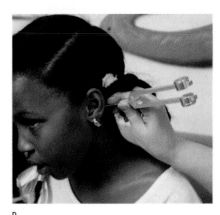

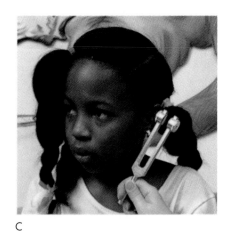

A

B

C

FIGURE 3–22. **A,** Weber test. Place vibrating tuning fork on midline of the child's head. **B,** Rinne test, step 1. Place vibrating tuning fork on mastoid process. **C,** Rinne test, step 2. Reposition still vibrating tines between 2.5 and 5 cm (1 and 2 in.) from ear.

To perform the *Rinne test* place the vibrating tuning fork handle on the mastoid process behind an ear. Ask the child to tell you when the sound is no longer heard. Immediately move the tuning fork, holding the vibrating tines about 2.5–5 cm (1–2 in.) from the same ear. Again, ask the child to indicate when the sound is no longer heard. The child normally hears the air-conducted sound twice as long as the bone-conducted sound. The Rinne test is repeated on the other ear. Table 3–11 provides an interpretation of the Weber and Rinne tests.

3-11	Interpretation of the Weber and Rinne Tests of Hearing

Test and Result	Associated Condition
Weber Test	
Sound heard equally in both ears	No hearing loss
Sound heard better in one ear (lateralized)	Conductive hearing loss if sound lateralized to deaf ear
	Sensorineural hearing loss if sound lateralized to good ear
Rinne Test	
Sound heard by air conduction twice as long as bone conduction	No hearing loss
Sound heard longer by bone conduction than air conduction	Conductive hearing loss in affected ear
Sound heard longer by air conduction than bone conduction, but less than twice as long	Sensorineural hearing loss in affected ear

► ASSESSING THE NOSE AND SINUSES FOR AIRWAY PATENCY AND DISCHARGE

What is the most common cause of a nasal obstruction in children? What does nasal flaring indicate? What signs indicate that a foreign body might be lodged in the nose? What does it mean if the child frequently wipes the nose upward with a hand?

INSPECTION OF THE EXTERNAL NOSE

The external nose characteristics and placement on the face are examined simultaneously with the facial features. Inspect the external nose for size, shape, symmetry, and midline placement on the face. The nose should be proportional in size to other facial features and positioned in the middle of the face. A flattened nasal bridge is the expected finding in Asian and black children.

The nasolabial folds are normally symmetric. Asymmetry of the nasolabial folds may be associated with injury to the facial nerve (cranial nerve VII). A saddle-shaped nose is associated with congenital defects such as cleft palate.

Inspect the external nose for the presence of unusual characteristics. For example, a crease across the nose between the cartilage and bone is often caused by the allergic child's wiping an itchy nose upward with a hand.

PALPATION OF THE EXTERNAL NOSE

When a deformity is noted, gently palpate the nose to detect any pain or break in contour. No tenderness or masses are expected. Pain and a contour deviation are usually the result of trauma.

Nasal Patency

The child's airway must be patent to ensure adequate oxygenation. To test for nasal patency, occlude one nostril and observe the child's effort to breathe through the open nostril with the mouth closed. Repeat the procedure with the other nostril. Breathing should be noiseless and effortless. *Nasal flaring,* an effort the child makes to widen the airway, is a sign of respiratory distress and should not be present.

If the child struggles to breathe, a nasal obstruction may be present. Nasal obstruction may be caused by a foreign body, congenital defect, dry mucus, discharge, polyp, or trauma. Newborns may have respiratory distress because of *choanal atresia,* a congenital membranous or bony obstruction between the nose and the nasopharynx. Young children commonly place objects up their nose, and unilateral nasal flaring is a sign of such an obstruction.

ASSESSMENT OF SMELL

The olfactory nerve (cranial nerve I) is rarely tested in preschool children, but it can be tested in school-age children and adolescents. When testing smell, choose scents the child will easily recognize such as orange, chocolate, and mint. When the child's eyes are closed, occlude one nostril and hold the scent under the nose. Ask the child to take a deep sniff and identify the scent. Alternate odors between the nares. The child can normally identify common scents.

GROWTH & DEVELOPMENT CONSIDERATIONS

Infants under 6 months of age will not automatically open their mouths to breathe when their nose is occluded, such as by mucus.

INSPECTION OF THE INTERNAL NOSE

Inspect the internal nose for color of the mucous membranes and the presence of any discharge, swelling, lesions, or other abnormalities. Use a bright light, such as an otoscope light or penlight. For infants and young children, push the tip of the nose upward and shine the light at the end of the nose (Fig. 3–23). The nasal speculum for the otoscope can be used in older children. Avoid touching the septum of the nose with the speculum. Injury to the septum can cause a nosebleed.

Mucous Membranes

The mucous membranes should be dark pink and glistening. A film of clear discharge may also be present. Turbinates, if visible, should be the

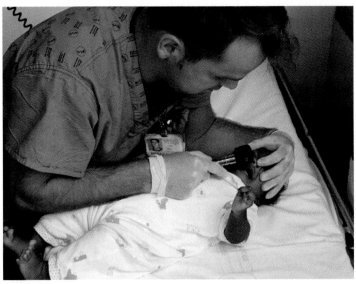

A

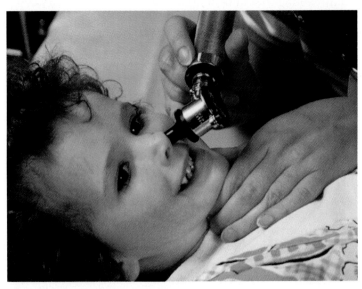

FIGURE 3–23. Techniques for examining nose. A, Technique for infant or small child. B, Technique for older child.

B

same color as the mucous membranes and have a firm consistency. When the turbinates are pale or bluish gray, the child may have allergies. A polyp, a rounded mass projecting from the turbinate, is also associated with allergies.

Nasal Septum

Inspect the nasal septum for alignment, perforations, bleeding, or crusting. The septum should be straight. Crusting will be noted over the site of a nosebleed.

Discharge

Observe for the presence of nasal discharge, noting if the drainage is from one or both nares. Nasal discharge is not a normal finding unless the child is crying. Discharge may be watery, mucoid, purulent, or bloody. The character of the discharge depends on the condition present. A foul-smelling discharge in only one nostril is often associated with a foreign body. Table 3–12 lists conditions associated with nasal discharge.

INSPECTION OF THE SINUSES

The maxillary and ethmoid sinuses develop during early childhood (Fig. 3–24). Sinus infections are rare in young children but occasionally can occur in school-age children. Suspect a sinus problem when the child has a headache or pain and swelling around one or both eyes.

Inspect the face for any puffiness around one or both eyes. Puffiness and swelling are not normally present. To palpate over the maxillary si-

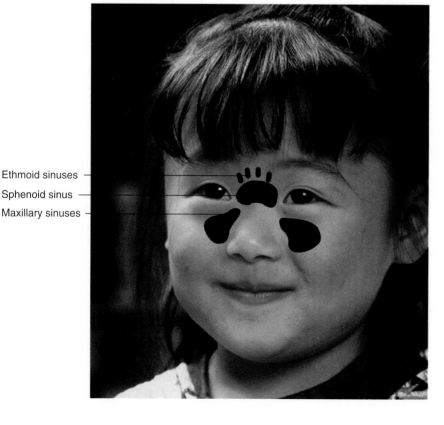

Ethmoid sinuses
Sphenoid sinus
Maxillary sinuses

FIGURE 3–24. Maxillary sinuses can be identified in 1-year-old children. Ethmoid sinuses have developed in children by 6 years of age. Sinus problems under age 7 years occur infrequently.

3-12	Nasal Discharge Characteristics and Associated Conditions	
Discharge Description		**Associated Condition**
Watery		
Clear, bilateral		Allergy
Serous, unilateral		Spinal fluid from fracture of cribriform plate
Mucoid or purulent		
Bilateral		Upper respiratory infection
Unilateral		Foreign body
Bloody		Nose bleed, trauma

nuses, press up under both zygomatic arches with the thumbs. To palpate the ethmoid sinuses, press up against the bone above both eyes with the thumbs. No swelling or tenderness is expected. Tenderness may be an indication of sinusitis.

► ASSESSING THE MOUTH AND THROAT FOR COLOR, FUNCTION, AND SIGNS OF ABNORMAL CONDITIONS

What is the best site to evaluate cyanosis in children? What is the expected sequence of tooth eruption? How is it determined that the tongue has adequate movement for all speech sounds? How can the throat be inspected without causing the child to gag?

INSPECTION OF THE MOUTH

Young children often need coaxing and simple explanations before they will cooperate with the mouth and throat examination. Most children readily show their teeth. If the child resists by clenching the teeth, they can be gently separated with a tongue blade. Wear gloves when examining the mouth because of contact with mucous membranes (Fig. 3–25).

Lips

Inspect the lips for color, shape, symmetry, moisture, and lesions. The lips are normally symmetric without drying, cracking, or other lesions. Lip color is normally pink in white children and more bluish in darker skinned children. Pale, cyanotic, or cherry-red lips are indicators of poor tissue perfusion caused by various conditions.

Teeth

Inspect and count the child's teeth. The timing of tooth eruption is often genetically determined, but there is a regular sequence of tooth eruption. Figure 3–26 presents the typical sequence of tooth eruption for both deciduous and permanent teeth.

Inspect the condition of the teeth, look for loose teeth, and note any spaces where teeth are missing. Compare empty tooth spaces with the

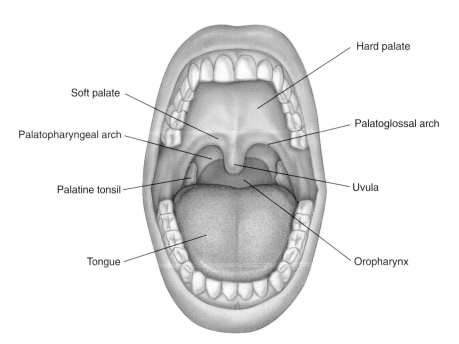

FIGURE 3-25. The structures of the mouth.

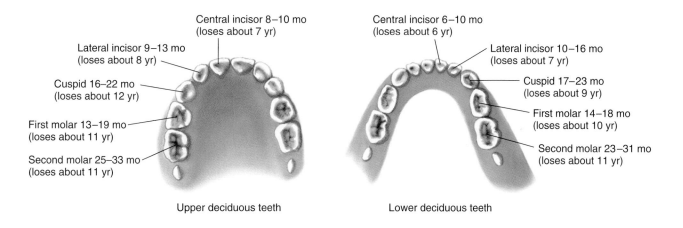

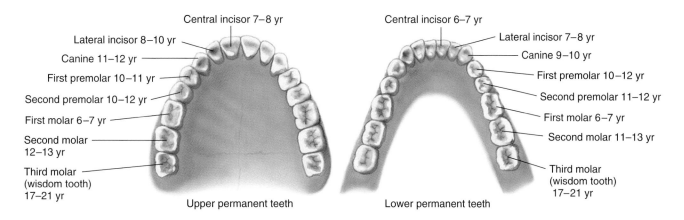

FIGURE 3-26. Typical sequence of tooth eruption for both deciduous and permanent teeth. Notice that bottom teeth come in first for each kind of tooth, incisors, cuspids, and molars. They are lost in the same pattern.

child's developmental stage of tooth eruption. Once the permanent teeth have erupted, none should be missing. Teeth are normally white, without a flattened, mottled, or pitted appearance. Discolorations on the crown of a tooth may indicate caries.

Mouth Odors

During inspection of the teeth, be alert to any abnormal odors that may indicate problems such as diabetic ketoacidosis, infection, or poor hygiene.

Gums

Inspect the gums for color and adherence to the teeth. The gums are normally pink, with a stippled or dotted appearance. Use a tongue blade to help visualize the gums around the upper and lower molars. No raised or receding gum areas should be apparent around the teeth. When inflammation, swelling, or bleeding is observed, palpate the gums to detect tenderness. Inflammation and tenderness are associated with infection and poor nutrition.

Buccal Mucosa

Inspect the mucous membrane lining the cheeks for color and moisture. The mucous membrane is usually pink, but patches of hyperpigmentation are commonly seen in darker skinned children. The Stensen duct, the parotid gland opening, is opposite the upper second molar bilaterally. Normally pink, the duct opening becomes red when the child is infected with mumps. Small pink sucking pads can be present in infants. No areas of redness, swelling, or ulcerative lesions should be present.

Tongue

Inspect the tongue for color, moistness, size, tremors, and lesions. The child's tongue is normally pink and moist, without a coating. The tongue's size permits it to fit easily into the mouth. A pattern of gray, irregular borders that form a design (geographic tongue) is often normal, but it may be associated with fever, allergies, or drug reactions. Tremors are abnormal. A white adherent coating on an infant's tongue may be caused by thrush, a *Candida* infection.

Observe the mobility of the tongue. The child should be able to touch the gums above the upper teeth with the tongue. This tongue movement is adequate to enunciate all speech sounds clearly. Ask the child to stick out the tongue and lift it so the underside of the tongue and the floor of the mouth can be inspected for distended veins.

Palate

Inspect the hard and soft palate to detect any clefts or masses or an unusually high arch. The palate is normally pink, with a dome-shaped arch and no cleft. The uvula hangs freely from the soft palate. Newborns often have Epstein pearls, white papules in the midline of the palate that disappear in a few weeks. A high-arched palate can be associated with sucking difficulties in young infants.

PALPATION OF THE MOUTH STRUCTURES

Palpate any masses seen in the mouth to determine their characteristics, such as size, shape, firmness, and tenderness. No masses should be found.

Tongue

To assess the tongue's strength, simultaneously testing the hypoglossal nerve (cranial nerve XII), place the index finger against the child's cheek and ask the child to push against your finger with the tongue. Some pressure against the finger is normally felt.

Palate

To palpate the palate, insert the little finger, with the fingerpad upward, into the mouth. While the infant sucks against your finger, palpate the entire palate. This procedure also tests the strength of the sucking reflex, innervated by the hypoglossal nerve (cranial nerve XII). No clefts should be palpated.

INSPECTION OF THE THROAT

Inspect the throat for color, swelling, lesions, and the condition of the tonsils. Ask the child to open the mouth wide and stick out the tongue. A flashlight is used to illuminate the throat. A tongue blade can be used, if needed, to visualize the posterior pharynx. Moistening the tongue blade may decrease the child's tendency to gag. The throat is normally pink without lesions, drainage, or swelling. Swelling or bulging in the posterior pharynx may be associated with a peritonsillar abscess.

Tonsils

During childhood the tonsils are large in proportion to the size of the pharynx because lymphoid tissue grows fastest in early childhood. The tonsils should be pink without exudate, but *crypts* (fissures) may be present as a result of prior infections.

Gag Reflex

Use a tongue blade when you are unable to see the posterior pharynx or need to test the gag reflex. The gag reflex is tested at the end of the examination because children dislike the gagging sensation. Prepare the child for what will happen. Ask the child to say "Ah" and watch for the symmetric rising movement of the uvula. This reflex tests the glossopharyngeal and vagal nerves (cranial nerves IX and X). If the uvula does not rise or rises to one side, cranial nerves IX and X may be paralyzed. The epiglottis lies behind the tongue and is normally pink like the rest of the buccal mucosa.

► ASSESSING THE NECK FOR CHARACTERISTICS, RANGE OF MOTION, AND LYMPH NODES

What does it mean when a child's head is tilting to one side? By what age should an infant be able to control his or her head? What does a lymph node feel like? What does an enlarged lymph node feel like?

INSPECTION OF THE NECK

Inspect the neck for size, symmetry, swelling, and any abnormalities. A short neck with skin folds is normal for infants. The neck is normally symmetric. No swelling should be present. Swelling may be caused by local infections such as mumps or a congenital defect. The neck lengthens between 3 and 4 years of age.

Inspect the child's neck for any *webbing*, an extra skin fold on each side of the neck. Webbing is commonly associated with Turner syndrome.

Infants develop head control by 2 months of age. By this age an infant can lift the head up and look around when lying on the stomach. A lack of head control can result from neurologic injury, such as an anoxic episode.

PALPATION OF THE NECK

Face the child and use the fingerpads to simultaneously palpate both sides of the neck for lymph nodes, as well as the trachea and thyroid.

Lymph Nodes

To palpate the lymph nodes, slide the fingerpads gently over the lymph node chains in the head and neck. The sequence for lymph node palpation is as follows: around the ears, under the jaw, the occipital area, and the cervical chain in the neck (Fig. 3–27). Firm, clearly defined, nontender, movable lymph nodes up to 1 cm (½ in.) in diameter are common in young children. Enlarged, firm, warm, tender lymph nodes indicate the presence of local infection.

Trachea

Palpate the trachea to determine its position and to detect the presence of any masses. The trachea is normally in the midline of the neck. It is difficult to palpate in children less than 3 years of age because of their short necks. To palpate the trachea, place the thumb and forefinger on each side of the

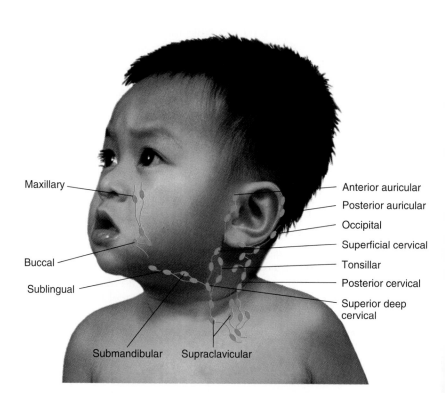

FIGURE 3–27. The neck is palpated for enlarged lymph nodes around the ears, under the jaw, in the occipital area, and in the cervical chain of the neck.

Maxillary

Buccal

Sublingual

Submandibular   Supraclavicular

Anterior auricular

Posterior auricular

Occipital

Superficial cervical

Tonsillar

Posterior cervical

Superior deep cervical

trachea near the chin and slowly slide them down the trachea. Any shift to the right or left of midline may indicate a tumor or a collapsed lung.

Thyroid

As the fingers slide over the trachea in the lower neck, attempt to feel the isthmus of the thyroid, a band of glandular tissue crossing over the trachea. The lobes of the thyroid wrap behind the trachea and are normally covered by the sternocleidomastoid muscle. Because of the anatomic position of the thyroid, the lobes of the thyroid are not usually palpable in the child unless they are enlarged.

RANGE OF MOTION ASSESSMENT

To test the neck's **range of motion,** ask the child to touch the chin to each shoulder and to the chest and then to look at the ceiling. Move a light or toy in all four directions when assessing infants. Children should freely move the neck and head in all four directions without pain.

When the child is unable to move the head voluntarily in all directions, passively move the child's neck through the expected range of motion. Limited horizontal range of motion may be a sign of *torticollis,* persistent head tilting. Torticollis results from a birth injury to the sternocleidomastoid muscle or from unilateral vision or hearing impairment. Pain with flexion of the neck toward the chest (Brudzinski sign) may indicate meningitis.

► ASSESSING THE CHEST FOR SHAPE, MOVEMENT, RESPIRATORY EFFORT, AND LUNG FUNCTION

What terms are used to describe the location of specific sounds heard when auscultating the chest? What does it mean when a child's chest is rounded in shape? What are retractions and what do they indicate? How can normal and adventitious breath sounds be distinguished when auscultating the lungs?

Examination of the chest includes the following procedures: inspecting the size and shape of the chest, palpating chest movement that occurs during respiration, observing the effort of breathing, and auscultating breath sounds.

TOPOGRAPHIC LANDMARKS OF THE CHEST

The chest skeleton provides most of the landmarks used to describe the location of findings during examination of the chest, lungs, and heart. The intercostal spaces are the horizontal markers used to describe the location of a finding on the chest. The sternum and spine are the vertical landmarks. When both a horizontal and a vertical landmark are used, the location of findings can be precisely described (Figs. 3–28 and 3–29). Be sure to indicate whether the finding is on the right or left side of the patient's chest (Table 3–13).

INSPECTION OF THE CHEST

Position the child on the parent's lap or on the examining table with all clothing above the waist removed to inspect the chest. The thoracic muscles

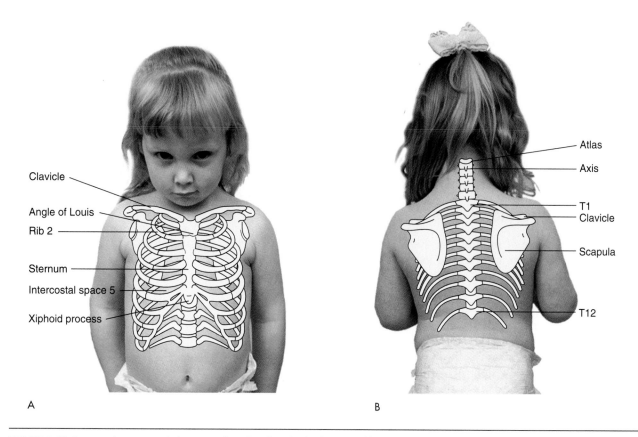

Clavicle

Angle of Louis

Rib 2

Sternum

Intercostal space 5

Xiphoid process

A

Atlas

Axis

T1
Clavicle

Scapula

T12

B

FIGURE 3–28. Intercostal spaces and ribs are numbered to describe the location of findings. **A,** To determine the rib number on the anterior chest, palpate down from the top of the sternum until a horizontal ridge, the Angle of Louis, is felt. Directly to the right and left of that ridge is the second rib. The second intercostal space is immediately below the second rib. Ribs 3–12 and the corresponding intercostal spaces can be counted as the fingers move toward the abdomen. **B,** To determine the rib number on the posterior chest, find the protruding spinal process of the seventh cervical vertebra at the shoulder level. The next spinal process belongs to the first thoracic vertebra, which attaches to the first rib.

and subcutaneous tissue are less developed in children than in adults, so the chest wall is thinner. As a result the rib cage is more prominent.

Size and Shape of the Chest

Inspect the chest for any irregularities in shape. A rounded chest is present when the anteroposterior diameter is approximately equal to the lateral di-

3-13	Vertical Landmarks of the Chest
Vertical Lines for Examining the Chest	**Location of Vertical Lines**
Midsternal	Through the middle of the sternum
Midclavicular	From the middle of the clavicle
Anterior axillary	From the anterior axillary fold
Midaxillary	From the middle of the axilla
Posterior axillary	From the posterior axillary fold
Spinal	Through the spinous processes of the vertebrae

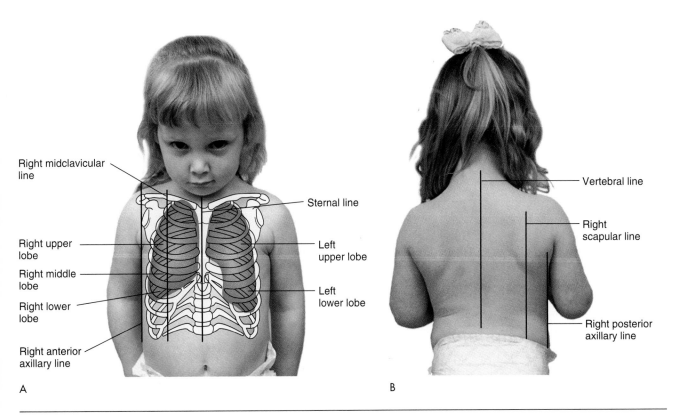

FIGURE 3–29. The sternum and spine are the vertical landmarks used to describe the anatomic location of findings. The distance between the finding and the center of the sternum (midsternal line) or the spinal line can be measured with a ruler. Imaginary vertical lines, parallel to the midsternal and spinal lines, are used to further describe the location of findings.

ameter. If a rounded chest is found in a child over 2 years of age, a chronic obstructive lung condition such as asthma or cystic fibrosis may be present.

An abnormal chest shape results from two different structural deformities (Fig. 3–30). If the sternum protrudes, increasing the anteroposterior diameter, pigeon chest (pectus carinatum) may be present. If the lower portion of the sternum is depressed, decreasing the anteroposterior diameter, funnel chest (pectus excavatum) may be present. *Scoliosis,* curvature of the spine, causes a lateral deviation of the chest. See Chapter 19.

Chest Movement and Respiratory Effort

Inspect for simultaneous chest expansion and abdominal rise. Chest movement is normally symmetric bilaterally, rising with inspiration and falling with expiration. The chest movement of infants and young children is less pronounced than the abdominal movement. The diaphragm is the primary breathing muscle in infants and children under 6 years old. The thoracic muscles are less developed and serve as accessory muscles in cases of respiratory distress. As the thoracic muscles develop, they become primarily responsible for ventilation. On inspiration the chest and abdomen should rise simultaneously. Asymmetric chest rise is associated with a collapsed lung. Retractions, depression of sections of the chest wall with each inspiration, are seen when the accessory muscles are used for breathing in cases of respiratory distress.

Respiratory Rate

Because young children use the diaphragm as the primary breathing muscle, observe or feel the rise and fall of the abdomen to count the respira-

GROWTH & DEVELOPMENT CONSIDERATIONS

In infants the chest is rounded with the anteroposterior diameter approximately equal to the lateral diameter. The chest becomes more oval with growth and by 2 years of age the lateral diameter is greater than the anteroposterior diameter.

GROWTH & DEVELOPMENT CONSIDERATIONS

Infants and children have a faster respiratory rate than adults because of a higher metabolic rate and need for oxygen. Young children are also unable to increase the depth of respirations because not all the alveoli are developed.[7]

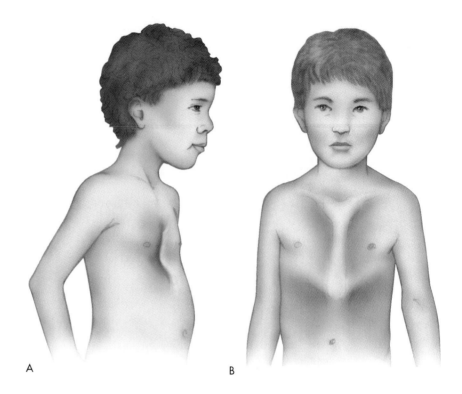

FIGURE 3–30. Two types of abnormal chest shape. **A,** Funnel chest. **B,** Pigeon chest.

A   B

tory rate in children under age 6 years. Table 3–14 gives the normal respiratory rates for each age group. Make every effort to count the respiratory rate when the child is quiet. The respiratory rate rises in response to excitement, fear, respiratory distress, fever, and other conditions that increase oxygen needs.

A sustained respiratory rate greater than 60 breaths per minute is an important sign in respiratory distress. At that rate, children develop hypoxemia if treatment is not started. The child's airway is very narrow, resulting in higher airway resistance than occurs in adults. When the respiratory rate exceeds 60 breaths per minute, inspired oxygen does not reach the alveoli for gas exchange because air moves no farther than the upper airway.[8]

PALPATION OF THE CHEST

Palpation is used to evaluate chest movement, respiratory effort, deformities of the chest wall, and tactile fremitus.

Chest Wall

To palpate the chest motion with respiration, place the palms of your hands with fingers spread on each side of the child's chest. Confirm the bilateral symmetry of chest motion. Use your fingerpads to palpate any depressions, bulges, or unusual chest wall shape that might indicate abnormal findings such as tenderness, cysts, other growths, crepitus, or fractures. None should be found. *Crepitus,* a crinkly sensation palpated on the chest surface, is caused by air escaping into the subcutaneous tissues. It often indicates a serious injury to the upper or lower airway. Crepitus may also be felt near a fracture.

Tactile Fremitus

Crying and talking produce vibrations, known as *tactile fremitus,* that can be palpated on the chest. Place the palms of your hands on each side of the

---

CLINICAL TIP

To get the most accurate reading of a newborn's respiratory rate, wait until the baby is sleeping or resting quietly. Use the stethoscope to auscultate the rate or place your hand on the abdomen. Count the number of breaths for an entire minute, because newborns often have irregular respirations.

3-14	Normal Respiratory Rate Ranges for Each Age Group	
Age	**Respiratory Rate per Minute**	
Newborn	30–80	
1 year	20–40	
3 years	20–30	
6 years	16–22	
10 years	16–20	
17 years	12–20	

chest to evaluate the quality and distribution of these vibrations. Ask the child to repeat a series of words or numbers, such as Mickey Mouse or ice cream. As the child repeats the words, move your hands systematically over the anterior and posterior chest, comparing the quality of findings side to side. The vibration or tingling sensation is normally palpated over the entire chest. Decreased sensations indicate that air is trapped in the lungs, as occurs with asthma. Increased sensations indicate lung consolidation, as occurs with pneumonia.

AUSCULTATION OF THE CHEST

Auscultate the chest with a stethoscope to assess the quality and characteristics of breath sounds, to identify abnormal breath sounds, and to evaluate vocal resonance. Use an infant or pediatric stethoscope when available to help you localize any unexpected breath sounds. Use the stethoscope diaphragm because it transmits the high-pitched breath sounds better.

Breath Sounds

Evaluate the quality and characteristics of breath sounds over the entire chest, comparing sounds between the sides. Select a routine sequence for auscultating the entire chest so you will consistently assess all lobes of the lungs. Figure 3–31 shows one suggested chest auscultation sequence. Listen to an entire inspiratory and expiratory phase at each spot on the chest before you move to the next site.

    Three types of normal breath sounds are usually heard when the chest is auscultated. *Vesicular* breath sounds are low-pitched, swishing, soft, short

CLINICAL TIP

Auscultation of breath sounds is difficult when an infant is crying. First, try to quiet the infant with a pacifier, bottle, or toy. If the infant continues to cry, all is not lost. At the end of each cry the infant takes a deep breath, which you can use to assess breath sounds, vocal resonance, and tactile fremitus. Encourage toddlers and preschoolers to take deep breaths by providing a pinwheel or mobile to blow.

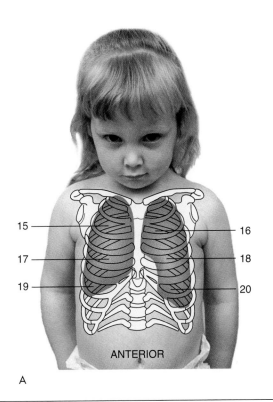

ANTERIOR

A

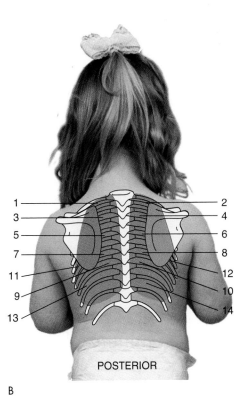

POSTERIOR

B

FIGURE 3–31. One example of a sequence for auscultation of the chest.

GROWTH & DEVELOPMENT CONSIDERATIONS

Infants and young children have a thin chest wall because of immature muscle development. The breath sounds of one lung are heard over the entire chest. It takes practice to accurately identify absent or diminished breath sounds in infants and young children. Because the distance between the lungs is greatest at the apices and midaxillary areas in young children, these sites are best for identifying absent or diminished breath sounds. Carefully auscultate, comparing the quality of breath sounds heard bilaterally.

CLINICAL TIP

When trying to get the child to breathe normally while auscultating the chest, use suggestive language to increase cooperation. "You certainly are good at breathing slowly. Have you been practicing?" The child will often deepen and slow the breathing pattern as you give praise and draw attention to it.

expiratory sounds. They are usually heard in older children but not in infants and young children. *Bronchovesicular* breath sounds are medium-pitched, hollow, blowing sounds heard equally on inspiration and expiration in all age groups. The location of these sounds on the chest is related to the child's age. *Bronchial/tracheal* breath sounds are hollow and higher pitched than vesicular breath sounds.

Breath sounds normally have equal intensity, pitch, and rhythm bilaterally. Absent or diminished breath sounds generally indicate a partial or total obstruction, such as from a foreign body or mucus, that does not permit airflow.

Vocal Resonance

Auscultate the chest to evaluate how well voice sounds are transmitted. Have the child repeat a series of words, either the same as or different from those used for evaluating tactile fremitus. Use the stethoscope to auscultate the chest, comparing the quality of sounds from side to side and over the entire chest. Voice sounds, with words and syllables muffled and indistinct, are normally heard throughout the chest.

If voice sounds are absent or more muffled than usual, an airway obstruction condition such as asthma may be present. When a lung consolidation condition such as pneumonia is present, the vocal resonance quality changes in characteristic ways. These abnormal characteristics are called whispered pectoriloquy, bronchophony, and egophony. *Whispered pectoriloquy* is present when syllables are heard distinctly in a whisper. *Bronchophony* is the increased intensity and clarity of sounds while the words remain indistinct. *Egophony* is the transmission of the "eee" sound as a nasal "ay" sound.

Abnormal Breath Sounds

Abnormal breath sounds, also called adventitious sounds, generally indicate the presence of a disease process. Examples of abnormal breath sounds are crackles, rhonchi, and friction rubs. To further assess abnormal breath sounds, the examiner determines their location, the respiratory phase in which they are present, and whether they change or disappear when the child coughs or shifts position. To routinely identify these adventitious sounds takes practice. Table 3–15 describes adventitious sounds.

Abnormal Voice Sounds

Observing the quality of the voice and other audible sounds is also important during an examination of the lungs. Examples of these sounds are hoarseness, stridor, and cough. Stridor is a noise resulting from air moving through a narrowed trachea and larynx; it is associated with croup. *Wheezing* is a noise resulting from the passage of air through mucus or fluids in a narrowed lower airway; it is associated with asthma. A *cough* is a reflexive clearing of the airway associated with a respiratory infection. *Hoarseness* is associated with inflammation of the larynx.

PERCUSSION OF THE CHEST

Percussion is a method sometimes used to assess the resonance of the lungs and the density of underlying organs, such as the heart and liver. Today there is less reliance on percussion to evaluate the lungs because of the frequent use of x-ray examination.

3-15	Description of Selected Adventitious Sounds and Their Cause	
Type	Description	Cause
Fine crackles	High-pitched, discrete, noncontinuous sound heard at end of inspiration (Rub pieces of hair together beside your ear to duplicate the sound.)	Air passing through watery secretions in the smaller airways (alveoli and bronchioles)
Sibilant rhonchi	Musical, squeaking, or hissing noise heard during inspiration or expiration, but generally louder on expiration	Bronchospasm or an anatomic narrowing of the trachea, bronchi, or bronchioles
Sonorous rhonchi	Coarse, low-pitched sound like a snore, heard during inspiration or expiration; may clear with coughing	Air passing through thick secretions that partially obstruct the larger bronchi and trachea

When percussing the anterior and posterior chest, choose a sequence that covers the entire chest and permits comparison bilaterally. The same sequence as that used for auscultation is effective. To perform *indirect percussion,* lay the middle finger of your nondominant hand on the child's chest at an intercostal space. Keep the other fingers off the chest. With a springlike motion, use the fingertip of your other hand to tap the finger in contact with the chest (Fig. 3–32A). *Direct percussion* is a technique effective for infants. Tap the chest at an intercostal space with a fingertip to elicit the quality of resonance (Fig. 3–32B).

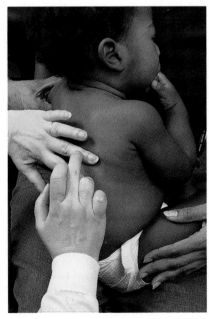
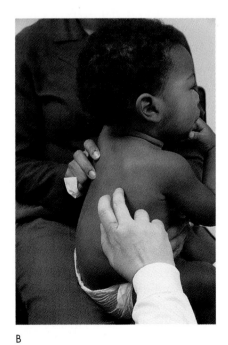

A   B

FIGURE 3–32. A, Indirect percussion. Place the middle finger on the child's chest at an intercostal space with the other fingers off of the chest. Tap the finger with a springlike motion with the fingertip of the other hand. B, Direct percussion. Tap the infant's chest with the fingertip directly at an intercostal space.

FIGURE 3–33. Normal resonance patterns expected over the chest. *Tympany* is a loud, high-pitched sound, like a drum. It is usually heard over an air-filled stomach. *Flatness* is a soft, dull sound, like the sound made when percussing your thigh. It is heard over dense muscles and bone. *Dullness* is a moderately loud, thudlike sound. It is heard when percussing over the liver and heart, and at the base of the lungs (at the level of the diaphragm). *Resonance* is a loud, low-pitched, hollow sound, like the sound made when percussing a table. It is heard over the lungs. *Hyperresonance* is a loud, very low-pitched, booming sound. It is usually heard over superinflated lungs. However, because of the thin chest wall in young children, hyperresonance may be a normal finding.

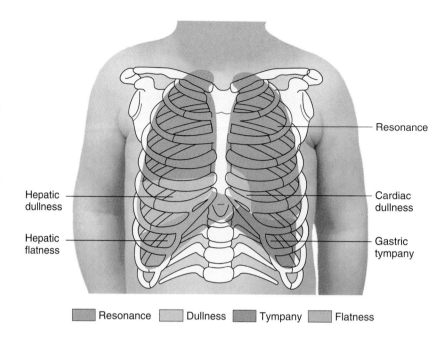

Characteristic patterns of percussion resonance are expected (Fig. 3–33). Characteristic descriptions of sounds heard with percussion of the chest include tympany, flatness, dullness, resonance, and hyperresonance.

► ASSESSING THE BREASTS FOR DEVELOPMENT AND MASSES

What is the first stage of breast development in girls? Do boys have breast development during puberty? What does breast tissue feel like?

INSPECTION OF THE BREASTS

Stages of Development

Inspect the breasts for stage of development. Breast development in girls precedes other pubertal changes. Breast budding, the first stage of pubertal development in girls, normally occurs between 10 and 14 years of age. Breast development before 8 years of age is abnormal. Figure 3–34 shows normal breast development. A girl's breasts may develop at different rates and appear asymmetric. Boys often have unilateral or bilateral breast enlargement during adolescence. This enlargement can occur as breast buds or actual breast tissue (gynecomastia). It generally disappears without treatment, usually within a year.

Nipples

The nipples of prepubertal boys and girls are symmetrically located near the midclavicular line at the fourth to sixth ribs. The areola is normally round and more darkly pigmented than the surrounding skin. Inspect the anterior chest for other dark spots that may be *supernumerary nipples*, which are small, undeveloped nipples and areola that may be mistaken for

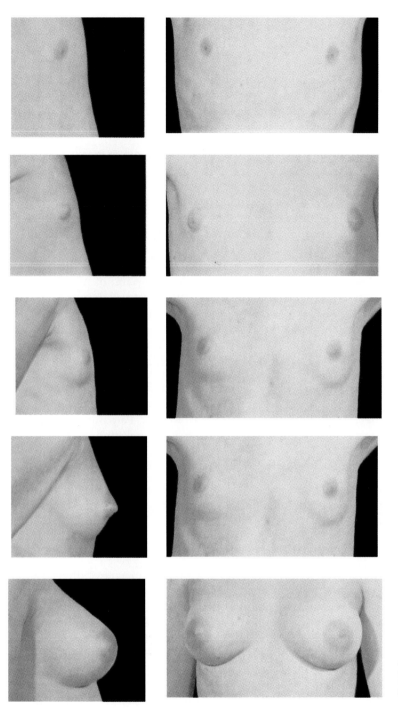

FIGURE 3–34. Normal stages of breast development.

moles. Their presence may be associated with congenital renal or cardiac anomalies.

PALPATION OF THE BREASTS

The developing breasts of adolescent females are palpated for abnormal masses or hard nodules. Breast tissue normally feels dense, firm, and elastic.

► ASSESSING THE HEART FOR HEART SOUNDS AND FUNCTION

What is the point of maximum intensity and where is it located? Where are the pulse points to assess pulse quality? What heart sounds are associated with systole and diastole? What is the normal heart rate of infants and children? What is the difference between heart sounds and murmurs?

INSPECTION OF THE PRECORDIUM

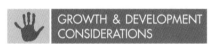
EQUIPMENT NEEDED

Stethoscope
Sphygmomanometer

Begin the heart examination by inspecting the *precordium,* or anterior chest. Place the child in a reclining or semi-Fowler's position, either on the parent's lap or on the examining table. Inspect the shape and symmetry of the anterior chest from the front and side views. The rib cage is normally symmetric. Bulging of the left side of the chest wall may indicate an enlarged heart.

Observe for any chest movement associated with the heart's contraction. The *apical impulse,* sometimes called the point of maximum intensity, is located where the left ventricle taps the chest wall during contraction. The apical impulse can normally be seen in thin children. A *heave,* an obvious lifting of the chest wall during contraction, may indicate an enlarged heart.

PALPATION OF THE PRECORDIUM

Place the entire palmar surface of the fingers together on the chest wall to palpate the precordium. Systematically palpate the entire precordium to detect any pulsations, heaves, or vibrations. Palpating with minimal pressure increases the chance of detecting abnormal findings.

GROWTH & DEVELOPMENT CONSIDERATIONS

The location of the apical impulse changes as the child's rib cage grows. In children under 7 years old, it is located in the fourth intercostal space just lateral to the left midclavicular line. In children over 7 years old, it is located in the fifth intercostal space at the left midclavicular line.

Apical Impulse

The apical impulse is normally felt as a slight tap against one fingertip. Use the topographic landmarks of the chest to describe its location (see Figs. 3–28 and 3–29). Any other sensation palpated is usually abnormal.

Abnormal Sensations

A *lift* is the sensation of the heart lifting up against the chest wall. It may be associated with an enlarged heart or a heart contracting with extra force. A *thrill* is a rushing vibration that feels like a cat's purr. It is caused by turbulent blood flow from a defective heart valve and a heart murmur. If present, the thrill is palpated in the right or left second intercostal space. To describe a thrill's location, use the topographic landmarks of the chest (see Figs. 3–28 and 3–29) and estimate the diameter of the thrill palpated.

PERCUSSION OF THE HEART BORDERS

Percussion of the heart borders is rarely performed during physical examination. The borders of the heart are better identified by x-ray examination. Percussion of the heart should be performed only by an experienced examiner.

AUSCULTATION OF THE HEART

Auscultation is used to count the apical pulse, to assess the characteristics of the heart sounds, and to detect abnormal heart sounds. Use the bell of the stethoscope to detect these higher pitched sounds.

To assess heart sounds completely, auscultate the heart with the child in both sitting and reclining positions. Differences in heart sounds caused by a change in the child's position or by a change in the position of the heart near the chest wall can then be detected. If differences in heart sounds are detected with a position change, place the child in the left lateral recumbent position and auscultate again.

Heart Rate and Rhythm

The apical heart rate can be counted at the site of the apical impulse, either by palpation or by auscultation. Count the apical rate for 1 minute in infants and in children who have an irregular rhythm. The brachial or radial pulse rate should be the same as the auscultated apical heart rate. Table 3–16 gives normal heart rates in children of different ages.

Listen carefully to the heart rate rhythm. Children often have a normal cycle of irregular rhythm associated with respiration called *sinus arrhythmia.* With sinus arrhythmia the child's heart rate is faster on inspiration and slower on expiration. When any rhythm irregularity is detected, ask the child to take a breath and hold it while you listen to the heart rate. The rhythm should become regular during inspiration and expiration. Other rhythm irregularities are abnormal.

Differentiation of Heart Sounds

Heart sounds are due to the closure of the valves and vibration or turbulence of blood produced by that valve closure. Two primary sounds, S_1 and S_2, are heard when the chest is auscultated.

S_1, the first heart sound, is produced by closure of the tricuspid and mitral valves when the ventricular contraction begins. The two valves close almost simultaneously, so only one sound is normally heard.

S_2, the second heart sound, is produced by the closure of the aortic and pulmonic valves. Once blood has reached the pulmonic and aortic arteries, the valves close to prevent leakage back into the ventricles during diastole. The timing of the valve closure varies with respirations. Sometimes S_2 is heard as a single sound and at other times as a *split sound,* that is, two sounds heard a fraction of a second apart.

Sound is easily transmitted in liquid, and it travels best in the direction of blood flow. Auscultate heart sounds at specific areas on the chest wall in the direction of blood flow, just beyond the valve (Fig. 3–35). The sounds produced by the heart valves or blood turbulence are heard throughout the chest in thin infants and children. Both S_1 and S_2 can be heard in all listening areas.

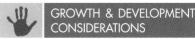

GROWTH & DEVELOPMENT CONSIDERATIONS

The child's heart rate varies with age, decreasing as the child grows older. The heart rate also increases in response to exercise, excitement, anxiety, and fever. Such stresses increase the child's metabolic rate, creating a simultaneous need for more oxygen. Children respond to the need for more oxygen by increasing their heart rate, a response called *sinus tachycardia.* They cannot increase their cardiac stroke volume to deliver more oxygen to the tissues as adults do.

3-16	Normal Heart Rates for Children of Different Ages	
Age	**Heart Rate Range (beats/min)**	**Average Heart Rate (beats/min)**
Newborns	100–170	120
Infants to 2 years	80–130	110
2–6 years	70–120	100
6–10 years	70–110	90
10–16 years	60–100	85

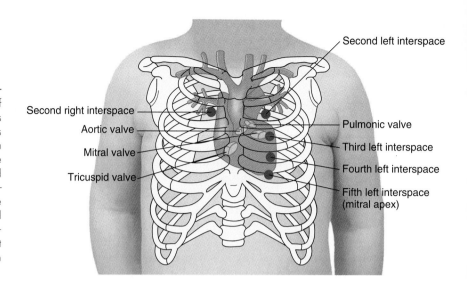

FIGURE 3–35. Sound travels in the direction of blood flow. Rather than listen for heart sounds over each heart valve, auscultate heart sounds at specific areas on the chest wall away from the valve itself. These areas are named for the valve producing the sound. *Aortic:* Second right intercostal space near the sternum. *Pulmonic:* Second left intercostal space near the sternum. *Tricuspid:* Fifth right or left intercostal space near the sternum. *Mitral (apical):* In infants—third or fourth intercostal space, just left of the left midclavicular line. In children—fifth intercostal space at the left midclavicular line.

CLINICAL TIP

Palpate the carotid pulse when auscultating the heart to distinguish between the two heart sounds. The heart sound heard simultaneously with the pulsation is S_1.

Auscultate heart sounds for quality (distinct versus muffled) and intensity (loud versus weak). First, distinguish between S_1 and S_2 in each listening area. Heart sounds are usually distinct and crisp in children because of their thin chest wall. Muffling or indistinct sounds may indicate a heart defect or congestive heart failure. Document the area where heart sounds are heard the best. Table 3–17 and Figure 3–35 review the location where each sound is normally best heard for assessment of quality and intensity.

Splitting of the Heart Sounds

After the first and second heart sounds are successfully distinguished, try to detect *physiologic splitting*. The split second heart sound is more apparent during inspiration when the child takes a deep breath. More blood returns to the right ventricle, causing the pulmonic valve to close a fraction of a second later than the aortic valve. To detect physiologic splitting, auscultate over the pulmonic area while the child breathes normally and then while the child takes a deep breath. Splitting is normally more easily detected after a deep breath. The splitting returns to a single

3-17	Identification of the Listening Sites for Auscultation of the Quality and Intensity of Heart Sounds	
Heart Sound	**Locations Best Heard**	**Where Heard Softly**
S_1	Apex of the heart Tricuspid area Mitral area	Base of the heart Aortic area Pulmonic area
S_2	Base of the heart Aortic area Pulmonic area	Apex of the heart Tricuspid area Mitral area
Physiologic splitting	Pulmonic area	
S_3	Mitral area	

sound with regular breathing. If splitting does not vary with respiration, it is called fixed splitting. This is an abnormal finding associated with an atrial septal defect.

Third Heart Sound

A third heart sound, S_3, is occasionally heard in children as a normal finding. S_3 is caused when blood rushes through the mitral valve and splashes into the left ventricle. It is heard in diastole, just after S_2. It is distinguished from a split S_2 because it is louder in the mitral area than in the pulmonic area.

Murmurs

Occasionally abnormal heart sounds are auscultated. These sounds are produced by blood passing through a defective valve, great vessel, or other heart structure.

To hear murmurs in children takes practice. Often murmurs must be very loud to be detected. For softer murmurs, normal heart sounds must be distinguished before an extra sound is recognized. Once a murmur is detected, define the characteristics of the extra sound.

Murmurs are classified by the following characteristics:

- *Intensity.* How loud is it? Can a thrill also be palpated?
- *Location.* Where is the murmur the loudest? Identify the listening area and precise topographic landmarks. Is the child sitting or lying down?
- *Radiation.* Is the sound transmitted over a larger area of the chest, to the axilla, or to the back?
- *Timing.* Is the murmur heard best after S_1 or S_2? Is it heard during the entire phase between S_1 and S_2?
- *Quality.* Describe what the murmur sounds like, for example, machine-like, musical, or blowing.

COMPLETING THE HEART EXAMINATION

A complete assessment of cardiac function also includes measuring the blood pressure, palpating the pulses, and evaluating signs from other systems.

Blood Pressure

Assessment of blood pressure is important to detect conditions of hypertension or hypovolemic shock. The technique for obtaining the blood pressure in children can be found in the *Quick Reference to Pediatric Clinical Skills* accompanying this text. Table 3–18 gives average blood pressure readings of children at different ages.

Palpation of the Pulses

Palpate the characteristics of the pulses in the extremities to assess the circulation. The technique and sites for palpating the pulse are the same as those used for adults (Fig. 3–36). Evaluate the pulsation for rate, regularity of rhythm, and strength in each extremity and compare your findings bilaterally. The femoral and brachial pulses are the most important pulses to evaluate.

GUIDELINES FOR GRADING THE INTENSITY OF A MURMUR	
Intensity	*Description*
Grade I	Barely heard in a quiet room
Grade II	Quiet, but clearly heard
Grade III	Moderately loud, no thrill palpated
Grade IV	Loud, a thrill is usually palpated
Grade V	Very loud, a thrill is easily palpated
Grade VI	Heard without the stethoscope in direct contact with the chest wall

GROWTH & DEVELOPMENT CONSIDERATIONS

Infants have a low systolic blood pressure, and detecting the distal pulses is often difficult. Use the brachial artery in the arms and the popliteal or femoral artery in the legs to evaluate the pulses. The radial and distal tibial pulses are normally palpated easily in older children.

Palpate the femoral arteries and compare their strength with the strength of the brachial pulse. The femoral pulsations are usually stronger than or as strong as the brachial pulsations. A weaker femoral pulse is associated with coarctation of the aorta.

Other Signs

To assess the heart and tissue perfusion, other signs should be considered. These signs include skin color, capillary refill, and respiratory distress. The mucous membranes are usually pink. Cyanosis is most commonly associated with a congenital heart defect in children. Capillary refill is normally less than 2 seconds, indicating good circulation and perfusion of the tissues. Signs of respiratory distress, such as tachypnea, flaring, and retractions, may be associated with the child's attempts to compensate for hypoxemia caused by a congenital heart defect.

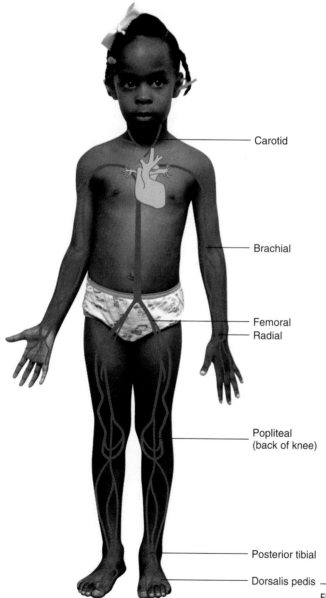

Carotid

Brachial

Femoral
Radial

Popliteal
(back of knee)

Posterior tibial

Dorsalis pedis

A

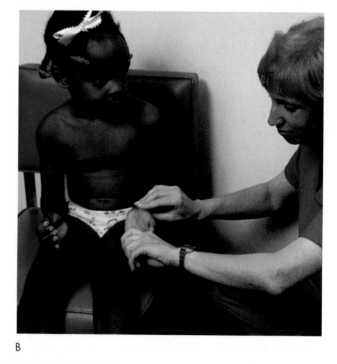

B

FIGURE 3–36. A, The sites used to assess pulses in children. B, Place your fingerpads firmly over each pulse point to evaluate the pulsation.

3-18	Median Systolic and Diastolic Blood Pressure Values for Children of Different Ages	
Age	Systolic (mm Hg) 50th Percentile Readings	Diastolic (mm Hg) 50th Percentile Readings
Newborn	73	55
1 month	86	52
6 months	90	53
1 year	90	56
3 years	92	55
6 years	96	57
9 years	100	61
12 years	107	64
15 years	114	65
18 years	121	70

Adapted from the Normal Blood Pressure Readings for Boys from the Second Task Force on Blood Pressure Control in Children, National Heart, Lung, and Blood Institute, Bethesda, MD, 1987. Normal blood pressure readings for girls are very similar to those for boys at all age groups.

► ASSESSING THE ABDOMEN FOR SHAPE, BOWEL SOUNDS, AND UNDERLYING ORGANS

What does a sunken abdomen indicate? What do bowel sounds normally sound like? How frequently should bowel sounds be heard in children? What do the various percussion tones indicate? What does a rigid abdomen indicate?

TOPOGRAPHIC LANDMARKS OF THE ABDOMEN

The location of underlying organs and structures of the abdomen must be considered when the abdomen is examined. The abdomen is commonly divided by imaginary lines into quadrants for the purpose of identifying underlying structures (Fig. 3–37).

INSPECTION OF THE ABDOMEN

Begin the examination of the abdomen by inspecting the shape and contour, condition of the umbilicus and rectus muscle, and abdominal movement. Inspect the child's abdomen from the front and side with good lighting.

Shape

Inspect the shape of the abdomen to identify an abnormal contour. The child's abdomen is normally symmetric and rounded or flat when the child is supine. A scaphoid or sunken abdomen is abnormal and may indicate dehydration.

EQUIPMENT NEEDED

Stethoscope

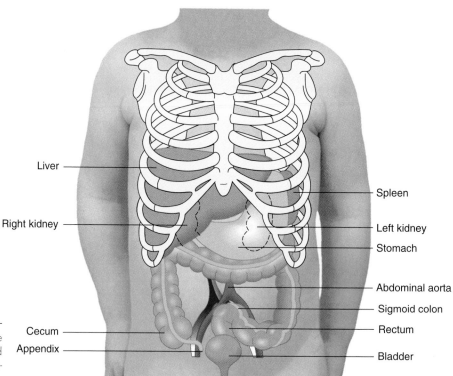

Liver
Spleen
Right kidney
Left kidney
Stomach
Abdominal aorta
Sigmoid colon
Cecum
Rectum
Appendix
Bladder

FIGURE 3–37. Topographic landmarks of the abdomen. The abdomen is commonly divided by imaginary lines into quadrants for the purposes of identifying underlying structures.

Umbilicus

Observe the newborn's umbilical stump for color, bleeding, odor, and drainage. The stump becomes black, dry, and hard within a couple of days after birth. It normally falls off between 7 and 14 days after birth. After the stump falls off, inspect the umbilicus for complete healing. Continued drainage may indicate an infection or a granuloma.

Inspect the umbilicus in older infants and toddlers. Children in these age groups often have an umbilical hernia, a protrusion of abdominal contents through an open umbilical muscle ring.

Rectus Muscle

Inspect the abdominal wall for any depression or bulging at midline above or below the umbilicus, indicating separation of the rectus abdominis muscles. The depression may be up to 5 cm (2 in.) wide. Measure the width of the separation to monitor change over time. As abdominal muscle strength develops, the separation usually becomes less prominent. However, the splitting may persist if congenital muscle weakness is present.

Abdominal Movement

Infants and children up to 6 years of age breathe with the diaphragm. The abdomen rises with inspiration and falls with expiration, simultaneously with the chest rise and fall. When the abdomen does not rise as expected, peritonitis may be present.

Other abdominal movements such as peristaltic waves are abnormal. *Peristaltic waves* are visible rhythmic contractions of the intestinal wall smooth muscle, which move food through the digestive tract. Their presence generally indicates an intestinal obstruction, such as pyloric stenosis.

AUSCULTATION OF THE ABDOMEN

To evaluate bowel sounds, auscultate the abdomen with the diaphragm of the stethoscope. Bowel sounds normally occur every 10–30 seconds. They have a high-pitched, tinkling, metallic quality. Loud gurgling *(borborygmi)* is heard when the child is hungry. Listen in each quadrant long enough to hear at least one bowel sound. Before determining that bowel sounds are absent, auscultate at least 5 minutes. Absence of bowel sounds may indicate peritonitis or a paralytic ileus. Hyperactive bowel sounds may indicate gastroenteritis or a bowel obstruction.

Next auscultate over the abdominal aorta and the renal arteries for a vascular hum or murmur. No murmur should be heard. A murmur may indicate a narrowed or defective artery.

PERCUSSION OF THE ABDOMEN

Use indirect percussion to evaluate borders and sizes of abdominal organs and masses. Percussion is performed with the child supine. Choose a sequence that permits you to systematically percuss the entire abdomen (Fig. 3–38).

Different tones are expected when the abdomen is percussed, depending on the underlying structures. Organ size can be identified by listening for a percussion tone change at the border of an organ. For example, when you percuss down the chest, the upper edge of the liver is usually detected by a tone change from resonant to dull near the fifth intercostal space at the right midclavicular line. The lower liver edge is usually detected 2–3 cm

CLINICAL TIP

Inspection and auscultation are performed before palpation and percussion because touching the abdomen may change the characteristics of bowel sounds.

CLINICAL TIP

Expected pattern of percussion tones over the abdomen: *Dullness* is found over organs such as the liver, spleen, and full bladder. *Tympany* is found over the stomach or the intestines when an obstruction is present. Tympany may be found over areas beyond the stomach in infants because of air swallowing. A *resonant tone* may be heard over other areas.

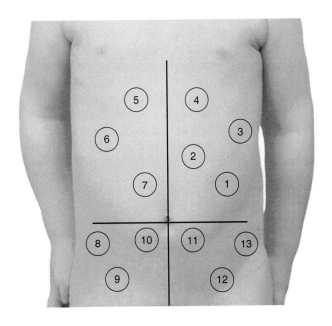

FIGURE 3–38. Sequence for indirect percussion of the abdomen.

(about 1 in.) below the right costal margin in infants and toddlers, but closer to the costal margin in older children.

PALPATION OF THE ABDOMEN

Both light and deep palpation are used to examine the abdomen's organs and to detect any masses. *Light palpation* is used to evaluate the tenseness of the abdomen (how soft or hard it is), the liver, the presence of any tenderness or masses, and any defects in the abdominal wall. *Deep palpation* is used to detect masses, define their shape and consistency, and identify tenderness in the abdomen.

To make the most accurate interpretation, perform the abdominal examination when the child is calm and cooperative. Organs and other masses are more easily palpated when the abdominal wall is relaxed. Infants and toddlers often feel more secure lying supine across both the parent's and the examiner's laps. A bottle, pacifier, or toy may distract the child and improve cooperation for the examination.

To begin palpation, position the child supine with knees flexed. Stand beside the child and place your warmed fingertips across the child's abdomen. Palpate with the edge of your fingers, not just your fingerpads, and palpate in a sequence to examine the entire abdomen. Watch the child's face as you palpate for a grimace or constriction of the pupils, which indicates the presence of pain.

Light Palpation

For light palpation, use a superficial, gentle touch that slightly depresses the abdomen. Usually the abdomen feels soft and no tenderness is detected. Palpate any bulging along the abdominal wall, especially along the rectus muscle and umbilical ring, which could indicate the presence of a hernia. Measure the diameter of the muscle ring, rather than the protrusion, to monitor change over time. The muscle ring normally becomes smaller and closes by 4 years of age. An umbilical hernia that persists beyond this age may need surgical repair.

Liver
Locate and lightly palpate the lower liver edge. Place the fingers in the right midclavicular line at the level of the umbilicus and gently move them toward the costal margin during expiration. As the liver edge descends with inspiration, a flat, narrow ridge is usually felt by your finger. Measure the distance of the liver edge from the right costal margin at the right midclavicular line. The liver edge is normally palpated 2–3 cm (1 in.) below the right costal margin in infants and toddlers. It may not be palpable in older children. The liver is enlarged when the edge is more than 3 cm (1 in.) below the right costal margin. An enlarged liver may be associated with congestive heart failure or hepatic disease.

Deep Palpation

To perform deep palpation, press the fingers of one hand (for small children) or two hands (for older children) more deeply into the abdomen. Because the abdominal muscles are most relaxed when the child takes a deep breath, ask the child to take regular deep breaths when each area of the abdomen is palpated.

CLINICAL TIP

Use suggestive words to help the child relax so you can palpate the abdomen. "How soft will your tummy get when my hand feels it? Does it get softer than this? Yes. See, it softens as you breathe out. Will it also be softer here?" In this way, the child learns to relax the abdomen and is challenged to do it better.

CLINICAL TIP

When children are ticklish, some special approaches are needed to gain their cooperation. Use a firm touch and do not pretend to tickle the child at any point in the examination. Alternatively, put the child's hand on the abdomen and place your hand over the child's. Let your fingertips slide over to touch the abdomen. The child has a sense of being in control, and you may be able to palpate directly.

CLINICAL TIP

Older children often need distraction, especially when there is a question of abdominal tenderness and guarding or when the child is ticklish. Have the child perform a task that requires some concentration, such as pressing the hands together or pulling locked hands apart.

Spleen

Palpate for the spleen at the left costal margin in the midclavicular line. The spleen tip may be felt when the child takes a deep breath. The spleen is enlarged when it can be easily palpated below the left costal margin.

Kidneys

Palpate for the kidneys deep in the abdomen along each side of the spinal column. The kidneys are difficult to palpate in all children, except newborns, because of the deep layer of abdominal muscles and intestines. If a kidney is actually palpated, an abnormal mass may be present.

Other Masses

Occasionally other masses, both normal and abnormal, can be palpated in the abdomen. A tubular mass commonly palpated in the lower left or right quadrant is often an intestine filled with feces. A distended bladder is often palpated as a firm, central, dome-shaped mass above the symphysis pubis in young children. Any fixed mass that moves laterally, pulsates, or is located along the vertebral column may be a neoplasm.

NURSING ALERT

If an enlarged kidney or mass is detected, do not continue to palpate the kidney. Pressure on the mass may release cancerous cells.

ASSESSMENT OF THE INGUINAL AREA

The inguinal area is inspected and palpated during the abdominal examination to detect enlarged lymph nodes or masses. The femoral pulse, a part of the heart examination, may be assessed simultaneously with the abdominal examination.

Inspection

Inspect the inguinal area for any change in contour, comparing sides. A small bulging noted over the femoral canal in girls may be associated with a femoral hernia. A bulging in the inguinal area in boys may be associated with an inguinal hernia.

Palpation

Palpate the inguinal area for lymph nodes and other masses. Small lymph nodes, less than 1 cm (½ in.) in diameter, are often present in the inguinal area because of minor injuries on the legs. Any tenderness, heat, or inflammation in these palpated lymph nodes could be associated with a local infection.

► ASSESSING THE GENITAL AND PERINEAL AREAS FOR PUBERTAL DEVELOPMENT AND EXTERNAL STRUCTURAL ABNORMALITIES

How is the stage of pubertal development determined in girls and boys? What can a vaginal discharge indicate in a preadolescent girl? Is swelling in a newborn's scrotum normal? Where is the proper location of the urethral meatus on the penis?

EQUIPMENT NEEDED

Gloves
Lubricant
Penlight

GROWTH & DEVELOPMENT CONSIDERATIONS

Preschool-age children are often taught that strangers are not permitted to touch their "private parts." When a child this age actively resists examination of the genital area, ask the parent to tell the child you have permission to look at and touch these parts of the body. Some children develop modesty during the preschool period. Briefly explain what you need to examine and why. Then calmly and efficiently examine the child.

PREPARATION OF CHILDREN FOR THE EXAMINATION

Examination of the genitalia and perineal area can cause stress in children because they sense their privacy has been invaded. To make young children feel more secure, position them on the parent's lap with their legs spread apart. Children can also be positioned on the examining table with their knees flexed and the legs spread apart like a frog.

In younger children the genital and perineal examination is performed immediately after assessment of the abdomen. The genitals and perineum may be examined last in older children and adolescents.

INSPECTION OF THE FEMALE GENITALIA

The external genitalia of girls are inspected for color, size, and symmetry of the mons pubis, labia, urethra, and vaginal opening (Fig. 3–39). The stage of pubertal maturation is also determined. Simultaneously look for any abnormal findings such as swelling, inflammation, masses, lacerations, or discharge.

Mons Pubis

Inspect the mons pubis for pubic hair. The presence, amount, and distribution of pubic hair indicates the sexual maturation stage in the girl. Preadolescent girls have no pubic hair. Initial pubic hair is lightly pigmented, sparse, and straight. Pubic hair develops in consistent stages for all girls, but the timing of pubic hair stages is individually determined.[9] Figure 3–40 illustrates the normal stages of female pubic hair development. Breast devel-

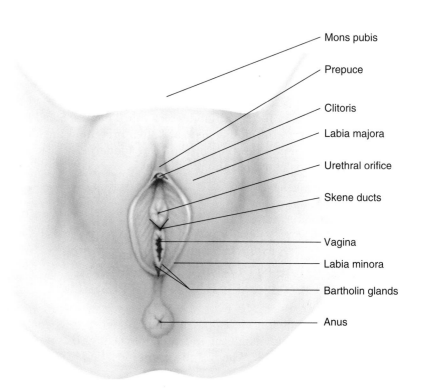

FIGURE 3–39. Anatomic structures of the female genital and perineal area.

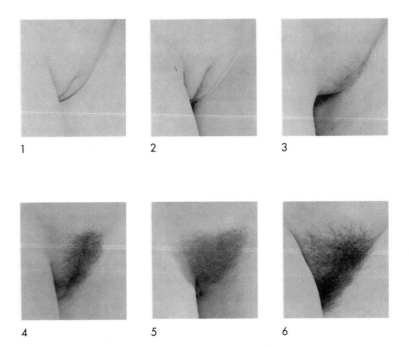

1   2   3

4   5   6

FIGURE 3–40. The stages of female public hair development with sexual maturation. Soft downy hair along the labia majora is an indication that sexual maturation is beginning. Hair grows progressively coarse an curly as development proceeds.
From Van Wieringen et al. (1971). Growth diagrams 1965 Nethelands. Groningen: Walters-Noardhof.

opment usually precedes pubic hair development. The presence of pubic hair before 8 years of age is unusual.

Labia

The labia minora are usually thin and pale in preadolescent girls but become dark pink and moist after puberty. In young infants the labia minora may be fused and cover the structures in the vestibule. These adhesions may need to be separated.

Hymen

Use the thumb and forefinger of one hand to separate the labia minora for viewing structures in the vestibule. The hymen is just inside the vaginal opening. In preadolescents it is usually a thin membrane with a crescent-shaped opening. The vaginal opening is usually about 1 cm (½ in.) in adolescents when the hymen is intact. Sexually active adolescents may have a vaginal opening with irregular edges.

Urethral and Vaginal Openings

Inspect the vestibule for lesions. No lesions or signs of inflammation are expected around the urethral or vaginal opening. Redness and excoriation are often associated with an irritant such as bubble bath.

Vaginal Discharge

Preadolescent girls do not normally have a vaginal discharge. Adolescents often have a clear discharge without a foul odor. Menses generally begin approximately 2 years after breast bud development. A foul-smelling discharge in preschool-age children may be associated with a foreign body. Various organisms may cause a vaginal infection in older children.

GROWTH & DEVELOPMENT CONSIDERATIONS

The newborn's external genital structures are strongly influenced by maternal hormones. The labia majora are swollen and the labia minora may be more prominent. The clitoris is relatively large. A white mucoid vaginal discharge can also be seen. As the hormonal influence decreases over a few weeks, these structures attain normal size.

NURSING ALERT

Signs of sexual abuse in young children include bruising or swelling of the vulva, foul-smelling vaginal discharge, enlarged opening of the vagina, and rash or sores in the perineal area.

An internal vaginal examination is indicated when abnormal findings such as a vaginal discharge or trauma to the external structures is noted. The vaginal examination of the child should be performed only by an experienced examiner.

PALPATION OF THE FEMALE GENITALIA

Palpate the vaginal opening with a finger of your free hand. The Bartholin and Skene glands are not usually palpable. Palpation of these glands in preadolescent children indicates enlargement because of an infection such as gonorrhea.

INSPECTION OF THE MALE GENITALIA

The male genitalia are inspected for the structural and pubertal development of the penis, scrotum, and testicles. Boys are placed in tailor position, seated with their legs crossed in front of them. This position puts pressure on the abdominal wall to push the testicles into the scrotum.

Penis

The penis is inspected for size, foreskin, hygiene, and position of the urethral meatus. The length of the nonerect penis in the newborn is normally 2–3 cm (1 in.). The penis enlarges in length and breadth during puberty. The penis is normally straight. A downward bowing of the penis may be caused by a *chordee*, a fibrous band of tissue associated with hypospadias.

When the penis is circumcised, the glans penis is exposed. To inspect the glans penis of an uncircumcised boy, ask the child or parent to pull the foreskin back. Alternatively, the examiner may retract the foreskin. The foreskin of children over 6 years of age normally retracts easily. If the foreskin is tight and cannot be retracted, phimosis is present.

The glans penis is normally clean and smooth without inflammation or ulceration. The urethral meatus is a slit-shaped opening near the tip of the glans. No discharge should be present. A round, pinpoint urethral meatus may indicate meatal stenosis. Location of the urethral meatus at another site on the penis is abnormal, indicating hypospadias or epispadias. Inspect the urinary stream. The stream is normally strong without dribbling.

Scrotum

Inspect the scrotum for size, symmetry, presence of the testicles, and any abnormalities. The scrotum is normally loose and pendulous with rugae, or wrinkles. The scrotum of infants often appears large in comparison to the penis. A small, undeveloped scrotum that has no rugae indicates that the testicles are undescended. Enlargement or swelling of the scrotum is abnormal. It may indicate an inguinal hernia, hydrocele, torsion of the spermatic cord, or testicular inflammation. A deep cleft in the scrotum may indicate ambiguous genitalia.

Pubic Hair

Inspect the presence, amount, and distribution of pubic hair. Straight, downy pubic hair first develops at the base of the penis. The hair becomes

GROWTH & DEVELOPMENT CONSIDERATIONS

The foreskin is usually not completely separated from the glans at birth. Separation is normally completed by 3–6 years of age. A foreskin opening large enough for a good urinary stream is normal, even when the foreskin does not fully retract.

SAFETY PRECAUTIONS

When the boy's foreskin does not easily retract, do not forcefully pull it back. Force may result in torn tissues that heal with adhesions between the foreskin and the glans.

GROWTH & DEVELOPMENT CONSIDERATIONS

The stage of pubertal maturation is determined by inspecting the amount of pubic hair, size of the penis, and development of the testicles and scrotum. Pubic hair usually appears after the scrotum and testicles start to grow but before the penis begins enlarging.[9]

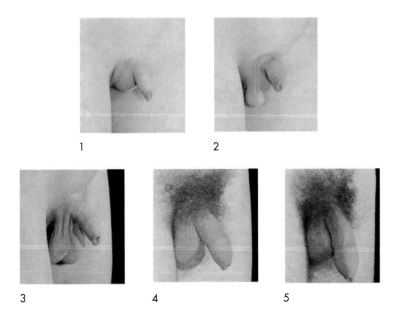

FIGURE 3-41. The stages of male pubic hair and external genital development with sexual maturation.
From Van Wieringen et al. (1971). Growth diagrams 1965 Netherlands. Groningen: Wolters-Noordhof.

darker, dense, and curly, extending over the pubic area in a diamond pattern by the completion of puberty. The presence of pubic hair before 9 years of age is uncommon. Stages of pubic hair development follow a standard pattern, as illustrated in Figure 3-41.

PALPATION OF THE MALE GENITALIA

Penis

Palpate the shaft of the penis for nodules and masses. None should be present.

Testicles

Palpate the scrotum for the presence of the testicles. Make sure your hands are warm to avoid stimulating the cremasteric reflex that causes the testicles to retract. Place your index finger and thumb over both inguinal canals on each side of the penis. This keeps the testicles from retracting into the abdomen (Fig. 3-42).

Gently palpate each testicle with only enough pressure to identify the shape and size. The testicles are normally smooth and equal in size. They are approximately 1–1.5 cm (½ in.) in diameter until puberty, when they increase in size. A hard, enlarged, painless testicle may indicate a tumor.

If a testicle is not palpated in the scrotum, the examiner palpates the inguinal canal for a soft mass. When the testicle is found in the inguinal canal, try to move it to the scrotum to palpate the size and shape. The testicle is descendable when it can be moved into the scrotum. An undescended testicle is one that does not descend into the scrotum or cannot be palpated in the inguinal canal.

Spermatic Cord

Palpate the length of the spermatic cord between the thumb and forefinger from the testicle to the inguinal canal. It normally feels solid and smooth. No tenderness is expected.

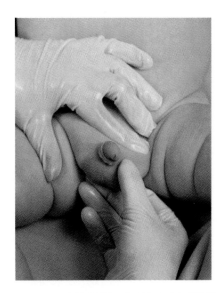

FIGURE 3-42. Palpating the scrotum for descended testicles and spermatic cords.

Enlarged Scrotum

When bulging or swelling of the scrotum is present, palpate the scrotum to identify the characteristics of the mass. Try to determine whether the mass is unilateral or bilateral and attempt to reduce the mass by pushing it back through the external inguinal ring. A mass that decreases may indicate an inguinal hernia. A mass that does not decrease may indicate a hydrocele or an incarcerated hernia.

Inguinal Canal

Attempt to insert your little finger into the external inguinal canal to determine whether the external inguinal ring is dilated. The inguinal ring is normally too small for the finger to pass into the canal. If the finger passes into the inguinal canal, ask the child to cough. A sensation of abdominal contents coming down to touch the fingertip may indicate an inguinal hernia.

Cremasteric Reflex

Stroke the inner thigh of each leg to stimulate the cremasteric reflex. The testicle and scrotum normally rise on the stroked side. This response indicates intact function of the spinal cord at the T12, L1, and L2 levels.

INSPECTION OF THE ANUS AND RECTUM

Inspect the anus for sphincter control and any abnormal findings such as inflammation, fissures, or lesions. The external sphincter is usually closed. Inflammation and scratch marks around the anus may be associated with pinworms. A protrusion from the rectum may be associated with a rectal wall prolapse or a hemorrhoid.

PALPATION OF THE ANUS AND RECTUM

Lightly touching the anal opening should stimulate an anal contraction or "wink." Absence of a contraction may indicate the presence of a lower spinal cord lesion.

Patency of the Anus

Passage of meconium by newborns indicates a patent anus. When passage of meconium is delayed, a lubricated catheter can be inserted 1 cm (½ in.) into the anus. Resistance in passage of the catheter may indicate an obstruction.

Rectal Examination

A rectal examination is not routinely performed on children. It is indicated for symptoms of intraabdominal, rectal, bowel, or stool abnormalities. The rectal examination should be performed only by an experienced examiner.

► ASSESSING THE MUSCULOSKELETAL SYSTEM FOR BONE AND JOINT STRUCTURE, MOVEMENT, AND MUSCLE STRENGTH

What do extra skin folds on an arm or leg indicate? What causes poor muscle tone? What condition does a rib hump indicate? At what age is it normal for children to be knock-kneed and bowlegged?

INSPECTION OF THE BONES, MUSCLES, AND JOINTS

Bones and Muscles

Inspect and compare the arms and then the legs for differences in alignment, contour, skin folds, length, and deformities. The extremities normally have equal length, circumference, and numbers of skin folds bilaterally. Extra skin folds and a larger circumference may indicate a shorter extremity.

Joints

Inspect and compare the joints bilaterally for size, discoloration, and ease of voluntary movement. Joints are normally the same color as surrounding skin, with no sign of swelling. Children should voluntarily flex and extend joints during normal activities without pain. Redness, swelling, and pain with movement may indicate injury or infection.

PALPATION OF THE BONES, MUSCLES, AND JOINTS

Bones and Muscles

Palpate the bones and muscles in each extremity for muscle tone, masses, or tenderness. Muscles normally feel firm, and bony masses are not normally present. Doughy muscles may indicate poor muscle tone. Rigid muscles, or *hypertonia,* may be associated with an active seizure or cerebral palsy. A mass over a long bone may indicate a recent fracture or a bone tumor.

GROWTH & DEVELOPMENT CONSIDERATIONS

Palpate the clavicles of the newborn from the sternum to the shoulder. These bones are often fractured during delivery. A mass and crepitus may indicate a fracture.

Joints

Palpate each joint and surrounding muscles to detect any swelling, masses, heat, or tenderness. None is expected when the joint is palpated. Tenderness, heat, swelling, and redness can result from injury or a chronic joint inflammation such as juvenile rheumatoid arthritis.

RANGE OF MOTION AND MUSCLE STRENGTH ASSESSMENT

Active Range of Motion

Observe the child during typical play activities, such as reaching for objects, climbing, and walking, to assess range of motion of all major joints. Children spontaneously move their joints through the full normal range of motion with play activities when no pain is present. Limited range of motion may indicate injury, inflammation of a joint, or a muscle abnormality.

Passive Range of Motion

When a joint is suspected of having limited active range of motion, perform passive range of motion. Flex and extend, abduct and adduct, or rotate the affected joint cautiously to avoid causing extra pain. Full range of motion without pain is normal. Limitations in movement may indicate injury, in-

GROWTH & DEVELOPMENT CONSIDERATIONS

Newborns typically have a limited extension of the hips, knees, and elbows, resulting from their flexed fetal position. When the newborn's arms and legs are extended and released, the extremities rapidly return to their flexed fetal position.

flammation, or malformation. Increased passive range of motion may indicate muscle weakness.

Muscle Strength

Observe the child's ability to climb onto an examining table, throw a ball, clap the hands, or move around on the bed. The child's ability to perform age-appropriate play activities indicates good muscle tone and strength. Attainment of age-appropriate motor development is another indicator of good muscle strength (Table 3–19).

To assess the strength of specific muscles in the extremities, engage the child in some games. Muscle strength is compared bilaterally to identify muscle weakness. For example, ask the child to squeeze your fingers tightly with each hand; push against and pull your hands with his or her hands, lower legs, and feet; and resist extension of a flexed elbow or knee. Children normally have good muscle strength bilaterally. Unilateral muscle weakness may be associated with a nerve injury. Bilateral muscle weakness may result from hypoxemia or a congenital disorder such as Down syndrome.

When generalized muscle weakness is suspected in a preschool- or school-age child, ask the child to stand up from the supine position. Children are normally able to rise to a standing position without using their arms as levers. Children who push their body upright using the arms and hands may have generalized muscle weakness, known as a *positive Gower sign*. This may indicate muscular dystrophy (see Figure 19–16.)

POSTURE AND SPINAL ALIGNMENT

Posture

Inspect the child's posture when standing from a front, side, and back view. The shoulders and hips are normally level. The head is held erect without a tilt, and the shoulder contour is symmetric. The spine has normal thoracic convex and lumbar concave curves after 6 years of age. Table 3–20 shows normal posture and spinal curvature development.

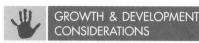

CLINICAL TIP

To check the muscle strength in a newborn, hold the infant upright with your hands under the infant's arms. An infant who is held lightly normally does not slip through the hands. Muscle weakness is present when the infant slides through the hands.

GROWTH & DEVELOPMENT CONSIDERATIONS

After beginning to walk, young children often have a pot-bellied stance because of a lumbar lordosis. This posture generally disappears by 5 years of age.

3-19	Selected Gross Motor Milestones for Age

Gross Motor Milestones	Age Attained
Rolls over from prone to supine position	4 months
Sits without support	8 months
Pulls self to standing position	10 months
Walks around room holding onto objects	11 months
Walks alone well	15 months
Kicks ball	24 months
Jumps in place	30 months
Throws ball overhand	36 months

From Frankenburg, W.K., Dodds J., Archer, P., Shapiro, H., and Bresnick, B. (1992). The Denver II: A major revision and restandardization of the Denver Developmental Screening Test. Pediatrics, 89, 91–97.

3-20   Normal Development of Posture and Spinal Curves

Infant
2–3 months

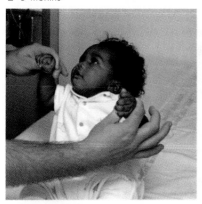

Holds head erect when held upright; thoracic kyphosis when sitting.

6–8 months

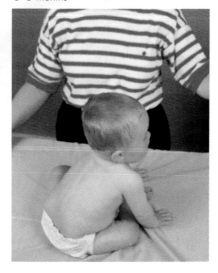

Sits without support; spine is straight.

10–15 months

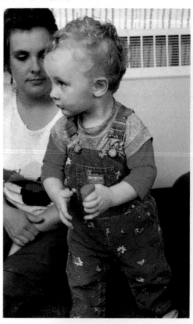

Walks independently; straight spine.

Toddler
Protruding abdomen; lumbar lordosis.

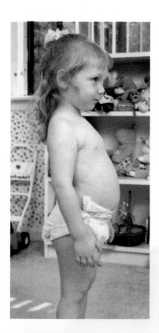

School-age child
Height of shoulders and hips is level; balanced thoracic convex and lumbar concave curves.

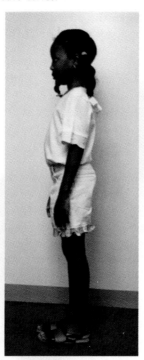

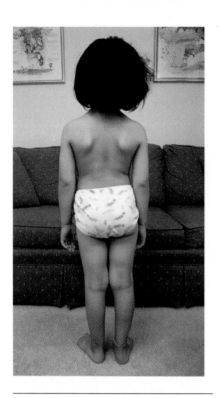

FIGURE 3–43. Does this child have legs of different lengths or scoliosis? Look at the level of the iliac crests and shoulders to see if they are level. See the more prominent crease at the waist on the right side? This child could have scoliosis.

Spinal Alignment

Assess the school-age child and adolescent for *scoliosis*, a lateral spine curvature. Stand behind the child, observing the height of the shoulders and hips (Fig 3–43). Ask the child to bend forward slowly at the waist, with arms extended toward the floor. No lateral curve should be present in either position. The ribs normally stay flat bilaterally. The lumbar concave curve should flatten with forward flexion (Fig. 3–44). A lateral curve to the spine or a one-sided rib hump is an indication of scoliosis (see also Chap. 19).

INSPECTION OF THE UPPER EXTREMITIES

Arms

The alignment of the arms is normally straight, with a minimal angle at the elbows, where the bones articulate.

Hands

Count the fingers. Extra finger digits *(polydactyly)* or webbed fingers *(syndactyly)* are abnormal. Inspect the creases on the palmar surface of each hand. Multiple creases across the palm are normal. A single crease that crosses the entire palm of the hand, a simian crease, is associated with Down syndrome (Fig. 3–45).

Nails

Inspect the nails for size, shape, and color. Nails are normally convex, smooth, and pink. *Clubbing,* widening of the nailbed with an increased angle between the proximal nail fold and nail, is abnormal (see Fig. 12–7). Clubbing is associated with chronic respiratory and cardiac conditions.

INSPECTION OF THE LOWER EXTREMITIES

Hips

Assess the hips of newborns and young infants for dislocation or subluxation. The skin folds on the upper legs are inspected first. The same number

FIGURE 3–44. Inspection of the spine for scoliosis. Ask the child to slowly bend forward at the waist, with arms extended toward the floor. Run your forefinger down the spinal processes, palpating each vertebra for a change in alignment. A lateral curve to the spine or a one-sided rib hump is an indication of scoliosis.

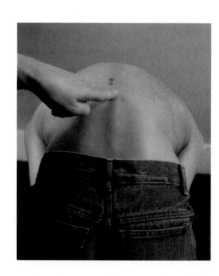

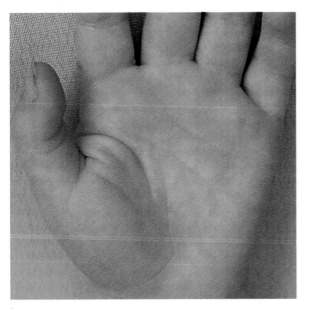
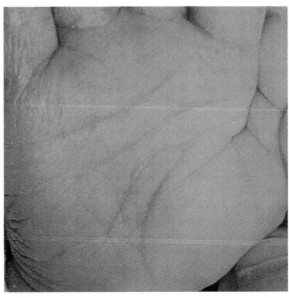

A   B

FIGURE 3–45. A, Normal palmar creases. **B,** Simian crease associated with Down syndrome.
Source **B:** *From Zitelli, B.J., & Davis, H.W. (Eds.). (1997). Atlas of pediatric physical diagnosis (3rd ed.). St. Louis: Mosby–Year Book.*

of skin folds should be present on each leg. Uneven skin folds may indicate a hip dislocation or difference in leg length (Allis sign). Then check for a difference in knee height symmetry (Fig. 3–46). The Ortolani–Barlow maneuver is used to assess an infant's hips for dislocation or subluxation (Fig. 3–47).

The child is asked to stand on one leg and then the other. The iliac crests should stay level. If the iliac crest opposite the weight-bearing leg appears lower, the hip bearing weight may be dislocated.

Legs

Inspect the alignment of the legs. After a child is 4 years of age, the alignment of the long bones is straight, with minimal angle at the knees and feet where the bones articulate. Alignment of the lower extremities in infants and toddlers is assessed to ensure that normal changes are occurring. To

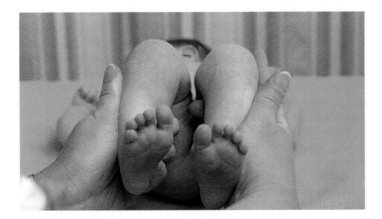

FIGURE 3–46. Flex the infant's hips and knees so the heels are as close to the buttocks as possible. Place the feet flat on the examining table. The knees are usually the same height. A difference in knee height (Allis sign) is an indicator of hip dislocation (see also Chap. 19).
Courtesy Dee Corbett, RN, Children's National Medical Center, Washington, DC.

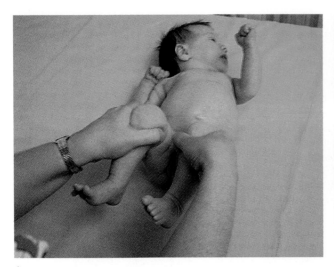

A

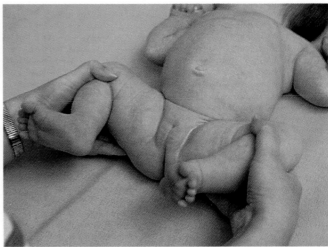

B

FIGURE 3–47. Ortolani–Barlow maneuver. **A,** Place the infant on his or her back and flex the hips and knees at a 90 degree angle. Place a hand over each knee with the thumb over the inner thigh, and the first two fingers over the upper margin of the femur. Move the infant's knees together until they touch, and then put downward pressure on both femurs to see if the hips easily slip out of their joints, or dislocate. **B,** Slowly abduct the hips, moving each knee toward the examining table. Keep pressure on the hip joints with the fingers in a lever type motion. Equal hip abduction, with the knees nearly touching the examining table, is normal. Any resistance to abduction or a clunk felt on palpation can be an indication of a congenital hip dislocation.

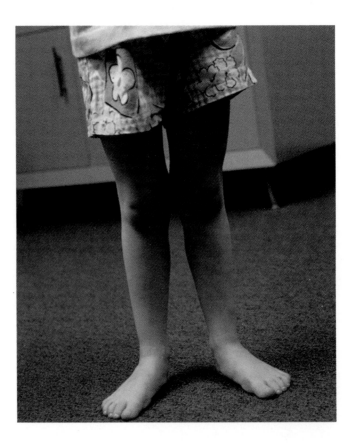

FIGURE 3–48. To evaluate the child with knock-knees, have the child stand on a firm surface. Measure the distance between the ankles when the child stands with the knees together. The normal distance is not more than 2 in. (5 cm) between the ankles.

evaluate the toddler with bowlegs, have the child stand on a firm surface. Measure the distance between the knees when the child's ankles are together. No more than 1.5 in. (3.5 cm) between the knees is normal. See Fig. 3–48 for assessment of knock-knees.

Feet

Inspect the feet for alignment, the presence of all toes, and any deformities. The weight-bearing line of the feet is usually in alignment with the legs. Many newborns have a flexible forefoot inversion (metatarsus adductus) that results from uterine positioning. Any fixed deformity is abnormal.

Inspect the feet for the presence of an arch when the child is standing. Children up to 3 years of age normally have a fat pad over the arch, giving the appearance of flat feet. Older children normally have a longitudinal arch. The arch is usually seen when the child stands on tiptoe or is sitting.

► ASSESSING THE NERVOUS SYSTEM FOR COGNITIVE FUNCTION, BALANCE, COORDINATION, CRANIAL NERVE FUNCTION, SENSATION, AND REFLEXES

What aspects of developmental information are useful for assessment of cognitive function? How is the infant's and child's level of consciousness evaluated? How are cranial nerves assessed in infants? A scissoring gait is associated with what condition? At what age does a Babinski response become abnormal? What response is expected when a deep tendon reflex is stimulated?

COGNITIVE FUNCTION

Observe the child's behavior, facial expressions, gestures, communication skills, activity level, and level of consciousness to assess cognitive functioning. Match the neurologic examination to the child's stage of development. For example, cognitive function is evaluated much differently in infants than in older children because infants cannot use words to communicate.

Behavior

The alertness of infants and children is indicated by their behavior during the assessment. Infants and toddlers are curious but seek the security of the parent, either by clinging or by making frequent eye contact. Older children are often anxious and watch all of the examiner's actions. Lack of interest in assessment or treatment procedures may indicate a serious illness. Excessive activity or an unusually short attention span may be associated with an attention deficit hyperactivity disorder.

Communication Skills

Speech, language development, and social skills provide good clues to cognitive functioning. Listen to speech articulation and words used,

GROWTH & DEVELOPMENT CONSIDERATIONS

Infants are often born with a twisting of the tibia caused by positioning in utero (tibial torsion). The infant's toes turn in as a result of the tibial torsion. Toddlers go through a skeletal alignment sequence of bowlegs (genu varum) and knock-knees (genu valgum) before the legs assume a straight alignment.

EQUIPMENT NEEDED

Reflex hammer
Cotton balls
Penlight
Tongue blades

CLINICAL TIP

The neurologic examination provides an opportunity to develop rapport with the child. Many of the procedures can be presented as games that young children enjoy. Cognitive function can be assessed by how well the child follows directions for the game. As the assessment proceeds, the child develops trust and is more likely to cooperate with examination of other systems.

3-21	Expected Language Development for Age

Language Milestones	Age Attained
Understands Mama and Dada	10 months
Says Mama, Dada, 2 other words; imitates animal sounds	12 months
4–6 word vocabulary, points to desired objects	13–15 months
7–20 word vocabulary, points to 5 body parts	18 months
2-word combinations	20 months
3-word sentences, plurals	36 months

From Capute, A.J., Shapiro, B.K., & Palmer, R.B. (1987). Marking the milestones of language development. Contemporary Pediatrics, 4, 24–41.

comparing the child's performance with standards of social development and speech articulation for the child's age (Table 3–21). Toddlers can normally follow simple directions such as "Show me your mouth." By 3 years of age the child's speech should be easily understood. Delay in language and social skill development may be associated with mental retardation.

Memory

Immediate, recent, and remote memory can be tested in children starting at approximately 4 years of age. To evaluate recent memory, ask the child to remember a special name or object. Then 5–10 minutes later during the examination, have the child recall the name or object. To evaluate remote memory, ask the child to repeat his or her address or birth date or a nursery rhyme. By 5 or 6 years of age, children are normally able to recall this information without difficulty.

Level of Consciousness

When approaching the infant or child, observe his or her level of consciousness and activity, including facial expressions, gestures, and interaction. Children are normally alert, and sleeping children arouse easily. The child who cannot be awakened is unconscious. A lowered level of con-

GROWTH & DEVELOPMENT CONSIDERATIONS

Immediate memory can be tested by asking the child to repeat a series of words or numbers, such as the names of Disney or Sesame Street characters. Children can remember more words or numbers with age.

Age	Recall Ability
4 years	3 words or numbers
5 years	4 words or numbers
6 years	5 words or numbers

3-22	Expected Balance Development for Age

Balance Milestones	Age Attained
Stands without support briefly	12 months
Walks alone well	15 months
Walks backwards	2 years
Balances on 1 foot for 5 seconds	4 years
Hops on 1 foot, heel-toe walking	5 years
Heel-toe walking backwards	6 years

sciousness may be associated with a number of neurologic conditions such as a head injury, seizure, infection, or brain tumor.

CEREBELLAR FUNCTION

Observe the young child at play to assess coordination and balance. Development of fine motor skills in infants and preschool children provides clues to cerebellar function.

Balance

Observe the child's balance during play activities such as walking, standing on one foot, and hopping (Table 3–22). The Romberg procedure can also be used to test balance in children over 3 years of age (Fig. 3–49). Once balance and other motor skills are attained, children do not normally stumble or fall when tested. Poor balance may indicate cerebellar dysfunction or an inner ear disturbance.

Coordination

Tests of coordination assess the smoothness and accuracy of movement. Development of fine motor skills can be used to assess coordination in young

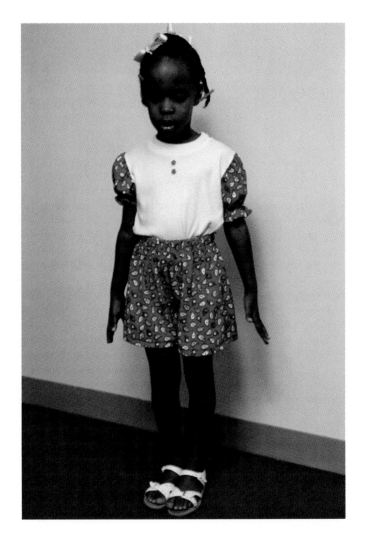

FIGURE 3–49. Romberg procedure. Ask the child to stand with feet together and eyes closed. Protect the child from falling by standing close. Preschool-age children may extend their arms to maintain balance, but older children can normally stand with their arms at their sides. Leaning or falling to one side is abnormal and indicates poor balance.

3-23	Expected Fine Motor Development for Age

Fine Motor Milestones	Age Attained
Transfers objects between hands	7 months
Picks up small objects	10 months
Feeds self with cup and spoon	12 months
Scribbles with crayon or pencil	18 months
Builds 2-block tower	24 months
Builds 4-block tower	30 months
Unfastens front buttons	36 months

From Frankenburg, W.K., Dodds J., Archer, P., Shapiro, H., and Bresnick, B. (1992). The Denver II: A major revision and restandardization of the Denver Developmental Screening Test. Pediatrics, 89, 91–97.

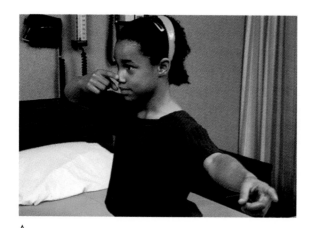

A

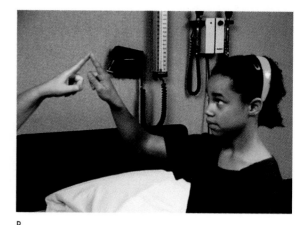

B

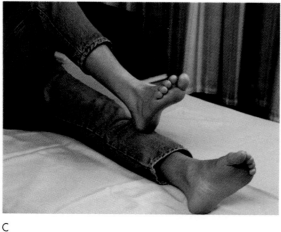

C

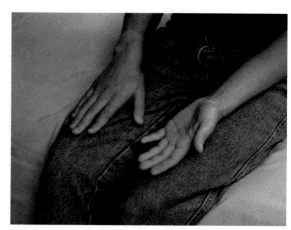

D

FIGURE 3–50. Tests of coordination. **A,** *Finger-to-nose test.* Ask the child to close the eyes and touch his or her nose, alternating the index fingers of the hands. **B,** *Finger-to-finger test.* Ask the child to alternately touch his or her nose and your index finger with his or her index finger. Move your hand to several positions within the child's reach to test pointing accuracy. Repeat the test with the child's other hand. **C,** *Heel-to-shin test.* Ask the child to rub his or her leg from the knee to the ankle with the heel of the other foot. Repeat the test with the other foot. This test is normally performed without hesitation or inappropriate placement of the foot. **D,** *Rapid alternating motion test.* Ask the child to rapidly rotate his or her wrist so the palm and dorsum of the hand alternately pat the thigh. Repeat the test with the other hand. Hesitating movements are abnormal. Mirroring movements of the hand not being tested indicates a delay in coordination skill refinement.

children (Table 3–23). After 6 years of age the tests for adults (finger-to-nose, finger-to-finger, heel-to-shin, and alternating motion) can be used (Fig. 3–50). The child usually responds enthusiastically when these tests are presented as games. Jerky movements or inaccurate pointing *(past pointing)* indicates poor coordination, which can be associated with delayed development or a cerebellar lesion.

Gait

A normal gait requires intact bones and joints, muscle strength, coordination, and balance. Inspect the child when walking from both a front and a rear view. The iliac crests are normally level during walking, and no limp is expected. A limp may indicate injury or joint disease. Staggering or falling may indicate cerebellar ataxia. *Scissoring*, in which the thighs tend to cross forward over each other with each step, may be associated with cerebral palsy or other spastic conditions.

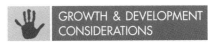

GROWTH & DEVELOPMENT CONSIDERATIONS

Gait is related to the motor development of the child. Toddlers beginning to walk have a wide-based gait and limited balance. With practice the toddler's balance improves and the gait develops a narrower base.

CRANIAL NERVE FUNCTION

To assess the cranial nerves in infants and young children, modifications can be made to the procedures used to assess school-age children and adults (Table 3–24). Abnormalities of cranial nerves may be associated with compression of an individual nerve, head injury, or infections.

SENSORY FUNCTION

To assess sensory function, compare the responses of both sides of the body to various types of stimulation. Equal responses bilaterally are normal. Loss of sensation may indicate a brain or spinal cord lesion.

Superficial Tactile Sensation

Stroke the skin on the lower leg or arm with a cotton ball or a finger while the child's eyes are closed. Cooperative children over 2 years of age can normally point to the location touched.

Superficial Pain Sensation

Break a tongue blade to get a sharp point. After asking the child to close the eyes, touch the child in various places on each arm and leg, alternating the sharp and dull ends of the tongue blade. Children over 4 years of age can normally distinguish between a sharp and dull sensation each time. To improve the child's accuracy with the test, let the child practice telling you the difference between the sharp and dull stimulation.

    An inability to identify superficial touch and pain sensation may indicate sensory loss. Identify the extent of sensory loss, such as all areas below the knee. Other sensory function tests (temperature, vibratory, deep pressure pain, and position sense) are performed when sensory loss is found. Refer to other texts for description of these procedures.

CLINICAL TIP

An infant's sensory function is not routinely assessed. Withdrawal responses to painful procedures indicate normal sensory function.

INFANT PRIMITIVE REFLEXES

Evaluate the movement and posture of newborns and young infants by the Moro, palmar grasp, plantar grasp, placing, stepping, and tonic neck prim-

3-24	Age-Specific Procedures for Assessment of Cranial Nerves in Infants and Children

Cranial Nerve[a]	Assessment Procedure and Normal Findings[b]
I Olfactory	Infant: Not tested. Child: Not routinely tested. Give familiar odors to child to smell, one naris at a time. *Identifies odors such as orange, peanut butter, and chocolate.*
II Optic	Infant: Shine a bright light in eyes. *A quick blink reflex and dorsal head flexion indicates light perception.* Child: Test vision and visual fields if cooperative. *Visual acuity appropriate for age.*
III Oculomotor IV Trochlear VI Abducens	Infant: Shine a penlight at the eyes and move it side to side. *Focuses on and tracks the light to each side.* Child: Move an object through the six cardinal points of gaze. *Tracks object through all fields of gaze.* All ages: Inspect eyelids for drooping. Inspect pupillary response to light. *Eyelids do not droop and pupils are equal sized and briskly respond to light.*
V Trigeminal	Infant: Stimulate the rooting and sucking reflex. *Turns head toward stimulation at side of mouth and sucking has good strength and pattern.* Child: Observe the child chewing a cracker. Touch forehead and cheeks with cotton ball when eyes are closed. *Bilateral jaw strength is good. Child pushes cotton ball away.*
VII Facial	All ages: Observe facial expressions when crying, smiling, frowning, etc. *Facial features stay symmetric bilaterally.*
VIII Acoustic	Infant: Produce a loud sound near the head. *Blinks in response to sound, moves head toward sound, or freezes position.* Child: Use a noisemaker near each ear or whisper words to be repeated. *Turns head toward sound and repeats words correctly.*
IX Glossopharyngeal X Vagus	Infant: Observe swallowing during feeding. *Good swallowing pattern.* All ages: Elicit gag reflex. *Gags with stimulation.*
XI Spinal accessory	Infant: Not tested. Child: Ask child to raise the shoulders and turn the head side to side against resistance. *Good strength in neck and shoulders.*
XII Hypoglossal	Infant: Observe feeding. *Sucking and swallowing are coordinated.* Child: Tell the child to stick out the tongue. Listen to speech. *Tongue is midline with no tremors. Words are clearly articulated.*

[a]Bracketed nerves are tested together.
[b]Italic indicates normal findings.

itive reflexes (Table 3–25). These reflexes appear and disappear at expected intervals in the first few months of life as the central nervous system develops. Movements are normally equal bilaterally. An asymmetric response may indicate a serious neurologic problem on the less responsive side.

SUPERFICIAL AND DEEP TENDON REFLEXES

Evaluate the superficial and deep tendon reflexes to assess the function of specific segments of the spine.

Superficial Reflexes

Assess superficial reflexes by stroking a specific area of the body. The plantar reflex, testing spine levels L4–S2, is routinely evaluated in children (Fig. 3–51). Assess the cremasteric reflex in boys (see p. 154).

Primitive Reflex	Technique and Normal Findings[a]	Normal Appearance and Disappearance

Moro

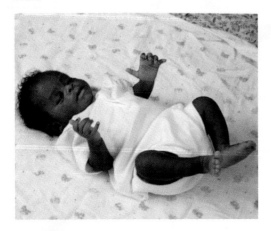

Startle the infant with a sudden noise or change in position.
The arms extend and the fingers form a C as they spread. The arms slowly move together as in a hug. The legs may make a similar motion.

Present at birth. Decreases in strength by 4 months of age. Disappears by 6 months of age.

Palmar grasp

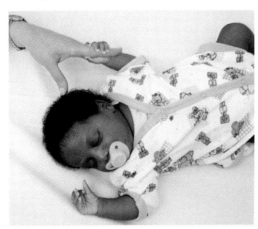

Place finger across the infant's palm and avoid touching the thumb.
A strong grip around the finger is normal.

Present at birth. Disappears by 3 months of age.

Plantar grasp

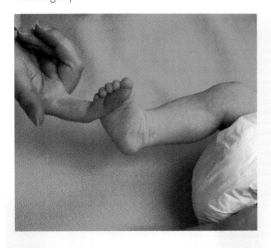

Place finger across the foot at the base of the toes.
The toes normally curl as if gripping the finger.

Present at birth. Disappears at about 8 months of age

[a]Italics indicate normal findings.

Continued . . .

Primitive Reflex	Technique and Normal Findings[a]	Normal Appearance and Disappearance
Placing 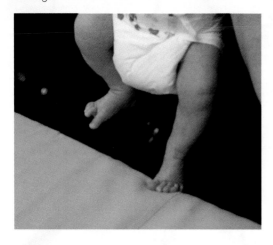	Hold the infant erect and touch the top of one foot with the edge of a table or chair. *The infant normally lifts the foot, as if to step up onto the surface.*	Present within days of birth. Disappears at various times.
Stepping 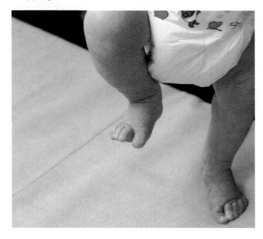	Hold the infant erect and touch the bottom of one foot on the surface of a table or chair. *The feet lift in an alternating pattern as if to walk.*	Present at birth. Disappears between 4 and 8 weeks of age.
Tonic neck 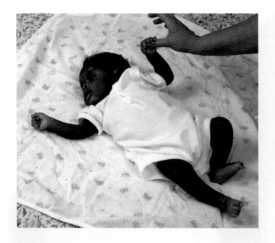	Place the infant in a supine position and, when relaxed, turn the head to one side. Repeat by turning the head to the opposite side. *The arm and leg on the face side normally extend and the opposite arm and leg flex, as if to assume a fencing position.*	Appears about 2 months of age. Deceases by 4 months of age. Disappears no later than 6 months of age. This reflex must disappear before the infant can turn over.

[a]Italics indicate normal findings.

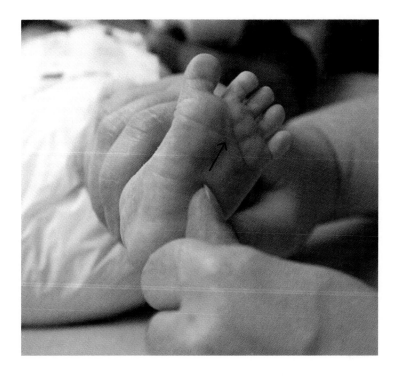

FIGURE 3–51. To assess the plantar reflex, stroke the bottom of the infant's or child's foot in the direction of the arrow. Watch the toes for plantar flexion or the Babinski response, fanning and dorsiflexion of the big toe. The Babinski response is normal in children under 2 years of age. Plantar flexion of the toes is the normal response in older children. A Babinski response in children over 2 years of age can indicate neurologic disease.

3-26	Assessment of Deep Tendon Reflexes and the Spinal Segment Tested With Each

Deep Tendon Reflex	Technique and Normal Findings[a]	Spine Segment Tested
Biceps		
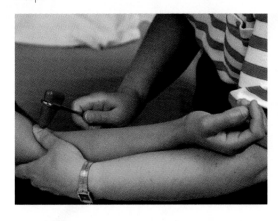	Flex the child's arm at the elbow, and place your thumb over the biceps tendon in the antecubital fossa. Tap your thumb. *Elbow flexes as the biceps muscle contracts.*	C5 and C6
Triceps		
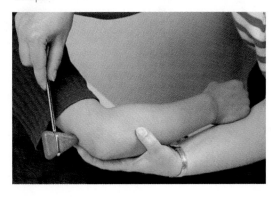	With the child's arm flexed, tap the triceps tendon above the elbow. *Elbow extends as the triceps muscle contracts.*	C6, C7, and C8

Continued . . .

Deep Tendon Reflex	Technique and Normal Findings[a]	Spine Segment Tested
Brachioradialis		

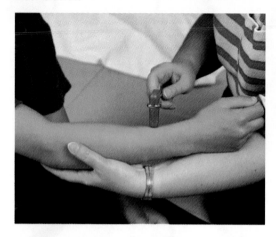

Lay the child's arm with the thumb upright over your arm. Tap the brachioradial tendon 2.5 cm (1 in.) above the wrist.
Forearm pronates (palm facing downward) and elbow flexes.

C5 and C6

Patellar

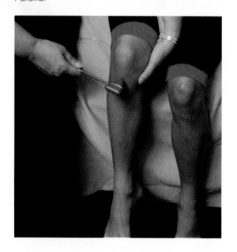

Flex the child's knees, and when the legs are relaxed, tap the patellar tendon just below the knee.
Knee extends (knee jerk) as the quadriceps muscle contracts.

L2, L3, and L4

Achilles

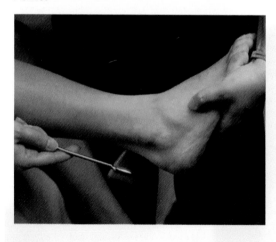

While the child's legs are flexed, support the foot and tap the Achilles tendon.
Plantar flexion (ankle jerk) as the gastrocnemius muscle contracts.

S1 and S2

[a]Italics indicate normal findings.

3-27	Numeric Scoring of Deep Tendon Reflex Responses
Grade	**Response Interpretation**
0	No response
1+	Slow, minimal response
2+	Expected response, active
3+	More active or pronounced than expected
4+	Hyperactive, clonus may be present

Deep Tendon Reflexes

To assess the deep tendon reflexes, tap a tendon near specific joints with a reflex hammer (or with the index finger for infants), comparing responses bilaterally. The biceps, triceps, brachioradialis, patellar, and Achilles tendons are usually evaluated in children. Inspect for movement in the associated joint and palpate the strength of the expected muscle contraction (Table 3–26). Table 3–27 outlines the numeric scoring of deep tendon reflexes. Responses are normally symmetric bilaterally. The absence of a response is associated with decreased muscle tone and strength. Hyperactive responses are associated with muscle spasticity.

► ASSESSING NUTRITIONAL STATUS BY MEASURING GROWTH AND EVALUATING DIETARY INTAKE

What is the best indication that the child's nutrition is adequate? Which data-collection tools provide good information about a child's dietary intake?

GROWTH MEASUREMENTS

The infant's weight, length, and head circumference are measured to assess growth. A standing height is substituted for the length measurement in children. The head circumference is routinely measured until 5 years of age. The *Quick Reference to Pediatric Clinical Skills* accompanying this text presents techniques used to measure weight, length, standing height, and head circumference.

Once the measurements are collected for the child, plot the readings on the appropriate standardized growth curves for weight, length or height, head circumference, and weight for length for the child's age and sex. For example, to plot the length measurement, mark an X on the spot where the child's age and length intersect. Appendix A gives standardized growth curves for infants, children, and adolescents by sex. Identify which percentile for weight, length or height, weight for length, and head circumference for age the child falls in. Children normally fall between the 10th and 90th percentiles for weight, length or height, and weight for length. A measurement below the 10th percentile of weight for length may indicate undernutrition, whereas a measurement over the 90th percentile may indicate overnutrition. Measurements of weight, length, or height below the 10th percentile may be normal in some cultural groups.

CLINICAL TIP

The best response to deep tendon reflex testing is achieved when the child is relaxed or distracted. Children often anticipate the knee jerk and either tighten up or exaggerate the response. Making the child focus on another set of muscles may provide a more accurate response. When testing the reflexes on the lower legs, have the child press his or her hands together or try to pull them apart when gripped together.

EQUIPMENT NEEDED

Scale
Height or length measuring device
Age-appropriate standardized
    growth curves
Forms of data collection tools

CULTURAL CONSIDERATIONS

Although growth curves have been standardized on the U.S. population, they can be used on children of different ethnic groups. Children of first- or second-generation immigrants to the United States follow patterns of growth similar to those of the children whose families have been in the United States longer, but often at a lower percentile.

When measurements of the child's weight and length at earlier ages are available, plot them on the same growth curve. Growth measurements following a same percentile curve for weight and length or height over time are normal, indicating that the child's nutrition is adequate. A sudden or sustained drop below a previously established percentile for weight or length may indicate inadequate dietary intake or a chronic disorder.

DIETARY INTAKE

CULTURAL CONSIDERATIONS

Each culture has eating practices that influence dietary intake. It is important to understand the foods commonly eaten by each cultural group and their contribution to the total nutrition of the child.

Obtain detailed information about the child's dietary intake when there is a potential for nutritional deficiency because of disease, knowledge deficit, or socioeconomic status. After the information is collected, compare the dietary intake to the energy and recommended daily nutritional and energy needs of the child (see Appendix B for Food Pyramid and Appendix C for the Recommended Dietary Allowances chart). The 24-hour recall of food intake and the dietary screening history provide a good overview of the infant's or child's dietary intake and eating patterns. A food diary provides information about the child's precise food intake.

24-Hour Recall of Food Intake

Ask the parent to list all foods eaten by the infant or child during the past 24 hours. Make sure the 24-hour period is an example of the child's typical dietary intake. For example, when the child is ill, food intake changes. In such a case a recent, more typical 24-hour period should be used for data collection. When obtaining the information, ask the parent specifically about the following food intake:

- All meals and between-meal snacks
- Approximate amounts (for example, tablespoon, half cup) of each food eaten at each meal
- What was added to foods, such as cereal mixed with formula
- How the food was prepared
- Vitamins or other food supplements (iron, fluoride) given

Dietary Screening History

Ask the parent about the infant's or child's eating habits using questions in Tables 3–28 and 3–29. These responses provide additional information about the family's eating habits and food beliefs beyond that collected on the 24-hour dietary recall.

Food Diary

CLINICAL TIP

Parents seldom control all of the food a child eats. To help parents record the most complete food diary, remind them about all the places a child might be fed or obtain food. Older children often get snacks independently. Younger children may be fed in day-care centers. Parents need to obtain information from the child as well as all persons feeding the child.

Parents are asked to keep a food diary when the child has a nutrition problem, such as malnutrition, obesity, or a disorder like diabetes mellitus that requires dietary management. All meals and snacks, with food preparation method and quantities eaten, over a 3–7-day period are recorded. Eating patterns change significantly for holidays or family gatherings, so ask parents to select typical days for the food diary or to record specific events affecting food intake.

Assessing the Adequacy of Intake

Review the overall pattern of food intake to ensure that the child is getting some foods from all the basic food groups (milk, meat, fruits, vegetables, and grains or bread). A good mix of protein, carbohydrates, and fats is also

Overview Questions

What was the infant's birth weight?
At what age did the birth weight double and triple?
Was the infant premature?
Does the infant have any feeding problems such as difficulty sucking and swallowing, spitting up, fatigue, or fussiness?

If Infant Is Breast-Fed

How long does the baby nurse at each breast?
What is the usual schedule for nursing?
Does the baby also take any milk or formula? Amount and frequency? What type?

If Infant Is Fed Other Foods

What formula is used? Is it iron fortified?
How is it prepared?
Do you hold or prop the bottle for feedings?
How much formula is taken at each feeding?
How many bottles are taken each day?
Does the baby take a bottle to bed for naps or nighttime? What is in the bottle?

If Infant Is Formula Fed

At what age did the baby start eating other foods?
    Cereal   Finger foods
    Fruit/juices   Meats
    Vegetables   Other protein sources
Do you use commercial baby food or make your own?
Does the baby eat any table foods?
How often does the baby take solid foods?
How is the baby's appetite?
Do you have any concerns about the baby's feeding habits?
Does the baby take a vitamin supplement?
Have there been any allergic reactions to foods? Which ones?
    Does the baby spit up frequently?
    Have there been any rashes?
What types of stools does the baby have? Frequency? Consistency?

What foods or beverages does the child dislike?
What types of food or beverage does the child especially like?
What is the child's typical eating schedule? Meals and snacks?
Does the child eat with the family or at separate times?
    Where does the child eat each meal?
Who prepares the food for the family?
    What method of cooking is used? Baking? Frying? Broiling?
    What ethnic foods are commonly eaten?
Does the family eat in a restaurant frequently? What type?
    What type of food does the child usually order?
Is the child on a special diet?
Does the child need to be fed, feed himself or herself, need assistance eating, or need any adaptive devices for eating?
What is the child's appetite like?
Does the child take any vitamin supplements (iron, fluoride)?
Does the child have any allergies? What types of symptoms?
What types of regular exercise does the child get?
Are there any concerns about the child's eating habits?

3-30	Signs of Inadequate Nutrition in Children

Nutrient Deficiency	Physical Signs of Malnutrition
Protein and calorie	Poor growth Hair: dull, dry, thin Mouth: enlarged parotid glands Skin: depigmentation, pretibial edema Musculoskeletal: muscle weakness Neurologic: listlessness Abdomen distended
Minerals	Enlarged thyroid Heart: murmur, tachycardia, arrhythmias Musculoskeletal: muscle weakness, bony overgrowth, skeletal bending
Vitamins	Skin: rough, dry, lesions, pallor Eyes: night blindness; light sensitivity; dull, dark circles Mouth: cracking, scaling lips; spongy, swollen, bleeding gums; smooth or fissured tongue; poor tooth development Musculoskeletal: soft bones, bowing or knock-knees, bony overgrowth Neurologic: depressed deep tendon reflexes, motor weakness, lethargy

important. Estimate the daily caloric intake by using a calorie chart. Various physical signs of malnutrition from protein, calorie, and specific nutrients may be detected in various body systems (Table 3–30). A nutritionist can perform a more detailed nutritional assessment.

► ANALYZING DATA FROM THE PHYSICAL EXAMINATION

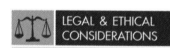

LEGAL & ETHICAL CONSIDERATIONS

Be sure to record all findings from the physical assessment legibly, in detail, and in the format approved by your institution.

Once the physical examination has been completed, any abnormal findings for each system should be grouped with those of other systems. **Clinical judgment** is used to identify common patterns of physiologic responses associated with medical conditions. Individual abnormal physiologic responses are also the basis of many nursing diagnoses.

Let's return to the vignette at the beginning of the chapter. Your thorough physical assessment of Latoya has revealed signs of respiratory distress and inadequate tissue perfusion from several body systems. These signs include mottled skin color, an increased resting respiratory rate, retractions, increased respiratory effort, nasal flaring, tachycardia, and lethargy. These signs represent the integumentary, respiratory, cardiac, and neurologic systems. Based on these findings, you would be able to select nursing diagnoses appropriate for an infant with bronchiolitis, for example, Altered Tissue Perfusion, Cardiopulmonary, related to lower airway obstruction and hypoxia; and Ineffective Breathing Pattern related to respiratory distress. These diagnoses, in turn, would direct your nursing care of this child.

REFERENCES

1. Spector, R.E. (1996). *Cultural diversity in health and illness* (4th ed.). Stamford, CT: Appleton & Lange.
2. Burns, C. (1992). A new assessment model and tool for pediatric nurse practitioners. *Journal of Pediatric Health Care, 6,* 73–81.
3. Byrnes, K. (1996). Conducting the pediatric health history: A guide. *Pediatric Nursing, 22,* 135–137.
4. Goldenring, J.M., & Cohen, E. (1988). Getting into adolescent heads. *Contemporary Pediatrics, 5,* 75–90.
5. Wilson, E.F. (1977). Estimation of the age of cutaneous contusions in child abuse. *Pediatrics, 60,* 750.
6. Seidel, H.M., Ball, J.W., Dains, J., & Benedict, G.W. (1995). *Mosby's guide to physical examination* (3rd ed.). St. Louis: Mosby–Year Book.
7. Smith, J. (1988). Big differences in little people. *American Journal of Nursing, 88,* 458–462.
8. Eichelberger, M.R., Ball, J.W., Pratsch, G.S., & Clark, J.R. (1998). *Pediatric emergencies: A manual for prehospital care providers* (2nd ed.). Upper Saddle River, NJ: Brady, Prentice Hall.
9. Tanner, J.M. (1962). *Growth at adolescence* (2nd ed.). Oxford: Blackwell Scientific Publications, Inc.

ADDITIONAL RESOURCES

Barness, L. (1991). *Manual of pediatric physical diagnosis* (6th ed.). St. Louis: Mosby–Year Book.

Bradley, J.C., & Edinberg, M.A. (1990). *Communication in the nursing context* (3rd ed.). Norwalk, CT: Appleton & Lange.

Calhoun, M. (1986). Providing health care to Vietnamese in America: What practitioners need to know. *Home and Healthcare Nurse, 4,* 14–19, 22.

Castiglia, P.T. (1989). Ambiguous genitalia. *Journal of Pediatric Health Care, 3,* 319–321.

Curry, L.C., & Gibson, L.Y. (1992). Congenital hip dislocation: The importance of early detection and comprehensive treatment. *Nurse Practitioner, 17,* 49–52, 55.

Elvik, S.L. (1990). Vaginal discharge in the prepubertal girl. *Journal of Pediatric Health Care, 4,* 181–185.

Engel, J.K. (1996). *Pocket guide to pediatric assessment* (3rd ed.). St. Louis: Mosby–Year Book.

Finelli, L. (1991). Evaluation of the child with acute abdominal pain. *Journal of Pediatric Health Care, 5,* 251–256.

Gessner, I.H. (1997). What makes a heart murmur innocent? *Pediatric Annals, 26*(2), 82–91.

Henry, J.J. (1992). Routine growth monitoring and assessment of growth disorders. *Journal of Pediatric Health Care, 6,* 291–301.

Lippe, B.M. (1987). Short stature in children: Evaluation and management. *Journal of Pediatric Health Care, 1,* 313–322.

Litt, I.F. (1990). *Evaluation of the adolescent patient.* Philadelphia: Hanley & Belfus, Inc.

Pipes, P.L., & Trahms, C.M. (1993). *Nutrition in infancy and childhood* (5th ed.). St. Louis: Mosby–Year Book.

Rosenthal, S.L., Burklow, K.A., Biro, F.M., Pace, L.C., & DeVellis, R.F. (1996). The reliability of high-risk adolescent girls' report of their sexual history. *Journal of Pediatric Health Care, 10,* 217–220.

Ruben, R.J. (1994). Communicative disorders: The first year of life. *Pediatric Clinics of North America, 41,* 1035–1045.

Rudy, E.C. (1991). Hair loss in children and adolescents. *Journal of Pediatric Health Care, 5,* 245–250.

Sifuentes, M. (1996). Talking to adolescents, In C.D. Berkowitz (Ed.), *Pediatrics: A primary care approach* (pp. 10–12). Philadelphia: W.B. Saunders.

Thomas, D. (1996). Assessing children—it's different. *RN, 59,* 38–44.

Unti, S.M. (1994). The critical first year of life: History, physical examination, and general developmental assessment. *Pediatric Clinics of North America, 41,* 859–873.

Vessey, J.A. (1995). Developmental approaches to examining young children. *Pediatric Nursing, 21,* 53–56.

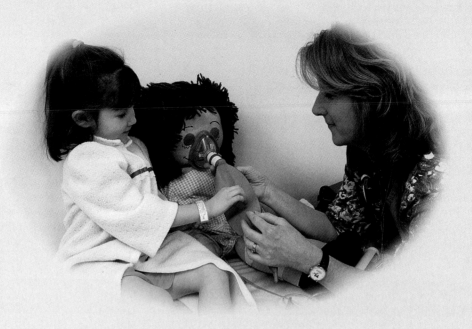

Four-year-old Sabrina has had several nosebleeds and fainting spells recently. After examination by her physician and a number of diagnostic studies such as chest x-ray examination, echocardiography, and electrocardiography, coarctation of the aorta is diagnosed. Sabrina will come in this week for a cardiac catheterization. In 2 weeks, she is scheduled to have open heart surgery.

Sabrina and her family live about 50 miles from the medical center. Her parents have three other children, ages 9, 7, and 2. The parents are both employed, but Sabrina's mother plans to take several days off at the time of surgery. Sabrina attends preschool, and she is used to spending time with other children.

Sabrina has had few health problems, and her experiences with health care professionals are limited. Her parents, who are anxious about the heart surgery, are concerned about how their daughter will adapt to hospitalization.

How should you prepare Sabrina for the cardiac catheterization and for the surgery? How far in advance should teaching take place? What teaching aids are helpful? How can Sabrina's parents be involved in and reinforce the teaching? What kind of support do her parents, siblings, and friends need during hospitalization?

NURSING CONSIDERATIONS FOR THE HOSPITALIZED CHILD

4

"Using a doll to demonstrate procedures is a helpful technique in preparing a child of Sabrina's age for surgery. Although she is anxious at first, playing with the doll helps her to feel more control over what will happen. She also understands that the surgery will help her feel better again."

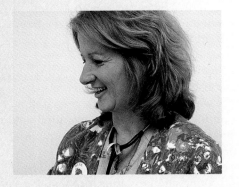

TERMINOLOGY

- **case manager** Person who coordinates health care to prevent gaps or overlaps.
- **child life specialist** Trained professional who plans therapeutic activities for hospitalized children.
- **Individualized Education Plan** Formulation of a specific learning approach for a child with a physical or mental handicap, following thorough assessment of the child's capabilities and areas of need.
- **rehabilitation** Assisting a child with physical or mental challenges to reach his or her fullest potential through therapy and education that considers the physiologic, psychologic, and environmental strengths and limitations of the child.

- **rooming in** Practice in which parents stay in the child's hospital room and care for the child.
- **separation anxiety** Distress behaviors observed in young children separated from familiar caregivers.
- **therapeutic play** Planned play techniques that provide an opportunity for children to deal with their fears and concerns related to illness or hospitalization.

Hospitalization, whether it is elective, planned in advance, or the result of an emergency or trauma, is stressful for children of all ages and their families. Today, children are infrequently hospitalized, because most pediatric conditions can be managed within the community. Hospitalized children are usually very ill. Hospitalized children are in an unknown environment, surrounded by strange people, equipment, and frightening sights and sounds. They are subjected to unfamiliar procedures, some of which are invasive, and may even have surgery. For both children and families, routines are disrupted and normal coping strategies are tested.

To minimize the stress of hospitalization, nurses need to provide support to children and their families before, during, and after hospitalization. Through preadmission preparation, children and their families are introduced to the acute care setting. During hospitalization, various strategies may be used to promote coping and adaptation and prepare children for procedures and surgery. Nurses are instrumental in ensuring that the developmental and educational needs of children are met, especially when hospitalization is prolonged. Nurses also help prepare children and their families for discharge or for transfer to a long-term care or rehabilitation facility.

▶ EFFECTS OF ILLNESS AND HOSPITALIZATION ON CHILDREN AND FAMILIES

CHILDREN'S UNDERSTANDING OF HEALTH AND ILLNESS

Can you remember as a child thinking that yelling at your mother caused your strep throat? Perhaps as an adolescent you believed that you would never become ill or have an accident. Maybe you feared being in a car crash like that of a friend. Children have limited knowledge about the body and its relation to health and illness. Their understanding is based primarily on their cognitive ability at various developmental stages and on previous experiences with health care professionals.

Infant

By about 6 months of age, infants have developed an awareness of themselves as separate from their mother or father. They are able to identify primary caretakers and to feel anxious when in contact with strangers. Hospitalization can be a traumatic time for an infant, particularly if the parents are not staying with the child.

Three phases of **separation anxiety** were first identified in young children who were separated from their parents for long periods or permanently and lacked a close relationship with one caretaker after separation.[1] Characteristic behaviors of children in the three phases of separation anxiety are listed in Table 4–1. Infants and young children who are hospitalized often display some of these behaviors.

Before the 1970s, health care professionals assumed that the despair and denial manifested by infants and young children after prolonged separation were signs of positive adaptation. Infants appeared to protest when their parents visited, and parents were sometimes advised not to visit often. However, the protest phase is now viewed as a healthy response to separation from loved ones and as an indication that the infant has meaningful,

4-1　Stages of Separation Anxiety in Young Children

Protest
Screaming, crying
Clinging to parents
Withdrawal from other adults

Despair
Sadness, depression
Withdrawal or compliant behavior
Crying when parents appear

Denial
Lack of protest when parents leave
Appearance of being happy and content with everyone
Close relationships not established
Developmental delay possible

Based on Bowlby, J. (1960). Separation anxiety. International Journal of Psychoanalysis, 41, 89–113.

close relationships. Parents should be encouraged to remain with and provide care to the hospitalized infant.

Toddler and Preschooler

Toddlers and preschoolers are beginning to understand illness but not its cause. Two unrelated events may appear to have a cause-and-effect relationship for young children, who may consider the sun, an animal, bad behavior, or even magic to be the cause of their illness. These children may blame other people, events, or themselves for an illness.[2] This is especially true if the other event occurs shortly before the illness.

The child's concept of the body usually is limited to names and locations of some body parts. While toddlers and preschoolers are not likely to understand how lungs, heart, bones, or other body parts function, they are learning concepts of safety and other health-related issues.[3,4]

Separation from parents remains the major stressor for the child. When a parent cannot be present, reminders can be left with the child. These might include a piece of cloth saturated with the mother's favorite perfume or father's cologne, an object belonging to the parent, or an audiotape with messages from the parents. Toddlers and preschoolers fear bodily mutilation and change. If, like Sabrina, the child is undergoing an operation, the nurse should explain to the child that surgery will fix the body. The nurse should encourage the parents to be present as much as possible for important rituals such as toileting, carrying out bedtime routines, and singing favorite nursery rhymes.

School-age Child

Older children have a more realistic understanding of the reasons for illness and are able to comprehend explanations. The child's concept of body parts and function is maturing. Concepts of time are well formed, and parents should be encouraged to tell the child when they will return. Parents should also be available for telephone calls to provide support and comfort. Stressful procedures can lead to regression or other behavioral changes.

GROWTH & DEVELOPMENT CONSIDERATIONS

School-age children between the ages of 5 and 8 years believe that the internal body consists of heart and bones. They view the digestive system as having two parts, the mouth and the stomach.

The child relies on parents and others for support and understanding during these events.

Adolescent

After 11 years of age, adolescents become increasingly aware of the physiologic, psychologic, and behavioral causes of illness and injury. Adolescents are concerned with appearance and perceive an illness or injury in terms of its effect on their body image. Allowing choices in clothing, hair, and music acknowledges the importance of their self-identity.[5] Privacy and modesty are major concerns of adolescents because their physical characteristics are rapidly changing. Nurses should respect their feelings. Adolescents are in the process of becoming independent of their parents' influence, and the peer group is a major influence in their lives. Separation from peers may be difficult.

FAMILY RESPONSES TO HOSPITALIZATION

The illness and hospitalization of a child disrupt a family's usual routines. Sometimes roles are altered as one parent stays at the hospital while the other parent or siblings take on additional tasks at home. Family members may be anxious and fearful, especially when the outcome is unknown or potentially serious. Watching a child in pain is difficult for a parent. Adjustment is made more difficult by a lengthy illness, chronic condition, poor prognosis, lack of family support, and lack of financial or community services.

The siblings of an ill child often receive little attention from the parents. Parents are preoccupied and may not think to take the siblings to visit the child in the hospital. The siblings may fantasize about the illness or injury and the appearance of their brother or sister. Siblings who are not adequately informed about the hospitalized child's condition may fear that the child will be disabled or even die, even when this is unlikely. They may feel guilty about fighting with or being mean to their brother or sister in the past and believe that they played a role in causing his or her illness.

As family roles and routines change, siblings may feel insecure and anxious. Behavioral problems may develop, or school performance may deteriorate. Siblings may feel jealous because the ill brother or sister seems to monopolize the parents' attention. Given support, however, the siblings of an ill child manage well. Chapter 7 describes strategies for working with the siblings of a hospitalized child.

▶ PREPARATION FOR HOSPITALIZATION

Hospitalization may be planned or unexpected. A child may be hospitalized for one of the following reasons:

- The child who has been ill at home gradually or suddenly becomes worse.
- The child needs diagnostic or treatment procedures or requires elective surgery.
- The child who was previously healthy suffers an injury, necessitating unexpected hospitalization.

When hospitalization is planned, both children and their parents have time to prepare for the experience. Assess the family's knowledge and expecta-

---

GROWTH & DEVELOPMENT CONSIDERATIONS

Young adolescents, aged 11–13 years, can describe the location and function of major organs such as the brain, nose, eyes, heart, and stomach.

tions and then provide information about what is likely to happen. A variety of approaches can be used to provide information and allay fears.

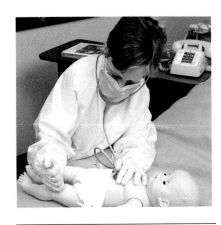

- Tours of the hospital unit or surgical area are helpful. During tours, preschoolers and school-age children should be allowed to see and touch items with which they will come in contact. The surgical team's attire is less frightening if the child has had a chance to try it on (Fig. 4–1). Medical equipment is not as scary when the child learns what it does and sees how it is used, for example, through demonstration on a doll (Fig. 4–2).

- If a tour is not possible, photographs or a videotape can be used to show the medical setting and procedures.

- Many hospitals offer health fairs to explain health procedures to children. The Association for the Care of Children's Health (ACCH) sponsors a National Children and Hospital Week each year.

- During a tour, while hospitalized, or at home, the child can be exposed to books or films that explain in age-appropriate terms what to expect during various procedures (Table 4–2). Use coloring books or other methods to reinforce teaching.

FIGURE 4–1. Allowing the child to dress up as a doctor or a nurse helps prepare the child for hospitalization. This helps the child adjust to treatment, care, and the recovery process. Why? What might the child's concerns be? Can you think of any concerns that could be related to cultural background?

Parents can be instrumental in preparing a child for hospitalization by reviewing material presented, being available to answer questions, and by being truthful and supportive (Table 4–3, Fig. 4–3).

Different approaches are useful when adolescents are being prepared for hospitalization. They learn not only from written materials, models, and videotapes, but also from talking with peers who have had similar experiences. A forum for asking questions without parents present should be provided.

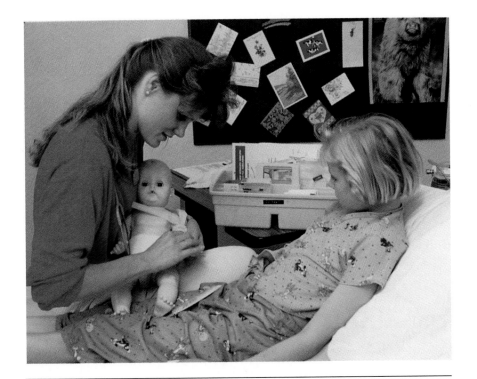

FIGURE 4–2. The child's anxiety and fear often will be reduced if the nurse explains what is going to happen and demonstrates how the procedure will be done by using a doll. Based on your experience, can you list five things you can do to prepare a school-age child for hospitalization?

4-2 Sample Teaching Materials for Children Requiring Hospitalization

Videotapes

Clean Intermittent Catheterization.	Learner Managed Designs, Inc.
I Have Epilepsy Too.	Epilepsy Foundation.
What Do I Tell My Children? How to Help a Child Cope With the Death of a Loved One	Life Cycle Productions.

Books

Barney Is Best. Carlstrom, L.	Barney Publications.
Becky's Story. Baznick, D.	Association for the Care of Children's Health.
Curious George Goes to the Hospital. Rey, M., & Rey, H.A.	Houghton Mifflin Company.
Doctors and Nurses: What Do They Do? Green, C.	Harper & Row Junior Books.
The Fall of Freddie the Leaf. Buscaglia, L.	Holt, Rinehart, & Winston.
First Time at the Hospital. Burton, N., & Burton, T.	Macdonald Educational Ltd.
Going to the Hospital. Rogers, F.	Random House Value.
Having an Operation. Greenwald, A., & Head, B.	Family Communications.
The Hospital Book. Howe, J.	Crown Publishers.
Hospitals. Fisher, L.E.	Holiday House.
A Night Without Stars. Howe, J.	Avon.
No Measles, No Mumps for Me. Showers, P.	Thomas Y. Crowell.
The Operation. Anderson, P.	Children's Press.
Richard Scarry's Nicky Goes to the Doctor. Scarry, R.	A Golden Book.
Rita Goes to the Hospital. Davison, M.	Random Books.
A Visit to the Sesame Street Hospital. Hautzig, D.	Random Books.
Wearing a Cast. Greenwald, A., & Head, B.	Family Communications.
When Molly Was in the Hospital: A Book for Brothers and Sisters of Hospitalized Children. Duncan, D.	Rayve Productions.
Why Am I Going to the Hospital? Cilliota, C., & Livingston, C.	Lyle Stuart.

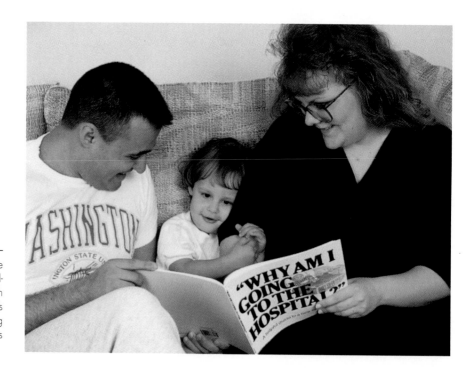

FIGURE 4–3. Jasmine's parents are taking the time to prepare her for hospitalization by reading a book recommended by the nurse. Such material should be appropriate to the child's age and culture. Why do you think that having the parents read this material to the child is valuable?

| 4-3 | Parental Preparation of Children for Hospitalization |

- Read stories to the child about the experience.
- Talk about going to the hospital, what it will be like. Talk about coming home.
- Encourage the child to ask questions.
- Encourage the child to draw pictures of what the hospital will be like.
- Visit the hospital unit if possible.
- Let the child touch or see equipment if possible.
- Plan for support via parents' presence, telephone calls, special items of the parents that child can keep during the stay.
- Be honest.

▶ ADAPTATION TO HOSPITALIZATION

SPECIAL UNITS AND TYPES OF CARE

Children who are admitted to a hospital may be cared for in one or more of the following units: emergency department, intensive care unit, or short stay unit. They may require surgical treatment involving preoperative and postoperative care. Children with infectious diseases may require isolation precautions. Other children may need rehabilitative care to achieve or restore maximum potential.

Emergency Care

When a child is brought to an emergency department, the parents are usually frightened and insecure and may even be in a state of shock. The fast pace and critical nature of the unit create an atmosphere in which parents are hesitant to ask questions and are anxious about the outcome. Keep both the child and the family informed about what is being done and when more news may be available. The parents and child should remain together as much as possible.

Intensive Care

Parents of a child in an intensive care unit are also likely to be anxious, particularly since the child's illness may be severe and the prognosis may be guarded. The unfamiliar equipment may create an atmosphere of fear. Numerous health care professionals come and go, and parents may not know whom to turn to or even what questions to ask. Provide emotional support, explain the purpose of treatments and machines, help parents to hold or touch their child, and provide support and referral to other services if appropriate. (See Chapter 6 for a discussion of stressors in parents and children in an intensive care unit and the nursing strategies intended to address these stressors.)

Preoperative and Postoperative Areas

Many hospitals now allow parents to be with their child right up until surgery begins and again in the postanesthesia recovery area. Parents often want to support their child before and immediately after a surgical procedure, and their presence may offer reassurance and comfort to the child.

Prepare family members for what will happen and what is expected of them. In some hospitals, only one or two close family members are allowed to see the child. They may need to wear special gowns, shoes, or hats, and they may be restricted to certain areas. Special equipment such as intravenous setups and monitoring devices should be explained.

Short Stay Units

Hospitalizations have generally become short, with minor surgery, diagnostic tests such as radiology studies, and treatments such as chemotherapy performed in 1 day. The child may be admitted in the morning and go home in the afternoon. These short stays are beneficial because they cause minimal disruption of family patterns. Nurses can help parents prepare the child properly for the admission, monitor the child during the procedures, and keep families well informed (Table 4–4).

Isolation

Children who are placed in isolation may suffer lack of stimulation because of limited contact with other children. Frequent family visits are important and should be encouraged. Family members may be reluctant to wear protective garments either out of fear of using them incorrectly or a belief that they are unnecessary. Be sure the family understands the reason for isolation and any special procedures. Having contact with and holding the child should be encouraged whenever possible. (Standard precautions are described in the *Quick Reference to Pediatric Clinical Skills* accompanying this text.)

Rehabilitation

Rehabilitation units provide children with ongoing care and support to continue recovery beyond the initial period of illness or injury. These may be separate units within a hospital or independent centers. The objective of **rehabilitation** is to help the child with physical or mental challenges reach his or her fullest potential and to promote achievement of developmentally appropriate skills. Parental involvement is essential.

FAMILY ASSESSMENT

To develop a plan of care that involves all family members, assess the impact of the child's illness or hospitalization on the family (Table 4–5). Teaching

4-4	Nursing Considerations in Preparing Parents and Child for Planned Short Stay Admission

- Are there special requirements, such as not being permitted food or drink or needing extra fluid intake?
- What time and where must the child appear?
- Are any special forms, insurance numbers, or previous records needed?
- How long will the child stay in the hospital?
- Are parents expected or encouraged to be with the child or stay in the health facility?
- Is there a chance the child may need to remain longer than expected?
- What will the child's condition be for transfer home?
- Will special equipment or care be needed?
- What symptoms can indicate problems?
- Where can the family go or whom can they call in case of problems or questions?

4-5   Family Assessment

Family Roles
- What changes will the child's illness create in the family?
- Will household tasks need to be reallocated?
- Will a burden be placed on certain family members?
- Will one parent room in or spend a great deal of time in the hospital?

Knowledge
- What knowledge does the family have about the child's condition and treatment? Do they need further information?
- Is there a need to start discharge planning and teaching early?

Support Systems
- Does the family have medical insurance? What percentage of costs will it cover? Will other financial support be needed?
- Are close friends or family available to provide child care for other children, assist with family tasks, or help in other ways?
- Are there community services such as support groups, camps for children with disabilities, education sessions, or equipment and financial resources to which the nurses can refer the family?

Siblings
- Have they been informed of the ill child's condition and the expected outcome?
- Have they been reassured that they did not cause the illness?
- Do they understand the change in roles and family routines?
- Are they able to visit the ill child?
- Have their teachers been informed of the family stress?
- If the hospitalized child's life is threatened, are the siblings involved in a therapy plan to assist them in dealing with that stress?

---

the child and family, providing support, and referring them to community resources are key elements of the plan.

The family's resources should be assessed frequently. These resources include the coping strategies of family members, financial resources, access to health care, and availability of community services. One family may manage quite well with limited financial support because they have good coping strategies, while another family with greater financial resources may have difficulty caring for an ill child.

It is important to assess the family dynamics. Evaluate the quality of communication, methods of handling problems, and sources of strength. Referrals to family service agencies or other community organizations may be needed. Support groups in the community or agencies that provide medical equipment can also be helpful.

CHILD AND FAMILY TEACHING

Teaching is an essential part of the nurse's role in care of hospitalized children and their parents. Teaching may be informal, as when the nurse provides an explanation during routine care, or structured, as when the nurse plans and implements a formal teaching program. Teaching about the behaviors seen in hospitalized children and strategies to deal with these behaviors are helpful for parents. For instance, it has been shown that providing information for parents of hospitalized toddlers on the typical behaviors of hospitalized children and on the strategies to assist children leads to less

LEGAL & ETHICAL CONSIDERATIONS

The American Nurses Association's 1996 *Statement on the Scope and Standards of Pediatric Clinical Nursing Practice* mandates teaching as a component of pediatric nursing care.

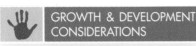

GROWTH & DEVELOPMENT CONSIDERATIONS

For children who can hear, touch, see a model or equipment, read, look at pictures, or even smell things like alcohol swabs, learning is more complete. This is particularly important for the school-age child in the stage of concrete operational thought, who must be able to manipulate materials in order to learn.

anxiety on the part of the parents and to greater parental involvement and support of the child during the hospitalization.[6] How can you plan to provide such information for parents?

Teaching directed at children must take into account their developmental level and cognitive abilities. Learning is easier when teaching involves more than one sense (such as hearing, vision, and touch). Teaching directed at parents must be geared to their level of understanding. If English is the parents' second language, a translator may be necessary.

Timing is a critical factor in teaching. Parents and children are less receptive to teaching when they are preoccupied with other thoughts or activities. Scheduling specific times for teaching sessions may be helpful.

Depending on the information to be presented, teaching may use the cognitive, psychomotor, or affective domains of learning. Teaching that includes all three domains is more effective.

Teaching Plans

A teaching plan is a written plan that includes outcome objectives, interventions needed to achieve specified goals, and a method and time for evaluation. The teaching plan may also specify teaching methods and types of materials to be used. Developing a teaching plan helps to ensure that all the necessary information is included and makes teaching more efficient.

The child's primary caretaker should participate in the teaching. The primary caretaker is most often a parent but may be a close family member (uncle, aunt, grandparent). The first step in establishing a teaching plan is to assess the child's or parent's knowledge, skills, and feelings by asking the following questions:

- What does the parent or child know about the health issue?
- What is the cognitive level or ability to learn?
- Is there a desire to learn?
- What previous experiences affect the learning experience, either positively or negatively?
- Are there feelings or beliefs that might interfere with the learning process?

The second step involves deciding what knowledge, skill, or change in attitude is desired. Outcome criteria or objectives are established for the parent and child.

- A learning objective for a parent might be: The parent states the importance of checking the child's toes in the casted leg twice daily for temperature, movement, sensations, color, and edema (cognitive domain).
- An objective for a child might be: The child self-catheterizes using correct technique and records the amount of urine in a log (psychomotor domain).
- An objective for an adolescent might be: The adolescent explores methods of managing feelings of loss of control related to diabetes management (affective domain).

Possible teaching methods and approaches should be explored. A variety of sources, including written materials (books, pamphlets, handouts, and stories), computer software, audiovisual presentations, and others, are available (see Table 4–2). In some settings, audiovisual and computer resources may be limited. Small-group teaching sessions (eg, for children with recently diagnosed diabetes or cystic fibrosis) may be another option. Gathering two or three parents or children together on a unit to learn and share experiences may be helpful.

For some conditions, standardized teaching plans are available in books and from health care agencies. These plans can serve as a guide in developing an individualized teaching plan.

Children With Special Needs

Children with disabilities may have special learning needs.[7] If they have visual impairment or visual perceptual difficulty, material must be presented in auditory and tactile ways. Children with hearing deficits need visual and tactile presentations. Children with learning disabilities may need more frequent reinforcement and shorter teaching sessions. They should be evaluated for comprehension often so teaching can be adjusted as necessary. When psychomotor skill performance is needed, special aids may be necessary so the child can hold a syringe, draw up a liquid, or perform other tasks. Adequate assessment of the child's strengths and disabilities, along with consultation with parents and the child's teachers, can help the nurse plan teaching methods.

STRATEGIES TO PROMOTE COPING AND NORMAL DEVELOPMENT

During hospitalization, care of the child focuses not only on meeting physiologic needs, but also on meeting psychosocial and developmental needs. Several strategies may be used to help children adapt to the hospital environment, promote effective coping, and provide developmentally appropriate activities (Fig. 4–4). These strategies include child life programs, rooming in, therapeutic play, and therapeutic recreation.

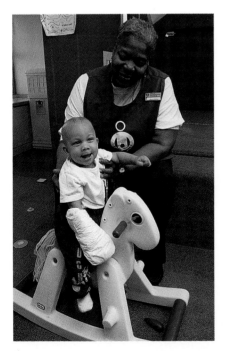

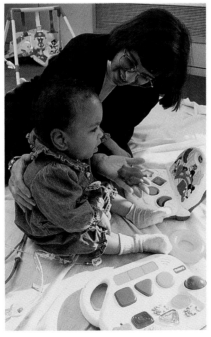

FIGURE 4–4. A, Volunteers such as this foster grandmother can provide stimulation and nurturing to help young children adapt to lengthy hospitalizations. **B,** Child life specialists plan activities for young children in the hospital to facilitate play and stress reduction.

A   B

Child Life Programs

Many hospitals have child life programs that focus on the psychosocial needs of hospitalized children. Professional child life specialists, paraprofessionals, and volunteers staff these departments. A **child life specialist** plans activities to provide age-appropriate playtime for children either in the child's room or in a playroom. Some of the planned activities are designed to assist children in working through feelings about illness. Examples include playing with medical equipment or drawing pictures about hospital treatments (Fig. 4–5). A trusted child life specialist may stay with a child during a particularly frightening procedure such as a venipuncture or bone marrow aspiration.

Both the child life department and the nursing staff focus on the emotional needs of hospitalized children. Child life specialists and nurses may formulate a plan together to assist children with particular needs.

Rooming In

Rooming in is the practice of having a parent stay in the child's hospital room and care for the hospitalized child. Some hospitals provide cots, others have special built-in beds on pediatric wards, and in some institutions a parent stays in a separate room on the unit. A parent who is rooming in may want to perform all of the child's basic care or help with some of the medical care. Communication between nurse and parent is important so that the parent's desire for involvement is supported.

Therapeutic Play

Play is an important part of childhood. The stress of illness and hospitalization increases the value of play. Not only is normal development facilitated by play, but play sessions can provide a means for the child to learn about health care, to express anxieties, to work through feelings, and to achieve a

---

CHANGING HEALTH CARE SYSTEM

Due to changes in the health care system, more children today are receiving care in outpatient centers, day surgery units, and other community centers. Pediatric inpatient units are consequently small, and play therapy programs are being curtailed. It is important for nurses to plan for provision of play in care, whatever the unit may be. Play therapists can become involved in the wide variety of units in which children receive health care.[8]

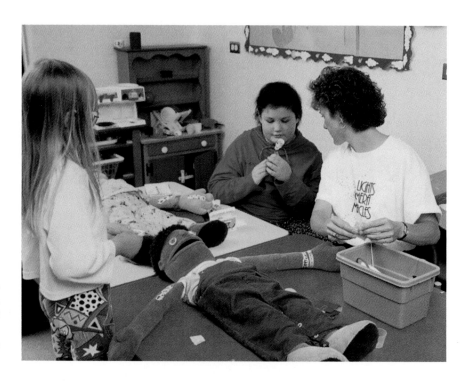

FIGURE 4–5. At Deaconess Hospital in Spokane, Washington, the child life specialist works with children being treated for cancer. Special dolls are used to familiarize children with the procedures that they will undergo.

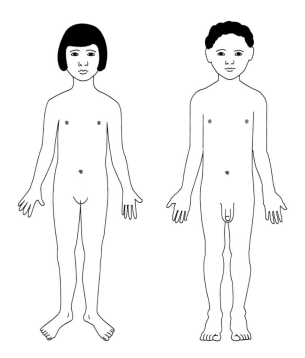

FIGURE 4–6. The nurse can use a simple gender-specific outline drawing of a child's body to encourage children to draw what they think about their medical problem. Such drawings reveal a child's interpretation, which the nurse can work with to provide appropriate care.

sense of mastery or control over frightening or little-understood situations. In the present era of cost containment, play programs may be minimized in hospitals. The nurse and others involved in caring for hospitalized children must document the needs and benefits of play.[8] Play that presents an opportunity to deal with the fears and concerns of health experiences is called **therapeutic play.**

Through therapeutic play the child's knowledge of his or her illness or injury can be assessed. A common technique involves using an outline drawing of the body (Fig. 4–6) or stories and asking the child to draw in or talk about what the illness or injury means to him or her.[9] Alternatively, the child may be asked to draw a picture or make up a story, enabling the nurse to assess fears and other emotions. The Goodenough Draw-A-Person test helps to assess the cognitive level of children between 3 and 13 years of age (Table 4–6). The Gellert Index is another tool that helps to assess the child's knowledge of the

4-6	Goodenough Draw-A-Person Test

- The child is asked to draw a picture of a person and to do so carefully and completely, taking his or her time. It is preferable to have the child take the test alone, away from parents.
- Points are assigned for specific details included in the drawing, for example, 1 point each for the presence of head, legs, arms, trunk, and eyes. Additional points are assigned depending on the complexity of details.
- For every 4 points assigned, another year is added to a baseline age of 3 years. For example, a child who scores 24 points (by including 24 details) would have a total score of 9 years (6 plus 3 baseline years). This number is compared to the child's chronologic age to determine his or her cognitive level.

The Goodenough Test may be obtained from the Psychological Corporation, 555 Academic Court, San Antonio, TX 78204.

body (Table 4–7). In addition to assessment, drawing can be used as a nursing intervention. Show the child on a drawing what will happen during surgery or a treatment. The child's drawings of health care experiences allow him or her to express fears and gain mastery over the situation.

A variety of techniques may be used to promote therapeutic play (Table 4–8). Specific techniques are chosen to reflect the child's developmental stage.

Toddler

Play is important for toddlers. Through play they explore the environment and learn to identify with significant people in their lives. Play is also an ac-

---

4-7   Gellert Index of Body Knowledge

Part A

What do you have inside you? Tell me as many things as you can think of that are inside you.

Part B

1. Show me the head. What is in the head? (Tell me all the things that are in the head.)
2. Make a circle showing where and about how big the heart is. What does the heart do? (What is it for?) What would happen if we didn't have a heart?
3. Show me some places where you have bones. (Try for a minimum of five locations.) What do we have bones for? What would happen if we didn't have bones?
4. Make a circle showing where and about how big the stomach is. What does the stomach do? Show me where the food goes after you swallow it. (Sketch in diagram.) And then? (If excretion is not mentioned spontaneously, ask: Does it ever come out anywhere? If the answer is affirmative, ask: Show me where it comes out.)
5. Make a circle showing about where and about how big the ribs are. Why do we have ribs? (What for?) What would happen if we didn't have ribs?
6. Make a circle showing about where and about how big the liver is. What does the liver do? What would happen if we didn't have a liver?
7. What do you think we have a skin for? What would happen if we didn't have a skin?
8. Make a circle showing where and about how big the lungs are. How many lungs are there? What do we have lungs for? What would happen if we didn't have lungs?
9. Do you have any nerves? (If no, ask: Does anybody else? If so, who?) What would happen if we didn't have any nerves?
10. Make a circle showing where and about how big the bladder is. What do we have a bladder for? What would happen if we didn't have a bladder?
11. How come we have bowel movements? (What for?) Where do bowel movements come from? (Probe for derivation from food, stomach, intestines.) Show me on the diagram. What would happen if we didn't have bowel movements? About how often (how many times) should people have bowel movements? About how often do you have bowel movements?

Part C

1. What do you think is the most important part of you? (If you picked one part of you as the most important, which one would you pick?)
2. Are there any parts of you that could live (get along) without? Which ones?

From Gellert, E. (1962). Children's conception of the content and functions of the human body. Genetic Psychology Monographs. Reprinted with permission of the Helen Dwight Reid Education Foundation. Published by Heldref Publications, 1319 18th St NW, Washington, DC 20036–1802

4-8	Therapeutic Play Techniques	
Technique	**Assessment**	**Intervention**
Stories	Have the child make up a story about a picture. Analyze content and emotional clues in the story. Have children tell a story about an important experience in a group of other children.	Read or make up stories to explain illness, hospitalization, or other specific aspects of health care. Emotions such as fear can be included.
Drawings	Administer Goodenough Draw-A-Person test (see Table 4–6) to evaluate cognitive level. Consider subject matter, size and placement of items in drawings, colors used, presence or absence of physical barriers, and general emotional feeling. Administer Gellert Index (Table 4–7) to learn about the child's knowledge of the body and its functioning before planning teaching.	Use the child's drawings or outlines of the body to explain care, procedures, or conditions. Provide an opportunity for the child to draw pictures of his or her choice or directed topics such as a picture of the child's family or health care encounter. Ask the child: "Tell me about your picture." Be alert to the child's emotions: "This child must be frightened by the big x-ray machine."
Music	Observe types of music chosen and effects of played music on behavior.	Encourage parents and children to bring favorite tapes to the hospital for stress relief. Have tapes playing during tests and procedures. Parents can tape their voices to play for infants and young children during separations. During longer hospitalizations children can tape messages for siblings or classmates, who are then encouraged to retape their responses. Playtime can include the opportunity to play instruments and sing.
Puppets	The puppets can ask questions of young children, who are often more likely to answer the puppet than a person.	Perform short skits to teach children necessary health care information. Include emotional content when appropriate.
Dramatic play	Provide dolls and medical equipment, and analyze the roles assigned to dolls by the child, the behavior demonstrated by the dolls in the child's play, and the apparent emotions. Dolls with handicaps like those of the child are especially helpful (see Fig. 4–7B).	Provide dolls and equipment for play sessions. To ensure safety, supervise closely when actual equipment is used. Respond to emotions and behavior shown. Use dolls and equipment such as casts, nebulizer, intravenous apparatus, and stethoscope to explain care. Use dolls with problems or handicaps similar to those of the child when available. Provide toys that foster expression of emotion, such as a pounding board and indoor darts.

Additional techniques, such as sand or water play or pet therapy, may be appropriate in specific situations.

ceptable way for toddlers to release tensions caused by stress or aggressive impulses.

Toddlers should be approached slowly, and the initial approach should be made in their parents' presence, if possible, to decrease feelings of stranger anxiety (wariness of strangers). Playing a variation of peek-a-boo or hide-and-seek using the curtain surrounding the toddler's crib or bed helps promote the realization that objects out of sight, such as parents, do return. The use of transitional objects, such as a familiar blanket or stuffed animal, can temporarily substitute for the security of parents. The toddler who is restrained can be read familiar stories. Repetition of stories promotes a sense of stability in the unfamiliar hospital environment.

A doll is a familiar toy that can be used to recreate a stressful environment, thereby providing an opportunity for the child to express and work through feelings. Other developmentally appropriate toys for toddlers include familiar objects from home such as measuring cups or spoons, wooden puzzles, building blocks, and push-and-pull toys. Playing with safe hospital equipment (bandages, syringes without needles, and stethoscopes) helps toddlers to overcome the anxiety associated with these items. Supervise these play sessions and remove hospital equipment when you leave.

Preschooler

The nurse can intervene to reduce the stress produced by preschoolers' fears through the use of some kinds of play. A simple outline of the body or a doll can be used to address the child's fantasies and fears of bodily harm. Playing with safe hospital equipment may help preschoolers to work through feelings such as aggression (Fig. 4–7).

Preschoolers like crayons and coloring books, puppets, felt and magnetic boards, play dough, books, and recorded stories. Both preschool and school-age children may enjoy playing with a toy hospital.

School-Age Child

Although play begins to lose its importance in the school-age years, the nurse can still use some techniques of therapeutic play to help the hospitalized child deal with stress. School-age children often regress developmentally during hospitalization, demonstrating behaviors characteristic of an earlier state, such as separation anxiety and fear of bodily injury. Outlines of the body and, occasionally, dolls can be used to illustrate the cause and treatment of the child's illness. Terms for body parts that are suitable for older children should be used. Drawings provide an outlet for expression of fears and anger.

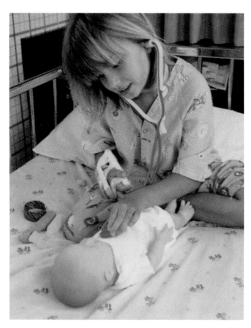

A

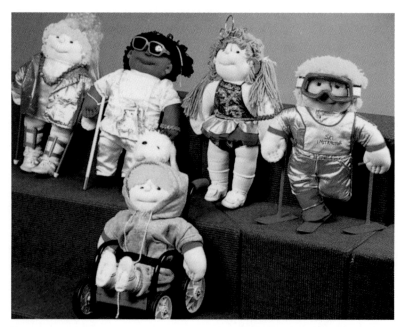

B

FIGURE 4–7. A, Age-appropriate play will help the child adjust to hospitalization and care. B, Having the child play with dolls that have "disabilities" similar to his or her own will help the child adjust. Such play helps the child realize what activities are possible.

School-age children enjoy collecting and organizing objects and often ask to keep disposable equipment that has been used in their care. They may use these items later to relive the experience with their friends. Games, books, schoolwork, crafts, tape recordings, and computers provide an outlet for aggression and increase self-esteem in the school-age child. The type of play used should promote a sense of mastery and achievement.

Therapeutic Recreation

Many of the special play techniques used with younger children are not suitable for adolescents. However, adolescents do need a planned recreation program to assist them in meeting developmental needs during hospitalization. Peers are important, and the isolation of hospitalization can be difficult. Telephone contact with other teenagers and visits from friends should be encouraged. Interactions with other teenagers at a pizza party, video game, or movie night or during other activities can help adolescents feel normal (Fig. 4–8). Physical activities that provide an outlet for stress are recommended. Even adolescents on bed rest or in wheelchairs can play a modified form of basketball.

The independence of adolescence is interrupted by illness. Nurses can provide choices for teenagers to assist them in regaining control. Giving them options and letting them choose an evening recreational activity can promote their feelings of independence. Passes to leave the hospital for special activities may be possible.

STRATEGIES TO MEET EDUCATIONAL NEEDS

Some hospitalizations are so short that the absence of the child or adolescent from school and peers is of minimal concern. However, if hospitaliza-

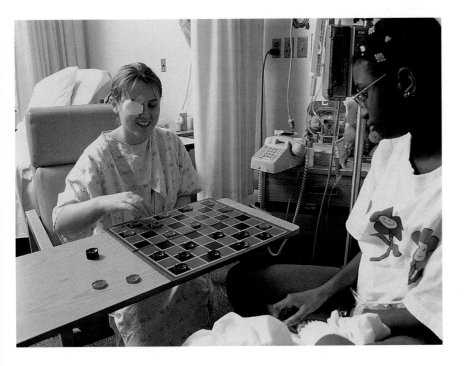

FIGURE 4–8. Having interaction with other hospitalized adolescents and maintaining contact with friends outside the hospital are very important so that the teenager does not feel isolated and alone. A friendly yet competitive checkers game helps to stimulate these teenagers and allows for self-expression. What are the other benefits?

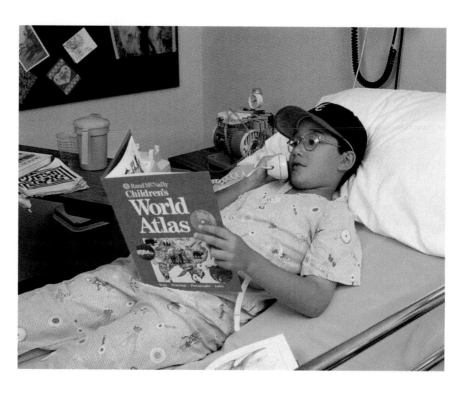

FIGURE 4–9. It is important that the hospital-ized child not fall behind in schoolwork. As soon as the child is able, schoolwork should be resumed. If the child is unable to get out of bed, all necessary study materials should be brought to the child.

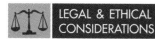

LEGAL & ETHICAL CONSIDERATIONS

The Joint Commission on Accreditation of Healthcare Organizations (1992) mandates provision for schooling of the child in a health care facility for an extended period.

tion is expected to last longer than a few days or if the child's condition will change, necessitating special school arrangements, the nurse should assess the effects of hospitalization on the child's education.

When an elective procedure occurs, families should be encouraged to arrange the extended school absence with teachers. The child can then be provided with schoolwork to do in the hospital or at home when well enough. This minimizes educational deficits and future problems for the child. Pencils, paper, comfortable work areas, and quiet work times should be provided (Fig.4–9). Telephone calls with teachers can be arranged as needed.

The social aspects of school and peers should also be considered. Peers can be encouraged to visit a hospitalized classmate, send cards and letters, or call on the phone. When the child returns to school, the nurse can visit the classroom to provide classmates with information about the child's med-ical condition.

The hospital nurse may contact the child's school nurse when special arrangements are necessary. For example, the child who is wearing a large cast or who needs medications or other treatments may offer challenges in a traditional school setting.

The child with chronic health problems or requiring long-term hos-pitalization has other needs with regard to school. Hospitals or reha-bilitation units may have classrooms, teachers, and facilities to pro-mote learning (Fig. 4–10). Many school districts provide tutors for stu-dents who are hospitalized or receiving home care for long periods. Telephone or computer contacts with the classroom may be neces-sary. Teachers can visit children at the hospital or at home. Parents are often pivotal in making arrangements to meet the child's educational needs, since they interact with the child, the school, and the health care team.

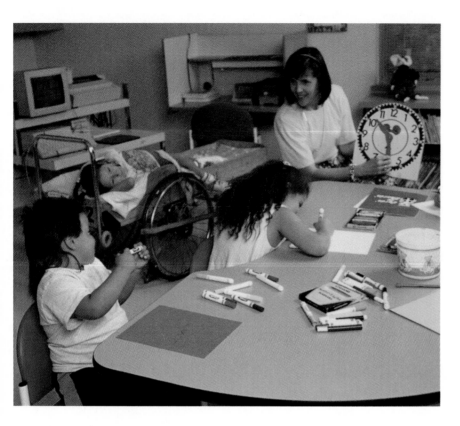

FIGURE 4-10. Shriners Hospital in Spokane, Washington, has a special classroom and teacher for children undergoing a lengthy hospital stay, enabling them to remain current with their schoolwork. The child who falls behind other students might not fit in when he or she returns to school or might be required to repeat a grade. What are the potential consequences of these situations?

PREPARATION FOR PROCEDURES

A number of procedures take place during hospitalization, from collection of urine or blood specimens to spinal taps and surgery. Special techniques can help the child to understand and cope with feelings about these procedures. Nurses should never assume that a procedure will not be traumatic for the child. Even providing urine in a specimen cup or undergoing x-ray examination can be frightening if the child does not understand the reason for the procedure or what to expect.

To assess the child's feelings about the procedure, ask the following questions:

- Does the child know the purpose of the procedure?
- Has the child experienced this procedure before? Was the experience painful, frightening, or reassuring?
- What does the child think will happen? Are the child's beliefs accurate?
- Is the procedure painful?
- What techniques does the child use to gain control in challenging situations?
- Will the parents or adult friends be present to provide support?

Preparation may begin a few moments to several days before the procedure, depending on the child's age. Use words that the child understands to describe the procedure and its purpose (refer to Chapter 2). Older children need explanations geared to their cognitive level and previous experiences

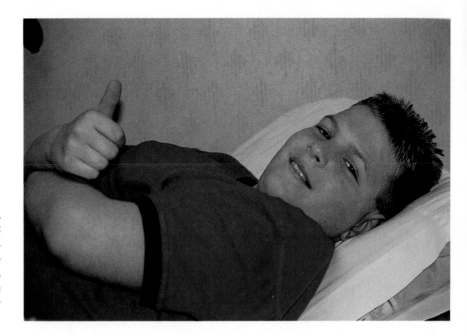

FIGURE 4-11. This boy was formerly afraid of blood draws but with the aid of health professionals has overcome his fear and can now have the procedure done calmly. He shows us his mastery over the situation. What can you do to help children afraid of procedures to develop coping mechanisms to assist them?

4-9 Assisting Children Through Procedures

Developmental Stage	Before Procedure	During Procedure
Infant	None for infant. Explain to parents the procedure, the reason for it, and their role.	Restrain infant securely and gently. Perform procedure quickly. Use touch, voice, pacifier, and bottle as distractions. Have parent hold, rock, and sing to infant after procedure.
Toddler	Give explanation just before procedure, since toddler's concept of time is limited. Explain that child did nothing wrong; the procedure is simply necessary.	Perform in treatment room. Give short explanations and directions in a positive manner. Avoid giving choices when none are available. For example, "We are going to do this now" is better than "Is it okay to do this now?" Allow child to cry or scream. Comfort child after procedure. Give child a choice of favorite drink or special sticker.
Preschool child	Give simple explanations of procedure. Basic drawings may be useful. While providing supervision, allow the child to touch and play with equipment to be used if possible. Since any entry into the body is viewed as a threat, state that the child's body will remain the same, and use adhesive bandages to reassure the child that the body is intact and parts will not "fall out."	Perform in treatment room. Restrain securely. Give short explanations and directions in a positive manner. Encourage control by having the child count to 10 or spell name. Allow child to cry. Give positive feedback for cooperation and getting through procedure. Encourage the child to draw afterward to explore the experience.
School-age child	Clear, thorough explanations are helpful. Use drawings, pictures, books, and contact with equipment. Teach stress reduction techniques such as deep breathing and visualization. Offer a choice of reward after procedure is completed.	Be ready to restrain child if needed. Allow child to remain in position by self if child is able to be still. Explain throughout procedure what is happening. Facilitate use of stress control techniques. Praise cooperative efforts.
Adolescent	Give clear explanations orally and in writing. Teach stress reduction techniques. Explore fear of certain procedures, such as staple removal or venipuncture.	Assist adolescent in self-control. Avoid using restraints. Assist with use of stress control techniques. Explain expected outcome and tell when results of test will be completed.

(Fig. 4–11). They will want to know what is happening, why, and what they can do to cope during the procedure (Table 4–9).

Provide written information for adolescents, and schedule time for questions and discussions. Adolescents can make many choices about their own health care. They can be asked such questions as, "Do you want a local or general anesthetic?" or "Do you want your hand numbed for the intravenous start?" Some adolescents want their parents involved in their care, while others prefer to minimize the parents' role.

The procedure should be performed as quickly and efficiently as possible. Parents may wish to be involved or may prefer to be available afterward to comfort the child. The parents or nurse can be designated to support the child. This may involve gentle touch, talking, singing, reassurance, or a stress-reduction technique.

Procedures on young children are generally performed in a treatment room so the child's own room is viewed as a "safe" and relatively pain-free site. After the procedure the child can be taken back to his or her room for comfort and reassurance. A choice of reward often soothes the young child. Table 4–10 describes strategies for preparing a toddler for venipuncture.

Preparation for Surgery

A child's surgical experience can be elective, planned in advance, or a result of an emergency or trauma. How a child responds to the experience depends on the psychologic and physical preparation he or she receives. The accompanying Nursing Care Plan for the Child Undergoing Surgery summarizes key elements of preoperative and postoperative care.

Preoperative Care

Preoperative care of the child includes both psychosocial and physical preparation for surgery.

4-10 **Communication Strategy: Preparing a Toddler for Venipuncture**

Twenty-eight-month-old Clarissa needs to have her blood drawn. How can the nurse best communicate with her?

1. Avoid telling Clarissa about the procedure in advance, since she has no concept of time and may become quite anxious. Tell her about the procedure just before it occurs and in simple terms: "We need to get a little blood from you arm. It will help us to find out if you are getting better. Your Mom will hold your arm real still so we can do it quickly."
2. Allow Clarissa to cry. Tell her it must be frightening and that you understand.
3. Perform the procedure in a treatment room so that Clarissa's bed and room are a safe haven.
4. Be sure Clarissa is restrained securely. Immobilize the joints above and below the area where blood is to be drawn. This way the procedure can be done quickly with the least trauma possible. Be sure the parent who is helping to restrain the child knows how to do this.
5. Use an adhesive bandage to cover up the site. This may reassure Clarissa that her body is still intact.
6. Praise Clarissa's cooperation and acknowledge that the venipuncture is difficult.
7. Comfort Clarissa by holding, rocking, offering a favorite drink, and playing music. If her parents are present, they can comfort her.

NURSING CARE PLAN
THE CHILD UNDERGOING SURGERY

GOAL	INTERVENTION	RATIONALE	EXPECTED OUTCOME

Preoperative Care

1. Knowledge Deficit related to preoperative and postoperative events

The child and family will verbalize procedures and events related to the operation.	• Ask questions of the parent and child about surgery.	• Prior knowledge and understanding can be reinforced and used to guide your presentation.	The child and family are able to verbalize details about expected preoperative and postoperative events. They ask questions that demonstrate understanding.
	• Teach about preoperative and postoperative events using appropriate developmental methods such as dolls, drawings, stories, and tours.	• Developmental level determines the cognitive approach that works best for teaching.	
	• Reinforce information the family has received about the purpose of surgery.	• The physician may have explained operation.	
	• Have the child demonstrate postoperative events that pertain to his or her case such as deep breathing, putting bandage on doll, taping intravenous line on doll, and pressing patient-controlled analgesia button.	• Concrete experience promotes learning.	The child demonstrates skills needed in the postoperative period.
	• Allow the parents and child to ask questions.	• Learners must have opportunity to ask questions.	

2. Anxiety related to preoperative and postoperative events

The child and family will show decreased behavior indicating anxiety.	• Question the child about expectations of hospitalization and previous experiences.	• Previous experiences can influence present anxiety level.	The child and family demonstrate less anxiety. They verbalize understanding and comfort in hospital routines.
	• Orient the child to the hospital setting, routines, staff, and other patients.	• Familiarity with the setting and people can decrease anxiety by removing unknown factors.	
	• Institute age-appropriate play and interactions with the child.	• Play can increase trust level and decrease anxiety.	Parents support the child for traumatic procedures.
	• Explain procedures and prepare for those that might cause trauma. Encourage parents to support the child.	• The child is more likely to trust caregivers if they are truthful and if parents are present.	

NURSING CARE PLAN
THE CHILD UNDERGOING SURGERY— *Continued*

GOAL	INTERVENTION	RATIONALE	EXPECTED OUTCOME
	• Allow the parents and child to ask questions.	• Questioning provides an opportunity to explain the unknown, which decreases anxiety.	

3. Risk for Injury related to exposure to nosocomial infection and use of preoperative medication

The child will show no signs of infection.	• Monitor vital signs at least every 4 hours. Inspect skin and respiratory status each shift.	• Increase in vital sign levels, skin lesions, nasal drainage, or adventitious breath sounds can indicate signs of infection in the child.	The child's vital signs and assessment are within normal limits.
The child will remain free of injury.	• Report any variations from expected vital signs.	• Symptoms are reported so surgery can be canceled if necessary.	
	• Keep side rails up after preoperative medication is given. Maintain NPO status when ordered. Transport the child to the operating room safely secured.	• Preoperative medication can alter level of consciousness. NPO status prevents aspiration.	The child is transported safely to the operating room.

Postoperative Care

4. Risk for Infection related to surgical procedure and intravenous line

The child will be free of infection.	• Monitor vital signs per hospital routine. Record and report changes from baseline.	• Changes in vital signs, especially increased temperature and pulse, can indicate infection.	The child shows no signs of infection.
	• Monitor surgical dressing and drains every hour.	• Excess drainage may indicate infection.	The surgical wound heals without infection.
	• Change or reinforce dressings when wet.	• Wet dressing can allow organisms to come into contact with surgical wound.	
	• Check the intravenous site every 2 hours for redness, swelling, pain, or pallor.	• Intravenous lines may become infiltrated or cause thrombophlebitis.	The intravenous line remains patent without signs of infection.
	• Teach parents signs of infection before discharge. Teach parents aseptic technique for dressing change and wound care.	• Parents report signs of infection and perform home care as needed.	The child continues to demonstrate no signs of infection at home.

Continued . . .

NURSING CARE PLAN
THE CHILD UNDERGOING SURGERY– *Continued*

GOAL	INTERVENTION	RATIONALE	EXPECTED OUTCOME

5. Alteration in Elimination: Constipation related to surgical procedure and anesthetics

GOAL	INTERVENTION	RATIONALE	EXPECTED OUTCOME
The child will achieve and maintain normal bowel functioning by the fourth postoperative day.	• Auscultate bowel sounds every 4 hours. Offer liquids only when bowel sounds are present. Assess the abdomen for distention.	• Restricting fluids avoids distention if peristalsis is not normal.	The child has bowel movement within 2 to 3 days after surgery with normal pattern by the fourth postoperative day.
	• Document the character and frequency of bowel movements.	• Knowledge of bowel status ensures early identification of constipation.	
	• Advance the diet as tolerated.	• Fluids and roughage promote normal bowel functioning.	
	• Increase activity as ordered and tolerated.	• Physical activity promotes peristalsis.	

6. Fluid Volume Excess or Deficit related to intravenous infusion and NPO status

GOAL	INTERVENTION	RATIONALE	EXPECTED OUTCOME
The child will achieve and maintain proper circulating volume.	• Monitor vital signs per hospital routines.	• Changes in vital signs, especially pulse or blood pressure, can indicate fluid imbalance.	The child remains in fluid balance with no vomiting in postoperative period.
The child will tolerate oral intake when started, with no nausea, vomiting, or dehydration present.	• Record intake and output. Be alert for fluid loss via dressings or watery stools. Evaluate hydration status by skin turgor and mucous membranes.	• Intake and output are roughly equivalent. Urinary retention sometimes occurs postoperatively as a result of anesthesia. Fluid status can be assessed by skin and mucous membrane hydration.	
	• Monitor laboratory values of hematocrit and hemoglobin.	• Increased hematocrit and hemoglobin can indicate hemoconcentration and underhydration. Decreased serum values can indicate hemodilution or overhydration.	
	• Begin oral intake after assessment of bowel sounds. Record vomiting. Administer antiemetics if indicated.	• Vomiting can cause fluid loss.	

NURSING CARE PLAN
THE CHILD UNDERGOING SURGERY— *Continued*

GOAL	INTERVENTION	RATIONALE	EXPECTED OUTCOME

7. *Ineffective Airway Clearance related to anesthetics and pain*

GOAL	INTERVENTION	RATIONALE	EXPECTED OUTCOME
The child will maintain adequate ventilation with no respiratory impairment.	• Auscultate lungs every 2 hours. Record rate, rhythm, and quality of respiration. Evaluate respiratory rate after analgesics.	• Early identification of respiratory difficulty aids early treatment. Analgesics, especially morphine, may slow respiratory rate.	The child remains free of respiratory complications.
	• Administer oxygen if ordered.	• Oxygen may facilitate breathing status postoperatively.	
	• Reposition the child every 2 hours.	• Repositioning ensures expansion of all lung fields.	
	• Encourage deep breathing and coughing every 2 hours. Use incentive spirometer, pinwheels, or other blow toys appropriate for the development level of the child.	• All areas of the lungs must be expanded. Mucus is expectorated.	
	• Ensure proper intake and output.	• Balanced fluid status ensures liquification of secretions and prevents excess fluid accumulation.	

8. *Pain related to surgical procedure*

GOAL	INTERVENTION	RATIONALE	EXPECTED OUTCOME
The child will maintain an adequate comfort level.	• Assess behavioral cues (eg, crying, movement, guarding).	• Behavior of preverbal children provides clues to pain experience.	The child's pain is controlled as demonstrated by a low number on the pain control scale (behavioral or verbal).
	• Use an appropriate pain scale with verbal children.	• Pain scales allow children to quantify the amount of pain (see Chap. 7).	
	• Administer prescribed pain medications on a regular basis.	• Narcotics and nonnarcotic analgesics alter pain perception.	
	• Use age-appropriate nonpharmacologic methods of pain control (eg, distraction, repositioning).	• Nonpharmacologic interventions interfere with pain perception.	

Continued . . .

NURSING CARE PLAN
THE CHILD UNDERGOING SURGERY– *Continued*

GOAL	INTERVENTION	RATIONALE	EXPECTED OUTCOME

9. Risk for Impaired Skin Integrity related to limited mobility after surgery

The child's skin will remain intact.	• Turn and reposition the child every 2 hours.	• Repositioning takes pressure off the skin and allows increased circulation.	The child develops no pressure areas.
	• Keep linens clean and dry.	• Clean linen decreases the chance of skin breakdown.	The wound heals without complication.
	• Check pressure areas when turning and rub erythematous areas with lotion.	• Rubbing increases circulation.	
	• Get the child up and ambulating when ordered.	• Movement decreases pressure on skin.	
	• Check the incision for drainage, redness, and intactness of staples or stitches every 4–8 hours.	• Early identification of infection or problems with wound healing can ensure fast treatment.	

10. Anxiety (Child and Family) related to equipment and surgical outcome

The child and family will verbalize comfort with postoperative care and outcome.	• Explain monitors, drains, dressings, intravenous lines, and procedures.	• Knowledge of purpose decreases anxiety.	The child and family demonstrate coping skills to deal with hospitalization.
	• Reassure the child and family that anxiety is a normal response to the stressful event of surgery.	• Knowledge of what is expected decreases anxiety.	
	• Encourage parental presence and care of the child.	• The child's anxiety decreases with parental presence.	

11. Knowledge Deficit (Child and Family) related to needed home care

The child and family will verbalize self-care required at home.	• Provide oral and written home care instructions regarding surgical wound care, medications, activities, and diet.	• Teaching regarding home care is necessary early in hospitalization.	The child and family demonstrate skills needed for home care following discharge. They verbalize plans for future care.
	• Provide a number to call for questions or concerns. Instruct on follow-up visits.	• Parents need to know emergency information and that follow-up care is required.	

Psychosocial Preparation

The goal of preoperative teaching is to reduce the fear associated with the unknown and decrease stress and anxiety associated with surgery. Teaching should be geared to the child's developmental level. If child life teachers are available, they can play an important role in preparing the child for surgery.

If the child will be in an intensive care unit or recovery room after surgery, a visit there before surgery can reduce the fear and anxiety associated with waking up in a strange environment filled with frightening sights, sounds, and smells. The use of tapes, anatomically correct puppets and dolls, drawings, and models is encouraged to teach the child about the surgical procedure. For example, a doll was used as a teaching aid in preparing Sabrina, the preschooler described in the opening vignette, for surgery. Playing with stethoscopes, gowns, masks, and syringes without needles also helps the child feel more in control. Children should be reassured that their parents can accompany them to the operating room floor and will be waiting when they awaken from surgery.

Physical Preparation

Preoperative procedures and guidelines vary among hospitals and outpatient surgical centers. Preoperative checklists are used in ambulatory and acute care settings to ensure proper physical preparation of patients for surgery. A sample checklist is provided in Table 4–11.

Postoperative Care

Postoperative care of the child includes both physical and psychologic care. The child's level of consciousness is evaluated, and vital signs are taken frequently. The surgical site is observed for drainage, and dressings are checked. The nurse monitors the child's intake and output and provides comfort and pain relief. (See Chapter 6 for details concerning pain management.) Parents should be allowed to visit with the child as soon after

---

4-11   Preoperative Checklist

_____ Check that consent forms are witnessed and signed and in the patient's chart.

_____ Be sure the child's name band is in place.

_____ Be sure any allergies are prominently noted in the child's chart.

_____ Remove any prosthetic devices, including orthodontic appliances.

_____ Check the child's mouth for loose teeth.

_____ Remove eyeglasses.

_____ Bathe and cleanse the operative site if ordered.

_____ Put the child in an operating room gown, allowing the child to wear underwear.

_____ Check that all special tests have been completed and the results are in the child's chart.

_____ Have the child void before surgery.

_____ Keep the child NPO before surgery.

_____ Give the child prescribed medications.

_____ Transport the child safely to the operating room.

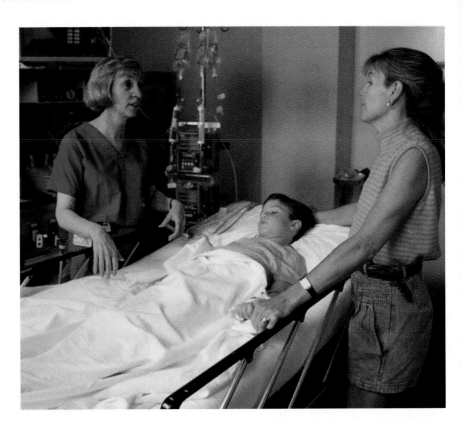

FIGURE 4–12. This child has just undergone cardiac surgery and is in the PICU. Although the child's physical care is immediate and important, remember that both the child and the family have strong psychosocial needs that must be addressed concurrently. It is important to reunite the family as soon as possible after surgery.

surgery as possible (Fig. 4–12). Refer to the Nursing Care Plan for the Child Undergoing Surgery.

▶ PREPARATION FOR LONG-TERM CARE

When ill or injured children require long-term care, they are often transferred from an acute care hospital to a rehabilitation center or other long-term care facility. The rehabilitation phase of the treatment does not begin at the time of discharge from the acute care hospital but, instead, early in the hospitalization phase. The plan of care is instituted in the hospital, interventions and therapies are begun, and plans are made for continued care.

When it becomes apparent that a child will need long-term care, the health care team explores with the family the options and resources available to provide such care:

- Home care with support services such as visiting nurses and physical therapists
- A long-term care facility
- A specialized rehabilitation center that can provide care for an extended period

The family should make the decision about which option will work best, considering the needs of the child, the financial implications, the roles and supports available to the family unit, and the resources available in the community. Guidelines to assist parents in evaluating rehabilitation centers are available from the The Brain Injury Association (see Appendix F).

Nurses in acute care hospitals frequently coordinate services when transfer to another facility occurs. This involves giving information about the child's history, plan of care, and treatment to the new facility. Forms are available to assist the person responsible for coordinating the transfer. Families will need support and assistance in dealing with the transfer from the acute care setting to another facility.

▶ PREPARATION FOR HOME CARE

Nurses play an important role in preparing the child and family for discharge home. When care will continue, the nurse works with the social service department, home care agencies, and the family to plan for equipment, procedures, and other home care needs. Home care nurses then take over the child's care and assist families to meet the child's health care needs.

ASSESSING THE CHILD IN PREPARATION FOR DISCHARGE

Discharge plans should begin early in the child's hospitalization. A health care team, including the physician, nurse, social worker, discharge planner, and family, works together to ensure a smooth transition home. An assessment of the family's ability to manage the child's care and of the appropriateness of the home for providing care should be made.[10]

Children with multisystem problems may require home care involving specialized equipment and personnel. Early planning gives the family time to investigate health insurance benefits, support services in the community, and other needs before discharge.

When a child is to be discharged home, the school district should be contacted and plans for education made. This involves an assessment of the child by the school district and formulation of an **Individualized Education Plan** (IEP). The IEP may include home tutors, specialized services from persons such as physical or speech therapists, or arrangements for transport of the handicapped child to the school and provisions for special medical care as needed.

Some common problems that interfere with successful discharge planning include financial concerns, the family's unavailability for teaching and planning, and poor communication and lack of teamwork among involved health care disciplines. Nurses should be alert to these potential problems from the initial contact with the child and family and should take precautions to solve them as soon as possible.[11]

HOME CARE TEACHING

The family may need to learn physical and rehabilitative procedures for the child's care. Short-term care may be necessary until the child regains full function. In other situations, care may be required throughout the child's life. This may involve measuring vital signs or determining blood glucose levels. For the child requiring complex long-term care, parents may need to learn about intravenous lines, medications, oxygen administration, or ventilators[12] (Fig. 4–13). Parents need to be taught how to use the equipment needed for the child's care and must show that they can use it correctly. They must be able to identify symptoms of distress and report them imme-

LEGAL & ETHICAL CONSIDERATIONS

The Education for All Handicapped Children Act, P.L. 94-142, mandates that public education be provided for all handicapped children from 2 to 21 years of age.

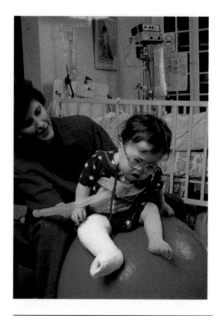

FIGURE 4–13. This child with chronic medical problems is being cared for at home. Are there any legal implications for the hospital and the nurse associated with the preparation of the child and family for home care?

diately to the health care provider. The education provided and the parents' ability to perform care are discussed with a visiting nurse or individual who manages the home care program. Parents should be encouraged to learn cardiopulmonary resuscitation. (Refer to Chapter 5, Nursing Considerations for the Child in the Community.)

Help parents explore options for respite. If they cannot provide daily care or need a break, they should be able to rely on others for a short period. Some agencies are available to provide respite care. Ongoing assistance may be needed to help families deal with financial, time, and other challenges.[13] Families with the greatest burdens in caring for their children will require the most interventions.[14]

PREPARING PARENTS TO ACT AS CASE MANAGERS

The family is an integral part of the plan of care for an ill or hospitalized child. The child with a chronic illness or an injury requiring long-term care will probably require the services of numerous health care personnel or health care agencies. One person needs to be identified as a **case manager** to coordinate health care and to prevent gaps and overlaps. In some hospitals nurses act as case managers. They may organize a patient care conference while the child with a chronic condition is hospitalized. Management goals are set and decisions are made about which health care provider or agency is responsible for helping the child meet each goal.

Parents can also be case managers. The parent as case manager coordinates medical care, hospital stays, and visits to specialists; meets with school district representatives to plan the individualized education program for the child; finds equipment, personnel, and other services for home care; and manages the child's overall care.

Nurses should strongly encourage parents who want to take over case management to do so. They can be assisted to learn the management skills required. Many communities have workshops for parents who are managing the complex care of their children.

REFERENCES

1. Bowlby, J. (1960). Separation anxiety. *International Journal of Psychoanalysis, 41*(2/3), 89–113.

2. Bibace, R., & Walsh, M. (1981). Children's conceptions of illness. In R. Bibace & M. Walsh. (Eds.), *Children's conceptions of health, illness, and bodily function.* San Francisco: Jossey-Bass.

3. Logsdon, D.A. (1991). Conceptions of health and health behaviors of preschool children. *Journal of Pediatric Nursing, 6*(6), 396–405.

4. Mobley, C.E. (1996). Assessment of health knowledge in preschoolers. *Children's Health Care, 25*(1), 11–18.

5. Rosenbaum, J.N., & Carty, L. (1996). The subculture of adolescence: Beliefs about care, health and individuation within Leininger's theory. *Journal of Advanced Nursing, 23*(4), 741–746.

6. Melnyk, B.M. (1995). Parental coping with childhood hospitalization: A theoretical framework to guide research and clinical interventions. *Maternal-Child Nursing Journal, 23*(4), 123–131.

7. Greenberg, L.A. (1991). Teaching children who are learning disabled about illness and hospitalization. *American Journal of Maternal-Child Nursing, 16*(5), 260–263.

8. Thompson, R.H. (1995). Documenting the value of play for hospitalized children: The challenge in playing the game. *The ACCH Advocate, 2*(1), 11–19.

9. Kreitmeyer, B., & Heiney, S. (1992). Storytelling as a therapeutic technique in a group for school-aged oncology patients. *Children's Health Care, 21*(1), 14–20.

10. Votroubek, W. & McCoy, P. (1990). *Pediatric home care: A comprehensive approach.* Rockville, MD: Aspen Publications.

11. Proctor, E.K., Morrow-Howell, N., Kitchen, A., & Wang, Y.T. (1995). Pediatric discharge planning: Complications, efficiency, and adequacy. *Social Work in Health Care, 22*(1), 1–18.

12. Feeney, D., & Kaufman, J. (1994). Caring for children with special health care needs. *Caring, 13*(12), 12–16.

13. Baginski, Y. (1994). Roadblocks to home care. *Caring, 13*(12), 18–24.

14. Jessop, D.J., & Stein, R.E.K. (1991). Who benefits from a pediatric home care program? *Pediatrics 88*(3), 497–505.

ADDITIONAL RESOURCES

Abbot, K. (1990). Therapeutic use of play in psychological preparation of preschool children undergoing cardiac therapy. *Issues in Comprehensive Pediatric Nursing, 13*(4), 265–277.

American Academy of Pediatrics. (1993). Child life programs. *Pediatrics, 91*(3), 671–673.

American Nurses Association (1996). *Statement on the scope and standards of pediatric clinical nursing practice.* Washington, DC: Author.

Azarnoff, P. (1990). Teaching materials for pediatric health professionals. *Journal of Pediatric Health, 4*(6), 282–289.

Azarnoff, P. (1983). *Health, illness, and disability: A guide to books for children and young adults.* New York: R.R. Bowker.

Azarnoff, P. (Ed.). (1983). *Preparation of young healthy children for possible hospitalization: The issues.* Santa Monica, CA: Pediatric Projects.

Byers, M.L. (1987). Same day surgery: A preschooler's experience. *American Journal of Maternal-Child Nursing, 16*(3), 277–282.

Coyne, I.T. (1996). Parent participation: A concept analysis. *Journal of Advanced Nursing, 23*(4), 733–740.

Darbyshire, P. (1993). Parents, nurses and paediatric nursing: A critical review. *Journal of Advanced Nursing, 18*(11), 1670–1680.

Fossin, A., Martin, J., & Haley, J.(1990). Anxiety among hospitalized latency-age children. *Journal of Developmental and Behavioral Pediatrics, 11,* 324–327.

Gottlieb, S.E. (1990). Documenting the efficacy of psychosocial care in the hospital setting. *Journal of Developmental and Behavioral Pediatrics, 11,* 328–329.

Jones, E., Badger, T., & Moore, I. (1992). Children's knowledge of internal anatomy: Conceptual orientation and review of research. *Journal of Pediatric Nursing, 7*(4), 262–268.

Oster, G., & Gould, P. (1987). *Using drawings in assessment and therapy.* New York: Brunner/Maazel.

Price, S. (1994). The special needs of children. *Journal of Advanced Nursing, 20*(2), 227–232.

Ramsey, A.M., & Siroky, A. (1988). The use of puppets to teach school-age children with asthma. *Pediatric Nursing, 14*(3), 187–190.

Redman, B.K. (1993). *The process of patient education* (7th ed.). St. Louis: Mosby–Year Book.

Riddle, I. (1990). Reflections on children's play. *American Journal of Maternal-Child Nursing, 19*(4), 271–279.

Santrock, P. (1997). *Children* (pp. 321–324). Madison, WI: Brown & Benchmark.

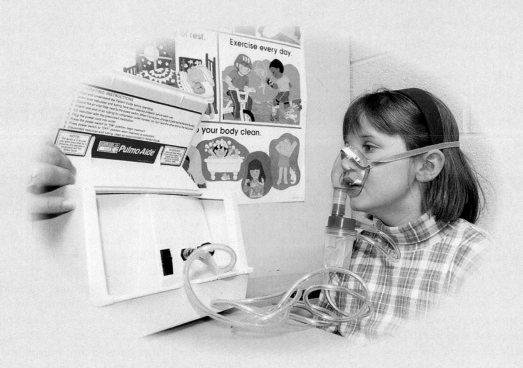

Jessica, 8 years old, is anxious because her asthma attack is getting worse. Her teacher sees that she is having trouble breathing, so she sends her to the school health office for treatment. Jessica has such severe asthma that a nebulizer is kept at school for her to use. This treatment will often relieve Jessica's symptoms and permit her to return to classes. However, in this case, the asthma attack does not respond to the treatment, and the school contacts her mother to come pick her up from school. This means another visit to the emergency department for treatment.

Jessica has had asthma since she was 2 years old and has needed to stay in the hospital for severe asthma attacks twice over the past 2 years. Fortunately, her asthma attack improves with the medications provided in the emergency department, and she can go home after a couple of hours. Jessica does not like to miss school or to worry her mother. Her mother wishes there were some way to reduce the number and severity of her asthma attacks.

What are some possible triggers of Jessica's asthma attacks at school? What measures can be taken to control her asthma on a daily basis and reduce the number of attacks? What special arrangements are needed to permit a child to receive care for asthma or another chronic situation while at school?

NURSING CONSIDERATIONS FOR THE CHILD IN THE COMMUNITY 5

"Sometimes Jessica's asthma attacks really frighten me because she struggles so hard to breathe. I don't like to send her out of class too soon, but I don't want to make her condition worse. I wish I knew what to do!"

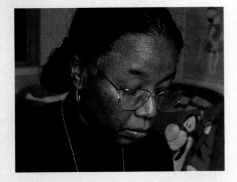

TERMINOLOGY

- **chronic condition** A health condition that lasts or is expected to last 3 months or more.
- **developmental surveillance** A continuous process of skilled observations of a child's fine and gross motor, language, and psychosocial behavior milestones throughout encounters during child health visits.
- **disability** Impairment in one or more of five categories of function— cognition, communication, motor abilities, social abilities, or patterns of interactions.
- **health supervision** The process of health promotion services, growth and development monitoring, and disease and injury prevention throughout the child's life.

- **medical home** A primary care provider or regular source of health care.
- **medically fragile** Children who need skilled nursing care with or without medical equipment to support vital functions.
- **screening tests** Procedures used to detect the presence of a health condition before symptoms are apparent.
- **sensitivity** Screening test value stated as the percentage of children testing positive for a condition who truly have that condition.
- **specificity** Screening test value stated as the percentage of children testing negative for a condition who do not have that condition.

Nurses care for children in a wide variety of community settings. Some of these settings include day-care centers, schools, camps, physician offices, hospital or public health clinics, and the home. The range of nursing care varies from monitoring the health and safety of children in day-care centers and schools to the provision of acute care to a child at home. Falling within this range are the provision of health supervision or well-child care, care for episodic illnesses and injuries, and assisting families to learn optimal management of their child's chronic conditions. Each of these nursing roles is important in promoting the health of children in the community.

Children receive most of their health care (health supervision and episodic health care for acute illnesses and injuries) in community settings. Depending on the community, health care resources, and age of the child, this care may be provided in any of the settings previously described.

During the past decade, the United States has begun to place a greater emphasis on health promotion and disease and injury prevention (health protection). The purpose is not only to promote optimal well-being and to reduce the pain and suffering of children and families, but also to reduce health care costs. Other patterns of health care delivery are also changing to reduce the costs of health care. Examples of these changes include day surgery in ambulatory surgical centers, newborn discharge after 24–48 hours, home care for long-term intravenous antibiotics, and short stay units associated with emergency departments. Managed care organizations and other health care providers continue to explore options to provide safe, high-quality care with fewer hospitalizations or shorter stays when hospitalization is needed. Home care services have developed to support families who now care for more acutely ill children.

This trend in out-of-hospital care is also seen among children with chronic health conditions and advanced disease states. Technologic advances, such as portable medical equipment, now make it possible to provide complex health care services in the home and other community settings (Fig. 5–1). Strategies to support families who provide care to their

---

LEGAL & ETHICAL CONSIDERATIONS

The 1975 Education for All Handicapped Children Act, P.L. 94-142, and the Education of the Handicapped Amendments of 1986, P.L. 99-457, guarantee a free and appropriate education for all children with disabilities between 3 and 11 years of age. This legislation was renamed the Individuals with Disabilities Education Act (IDEA) in 1991 and reauthorized by Congress in 1997. As a result of these laws, children with complex health conditions must be managed in school settings in the least restrictive educational environment.

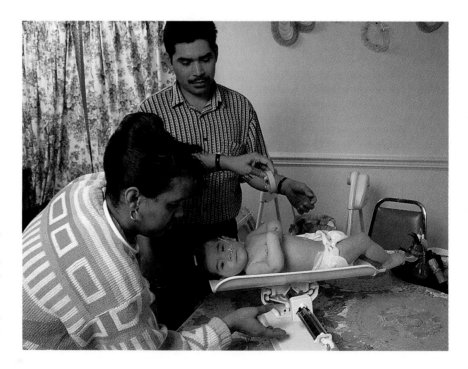

FIGURE 5–1. Nurses provide both short-term and long-term services to families in the home setting. In some cases, families need support for a short time after the child is discharged from the hospital following an acute illness. In other cases, families need assistance with complex nursing care for the child dependent on technology for survival.

children in the home have developed. Additionally, federal law mandates that education be provided to all disabled children, and there are no exceptions based on health care status. As a result, schools are now obligated to provide complex health care to children.

Care of children continues to shift from the hospital to community settings at a rapid rate. The nurse working with families in a community setting must use the knowledge of how the larger environment influences the child's health and development and the family's activities. To work effectively in the community the nurse's role includes:

- Making assessments, planning strategies, and implementing and evaluating approaches to care that match the family's economic and social situation, and available resources.
- Working with others in the community to make assessments, plan strategies, and implement and evaluate approaches addressed to the health care needs of the community's children.[1]

► HEALTH SUPERVISION

How often do children need health supervision visits? What are the elements of a health supervision visit? Why are children screened for health conditions at certain times?

All children need a regular source of health care, a primary care provider or **medical home** that supports the family and child during the important developmental years. When a family has an established relationship with a primary care provider, comprehensive, family-centered health services can be provided based on the provider's knowledge of the family's strengths and weaknesses.

Health supervision is the provision of services that focus on disease and injury prevention, growth and developmental surveillance, and health promotion at key intervals during the child's life (Fig. 5–2). It is not just a periodic visit for health care services. National guidelines for preventive health services have been developed for infants, children, and

Health supervision

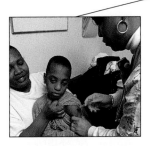

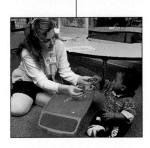

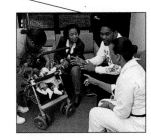

Disease and injury prevention
Screening tests
Immunizations
Safety teaching
Anticipatory guidance

Developmental surveillance
Observation of progress in areas of fine motor, gross motor, language, adaptive skills, and cognition.

Health promotion
Child and family guidance to promote family strengths in areas of healthy life styles, social development, coping, and family interactions.

FIGURE 5–2. Model of pediatric health supervision visits.

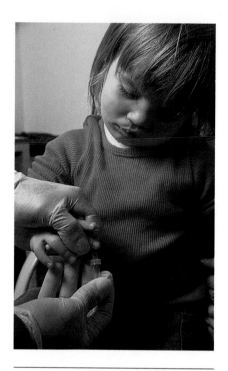

FIGURE 5–3. This 18-month toddler is having a blood screening test to detect iron deficiency anemia. Children are often screened for adequate levels of iron in the latter stages of infancy and during toddlerhood.

adolescents by the U.S. Department of Health and Human Services (DHHS) and the American Medical Association. Settings for health supervision visits vary widely within a community and include physician offices, community health centers, the home, schools or child-care centers, or shelters.

The health supervision visit must be individualized to the family and child. Every health visit, including an episodic illness visit or maintenance care for a chronic condition, is a potential health promotion visit. A tracking system in the primary care setting helps to identify appropriate health supervision activities for each child at every visit. For example, needed immunizations may sometimes be given during a visit for an acute condition if the child has missed a prior health supervision visit. Refer to Chapter 10 for guidelines.

Nurses play an important role in managing these health supervision visits. Depending on the setting, the nurse may provide all services or support the physician by obtaining an updated health history, screening for diseases and other conditions, conducting a developmental assessment, and providing immunizations, anticipatory guidance, and health education.

NURSING ASSESSMENT

Nursing assessment of the child and family at each visit for health supervision focuses on the following:

- Interviewing the family and child to update the health history, assessing the child's developmental or educational progress, identifying nutritional status and dietary habits, and discussing any concerns the parent or child has (see Chap. 3)
- Observing the family–child relationships
- Conducting developmental surveillance assessments
- Performing age-appropriate screening tests (Fig. 5–3)
- Performing a physical assessment

Disease and Injury Prevention

Screening tests are procedures used to detect the presence of a health condition before symptoms are apparent. Once a screening test identifies the existence of a health condition, early intervention can begin, with the goal of reducing the severity or complications of the condition. For example, all newborns are screened within 1 week of birth for at least two genetic diseases, congenital hypothyroidism and phenylketonuria. Appropriate interventions (medication or diet therapy) reduce the chances or severity of mental retardation if either of these conditions is present. (See Chap. 20 for more information about newborn screening.)

Screening tests are administered at times when children are most likely to develop a condition or to identify the greatest number of children at highest risk for the condition. Screening tests are also expected to correctly identify children who truly have the condition. Some children are at greater risk of contracting certain conditions because of their environment (Fig. 5–4). For example, young children living in housing built before 1960 are screened more frequently for lead poisoning than children who live in newer houses where only lead-free paints have been used. Table 5–1 outlines the recommended screening tests by age for infants, children, and adolescents.

SCREENING TEST INTERPRETATION

Sensitivity is the proportion of children with a condition who test positive for that condition. Some children who test positive do not have the condition; they are false positives.

Specificity is the proportion of children who do not have a condition who test negative for that condition. Some children who test negative actually have the condition; they are false negatives.

The best screening tests have both a high sensitivity and high specificity. If a child tests positive on a screening test, additional tests are usually performed to confirm the presence of the condition.[2]

Developmental Surveillance

Developmental surveillance is a flexible, continuous process of skilled observations of children's fine and gross motor skills, language, and psychosocial behavior milestones throughout encounters during child health visits. Information may be collected from several sources; for instance, a questionnaire that the parent completes, trigger questions asked during the interview, or observation of the child during the visit. Parents can also be interviewed to identify any developmental concerns they may have about the child. To initiate general health supervision and developmental surveillance, questions such as the following may be used.[3]

- Do you have any concerns about Sam's vision and hearing?
- What changes have you seen in Hannah's development?
- What kind of baby is Jamal?
- What do you and Brianna enjoy doing together?
- What are Brandon's favorite play activities?

Standardized developmental questionnaires are effective for developmental surveillance of most children, especially when time for health supervision visits is limited. These questionnaires are easy to administer, do not require the child's cooperation, and can be completed by parents in the waiting

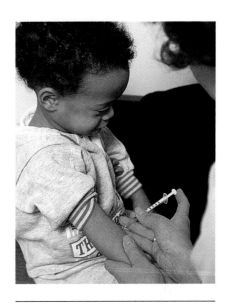

FIGURE 5–4. Children who live in an area where active tuberculosis has been detected or is epidemic need tuberculosis screening more frequently.

5-1   Schedule of Recommended Screening Tests for Infants, Children, and Adolescents[a]

Screening Tests	Year of Age																		
	0	1	2	3	4	5	6	7	8	9	10	11	12	13	14	15	16	17	18
Newborn screening																			
Head size																			
Height and weight																			
Blood pressure																			
Anemia																			
Lead																			
Tuberculosis																			
Hearing																			
Vision																			
Eye examinations																			
Dental examinations																			

[a]Recommended by most major authorities.
Modified from Office of Disease Prevention and Health Promotion, DHHS, Public Health Service. (1994). Clinician's handbook of preventive services: Put prevention into practice. Washington, DC: Government Printing Office, p. xviii.

5-2	Developmental Surveillance Questionnaires
Questionnaire	**Guidelines for Administration**
Parents' Evaluation of Developmental Status[a] birth to 4 years.	Consists of 10 questions for parents to answer in interview; based on research on parents' concerns.
	Requires less than 5 minutes to complete.
Prescreening Development Questionnaire (PDQ and Revised-PDQ)[b] birth to 6 years	Parents complete one of age-specific forms. Helps identify children who need Denver II assessment.
	Requires less than 10 minutes to complete.
	PDQ is available in English, Spanish, and French versions; R-PDQ in English only.
Ages and Stages Questionnaire[c] 4–48 months	Questionnaires for 11 specific ages, with 30 items each in areas of fine motor, gross motor, communication, adaptive, personal, and social skills. Parents try each activity with the child.
	Requires 10–15 minutes to complete.
	English and Spanish versions are available.

[a]Frances P. Glascoe, Radcliffe Medical Press Ltd., Oxon, England
[b]Denver Developmental Materials, Inc., P.O. Box 6919, Denver, CO 80206-0919
[c]Brookes Publishing Co., P.O. Box 10624, Baltimore, MD 21285-0625

RESEARCH CONSIDERATIONS

Past research has indicated that carefully eliciting parents' concerns about their child's development can be as accurate as screening tests in identifying true developmental problems.[4]

area. Children in need of more extensive developmental surveillance can be identified. See Table 5–2 for a list of commonly used developmental screening questionnaires that have been tested for validity and reliability.

When talking with parents, review physical, social, and communication milestones for infants and young children. Be aware that parents' recall of past developmental milestones is often faulty. The child is often reported to have achieved milestones at ages earlier than actually occurred. When accuracy of developmental milestones is critical, ask to see the child's baby diary or review the past health history at ages closer to the milestone achievement. The parent's report of current skills and achievements is usually accurate.

Review school performance for older children and adolescents. Review report cards, school achievement records, and any performance on psychoeducational tests when indicated. Inquire about the child's participation in sports and other activities, as well as noted abilities.

If a developmental delay or abnormality is suspected, a specific developmental screening test is needed to document developmental progress. See Table 5–3 for a list of commonly used developmental screening tests. Some health care providers actually use the Denver II as a developmental chart, like a growth curve to monitor the child's developmental progress (see Figs. 5–5 and 5–6). Remember: developmental screening tests are not diagnostic tests. They simply help to confirm that most children are progressing along an age-appropriate norm, and they help document suspicions or patterns of developmental problems.

To perform developmental screening with any of the standardized screening tools, make sure all directions are followed.

Screening Test	Guidelines for Administration
Denver II[a] birth to 6 years	Consists of observation of the child in four domains: personal–social, fine motor–adaptive, language, and gross motor. Requires 30 minutes to complete. A training video is available.
Bayley Infant Neurodevelopmental Screener (BINS)[b] 3–24 months	Consists of observation of child with 10–12 items for each of six age-specific scales. Requires 10–15 minutes to complete.
McCarthy Scales of Children's Abilities[b] 2.5–8.5 years	Consists of observation of child in domains of motor, verbal, perceptual–performance, quantitative, general cognition, and memory. Requires 45 minutes to complete.
Denver Articulation Screening Exam (DASE) 2.5–6 years[a]	Consists of observation of child's articulation of 30 sound elements and intelligibility. Requires 5 minutes to complete.
Early Language Milestone Scale—2 (ELM)[c] birth to 36 months	Consists of observation of child to assess auditory expressive, auditory receptive, and visual components of speech. Requires 5–10 minutes to complete.

[a]Denver Development Materials, Inc., P.O. Box 6919, Denver, CO 80206-0919
[b]Psychological Corporation, 304 E. 45th Street, New York, NY 10017-3425
[c]PRO-ED, Inc., 8700 Shoal Creek Blvd., Austin, TX 78758-6897

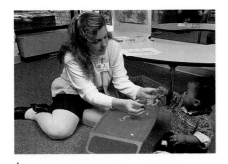

A

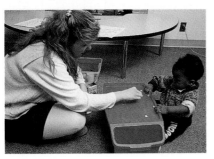

C

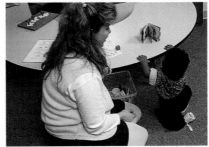

D

FIGURE 5–5. Follow all directions for performing the Denver II assessment and for interpreting responses. Develop rapport with the child and approach the assessment as fun. This often helps the child participate more actively during entire Denver II assessment. The 9-month-old boy in this sequence is able to perform the following age-appropriate behaviors: Banging two cubes **(A)**; playing ball with the examiner **(B)**; using a thumb-finger grasp **(C)**; and pulling to stand **(D)**.

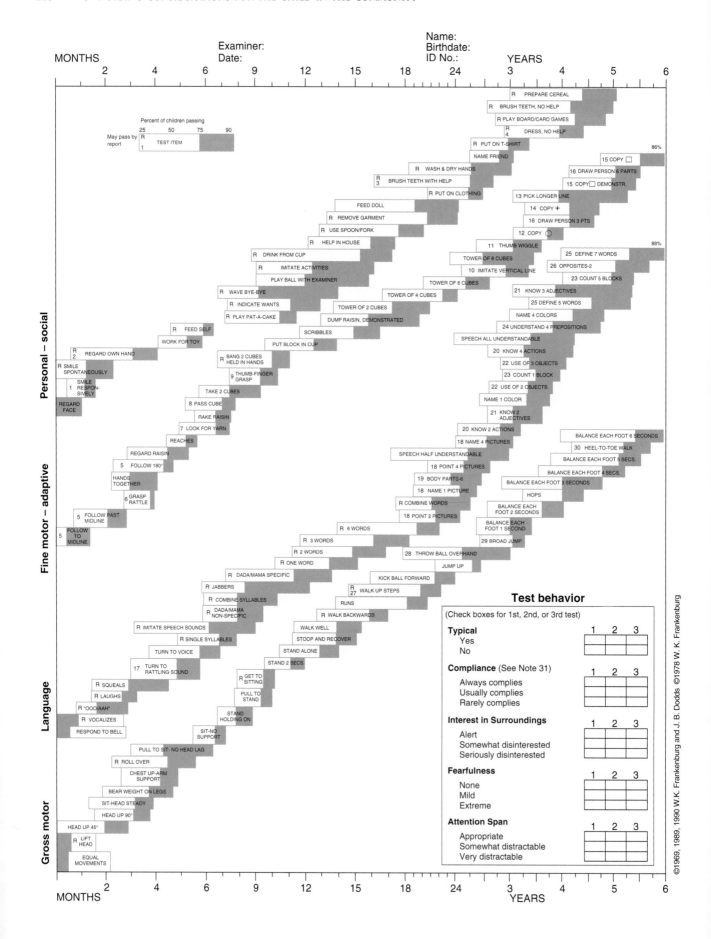

DIRECTIONS FOR ADMINISTRATION

1. Try to get child to smile by smiling, talking or waving. Do not touch him/her.
2. Child must stare at hand several seconds.
3. Parent may help guide toothbrush and put toothpaste on brush.
4. Child does not have to be able to tie shoes or button/zip in the back.
5. Move yarn slowly in an arc from one side to the other, about 8" above child's face.
6. Pass if child grasps rattle when it is touched to the backs or tips of fingers.
7. Pass if child tries to see where yarn went. Yarn should be dropped quickly from sight from tester's hand without arm movement.
8. Child must transfer cube from hand to hand without help of body, mouth, or table.
9. Pass if child picks up raisin with any part of thumb and finger.
10. Line can vary only 30 degrees or less from tester's line.
11. Make a fist with thumb pointing upward and wiggle only the thumb. Pass if child imitates and does not move any fingers other than the thumb.

  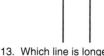   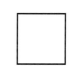

12. Pass any enclosed form. Fail continuous round motions.
13. Which line is longer? (Not bigger.) Turn paper upside down and repeat. (pass 3 of 3 or 5 of 6).
14. Pass any lines crossing near midpoint.
15. Have child copy first. If failed, demonstrate.

When giving items 12, 14, and 15, do not name the forms. Do not demonstrate 12 and 14.

16. When scoring, each pair (2 arms, 2 legs, etc.) counts as one part.
17. Place one cube in cup and shake gently near child's ear, but out of sight. Repeat for other ear.
18. Point to picture and have child name it. (No credit is given for sounds only.)
    If less than 4 pictures are named correctly, have child point to picture as each is named by tester.

  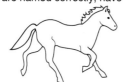   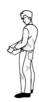

19. Using doll, tell child: Show me the nose, eyes, ears, mouth, hands, feet, tummy, hair. Pass 6 of 8.
20. Using pictures, ask child: Which one flies?... says meow?... talks?... barks?... gallops? Pass 2 of 5, 4 of 5.
21. Ask child: What do you do when you are cold?... tired?... hungry? Pass 2 of 3, 3 of 3.
22. Ask child: What do you do with a cup? What is a chair used for? What is a pencil used for?
    Action words must be included in answers.
23. Pass if child correctly places and says how many blocks are on paper. (1, 5).
24. Tell child: Put block **on** table; **under** table: **in front of** me, **behind** me. Pass 4 of 4.
    (Do not help child by pointing, moving head or eyes.)
25. Ask child: What is a ball?... lake?... desk?... house?... banana?... curtain?... fence?... ceiling? Pass if defined in terms of use, shape, what it is made of, or general category (such as banana is fruit, not just yellow). Pass 5 of 8, 7 of 8.
26. Ask child: If a horse is big, a mouse is_____? If fire is hot, ice is_____? If sun shines during the day, the moon shines during the ____? Pass 2 of 3.
27. Child may use wall or rail only, not person. May not crawl.
28. Child must throw ball overhand 3 feet to within arm's reach of tester.
29. Child must perform standing broad jump over width of test sheet (8 1/2 inches).
30. Tell child to walk forward, ⊂⊃⊂⊃⊂⊃ → heel within 1 inch of toe. Tester may demonstrate.
    Child must walk 4 consecutive steps.
31. In the second year, half of normal children are non-compliant.

OBSERVATIONS:

FIGURE 5–6. Denver II, page 216. Directions for administration of Denver II, page 217.
From W.K. Frankenburg, Denver, CO.

- Read directions thoroughly or utilize specific training tools available.
- Calculate the infant's age correctly, especially if premature.
- Attempt to develop rapport with the infant or child to get the best performance.
- In some cases, parents can be asked if a child demonstrates specific skills at home, especially if the child is not cooperative.
- Note the behavior and cooperativeness of the child during the screening process.
- Analyze the findings to make the correct interpretation.

Failure to perform a single item in a single domain does not mean the child has failed the test. The child should be reevaluated at a future visit. Provide parents with guidance on specific methods for stimulating the child. Failure of multiple items within one domain or across multiple domains is of greatest concern. When poor development patterns in one or more domains are revealed, referral for diagnostic developmental assessment is needed.

NURSING DIAGNOSES

Examples of nursing diagnoses for an 18-month-old child who is brought by parents for regular health supervision and immunizations may include:

- Altered Nutrition: More Than Body Requirements related to excessive amount of milk given to child daily
- Risk for Poisoning related to natural curiosity of toddler and increased mobility to reach and climb
- Altered Health Maintenance related to inadequate immunization
- Risk for Altered Parenting related to mother's plans to return to full-time work

NURSING MANAGEMENT

Nursing management for health supervision visits includes providing immunizations, offering anticipatory guidance, educating parents and children about healthy behaviors, carrying out collaborative nurse–family planning for health promotion, and providing referrals for follow-up care. For more information about the recommended schedule for immunizations and the nurse's role in ensuring full immunization status for children, refer to Chapter 10.

Most parents want to know how to contribute to their child's growth and development. Discussions at the conclusion of the health supervision assessments should focus on building family strengths by promoting the development of competence, confidence, and self-esteem in their growing child.

Although some specific interventions are most likely to take place only in a health care facility or physician office, most of the nursing management for health supervision can occur in any setting.

Provide Anticipatory Guidance

Anticipatory guidance provides the family with information on what to expect during the child's current and next stage of development. Topics for

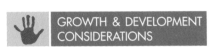

GROWTH & DEVELOPMENT CONSIDERATIONS

Community challenges that need to be considered during health supervision visits include:
- Poverty; inadequate housing; limited opportunities for employment; lack of affordable, high-quality child care
- Environmental hazards; unsafe neighborhood; community violence
- Isolation in a rural community; lack of programs for families with special needs; lack of social support; inadequate public services
- Lack of educational programs and social services for adolescent parents; lack of social, educational, cultural, and recreational opportunities
- Lack of access to medical or dental services; inadequate fluoride levels in community water

Parents who are experiencing more than two of these problems in their community may need extra assistance or guidance to provide a supportive environment for their child that fosters growth and development.

each visit should include age-appropriate information about healthy habits, prevention of illness and injury, prevention of poisoning, nutrition, oral health, and sexuality. Health promotion guidance also helps the child and family to develop strategies to support and enhance social development, family relationships, parental health, community interactions, self-responsibility, and school or vocational achievement.

Because the time for each visit is limited, build upon the parent's current knowledge and care practices. Time can be used to focus anticipatory guidance to introduce new information, to reinforce what the family is doing well, and to clear up any poorly understood concepts.

Take advantage of other sources of information in the community to enhance the guidance provided. For example, state and local SAFE KIDS Coalitions help inform families about injury-prevention strategies. School health programs may educate students about smoking and drug avoidance. Keep informed about the types of health education provided in different community settings so it is easier to reinforce the concepts already being taught.[4]

Encourage Health Promotion Activities

Often the family needs health education and counseling to promote healthy behaviors in their child. Examples of focused health education and counseling may be information about environmental control to reduce lead exposure; dietary changes to increase iron-rich foods; and reduction of milk intake for weight control or loss strategies. Counseling in the case of the 18-month-old toddler for whom nursing diagnoses were previously stated could focus on day-care arrangements and the anticipation and management of potential behavior problems.

Patient education and counseling are most effective when the family understands the relationship between the behavior change needed and the health outcome. The parents and child then work in partnership with the nurse or health care provider and make a commitment to the change or changes needed. Steps in promoting patient education and counseling include:[2]

- Working with families to assess barriers to behavior change.
- Involving patients in selecting a risk factor to change and the outcome goal.
- Gaining commitment from the parents and child to change.
- Using a combination of strategies.
- Designing a behavior modification program.
- Monitoring progress through follow-up contact.

Perform Health Supervision Interventions

After all of the information from the interviews, physical assessment, and screening tests is collected and analyzed, specific health and developmental achievements should be summarized for the parents and child. Immunizations are provided as appropriate. (See Chap. 10 for the recommended immunization schedule.) Anticipatory guidance may be offered at various points during the health supervision visit.

When a child is found to be at risk for a health condition or an actual health problem is detected, follow-up care must be arranged. The child may need to return for another visit to the primary care provider for further evaluation, or referral to another provider may be needed. The nurse needs to learn about all of the available community resources to make appropriate referrals. The range of such services may include:

- Hospital and community-based health care specialists from many disciplines (dentists, physicians, physical therapists, speech therapists, nutritionists, social workers)
- Community-based programs (child-care centers, developmental stimulation programs, home visitor programs, early intervention programs, mental health centers, diagnostic and evaluation centers, schools, family support centers, food and nutrition referral centers, public health clinics, churches, and other organizations that support families and children)

After appropriate education and counseling, the family and child need to collaborate with the health care provider in joint problem solving and decision making regarding the management of the child's condition.

Encourage parents to prepare for future health supervision visits by thinking about any questions or concerns they want to discuss. The success of the health supervision visit is largely based on how well the agenda of the family and child or adolescent has been addressed, as well as how adaptable they are to advice and change.

HEALTH SUPERVISION BY AGE GROUP

Infancy (Birth to 1 Year)

Health supervision visits occur frequently during the first year of life because growth and developmental changes are so rapid. Examples of developmental surveillance questions to use during infancy include the following:

- Do you have any specific concerns about Colin's development or behavior?
- How does Taneka communicate what she wants?
- What do you think Joshua understands?
- How does Tasha act around family members?
- Tell me about Emily's typical play.

Anticipatory guidance should focus on the infant's stages of rapid growth and development, injury prevention (see Chap. 2, pages 63–64), and nutrition (eg, adequate amounts of formula or breast milk, when to start solid foods, and avoidance of honey). Make sure the parents recognize their strengths in caring for the infant and other family members.

Health education focuses on issues such as colic, normal sleep patterns, bowel movements, skin and hair care, appropriate dress for weather, and prevention of sunburn. Teach parents how to recognize signs of early illness in their children, including fever, failure to eat, vomiting, diarrhea, dehydration, unusual irritability or sleepiness, and skin rash.

Early Childhood (1–5 Years)

Health supervision visits are needed frequently during early childhood for developmental surveillance, screening for health problems, and immunizations. Examples of developmental surveillance questions to ask during these visits include:

- Do you have any specific concerns about Jawan's development or behavior?

RECOMMENDED SCHEDULE FOR HEALTH SUPERVISION VISITS DURING INFANCY[5]

Prenatal
Newborn
First week
1 month
2 months
4 months
6 months
9 months

RECOMMENDED SCHEDULE FOR HEALTH SUPERVISION VISITS DURING EARLY CHILDHOOD[5]

1 year
15 months
18 months
2 years
3 years
4 years

- How does Nicki communicate what she wants?
- What do you think Jerry understands?
- How does Penny get from one place to another?
- How does Kevin act around family members?
- How does Lataye react to strangers?
- To what extent does Chris eat independently?
- Tell me about Jodie's typical play.

Anticipatory guidance should focus on promoting growth and development, nutrition, setting limits and discipline, toilet training, injury prevention (see Chap. 2, pages 69–70), family activities, conflict with siblings, day care or play groups, and showing interest in the child's achievements.

Health education should focus on good nutrition; feeding and mealtime strategies; tooth brushing, fluoride supplements (as needed), and dental visits; the child's natural curiosity about genital differences and masturbation; and management of common minor illnesses.

Middle Childhood (5–12 Years)

Health supervision visits occur less frequently during middle childhood as the health of most children is stable, growth has slowed, and screening for health conditions is needed less frequently. Examples of developmental surveillance questions to use at visits for children in this age range include:

RECOMMENDED SCHEDULE FOR HEALTH SUPERVISION VISITS DURING MIDDLE CHILDHOOD[5]
5 years
6 years
8 years
10 years

- Do you have any specific concerns about Shanelle's development or behavior?
- How do you think Ben is performing in school? How is his attendance?
- Does Shawn seem able to follow the rules at school?
- When Richie plays with other children, can he keep up with them?
- Is Marta proud of her achievements at school? Does she talk with you about what goes on at school? How do you acknowledge or praise these achievements?
- Have you visited Jorge's classroom? Do you participate in activities at his school? What does the teacher say about him during your parent–teacher conference?

Anticipatory guidance should focus on issues such as growth and development, school entry and educational progress, the growing influence of peers, injury prevention (see Chap. 2, page 84), setting reasonable expectations, recognition of achievements, setting limits and discipline, respecting authority, promoting independence, and beginning to have responsibility for chores.

Health education should focus on oral health, nutrition, need for regular physical activity, and teaching the child about personal care and hygiene, preparation for puberty and sexual development, and managing conflict.

Adolescence (12–18 Years)

Health supervision visits should occur annually during adolescence because of the dramatic changes occurring in physical, social, and emotional development. Adolescents need comprehensive clinical preventive services to deter them from participating in behaviors that jeopardize their health; to detect physical, emotional, and behavioral problems early; and to encourage behaviors that will promote healthy lifestyles.[6] See Table 5–4 for recommended health supervision activities by age.

5-4   Recommended Adolescent Preventive Health Services by Age and Procedure

| | Age of Adolescent | | | | | | | | | | |
| | Early | | | | Middle | | | Late | | | |
Procedure	11	12	13	14	15	16	17	18	19	20	21
Health guidance											
Parenting^a			■———			■———					
Development	■	■	■	■	■	■	■	■	■	■	■
Diet and physical activity	■	■	■	■	■	■	■	■	■	■	■
Healthy lifestyles^b	■	■	■	■	■	■	■	■	■	■	■
Injury prevention	■	■	■	■	■	■	■	■	■	■	■
Screening history											
Eating disorders	■	■	■	■	■	■	■	■	■	■	■
Sexual activity^c	■	■	■	■	■	■	■	■	■	■	■
Alcohol and other drug use	■	■	■	■	■	■	■	■	■	■	■
Tobacco use	■	■	■	■	■	■	■	■	■	■	■
Abuse	■	■	■	■	■	■	■	■	■	■	■
School performance	■	■	■	■	■	■	■	■	■	■	■
Depression	■	■	■	■	■	■	■	■	■	■	■
Risk for suicide	■	■	■	■	■	■	■	■	■	■	■
Physical assessment											
Blood pressure	■	■	■	■	■	■	■	■	■	■	■
Body Mass Index	■	■	■	■	■	■	■	■	■	■	■
Comprehensive examination	————	—■—	————		————	—■—	————	————	—■—	————	
Tests											
Cholesterol	———	—1—	———		———	—1—	———	———	—1—	———	
TB	———	—2—	———		———	—2—	———	———	—2—	———	
GC, chlamydia, syphilis, and HPV	———	—3—	———		———	—3—	———	———	—3—	———	
HIV	———	—4—	———		———	—4—	———	———	—4—	———	
Pap smear	———	—5—	———		———	—5—	———	———	—5—	———	
Immunizations											
MMR	——■—										
Td	——■—					○					
Hepatitis B	——■—					6				6	
Hepatitis A	———	—7—	———		———	—7—	———	———	—7—	———	
Varicella	———	—8—	———		———	—8—	———	———	—8—	———	

^aA parent health guidance visit is recommended during early and middle adolescence.

^bIncludes counseling regarding sexual behavior and avoidance of tobacco, alcohol, and other drug use.

^cIncludes history of unintended pregnancy and STD.

1. Screening test performed once if family history is positive for early cardiovascular disease or hyperlipidemia.
2. Screen if positive for exposure to active TB or lives/works in high-risk situation, eg, homeless shelter, health care facility.
3. Screen at least annually if sexually active.
4. Screen if high risk for infection.
5. Screen annually if sexually active or if 18 years or older.
6. Vaccinate if high risk for hepatitis B infection.
7. Vaccinate if at risk for hepatitis A infection.
8. Vaccinate if no reliable history of chicken pox.
○ Do not give if administered in last 5 years.

From Department of Adolescent Health. (1996). Guidelines for Adolescent Preventive Services (GAPS). *Chicago, IL: American Medical Association.*

Developmental surveillance questions should focus on physical, social, and emotional development (Fig. 5–7). The assessment of health behaviors and developmental surveillance become more closely related as the adolescent becomes more heavily influenced by peers. Examples of questions to ask include the following:

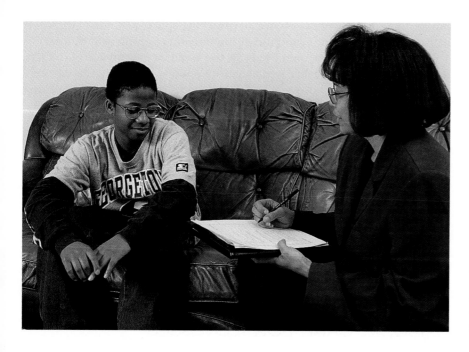

FIGURE 5–7. With adolescents, in contrast to the earlier developmental stages, developmental surveillance questions should be directed to the child rather than the parent.

- Who is your best friend? What do you do together? About how many friends do you have? How old are your friends? What do you and your friends do outside of school?

- What are some of the things that worry you? Make you sad? Make you angry? What do you do about these things? Whom do you talk to about them?

- Tell me some things you are really good at.

- Have you ever been in trouble at school or with the law? Have you thought about running away? Have you ever thought about hurting yourself or killing yourself?

- Do you think you are developing pretty much like the rest of your friends? How do you feel about the way you look? Has anyone talked with you about what to expect as your body develops? Have you read about it?

- Compared with others in your class, how well do you think you are doing? Average? Better than average? Below average?

- What types of activities are you involved in?

- What type of responsibilities do you have at home?

- Have you drunk alcohol in the last month? How much? What is the most you have ever had to drink? Have you ever tried other drugs? How often have you taken them in the past month?

- Do your friends pressure you to do things you don't want to do? How do you handle that?

- Do you date? Do you have a steady partner? Are you happy with dating or with this relationship?

- Have you ever been frightened by violent or sexual things someone has said to you? Has anyone ever tried to harm you physically? Has anyone ever touched you in a way you don't like? Forced you to have sex?

- What would you like to change about your family if you could?

Anticipatory guidance should focus on future healthy behaviors such as the following: school achievement, identification of talents and interests to pursue, how to deal with stress, use of protective sports gear, use of car safety belts, violence prevention, and use of sun screen to prevent skin cancer.

Health education should focus on the avoidance of tobacco products, drugs and alcohol; sexuality, sexual activity options (abstinence, contraception, and safe sex); and good health behaviors including nutrition, oral health, exercise, and sleep.

► HEALTH PROMOTION FOR CHILDREN IN COMMUNITY SETTINGS

What nursing care does the child with a chronic illness need in different community health care settings? How can you ease the transition back to school for the child with a chronic condition? How do you identify families that need extra support to care for their child at home? Nursing care in all community health care settings (home, school, specialty clinic, primary care office) is focused on minimizing the impact of the health condition on the child's physical and emotional development and functioning.

EPISODIC CARE FOR ILLNESSES AND INJURIES

During childhood, most children have several episodes of illnesses and injuries that require health care. In most cases, care is provided by the primary care provider. At other times, the urgency of the condition requires that the child go to an urgent care center or emergency department. The nurse's role in the cases of these episodic health care visits includes the following:

- Collecting health information about the condition
- Performing an assessment
- Assisting the primary care provider with any diagnostic or therapeutic procedures
- Educating the child and family about care of the child at home and how to identify any signs that the health problem is getting more serious

CARE OF THE CHILD WITH SPECIAL HEALTH CARE NEEDS

Children with a **chronic condition,** a condition that lasts or is expected to last 3 months or more, are also defined as *children with special health care needs.* Many of these children have **disabilities,** impairment in one or more of five categories of function (cognition, communication, motor abilities, social abilities, or patterns of interactions). Most children with chronic conditions are cared for in the home without home nursing or other health care services. Children with chronic health conditions need regular health supervision, as well as additional health services to help the child and family manage the condition.

Health promotion is as important for the child with a chronic condition as for other children. The child with special health care needs already has a condition that places him or her at higher risk for other problems, such as infectious diseases, injury, or developmental delay. The goal is to permit the child, such as Jessica in the opening scenario, to have as normal a childhood as possible.

The provider of care for children with chronic conditions varies by the type of condition, type of health insurance coverage, preferences of the family, and availability of pediatric specialty resources. Most children with chronic conditions, such as asthma, have a primary care provider. The primary care provider is usually the most knowledgeable about local community resources that may help the child and family. The child is often referred to pediatric specialists, as needed, for a review of the management of the child's health condition, and to make new recommendations according to the child's health status.

A pediatric specialist and advanced practice nurses may collaborate with the primary care provider to coordinate care of the child with chronic conditions, such as spina bifida, cystic fibrosis, or diabetes mellitus. In this manner, the child benefits from the most current health care guidelines and expertise in care for the specific condition. The child and family usually retain a primary care provider, who provides health supervision care and episodic illness care while serving as the child's advocate in the larger health care system. Sometimes a pediatric specialist serves as the child's primary care provider, but it is important to make sure regular health supervision services are not forgotten during the care of acute exacerbations of the chronic condition. Some children with chronic conditions may even require additional health supervision visits for added immunizations, such as the pneumococcal, meningococcal, and influenza vaccines.

Nurses working in hospital specialty clinics and other community settings can help assure that these children receive the appropriate health supervision services. The nurse in a tertiary care facility needs to identify appropriate resources and to help the family establish linkages with those existing in the child's community. This is a greater challenge if the child and family have traveled a distance to obtain the specialty services. It is often best to make sure the child has a primary care provider in the home community to provide regular care and to help with the coordination of local community resources.

The role of the nurse in caring for the chronically ill child in a community setting includes providing health supervision, teaching the parents to manage the child's care at home, providing guidelines to promote the child's growth and development, monitoring the child's health status, and referring the family to appropriate community services. Nurses providing care to children with specific chronic conditions need the following knowledge and skills:[5]

- Knowledge of the pathophysiology of the chronic condition and anticipated disease trajectory
- Knowledge of child and family reactions to the stress of the chronic condition
- The ability to work with the family in their efforts to manage the child's normal growth and development
- Assessment skills to identify any changes in the child's condition requiring referral or consultation
- The ability to communicate effectively with appropriate health professionals regarding any changes in the child's physical or psychosocial health
- The ability to work collaboratively with other health professionals
- Knowledge of resources (community agencies, tertiary care centers, specialty professionals) appropriate for the child and family with a chronic condition
- The ability to identify a dysfunctional family needing intervention

In Jessica's case, a nurse with some of the above knowledge and skills could collaborate with the primary care provider to help Jessica improve her asthma control. The recommended care of children with asthma has changed from episodic care for acute asthma attacks with minimal daily management to guidelines for aggressive daily management by the child and family (Fig. 5–8). Recognition of early warning signs of an asthma at-

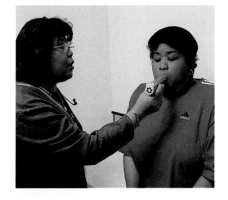

FIGURE 5–8. Nurses provide patient education to help families learn to recognize the early stages of an asthma attack by using a peak flow meter. The child learns the proper method for taking a deep breath and blowing into the peak flow meter so the best reading is obtained.

tack can lead to the initiation of extra medications in an effort to avert a severe attack. (See Chap. 11 for a discussion of asthma management.) The accompanying Nursing Care Plan outlines community-based strategies that can be used when working with a child such as Jessica and her family to improve asthma management.

NURSING CARE PLAN
THE CHILD WITH ASTHMA IN THE COMMUNITY SETTING

GOAL	INTERVENTION	RATIONALE	EXPECTED OUTCOME

1. Family Coping: Potential for Growth related to increased control of asthma with daily therapeutic care

GOAL	INTERVENTION	RATIONALE	EXPECTED OUTCOME
The child and parents will work in partnership with the nurse to improve the child's asthma management.	• Listen to the family's concerns about asthma management and respond with information to correct any misconceptions. • Teach the family skills (assessment, use of equipment, and giving medications) for managing the child's asthma attack. • Provide telephone consultation to the parents during management of the first few asthma attacks. • Educate the parents about when to call for future medical advice or to seek emergency treatment.	• The parents' concerns may not be the same as the nurse's. If the parents' concerns are not addressed, the parents may not comply with recommended care. • Proper use of equipment and appropriate medication dosage will help alleviate asthma symptoms. • Support and reinforcement of learning during an asthma attack will increase the parents' confidence in managing future attacks. • Parents need guidelines for judging the severity of asthma attacks.	The parents express greater confidence in averting and managing their child's asthma attacks.

2. Knowledge Deficit (Recognition of Early Asthma Signs) related to changing asthma care guidelines

GOAL	INTERVENTION	RATIONALE	EXPECTED OUTCOME
The child and parents will recognize early signs of an asthma attack and begin taking additional medications.	• Teach the child and parents to use a peak flow meter. • Help the child recognize his or her personal best peak flow and range indicating development of asthma symptoms. • Teach the family and child to give medications when the peak flow falls to the yellow range.	• The peak flow meter helps quantify changes in respiratory status before symptoms are detected. • Identifying a personal best peak flow helps establish the ranges to be used for future symptom identification. • Giving medications before an asthma attack becomes established may help avert the actual attack.	The number of asthma attacks requiring medical intervention is reduced.

GOAL	INTERVENTION	RATIONALE	EXPECTED OUTCOME

2. Knowledge Deficit (Recognition of Early Asthma Signs) related to changing asthma care guidelines (continued)

| | • Teach the child and family to monitor the child's response to medications with the peak flow meter. | • Monitoring the response gives the family information to determine when home care is inadequate and medical intervention is needed. | |

3. Ineffective Management of Therapeutic Regimen: Community, related to lack of school asthma management plan

| An Individual School Health Plan will be developed to help control and manage the child's asthma symptoms. | • Provide the family with educational materials to give to the school nurse and school administrators.
• Advocate for all children to have an asthma management plan developed.

• Support the family to have a school health plan that includes the physician's written orders customized for the child.
• Help the family to obtain extra equipment and medications that can be provided to the school.
• Work with the parents and school nurse to teach the specific asthma interventions to a designated person in the school nurse's absence. | • School personnel need the latest information about effective asthma management in school settings.
• Establishing a school policy will help all children with asthma receive appropriate care.
• The child with severe asthma needs a personalized care plan to be most successful in controlling asthma attacks.
• Schools will provide care, but the families must provide all supplies, equipment, and medications.
• School nurses often travel between several schools. The school administrator or secretary often serves as the backup care provider. | Implementation of the school health plan reduces the number of school absences for asthma attacks that occur during school hours. |

4. Body Image Disturbance (Child) related to need to seek special care during school hours

| The child's improved control over asthma will increase his or her self-esteem and peer relationships. | • Assess the child's peer relationships and opportunities for age-appropriate interactions.
• Motivate the child and family to gain increased control of asthma so the child can participate in normal childhood activities.
• Identify types of conflict and teasing the child experiences with peers, and teach the child defense tactics to deal with them. | • Assessment is important to identify the best strategies to support the child and family.
• Motivation may increase compliance with recommended daily asthma control interventions.

• If the child is able to gain some control over these situations, his or her self-esteem will be improved. | The child establishes friendships and engages in activities with peers. |

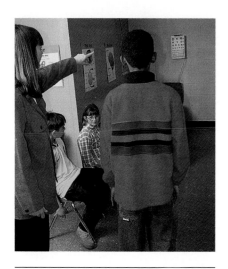

FIGURE 5–9. The school is often the setting for screening tests of large groups of students at risk for a problem. Screening tests are often organized so all children in a particular grade are assessed, as in this test to detect vision problems.

NURSING IN A SCHOOL SETTING

School nurses work to remove or minimize the health barriers to learning so students can perform academically. Nursing actions for all children focus on the following strategies:

- Reducing infectious disease transmission so school attendance is improved
- Promoting healthy behaviors through health education
- Providing safe school facilities by inspecting the school environment for hazards
- Screening children for health conditions that are common among school-age children (such as vision and hearing impairments, and scoliosis) (Fig. 5–9)
- Planning health promotion strategies
- Building effective student–family–school–community support systems

Table 5–5 presents Standards of School Nursing Care.

Emergency preparedness is important and a plan of managing the emergency care of all students should be developed. Injuries and acute illnesses occur frequently during school hours. School personnel (administrators, secretaries, and health aides in the absence of the school nurse) need to be trained to distinguish between an emergency and an urgent problem that parents should be called to manage. Guidelines for activation of the community's emergency medical services (EMS) should be developed in collaboration with the local EMS agency.

5-5	Standards of School Nursing Care

1. The school nurse uses a distinct clinical knowledge base for decision making in nursing practice.
2. The school nurse uses a systematic approach to problem solving in nursing practice.
3. The school nurse contributes to the education of the patient with special health needs by assessing the patient, planning and providing appropriate nursing care, and evaluating the identified outcomes of care.
4. The school nurse uses effective written, verbal, and nonverbal communication skills.
5. The school nurse establishes and maintains a comprehensive school program.
6. The school nurse collaborates with other school professionals, parents, and caregivers to meet the health, developmental, and educational needs of patients.
7. The school nurse collaborates with members of the community in the delivery of health and social services and uses knowledge of community health systems and resources to function as a school–community liaison.
8. The school nurse assists students, families, and the school community to achieve optimal levels of wellness through appropriately designed and delivered health education.
9. The school nurse contributes to nursing and school health through innovations in practice and participation in research or research-related activities.
10. The school nurse identifies, delineates, and clarifies the nursing role, promotes quality of care, pursues continued professional enhancement, and demonstrates professional conduct.

Proctor, S., Lordi, S., & Zaiger, D. (1993). School nursing practice—Roles and standards. Scarborough, ME: National Association of School Nurses.

Children with chronic conditions may have special challenges when attending school. An Individual School Health Plan, developed collaboratively by the parent, child, school nurse, school administrator, and teachers, is a formal mechanism to assure that the child's health needs are managed (Fig. 5–10). In some cases the health plan is integrated into the child's Individualized Education Plan or Individual Family Service Plan. The information in this plan is treated confidentially, but stored in an easily accessible area for personnel who may have to provide care. The parent provides medications, supplies, and equipment along with the physician's written instructions for care. In some cases, school personnel must be trained to care for the child who has special equipment, including special precautions when providing care. The school nurse often provides the training to school personnel who will be responsible for providing care.

When a child returns to school following the diagnosis of a chronic condition or a significant change in condition, the child's nurse (in either the hospital or community setting) can help with the transition of the child back to the classroom. Contact the school administrators and school nurse. Work with the family to begin preparing teachers and school administrators for the child's special needs. Send educational materials about the child's condition to the school. Often an Individual School Health Plan must be developed or modified. Work with the child's family and teachers to prepare classmates for the visible changes they will see in the child. Help them understand more about the child's condition.

NURSE'S ROLE IN OTHER COMMUNITY SETTINGS

In several other settings in the community, the nurse's role may parallel that in a school setting. Promoting health and preventing disease and injury are equally important in day-care centers, camps, health department clinics, and shelters. For example, nurses work with day-care center admin-

CLINICAL TIP

Make sure the Individual School Health Plan includes directions for care of the child on the bus, on field trips, and during extracurricular activities.

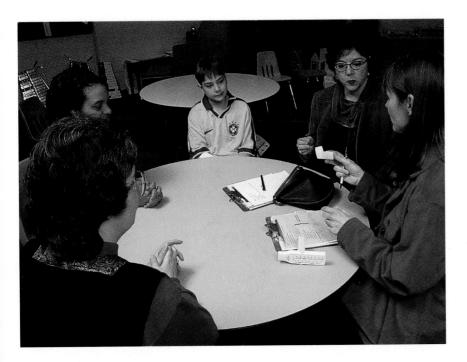

FIGURE 5–10. Because some children need medications or other therapies during school hours, the parents and child, school nurse, teacher, and school administrators develop a plan to manage the child's condition during school hours. This document is the child's Individual School Health Plan.

istrators to address infection control issues and to assess the safety of the children's environment. Nurses in camps assess the safety of the children's environment, but also provide nursing care to children with acute illnesses and injuries and plan activities to promote health. Some special camps for children with chronic conditions must have trained personnel to provide needed medical and nursing care while children are participating in recreational activities. Children in health department clinics and shelters need health supervision services as well as linkage with other community resources to promote health.

▶ FAMILY ASSESSMENT

The strength, resilience, coping skills, and resources of a child's family plays a major role in fostering the child's growth and development, as well as managing the child's health problems. When providing care to children in all settings, taking time to assess the family will help you to plan and provide nursing care that corresponds to the family's values, resources, and abilities. Information about the family's structure, home and community environments, occupation and education, and cultural characteristics should be collected. Information about the way the family functions in nurturing its members, problem solving, and communicating may help identify strategies that are potentially more effective for management of the child's health care. Tables 3–4 and 3–7, in Chapter 3, provide suggestions for information that should be collected for the family assessment.

The presence of a chronic illness or disability adds a dimension of developmental risk for an infant, child, or youth. The child and family members can respond with either psychologic or behavioral problems. Families need support to increase their resources and coping behaviors so they can successfully manage the multiple stressors, strains, and hassles of daily living along with the child's chronic condition.

Resilient families are able to bounce back from the stresses and challenges while adapting to successfully manage the child's chronic illness or disability. These families have effective coping behaviors and the ability to acquire and maintain needed resources for managing the demands of the child's condition. Characteristics of a resilient family include:[7]

- Balancing the child's illness with other family needs
- Forming collaborative relationships with health care professionals
- Maintaining a professional relationship rather than a friendship relationship with providers
- Developing competence in communication skills
- Maintaining family flexibility and adapting to changing circumstances
- Maintaining a commitment to the family as a unit
- Attributing positive meaning to the situation
- Maintaining supportive relationships outside the family
- Engaging in active coping efforts with effective and efficient problem-solving abilities

Most families do not naturally develop resilience. Often nursing support is needed to help family members learn new skills, make adaptations, and gain confidence in their abilities to manage the challenges they face. Nurses need to help families identify their strengths and areas for improvement that will lead to increased resiliency.

NURSING ASSESSMENT

Family Assessment Tools

Several family assessment tools have been developed that help measure family coping and functioning. Identification of family strengths and deficits gives nurses information that can be used to support family development—to reinforce family functioning, for family education, for intervention directed to meet special needs, and for referrals to community resources for long-term follow-up.

The Family APGAR is a good initial screening tool that focuses on the family's *a*daptation, *p*artnership, *g*rowth, *a*ffection, and *r*esolve (Table 5–6). The five-item questionnaire can be administered quickly. All family members

---

5-6   The Family APGAR Questionnaire

PART I

The following questions have been designed to help us better understand you and your family. You should feel free to ask questions about any item in the questionnaire.

The space for comments should be used when you wish to give additional information or if you wish to discuss the way the question is applied to your family. Please try to answer all questions.

Family is defined as the individual(s) with whom you usually live. If you live alone, your "family" consists of persons with whom you now have the strongest emotional ties.[a]

For each question, check only one box

	Almost always	Some of the time	Hardly ever
I am satisfied that I can turn to my family for help when something is troubling me. Comments:	☐	☐	☐
I am satisfied with the way my family talks over things with me and shares problems with me. Comments:	☐	☐	☐
I am satisfied that my family accepts and supports my wishes to take on new activities or directions. Comments:	☐	☐	☐
I am satisfied with the way my family expresses affection and responds to my emotions, such as anger, sorrow, and love. Comments:	☐	☐	☐
I am satisfied with the way my family and I share time together. Comments:	☐	☐	☐

---

[a]According to which member of the family is being interviewed the interviewer may substitute for the word "family" either spouse, significant other, parents, or children.
From Smilkstein, G. (1978). The family APGAR: A proposal for a family function test and its use by physicians. Journal of Family Practice, 6(6), 1231–1239.

are asked to complete the questionnaire, so the nurse gains a picture of the family's perspective on family functioning. Be more concerned if the majority of responses fall in the "hardly ever" category or responses vary a lot among family members. This may indicate a family that needs much more support to cope with the demands of daily life and management of the child's condition. Discuss the findings with the family members.

The Family Profile (Table 5–7) is another family assessment tool that will be of help when parents are caring for a child with special health care needs in the home. The parents complete this survey of their resources and current use of community services. This assessment may set the stage for the family to become a fully collaborative partner in caring for the child with a serious chronic condition.

5-7   Questions from the Family Profile

Family Structure/Roles

Do you want to care for your child at home?

Are you aware of any alternatives to home care?

Who are your child's primary caregivers?

Who are the other members of your household?

Can you identify another person to act as backup caregiver for your child.

Are there others (friends/family members) who can assist you with your child with special needs, with your other children, or with your family obligations?

Medical Management

Have you completed the hospital training in your child's care? If no, what is left to learn?

Has your child's backup caregiver completed training? If no, what is left to learn?

Do you or your backup caregiver need refresher training for anything?

Do you have transportation to medical appointments?

Do you need help in selecting a nursing provider?

Do you need help in selecting a vendor?

Nutrition

How is your child fed?

If formula, will you need help to buy/locate the formula?

Have you applied for WIC?

Does your child have a special need for diapers that is greater than the norm?

Education

Will your child be going out to school?

Do you know which school your child will attend?

Has your child been referred for the Infant and Toddler program?

Do you have an IFSP for your child? An IEP?

Do you have a contact person in the school program?

Will your child need adaptive equipment at home?

Parenting/Child Care

What hours/shifts do you think you will need nursing for your child?

In the event you need to leave home quickly or if you become in-

capacitated, who will watch your child with special needs? Your other children?

What is your plan for child care in the event of the nurse's absence?

Will you need help in finding day care for your other children?

Do you work outside the home? Any plans for the future?

Do you go to school? Any plans for the future?

Financial Resources

Does your child have medical insurance? Are your other children covered under a family insurance plan?

Do you need more information about or referrals to WIC, SSI, TANF, Food Stamps, Housing, Respite Care?

Do you need help in obtaining everyday supplies for your child?

Do you need a referral for help in obtaining other items for your child, such as furniture, clothing, toys?

Do you need help with budgeting?

Community Resources

Are you involved with any other helping agencies or persons, especially those you would like to include in this planning process?

Do you or other family members belong to a church? Social groups? Clubs? Associations?

Would you like to talk to another parent who has a child with special needs?

Would you like a referral to a support group?

Do you want a referral for counseling? Individual? Marital? Family? Child? Sibling?

Family Life

Do you see your child's homecoming as making a significant change in your lifestyle, and if so, how?

Do you have concerns about your other children?

Can you describe how you see your child in a few months? What are your short-term goals for your child?

Can you describe how you see your child in a few years? What are your long-term goals for your child?

How would you describe your family strengths?

What are your family's needs at this time?

From McCord, B. (1993). Family Profile. Millersville, MD: Coordinating Center for Home and Community Care.

Home Assessment Tools

Assess the home environment to determine factors that promote the child's growth and development. Both assessments will help the nurse plan care that will promote safety for the child and strategies to promote the child's development.

The Home Observation for Measurement of the Environment (HOME) is an assessment tool developed to measure the quality and quantity of stimulation and support available to the child in the home environment[8] (Fig. 5–11). Four age-specific scales are available (birth to 3 years, 3–6 years, 6–10 years, and 10–15 years). Examples of subscales within each age-specific scale include parental responsivity, acceptance of child, the physical environment, learning materials, variety in experience, and parental involvement. Data are collected during an informal, low-stress interview and observation over approximately an hour. The child must be awake during the majority of the interview. Observation of the parent–child interaction is an essential part of the assessment. The intent is to allow family members to act normally.

NURSING DIAGNOSES

Several nursing diagnoses may result from the family and home assessment, among them:

- Risk for Caregiver Role Strain related to child with a newly diagnosed chronic condition
- Impaired Social Interaction (Parents and Child) related to child's chronic condition and lack of family or respite support for community interaction
- Family Coping: Potential for Growth related to strong family communication, commitment to family unit, and social support system
- Ineffective Family Coping: Compromised, related to multiple burdens of inadequate finances and demands to meet other family member needs

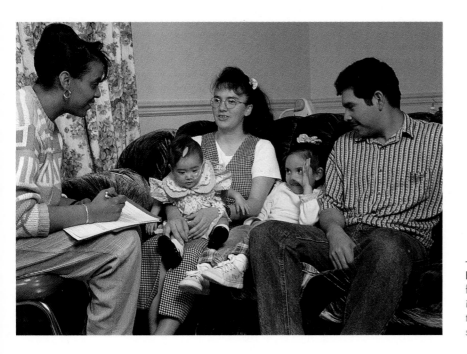

FIGURE 5–11. A visit to the home when all family members are present provides the best information for completion of an assessment tool such as the Home Observation for Measurement of the Environment (HOME).

• Risk for Altered Parent/Infant Attachment related to dependence on technology and stress of home care

NURSING MANAGEMENT

Work to establish a therapeutic relationship with the family. This relationship should be characterized by empathy and trust, as well as the development of mutually identified goals for the child's care. To help families develop resiliency, focus on family competence and strengths. Acknowledge and validate their emotions. Provide information in a clear, timely, and sensitive manner. Ask questions that help direct the family's thinking rather than providing them with all of the answers. Work with families to create solutions until they are able to solve problems independently.[9] Linkage with other families who have faced similar situations may be helpful.

Refer families with moderate or severe dysfunctioning to community resources for social support and counseling as appropriate. Make sure the family has a coordinator of care, especially when a family member seems to be unable to assume the case management role initially. When families seem unable to use referrals and recommendations for identifying and obtaining community assistance, the nurse can help in some additional ways:[10]

• Call and act as the family's advocate.

• Help with role rehearsal.

• Provide instructions and support.

• Connect the family with a volunteer who can accompany the family to services.

• Perform or refer the family for case management services.

▶ HOME HEALTH CARE NURSING

• Children with prolonged dependence on a medical device that is required to sustain life (mechanical ventilators, intravenous nutrition or drugs, tracheostomy, suctioning, oxygen, or tube feedings)
• Children with prolonged dependence on other medical devices that compensate for vital body functions who require daily or near daily nursing care (apnea monitors, renal dialysis, urinary catheters, and colostomies)

Home health care is a component of the continuum of comprehensive health care provided to individuals and families in their home. Many of the children needing home health care are **medically fragile,** children who need skilled nursing care with or without medical equipment to support vital functions. Only 2–5% of these children have chronic conditions serious enough to need regular home health care services.[12] Home health care services may also be provided for short intervals to help families during their child's acute recovery, such as a child with a fractured femur being cared for at home in traction or in a spica cast. There are two major goals of working with families in the home care setting:

• Promoting or restoring health while attempting to minimize the effects of the disability and illness, including terminal illness

• Promoting child or family self-care capacity in the home

Home care nursing is focused on assisting a family to gain a greater ability to manage the care of a child with a chronic condition more independently. The home is also seen as a much better environment to promote the child's growth and development.

Parents and other care providers without backgrounds in health care are given tremendous responsibilities to provide technology-assisted health care to their child. Technology assistance includes any of the following: ventilators; tracheostomies; suctioning; nasogastric, gastrostomy, or parenteral feeding with feeding pumps; intravenous fluids and medications with intravenous pumps. In some cases, families have created mini-intensive care units in their home. Examples of some serious chronic conditions cared for by families in the home include children with congenital heart defects before corrective surgery, bronchopulmonary dysplasia, and cancer in its terminal stage.

Health care systems (health care providers and insurers) are challenged to simultaneously address the child's illness and developmental needs while providing the support needed by these families so that children do well in their environments. The family also needs help to support the growing child in the school and other peer settings.

To work in the home care setting, nurses need a variety of skills:

- Knowledge and experience in acute care practice with various medical technologies to work with these children. These skills enable nurses to provide direct care, teach the family and child self-care practices, and monitor the child's progress.
- Community assessment skills; an understanding of community resources, financing mechanisms, and multi-agency collaboration; and good communication skills.[13]
- Understanding these resources helps nurses to assist families to find the most supportive services to match the child's and family's needs.

NURSING ASSESSMENT

Assessment in the home is focused on the child being cared for, the family's strengths and coping, and utilization of community resources.

Transition from the Hospital

For most children, home health care is initiated after an acute hospitalization. The hospital or home care nurse can be responsible for coordinating and linking the transition steps. Critical pathways or case management are methods for promoting a smooth transition. Expected outcomes for the child are documented. The home care nurse works in collaboration with hospital nurses by assessing the following:

- Caregiver readiness
- Home readiness (safe sleeping arrangements, adequate supplies, ability to meet nutritional and fluid needs, telephone access, heat, electricity, refrigeration, and lack of any communicable diseases in the home)

NURSING MANAGEMENT

Nurses help families in the home setting in the following ways:[11]

- Assuring competent care to the child
- Providing information about the child's condition and community resources
- Assisting families in time management skills and patient care management

SAFETY PRECAUTIONS

Assess the home environment for potential hazards related to the child's age, condition, and requirements for technology-assisted care. For example, are extension cords needed to reach electric outlets? The equipment may lose power if someone trips over the cord and disconnects it by mistake.

SAFETY PRECAUTIONS

Consider any features of the child's home environment that could cause an acute illness. For example, use of a woodstove or fireplace for heating could cause respiratory distress; renovation of a house built before 1960 could expose the child to lead dust.

CULTURAL CONSIDERATIONS

When providing care in the home, recognize potential conflicts between "mainstream" medical care and the family's cultural preferences after carefully listening to the parents' perspectives. Learn and use the family's perspectives of health and disease in discussions and in development of the plan of care.[14]

LEGAL & ETHICAL CONSIDERATIONS

Home care assumes the presence of the child's primary caregiver. Invasive treatments and decisions for provision of emergency care to avoid serious risk to life and limb require informed consent. When the caregiver is not present and the home care nurse provides such care, the home health care agency and the nurse are at significant liability risk.[15]

EMERGENCY MEDICAL DATA

Special medical problems can develop quickly in a child with severe and complex medical problems. An Emergency Data Set should provide a summary of the child's medical history, baseline physical findings, and important and unique management requirements.[16]

- Advocating for increased insurance coverage or locating other sources of financial assistance
- Identifying appropriate programs in the community such as respite care, therapeutic recreation, or educational opportunities

Recognize that control belongs to the family in the home care setting. The parents are the employer with the ability to hire and fire. Every interaction is negotiated with the family, or between the family and child if there are differences in what they want. The nurse must be flexible and able to set aside power. House rules for such things as parking, private areas in the home, routines, and discipline of the child must all be followed. Role expectations of the nurse must be clearly understood to reduce stress in the family. The success of home care is also based upon effective cultural communication.

The range of nursing care activities that may be included in a child's care plan in the home setting include sensory stimulation, routines of daily living (integrating the child into the family's routines whenever possible), positioning and skin care with gentle handling, respiratory care, nutrition and elimination, medications, and other supportive therapies. A plan for safe evacuation of the home is needed in case of fire. An emergency care plan should be developed for the child that includes an emergency medical history readily available to emergency care providers. The emergency health care provider needs enough information to understand the basics of the child's problem, to prevent delays in disease-specific treatment, and to minimize unnecessary interventions until the child's personal physician can be consulted. The family also needs to notify the emergency medical services agency and the power company about the presence of a technology-assisted child in the home. Back-up generators may be needed if electrical power for life-sustaining equipment is essential.

REFERENCES

1. Pridham, K.F., Broome, M., & Woodring, B. (1996). Education for the nursing of children and their families: Standards and guidelines for prelicensure and early professional education. *Journal of Pediatric Nursing, 11*(5), 273–280.

2. Curry, D.M., & Duby, J.C. (1994). Developmental surveillance by pediatric nurses. *Pediatric Nursing, 20*(1), 40–44.

3. Deloian, B.J. (1997). Screening tests. In J.A. Fox (Ed.), *Primary health care of children* (pp. 148–157). St. Louis: Mosby.

4. Glascoe, F.P. (1997). Parents' concerns about children's development: Prescreening technique or screening test? *Pediatrics, 99*(4), 522–528.

5. Office of Disease Prevention and Health Promotion, DHHS, Public Health Service. (1994). *Clinician's handbook of preventive services: Put prevention into practice.* Washington, DC: Government Printing Office.

6. Green, M. (Ed.). (1994). *Bright futures: Guidelines for health supervision of infants, children, and adolescents.* Arlington, VA: National Center for Education in Maternal and Child Health.

7. Department of Adolescent Health. (1996). *Guidelines for adolescent preventive services (GAPS).* Chicago, IL: American Medical Association.

8. Jackson, P.L. (1996). The primary care provider and children with chronic conditions. In P.L. Jackson & J.A. Vessey (Eds.), *Primary care of the child with a chronic condition* (2nd ed.). St. Louis: Mosby.

9. Patterson, J.M. (1991). Family resilience to the challenge of a child's disability. *Pediatric Annals, 20*(9), 491–499.

10. Caldwell, B.M., & Bradley, R.H. (1984). *The Home Observation for Measurement of the Environment.* Little Rock, AR: University of Arkansas.

11. Office of Technology Assessment. (1987). *Technology-dependent children: Hospital vs. home care. A technical*

memorandum. Washington, DC: Congress of the United States.

12. Patterson, J.M. (1995). Promoting resilience in families experiencing stress. *Pediatric Clinics of North America, 42*(1), 47–63.

13. Taylor, E.H., & Edwards, R.L. (1995). When community resources fail: Assisting the frightened and angry parent. *Pediatric Clinics of North America, 42*(1), 209–216.

14. Ahmann, E. (1996). *Home care for the high risk infant: A family centered approach* (2nd ed.). Gaithersburg, MD: Aspen Publishers.

15. Hogue, E. (1993). Care in the absence of primary caregivers. *Pediatric Nursing, 19*(1), 49–50.

16. Sacchetti, A., Gerardi, M., Barkin, R., et al. (1996). Emergency data set for children with special needs. *Annals of Emergency Medicine, 28,* 324–327.

ADDITIONAL RESOURCES

Ahmann, E., & Lierman, C. (1992). Promoting normal development in technology-dependent children: An introduction to the issues. *Pediatric Nursing, 18*(2), 143–148.

Ahmann, E., & Lipsi, K. (1992). Developmental assessment of the technology-dependent infant and young child. *Pediatric Nursing, 18*(3), 299–305.

Coplan, J., & Gleason, J.R., (1993). Test-retest and interobserver reliability of the Early Language Milestone Scale (2nd ed.). *Journal of Pediatric Health Care, 7*(5), 212–219.

Dworkin, P.H., & Glascoe, F.P. (1997). Early detection of developmental delays: How do you measure up? *Contemporary Pediatrics, 14*(4), 158–168.

Friedman, M.M. (1998). *Family nursing: Research theory & practice* (4th ed.), Stamford, CT: Appleton & Lange.

Garwick, A.E., & Millar, H.E.C. (1996). *Promoting resilience in youth with chronic conditions and their families.* Washington, DC: DHHS Health Resources and Services Administration, Maternal and Child Health.

Gellerstedt, M.E., & leRoux, P. (1995). Beyond anticipatory guidance: Parenting and the family life cycle. *Pediatric Clinics of North America, 42*(1), 65–78.

Green, M. (1996). Task of the times. *Contemporary Pediatrics, 13*(6), 94–104.

Green, M. (1995). No child is an island: Contextual pediatrics and the "new" health supervision. *Pediatric Clinics of North America, 42*(1), 79–87.

Jackson, P.L., & Vessey, J.A. (1996). *Primary care of the child with a chronic condition* (2nd ed.). St. Louis: Mosby.

Knafl, K., Breitmayer, B., Gallo, A., & Zoeller, L. (1996). Family response to childhood chronic illness: Description of management styles. *Journal of Pediatric Nursing, 11*(5), 315–326.

Pender, N.J. (1996). *Health promotion in nursing practice* (3rd ed.). Stamford, CT: Appleton & Lange.

Perrin, E.C., Newacheck, P., Pless, I.B., et al. (1993). Issues involved in the definition and classification of chronic health conditions. *Pediatrics, 91,* 787–793.

Rabin, N.B. (1994). School reentry and the child with a chronic illness: The role of the pediatric nurse practitioner. *Journal of Pediatric Health Care, 8*(5), 227–232.

Thurber, F. Berry, B., & Cameron, M.E. (1991). The role of school nursing in the United States. *Journal of Pediatric Health Care, 5*(3), 135–140.

Vessey, J.A. (1994). Improving the primary care pediatric nurses provide to children and their families. *Pediatric Nursing, 20*(1), 64–65.

Worthington, R.C. (1995). Effective transitions for families: Life beyond the hospital. *Pediatric Nursing, 21*(1), 86–87.

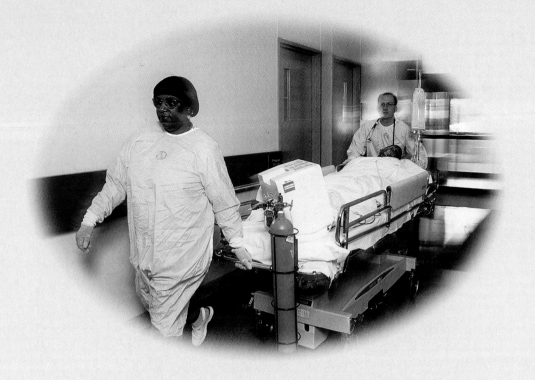

The telephone in the pediatric intensive care unit (PICU) rings at 8:30 AM. A referring hospital is calling to request the transport of an unstable 12-year-old boy, Jeremiah, who is in status epilepticus. Jeremiah has a seizure disorder that is usually controlled with medications, but several days ago he decided to stop taking his medications. So many seizure medications have been given in the emergency department at the referring hospital to try to stop the seizures that Jeremiah is now unconscious and must be intubated to maintain his airway until the medications wear off.

The transport team is in the air within minutes and arrives at the rural community hospital 25 minutes later. After stabilizing Jeremiah and receiving reports from the medical and nursing teams, the transport team meets briefly with his parents, answers a few questions, and is back in the air.

Jeremiah is admitted directly to the PICU, where the unit team has been preparing for his arrival. He is connected to cardiorespiratory and noninvasive blood pressure monitors, while his existing intravenous lines and endotracheal tube are evaluated for patency. Team members quickly complete a head-to-toe assessment. The unit clerk enters Jeremiah's room to say that his parents have arrived in the emergency department and are being escorted to the PICU.

THE CHILD WITH A LIFE-THREATENING ILLNESS OR INJURY

6

"Continuous, careful assessment is needed to make sure the child admitted into the intensive care unit has the best nursing care planned. In Jeremiah's case, it is so important to maintain the airway and oxygenation to prevent him from developing major complications."

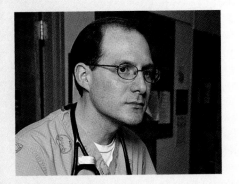

TERMINOLOGY

- **death anxiety** A feeling of apprehension or fear of death.
- **death imagery** Any reference to death or death-related topics, such as going away, separation, funerals, and dying, given in response to a picture or story that would not usually stimulate other children to discuss death-related topics.
- **family crisis** An event occurring when a family encounters problems that for a time seem insurmountable and with which the family is unable to cope in its usual ways.

- **hospice** A philosophy of care that focuses on helping persons with short life expectancies to live their remaining lives to the fullest—without pain and with choices and dignity.
- **stranger anxiety** Wariness of strange people and places, often shown by infants between 6 and 18 months of age.
- **support systems** The extended network of family, friends, and religious and community contacts that provide nurturance, emotional support, and direct assistance to parents.

What stressors do children like Jeremiah face after admission to the PICU? What strategies can you use to help such critically ill or injured children cope with the experience? What stressors will parents face during the initial period when you work with them? How can you intervene to help them in this crisis? What strategies should be used to help siblings understand what has happened to their brother or sister? This chapter will enable you to answer these questions and will assist you to provide supportive care to critically ill and injured children like Jeremiah and to their families.

The intense emotional and physical demands placed on the critically ill or injured child present a challenge to nurses' attempts to provide developmentally appropriate care. The child's parents and siblings are confronted with a stressful situation. A family-centered model of nursing practice offers a framework for performing interventions that help to minimize stress and enhance coping by parents, siblings, and the ill or injured child.

► LIFE-THREATENING ILLNESS OR INJURY

A threat to a child's life may be expected, as in a chronic illness or progressive disabling disease, or unexpected, as in an unintentional injury. How children, parents, and siblings cope with the threat will depend on the anticipated or unanticipated nature of the event and the conditions surrounding the child's admission to the hospital.

When death results from a chronic disease or terminal illness, the child and family have time to adjust to the impending death. Parents can become involved in the child's therapy as integral members of the treatment team. Emergency admission for an acute illness or unintentional injury, on the other hand, brings with it sudden stressors as the child and family are thrust into an unfamiliar environment, confronted with frightening or invasive procedures, and faced with an uncertain outcome.

Nursing care of children and families coping with specific chronic diseases or terminal illnesses such as cancer, cystic fibrosis, or muscular dystrophy is discussed elsewhere in this book. The following discussion focuses on care of children with life-threatening illnesses or injuries and care of the dying child.

► CHILD'S EXPERIENCE

Admission to the hospital, emergency department, or PICU is one of the most frightening experiences a child can have. The critically ill child may appear extremely anxious and fearful, or withdrawn, solemn, and preoccupied with his or her physical condition. The illness or injury often brings pain, decreases energy, and changes the child's level of consciousness. Younger children may be unable to understand what is happening to them. The environment appears overwhelming, fast paced, and frightening. The child's normal sleep patterns can be disrupted because of the lack of day–night patterns in many intensive care units. Being cared for by strangers produces anxiety in the child. The child's limited ability to move intensifies feelings of powerlessness and vulnerability.

Children's responses to stress are influenced by their developmental levels, past experiences, types of illness, coping mechanisms, and available emotional support. Nurses need to take into consideration how the child's developmental level and coping skills will influence his or her ability to deal with the PICU experience. Successful coping can provide the child with the skills to handle difficult situations in the future.

STRESSORS TO THE CHILD

The four most significant stressors for hospitalized children of all ages are (1) separation from parents or the primary caretaker, (2) loss of self-control, autonomy, and privacy, (3) being subjected to painful and invasive procedures, and (4) fear of bodily injury and disfigurement. Table 6–1 highlights key stressors of hospitalization for children at each developmental stage.

In addition to dealing with these stressors, the critically ill child experiences an intense emotional and physical threat to his or her well-being.

An unanticipated admission places the child at emotional risk for several reasons, including the lack of preparation for the experience, the uncertainty and unpredictability of events that follow, the unfamiliarity of the environment, and the heightened anxiety of parents. An admission for exacerbation of a disease such as cystic fibrosis or leukemia can provoke feelings of depression or hopelessness.

6-1 Stressors of Hospitalization for Children in Various Developmental Stages

Infant
Separation anxiety
Stranger anxiety
Painful, invasive procedures
Immobilization
Sleep deprivation

Toddler
Separation anxiety
Loss of self-control
Immobilization
Painful, invasive procedures
Bodily injury or mutilation
Fear of the dark

Preschooler
Separation anxiety and fear of abandonment
Loss of self-control
Bodily injury or mutilation
Painful, invasive procedures
Fear of the dark, ghosts, and monsters

School-Age Child
Loss of control
Loss of privacy and control over bodily functions
Bodily injury
Painful, invasive procedures
Fear of death

Adolescent
Loss of control
Fear of altered body image, disfigurement, disability, and death
Separation from peer group

Modified from Smith, J.B. (1983). Pediatric critical care. New York: Wiley & Sons; and Stevens, K.R. (1981). Humanistic nursing care for critically ill children. Nursing Clinics of North America, 16 (14), 611–622. Reproduced by permission. Pediatric Clinical Care, Smith, J. B. Delmar Publishers, Albany, NY, 1989.

Infant

After 3 months of age, most infants have started to develop a sense of object permanence (the knowledge that an object or person continues to exist when not seen, felt, or heard) and corresponding trust in parents and familiar caretakers. This makes separation from parents an anxiety-producing experience (see Chap. 4). In addition to separation anxiety, infants between 6 and 18 months of age may display **stranger anxiety** (wariness of strangers) when confronted with health care professionals. Other stressors to the infant include painful procedures, immobilization of extremities, and sleep deprivation caused by disruption of normal rhythms and patterns (Fig. 6–1).

Toddler

Toddlers are the group most at risk for a stressful experience as a result of illness. Separation from parents is extremely distressing to toddlers, and they protest vigorously when their parents depart. The toddler often becomes upset when known routines are altered. Being placed in restraints and confined is especially threatening to children in this age group. Fear of pain, fear of the dark, and fear of invasive procedures and mutilation are common.

Preschooler

The greatest stressors to preschoolers are fear of being alone, fear of the dark, fear of abandonment, fear of loss of self-control related to the body and emotions, and fear of bodily injury or mutilation. Waking up restrained in the PICU and feeling the presence of an endotracheal, nasogastric, or chest tube, along with intravenous, arterial, and urinary catheters, are terrifying to the preschooler.

School-Age Child

Major sources of stress for school-age children are loss of control related to bodily functions, privacy issues, fear of bodily injury, and concerns related

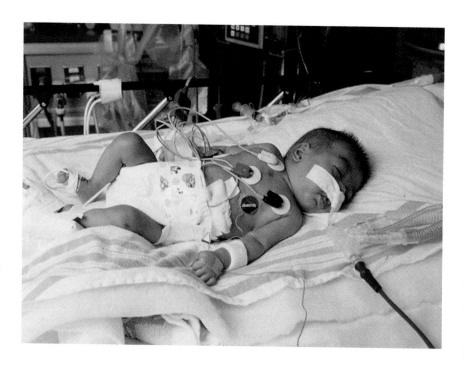

FIGURE 6–1. Jooti feels pain, hears noises, has her sleep disrupted, and has limited mobility because of all the equipment attached to her. What care and comfort can you offer parents who see their child like this?

to death. School-age children attempt to maintain their composure during painful or invasive procedures but generally still require a great deal of support.

Adolescent

Major stressors to adolescents are separation from the peer group, issues of control and related dependency, privacy, changes in body image, disability, and death. Adolescents often try to maintain rigid self-control when undergoing painful and invasive procedures.

COPING MECHANISMS

The child may mirror the parents' behaviors and responses, which may help or hinder the child's response to stress. The child's temperament, previous coping experiences, and availability of support systems all combine to influence his or her ability to cope with the current experience.

The nature and severity of the illness and an emergency admission to the hospital stress a child's coping capabilities. Defense mechanisms displayed by children in these situations include regression, or return to an earlier behavior (a common reaction to stress), denial, repression (involuntary forgetting), postponement, and bargaining.

NURSING ASSESSMENT

Nursing assessment involves, in addition to physiologic parameters, skilled observation of the child's psychosocial and emotional needs. It is important for the nurse to understand normal psychosocial and cognitive development in order to plan developmentally appropriate interventions. Assessment should include the child's response to illness, the environment, coping strategies, and the need for information and support.

NURSING DIAGNOSIS

The accompanying Nursing Care Plan includes common nursing diagnoses for the child coping with a critical illness or injury. The following nursing diagnoses may also be appropriate:

- Impaired Verbal Communication related to the effects of mechanical ventilation
- Impaired Social Interaction related to separation from family and friends
- Social Isolation related to the critical care environment
- Altered Sexuality Patterns related to the effects of acute illness or change in a body part
- Spiritual Distress related to the crisis of illness or suffering
- Ineffective Individual Coping related to changes in body integrity, separation from family and friends, or critical illness
- Impaired Physical Mobility related to trauma, pain, or use of physical restraints
- Fatigue related to illness, crisis, or sensory overload
- Sleep Pattern Disturbance related to medications, pain, fear, or critical care unit environment
- Diversional Activity Deficit related to the monotony of confinement

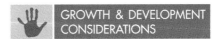

GROWTH & DEVELOPMENT CONSIDERATIONS

Coping behavior is influenced by maturation, cognitive development (increased attention span, problem-solving ability, and understanding of cause and effect), and increased impulse control. Young children use more behavioral strategies and ventilate feelings.[1]

- Altered Growth and Development related to critical illness or injury, the critical care environment, or separation from family and friends
- Body Image Disturbance related to loss of body function, severe trauma, or invasive procedures
- Self-Esteem Disturbance related to loss of body function, hospitalization, or loss of independence and autonomy
- Hopelessness related to critical illness, deteriorating condition, prolonged pain, altered body image, or separation from family and friends
- Anticipatory Grieving related to actual or perceived loss of function or impending death

NURSING MANAGEMENT

Nursing care focuses on promoting a sense of trust, providing education about the illness or injury, preparing the child for procedures, facilitating the use of play, and promoting a sense of control. Children admitted to a PICU are presented with a traumatic experience for which they need support. Nurses play a key role in providing developmentally appropriate support to the child. Nursing interventions are directed at building a trusting relationship, minimizing the stressors experienced by the child, and promoting coping. Ongoing reassessment of progress in meeting the child's needs is critical. Honesty in all discussions is key to building trust with the child. The accompanying Nursing Care Plan summarizes nursing care for the child coping with a life-threatening illness or injury.

Promote a Sense of Security

For children of all ages, feeling secure depends on a sense of physical and psychologic safety. A sense of physical safety is difficult to attain within the PICU because of the constant barrage of procedures that are part of the child's treatment plan. A sense of psychologic safety is best achieved by the presence of parents. An open visitation policy that enables parents to be at the bedside is optimal. Including parents as partners in the child's care provides comfort and reassurance to the child. Children whose parents have high anxiety levels pick up their parents' emotional cues and become more anxious. Interventions to lower the parents' anxiety may benefit the child.[2] Consistency of staff is invaluable in developing familiarity and a trusting relationship with the child.

Personalizing the child's bedside can promote comfort and a sense of security for the child. Pictures from home, a favorite blanket or toy, music tapes, or posters can make the environment friendlier and more familiar to the child (Fig. 6–2).

Provide Education About the Illness or Injury and Prepare the Child for Procedures

A child's ability to understand the cause of the illness and its therapy depends on his or her cognitive abilities. Help younger children to understand that illness and hospitalization are not a punishment.

Preparation for procedures is important at all ages, even for the unconscious or sedated child. The timing of this preparation depends on the child's cognitive level. Generally, the younger the child, the shorter the interval should be between the time of the teaching and the actual procedure (see Chap. 4).

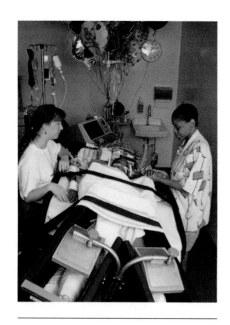

FIGURE 6–2. By their very nature, PICUs are ominous and sterile. To lessen this effect, it can help to personalize the child's space. Being there with the child and parent, answering questions, or just talking can be a comfort to both.

NURSING CARE PLAN
THE CHILD COPING WITH A
LIFE-THREATENING ILLNESS OR INJURY

GOAL	INTERVENTION	RATIONALE	EXPECTED OUTCOME

1. Fear or Anxiety (Child) related to separation from parents, foreign environment, strangers as caretakers, invasive procedures

The child will exhibit or express an increased sense of security.	• Encourage parents to remain at the bedside (open visitation) and to participate in the child's care by touching, talking to, reading to, and singing to the child.	• Presence of parents is comforting to the child.	The child appears more relaxed, acknowledges parents' presence, and allows staff to be supportive.
	• Talk with the child. Avoid discussions at bedside that the child should not overhear.	• The child may overhear and remember, even if unconscious.	
	• Provide the child with developmentally appropriate explanations when possible, encourage the child to ask questions, and express concerns	• Information reduces anxiety and builds trust.	
	• Prepare the child in advance for procedures using developmentally appropriate techniques.	• Preparation decreases anxiety related to the unknown.	
	• Make the child's bedside more personal and familiar by encouraging parents to bring in security objects, family photos, and favorite toys from home.	• Security objects decrease foreignness of hospital environment. The child derives comfort from presence of personal items.	
	• Involve the child in play appropriate to developmental age (see Chap. 4).	• Play provides familiarity, decreases fantasy, and provides motor activity.	
	• Provide care using a primary nursing care model.	• Consistency in caregivers helps to build the child's trust.	

2. Powerlessness related to inability to communicate, lack of privacy, control relinquished to the health care team

The child or adolescent will have an increased sense of control over the situation.	• Provide opportunities for choices when possible. • Encourage participation in self-care.	• Such opportunities provide sense of control and autonomy through decision making.	The child or adolescent expresses satisfaction over ability to control some element of situation.

Continued . . .

NURSING CARE PLAN
THE CHILD COPING WITH A
LIFE-THREATENING ILLNESS OR INJURY– *Continued*

GOAL	INTERVENTION	RATIONALE	EXPECTED OUTCOME

2. *Powerlessness related to inability to communicate, lack of privacy, control relinquished to the health care team (continued)*

- Prepare the child or adolescent in advance (timing dependent on developmental level) for procedures. Describe the sensations that will be experienced. Allow some choice in timing or method of pain relief.
- Provide coverage of private body areas. Use curtains around bed when feasible.
- Provide routines for the child both within a 24-hour period and for scheduled care. Tell the child before (timing dependent on developmental level), repeat explanation of why procedure is necessary, complete procedure in a consistent manner, and offer praise or a special story when completed. When possible, incorporate rituals from home.
- Encourage play as a means of expressing feelings.
- Provide other means of communication to the intubated child (eg, a word board or finger board).
- For the child requiring restraints, use as seldom as possible, provide appropriate explanations, and release at regular intervals. Wrapping IV lines well and using armboards can help maintain lines and avoid restraints.

- Information provides anticipatory guidance and a sense of involvement and value to the child.

- Privacy lessens feelings of vulnerability.

- Self-control is maintained through rituals.

- Play is a normal activity for children and provides freedom of expression.
- Maintaining communication provides autonomy and independence for the child.
- Release from restraints helps to diminish the sense of powerlessness that accompanies their use.

NURSING CARE PLAN
THE CHILD COPING WITH A LIFE-THREATENING ILLNESS OR INJURY— *Continued*

GOAL	INTERVENTION	RATIONALE	EXPECTED OUTCOME

3. Pain related to injuries, invasive procedures, surgery

GOAL	INTERVENTION	RATIONALE	EXPECTED OUTCOME
The child will experience reduced pain and improved comfort.	• Assess the child's pain: location, intensity, what makes it better or worse.	• Assessment provides baseline information from which a plan of care can be developed.	The child experiences a perceived or actual improvement in comfort level.
	• If appropriate, use pain assessment scale (see Chap. 7).	• Use of scale provides continuity and consistency in monitoring of the child's pain.	
	• Prepare the child for procedures. Be honest in explanations and use developmentally appropriate language and format. Describe the sensations that the child will feel, smell, taste, or see. Comfort the child after the procedure. Provide rest periods between procedures.	• Information reduces anxiety and fear associated with the unknown and helps child maintain self-control.	
	• Provide optimal pain relief with prescribed analgesics. Provide diversional activities as appropriate or possible.	• Physiologic and psychologic methods of pain control can be used in combination to maximally improve outcome.	

Children often feel and hear even when unconscious, so touch and verbal interchanges are important. Toddlers will benefit from being talked to, soothed, and touched during and after the procedure. Provide preschoolers, school-age children, and adolescents with an explanation of the sensations they can expect to experience (temperature, vibrations, sounds, smells, tastes, sight). This information may reduce their stress more than complete details about the procedures.[3] In any explanations to the child, avoid medical jargon and use simple language appropriate to the child's developmental level.

Facilitate the Use of Play

The use of play is important in alleviating stress and helping children to prepare for procedures. It is also another way for the nurse to assess the child's developmental level. Therapeutic play adds familiarity, diminishes fantasies, provides motor activity, and helps the child develop a sense of mastery (see Chap. 4). Children who are immobilized by tubes and restraints can still feel a sense of accomplishment, for example, by completing a puzzle, even if the nurse points to each piece and, through nods and gestures, indicates where it should be placed. Play can help children work through a painful situation, making it more tolerable.

Promote a Sense of Control

Children between toddlerhood and adolescence experience a loss of control during a life-threatening illness. This loss of control may be related to the body, emotions, normal routines, or privacy. Nursing interventions should promote a sense of control over these areas.

Give choices to the child whenever possible. Even the simple choice of which arm will receive a new intravenous line can help the child feel in control. Scheduling routine activities and treatments at the same time each day adds predictability and lessens anxiety. Limited mobility and the use of restraints, although sometimes necessary, contribute to the child's sense of powerlessness. Plan to release the child's restraints regularly for short periods. Restrain the toddler and preschooler as little as possible, and explain the rationale for restraints, emphasizing that they are not a punishment. Provide diversional activities for the child, for example, by reading stories, playing music, or watching videotapes (see Chap. 4).

Enhance the child's coping skills by teaching the child and family a combination of relaxation, visual imagery, or distraction techniques, and comforting self-talk phrases, such as "This will be over soon. If I stay calm, it will be all right. It will be over faster and then I can do something fun." Help the parents become the child's coping coaches.

▶ PARENTS' EXPERIENCE

Families have different reactions and coping mechanisms when challenged. Children who are hospitalized for a critical illness cannot be adequately cared for if their families' needs are not met. Not only will parents find it difficult to support the child if their own needs are not met, but they also can transmit their anxiety to the child, who then becomes even more anxious.

WHAT MAKES A PROBLEM A CRISIS?

A **family crisis** occurs when a family encounters a problem that seems insurmountable and with which the family cannot cope in its usual ways. The critical care environment and the implications of a life-threatening illness or injury are far removed from the everyday experiences of most families. The unfamiliarity of the environment and the uncertainty and seriousness of the illness or injury create a crisis for the family.

Unexpected illness or injury adds another dimension of stress, since families have little time to prepare for the experience. A sudden admission threatens family integrity, causing enormous stress and separation from loved ones.

REACTIONS TO LIFE-THREATENING ILLNESS OR INJURY

How do parents react to a threat to their child's life? What parental behaviors might nurses see when a child is critically ill or injured? Parents typically progress through stages that might include shock and disbelief; anger and guilt; deprivation and loss; anticipatory waiting; and readjustment or mourning.

Shock and Disbelief

The universal reaction of parents is shock and disbelief. As the familiar is disrupted, parents experience a loss of control, inability to regain their bearings, and feelings of immobility. The hospital environment, emergency department, or PICU may seem unreal. The emotions parents experience initially are intensified by the physical appearance of their child (particularly after traumatic injury); the presence of monitors, tubing, and equipment; and the actual injury or illness (Fig. 6–3). As the mother of a 5-year-old trauma patient said, "I felt distanced, in a daze, in and out of it that first day after the accident."

The stage of shock and disbelief begins in the first few moments after hearing the "news" and can last for days. For most parents, however, the overwhelming sense of shock passes during the first 24 hours. During this period, parents grope for answers and explanations about the illness or injury. Information must be repeated many times to parents, since in this stage they are often unable to assimilate information easily.

Anger and Guilt

Anger and guilt surface as parents become more aware of their child's illness or injury. Their anger may be directed toward themselves, each other, health care providers, or other children or parents, as in the case of a motor vehicle crash involving a group of teenagers. Parents may also be angry with their child. This anger may be a result of injuries the child sustained when breaking known rules such as drinking and driving, playing with matches, or riding a bike without a helmet. Lastly, the anger may not be directed at anyone specifically. Injuries caused by natural disasters such as an earthquake, flood, or hurricane provoke just as much anger as those that result from the actions of people. This may create a challenge to the parents' spiritual beliefs.

Parents typically react to their child's illness or injury with some degree of guilt. This reaction may be magnified in the intensive care environment. The fact that the guilt usually has no basis in real events does not lessen the feeling. A question parents frequently ask at this stage is, "Why not me instead of my child?" Parents' feelings of guilt may have one of two causes:

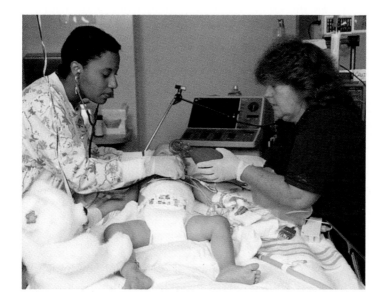

FIGURE 6–3. Procedures done in the PICU, such as mechanical ventilation, are frightening for parents. Treat the child first, but also remember the needs, fears, and anxieties of the parents and other family members. Anticipating the family's needs and keeping them informed will help them adjust.

1. *They may feel responsible for causing the illness or injury.* Statements such as, "If only I hadn't sent him to the store on his bike, this wouldn't have happened," or, from the father of a 2-year-old who nearly drowned, "Maybe if I hadn't been working, he would have been in my care and this wouldn't have happened," reflect feelings of guilt for causing or failing to prevent the injury.
2. *They may feel guilty about not noticing the onset of an illness or disregarding earlier symptoms of an illness.* The mother of a 1-year-old with *Haemophilus influenzae* meningitis repeatedly said, "I shouldn't have waited so long to take her to the doctor!"

Deprivation and Loss

As the shock slowly recedes, parents enter a stage of deprivation and loss related to their parental role. Within minutes or hours, parents have gone from the familiar role of being a parent of a healthy child to the unexpected and unfamiliar role of being a parent of a critically ill child. Parents have compared this deprivation and loss to that experienced when a family member dies.

Parents' difficulties and ambivalence in releasing to strangers a part of their responsibility as the child's primary caretakers can threaten their self-esteem and self-control. Moreover, if parents cannot participate in the child's care, they may feel helpless or worthless.

Anticipatory Waiting

Once the child's condition is stabilized and survival seems likely, parents often move into a period of anticipatory waiting. This stage is characterized as "life suspended in time." Parents spend a great deal of time waiting: for test results, for explanations, for their child to become conscious, or for surgery to be over. Parents may fear leaving the area because they may miss an important procedure, physician visit, or decisions or changes in treatment. Lack of mobility decreases the parents' use of typical coping mechanisms, so anxiety and the sense of powerlessness may increase. A pager system has been adopted in some facilities to give parents freedom to take breaks away from the child's bedside, knowing they will be alerted to important events.[4]

Parents may have a preoccupation with medical details. During this period, parents may ask questions about the long-term effects of the illness or injury on the child, about the potential for brain damage, or about the need for additional surgeries. Parents may place demands on staff and be frustrated when the child's progress is slow.

Readjustment or Mourning

The last stage that parents experience is readjustment or mourning. Readjustment is experienced as the child recovers, improves steadily, and prepares for transfer and discharge. In contrast, parents of the child who dies reenter the cycle of emotions characteristic of grief. Mourning also occurs when the child remains seriously ill or unresponsive, when the outcome remains uncertain for an extended period, or when long-term care is required.

Table 6–2 lists the most important needs of parents during a child's critical illness or injury.

NURSING ASSESSMENT

Nurses who work with families of critically ill children have a unique opportunity to help them adapt and to promote family functioning. They begin by assessing the family's reaction to the illness, coping skills, stressors,

6-2	Parental Needs During Hospitalization of a Critically Ill or Injured Child

Information (the most important identified need)
- Information and frequent updates about the child's condition
- Explanations they can understand about the child's condition, equipment being used, and procedures of care
- Discussion with a physician daily
- General information about unit policies, team members, phone numbers, etc

Proximity
- Permission to remain at the bedside
- Permission to touch and speak with the child
- Open, flexible visiting hours

Reestablishment of the parental control
- Recognition as important to the child's recovery
- Recognition as the decision maker of the child's treatment options

Participation in the child's care
- Performance of care (bathing, diaper changes, feeding, range of motion exercises, massages, hair care)
- Provision of comfort measures (reading, singing, telling stories, touching, talking)

Confidence in the treatment plan and caregivers
- Continuity in staffing and health care contacts
- Evidence that staff care about the child
- Knowledge that the child is receiving the best care possible

Psychologic support
- Acknowledgement that the situation is difficult
- Help to focus on the positive or unchanged aspects of the child's appearance
- Rest and nutrition to maintain physical resources necessary for coping
- Space and privacy as needed
- Hope—an essential component of coping
- Choice of other family members to be present

and needs. This initial assessment provides a baseline of information for developing a care plan and strategies to meet the psychosocial as well as physiologic needs of families.

NURSING DIAGNOSIS

Several nursing diagnoses may apply to parents who are dealing with their child's critical illness or injury. They include:

- Knowledge Deficit related to the child's critical condition and uncertain prognosis
- Altered Parenting related to the child's critical illness or injury
- Altered Family Processes related to the impact of a critically ill child on the family system
- Parental Role Conflict related to the child's critical illness or injury
- Spiritual Distress related to the child's critical illness, suffering, or death
- Ineffective Individual or Family Coping related to the child's severe or fatal illness
- Family Coping: Potential for Growth related to constructive crisis management

- Fatigue related to extreme stress, crisis, and sensory overload
- Hopelessness related to the child's deteriorating physiologic condition
- Powerlessness related to relinquishment of control to the health care team
- Anticipatory Grieving related to perceived loss of the child or the child's impending death

NURSING MANAGEMENT

Nursing care focuses on providing information and building trust, promoting parental involvement, providing for physical and emotional needs, facilitating positive staff–parent relationships and communication, and maintaining or strengthening family support systems. Ongoing reassessment provides a measure with which to evaluate the family's ability to manage the crisis. The best way to meet the needs of families, minimize stress, and enhance family coping is to provide care using a family-centered approach[5] (see Table 1–1, page 10). The challenge to nurses is to blend and balance technology with caring.

Provide Information and Build Trust

The information given to parents must be provided frequently and accurately. Information on the child's illness, condition, and plan of care should be delivered in a manner and language readily understandable to parents. Upon admission, parents need to be given an idea of what to expect in the days ahead and prepared for special procedures or major changes in therapy that may become necessary.

Honesty in discussions with parents is extremely important. If parents feel misled or that information is being withheld, a trusting relationship will be impossible. Informed parents, on the other hand, will feel that they are active participants in decision making and care planning for their child. Trust is facilitated when parents believe that the staff truly cares about the child and sees him or her as an individual, special child.

Parents also need a sense of hope regarding their child's illness to help them cope. Focus on the positives as the child progresses through the different phases of the critical illness.

Promote Parental Involvement

An important role of nurses is to encourage and strengthen parents in their parenting role. The parents' place when possible is at the bedside—their very presence can comfort the child, minimize fears, and reduce the child's experiences with pain during invasive procedures.[6,7] Parents' needs are best met when they are encouraged to participate in their child's care.

If the child is in the PICU, parents need to be prepared before they see their child for the first time. Throughout the child's hospitalization, parents will continue to need reassurance and encouragement. Open visitation by parents is important to maintain their parenting role.[8]

Provide for Physical and Emotional Needs

The experience of having a child with a critical illness drains parents' physical and emotional reserves. Parents often need encouragement to take care of themselves. A statement such as, "It is important for you to eat and rest because Jeremiah is really going to need you when he wakes up," helps

CLINICAL TIP

Explain to the child and parents, in easy-to-understand terms, the purpose of equipment that is being used. Answer alarms quickly. Follow with an explanation of why alarms sound.

CLINICAL TIP

Encourage parents to take time for themselves to be alone. Provide parents with a beeper, if possible, to reduce anxiety when they are away from the unit.

parents to realize that becoming exhausted benefits neither them nor the child.

Orienting parents to the hospital, as well as to the unit routines, helps them to adapt to their surroundings. Many communities now have Ronald McDonald houses—an inexpensive but warm and supportive environment for parents of ill children (Fig. 6–4) (see Appendix F). When financial burdens are a consideration, family and social service referrals may be needed.

Parents are often at different levels of coping during a crisis. The child's critical illness may foster cohesion between the couple and build a stronger relationship. Unfortunately, the reverse may also be true—differences in styles or levels of coping may foster a sense of isolation, placing a strain on the couple's relationship. Nurses should be alert to family dynamics and refer the family for counseling or therapy, if indicated.

Facilitate Positive Staff–Parent Relationships and Communication

Given the intensity of the parents' experience when their child is critically ill, it is easy to see how problems can arise between staff and parents. Each health care team member must be aware of the child's current status so that parents receive the same information from all staff. Consistency in the message can instill confidence. Provide explanations geared to the parents' level of understanding, using language the parents can understand.

Parents need to know who has the overall responsibility for the care of their child. They should be introduced to the nurse and physician responsible for the child's care. This is especially important in teaching hospitals that have rotating staff. The staff physician with the overall responsibility should meet with parents as often as necessary to talk about changes in the child's condition or treatment plan and to allow time for parents to ask questions (Fig. 6–5). Encourage parents to keep a daily log or notebook to record information on the child's care, progress, and

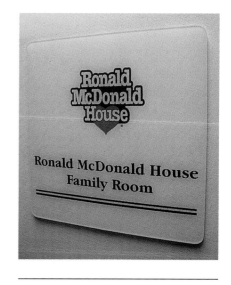

FIGURE 6–4. A Ronald McDonald family room in a large metropolitan hospital provides a comfortable setting where families of seriously ill children can go to get away from the high-tech hospital atmosphere while remaining near the ill child.

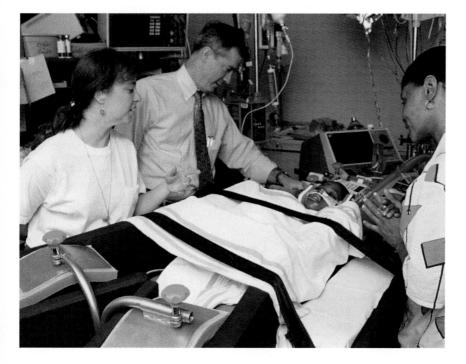

FIGURE 6–5. In times of crisis, everyone likes to know that someone is in charge and who that person is. The parents should meet and talk with the staff physician in charge and the nurses as often as possible. Parents need to know that someone is responsible, even if different people are providing care.

needs. Family care conferences can be helpful when a large number of team members provide care.

Maintain or Strengthen Family Support Systems

Support systems are the extended network of family, friends, and religious and community contacts that provide nurturance, emotional support, and direct assistance to parents, enabling them to cope with overwhelming problems and crises. Most parents indicate that having family or friends nearby is crucial as a support system.

Parents may need to be reassured that it is all right to ask for help from family, friends, or community services. They may be uncomfortable asking for help, instead attempting to handle multiple responsibilities themselves, often to the point of exhaustion. Some parents are unable to respond to offers of help because it requires too great a mental effort on their part.

Nurses may need to intervene on parents' behalf when they have inappropriate support.[9] Parents may be frustrated by people who come to visit unannounced, stay too long, or visit too often, and may find it difficult to tell well-meaning but insensitive friends that they cannot deal with visitors right now. In these situations, offering to serve as a gatekeeper may be helpful.

Families of critically ill or dying children often have emotional needs beyond the support capabilities of the nurse caring for the child. Referrals to family and support services or pastoral care may be beneficial in these instances.

► SIBLINGS' EXPERIENCE

As the parents' focus shifts to the critically ill child, they may need support in dealing with the healthy siblings. Siblings also need care and may feel left out when everyone's attention is focused on the ill child. Siblings of critically ill children may demonstrate behaviors ranging from jealousy or envy to resentment, guilt and hostility, anger, insecurity, and fear. Recognize that siblings may fear becoming ill themselves or believe that they played a role in the child's illness. Siblings often have nightmares about the illness or injury their brother or sister has sustained and about the ill child dying.

Tell siblings about their brother or sister using language and concepts appropriate to their ages and developmental levels. As appropriate, siblings should be allowed to visit. These visits often help to lift the spirits of the ill child. Because children's fantasies are often worse than reality, unfounded fears may be relieved by a visit.

Preparation for the visit is important. Before the visit, talk with the siblings about what to expect and describe how their brother or sister will look. If the ill child acts, moves, talks, or looks different than usual, provide an explanation beforehand. Describe the hospital environment, including equipment, sounds, and smells. Using a doll, drawing pictures, or showing an actual picture of the child can help prepare the siblings. Table 6–3 summarizes strategies for working with siblings of an ill or injured child.

During the visit, demonstrate how to talk to and touch the ill child and encourage the siblings to do the same (Fig. 6–6). After the visit, discuss with siblings what they saw and felt, and answer any questions they may have.

CULTURAL CONSIDERATIONS

As in many other cultural groups, Mexican-American families have close kinship ties with an extended network of relatives, including grandparents, uncles, aunts, cousins, and *compadres* (children's godparents). The extended family is a source of strength and can provide much-needed emotional and physical support during crises.

6-3 Strategies for Working With Siblings of an Ill or Injured Child

- Be truthful. Tell why the child is hospitalized, what the treatment involves, and how long the hospitalization is expected to last.
- Assure siblings that they did not cause the illness and that the ill child did nothing wrong.
- Allow siblings to ask questions and state fears and other feelings.
- Allow siblings to visit if possible. Prepare them for any equipment, dressing, and procedures they might see. Warn them if the ill child is not speaking. Say something like, "John can't talk now. He seems to be sleeping deeply. He may be able to hear, though, so you can touch him and talk to him."
- Encourage siblings to express their feelings related to the disruptive effect of the child's hospitalization on family life.

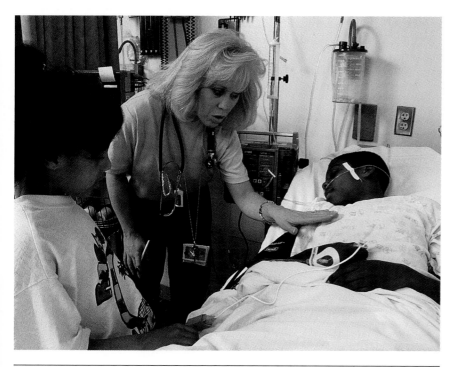

FIGURE 6–6. During the sibling's visit to the ill child, it is important to talk with the sibling and answer any questions asked in an honest manner at a level the child can understand.

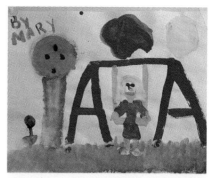

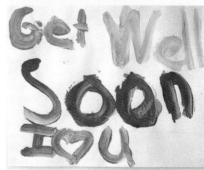

FIGURE 6–7. It is important that parents and siblings feel comfortable communicating with the seriously ill child. If siblings cannot visit, they should be encouraged to paint or record messages. They need to be able to express themselves and to feel that they are helping.

When a sibling cannot visit, contact with the ill child can be maintained by sending pictures, drawings, cards, and messages recorded on audiotapes or videotapes (Fig. 6–7).

If parents are staying at the hospital with the ill child, encourage them to call the siblings at home at a regular time each night. Allowing the siblings at home the opportunity to share their day as well as to receive an update on the ill child provides a feeling of connectedness. The phone call offers siblings a consistent link to the parent as well as the reassurance that they are important and loved.

▶ BEREAVEMENT

PARENTS' REACTIONS

The death of one's child is probably the most painful experience for a parent. When the loss is sudden and unexpected, the abruptness adds a dimension of shock that may last for 4–5 weeks. The goal of the nurse in these situations is to provide comfort and support for the dying child and the family (Table 6–4). Staff education must be built on the premise that grief and mourning are normal, necessary processes.

Grief is painful, individualized, and exhausting. Many factors influence the parents' grief responses, including their perception of the preventability of the illness or injury, the suddenness and other circumstances of the death, the nature of their attachment to the child, previous losses, spiritual or religious orientation, and culture.

Although parents progress through distinct stages of grief, the time line and nature of the grief process differ for each individual. The intense pain and shock initially felt by parents gradually give way to feelings of anger, guilt, depression, and loneliness. Very slowly, and with much support, energy returns and parents again begin to enjoy life experiences. Spouses may need additional support when they are at different levels of grieving to prevent a sense of loneliness and isolation.

Work closely with the family when the child's death is imminent, since they will remember the experience for the rest of their lives. Prepare the family for changes in the child's appearance and the events to follow. Providing parents with a room in which to be alone with the child ensures privacy at this extremely personal time. Ask the family what is important to them in the last moments or hours of their child's life. Certain religious or cultural practices may need to be planned. Holding the child is a universal request and should be permitted. Many families find that saying good-bye as a group is helpful. Allowing the family to hold, kiss, and talk to the dying child can help grieving.[10] Encourage parents to continue in their parental

CULTURAL CONSIDERATIONS

Many culturally influenced rules and customs surround dying. For instance, the Hmong belief system holds that children will live in eternity in the same state in which they existed at the time of death. Therefore it is important that the child's body be intact at death.

6-4	**Strategies for Working with Parents Whose Child Dies Suddenly**

- Identify a spokesperson for the medical team to keep the family informed during resuscitation efforts.
- Provide private space with telephone access.
- Create time for families to assimilate the child's worsening status by providing several updates during the resuscitation. Prepare them for what is to come.
- Offer to telephone clergy, family, and friends.
- After the death, prepare the body for viewing.
- Provide time and a place for the family to say good-bye.
- Share your emotions with the family.
- Convey information to the family about the cause of death, autopsy, funeral preparations, and the normal grief process.
- Arrange for family follow-up.

Modified from Anderson, J.E. (1996). Helping parents cope with sudden death. Contemporary Pediatrics, 13(12), 42–57.

role by continuing with caregiving activities such as bathing or dressing the child for the last time.

After the child's death, allow the family to spend as much time as they need with the child's body. Never rush family members who are saying good-bye to the child. Save all of the child's personal items—especially in the case of an infant, whose parents may have few mementos. A lock of hair, hand or foot prints, the infant's identification band, the child's weight and height, the last clothes or patient gown worn by the child sealed in a plastic bag to retain the child's scent, or a picture of the infant can be sources of comfort and remembrance for families.

Parents may need direction about resources available to help with a memorial service or funeral. Information about organ and tissue donation, as well as the need for an autopsy, if required, needs to be discussed. Acknowledge with parents that certain dates—such as the day of the week the child died, the child's birthday, or family holidays—will be difficult and may trigger intense sadness again. Parents may benefit from keeping a journal of their thoughts and memories, or writing letters or poems to or about their child.

Emphasize to parents that although the period surrounding their child's death is difficult, caring for themselves physically and mentally is important. A list of appropriate support groups, books, and articles can be given to parents for later use. Parents can be referred to national organizations, such as the Candlelighters Foundation or Compassionate Friends, and to local support groups for bereaved parents or siblings (refer to Appendix F). Some institutions have formal follow-up programs for bereaved parents to encourage a healthy progression through the grieving process.

SIBLINGS' REACTIONS

Siblings experiencing the death of a brother or sister require supportive and compassionate care. In the course of the child's illness the siblings probably will have received less attention from parents. They may fear that they caused their brother or sister to be injured or become ill, or worry that bad thoughts on their part brought on the illness. They need help in adapting to their parents' distraction, grief, and increased protectiveness of them.[11, 12] Table 6–5 highlights children's understanding of death at different developmental stages and some of the possible behavioral responses.

When talking to the siblings of a dying child, honesty is most important. Provide explanations in language that is developmentally appropriate. Reassure siblings that they did not cause their brother or sister to die and that death was not a punishment for wrongdoing. Allow the siblings to ask questions. Acknowledge the emotions they are feeling, and emphasize that it is all right for them to be sad, angry, frightened, or tearful. Ask how they feel about saying good-bye to the dying child, and provide physical and emotional support. Preparation of the siblings before seeing the dying child involves a brief explanation of what they will see, feel, hear, and smell. Answer questions truthfully. You may have to repeat information several times.

As appropriate and comfortable, siblings should be permitted to participate in planning the child's memorial or funeral service. Being able to grieve as a family provides siblings with a sense of connectedness to parents and provides security at a vulnerable time.

CULTURAL CONSIDERATIONS

Always ask the parent before cutting a lock of the child's hair. Some cultures and religions, including Native American groups, forbid it.[10]

GROWTH & DEVELOPMENT CONSIDERATIONS

Children need to understand the finality of death—that all body functions have stopped. Simple statements that can be told to children include, "Adam's heart will never beat again," "He will never get cold or hungry," and "He will never come home again." These simple statements may need to be repeated several times since young children will test to see if the same answers are given each time.[13]

GROWTH & DEVELOPMENT CONSIDERATIONS

Children must also complete a grieving process. This is usually accomplished in three stages.[14]

- *Early stage:* They understand the death occurred, while using self-protective mechanisms to block the full emotional impact of the loss.
- *Middle stage:* They accept and rework the loss while experiencing the intense psychologic pain.
- *Late stage:* They integrate the loss experience into their identity and resume age-appropriate developmental progress.

6-5   Children's Understanding of Death and Possible Behavioral Responses

Understanding of Death	Possible Behaviors
Infant • Lacks understanding of concept of death • May sense caregivers are tense, routines are altered	• May show sadness by turning away from your gaze • Resists cuddling and eats less • Sleeping more
Toddler • Unable to distinguish fact from fantasy • No understanding of true concept of death • Aware someone is missing—separation anxiety	• Clingy, refuses to let parent out of sight • Stops walking and talking • Shows distress by biting, hitting, tears • Fearfulness • Problems eating and sleeping
Preschooler • Believes death is reversible, temporary • Believes bad thoughts cause death • Believes magical thinking can bring the dead person back • May see death as punishment • Is developing a sense of past, present, future • Has beginning experience with death of animals and plants	• May fear going to sleep, has nightmares • Out-of-control behavior, hyperactivity, tantrums • Problems with bowel and bladder control • Crying spells • Seems morbidly fascinated with death • Asks lots of questions • Displays anger at failure to keep person "alive"
School-Age Child • Acquires more realistic understanding of death • By 8–10 years, understands that death is permanent and irreversible • Believes that death is universal and will happen to him or her • May have exaggerated concerns about death	• May deny sadness by hiding tears and acting more like adults • Difficulty concentrating on school work • Psychosomatic complaints—tummy ache or headache • Acting-out behavior • May try to comfort parents by taking over tasks
Adolescent • Intellectually capable of understanding death • Has a better grasp of association between illness and death • Sense of invincibility conflicts with fear of death	• Same as school-age child • May have severe depression • Acting-out behavior—risk-taking behavior, delinquency, suicide attempts, promiscuity

Modified from Krulik, T., Holaday, B., & Martinson, I.M. (Eds.). (1987). The child and family facing life-threatening illness. Philadelphia: Lippincott; McIntier, T.M., Sr. (1995). Nursing the family when the child dies, RN, 58, 50–54; and Anderson, J.E. (1996). Helping parents cope with sudden death. Contemporary Pediatrics, 13, 42–55.

▶ DYING CHILD

Care of the dying child presents one of the greatest challenges to the nurse, requiring the utmost sensitivity and compassion. A child's understanding of death varies according to developmental stages, as described in Table 6–5.

Children as young as 5 years of age can sense when they are seriously ill. A child's awareness of death develops more rapidly when he or she is experiencing the progression of a disease and related medical treatment. Children with life-threatening illnesses often learn about death and their own illness from exposure to other seriously ill and dying children when they are receiving treatment during hospitalization or clinic visits.

Preschool children can see their body deteriorate and feel the toxic effects of chemicals during disease progression and treatment. Changes in self-concept occur as they perceive these body changes. They often describe their illness in terms of mutilation to their body. They may realize that they are dying because of these physical changes.

School-age children also have subtle fears about body integrity and anxieties about the seriousness of their illness. This greater preoccupation with illness is considered by many professionals as the child's version of **death anxiety,** a feeling of apprehension or fear of death. Death anxiety occurs in children even though they are unable to conceptualize or describe death at an adult's level of understanding. It can develop from the perception of loneliness associated with a separation from the known world. Children may express death anxiety as a concern with treatments that invade the body or interfere with normal body functions.

Children intuitively know when they are dying, and they usually do not have the same fears that adults do. Some children keep most of their thoughts about death to themselves. They may fear that the family members will abandon them emotionally. Displays of anger often are avoided, since children fear desertion more than death. They may also believe that expressing their awareness of death and their fears will place added emotional burdens on family members that could be unbearable to the family. Parents may not recognize the child's death anxiety because of their own fears, concerns, and feelings of helplessness.

Waechter's study of hospitalized and fatally ill children revealed that children who were given an opportunity to discuss issues related to death openly did not have greater anxiety about death. The permission to discuss any aspect of the illness made the child feel less isolated and alienated from the parents. The child felt that the illness was not too terrible to discuss.[15]

Adolescents have a mature understanding of death, but the normal developmental milestones of adolescence add to their problems in facing a terminal illness. They are struggling to establish their own identity and plans for the future. At a time when body image is extremely important, they may be faced with the possibility of mutilation and disfigurement. Dying teens are often isolated from their peers during a period when peers are the most essential social group. Adolescents with terminal illnesses may be angry because they recognize their loss when the whole world is opening up to them.

Do not expect adolescents to handle feelings in the same way that adults do. Adolescents often avoid expressing anger against the family, seeking to control and direct these feelings elsewhere. They often become angry at changes in treatment procedures, lack of explanations, and threats to their independence. As death nears, the adolescent may permit comforting and support and may accept care from warm and loving family members, as long as he or she is not treated condescendingly.

CULTURAL CONSIDERATIONS

Depending on the family's cultural and religious beliefs, a chaplain or other health care professional who specializes in working with terminally ill children and families may help reduce a child's spiritual fears and promote peace and comfort among family members.

NURSING MANAGEMENT

Make a commitment to children while they are living—to promote growth and development and to foster relationships with family and peers. Help children maintain contact with peers on the hospital unit as long as the child has energy to benefit from the companionship. The comfort of peers reduces the child's feelings of isolation.

Provide opportunities for fantasy play, drawings, and storytelling, without emphasizing or reinforcing death themes. Listen to what children tell you about themselves and their lives. **Death imagery,** references to death or death-related topics (going away, separation, and funerals), or anticipated experiences with treatment may be themes of their stories. These themes are expected and do not reflect repression or other pathology.

LEGAL & ETHICAL CONSIDERATIONS

Some parents ask that their child not be told he or she is dying. Do you abide by their wishes when the child asks you if he or she is dying? Tell the parents that the child asked the question. Offer to set up a meeting with the care team to discuss their fears and concerns about telling their child the truth. Offer words and phrases they can use to talk with their child about his or her death.

LEGAL & ETHICAL CONSIDERATIONS

The Patient Self-Determination Act of 1990 (PSDA) supports the rights of persons 18 years of age or older in decisions about their medical care and when they should be admitted to a medical facility. Although many adolescents younger than age 18 have the cognitive skills necessary for decision making and are involved in decisions concerning their care, the PSDA limits their legal rights. Creative strategies are needed to develop a model of decision-making rights and responsibilities for adolescents built on the PSDA.

Parents may feel incapable of dealing directly with the child's questions about dying. They may fear that they will be unable to cope with their own feelings during a frank discussion of the possibility of the child's imminent death. The types of questions that children most frequently ask include the following:

- What will death be like?
- What will happen to me when I die?
- Will I be punished for the bad things I have done?
- When will I be with [person(s) closest to child] again?
- Will my parents be all right?
- Will I experience much pain?

Some parents need help in understanding and answering the child's questions at a developmentally appropriate level for the child. Provide guidance about appropriate methods and words to use that will support the child. Some parents may prefer that the child's questions be answered honestly by another professional. A professional who has special bereavement counseling trainig can assist children and families with discussions.

When caring for adolescents, remember that outbursts of anger are common but not personally directed at you. Provide activities to help teens channel their feelings. Continue providing support in spite of their behavior. This approach may encourage teens to accept comforting without losing face. Be available to listen when the teen wants to talk and express feelings and frustrations. Promote friendships with other teens having similar interests or problems.

Provide teens with as much independence and control over their situation as possible. Give them a voice in decisions. Answer questions honestly without using a condescending tone.

Hospice care helps persons with short life expectancies to live their remaining lives to the fullest—without pain and with choices and dignity. Families may need help to focus on the time left with the child. In pediatric hospice, the family is helped to focus on the quality of life by facilitating communication between the child and family. Encourage the family to participate in the child's physical and emotional care. Families need to cry together and to tell each other how much they will miss each other. They need to be assured that the vigil with the child is important so the child does not feel isolated or abandoned as death approaches.

► STAFF REACTIONS TO THE DEATH OF A CHILD

Children are highly valued by society because of their potential future contributions. Children are expected to have a normal life span, and the death of a child is often viewed as a tragedy. Caring for dying children is especially stressful and demanding for health care professionals. Nurses involved in long-term relationships with children experience severe grief when these children die.[16] Nurses often cope by distancing themselves socially from the dying child and family to maintain composure and a professional demeanor. Waechter reported that the total time nurses spent with children decreased as death became more imminent.[17]

Caring for the dying child may be especially difficult for nurses with young children of their own. They tend to identify with the child, making it more likely that they will have difficulty dealing with the death in a professional manner. Nurses may not be able to recognize the dying child's anxi-

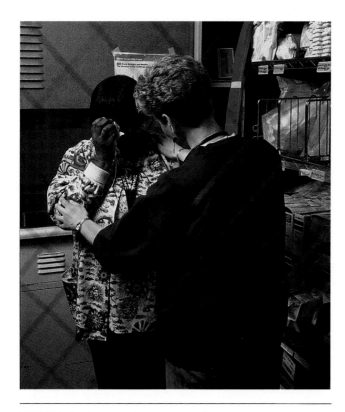

FIGURE 6–8. Nurses need to express grief in a supportive environment after a child's death. Sharing the sadness and grief or futility of resuscitation efforts with colleagues can often help nurses continue to provide supportive care to the next families who need compassionate care.

ety and fears because of their own personal defenses against their sense of helplessness to alter the course of the child's disease.

Nurses who work with terminally ill children and their families need special preparation to meet the needs of these individuals and to manage personal stress simultaneously. Mentorship with experienced hospice nurses, as well as additional educational experiences, may help promote professional nursing care. Nurses who work with dying children and families must learn to cope effectively with grief and develop empathy, competence, and confidence, in their ability to provide more humane and effective nursing care.

Nurses working in hospice settings or hospital units that care for terminally ill children need support systems to help balance the stresses of working with dying children. The workplace should acknowledge the stress nurses experience when working with terminally ill children. Support systems may include discussions with peers or debriefing group sessions with mental health professionals that provide an opportunity to discuss their feelings and concerns (Fig. 6–8). Participating in team decisions regarding the dying child's plan of care (palliative rather than curative) helps many nurses manage their distress.

 LEGAL & ETHICAL CONSIDERATIONS

Nurses who have recognized the inevitability of a child's death experience moral distress with feelings of anger, frustration, sadness, and powerlessness when asked to carry out treatments that cause pain and suffering to the child. Discuss these feelings with members of the care team to determine when curative efforts will stop and the focus of attention will shift to palliative care.[16]

REFERENCES

1. Ryan-Wenger, N.A. (1996). Children, coping, and the stress of illness: A synthesis of research. *Journal of the Society of Pediatric Nurses, 1*(3), 126–138.

2. LaMontagne, L.L., Hepworth, J.T., Johnson, B.D., & Cohen, F. (1996). Children's preoperative coping and its effects on postoperative anxiety and

return to normal activity. *Nursing Research, 45*(3), 141–147.

3. LaMontagne, L.L. (1993). Bolstering personal control in child patients through coping mechanisms. *Pediatric Nursing, 19*(3), 235–237.

4. Ashenberg, M.D., Lambert, S.A., Maier, N.P., & McAliley, L.G. (1996). Easing the wait: Development of a pager program for families. *Pediatric Nursing, 22*(2), 103–107.

5. Ahman, E. (1994). Family-centered care: Shifting orientation. *Pediatric Nursing, 20*(2), 113–117.

6. Evans, M. (1994). An investigation into the feasibility of parental participation in the nursing care of their children. *Journal of Advanced Nursing, 203*(3), 477–482.

7. George, A., & Hancock, J. (1993). Reducing pediatric burn pain with parent participation. *Journal of Burn Care and Rehabilitation, 14*(1), 104–107.

8. Henneman, E.A., McKenzie, J.B., & Dewa, C.S. (1992). An evaluation of interventions for meeting the information needs of families of critically ill patients. *American Journal of Critical Care, 1*(3), 85–93.

9. Tomlinson, P.S., & Mitchell, K.E. (1992). On the nature of social support for families of critically ill children. *Journal of Pediatric Nursing, 7*(6), 386–394.

10. Nelson, L. (1995). When a child dies: Practical, sensitive advice for helping parents through their worst nightmare. *American Journal of Nursing, 95*(3), 61–64.

11. McIntier, T.M., Sr. (1995). Nursing the family when a child dies. *RN, 58*(2), 50–54.

12. Schonfeld, D.J. (1993). Talking with children about death. *Journal of Pediatric Health Care, 7*(6), 269–274.

13. Mahan, M.M. (1994). Death of a sibling: Primary care interventions. *Pediatric Nursing, 20*(3), 293–295, 328.

14. Baker, J.E., Sedney, M.A., & Gross, E. (1992). Psychological tasks for bereaved children. *American Journal of Orthopsychiatry, 62*(1), 105–116.

15. Waechter, E.H. (1987). Children's reactions to fatal illness. In T. Krulik, B. Holaday, & I.M. Martinson, (Eds.), *The child and family facing life-threatening illness.* Philadelphia: Lippincott.

16. Davies, B., Cook, K., O'Loane, M., Clarke, D., MacKenzie, B., Stutzer, C., Connaughty, S., & McCormick, J. (1996). Caring for dying children: Nurses' experiences. *Pediatric Nursing, 22*(6), 500–507.

17. Davies, B., & Eng, B. (1993). Factors influencing nursing care of children who are terminally ill: A selective review. *Pediatric Nursing, 19*, 9–14.

ADDITIONAL RESOURCES

Anderson, J.E. (1996). Helping parents cope with sudden death. *Contemporary Pediatrics, 13*(12), 42–57.

Anderson, A.H., Bateman, L.H., Ingallinera, K.L., & Woolf, P.J. (1991). Our caring continues: A bereavement follow-up program. *Focus on Critical Care, 18*(6), 523–526.

Armstrong-Dailey, A. (1990). Children's hospice care. *Pediatric Nursing, 16*, 337–339, 409.

Back, K.J. (1991). Sudden, unexpected pediatric death: Caring for families. *Pediatric Nursing, 17*(6), 571–575.

Brown, P.S., & Sefansky, S. (1995). Enhancing bereavement care in the pediatric ICU. *Critical Care Nurse, 15*(5), 59–64.

Curley, A.Q. (1988). Effects of the nursing mutual participation model of care on parental stress in the pediatric intensive care unit. *Heart & Lung, 17*(6), 682–688.

Fina, D.K. (1994). A chance to say goodbye. *American Journal of Nursing, 94*(5), 42–45.

Gibbons, M.B. (1992). A child dies: The impact on siblings. *Journal of Pediatric Health Care, 6*(2), 65–72.

Hazinski, M.F. (1992). *Nursing care of the critically ill child* (2nd ed.). St. Louis: Mosby–Year Book.

Hersch, S.P., & Wiener, L.S. (1997). Psychosocial support for the family of the child with cancer. In P.A. Pizzo, &

D.G. Poplack, (Eds.), *Principles and practice of pediatric oncology* (3rd ed.). Philadelphia: Lippincott.

Krulik, T., Holaday, B., & Martinson, I.M. (Eds.). (1987). *The child and family facing life-threatening illness.* Philadelphia: Lippincott.

Kübler-Ross, E. (1983). *On children and death.* New York: Collier/Macmillan.

LaMontagne, L.L., Hepworth, J.T., Pawlak, R., & Chiafery, M. (1992). Parental coping and activities during pediatric critical care. *American Journal of Critical Care, 1*(2), 76–80.

Leske, J.S. (Ed.). (1991). Family interventions. *AACN Clinical Issues in Critical Care Nursing, 2*(2), 181–355.

Miles, A. (1994). Am I going to die? *American Journal of Nursing, 94*, 20.

Miles, M.S., & Carter, M.C. (1985). Coping strategies used by parents during their child's hospitalization in an intensive care unit. *Children's Health Care, 14*(1), 14–21.

Miles, M.S., & Carter, M.C. (1983). Assessing parental stress in intensive care units. *American Journal of Maternal-Child Nursing, 8*(5), 354–359.

Mishel, M. (1983). Parents' perceptions of uncertainty concerning their hospitalized child. *Nursing Research, 32*, 324–330.

Parkman, S.E. (1992). Helping families say good-bye. *American Journal of Maternal-Child Nursing, 17,* 14–17.

Philichi, L.M. (1989). Family adaptation during a pediatric intensive care hospitalization. *Journal of Pediatric Nursing, 4*(4), 268–276.

Rushton, C.H. (1990). Family-centered care in the critical care unit: Myth or reality? *Children's Health Care, 19*(2), 68–70.

Rushton, C.H. (1990). Strategies for family-centered care in the critical care setting. *Pediatric Nursing, 16*(2), 195–199.

Rushton, C.H., & Lynch, M.E. (1992). Dealing with advance directives for critically ill adolescents. *Critical Care Nurse, 12*(5), 31–37.

Stewart, E.S. (1995). Family-centered care for the bereaved. *Pediatric Nursing, 21*(2), 181–184, 187.

Tichy, A.M., Braam, C.A., Meyer, T.A., & Rattan, N.S. (1988). Stressors in pediatric intensive care units. *Pediatric Nursing, 14*(1), 40–42.

Todres, I.D., Earle, M., & Jellinek, M.S. (1994). Enhancing communication: The physician and family in the pediatric intensive care unit. *Pediatric Clinics of North America, 41*(6), 1395–1404.

Tse, A.M., Perez-Woods, R.C., & Opie, N.D. (1987). Children's admissions to the intensive care unit: Parents' attitudes and expectations of outcome. *Children's Health Care, 16*(2), 68–75.

Vachon, M.L.S., & Pakes, E. (1985). Staff stress in the care of the critically ill and dying child. *Issues in Comprehensive Pediatric Nursing, 8,* 151–182.

Wyckoff, P.M., & Erickson, M.T. (1987). Mediating factors of stress on mothers of seriously ill, hospitalized children. *Children's Health Care, 16*(1), 4–12.

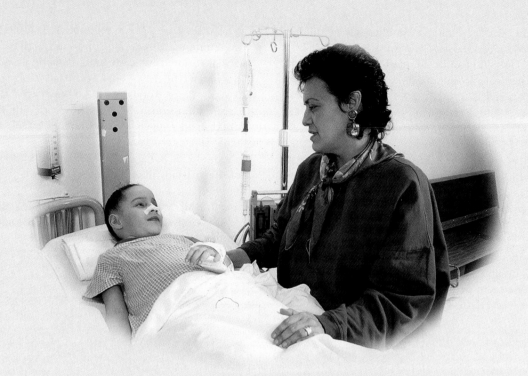

Felicia, who is 5 years old, was struck by a car. Six hours ago she had surgery to repair a liver laceration. After spending 3 hours in the postanesthesia unit, she was moved to the pediatric inpatient unit. She has an intravenous line in place, as well as a nasogastric tube for suction. Her abdominal dressing is clean and dry.

Felicia's mother is rooming in with her during her hospital stay. Because Felicia is thrashing around, her mother thinks she is in pain. She asks the nurse to give her some pain medication. When the nurse enters Felicia's room, she is napping and her facial expression indicates that she is not in pain. When the nurse attempts to straighten her position in bed, she moans. The nurse asks Felicia if she hurts, and she shakes her head no. According to Felicia's chart, she received pain medication just before her transfer from the postanesthesia unit 3 hours ago. Her physician has ordered pain medication every 3–4 hours as needed.

How do you know whether Felicia is in pain? Can you expect her to tell you if she feels pain? Is any additional assessment needed to justify giving Felicia more pain medication? What other pain relief measures could reduce or help to control her pain?

PAIN ASSESSMENT AND MANAGEMENT 7

"Felicia must be in pain so soon after her surgery. I know I would have pain if it were me. Can she get pain medicine without getting another needle?"

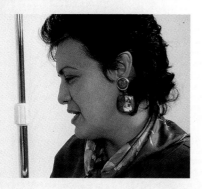

TERMINOLOGY

- **acute pain** Sudden pain of short duration, associated with a tissue-damaging stimulus.
- **anxiolysis** Sedation by medication.
- **chronic pain** Persistent pain lasting longer than 6 months, generally associated with a prolonged disease process.
- **conscious sedation** Light sedation during which the child maintains airway reflexes and responds to verbal stimuli.
- **deep sedation** A controlled state of depressed consciousness or unconsciousness in which the child may experience partial or complete loss of protective reflexes.
- **distraction** The ability to focus attention on something other than pain, such as an activity, music, or a story.
- **electroanalgesia** A method of delivering electrical stimulation to the skin, to compete with pain stimuli for transmission to the spinal cord; also known as transcutaneous electrical nerve stimulation (TENS).
- **equianalgesic dose** The amount of a drug, whether administered orally or parenterally, needed to produce the same analgesic effect.
- **NSAIDs** Nonsteroidal antiinflammatory drugs, used for the treatment of pain.
- **opioids** Synthetic narcotic drugs used for the treatment of pain.
- **pain** An unpleasant sensory and emotional experience associated with actual or potential tissue damage. Pain exists when the patient says it does.
- **patient-controlled analgesia (PCA)** A method for administering an intravenous analgesic, such as morphine, using a computerized pump that the patient controls.
- **tolerance** An altered state of response to an opioid or other pain agent in which increasing amounts of the drug are needed to produce or maintain the same level of pain relief.

Everyone has his or her own perception of pain. A neurologic response to tissue injury, **pain** is an unpleasant sensory and emotional experience associated with actual or potential tissue damage. It exists when the patient says it does (Fig. 7–1).

Pain may be either acute or chronic. **Acute pain** is sudden pain of short duration that may be associated with a single event, such as surgery, or an acute exacerbation of a condition such as a sickle cell crisis. **Chronic pain** is persistent pain lasting longer than 6 months that is generally associated with a prolonged disease process such as juvenile rheumatoid arthritis.

▶ OUTDATED BELIEFS ABOUT PAIN IN CHILDREN

In the past, children did not receive adequate treatment for pain. Undertreatment still occurs.[1] Health care professionals once believed that children feel less pain than adults (Table 7–1). In fact, most physicians did not prescribe pain medication for children or ordered it only as needed. This undertreatment was based on the attitudes of health care professionals about pain, the difficulty and complexity of pain assessment in children, and inadequate research.

Research has shown that past beliefs about children's perception of pain were incorrect. Neonates and infants do feel and remember pain. By 6 months of age, children demonstrate anticipatory fear of pain when taken to

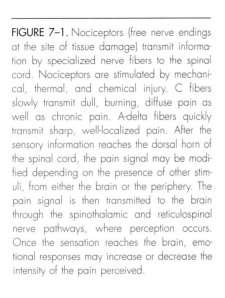

CULTURAL CONSIDERATIONS

The cultural experiences of health care professionals often contribute to their outdated attitudes about pain experienced by children. For example, health care workers may believe that being in pain for a little while is not so bad, that pain helps build character, or that using pain medication is a sign of a weak character.

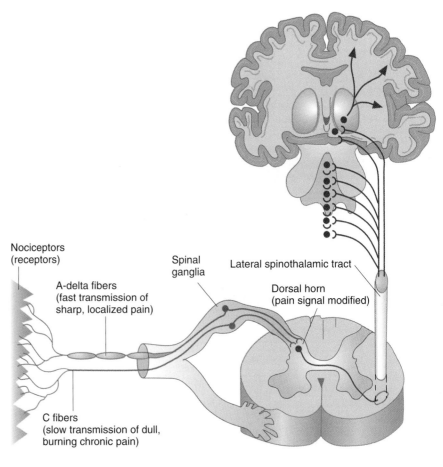

FIGURE 7–1. Nociceptors (free nerve endings at the site of tissue damage) transmit information by specialized nerve fibers to the spinal cord. Nociceptors are stimulated by mechanical, thermal, and chemical injury. C fibers slowly transmit dull, burning, diffuse pain as well as chronic pain. A-delta fibers quickly transmit sharp, well-localized pain. After the sensory information reaches the dorsal horn of the spinal cord, the pain signal may be modified depending on the presence of other stimuli, from either the brain or the periphery. The pain signal is then transmitted to the brain through the spinothalamic and reticulospinal nerve pathways, where perception occurs. Once the sensation reaches the brain, emotional responses may increase or decrease the intensity of the pain perceived.

Nociceptors (receptors)

A-delta fibers (fast transmission of sharp, localized pain)

Spinal ganglia

Lateral spinothalamic tract

Dorsal horn (pain signal modified)

C fibers (slow transmission of dull, burning chronic pain)

7-1	Outdated Beliefs About Pain and Pain Medication in Children

- Children without obvious physical reasons for pain are not likely to have pain.
- Neonates do not feel pain.
- Children do not feel pain with the same intensity as adults because a child's nervous system is immature.
- Children tolerate discomfort well. They become accustomed to pain after having it for a while.
- Children tell you if they are in pain. They do not need medication unless they appear to be in pain.
- Children are not in pain if they can be distracted or they are sleeping.
- Children recover more quickly than adults from painful experiences such as surgery.
- Parents exaggerate or aggravate their child's pain.
- Children have no memory of pain.
- Narcotics are dangerous for children because they can cause respiratory depression and addiction.
- The best route for giving analgesics is intramuscular.
- After surgery, children should not receive the next analgesic dose until they show obvious signs of pain.
- As-needed medication orders mean that medication should be given as infrequently as possible.

a location where they once experienced pain.[3] Health care professionals now recognize that children do not complain of pain because they are afraid that the injection to relieve pain will hurt more than the pain already does.

▶ PAIN INDICATORS

PHYSIOLOGIC INDICATORS

Acute pain stimulates the adrenergic nervous system and results in physiologic changes, including tachycardia, tachypnea, hypertension, pupil dilation, pallor, and increased perspiration. Changes in these signs demonstrates a complex stress response. As the body adapts physiologically, vital signs return to near normal and perspiration decreases after several minutes. Thus changes in vital signs are not a reliable indicator of pain in children because they last such a short time.

Chronic pain of long duration permits physiologic adaptation so normal heart rate, respiratory rate, and blood pressure levels are often seen.[4]

BEHAVIORAL INDICATORS

Children in acute pain behave in many of the same ways as children who show signs of fear and anxiety.[5,6] These behaviors include the following:

- Restless and agitated or hyperalert and vigilant
- Short attention span (child is difficult to distract)
- Irritability (child is difficult to comfort)
- Facial grimacing, posturing (guarding a painful joint by avoiding movement), or protecting the painful area (Fig. 7–2)

 GROWTH & DEVELOPMENT CONSIDERATIONS

Even neonates feel pain. Cutaneous sensation is actually present by 20 weeks' gestation. Brain centers necessary for pain perception develop toward the end of gestation. Nerve pathways associated with pain transmission are functional at birth, but myelination (further development of the myelin sheath) continues during infancy. Although pain conduction may be slower in neonates, the distance that pain stimuli must travel is much shorter than in adults. Because of their immature nervous systems, young children may actually have a lower pain threshold and pain tolerance. Premature infants may be even more sensitive to pain than full-term infants.[2]

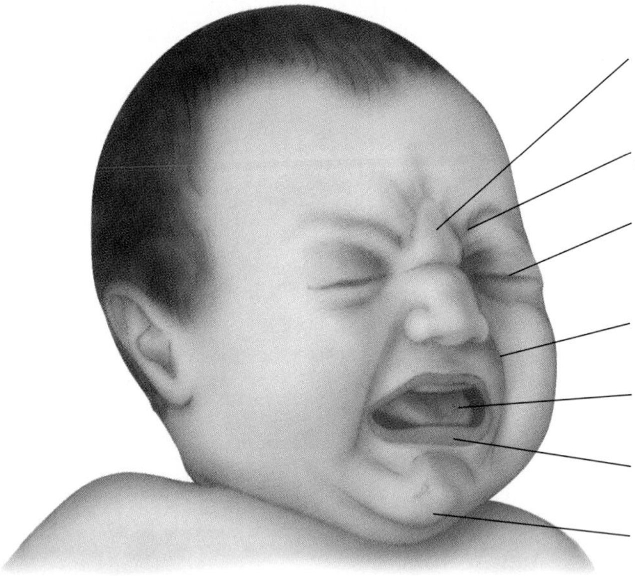

FIGURE 7–2. Neonatal characteristic facial responses to pain include: bulged brow, eyes squeezed shut, furrowed nasolabial creases, open lips, pursed lips, stretched mouth, taut tongue, and a quivering chin.
Redrawn from Carlson, K.L., Clement, B.A., & Nash, P. (1996). Neonatal pain: From concept to research questions and the role of the advanced practice nurse. Journal of Perinatal Neonatal Nursing, 10(1), 64–71.

- Bulged brows
- Brows lowered, drawn together
- Eyes squeezed shut
- Furrowed nasolabial creases
- Taut tongue
- Open, angular, squarish lips and mouth
- Quivering chin

- Anorexia
- Lethargy
- Sleep disturbances

The nurse evaluating Felicia, the 5-year-old girl described in the opening vignette, would observe for such behavioral indicators of pain.

Children often suffer additional emotional distress and fear that the discomfort will worsen. Depression and aggressive behavior are frequently overlooked as indicators of pain.

7-2	Physiologic Consequences of Unrelieved Pain in Children
Responses to Pain	**Potential Physiologic Consequences**
Respiratory Changes	
Rapid shallow breathing	Alkalosis
Inadequate lung expansion	Decreased oxygen saturation
Inadequate cough	Retention of secretions
Neurologic Changes	
Increased sympathetic nervous system activity	Tachycardia, change in sleep patterns, increased blood glucose and cortisol levels
Metabolic Changes	
Increased metabolic rate with increased perspiration	Increased fluid and electrolyte losses

Modified from Eland, J.M. (1990). Pain in children. Nursing Clinics of North America, 25, 871–884, and Altimier, L., Norwood, S., Dick, M.J., et al. (1994). Postoperative pain management in preverbal children: The prescription and administration of analgesia with and without caudal analgesia. Journal of Pediatric Nursing, 9(4), 226–232.

Behavioral indicators of chronic pain and pain of long duration include posturing and inactivity to avoid pain, depression, difficulty sleeping, and an inability to concentrate.[7]

CONSEQUENCES OF PAIN

Unrelieved pain is stressful and has many undesirable physiologic consequences (Table 7–2). For example, the child with acute postoperative pain takes shallow breaths and suppresses coughing to avoid more pain. These self-protective actions increase the potential for respiratory complications. Unrelieved pain may also delay the return of normal gastric and bowel functions. Anorexia associated with pain may delay the healing process. The long-term effects of pain on the child's physical or psychologic condition are unknown.

▶ PAIN ASSESSMENT

No laboratory tests are routinely used to assess pain. Prolonged, severe pain produces a physiologic stress response that includes the chemical release of catecholamines, cortisol, aldosterone, and other corticosteroids. Insulin secretion also decreases, leading to increased amounts of glucose and severe hyperglycemia.[5] Existing conditions such as infection, trauma, and anemia can cause the vital sign changes seen with sudden pain.

The goal of pain assessment is to provide accurate information about the location and intensity of pain and its effects on the child's functioning. When assessing pain in children, keep the following questions in mind:

- What is happening in tissues that might cause pain? Assume that children who have had surgery, injury, or illness are experiencing pain, since these events also cause pain in adults.

- What external factors could be causing pain? For example, is the cast too tight or is the child poorly positioned in bed?

- Are there any indicators of pain, either physiologic or behavioral?

- How is the child responding emotionally?

- How does the child or parent rate the pain?

PAIN HISTORY

Parents can provide a great deal of information about the child's response to pain, such as the following:

- How the child typically expresses pain, both verbally and behaviorally. Children and parents use similar terms to describe pain.[8] Some examples of words used are a hurt, owie, boo-boo, stinging, sore, cutting, burning, itching, hot, and tight. Knowing the appropriate word to use makes communicating with the child easier.

- The child's previous experiences with painful situations.

- How the child copes with pain. The child with several past pain experiences may not exhibit the same types of stressful behaviors as the child with few pain experiences.

- The parent's and child's preferences for analgesic use.

Older children may be able to give a history of painful procedures. When attempting to obtain information about the child's pain experiences

CLINICAL TIP

The presence of physiologic symptoms such as nausea, fatigue, dyspnea, bladder and bowel distention, and fever may influence the intensity of pain felt by a child. The child's behavior or responses to pain stimuli may also be affected by fear, anxiety, separation from parents, anger, culture, age, or a previous pain experience.

7-3 Pediatric Pain History for Children and Parents	
Questions for Children	Questions for Parents
Past Pain Experiences	
Tell me what pain is.	What word(s) does your child use to describe
Tell me about the hurt you have had	pain?
before.	Describe pain experiences your child has pre-
Do you tell others when you hurt?	viously had.
Who?	Does your child tell you or others when he or
What do you do for yourself when	she is in pain?
you are hurting?	How do you know when your child is in
What helps the most to take your hurt	pain?
away?	How does your child usually react to pain?
What do you want others to do for	What do you do for your child when he or
you when you hurt?	she is in pain?
What don't you want others to do for	What does your child do to manage pain?
you when you hurt?	What works best to reduce or take away your
Is there anything special you want me	child's pain?
to know about when you hurt?	Is there anything special you would like me to
What?	know about your child and pain?
Present Pain Experiences	
Where is the pain?	Tell me about the pain your child is having
What does it feel like?	now. Where is it and what does it feel
What do you think is causing the pain?	like?
What would you like me to do for you?	What would you like me to do for your child?

Modified from Hester, N.O., & Barcus, C.S. (1986). Assessment and management of pain in children. Pediatrics: Nursing Update, 1, 2–8.

CLINICAL TIP

When help in describing pain is needed, give the child over 6 years of age some words to select from, such as sharp, dull, aching, pounding, cold, hot, burning, throbbing, stinging, tingling, or cutting.

CULTURAL CONSIDERATIONS

Some ethnic groups, such as Asian, Anglo-Saxon–Germanic, and Irish, do not openly express pain. People of Italian and Jewish descent are more likely to use both verbal and nonverbal methods to express pain freely. However, children have individualized responses, and younger children have had less time to acquire culturally learned behaviors.

and present level of pain, ask the child and parent similar open-ended questions. Sample questions are given in Table 7–3. Many children modify their pain descriptions depending on the type of questions asked and what they expect will happen as a result of their response.

Children with recurrent episodes of pain can be asked to keep a diary or log to describe the characteristics, timing, activities, and potential triggers of their pain, as well as their response to pain treatment measures. This record can help improve pain management.

CULTURAL INFLUENCES ON PAIN

Children's culture and social learning have a tremendous influence on their expression of pain. Cultural traditions often guide children about self-control, coping, and enlisting the assistance of others.[4] Children learn directly and indirectly from their parents about how to respond to pain. By showing approval and disapproval, parents teach their children how to behave when in pain. This instruction includes the following:

- How much discomfort justifies a complaint
- How to express the complaint
- How and when to stop complaining
- Whom to approach for pain relief

7-4	Behavioral Responses and Verbal Descriptions of Pain by Children of Different Developmental Stages	
Age Group	**Behavioral Response**	**Verbal Description**
Infants		
< 6 months	Generalized body movements, chin quivering, facial grimacing, poor feeding	Cries
6–12 months	Reflex withdrawal to stimulus, facial grimacing, disturbed sleep, irritability, restlessness	Cries
Toddlers		
1–3 years	Localized withdrawal, resistance of entire body, aggressive behavior, disturbed sleep	Cries and screams, cannot describe intensity or type of pain
Preschoolers		
3–6 years (preoperational)	Active physical resistance, directed aggressive behavior, strikes out physically and verbally when hurt, low frustration level	Can identify location and intensity of pain, denies pain, may believe his or her pain is obvious to others
School-Age Children		
7–9 years (concrete operations)	Passive resistance, clenches fists, holds body rigidly still, suffers emotional withdrawal, engages in plea bargaining	Can specify location and intensity of pain and describe its physical characteristics
10–12 years (transitional)	May pretend comfort to project bravery, may regress with stress and anxiety	Able to describe intensity and location with more characteristics, able to describe psychologic pain
Adolescents		
13–18 years (formal operations)	Want to behave in a socially acceptable manner (like adults), show a controlled behavioral response	More sophisticated descriptions as experience is gained

For example, boys in the United States are usually encouraged to hide their pain by acting brave and not crying. Girls are often encouraged to express their pain openly. Children also observe other family members in pain and imitate their responses.[9]

PAIN ASSESSMENT SCALES

A child's responses to and understanding of pain depend on the child's age, stage of development, and other situational factors[10] (Tables 7–4, 7–5, and 7–6). For example, neonates cannot anticipate pain and may not demonstrate typical behavior associated with a painful response. Young children are unable to give a detailed description of their pain because of their limited vocabulary and pain experiences. Depending on their developmental stage, children use different coping strategies, such as escape, postponement or avoidance, diversion, and imagery, to deal with pain.

Various pain scales have been developed to assess pain in children (see Figs. 7–3 to 7–7 in Table 7–7). Physical and behavioral indicators are used to quantify pain in children. Some pain assessment scales rely on the nurse's observation of the child's behavior if the child is nonverbal, for example, the Children's Hospital of Eastern Ontario Pain Scale (CHEOPS) (see Table 7–7) and Neonatal Infant Pain Scale (NIPS) (Table 7–8).[11] These scales can provide only an indirect estimate of pain strength from the child's behaviors or physical states. Most scales depend on the child's report of pain intensity (Table 7–7). Facial scales may be a measure of

GROWTH & DEVELOPMENT CONSIDERATIONS

Preverbal children may show conflicting signs of pain (increased or decreased vital signs, agitation or withdrawal, increased or decreased activity, grimacing, crying, or anger), making assessment and monitoring pain management more challenging.

CLINICAL TIP

Children do not exhibit distress in direct proportion to their pain intensity. Thus, behavioral measures may not match the child's self-report of pain intensity.[10]

Text continues on page 275.

7-5   Children's Understanding of Pain by Developmental Stage

Developmental Stage	Understanding of Pain
Infants	
< 6 months	No apparent understanding of pain; infants do have memory of pain; neonates exposed to repeated painful experiences in intensive care unit demonstrate memory of pain by breathholding when approached by care providers
6–12 months	Anticipate a painful event such as an immunization with fear
Toddlers	
1–3 years	Demonstrate a fear of painful situations; use common words for pain such as "owie" and "boo-boo"
Preschoolers	
3–6 years (preoperational)	Pain is a hurt; do not relate pain to illness but may relate pain to an injury; often believe pain is punishment; do not believe an injection takes pain away
School-Age Children	
7–9 years (concrete operations)	Can understand simple relationships between pain and disease but have no clear understanding of the cause of pain; can understand the need for painful procedures to monitor or treat disease; may recognize psychologic pain related to grief and hurt feelings
10–12 years (transitional)	Have a more complex awareness of physical and psychologic pain, such as moral dilemmas and mental pain
Adolescents	
13–18 years (formal operations)	Have a capacity for sophisticated and complex understanding of the causes of physical and mental pain; can relate to the pain experienced by others; pain has both qualitative and quantitative characteristics

7-6   Situational Factors Influencing Pain in Children

Cognitive Factors
- Understanding of pain source
- Ability to control what will happen
- Expectations about the quality and strength of pain
- Whether attention is focused on painful event or distractor

Behavioral Factors
- Use of a pain-control strategy
- Response of parents and health care personnel
- Whether or not restrained
- Ability to continue usual activities

Emotional Factors
- Fear
- Anxiety
- Frustration
- Anger
- Depression

Adapted from McGrath, P.A. (1995). Pain in the pediatric patient: Practical aspects of assessment. Pediatric Annals, 24(3), 126–138.

Scale and Age Group	Administration	Use
NIPS Preterm and full-term infant to 6 weeks after birth (see Table 7–8)	Observe the neonate's facial expression, cry quality, breathing patterns, arm and leg position, and state of arousal	Useful in measuring pain or pain-elicited distress in infants; overall status of infant and the infant's environment must be factored into the assessment
CHEOPS 1–7 years	Observe the child's cry, facial expression, torso position, leg position, touch-painful area, and verbal complaints; select the numerical score for each category after 5 seconds	Primarily behavioral assessment for postoperative pain or following painful procedures; researchers have no specific score indicating pain in need of medication; in preverbal children scale may measure nonspecific stress rather than only pain
Eland Color Tool 4–9 years	Child picks a crayon color to represent the most severe pain, then a color for the next most severe pain, until four crayons have been selected; child then colors in an outline of the body to indicate the location of the areas that hurt by level of pain	You need six crayons: black, purple, blue, red, green, and orange; no one color is most often selected by children as representing the most pain; limited reliability and validity of data[a]
Oucher Scale 3–7 years	Child selects a face that best fits his or her level of pain; older child can select a number between 0 and 100	Useful in hospital settings; child must understand concepts of higher/lower and more/less; cultural versions available; tool has been successfully tested for reliability and validity in some age groups[a,b]

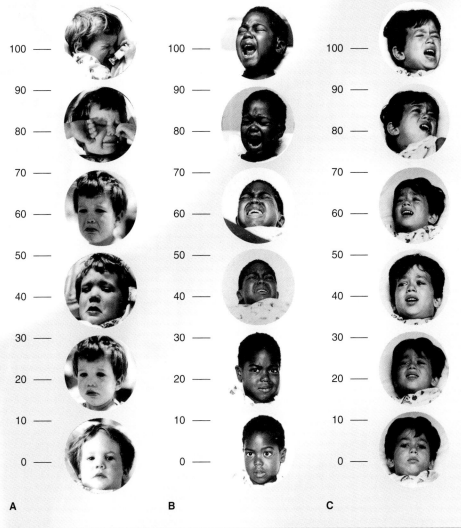

A   B   C

[a] Reliability is the extent to which the same score is obtained when an instrument or scale is used either by different persons or by the same person at different times. Validity is the extent to which an instrument or scale measures what it is supposed to measure.
[b] **A,** The Caucasian version of the Oucher, developed and copyrighted by Judith E. Beyer, RN, PhD, 1983. **B,** The African-American version of the Oucher, developed and copyrighted by Mary J. Denyes, RN, PhD, and Antonia M. Villarruel, RN, PhD, 1990. **C,** The Hispanic version of the Oucher, developed and copyrighted by Antonia M. Villarruel, RN, PhD, and Mary J. Denyes, RN, PhD, 1990.

Scale and Age Group	Administration	Use
Poker Chip Scale 3–7 years	Child selects the number of chips or checkers that matches level of hurt (1 = a little hurt, 5 = the most hurt)	Useful in hospital settings; child must have number concepts from 1 to 5; you can then obtain a measure of child's perception of pain

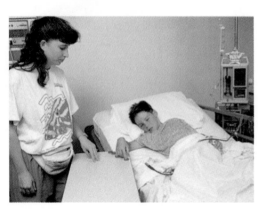

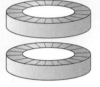 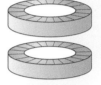 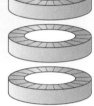

A tiny bit of hurt   Little more pain   Still more pain   Most hurt of all

Faces Pain Scale[c] (preschool children)	Child selects from one of several pictures of faces from happy to sad; child selects the one that is most like his or her pain	Provides a global index of how the child perceives pain; reliable and valid for children over 5 years of age

0: No hurt	1: Hurts a little	2: Hurts a little more	3: Hurts even more	4: Hurts a whole lot	5: Hurts worst

Numeric Pain Scale 9 years–adult	Ask child to rate pain felt on a line with 10 marks (1 = a little pain, 10 = the most pain)	Child must be verbal; easy to carry tool to patient

0   1   2   3   4   5   6   7   8   9   10

Pediatric Pain Questionnaire[d]	Child selects pain descriptors from checklist, rates current and average pain intensity with visual analog scale and uses own color choices to identify different pain intensities on pain map of body	Parent, child, and adolescent forms exist; parent form provides information about history of pain problem and its management; useful for chronic pain

[c]From Wong, D. (1997). Whaley & Wong's Essentials of pediatric nursing (5th ed., p. 1215). Copyrighted by Mosby-Yearbook Inc. Reprinted by permission.
[d]From Varni, J.W., Thompson, K.L., & Hanson V. (1987). The Varni/Thompson pediatric pain questionnaire: Chronic musculoskeletal pain in juvenile rheumatoid arthritis. Pain, 28, 27–38.

7-8   Neonatal Infant Pain Scale (NIPS)

Characteristic	Scoring Criteria
Facial Expression 0 = Relaxed muscles 1 = Grimace	• Restful face with neutral expression • Tight facial muscles; furrowed brow, chin, and jaw (Note: At low gestational ages, infants may have no facial expression)
Cry 0 = No cry 1 = Whimper 2 = Vigorous cry	• Quiet, not crying • Mild moaning, intermittent • Loud screaming, rising, shrill, and continuous (Note: silent cry may be scored if infant is intubated, as indicated by obvious mouth or facial movements)
Breathing Patterns 0 = Relaxed 1 = Change in breathing	• Usual breathing pattern maintained • Indrawing (retraction of chest), irregular, faster than usual, gagging, or holding breath
Arm Movements 0 = Relaxed/restrained (with soft restraints) 1 = Flexed/extended	• No muscle rigidity, occasional random movements (not fighting restraints) • Tense, straightened arms; rigidity; or rapid extension and flexion
Leg Movements 0 = Relaxed/restrained (with soft restraints) 1 = Flexed/extended	• No muscle rigidity, occasional random movements (not fighting restraints) • Tense, straightened arms; rigidity; or rapid extension and flexion
State of Arousal 0 = Sleeping/awake 1 = Fussy	• Quiet, peaceful sleeping; or alert and settled • Alert and restless or thrashing

From Lawrence, J., Alcock, D., McGrath, P., et al. (1993). The development of a tool to assess neonatal pain. Neonatal Network, 12(6), 61.

emotional distress because they reflect the unpleasantness of pain. The nurse caring for Felicia might use a pain scale such as the CHEOPS, Eland, Oucher, poker chip, or faces scale to help determine whether Felicia requires additional pain medication. Because adults cannot experience the child's pain, it is not possible to compare the pain felt by children and adults using these assessment tools, even when undergoing the same procedures.

▶ MEDICAL MANAGEMENT OF PAIN

The U.S. government has published guidelines for management of pain in all age groups, including children.[12] The recommendations for pain management include both drug and nondrug measures. Drug interventions include the use of **opioids** (narcotics) and nonsteroidal antiinflammatory drugs **(NSAIDs).**

GROWTH & DEVELOPMENT CONSIDERATIONS

Identify the child's stage of development for readiness to use pain scales.
• Assess the child's language skills (ability to use words in sequence, follow simple directions, and answer simple questions).
• Ask the child to count his or her fingers or up to 10.
• Determine whether the child can understand concepts such as more or less and higher or lower.

CLINICAL TIP

Surgery and trauma can result in multiple sites of pain (incision or laceration, cut or bruised muscles, interrupted blood supply, nasogastric tube placement, insertion sites of intravenous lines). When using pain scales in the assessment of a verbal child, attempt to identify all sites of pain. Then evaluate the intensity of pain at each site.

7-9   Opioid Analgesics and Recommended Doses for Children and Adolescents

Drug	Approximate Equianalgesic Oral Dose	Approximate Equianalgesic Parenteral Dose	Recommended Starting Dose (Adults >50 kg Body Weight)		Recommended Starting Dose (Children and Adults <50 kg Body Weight[a])	
			Oral	Parenteral	Oral	Parenteral
Opioid Agonist						
Morphine[b]	30 mg q 3–4 hr (around-the-clock-dosing) 60 mg q 3–4 hr (single dose or intermittent dosing)	10 mg q 3–4 hr	30 mg q 3–4 hr	10 mg q 3–4 hr	0.3 mg/kg q 3–4 hr	0.1 mg/kg q 3–4 hr
Codeine[c]	130 mg q 3–4 hr	75 mg q 3–4 hr (intramuscular/subcutaneous)	60 mg q 3–4 hr	60 mg q 2 hr	1 mg/kg q 3–4 hr[d]	NR
Hydromorphone[b] (Dilaudid)	7.5 mg q 3–4 hr	1.5 mg q 3–4 hr	6 mg q 3–4 hr	1.5 mg q 3–4 hr	0.06 mg/kg q 3–4 hr	0.015 mg/kg q 3–4 hr
Hydrocodone (in Lorcet, Lortab, Vicodin, others)	30 mg q 3–4 hr	NA	10 mg q 3–4 hr	NA	0.2 mg/kg q 3–4 hr[d]	NA
Levorphanol (Levo-Dromoran)	4 mg q 6–8 hr	2 mg q 6–8 hr	4 mg q 6–8 hr	2 mg q 6–8 hr	0.04 mg/kg q 6–8 hr	0.02 mg/kg q 6–8 hr
Meperidine (Demerol)	300 mg q 2–3 hr	100 mg q 3 hr	NR	100 mg q 3 hr	NR	0.75 mg/kg q 2–3 hr
Methadone (Dolophine, others)	20 mg q 6–8 hr	10 mg q 6–8 hr	20 mg q 6–8 hr	10 mg q 6–8 hr	0.2 mg/kg q 6–8 hr	0.1 mg/kg q 6–8 hr
Oxycodone (Roxicodone, also in Percocet, Percodan, Tylox, others)	30 mg q 3–4 hr	NA	10 mg q 3–4 hr	NA	0.2 mg/kg q 3–4 hr[d]	NA
Oxymorphone[b] (Numorphan)	NA	1 mg q 3–4 hr	NA	1 mg q 3–4 hr	NR	NR

OPIOIDS

Narcotics such as morphine and codeine may be administered by oral, subcutaneous, intramuscular, and intravenous routes. Administration of opioids by an oral route is as effective as by intramuscular and intravenous routes when the drug is given in an **equianalgesic dose** (the amount of drug, whether given by oral or parenteral routes, needed to produce the same analgesic effect) (Table 7–9). Rectal preparations of some opioids are also available.

Common side effects include sedation, nausea, vomiting, constipation, and itching. Potential complications of opioids include respiratory depres-

7-9 | Opioid Analgesics and Recommended Doses for Children and Adolescents (continued)

Drug	Approximate Equianalgesic Oral Dose	Approximate Equianalgesic Parenteral Dose	Recommended Starting Dose (Adults >50 kg Body Weight)		Recommended Starting Dose (Children and Adults <50 kg Body Weight[a])	
			Oral	Parenteral	Oral	Parenteral
Opioid Agonist-Antagonist and Partial Agonist						
Buprenorphine (Buprenex)	NA	0.3–0.4 mg q 6–8 hr	NA	0.4 mg q 6–8 hr	NA	0.004 mg/kg q 6–8 hr
Butorphanol (Stadol)	NA	2 mg q 3–4 hr	NA	2 mg q 3–4 hr	NA	NR
Nalbuphine (Nubain)	NA	10 mg q 3–4 hr	NA	10 mg q 3–4 hr	NA	0.1 mg/kg q 3–4 hr
Pentazocine (Talwin, other)	150 mg q 3–4 hr	60 mg q 3–4 hr	50 mg q 4–6 hr	NR	NR	NR

Note: Published tables vary in the suggested doses that are equianalgesic to morphine. Clinical response is the criterion that must be applied for each patient; titration to clinical response is necessary. Because there is not complete cross-tolerance among these drugs, it is usually necessary to use a lower than equianalgesic dose when changing drugs to retitrate to response.
NA, not available; NR, not recommended.
Caution: Recommended doses do not apply to patients with renal or hepatic insufficiency or other conditions affecting drug metabolism and kinetics.
[a]*Caution:* Doses listed for patients with body weight less than 50 kg cannot be used as initial starting doses in babies less than 6 months of age. Consult the *Clinical Practice Guideline for Acute Pain Management: Operative or Medical Procedures and Trauma* section on management of pain in neonates for recommendations.
[b]For morphine, hydromorphone, and oxymorphone, rectal administration is an alternate route for patients unable to take oral medications, but equianalgesic doses may differ from oral and parental doses because of pharmacokinetic differences.
[c]*Caution:* Codeine doses above 65 mg often are not appropriate because of diminishing incremental analgesia with increasing doses but continually increasing constipation and other side effects.
[d]*Caution:* Doses of aspirin and acetaminophen in combination opioid/NSAID preparation must also be adjusted to the patient's body weight.
From Acute Pain Management Guideline Panel. (1992). Acute pain management in infants, children, and adolescents: Operative and medical procedures. Quick reference guide for clinicians. (AHCPR Pub. No. 92-0020). Rockville, MD: Agency for Health Care Policy and Research, U.S. Public Health Service, Department of Health and Human Services.

sion, cardiovascular collapse, and addiction. When the child's condition is unstable, as in trauma or critical illness, the dosage of opioids must be carefully calculated to match the child's cardiorespiratory status, although infants and children are no more likely than adults to develop respiratory depression following administration of a weight-specific dose of narcotics.[13] Addiction is a rare complication in adults treated for painful conditions, and the same holds true for children.

NONSTEROIDAL ANTIINFLAMMATORY DRUGS

NSAIDs such as aspirin and acetaminophen, which are primarily given orally, are effective for the relief of mild to moderate pain and chronic pain. Table 7–10 presents recommended dosages of these drugs. They are most commonly used for bone, inflammatory, and rheumatoid conditions. A, NSAID may be prescribed in combination with an opioid to increase the effectiveness of the narcotic drug. This combination may ultimately reduce the amount of opioids needed for pain relief.

DRUG ADMINISTRATION

Pain from surgery, major trauma, or cancer will be present for predictable periods because of the effects of tissue damage. Pain relief should be pro-

 NURSING ALERT

Respiratory depression (a respiratory rate less than 20 breaths/min in infants, 16 breaths/min in children, and 12 breaths/min in adolescents) may progress to respiratory arrest and is the major life-threatening complication of opioid administration. Identify the time interval before drug-specific peak respiratory depression occurs, and then carefully monitor the child's vital signs during that period.

7-10   Recommended Doses of NSAIDs for Children and Adolescents

Oral NSAID	Usual Adult Dose	Usual Pediatric Dose[a]	Comments
Acetaminophen	650–975 mg q 4 hr	10–15 mg/kg q 4 hr po	Lacks the peripheral antiinflammatory activity of other NSAIDs
Aspirin	650–975 mg q 4 hr	10–15 mg/kg q 4 hr po[b]	Standard against which other NSAIDs are compared; inhibits platelet aggregation; may cause postoperative bleeding
Choline magnesium trisalicylate (Trilisate)	1000–1500 mg bid	15–20 mg/kg tid po[b]	May have minimal antiplatelet activity; also available as oral liquid
Ibuprofen (Motrin, others)	400 mg q 4–6 hr	4–10 mg/kg q 6–8 hr po	Available as several brand names and as generic; also available as oral suspension
Naproxen (Naprosyn)	500 mg initial dose followed by 250 mg q 6–8 hr	5–7 mg/kg q 12 hr po	Also available as oral liquid
Tolmetin (Tolectin)	600 mg–1.8 g qd po in 3 divided doses	6–8 mg/kg qid po	Available in scored 200-mg tablets
Ketorolac (Toradol)	30 mg q 6 hr IV or 10 mg q 4–6 hr po	0.5 mg/kg q 8 hr IV	Not yet approved for use in those under 16 years, but is sometimes used in children

[a]Drug recommendations are limited to NSAIDs where pediatric dose experience is available.
[b]Contraindicated in presence of fever or other evidence of viral illness.
Modified from Acute Pain Management Guideline Panel. (1992). Acute pain management in infants, children, and adolescents: Operative and medical procedures. Quick reference guide for clinicians. (AHCPR Pub. No. 92-0020). Rockville, MD: Agency for Health Care Policy and Research, U.S. Public Health Service, Department of Health and Human Services, and Holder, K.A., & Pratt, R.B. (1995). Taming the pain monster: Pediatric postoperative pain management. Pediatric Annals, 24(3), 164–168.

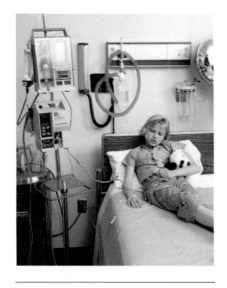

FIGURE 7–3. By using patient-controlled analgesia, the older child is able to regulate the intake of an intravenous analgesic such as morphine.

vided around the clock. Every effort should be made to give the child analgesics without causing more pain. The preferred routes of administration are intravenous and oral.

Continuous-infusion analgesia, which eliminates the peaks and valleys in pain control, is recommended to keep drug levels constant in children with continuous or persistent severe pain. Analgesics may also be given intravenously on a scheduled basis (eg, every 3–4 hours). Delays in giving analgesics on a scheduled basis increase the chances of breakthrough pain and the subsequent anticipation of pain. Giving analgesics on an as-needed basis for acute pain also results in the *loss of pain control*. More medications are often needed to restore pain control than would have been required for continuous infusion analgesia.

Patient-controlled analgesia (PCA) is a method of administering an intravenous analgesic, such as morphine, using a computerized pump that is programmed by the health care professional and controlled by the child (Fig. 7–3). This technique is especially useful for pain control in the first 48 hours after surgery. PCA is prescribed mostly for children 5 years old and older.[13] Children selected for PCA should be able to push the injection button and should understand that pushing the button will give them medication to relieve pain (Table 7–11).

After initial pain control has been achieved with an IV infusion by the nurse, the child presses a button to receive a smaller analgesic dose for episodic pain relief. The PCA monitor can be set up with or without a con-

7-11	Patient Education Guidelines for Patient-Controlled Analgesia (PCA)

- What is PCA? Analgesia means pain relief: you get to control the amount of medicine you receive by using the machine.
- The machine gives the medicine by passing it through the tube that is connected to your intravenous line. When you push the button, the machine pumps pain medicine into the intravenous line to make you feel better.
- The machine limits the amount of medicine you can get to what the doctor orders. You can get any amount up to the maximum by pushing the button repeatedly. The push button will not let you make a mistake if you drop it or roll on it.
- Whenever you feel pain, hurt, or discomfort, push the button to get more medicine. You should be the only one to push the button.
- No needles for pain shots are needed as long as the intravenous line is in place.
- The PCA may not relieve all of your pain, but it should make you feel comfortable. Let the nurse know if you think your PCA is not working.
- The PCA will be used until you can take pills or drink liquid pain medicine.

tinuous infusion of opioid drug in addition to the dose administered when the child pushes the button. A continuous infusion prevents a recurrence of pain during long sleeping periods. Additional pain medication is often ordered as needed to supplement the continuous and patient-administered infusion when pain control is not maintained.

Children and adolescents benefit from PCA by receiving continuous pain control and having the ability to control their comfort level with no trauma from injections. Several studies have documented the maintenance of pain relief without an increase in narcotic side effects.[14] Once children can take oral analgesics, PCA is discontinued.

Epidural pain control provides selective analgesia and is becoming more common for postoperative pain management. A catheter is inserted into either the lumbar or the caudal space. Only minute doses of drugs are needed because of the high concentration achieved at the opioid receptors in the spinal cord's dorsal horn.[13]

 SAFETY PRECAUTIONS

To prevent overdoses, the PCA computerized pump has safety features that include the ability to set the maximum number of infusions per hour and the maximum amount of drug received in a given time period.

► NURSING MANAGEMENT OF PAIN

Nurses have an ethical obligation to relieve a child's suffering not only because of the consequences of unrelieved pain but also because appropriate pain management may have benefits such as earlier mobilization, shortened hospital stays, and reduced costs. To provide effective nursing management of children in pain, anticipate the presence of pain and recognize the child's right to pain control.

Examples of nursing diagnoses for children in pain include the following:

- Pain related to surgery, injury, invasive procedure, or nerve compression from tumor growth
- Chronic Pain related to joint degeneration, inflammatory process
- Anxiety related to anticipation of pain from an invasive procedure, or pain recurrence
- Sleep Pattern Disturbance related to inadequate pain control

 LEGAL & ETHICAL CONSIDERATIONS

Most children are unaware of their right to pain relief. Nurses and health care institutions have a duty to prevent and alleviate suffering. Pain management should be an institutional priority with a standard of care. Nurses have an ethical responsibility to monitor implementation of that standard.[1]

NURSING CARE PLAN
THE CHILD WITH POSTOPERATIVE PAIN

GOAL	INTERVENTION	RATIONALE	EXPECTED OUTCOME

1. Pain related to surgery and injury

The child will report reduced pain.	• Give analgesic by a pain-free method. • Have the child select a pain scale and rate the amount of pain perceived before and 30–60 minutes after analgesic is given to ensure pain relief.	• The child may deny pain to avoid analgesia by painful route. • The child's pain rating is the best indicator of pain. Maintenance of pain control requires less analgesia than treating each acute pain episode.	The child reports reduced pain after administration of analgesia. The child's rating of pain stays at 0 or a low level.

2. Sleep Pattern Disturbance related to inadequate pain control

The child will experience fewer disruptions of sleep by pain.	• Give analgesia by continuous infusion or every 3–4 hr around the clock.	• Pain breakthrough occurs even during sleep	The child's sleep is undisturbed by pain. Child sleeps for age-appropriate number of hours per day.

3. Anxiety related to anticipation of a pain recurrence

The child will report reduced concern about pain recurrence.	• Reposition the child every 2 hr and maintain good body alignment. Provide therapeutic touch or massage.	• Anxiety increases perception of pain. New positions decrease muscle cramping and skin pressure.	The child expresses no anxiety about pain management.

- Knowledge Deficit related to self-management of pain control, and use of nonpharmacologic pain-control measures
- Inability to Sustain Spontaneous Ventilation: Potential for, related to opioid overdose
- Constipation: Potential for, related to side effect of pain medication and limited activity

Nursing management involves the following actions:

- Recognition of pain and formulation of a nursing diagnosis
- Pharmacologic intervention
- Nonpharmacologic intervention
- Monitoring the effectiveness of pain-control measures to provide optimal comfort
- Patient education

The accompanying Nursing Care Plan summarizes nursing care for the child with postoperative pain.

NURSING CARE PLAN
THE CHILD WITH POSTOPERATIVE PAIN– *Continued*

GOAL	INTERVENTION	RATIONALE	EXPECTED OUTCOME

4. Knowledge Deficit related to self-management of pain control and use of nondrug pain-control measures

The child and family will understand use of patient-controlled analgesia (PCA) and what nondrug pain control measures patient and family can use.	• Teach the child how the PCA works and when to push the button. • Teach the family and the child how to use age-appropriate imagery, distraction, relaxation techniques, and other nondrug pain-relief measures.	• The child must know that pushing the PCA button will keep pain under control. • Nondrug pain-control measures reduce amount of analgesia needed.	The child's pain rating stays low. The child and family independently use nondrug pain control measures.
The child and family will use appropriate analgesia after discharge.	• Discuss appropriate pain control for use at home after discharge.	• The family and the child may be anxious about pain management at home.	The family understands pain-relief measures for use at home and knows where to call if help is needed.

5. Risk for Inability to Sustain Spontaneous Ventilation related to opioid overdose

The child will maintain adequate respirations.	• Verify that correct dose of opioid analgesic is given. Monitor vital signs before analgesic is administered and at time of peak drug action. Calculate antagonist dose ordered by the physician to be sure it will reverse respiratory depression, not counteract effect of analgesia.	• Respiratory depression is a significant complication of opioid analgesics. Respiratory depression episode must not progress to respiratory arrest.	There is no episode of respiratory depression associated with analgesic.

INCREASE AND MAINTENANCE OF PATIENT COMFORT

Pharmacologic Intervention

Give analgesics as ordered by the physician, ensuring that the dose is appropriate for the child's weight. When administering an opioid by intravenous infusion or PCA, monitor the flow rate and the site for infiltration. Make sure analgesic antagonists such as naloxone are available should complications develop.

Monitor the child's vital signs for complications related to opioids, such as respiratory depression. Naloxone may be used to treat respiratory depression caused by an opioid drug at a dose that does not reverse the pain control effects of the narcotic. Other vital signs (heart rate and blood

CLINICAL TIP

Clinical signs that predict the development of respiratory depression include sleepiness, small pupils, and shallow breathing. Children at particular risk for respiratory depression induced by a narcotic are those with an altered level of consciousness, an unstable circulatory status, a history of apnea, or a known airway problem.

pressure) may not change in response to effective analgesia when infection, trauma, or other stressors keep them elevated. Check for the presence of other side effects of analgesics, such as sedation, nausea, vomiting, itching, and constipation.

Evaluate the child's level of pain at frequent intervals to determine whether the analgesic eliminated the pain and to identify any increase in pain intensity. Use information collected from the child and parent, as well as from an appropriate pain scale. Dramatic reductions in pain should occur, although not all pain may disappear. Many children sleep after receiving an analgesic. This sleep is not a side effect of the drug or a sign of an overdose, but the result of pain relief. Pain interrupts sleep, and once pain is relieved, the child can sleep comfortably. On the other hand, sleep does not always indicate pain control. A child in pain may fall asleep in exhaustion. Look for other symptoms of pain, such as excess movement or moaning. A flowsheet may be used to document assessments and medication administration during the postoperative period.

Become an advocate for children when the dose or type of analgesic ordered is inadequate. **Tolerance,** the altered state of response to an opioid or other pain agent in which increasing amounts of the drug are needed to produce or maintain the same level of pain relief, may occur when children with severe pain have been taking narcotics for several days. Breakthrough pain occurs, and an increase in dosage is needed to achieve the previous level of pain relief. Before asking the physician to change the analgesia, review the child's record for documentation that the prescribed drug has been given at the appropriate dose and frequency and that the child's pain relief is ineffective despite the drug administration. After verifying the record, provide the physician with information about the characteristics of the child's pain and ask that the medication be changed.

Oral NSAIDs are generally ordered for less severe pain or chronic pain. These drugs may mask fever. Be alert to the potential complication of gastrointestinal hemorrhage in critically ill children who have a physiologic stress response of increased gastric acids.

Nonpharmacologic Intervention

Use nonpharmacologic methods of pain control with or without analgesics. One or more of these methods may provide adequate pain relief when the child has low levels of pain. When used with analgesics, nonpharmacologic techniques often increase the effectiveness of the analgesic or reduce the dosage required. When used in association with a medical procedure, remember to use an intervention before, during, and after the procedure. This gives the child a chance to recover, feel mastery, and remember coping.[16]

Parental Involvement

Parents are the single most powerful nonpharmacologic method of pain relief available to children.[5] A parent's presence greatly reduces the anxiety associated with pain and hospitalization. Children often feel more secure telling their parents about their pain and anxiety.

Distraction

Distraction involves engaging a child in a wide variety of activities to help him or her focus attention on something other than pain and the anxiety associated with the procedure. Examples of distracting activities are listening to music, singing a song, playing a game, watching television or a video, and focusing on a picture while counting. Select activities that are develop-

LEGAL & ETHICAL CONSIDERATIONS

There is growing consensus that placebo use to assess and manage pain should be avoided, especially without consent. Studies suggest that placebos tend to be used for patients who are disliked, with whom staff have conflicts, or who have failed to respond to standard treatment. Placebo use involves deception. You must respect the patient's right to be informed of treatment.[15]

CLINICAL TIP

Assemble a pain management kit to promote distraction, imagery, and relaxation in children. Items that might be included are magic wands, pinwheels, bubble liquid, a slinky spring toy, a foam ball, party noisemakers, and pop-up books. It may also be helpful to include items for therapeutic play such as syringes, adhesive bandages, alcohol swabs, and other supplies from a medical kit. The pain management kit may be especially helpful for children who are being prepared for surgery or for painful procedures and need to be distracted.

mentally appropriate for the child. Children in severe pain cannot be distracted, but do not assume the pain is gone if a child can be distracted.

Cutaneous Stimulation

Cutaneous stimulation involves rubbing the painful area, massaging the skin gently, and holding or rocking the child. Infants require firm stroking to soothe their pain. Touching provides a stimulus to compete with the pain stimuli that are transmitted from the peripheral nerves to the spinal cord. These actions may reduce the pain felt by the child.

Electroanalgesia

Also known as transcutaneous electrical nerve stimulation (TENS), **electroanalgesia** delivers small amounts of electrical stimulation to the skin by electrodes. This stimulation may interfere with the transmission of pain from the peripheral nerves to the spinal cord. TENS may be used for both acute and chronic pain management.

Relaxation Techniques

Relaxation techniques are used to reduce muscle tension. Pain is often aggravated when muscles are tensed. Relaxation methods include rhythmic breathing (repeatedly taking a deep breath and slowly releasing it), alternately tensing and relaxing selected muscle groups, and focusing attention on something the child likes.

Hypnosis

An altered state of consciousness occurs when appropriate suggestions distort perception, memory, and mood in the child. Children who respond to hypnotic suggestions are often more relaxed and experience less pain.

Imagery

Imagery is a cognitive process that encourages the child to focus on and explore a favorite place, event, or funny story unrelated to the pain process. This method is most effective in children over 6 years of age. Ask the child to think about all the sights, sounds, smells, tastes, and feelings that will help him or her to experience the favorite place. Imagery is a form of self-hypnosis, and it is most effective when preceded by a relaxation exercise.

Application of Heat and Cold

Heat application promotes dilation of blood vessels. The increased blood circulation permits the removal of debris of cell breakdown from the site. Heat also promotes muscle relaxation, breaking the pain–spasm–pain cycle. To reduce edema, do not apply heat in the first 24 hours after an injury. The application of cold is believed to slow the ability of pain fibers to transmit pain impulses. Cold also controls pain by decreasing edema and inflammation. When cold is applied, care should be taken to avoid causing thermal injury.

DISCHARGE PLANNING AND HOME CARE TEACHING

Children are frequently discharged from the hospital with oral analgesics following surgery, injury, or treatment of acute medical conditions. Teach parents and children about the dosage and frequency of administration and the side effects of the analgesic ordered. Make sure parents know that a sudden increase in pain intensity indicates the development of a complication requiring medical attention.

GROWTH & DEVELOPMENT CONSIDERATIONS

Methods of distraction for pain control vary according to the child's developmental stage and individual interests.

- Infants: holding, cuddling, sucking a pacifier
- Preschoolers: engaging in therapeutic play, watching television or a video
- School-age children: talking about pleasant experiences, listening to radio, watching television or a video
- Adolescents: having visitors, playing games, watching television, listening to radio or tape player

HOME CARE CONSIDERATIONS

Parents have the responsibility to provide adequate pain control for their child after day surgery. Because of cultural values, some parents may feel the child should learn to tolerate some amount of pain. Provide guidance to help parents assess their child's pain and directions for giving pain medications. Take the time to discuss the importance of pain management and its benefits in promoting the child's healing.[17]

7-12	Strategies for Chronic Pain Management

- Explain and validate the pain and its causes.
- Define treatment goals, including medications.
- Use distraction, relaxation, self-hypnosis, TENS, and exercise.
- Develop strategies for functional restoration.
- Give guidelines for a gradual increase in activity.
- Have a plan for sudden painful episodes.
- Explore stressors and potential pain triggers.
- Consider whether the child uses manipulatory behaviors for attention or secondary gain.
- Refer to a mental health professional or pain management team as needed.

Adapted from Shapiro, B.S. (1995). Treatment of chronic pain in children and adolescents. Pediatric Annals, 24(3), 148–156.

Educate school-age children and adolescents about pain that may occur with elective procedures, the use of pain scales, and the methods available for pain relief, both pharmacologic and nonpharmacologic. Encourage children and parents to use the techniques that work best for them.

Children with chronic conditions (arthritis, sickle cell disease) or recurrent painful episodes (headaches, recurrent abdominal pain) often need long-term pain management (Table 7–12). For example, children with severe, long-term pain that is associated with cancer may be cared for at home with intravenous analgesics. Care of these children is usually managed by a home health care team. Educate parents thoroughly regarding intravenous care and analgesic administration.

Remember that many common health problems (otitis media, pharyngitis, and urinary tract infection) have pain as one of their presenting symptoms. Often the only medication prescribed is an antibiotic to clear the infection. This may leave the child in pain for 48–72 hours until the antibiotic brings the infection under control. Give parents recommendations for pain control and comfort measures during this period.

► PAIN ASSOCIATED WITH MEDICAL PROCEDURES

Children undergo a wide variety of painful diagnostic and treatment procedures in the hospital and in outpatient settings. Procedures rated the most painful by children in one study included chest tube insertion, arterial puncture, lumbar puncture, bone marrow aspiration, insertion of an intravenous line, and venipuncture.[17] The anticipation of these procedures causes anxiety and emotional distress that can lead to greater intensity of pain. Children who have experienced severe pain in the past may be unwilling to cooperate with health care personnel.

MEDICAL MANAGEMENT

Procedures such as burn debridement, laceration repair, bone marrow aspiration, and fracture reduction are associated with so much pain and anxiety that children need premedication with analgesia and **anxiolysis,** or administration of sedatives.

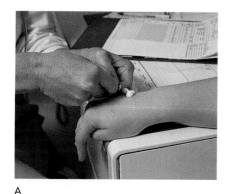
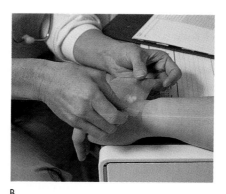

A   B

FIGURE 7–4. When painful procedures are planned, use EMLA cream to anesthetize the skin where the painful stick will be made. **A,** Apply a thick layer of cream over intact skin (½ of a 5-g tube). **B,** Cover the cream with a transparent adhesive dressing, sealing all the sides. The cream anesthetizes the dermal surface in 45–60 minutes.

A local anesthetic such as lidocaine is often injected subcutaneously in a small area to reduce the pain of deeper needle insertion. Topical anesthetics in the form of a EMLA (eutetic mixture of local anesthetics) cream, a mixture of lidocaine 2.5% and prilocaine 2.5% in an emulsion, can be used to reduce the pain associated with the first needle stick (Fig. 7–4).

Conscious sedation is a light sedation during which the child maintains airway reflexes and responds to verbal stimuli (Table 7–13). It can be used on a cooperative child. With conscious sedation, children have minimal anxiety, less pain, and often no memory of the procedure.[18] Conscious sedation is produced with various drugs, including midazolam, fentanyl, and a combination of Demerol (meperidine), Phenergan (promethazine), and Thorazine (chlorpromazine) (DPT). DPT is used less often because other drugs have a shorter action, are more predictable, and have fewer side effects.[18]

NURSING MANAGEMENT

Increase Comfort During Painful Procedures

Help the child cope with a painful procedure by telling the child what sensations to expect and what will happen during the procedure. This reduces stress more effectively than just providing information about the procedure.[19] Chapter 4 gives methods for preparing children of different developmental ages for procedures.

SAFETY PRECAUTIONS

Whenever conscious sedation is given, be sure to have the resources available to monitor the child's vital signs and to provide advanced life support if the child should progress to deep sedation. In case complications occur, the following equipment should be immediately available: suction apparatus, a bag-valve mask for assisted ventilation with capability of 90%–100% oxygen delivery, an oxygen supply (5 L/min for more than 60 minutes), and antagonists to sedative medication.

7-13	Characteristics of Conscious Sedation and Deep Sedation	
Assessment Factors	**Conscious Sedation**	**Deep Sedation**
Airway	Able to maintain airway independently and continuously	Unable to maintain airway independently or continuously
Cough and gag reflexes	Reflexes intact	Partial or complete loss of reflexes
Level of consciousness	Easily aroused with verbal or gentle physical stimulation	Not easily aroused, may not respond purposefully to verbal or gentle physical stimulation

From Zimmerman, S. (1993). Conscious sedation in the Emergency Medical Trauma Center. Washington, DC: Children's National Medical Center.

Help children manage the pain from immunizations by "blowing away the shot pain." As a form of distraction and imagery have the child repeatedly blow out air during the injection as if blowing bubbles.

Drugs may not be used for quick procedures, such as a dressing change, or an unexpected intravenous insertion, injection, or venipuncture. For a planned injection, intravenous insertion, or venipuncture, EMLA can be placed on the skin (see Fig. 7–4). Nonpharmacologic measures, especially imagery, relaxation techniques, and distraction, may reduce the anxiety associated with the anticipation of the procedure. Teach parents and children to use these interventions before procedures. Help children to control their anxiety through therapeutic play.

When pharmacologic pain management is used for a procedure, the nurse's responsibilities include the following:

- Treat anticipated procedure-related pain prophylactically. For example, give an analgesic before a bone marrow aspiration or fracture reduction. Permit time for the drug to become effective.

- Manage preexisting pain before beginning a procedure such as scrubbing a burn.

- Whenever possible, administer drugs by a nonpainful route (oral, transmucosal, intravenous). Avoid intramuscular injections.

- When procedures must be repeated (for example, bone marrow aspirations for children with leukemia), give optimal analgesia for the first procedure to reduce anxiety about future procedures.

- To prevent increased anxiety, avoid delays in performing procedures.

When the child receives conscious sedation, monitoring the child's status is important. Nursing assessments include heart and respiratory rates, blood pressure, pulse oximetry, level of consciousness (response to verbal and physical stimulation), and color. Vital signs must be checked every 15 minutes until the child regains full consciousness and level of functioning. If conscious sedation progresses to **deep sedation** (a controlled state of depressed consciousness or unconsciousness), vital signs should be checked every 5 minutes.

REFERENCES

1. Kachoyeanos, M.K., & Zollok, M.B. (1995). Ethics in pain management of infants and children. *American Journal of Maternal Child Nursing, 20,* 142–147.

2. Anand, K.J.S., & Carr, D.B. (1989). The neuroanatomy, neurophysiology, and neurochemistry of pain, stress, and analgesia in newborns and children. *Pediatric Clinics of North America, 36*(4), 795–822.

3. Lutz, W.J. (1986). Helping hospitalized children and their parents cope with painful procedures. *Journal of Pediatric Nursing, 1,* 24–32.

4. Ludwig-Beymer, P., Huether, S.E., & Schoessler, M. (1994). Pain, temperature regulation, sleep, and sensory function. In K.L. McCance, & S.E. Huether, (Eds.), *Pathophysiology: The biologic basis for disease in adults and children* (2nd ed.). St. Louis: Mosby–Year Book.

5. Eland, J.M., & Banner, W., Jr. (1992). Assessment and management of pain in children. In M.F. Hazinski,

(Ed.), *Nursing care of the critically ill child* (2nd ed., pp. 79–100). St. Louis: Mosby–Year Book.

6. Carlson, K.L., Clement, B.A., & Nash, P. (1996). Neonatal pain: From concept to research questions and the role of the advanced practice nurse. *Journal of Perinatal Neonatal Nursing, 10*(1), 64–71.

7. Shapiro, B.S. (1995). Treatment of chronic pain in children and adolescents. *Pediatric Annals, 24*(3), 148–156.

8. Varni, J.W., Thompson, K.L., & Hanson, V. (1987). The Varni/Thompson pediatric pain questionnaire: Chronic musculoskeletal pain in juvenile rheumatoid arthritis. *Pain, 28,* 27–38.

9. Abu-Saad, H. (1984). Cultural components of pain: The Asian-American child. *Children's Health Care, 13,* 11–14.

10. McGrath, P.A. (1995). Pain in the pediatric patient: Practical aspects of assessment. *Pediatric Annals, 24*(3), 126–138.

11. Lawrence, J., Alcock, D., McGrath, P.A., Kay, J., Mac-Murray, S.B., & Dulberg, C. (1993). The development of a tool to assess neonatal pain. *Neonatal Network, 12*(6), 59–66.

12. Acute Pain Management Guideline Panel. (1992). *Acute pain management in infants, children, and adolescents: Operative and medical procedures. Quick reference guide for clinicians.* (AHCPR Pub. No. 92-0020). Rockville, MD: Agency of Health Care Policy and Research, Public Health Service, U.S. Department of Health and Human Services.

13. Holder, K.A., & Patt, R.B. (1995). Taming the pain monster: Pediatric postoperative pain management. *Pediatric Annals, 24*(3), 164–168.

14. Berde, C.B., Lehn, B.M., Yee, J.D., Sethna, N.F., & Russo, D. (1991). Patient-controlled analgesia in children and adolescents: A randomized, prospective comparison with intramuscular administration of morphine for postoperative analgesia. *Journal of Pediatrics, 118,* 460–466.

15. Rushton, C.H. (1995). Placebo pain medication: Ethical and legal issues. *Pediatric Nursing, 21*(2), 166–168.

16. Fanurik, D., Koh, J., Schitz, M., & Brown, R. (1997). Pharmacobehavioral intervention: Integrating pharmacologic and behavioral techniques for pediatric procedures. *Children's Health Care, 26*(1), 1–13.

17. Wong, D.L., & Baker, C.M. (1988). Pain in children: Comparison of assessment scales. *Pediatric Nursing, 14,* 9–16.

18. Litman, R.S. (1995). Recent trends in management of pain during medical procedures in children. *Pediatric Annals, 24*(3), 158–163.

19. Broome, M.E. (1990). Preparation of children for painful procedures. *Pediatric Nursing, 16,* 537–541.

 ## ADDITIONAL RESOURCES

Abu-Saad, H. (1984). Cultural group indicators of pain in children. *American Journal of Maternal-Child Nursing, 13,* 187–196.

Adrian, E.R. (1994). Intranasal Versed: The future of pediatric conscious sedation. *Pediatric Nursing, 20*(3), 287–292.

Altimier, L., Norwood, S., Dick, M.J., Holditch-Davis, D., & Lawless, S. (1994). Postoperative pain management in preverbal children: The prescription and administration of analgesia with and without caudal analgesia. *Journal of Pediatric Nursing, 9*(4), 226–232.

Bender, L.H., Weaver, K., & Edwards, K. (1990). Postoperative patient-controlled analgesia in children. *Pediatric Nursing, 16,* 549–554.

Beyer, J.E., & Wells, N. (1989). The assessment of pain in children. *Pediatric Clinics of North America, 36,* 837–854.

French, G.M., Painter, E.C., & Coury, D.L. (1994). Blowing away shot pain: A technique for pain management during immunization. *Pediatrics, 93*(3), 384–388.

Gureno, M.A., & Reisinger, C.L. (1991). Patient controlled analgesia for the young pediatric patient. *Pediatric Nursing, 17,* 251–254.

Jones, M.A. (1989). Identifying signs that nurses interpret indicating pain in newborns. *Pediatric Nursing, 15,* 76–79.

Lau, N. (1992). Pediatric pain management, Part 1. *Journal of Pediatric Health Care, 6,* 87–92.

McCready, M., MacDavitt, K., & O'Sullivan, K.K. (1991). Children and pain: Easing the hurt. *Orthopaedic Nursing, 10,* 33–42.

McGrath, P.A. (1987). An assessment of children's pain: A review of behavioral, physiological and direct scaling techniques. *Pain, 31,* 147–176.

McGrath, P.J., & Craig, K.D. (1989). Developmental and psychological factors in children's pain. *Pediatric Clinics of North America, 36,* 823–836.

Morrison, R.A., & Vedro, D.A. (1989). Pain management in the child with sickle cell disease. *Pediatric Nursing, 15,* 595–599.

Schecter, N.L. (1995). Common pain problems in the general pediatric setting. *Pediatric Annals, 24*(3), 139–146.

Schecter, N.L. (1989). The undertreatment of pain in children: An overview. *Pediatric Clinics of North America, 36,* 781–794.

Stroud, S., & Dyer, J. (1992). Premedication takes the pain out of painful procedures for children. *American Journal of Nursing, 92,* 66.

Tyler, D.C. (1994). Pharmacology of pain management. *Pediatric Clinics of North America, 41*(1), 59–71.

Tyler, D.C., Tu, A., Douthit, J., & Chapman, C.R. (1993). Toward validation of pain measurement tools for children: A pilot study. *Pain, 52,* 301–309.

Yaster, M., Bean, J.D., Schulman, S.R., & Rogers, M.C. (1996). Pain, sedation, and postoperative anesthetic management in the pediatric intensive care unit. In Rogers, M.C. (Ed.), *Textbook of pediatric intensive care* (3rd ed., pp. 1547–1593). Baltimore: Williams & Wilkins.

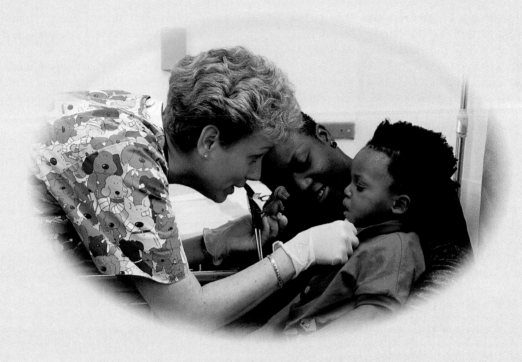

Vernon is 18 months old. Several days ago he developed vomiting and diarrhea. His parents tried to get him to eat, but he had little appetite. He drank a little water and a few sips of juice, but the next morning he was listless and would not drink anything. The diarrhea continued.

His mother has brought him to the urgent care center. Vernon is irritable on arrival, and his mother reports that he has been alternately irritable and lethargic. His mucous membranes and tongue appear dry, and skin turgor over the abdomen is slightly decreased. His mother notes that Vernon has had only two wet diapers today and says the urine in his diaper was dark in color. She also reports that he weighed 12 kg (26 lb) at the clinic last week. However, when the nurse weighs him, the scale reads only 11 kg (24½ lb). Vernon is moderately dehydrated. He needs rapid replacement of the proper type of fluids.

What happens inside the body when dehydration occurs? How can a nurse recognize dehydration? What types of fluid does Vernon need? What nursing management is important for his recovery? Why are young children at greater risk for dehydration than adults? What do parents need to be taught to prevent and manage dehydration? This chapter presents information that will enable you to answer these questions.

ALTERATIONS IN FLUID, ELECTROLYTE, AND ACID–BASE BALANCE

8

> *"So few parents realize how important proper hydration is in children. Such a large percentage of children's body weight is water that when they become dehydrated it can cause serious problems."*

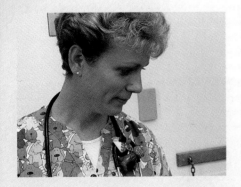

TERMINOLOGY

- **acidemia** Decreased blood pH.
- **acidosis** Condition caused by excess acid in the blood.
- **alkalemia** Increased blood pH.
- **alkalosis** Condition caused by too little acid in the blood.
- **body fluid** Body water that has substances (solutes) dissolved in it.
- **buffer** Related acid–base pair that gives up or takes up hydrogen ions as needed to prevent large changes in the pH of a solution.
- **dehydration** The state of body water deficit.
- **electrolytes** Charged particles (ions) dissolved in body fluid.
- **extracellular fluid** The fluid in the body that is outside the cells.
- **filtration** Movement into or out of capillaries as the net result of several opposing forces.
- **hypertonic fluid** Fluid that is more concentrated than normal body fluid.
- **hypotonic fluid** Fluid that is more dilute than normal body fluid.
- **interstitial fluid** That portion of the extracellular fluid that is between the cells and outside the blood and lymphatic vessels.
- **intracellular fluid** The fluid in the body that is inside the cells.
- **intravascular fluid** That portion of the extracellular fluid that is in the blood vessels.
- **isotonic fluid** Fluid that has the same osmolality as normal body fluid.
- **oncotic pressure** The part of the blood osmotic pressure that is due to plasma proteins; also called blood colloid osmotic pressure.
- **osmolality** The amount of concentration of a fluid; technically, the number of moles of particles per kilogram of water in the solution.
- **osmosis** Movement of water across a semipermeable membrane into an area of higher particle concentration.
- **pH** Negative logarithm of the hydrogen ion concentration; used to monitor the acidity of body fluid.
- **saline** A mixture of salt and water; *normal saline* refers to the mixture of salt and water in equal concentration in body fluids.

A thorough understanding of fluid, electrolyte, and acid–base homeostasis and imbalances is essential when providing nursing care to pediatric patients like Vernon, in the preceding scenario. This chapter presents information about the processes that maintain fluid and electrolyte balance, and describes the common imbalances that may occur in children. It also describes how the body regulates acid–base status and explains the management of acid–base imbalances.

Many health conditions cause changes in body fluids that must be regulated and managed. Sometimes management of fluid status in the home can prevent hospitalization and serious illness.

► ANATOMY AND PHYSIOLOGY OF PEDIATRIC DIFFERENCES

Infants and young children differ physiologically from adults in ways that make them vulnerable to fluid, electrolyte, and acid–base imbalances.

Fluid in the body is in a dynamic state. In persons of all ages, fluid continuously leaves the body through the skin, in feces and urine, and during respiration. Much of the human body is composed of water. **Body fluid** is body water that has solutes dissolved in it. Some of the solutes are **electrolytes,** or charged particles (ions). Electrolytes such as sodium (Na^+), potassium (K^+), calcium (Ca^{++}), magnesium (Mg^{++}), chloride (Cl^-), and inorganic phosphorus (Pi) ions must be present in the proper concentrations for cells to function effectively.

In persons of all ages, body fluid is located in several compartments. The two major fluid compartments contain the **intracellular fluid** (fluid inside the cells) and the **extracellular fluid** (fluid outside the cells). The extracellular fluid is made up of **intravascular fluid** (the fluid within the blood vessels) and **interstitial fluid** (the fluid between the cells and outside the blood and lymphatic vessels) (Fig. 8–1). Extracellular fluid accounts for about one third of total body water and intracellular fluid for about two thirds.[1] The concentrations of electrolytes in the fluid differ depending on the fluid compartment. For example, extracellular fluid is rich in sodium ions; intracellular fluid, by contrast, is low in sodium ions but rich in potassium ions (Table 8–1).

Fluid moves between the intravascular and interstitial compartments by a process called filtration. Water moves into and out of the cells by the process of osmosis. These processes are discussed later in the chapter.

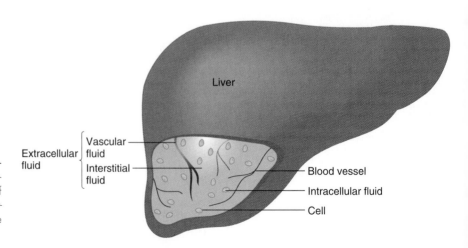

FIGURE 8–1. The major body fluid compartments. Extracellular fluid is composed mainly of *vascular fluid* (fluid in blood vessels) and *interstitial fluid* (fluid between the cells and outside the blood and lymphatic vessels).

8-1 | Electrolyte Concentrations in Body Fluid Compartments

| Components | Extracellular Fluid (ECF) | | Intracellular Fluid |
	Vascular	Interstitial	
Na⁺	High	High	Low
K⁺	Low	Low	High
Ca⁺⁺	Low	Low	Low (higher than ECF)
Mg⁺⁺	Low	Low	High
Pi	Low	Low	High
Cl⁻	High	High	Low
Proteins	High	Low	High

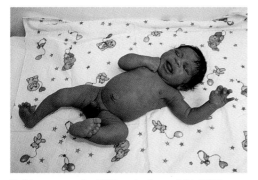

Full-term neonate, 75% water by weight: ECF = 45%, ICF = 30%

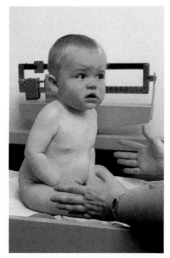

6-month infant, 65% water by weight: ECF = 25%, ICF = 40%

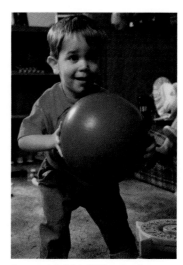

2-year-old child, 60% water by weight: ECF = 20%, ICF = 40%

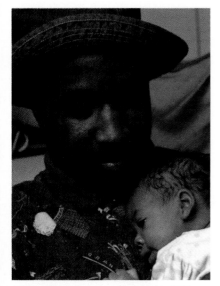

Adult male, 55% water by weight: ECF = 10–15%, ICF = 40%

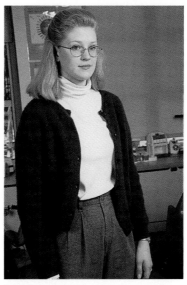

Adult female, 50% water by weight: ECF = 10–15%, ICF = 40%

FIGURE 8–2. The percentage of water in the body varies with age. (ECF = extracellular water; ICF = intracellular fluid.)

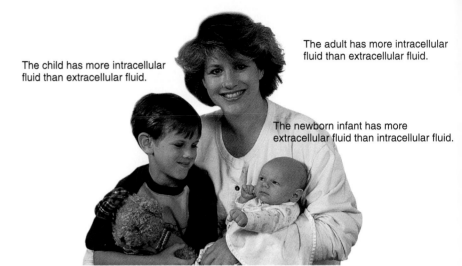

The child has more intracellular fluid than extracellular fluid.

The adult has more intracellular fluid than extracellular fluid.

The newborn infant has more extracellular fluid than intracellular fluid.

FIGURE 8–3. The proportion of extracellular fluid and intracellular fluid varies with age.

The percentage of body weight that is composed of water varies with age. The percentage is highest at birth (and higher in premature than in full-term infants) and decreases with age (Fig. 8–2). Neonates and young infants have a proportionately larger extracellular fluid volume than older children and adults because their brain and skin (both rich in interstitial fluid) occupy a greater proportion of their body weight. Much of our extracellular fluid is exchanged each day.[2] During infancy, there is a high daily fluid requirement with little fluid volume reserve; this makes the infant vulnerable to dehydration. As an infant grows, the proportion of water inside the cells increases (Fig. 8–3).

Infants and children under 2 years of age lose a greater proportion of fluid each day than older children and adults and are thus more dependent on adequate intake. They have a greater amount of skin surface or body surface area (BSA) and thus have greater insensible water losses through the skin. Because of this large BSA, they are also at greater risk when burned. In addition, respiratory and metabolic rates are high during early childhood. These factors lead to greater water loss from the lungs and greater water demand to fuel the body's metabolic processes (Fig. 8–4).

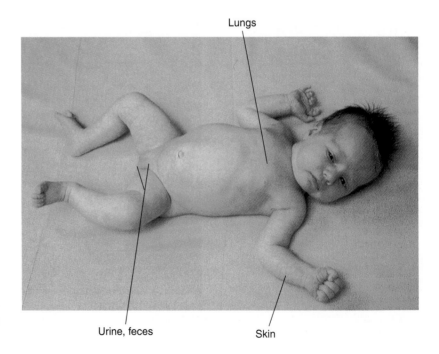

Lungs

Urine, feces

Skin

FIGURE 8–4. Normal routes of fluid excretion from infants and children.

| 8-2 | Health Conditions Contributing to Fluid Imbalance |

- Radiant heat (phototherapy) used to treat hyperbilirubinemia increases insensible water loss through the skin.
- The increased respiratory rate in some illnesses leads to excessive water loss from lungs.
- Fever increases the metabolic rate and, therefore, water demands of metabolism (for each degree of Celsius increase, 50–70 mL of fluid are lost).
- Vomiting and diarrhea increase fluid and electrolyte losses from the gastrointestinal system.
- Fistulas, blood loss, and drainage tubes contribute to fluid deficits.

When fluid status is compromised, a number of body mechanisms are activated to help restore balance. Several of these mechanisms occur in the kidney. The kidneys conserve water and needed electrolytes while excreting waste products and drug metabolites. In children under 2 years of age, however, the glomeruli, tubules, and nephrons of the kidneys are immature. They are thus unable to conserve water effectively[3] (see Chap. 16). Because more water is lost in the urine, the infant and young child can become dehydrated quickly or develop electrolyte imbalances. In addition, infants have a weaker transport system for ions and bicarbonate, placing them at greater risk for acidosis and acid–base imbalances. Children under 2 years of age also have difficulty regulating electrolytes such as sodium and calcium. Renal response to high solute loads is slower and less developed, with function improving gradually during the first year of life.[4]

Finally, in addition to the immaturity of physiologic processes, many health conditions make young children more vulnerable to fluid deficit (Table 8–2).

► FLUID VOLUME IMBALANCES

When fluid excretion and losses are balanced by the proper volume and type of fluid intake, fluid balance will be maintained. If, however, fluid output and intake are not matched, fluid imbalance may occur rapidly. The major types of fluid imbalances are extracellular fluid volume deficit (dehydration), extracellular fluid volume excess, and interstitial fluid volume excess (edema).

EXTRACELLULAR FLUID VOLUME IMBALANCES

Extracellular Fluid Volume Deficit (Dehydration)

Extracellular fluid volume deficit occurs when there is not enough fluid in the extracellular compartment (vascular and interstitial). Because sodium is generally lost along with water, hyponatremia can also be present. (Hyponatremia is described later, on p. 308.) The state of body water deficit is called **dehydration.**

Clinical Manifestations
The signs of dehydration relate to the severity or degree of the body water deficit (Table 8–3). They are a result of both the decreased fluid (eg, di-

8-3 Severity of Clinical Dehydration			
	Mild	Moderate	Severe
Percent of body weight lost	Up to 5%	6%–9%	10% or more
Level of consciousness	Alert, restless, thirsty	Restless or lethargic (infants and very young children); alert, thirsty, restless (older children and adolescents)	Lethargic to comatose (infants and young children); often conscious, apprehensive (older children and adolescents)
Blood pressure	Normal	Normal or low; postural hypotension (older children and adolescents)	Low to undetectable
Pulse	Normal	Rapid	Rapid, weak to nonpalpable
Skin turgor	Normal	Poor	Very poor
Mucous membranes	Moist	Dry	Parched
Urine	May appear normal	Decreased output (<1 mL/kg/hr) dark color	Very decreased or absent output
Thirst	Slightly increased	Moderately increased	Greatly increased unless lethargic
Fontanel	Normal	Sunken	Sunken
Extremities	Warm; normal capillary refill	Delayed capillary refill (>2 sec)	Cool, discolored; delayed capillary refill (>3–4 sec)

minished turgor and mucous membrane moisture) and the body's response to the fluid deficit (eg, pulse and blood pressure changes) (Table 8–4).

Mild dehydration is hard to detect, because children appear alert and have moist mucous membranes. Infants may be irritable and older children are thirsty. In moderate dehydration, the child is often lethargic and sleepy,

8-4 Clinical Manifestations of Extracellular Fluid Volume Deficit	
Signs and Symptoms	Physiologic Basis
Weight loss	Decreased fluid volume; 1 L of fluid weighs 1 kg
Postural blood pressure drop (older children)	Inadequate circulating blood volume to offset the force of gravity when in upright position
Increased small vein filling time	Decreased vascular volume
Delayed capillary refill time	Decreased vascular volume
Flat neck veins when supine (older children)	Decreased vascular volume
Dizziness, syncope	Inadequate circulation to brain
Oliguria	Inadequate circulation to kidneys
Thready, rapid pulse	Cardiac reflex response to decreased vascular volume
Sunken fontanel (infants)	Decreased fluid volume
Decreased skin turgor	Decreased interstitial fluid volume

but there may be periods of restlessness and irritability, especially in infants. Skin turgor is diminished, mucous membranes appear dry, and urine is dark in color and diminished in amount. Pulse rate is usually increased and blood pressure can be normal or low. Vernon, described at the beginning of this chapter, was displaying symptoms of moderate dehydration. His urine output was decreased, and he had lost about 8% of his body weight. What other signs and symptoms of moderate dehydration can you identify in the opening scenario? What additional assessments would you want to perform on Vernon?

Severe dehydration is manifested by increasing lethargy or nonresponsiveness, markedly decreased blood pressure, rapid pulse, poor skin turgor, dry mucous membranes, and markedly decreased or absent urinary output.

Etiology and Pathophysiology

Extracellular fluid volume deficit is usually caused by the loss of sodium-containing fluid from the body. The situations that most often cause loss of fluid containing sodium are vomiting, diarrhea, nasogastric suction, hemorrhage, and burns. Vomiting and diarrhea are common manifestations of disease in children throughout the world, and each year 5 million children die from dehydration related to diarrhea.[5]

Another cause of extracellular fluid volume deficit in infants is increased water loss in low birthweight infants kept under radiant warmers to maintain heat[1] (Fig. 8–5). Less frequently, adrenal insufficiency, accumulation of extracellular fluid in a "third space" such as the peritoneal cavity, and overuse of diuretics may be the cause. The latter etiology is most often seen in bulimic adolescents who are trying to control their weights (see Chap. 22).

 CLINICAL TIP

Assessing skin turgor takes skill and practice. In moderate dehydration, the skin may have a doughy texture and appearance. Later, in severe dehydration, the more typical "tenting" of skin is observed. Diminished turgor is most easily assessed in infants or children with little subcutaneous fat; it is more difficult to assess in those with larger amounts of fat.

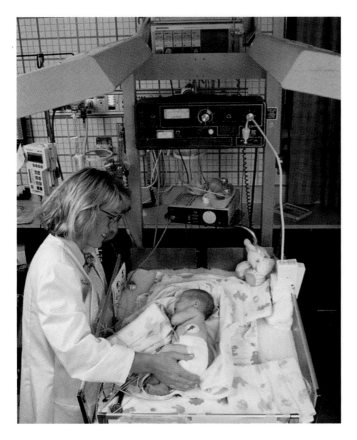

FIGURE 8–5. Use of an overhead warmer or phototherapy increases insensible fluid excretion through the skin and thus increases the fluid intake needed.

8-5 Oral Rehydration and Maintenance Fluids for Mild and Moderate Dehydration

Pedialyte

Infalyte

Resol

Nutralyte

NutraMax

Rehydralyte

WHO/UNICEF oral rehydration salts

Medical Management

The treatment of extracellular fluid volume deficit is administration of fluid containing sodium. This may be accomplished by oral rehydration therapy or by intravenous fluids.

Oral rehydration therapy has been used for a number of years in developing countries without an accessible supply of intravenous fluids. More recently, the benefits of using this therapy early to prevent severe dehydration and to treat mild and moderate dehydration in children in developed countries has been recognized. The therapy is successful in treating the dehydration caused by many gastrointestinal illnesses and prevents hospitalization for many infants and young children.[6] Solutions are available commercially that contain water, carbohydrate (sugar), sodium, potassium, chloride, and lactate (Table 8–5). Some clinicians allow lactose-free milk, breast milk, or half-strength milk to be given in addition to oral rehydration therapy solution. The WHO/UNICEF solution was developed for use with cholera and is not generally used for diarrhea treatment in the United States, as its sodium load is higher than that of other commercial solutions.

When the child is severely dehydrated, intravenous fluid will be given. The fluid is often Ringer's lactate followed or accompanied by dilute saline, such as one half or one quarter normal saline. The fluid combination replenishes the extracellular fluid volume and adds solutes to return the body fluid back to normal. The child may be hospitalized in a short-stay unit until the dehydration is controlled.

Nursing Assessment

Weigh the child daily with the same scale and without clothing. Compare to past weights and calculate weight loss. Carefully measure intake and output, urine specific gravity, level of consciousness, pulse rate and quality, skin turgor, mucous membrane moisture, and blood pressure. Compare the blood pressure when the child is supine with the pressure when the child is sitting with legs hanging down or standing. If the child is dehydrated, the sitting or standing blood pressure will be lower than the supine blood pressure, because blood accumulates in the dependent legs.

Nursing Diagnosis

The nursing diagnosis Fluid Volume Deficit applies to all children who have an extracellular fluid volume deficit. Other diagnoses depend on the severity of the condition and the age of the child. Several nursing diagnoses that might be appropriate for the mildly to severely dehydrated child are included in the accompanying Nursing Care Plans. Other specific examples might include:

• Fluid Volume Deficit related to fluid loss from gastrointestinal disease, hemorrhage, or burn
• Risk for Altered Peripheral Tissue Perfusion related to fluid volume deficit
• Risk for Injury related to postural hypotension

Nursing Management

Nursing care of the dehydrated child focuses on providing oral rehydration fluids, teaching parents oral rehydration methods, and, if necessary, admin-

Text continues on page 299.

NURSING CARE PLAN
THE CHILD WITH MILD OR MODERATE DEHYDRATION

GOAL	INTERVENTION	RATIONALE	EXPECTED OUTCOME

1. Knowledge Deficit (Parent) related to home management of diarrhea and vomiting

GOAL	INTERVENTION	RATIONALE	EXPECTED OUTCOME
Parents will describe appropriate home management of fluid replacement for diarrhea and vomiting.	• Explain how to replace body fluid with an oral rehydration solution. Encourage parents to keep the solution at home and begin use with the first sign of diarrhea.	• Use of an oral rehydration solution can enable successful treatment of vomiting and diarrhea at home.	Parents are successfully able to treat the child's diarrhea and vomiting at home.
	• Teach parents to continue the child's normal diet in addition to providing replacement fluids for diarrhea.	• Diet plus fluid supplementation leads to faster recovery.	
	• Provide verbal and written instructions to parents at each well-child visit.	• Parents are provided with a reference for later use.	

2. Knowledge Deficit (Parent) related to causes of dehydration

GOAL	INTERVENTION	RATIONALE	EXPECTED OUTCOME
Parents will state common causes of childhood dehydration.	• Teach parents childhood conditions that commonly lead to dehydration.	• If parents recognize situations that can lead to dehydration, they will be more alert to its appearance.	Parents recognize conditions of risk for dehydration in children.

3. Risk for Fluid Volume Deficit related to worsening of child's condition

GOAL	INTERVENTION	RATIONALE	EXPECTED OUTCOME
Parents will seek health care for the child's worsening condition.	• Teach parents to seek care when the child's vomiting or diarrhea worsens, or the child's mental alertness changes.	• Severe dehydration may occur if milder forms are not successfully treated.	Parents seek prompt attention for the child's worsening condition, preventing the development of severe dehydration.

NURSING CARE PLAN
THE CHILD WITH SEVERE DEHYDRATION

GOAL	INTERVENTION	RATIONALE	EXPECTED OUTCOME

1. Fluid Volume Deficit related to excess losses and inadequate intake

The child will return to normal hydration status and will not develop hypovolemic shock.	• Monitor weight daily. Assess intake and output every shift. Assess heart rate, postural blood pressure, skin turgor, small vein filling time, capillary refill time, fontanel (infant), and urine specific gravity every 4 hours or more frequently as indicated.	• Frequent assessment of hydration status facilitates rapid intervention and evaluation of the effectiveness of fluid replacement.	The child has signs of normal hydration.
	• Administer intravenous fluids as ordered. Monitor for crackles in dependent portions of the lungs.	• Replace fluid lost from the body. Excessive replacement of sodium-containing fluids could cause extracellular fluid volume excess.	

2. Risk for Injury related to decreased level of consciousness

The child will not experience injury.	• Raise the side rails of the bed. Ensure that a small child does not become tangled in bed covers.	• Safety measures protect the child.	The child does not fall or suffer other injury.
	• Monitor level of consciousness every 2–4 hours or more often as indicated.	• Frequent assessment provides evidence of the need for safety interventions and of the effectiveness of therapy.	
	• Monitor serum sodium concentration daily or more often.	• Elevated serum sodium concentration causes brain cell shrinkage and decreased level of consciousness.	
	• Have the child sit before rising from bed and assist to stand slowly.	• Slow adjustment to upright posture reduces light-headedness from decreased blood volume.	

NURSING CARE PLAN
THE CHILD WITH SEVERE DEHYDRATION– *Continued*

GOAL	INTERVENTION	RATIONALE	EXPECTED OUTCOME

3. Activity Intolerance related to weakness and dizziness

The child will engage in normal activity for age.	• Plan activities appropriate for the age of the child that can be done in bed. • Group nursing interventions to provide time for the child to rest. • Provide assistance during meals and other activities as needed.	• Activities will provide distraction and promote recovery. • The child will require more rest than usual. • Prevention of overexertion will conserve body fluid and promote healing.	The child engages in normal developmental activities and receives adequate rest.

istering intravenous fluids to restore fluid balance. The accompanying Nursing Care Plans summarize care of the child with mild to severe dehydration.

Provide Oral Rehydration Fluids. In mild or moderate dehydration, oral rehydration fluid is the first intervention (see Table 8–5). It is given in frequent small amounts; for example, 1–3 teaspoons of fluid every 10–15 minutes is a useful guideline for starting oral rehydration.[7] Instruct parents to continue to administer the 1 teaspoon every 2–3 minutes even if the child vomits, as small amounts of the fluid may still be absorbed.[8, 9] Table 8–6 outlines guidelines for oral rehydration therapy.

 SAFETY PRECAUTIONS

Sugar facilitates the absorption of sodium in oral rehydration fluids. Tell parents not to give diet beverages for oral rehydration because they contain no sugar and will not be effectively absorbed.

8-6 Oral Rehydration Therapy Guidelines

- Children with diarrhea and no dehydration should be continued on age-appropriate diets.
- For mild dehydration, give 50 mL/kg oral rehydration therapy in 4 hours in addition to replacing fluids lost in stool and emesis. (Measure emesis and give 10 mL/kg of fluid for each diarrheal stool.)
- For moderate dehydration, give 100 mL/kg oral rehydration therapy in 4 hours in addition to replacing fluids lost as described above.
- For severe dehydration, the child is hospitalized and treated with intravenous fluids. When hydrated adequately, begin oral rehydration therapy with 50–100 mL/kg of fluid in 4 hours and stool replacement as described above.
- When rehydration is complete, resume normal diet.

Adapted from Provisional Committee on Quality Improvement, Subcommittee on Acute Gastroenteritis. (1996). Practice parameter: The management of acute gastroenteritis in young children. Pediatrics, 97(3), 424–433; and Duggan, C. (1992). The management of acute diarrhea in children: Oral rehydration, maintenance, and nutritional therapy, Morbidity and Mortality Weekly Report, 41(RR-16), 1–20.

NURSING ALERT

If an oral rehydration solution is too concentrated, it can make diarrhea worse. Juice and cola are very concentrated and should be diluted to half strength if they are given to a child who has diarrhea. Encourage parents to keep an oral rehydration solution (see Table 8–5 for types of solutions) in liquid or powder form on hand at all times and to use these solutions rather than juice or soda when the child first develops diarrhea.

NURSING ALERT

Dizziness and lethargy can be manifestations of dehydration, so interventions to promote safety are important. Keep side rails up, and supervise the child when he or she is getting out of bed.

Teach Parents Oral Rehydration Methods. Instruct parents about the types of fluids and amounts to be given. Begin teaching with parents of all newborns and reinforce teaching at each well-child visit. Advise parents to continue the child's normal diet in addition to providing the rehydration solution. Cereal, starches, soup, fruits, and vegetables are all allowed. Tell parents to avoid simple sugars, which can worsen diarrhea because of osmotic effects. This includes soft drinks (if used, they should be diluted with equal parts of water), undiluted juice, Jell-O, and sweetened cereal.

Repeated vomiting of large volumes of fluid or a worsening of the child's condition can indicate the need for intravenous therapy. Teach parents when to seek further medical care. If the child's condition worsens or does not improve after 4 hours of oral rehydration therapy, parents should contact a health care professional.

Monitor Intravenous Fluid Administration. The hospitalized child usually requires administration of intravenous fluids. Be sure that the amount and type of fluid administered correspond with the diagnosed dehydration state of the child (Table 8–7). Usually, about one-half of the 24-hour total maintenance and replacement needs will be given in the first 6–8 hours, with a slower rate infused for the remainder of the 24 hours. During the first 1–3 hours, the infusion rate may be highest to rapidly expand the vascular space.[10]

Maintain the intravenous line carefully so fluid infusion can be kept on schedule (refer to the *Quick Reference to Pediatric Clinical Skills* accompanying this text). Use a pump to prevent inadvertent, rapid infusion, which can lead to fluid overload and electrolyte imbalance. Play with the toddler and preschool child frequently and use diversionary methods, as necessary, to distract the child from the intravenous line. Monitor the child carefully and implement safety precautions as necessary. Once the child begins to tolerate some oral fluids, oral rehydration therapy is substituted for intravenous fluid administration.

8-7	Calculation of Intravenous Fluid Needs

1. First, calculate the *maintenance* fluid needs of the child, according to the following guideline:

Usual Weight	Maintenance Amount
Up to 10 kg	100 mL/kg/24 hr
11–20 kg	1000 mL + (50 mL/kg for weight above 10 kg)/24 hr
>20 kg	1000 mL + (20 mL/kg for weight above 20 kg)/24 hr

   Example: Vernon's weight is 12 kg. He needs 1000 mL + (50 × 2), or 1100 mL/24 hr for maintenance fluid.

2. Next, calculate *replacement* fluid for that lost:

   Example: Vernon has lost 1 kg (8%) of his body weight. Multiplying the percentage of body weight × 10 yields the mL/kg/24 hr required:

   $$8 \times 10 = 80 \text{ mL/kg/24 hr}$$
   $$80 \text{ mL/kg} \times 12 \text{ kg} = 960 \text{ mL}$$

   Thus, Vernon's replacement fluid needs are 960 mL/24 hr.

3. Finally, continued *losses* must be calculated and added to the total of maintenance and replacement needs.

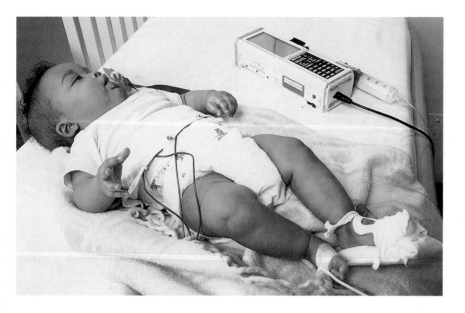

FIGURE 8–6. If isotonic fluid containing sodium is given too rapidly or in too great an amount, an extracellular fluid volume excess will develop. It is important to monitor fluid intake, excretion, and retention in children.

Discharge Planning and Home Care Teaching. Prior to discharge, parents need instructions about types of fluids and amounts to encourage. Teach the signs of dehydration (see Table 8–3) so that if the child does not take in adequate fluids, parents can seek help immediately. Encourage them to keep appropriate fluids at home to deal with mild dehydration. Review methods of minimizing the child's chance of acquiring gastrointestinal infections (eg, avoiding contact with other children who are infected; using careful handwashing and dish-washing procedures when another child in the home is affected).

Extracellular Fluid Volume Excess

Extracellular fluid volume excess occurs when there is too much fluid in the extracellular compartment (vascular and interstitial). This imbalance may also be called saline excess or extracellular volume overload. If this disorder occurs by itself (without saline disturbance), the serum sodium concentration is normal. There is simply too much extracellular fluid, even though it has a normal concentration.

Since fluid has weight, extracellular fluid volume excess is characterized by weight gain. An overload of fluid in the blood vessels and interstitial spaces can cause clinical manifestations such as bounding pulse, distended neck veins in children (not usually evident in infants), hepatomegaly, dyspnea, orthopnea, and lung crackles. Edema is the sign of overload of the interstitial fluid compartment. In an infant, edema is often generalized. Edema in children with extracellular fluid volume excess occurs in the dependent parts of the body, that is, in the parts closest to the ground. Thus, edema is evident in sacral areas in a child supine in bed. (Edema that develops from other causes is described in the next section of this chapter.)

Infants and children who develop an extracellular fluid volume excess have a condition that causes them to retain **saline** (sodium and water) or they have been given an overload of sodium-containing isotonic intravenous fluid (Fig. 8–6). What conditions cause retention of saline? The hormone aldosterone is secreted by the adrenal cortex. One of its normal functions is to cause the kidneys to retain saline in the body (Fig. 8–7). Saline excess can be caused by any condition that results in excessive aldosterone

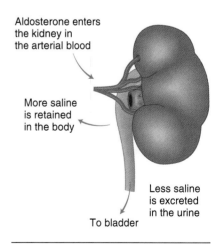

Aldosterone enters the kidney in the arterial blood

More saline is retained in the body

Less saline is excreted in the urine

To bladder

FIGURE 8–7. Aldosterone has a saline-retaining effect. Increased aldosterone secretion can be caused by adrenal tumors or congestive heart failure.

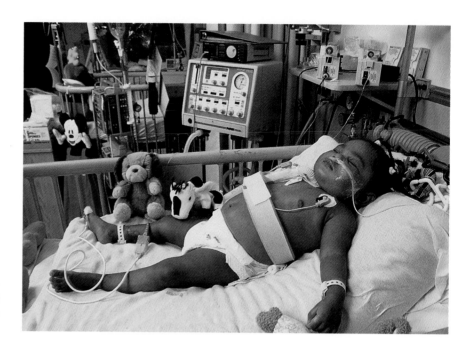

FIGURE 8-8. This infant with congenital heart disease has signs of generalized edema. Note the fluid retention in the face and abdomen.

 CLINICAL TIP

An infant's urine output can be approximated by weighing diapers before and after use. The difference in grams is the urine volume in milliliters. Change the diaper frequently to minimize loss from evaporation.

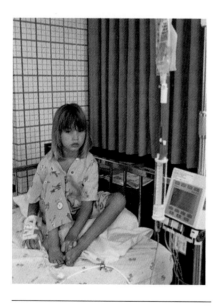

FIGURE 8-9. The use of a volume control device with an intravenous saline infusion is important to prevent a sudden extracellular fluid volume overload.

secretion, such as adrenal tumors that secrete aldosterone, congestive heart failure, liver cirrhosis, and chronic renal failure (Fig 8-8). Most glucocorticoid medications (such as prednisone) have a mild saline-retaining effect when taken on a long-term basis.

Intravenous fluid volume regulation is important, especially in young children. Either inaccurate calculation of needed fluid or inadvertent infusion of excess fluids can cause overload.

The medical management of extracellular fluid volume excess focuses on treating the underlying cause of the disorder. For example, a child who has congestive heart failure is given medications to strengthen the heart's ability to contract. Managing the cause also helps to reduce the extracellular fluid volume excess. Diuretics may be given to remove fluid from the body, thus reducing the extracellular fluid volume directly.

Nursing Management

Rapid weight gain is the most sensitive index of extracellular fluid volume excess. Therefore, daily weighing is an important nursing assessment. Measure the child's intake and output. When treatment is successful, output is greater than intake. Assess the character of the pulse and observe for neck vein distention when the child is sitting (usually visible only in older children). Monitor for signs of pulmonary edema (an indication of severe imbalance) by listening to lung sounds in the dependent lung fields (crackles) and assessing for respiratory distress (rapid respiratory rate, use of accessory muscles of respiration). Observe for edema.

The potential for a child to develop a fluid overload is present whenever an isotonic intravenous solution containing sodium is being administered. Therefore, monitor the infusion rate frequently and carefully (Fig. 8-9).

If an excess of fluid has already developed, administer the medical therapy as prescribed and monitor for any complications of the medical therapy. For example, many diuretics increase potassium excretion in the urine, an increase that may lead to an abnormally low plasma potassium concentration unless potassium intake is increased. (Refer to the discussion of hypokalemia later in this chapter.) It is also important to monitor for the development of extracellular fluid volume deficit as a result of diuretic therapy.

If edema is present, provide careful skin care and protection for edematous areas. Teach parents how to provide skin care and perform position changes at home. See the following section for additional interventions related to edema.

If a child has a long-term condition such as chronic renal failure that predisposes to extracellular fluid volume excess, a dietary sodium restriction may be prescribed. Teach parents how to manage sodium restriction. Plan low-sodium meals that fit the family's cultural practices. If the child is old enough to participate, incorporate games into the teaching. If a scale is available, teach parents to take and record an accurate daily weight.

INTERSTITIAL FLUID VOLUME EXCESS (EDEMA)

Edema is an abnormal increase in the volume of the interstitial fluid. It may be caused by an extracellular fluid volume excess or it may be due to other causes.

Edema causes swelling, which may be localized or generalized. The swelling of tissue may cause pain and restrict motion. Edema that is due to extracellular fluid volume excess or right-sided heart failure usually occurs in the dependent portion of the body. In a child who is walking, dependent edema is observed in the ankles; in a bedfast supine child, it is seen in the sacral area. The skin over an edematous area often appears thin and shiny.

The causes of edema are best understood in the context of normal capillary dynamics. Fluid moves between the vascular and interstitial compartment by the process of **filtration.** Filtration is the net result of forces that tend to move fluid in opposing directions. The strongest forces will determine the direction of fluid movement.

At the capillary level, two forces (blood hydrostatic pressure and interstitial osmotic pressure) tend to move fluid from the capillaries into the interstitial fluid, while two other forces (blood colloid osmotic pressure and interstitial fluid hydrostatic pressure) tend to move fluid in the opposite direction (from the interstitial fluid into the capillaries). The net result of these forces usually moves fluid from the capillaries into the interstitial compartment at the arterial end of the capillaries and fluid from the interstitial compartment back into the capillaries at the venous end of the capillaries. This process brings oxygen and nutrients to the cells and removes carbon dioxide and other waste products.

Edema occurs if the balance of these four forces is altered so that excess fluid either enters or leaves the interstitial compartment (Fig. 8–10). This may occur through (1) increased blood hydrostatic pressure, (2) decreased blood colloid osmotic pressure, (3) increased interstitial fluid osmotic pressure, or (4) blocked lymphatic drainage. Many different clinical conditions are associated with these altered forces (Table 8–8), which are described below.

1. *Increased blood hydrostatic pressure.* When extracellular fluid volume excess occurs, the increased fluid volume in the vascular compartment congests the veins. The pressure against the sides of the capillary is increased and more fluid then enters the interstitial compartment.
2. *Decreased blood colloid osmotic pressure.* Much of the osmotic pressure that pulls fluid into the capillaries is due to the presence of albumin

ISOTONIC INTRAVENOUS FLUIDS CONTAINING SODIUM

Normal saline (0.9% NaCl)
Ringer's solution
Lactated Ringer's solution

CULTURAL CONSIDERATIONS

To adapt teaching about low-sodium diets to the cultural practices of a family, ask them what types of food they usually eat. Help them to choose low-sodium foods from their diets and to avoid high-sodium foods. This approach is more effective than giving the same list of restricted foods to each family.

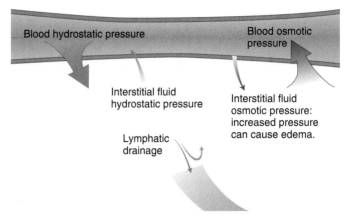

Hydrostatic pressure pushes fluid out of a compartment.

Osmotic pressure pulls fluid into a compartment.

Blood hydrostatic pressure

Blood osmotic pressure

Interstitial fluid hydrostatic pressure

Interstitial fluid osmotic pressure: increased pressure can cause edema.

Lymphatic drainage

Normally, lymphatic drainage removes small proteins and excess interstitial fluid. Blocked lymphatic drainage can cause edema.

FIGURE 8–10. With normal capillary dynamics, fluid moves out of the compartment by the force of hydrostatic pressure in the blood vessel and is pulled out by interstitial osmotic pressure. Fluid is forced into the compartment by interstitial hydrostatic pressure and pulled in by compartment osmotic pressure. Abnormal capillary dynamics cause edema.

8-8 Clinical Conditions That Cause Edema

Edema Due to Increased Blood Hydrostatic Pressure

Increased Capillary Blood Flow
Inflammation
Local infection

Venous Congestion
Extracellular fluid volume excess
Right heart failure
Venous thrombosis
External pressure on vein
Muscle paralysis

Edema Due to Decreased Blood Osmotic Pressure

Increased Albumin Excretion
Nephrotic syndrome (albumin leaks into urine)
Protein-losing enteropathies (excess albumin in feces)

Decreased Albumin Synthesis
Kwashiorkor (low-protein, high-carbohydrate starvation diet provides too few amino acids for liver to make albumin)
Liver cirrhosis (diseased liver unable to make enough albumin)

Edema Due to Increased Interstitial Fluid Osmotic Pressure

Increased Capillary Permeability
Inflammation
Toxins
Hypersensitivity reactions
Burns

Edema Due to Blocked Lymphatic Drainage
Tumors
Goiter
Parasites that obstruct lymph nodes
Surgery that removes lymph nodes

and other plasma proteins made by the liver. The part of the blood osmotic pressure that is due to plasma proteins is often called **oncotic pressure** or blood colloid osmotic pressure. Any condition that decreases plasma proteins will decrease blood colloid osmotic pressure and cause edema. For example, if a clinical condition causes large amounts of albumin to leak into the urine, the liver will not be able to make albumin fast enough to replace it. As a result, the plasma protein level will fall, decreasing the blood osmotic pressure. Without this pulling force to return fluid to the capillaries, edema will occur. This is the cause of the edema that occurs in children who have nephrotic syndrome (see Chap. 16).

3. *Increased interstitial fluid osmotic pressure.* Ordinarily, only a few small proteins enter the interstitial fluid and the interstitial fluid osmotic pressure is small. If the capillary becomes abnormally permeable to proteins, however, the influx of large amounts of proteins into the interstitial fluid causes a dramatic increase in interstitial fluid osmotic pressure. This increased pulling force keeps an abnormal amount of fluid in the interstitial compartment. This mechanism plays an important part in the edema caused by a bee sting or a sprained ankle. It occurs to a greater extent in burns, leading to swelling at the same time that there is a great loss of fluid volume through the burned skin (see Chap. 21).

4. *Blocked lymphatic drainage.* The lymph vessels normally drain small proteins and excess fluid from the interstitial compartment and return them to the blood vessels. If this process is blocked, fluid accumulates in the interstitial compartment. This may occur when a tumor blocks lymphatic drainage.

The main focus of medical management of edema is to treat the underlying condition that caused the edema. Such conditions are discussed throughout this book. The edema from inflammation of an injury is initially treated with cold to reduce capillary blood flow and thus reduce blood hydrostatic pressure.

Nursing Management

A child or parent may make comments that alert the nurse to the development of edema. Shoes may become tight by the end of the day (dependent edema); the waistband of pants or skirt may be "outgrown" suddenly (generalized edema or ascites [accumulation of fluid in the peritoneal cavity]); the eyes may be puffy (periorbital edema); a ring may be too tight; fingers may "feel like sausages." In many cases visual inspection is sufficient to recognize edema. Observe for the presence of pitting edema. To detect changes in the amount of swelling, measure around the edematous part (Fig. 8–11). If the edema is caused by extracellular fluid volume excess, daily measurements of weight and intake and output are a necessary part of the daily assessment. Nursing assessment should also focus on the integrity of the skin, presence of pain, restricted motion, and alterations in the child's body image.

Elevation of an area of localized edema helps to reduce the swelling. The skin over an edematous area needs extra care because it is fragile (Fig. 8–12). Carefully position an infant or child on bedrest and turn frequently to prevent pressure sores. Turning must be performed carefully to avoid skin abrasion by rubbing against the sheets. Pat the skin dry after cleansing rather than rubbing it. Trim the child's fingernails smooth to prevent scratching. Teach parents skin care for the child at home. Teach older children to inspect their skin carefully to identify areas needing special care.

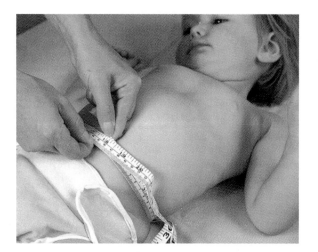

FIGURE 8–11. Finding the same location each day for measuring circumference to assess edema can be accomplished by use of a reference point. An indelible marker may be used to mark the measurement location on the skin, if this is acceptable to the child and parents.

If restricted mobility is a problem, specific plans to help the child manage activities are needed. For example, if an edematous finger restricts the motion of a hand, food can be cut into bite-sized portions before the meal is served, so that the child can still eat independently.

Discomfort from edema may require creative interventions by the nurse. Distraction with toys or activities appropriate to the child's developmental level can be useful. Interventions to treat the underlying problem can also reduce the edema and its accompanying discomfort. Interventions for edema should be added to the nursing management of the underlying condition that causes the edema. Administration of the prescribed medical therapy and observation for the complications of therapy are nursing responsibilities.

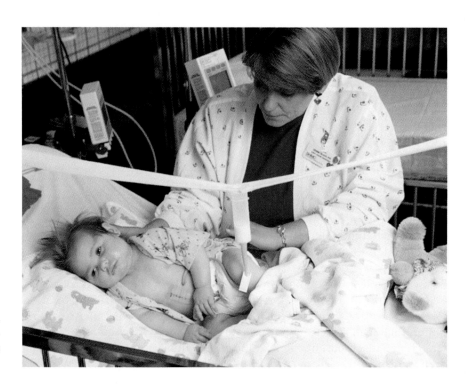

FIGURE 8–12. Edematous tissue is easily damaged. It must be kept clean and dry and free of pressure.

Discuss with school-age children and adolescents feelings of embarrassment about the edematous appearance. They need to understand the reason for edema and be able to explain it to peers. Arrange for the child to meet other children with similar concerns.

► ELECTROLYTE IMBALANCES

All body fluids contain electrolytes, although the concentration of those electrolytes varies, depending on the type and location of the fluid. When a serum electrolyte value is reported from the laboratory, it provides information about the concentration of that electrolyte in the blood. It may not necessarily reflect the concentration of the electrolyte in other body compartments.

Electrolytes are normally gained and lost in relatively equal amounts so the body remains in balance. However, when a child has an abnormal route of loss, such as vomiting, wound drainage, or nasogastric suction, electrolyte balance can be disturbed. Monitoring for signs of imbalance becomes important.

SODIUM IMBALANCES

The serum sodium concentration reflects the **osmolality** of body fluids; that is, their degree of concentration or dilution. It refers to the number of moles of particles per kilogram of water in the solution. Serum sodium concentration reflects the proportion of water and sodium in the extracellular compartment. When the osmolality of body fluids becomes abnormal, the cells swell or shrink. These cell size changes are due to **osmosis,** the movement of water across a semipermeable membrane into an area of higher particle concentration.

NORMAL SERUM SODIUM CONCENTRATION
Newborns: 133–146 mmol/L
Children: 135–148 mmol/L

Hypernatremia

Hypernatremia is a condition of increased osmolality of the blood. The body fluids are too concentrated, containing excess sodium relative to water. A serum sodium level above 148 mmol/L in children (146 mmol/L in newborns) is diagnostic of hypernatremia.

An infant or child who has hypernatremia is thirsty. The urine output is small unless the hypernatremia is caused by diabetes insipidus. A decreased level of consciousness manifested by confusion, lethargy, or coma results from shrinking of the brain cells. Seizures can occur when hypernatremia occurs rapidly or is severe. Severe hypernatremia can be fatal.

Hypernatremia is caused by conditions that cause the body to lose relatively more water than sodium or to gain relatively more sodium than water (Table 8–9). Special circumstances in which a high solute intake may occur without adequate water include an infant formula that is too concentrated or one that is prepared with salt instead of sugar.

Hypernatremia is treated by intravenous administration of **hypotonic fluid,** or fluid that is more dilute than normal body fluid. This therapy dilutes the body fluids back to normal concentration. If a child is dehydrated, **isotonic fluids** (those with the osmolality of body fluids) may be ordered first to replenish the volume, followed by hypotonic fluid to correct the osmolality.

Nursing Management

Monitor serum sodium level and measure intake and output and urine specific gravity. Specific gravity changes toward normal levels as therapy

8-9 Causes of Hypernatremia

Loss of Relatively More Water than Sodium	Gain of Relatively More Sodium Than Water
Diabetes insipidus (not enough antidiuretic hormone)	Inability to communicate thirst
Diarrhea or vomiting without fluid replacement	Limited or no access to water
Excessive sweating without fluid replacement	High solute intake without adequate water (eg, tube feedings)
High solute intake without adequate water (causes kidneys to excrete water)	Intravenous hypertonic saline

progresses. Frequently assess responsiveness to monitor the effect of hypernatremia on brain cells. As the concentration of body fluids returns to normal, the child will become more alert and responsive. Watch for rebound hyponatremia while monitoring the fluid replacement. Implement safety interventions such as raised bed rails for protection. Ensure adequate rest and introduce developmentally appropriate activities when the child is alert.

Water deprivation is a form of child neglect or abuse. In neglect, the parents simply do not provide adequate water for the child. A form of child abuse that sometimes includes water deprivation is Munchausen syndrome by proxy (see Chap. 22). A small child who is hospitalized with hypernatremia that does not have a detectable cause may be subject to water deprivation. Assess the child's general condition, developmental tasks, the family dynamics, and parent's understanding of formula preparation and the child's fluid intake needs.

Teaching can prevent many cases of hypernatremia. When an infant is sick or developing slowly, parents sometimes want to feed the infant more-concentrated formula to make him or her stronger. Parents and caregivers of bottle-fed babies should be taught never to give undiluted formula concentrate or evaporated milk. Parents should be cautioned to keep salt out of reach, since eating handfuls of salt has caused hypernatremia. Teach parents to offer extra fluids during hot weather. Teach oral rehydration therapy for use at home during mild vomiting and diarrhea (see p. 299).

Nurses can prevent hypernatremia in hospitalized infants and children by administering water between tube feedings, keeping water available, and offering it frequently. Offering frequent small amounts and using popsicles and other creative interventions can increase children's intake.

Hyponatremia

In hyponatremia, the osmolality of the blood is decreased. The body fluids are too dilute, containing excess water relative to sodium. Hyponatremia is the most common sodium imbalance in children.[4] A serum sodium level below 135 mmol/L in children (133 mmol/L in newborns) is diagnostic of hyponatremia.

8-10	Causes of Hyponatremia
Gain of Relatively More Water Than Sodium	**Loss of Relatively More Sodium Than Water**
Excessive intravenous D5W (5% dextrose in water) Excessive tap water enemas Irrigation of body cavities with distilled water Excessive antidiuretic hormone Forced excessive oral intake of tap water	Diarrhea or vomiting with replacement by tap water only instead of fluid containing sodium

Clinical Manifestations

The child who has hyponatremia has a decreased level of consciousness, which results from swelling of brain cells. This can be manifested as anorexia, headache, muscle weakness, decreased deep tendon reflexes, lethargy, confusion, or coma. If hyponatremia arises rapidly or is extreme, seizures may occur. Hyponatremia is a frequent cause of seizures in infants under 6 months of age who have a low body temperature.[11] Nausea and vomiting also occur in some children. Severe hyponatremia can be fatal.

Etiology and Pathophysiology

Hyponatremia is caused by conditions that cause gain of relatively more water than sodium or loss of relatively more sodium than water (Table 8–10). Oral intake of water causes hyponatremia in unusual conditions such as forced fluid intake. More commonly, parents feed an infant only water or dilute formula to save money instead of regular-strength formula or breast milk. Excessive swallowing of swimming pool water by an infant can have the same effect.

Medical Management

In most cases, hyponatremia is treated by restricting the intake of water. This therapy allows the kidneys to correct the imbalance by excreting excess water from the body. If a child is having seizures from hyponatremia, intravenous **hypertonic** saline (more concentrated than body fluid) may be administered. Use of this concentrated fluid is a way to rapidly increase body fluid concentration, but it must be monitored carefully because it can easily cause rebound hypernatremia.

Nursing Assessment

Monitor serum sodium level and measure intake and output. If an infant with hyponatremia has normal antidiuretic hormone (ADH) levels, and other causes have been ruled out, careful questioning about proper preparation of formula and feeding practices is needed. A toddler or school-age child may be subjected to forced fluid intake as a form of child abuse. Sensitive interviewing and a caring manner on the part of the nurse can help identify such problems in a family.

Since hyponatremia is characterized by decreased level of consciousness, frequent assessment of responsiveness will be necessary to monitor the

8-11	Nursing Interventions for a Child Who Has a Fluid Restriction

(Modify according to child's developmental level)
- Give cold rather than lukewarm fluids.
- Use an insulated glass that looks bigger than it is.
- Be sure that extra fluids are removed from meal trays before the child sees them.
- Have the child swish fluids around in the mouth before swallowing, to relieve thirst.
- Provide frequent oral care.
- Suggest eating meals dry and drinking between meals.
- Provide a chart so an older child can keep intake records.

response to therapy. The child will become more alert and responsive as the concentration of body fluids returns to normal.

Nursing Diagnosis
The highest priority nursing diagnosis for hyponatremia addresses the Risk for Injury related to the child's decreased level of consciousness. The following diagnoses might also apply:

- Self-Care Deficit related to lethargy
- Knowledge Deficit (Parents) related to proper preparation of infant formula

Nursing Management
Nurses can prevent hyponatremia in hospitalized children by using normal saline instead of distilled water for irrigations and by avoiding tap water enemas. It is important to help the child comply with prescribed fluid restrictions (Table 8–11). Allow the child to choose favorite fluids to drink.

Teach parents to replace body fluids lost through diarrhea or vomiting with oral electrolyte solutions (see p. 296).

POTASSIUM IMBALANCES

Potassium is an essential electrolyte that performs many necessary functions in the body. Potassium intake in healthy children comes from potassium-rich foods such as fruits and vegetables. Potassium is absorbed easily from the intestine. A normal potassium distribution is important for proper function.

Most of the potassium ions in the body are found inside the cells. The sodium-potassium pump in cell membranes moves potassium ions into cells to maintain the high intracellular potassium concentration. Potassium ions can be shifted into or out of cells by various physiologic factors (Fig. 8–13). Potassium is excreted from the body through urine, feces, and sweat. The hormone aldosterone increases potassium excretion in the urine.

A potassium imbalance arises when the serum potassium concentration rises or falls outside the normal range. Potassium imbalances are caused by alterations in potassium intake, distribution, or excretion; or by loss of potassium through an abnormal route such as burns, emesis, or renal failure.

NORMAL SERUM POTASSIUM CONCENTRATION

Premature infants: 4.5–7.2 mmol/L
Full-term newborns: 3.7–5.2 mmol/L
Children: 3.5–5.8 mmol/L

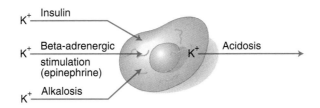

FIGURE 8–13. Factors that shift potassium ions into or out of cells.

Hyperkalemia

Hyperkalemia is an excess of potassium in the blood. It is reflected by a level above 5.8 mmol/L in children or above 5.2 mmol/L in newborns.

Clinical Manifestations

The clinical manifestations of hyperkalemia are all related to muscle dysfunction since potassium plays a vital role in muscle activity. Hyperactivity of gastrointestinal smooth muscle causes intestinal cramping and diarrhea in some children. The skeletal muscles become weak, beginning typically with leg weakness and ascending. Weakness can progress to flaccid paralysis. The child is often lethargic. Dysfunction of cardiac muscle causes cardiac arrhythmias such as tachycardia and may result in heart failure and cardiac arrest. Abnormalities in the electrocardiogram include a prolonged QRS complex, a peak in T waves, and prolonged PR intervals.[12]

Etiology and Pathophysiology

Hyperkalemia is caused by conditions that involve increased potassium intake, shift of potassium from cells into the extracellular fluid, and decreased potassium excretion. Increased potassium intake is usually due to intravenous potassium overload. Excessive or too rapid intravenous administration of potassium-containing solutions can occur if potassium requirement is overestimated or if the intravenous infusion runs in too fast.

Blood transfusion is another source of potassium intake that may cause hyperkalemia. Potassium ions leak out of red blood cells that are stored in a blood bank. The longer the blood is stored, the more potassium leaks out of cells and accumulates in the fluid portion of the transfusion. Hyperkalemia from administration of stored blood arises when multiple units are transfused, as when infants receive exchange transfusions or children receive multiple blood transfusions after a serious injury or in surgery.

Shift of potassium from cells into the extracellular fluid occurs when there is massive cell death, as with a crush injury, in sickle cell anemia (hemolytic crisis), or when chemotherapy for a malignancy is rapidly effective. In these situations, the dead cells release their high-potassium contents into the extracellular fluid. Potassium ions also shift out of cells in metabolic acidosis caused by diarrhea and in diabetes mellitus when insulin levels are low.

Decreased potassium excretion occurs with acute or chronic oliguria during renal failure, severe hypovolemia, and conditions that decrease the secretion of aldosterone by the adrenal cortex (lead poisoning, Addison's disease, hypoaldosteronism). Several medications can cause hyperkalemia.

> **DRUGS THAT MAY CAUSE HYPERKALEMIA**
>
> Potassium-containing preparations
> Cytotoxic agents
> Potassium-sparing diuretics
> Angiotensin-converting enzyme inhibitors
> Nonsteroidal antiinflammatory analgesics

Medical Management

Hyperkalemia is treated by management of the underlying condition that caused the imbalance. If the serum potassium concentration is very high or is causing dangerous cardiac arrhythmias, treatment to decrease the serum

CLINICAL TIP

If an infant's hyperkalemia was diagnosed using blood obtained from a heel stick, intracellular fluid may have contaminated the sample. A venous sample should be obtained.

GROWTH & DEVELOPMENT CONSIDERATIONS

The nursing diagnoses for hyperkalemic children will prompt a nurse to provide safety measures appropriate to the child's developmental level and to assist the child with activities that muscle weakness makes difficult. It is important to provide play and diversional activities that take into account the child's degree of muscle strength as well as the appropriate developmental level.

potassium level may be ordered. These treatments may remove potassium from the body or drive it from the extracellular fluid into the cells. Potassium is removed from the body by peritoneal dialysis or hemodialysis, by potassium-wasting diuretics, or with a cation exchange resin (Kayexalate) that is administered orally or rectally. Medical treatments that drive potassium ions into cells are intravenous bicarbonate, intravenous insulin, and glucose.

Nursing Assessment

Monitor serum potassium levels. Ongoing assessment of muscle strength is important because the muscle weakness may progress to flaccid paralysis. (This paralysis is reversible on correction of the potassium imbalance.) Diarrhea can occur in infants and children. An older child may complain of intestinal cramping. Monitor the pulse rate carefully.

Nursing Diagnosis

Nursing diagnoses for a child who has hyperkalemia depend on the severity of the clinical manifestations. The cause of the imbalance may also lead to useful diagnoses that guide teaching for the child and the parents. The following nursing diagnoses may apply:

- Risk for Decreased Cardiac Output related to cardiac arrhythmias
- Risk for Injury related to muscle weakness
- Self-Care Deficit related to severe muscle weakness
- Anxiety related to decreased muscle function
- Knowledge Deficit (Parents) related to management of potassium intake in chronic renal failure
- Ineffective Management of Therapeutic Regimen related to dietary potassium restriction

Nursing Management

Nursing care includes measures to prevent hyperkalemia from developing in hospitalized children. If hyperkalemia does develop, care shifts to administering intravenous solutions, monitoring cardiopulmonary status, ensuring safety, promoting adequate nutrition, and preparing the child and family for discharge.

Prevent Hyperkalemia. Any child who is receiving an intravenous infusion that contains potassium is at risk for hyperkalemia. Check that urine output is normal before administering intravenous potassium solutions. Intravenous solutions to which potassium has been added should be turned over several times to mix the contents thoroughly before they are connected to the infusion tubing.

Be sure blood or packed red blood cells are fresh, especially for the child receiving multiple transfusions. Use a cardiac monitor during infusion of these products to watch for arrhythmias.

Administer Intravenous Solutions. Once a child is diagnosed as hyperkalemic, ensure that any infusions with added potassium are stopped. Several infusions may need to be managed, including glucose, bicarbonate, and calcium gluconate. Maintain the infusion at the ordered rate and monitor the child's condition frequently.

Monitor Cardiopulmonary Status. Upon diagnosis of hyperkalemia, an electrocardiogram is performed and a cardiac monitor applied. Monitor for any changes in cardiac status and for cardiac arrhythmias. Report abnormal rate and character of pulse as well as shortness of breath.

Ensure Safety. Since the child is weak, side rails should be raised. Position the child carefully. Assist the child with activities requiring leg muscle strength, such as climbing into bed or pushing up in bed. Encourage quiet activities with frequent rest periods. Document and report any change in muscle weakness.

Promote Adequate Nutritional Intake. Adequate caloric intake is necessary to prevent tissue breakdown and the resultant potassium release from cells. Offer the child nourishing snacks if his or her appetite is decreased. Restrict potassium-rich foods.

Discharge Planning and Home Care Teaching. If the child has chronic renal failure or another condition that decreases aldosterone secretion, parents and children need to be taught to restrict foods that are high in potassium. Most oral rehydration solutions, including Pedialyte, contain potassium and should not be used to provide fluid for the child. Instruct the family not to use salt substitutes, which commonly contain potassium. Parents should check with the care provider and pharmacist before giving even over-the-counter products to the child, as some of these medications contain potassium. Management of renal failure at home with frequent visits for dialysis and other treatments can be challenging. Refer to Chapter 16 for further suggestions to help parents handle this condition.

Hypokalemia

Hypokalemia occurs when the serum potassium concentration is too low. Total body potassium may be decreased, normal, or even increased when the serum level is low, depending on the cause of the imbalance. Serum potassium levels below 3.5 mmol/L in children (3.7 mmol/L for newborns) are diagnostic of hypokalemia.

Clinical Manifestations

Since the ratio of intracellular to extracellular potassium determines the responsiveness of muscle cells to neural stimuli, it is not surprising that the clinical manifestations of hypokalemia involve muscle dysfunction. Gastrointestinal smooth muscle activity is slowed, leading to abdominal distention, constipation, or paralytic ileus. Skeletal muscles are weak and unresponsive to stimuli, and weakness may progress to flaccid paralysis. The respiratory muscles may be impaired. Cardiac arrhythmias can occur. Polyuria results from changes in the kidney caused by hypokalemia.

Etiology and Pathophysiology

Hypokalemia is caused by conditions that involve increased potassium excretion, decreased potassium intake, shift of potassium from the extracellular fluid into cells, and loss of potassium by an abnormal route.

Increased potassium excretion is a major cause of hypokalemia in children. In addition to diuretics and other medications, causes of increased urinary potassium excretion are osmotic diuresis (glucose present in urine), hypomagnesemia, increased aldosterone (hyperaldosteronism, congestive heart failure, nephrotic syndrome, cirrhosis), and increased cortisol (Cushing's disease and syndrome). Eating large amounts of black licorice increases renal excretion of potassium. Diarrhea causes potassium to be excreted in the feces. In the case study at the beginning of the chapter, Vernon had increased potassium excretion through diarrhea.

Decreased potassium intake will lead to hypokalemia slowly, or more rapidly if combined with increased excretion or loss of potassium. Hospitalized children may be placed on NPO status and receive prolonged intra-

POTASSIUM-RICH FOODS	
Apricots	Orange juice
Bananas	Peaches
Cantaloupe	Potatoes
Cherries	Prunes
Dates	Raisins
Figs	Strawberries
Molasses	Tomato juice

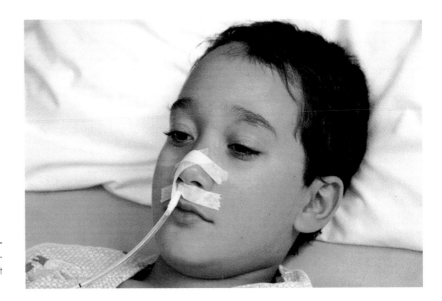

FIGURE 8–14. Because this child has a nasogastric tube in place that requires suctioning, it is important to monitor his potassium levels.

DRUGS THAT MAY CAUSE HYPOKALEMIA

Beta-adrenergic agonists
Insulin
Potassium-wasting diuretics
Parenteral penicillins
Glucocorticoids
Aminoglycoside antimicrobials
Systemic antifungals
Antineoplastics
Laxatives

venous therapy without potassium. Adolescents concerned about weight loss or those with anorexia nervosa may embark on fad diets low in potassium.

Shift of potassium from the extracellular fluid into cells occurs in alkalosis and hypothermia (unintentional or induced for surgery). Hyperalimentation often causes hypersecretion of insulin, which also shifts potassium into cells.

Loss of potassium by an abnormal route occurs through vomiting. Self-induced vomiting in bulimia is an example of this cause. Nasogastric suctioning (Fig. 8–14) and intestinal decompression can cause potassium loss. Hypokalemia can also be caused by several medications.

Medical Management

Medical management of hypokalemia focuses on replacement of potassium while treating the cause of the imbalance. Potassium replacement may be given intravenously or orally.

Nursing Assessment

Monitor serum potassium levels. Observe for muscle weakness, which is frequently detected first in the legs. Parents may report that muscle weakness restricts the child's activities and impairs interactions with peers. Skeletal muscle strength can be difficult to assess if the child is lethargic, as was seen with Vernon at the beginning of the chapter.

Muscle weakness may affect the respiratory muscles. Assess the child frequently to determine the need for assisted ventilation. Cardiac monitoring is important for continued assessment of hypokalemia-associated arrhythmias.

Assess for diminished bowel sounds. Ask the parents if the child has recently been awakening to use the toilet at night or has begun bedwetting after previously being dry at night. These may be symptoms of polyuria associated with chronic hypokalemia.

Nursing Diagnosis

The most important nursing diagnoses in the child with severe hypokalemia are related to cardiac arrhythmias and respiratory muscle weakness. The following nursing diagnoses may apply:

- Risk for Decreased Cardiac Output related to cardiac arrhythmias
- Ineffective Breathing Pattern related to respiratory muscle weakness
- Risk for Injury related to muscle weakness
- Self-Care Deficit related to severe muscle weakness
- Constipation related to decreased bowel function
- Anxiety related to decreased muscle function
- Knowledge Deficit (Parent) regarding management of potassium supplements or high-potassium diet
- Ineffective Management of Therapeutic Regimen related to prescribed potassium therapy
- Knowledge Deficit (Adolescent) regarding safe weight-loss diet

Nursing Management

Nursing care of the child with hypokalemia focuses on ensuring adequate potassium intake, monitoring cardiopulmonary status, promoting normal bowel function, ensuring safety, providing dietary counseling, and preparing the child and family for discharge.

Ensure Adequate Potassium Intake. Since potassium is excreted from the body every day, daily potassium intake is necessary to prevent hypokalemia. A hypokalemic child who is able to eat should be given a high-potassium diet. Teach parents (and the child if old enough) which foods are high in potassium and how to incorporate them into the daily diet (see p. 313).

Children who have no oral intake for a period of time should receive intravenous fluids that contain potassium. Calculate the dosage to be sure it is accurate. Ensure that the infusion runs on schedule. Sometimes the child will complain of burning along the vein when potassium is infused. The infusion may need to be slowed temporarily to allow it to continue. Check serum potassium to watch for high or low potassium levels. Monitor urine output. An oliguric child can develop hyperkalemia when receiving supplements.

Monitor Cardiopulmonary Status. Hypokalemia potentiates digitalis toxicity. A hypokalemic child who is receiving digitalis needs careful surveillance for digitalis toxicity, which is manifested as anorexia, nausea, vomiting, and bradycardia. Observe for these effects. Take the pulse rate and rhythm regularly. Monitor respirations and ease of breathing to watch for decreased respiratory muscle activity.

Promote Normal Bowel Function. Ensure adequate fluids and fiber in the diet. Monitor and record the number of stools and report inadequate stools.

Ensure Safety. Keep side rails up. Assist the child as needed to move into and out of bed. Reposition the child frequently to preserve skin integrity of limbs that are not moved regularly. Perform passive range of motion if the child is not moving. Use supportive pillows to position the child properly.

Provide Dietary Counseling. The adolescent who is trying to lose weight and not consuming a nutritious diet needs dietary teaching. More intensive treatment will be needed for teens who are anorexic or bulimic (see Chapter 22 for interventions in these cases).

Discharge Planning and Home Care Teaching. Teach parents how to give potassium supplements, if prescribed. Liquid or powdered potassium supplements can be mixed with juice or sherbet to im-

CLINICAL TIP

Bradycardia occurs at a different level for children of various ages. For infants, a pulse rate below 100 is considered bradycardia. For young children, 80 may be the identified number, whereas for adolescents, a pulse below 60 is bradycardia. Look at the child's age and normal pulse range to find changes that indicate bradycardia.

NORMAL SERUM CALCIUM CONCENTRATION
Premature infants: 3.5–4.5 mEq/L (1.7–2.3 mmol/L)
Full-term newborns: 4–5 mEq/L (2–2.5 mmol/L)
Children: 4.4–5.3 mEq/L (2.2–2.7 mmol/L)

THE THREE FORMS OF CALCIUM IN PLASMA
Calcium bound to protein
Calcium bound to small organic ions (eg, citrate)
Free ionized calcium (Ca⁺⁺), the only physiologically active form

prove the bitter taste. The parent should call the mixture "medicine" so that the child does not learn to dislike all juices. Teach the parents signs of hypokalemia and hyperkalemia and whom to call to report these symptoms. These signs must be reported promptly so medications can be adjusted.

CALCIUM IMBALANCES

A normal serum calcium concentration is important for many physiologic functions, including muscle and nerve function, secretion of hormones, bone formation and strength, and clotting of the blood.

Calcium imbalances are caused by alterations in calcium intake, absorption, distribution, or excretion. Calcium absorption requires vitamin D for maximum efficiency and is greatest in the duodenum. Calcium distribution involves calcium entry into and exit from bones and the distribution of different forms of calcium in the plasma. Excretion of calcium occurs in urine, feces, and sweat (Fig. 8–15).

Parathyroid hormone is the major regulator of the plasma calcium concentration. It increases the plasma calcium concentration by increasing calcium absorption, increasing calcium withdrawal from bones, and decreasing calcium excretion in the urine. The plasma calcium concentration has an important influence on cell membrane permeability and influences the threshold potential of excitable cells. For this reason, calcium imbalances alter neuromuscular irritability.

Some causes of excess calcium in the blood (hypercalcemia)

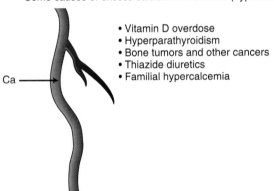

Ca

- Vitamin D overdose
- Hyperparathyroidism
- Bone tumors and other cancers
- Thiazide diuretics
- Familial hypercalcemia

Some causes of decreased calcium in the blood (hypocalcemia)

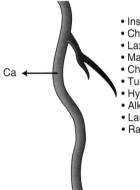

Ca

- Insufficient dietary calcium & vitamin D intake
- Chronic diarrhea
- Laxative abuse
- Malabsorption
- Chronic renal insufficiency
- Tumor lysis syndrome
- Hypoparathyroidism
- Alkalosis
- Large transfusion of citrated blood
- Rapid infusion of plasma expanders

FIGURE 8–15. Factors that cause calcium imbalances

Hypercalcemia

Hypercalcemia refers to a plasma excess of calcium (above 5.3 mEq/L [2.7 mmol/L] in children or 5 mEq/L [2.5 mmol/L] in newborns). Because so much calcium is stored in the bones, however, the serum levels of calcium may not reflect body stores.

Clinical Manifestations

Hypercalcemia may have nonspecific symptoms, making diagnosis difficult.[4] Many of the signs and symptoms of hypercalcemia are manifestations of decreased neuromuscular excitability. Constipation, anorexia, nausea, and vomiting can occur. Fatigue and skeletal muscle weakness predominate. Confusion, lethargy, and decreased attention span are common. Polyuria develops. Severe hypercalcemia may cause cardiac arrhythmias and arrest. Neonates with hypercalcemia have flaccid muscles and exhibit failure to thrive. Hypercalcemia increases sodium and potassium excretion by the kidneys and can lead to polyuria and polydipsia.

Etiology and Pathophysiology

Hypercalcemia is caused by conditions that involve increased calcium intake or absorption, shift of calcium from bones into the extracellular fluid, and decreased calcium excretion. Hypercalcemia due to increased calcium intake or absorption may occur if an infant is fed large amounts of chicken liver (source of vitamin A) or is given megadoses of vitamin D or vitamin A, or if a child or adolescent consumes large amounts of calcium-rich foods concurrently with antacids (milk-alkali syndrome). Infants with very low birthweight can develop hypercalcemia if they have inadequate phosphorus intake, as bone phosphorus and calcium will be resorbed. Hypercalcemia may also occur when children receiving total parenteral nutrition are given doses of calcium that are too high.

Most cases of hypercalcemia in children are due to a shift of calcium from bones into the extracellular fluid. The excessive amounts of parathyroid hormone produced in hyperparathyroidism cause calcium withdrawal from bones. Prolonged immobilization also causes withdrawal of calcium from bones. Often, the excess calcium ions are excreted in the urine. However, if calcium is withdrawn from bones faster than the kidneys can excrete it, hypercalcemia results. Hypercalcemia also occurs with many types of malignancies such as leukemias. The malignant cells produce substances that circulate in the blood to the bones and cause bone resorption. The calcium from the bones then enters the extracellular fluid, causing hypercalcemia. Bone tumors destroy bone directly, leading to the release of calcium. Familial hypercalcemia and infantile hypercalcemia are rare congenital disorders.

Thiazide diuretics (eg, thiazide and hydrochlorthiazide) decrease calcium excretion in the urine and may contribute to development of hypercalcemia.

Medical Management

Hypercalcemia is treated by increasing fluids and administering the diuretic furosemide (Lasix) to increase excretion of calcium in the urine. Treatment to decrease intestinal absorption of calcium involves effective use of glucocorticoids. Bone resorption can be decreased by administration of glucocorticoids and calcitonin. Phosphate is sometimes given to treat hypercalcemia, but it may cause dangerous precipitation of calcium phosphate salts in body tissues. Dialysis may be used, if necessary.

Nursing Assessment

Nursing assessment of a child with hypercalcemia includes monitoring serum calcium levels, level of consciousness, gastrointestinal function, urine volume, specific gravity, cardiac rhythm, and pH. With chronic hypercalcemia, assessment of activity tolerance and developmental level becomes important.

Nursing Diagnosis

Many nursing diagnoses are appropriate for children who have hypercalcemia. Diagnoses that address cardiac and neuromuscular manifestation are especially important. The following nursing diagnoses may apply:

- Risk for Decreased Cardiac Output related to cardiac arrest
- Risk for Injury related to decreased level of consciousness
- Risk for Injury related to muscle weakness
- Risk for Injury related to possibility of spontaneous fractures
- Self-Care Deficit related to fatigue and muscle weakness
- Anxiety related to decreased muscle function
- Constipation related to decreased bowel function
- Risk for Altered Nutrition: Less Than Body Requirements related to anorexia and nausea
- Risk for Altered Urinary Elimination related to renal calculi

Nursing Management

Carefully calculate calcium in total parenteral nutrition and other solutions, administer these solutions with caution, and use cardiac monitoring to prevent hypercalcemia in hospitalized children.

Interventions to increase fluid intake are important for children with hypercalcemia or those who are immobilized. A large fluid intake, appropriate to the child's age is necessary to keep the urine dilute and to help reduce constipation (a common symptom of hypercalcemia). An acidic urine helps to keep calcium from forming stones. Because urinary tract infections may cause the urine to be alkaline, nursing interventions to prevent urinary tract infection are necessary. Thiazide diuretics, which decrease calcium excretion, should not be given to the hypercalcemic child. Provide a high-fiber diet to help reduce constipation.

Increasing mobility through assisted weight-bearing helps to decrease the withdrawal of calcium from bones that is caused by immobility. If the hypercalcemia is caused by withdrawal of calcium from bones, the child is at risk for fractures with minor trauma and must be handled with special care.

Teach parents to avoid giving calcium-rich roods and calcium antacids (eg, Tums) to children with hypercalcemia. Vitamin D supplements also should be avoided as they increase calcium absorption from the gastrointestinal tract.

CLINICAL TIP

To decrease calcium intake in hypercalcemia, milk, ice cream, and other dairy products should be restricted. Nondairy fruit-based desserts are acceptable alternatives.

Hypocalcemia

Hypocalcemia is a serum deficit of calcium (below 4.4 mEq/L [2.2 mmol/L] in children or 4 mEq/L [2 mmol/L] in newborns]). (Remember that serum calcium levels may not reflect body stores of this mineral, as most of the body's calcium is stored in bone.)

Clinical Manifestations

The signs and symptoms of hypocalcemia are manifestations of increased muscular excitability (tetany). In children they include twitching and cramping, tingling around the mouth or in the fingers, carpal spasm, and pedal spasm. Laryngospasm, seizures, and cardiac arrhythmias are more severe manifestations of hypocalcemia and may be fatal. Hypocalcemia may cause congestive heart failure, especially in neonates.

Although these symptoms are diagnostic of acute calcium deficiency, a more common state in children and adolescents is chronic low intake of calcium. This may be manifested by spontaneous fractures in infants and in adolescents who exercise excessively.

Etiology and Pathophysiology

Hypocalcemia is caused by conditions that involve decreased calcium intake or absorption, shift of calcium to a physiologically unavailable form, increased calcium excretion, and loss of calcium by an abnormal route.

Decreased calcium intake or absorption causes hypocalcemia in children with chronic generalized malnutrition, or with a diet that is low in vitamin D and calcium. Female athletes and adolescents trying to lose weight often decrease foods that contain calcium and may develop chronic hypocalcemia. In these cases, premature bone loss and inadequate bone formation occur.[13] This deficit cannot be made up later in life, increasing the risk of osteoporosis.

Even with a normal calcium intake, hypocalcemia occurs if the mineral is not absorbed. If a child does not have enough vitamin D, calcium is not absorbed efficiently from the duodenum. Sunlight speeds formation of vitamin D in the skin. Children who are institutionalized without access to sunlight (eg, severely developmentally delayed children) may become hypocalcemic because of the lack of vitamin D. Uremic syndrome is another cause of vitamin D deficiency. It interferes with the kidney's ability to activate vitamin D. High phosphate intake can cause hypocalcemia. Chronic diarrhea and steatorrhea (fatty stools) also reduce calcium absorption from the gastrointestinal tract.

The shift of calcium into a physiologically unavailable form occurs when calcium shifts into bone or free ionized calcium in plasma binds to proteins or small organic ions in the plasma. Too much calcium shifts into bones in various types of hypoparathyroidism, including DiGeorge syndrome (congenital absence of the parathyroid glands). Hypomagnesemia impairs parathyroid hormone function and may cause hypocalcemia. Some types of neonatal hypocalcemia are associated with delayed parathyroid hormone function or hypomagnesemia. Calcium shifts rapidly into bone when rickets is treated. A high plasma phosphate concentration causes plasma calcium to decrease. Ionized hypocalcemia, which is due to an increased binding of plasma ionized calcium, occurs very rapidly. The ionized hypocalcemia persists until the alkalosis resolves or the citrate is metabolized by the liver. Children who receive liver transplants are hypocalcemic for several days because of impaired citrate metabolism.[14]

Increased calcium excretion occurs in steatorrhea, when calcium secreted into the gastrointestinal fluid binds to the fecal fat in addition to the dietary calcium that is bound in the feces. A similar situation occurs in acute pancreatitis.

Loss of calcium by an abnormal route may contribute to hypocalcemia as calcium is lost from the body through burn or wound drainage or sequestered in acute pancreatitis. Many different medications can cause hypocalcemia.

Medical Management

Hypocalcemia is treated by oral or intravenous administration of calcium. The original cause of the imbalance is also treated. If the hypocalcemia is

GROWTH & DEVELOPMENT CONSIDERATIONS

Hypocalcemia in infants is more frequently manifested as tremors, muscle twitches, and brief tonic–clonic seizures.

GROWTH & DEVELOPMENT CONSIDERATIONS

The term "female athlete triad" has been used to describe the female who exercises a great deal, tries to maintain weight at a low level by dieting, and has abnormal menstrual periods. Often calcium intake is low and bone formation is impaired. This is of great importance during the pubertal growth spurt, when about 60% of bone mass is deposited.

CAUSES OF IONIZED HYPOCALCEMIA

Alkalosis, which causes more calcium to bind to plasma proteins
Citrate in transfused blood products, which binds calcium

DRUGS THAT MAY CAUSE HYPOCALCEMIA

Antacids (if overused)
Laxatives (if overused)
Oil-based bowel lubricants
Anticonvulsants
Phosphate-containing preparations
Protein-type plasma expanders during rapid infusion
Antineoplastics

due to hypomagnesemia, the magnesium must be replenished before the calcium replacement can be successful. When the cause is chronic low dietary intake, counseling is needed about high-calcium foods.

Nursing Assessment

Carefully assess growth in the young female athlete who is trying to diet. Whenever an adolescent female is very thin, be sure to ask about sports and other activities, and about regularity of menstrual periods. If periods are irregular or not occurring, collect additional dietary information to help determine whether the girl is lacking in intake of calcium, calories, and other nutrients. These assessments are needed even if serum calcium values are normal. Look for signs of inadequate nutrition such as fat and muscle wasting, dry hair, and cold hands and feet.[15] Assess for muscle cramps, stiffness, and clumsiness; grimacing caused by spasms of facial muscles and twitching of arm muscles; and laryngospasm. Increased neuromuscular excitability may be detected by testing for Trousseau's sign or Chvostek's sign. Many healthy newborns have a positive Chvostek's sign; however, this assessment should be reserved for children over several months of age. Monitor serum calcium levels and perform cardiac monitoring to observe for cardiac arrhythmias.

Nursing Diagnosis

The effects of increased neuromuscular excitability in the child with hypocalcemia are the basis for several nursing diagnoses. These include:

- Risk for Injury related to potential for fractures
- Risk for Injury related to increased neuromuscular excitability
- Risk for Ineffective Breathing Pattern related to laryngospasm
- Risk for Decreased Cardiac Output related to cardiac arrhythmias
- Sensory/Perceptual Alteration related to paresthesia
- Anxiety related to increased neuromuscular excitability
- Knowledge Deficit related to necessity for and sources of calcium intake

Nursing Management

To correct calcium deficiency in the hospitalized child, give oral or intravenous calcium as ordered. Monitor for complications of calcium supplementation. A 10% calcium gluconate solution should be readily available for emergency use in severe hypocalcemia. Calcium is never given intramuscularly because it causes tissue necrosis.

Take measures to ensure safety for the child who is hospitalized with hypocalcemia. Seizure precautions may be necessary. Explain the cause of muscle cramps to parents and older children.

Counsel the family about dairy products and nondairy foods rich in calcium (see adjacent box). For the young female athlete whose weight and menstrual patterns show irregularities, total calories and calcium intake should be increased. Teaching may also be needed about proper calcium intake and its importance both to athletic performance and to prevention of osteoporosis. Encourage three glasses of nonfat milk per day.[16] Teach ways to use milk in the diet. For example, sprinkle nonfat dry milk on cereal and other foods. If the child is lactose-intolerant, emphasize nondairy sources of calcium and advise parents to purchase special milk treated with lactase. This milk is more costly, and inadequate family finances may be an impediment to its use. If a child has a health condition leading to chronic

CLINICAL TIP

To test for Trousseau's sign, apply a blood pressure cuff to the arm and leave inflated for 3 min. If a carpal spasm occurs, the Trousseau's sign is positive. To test for Chvostek's sign, tap the skin lightly just in front of the ear (over the facial nerve). If the corner of the mouth draws up because of muscle contraction, the Chvostek's sign is positive.

COMPLICATIONS OF CALCIUM SUPPLEMENTS

Oral Calcium
Constipation
Intravenous Calcium
Tissue sloughing with infiltration
Elevated serum calcium
Decreased serum phosphate

HIGH-CALCIUM FOODS

Milk	Legumes
Cheese	Nuts
Yogurt	Figs
Pudding	Chicken
Egg yolks	Salmon
Grains	(canned with
(cream of	bones)
wheat,	Sardines (canned)
farina, bran	Tofu
muffins)	

diarrhea, encourage increased intake of calcium-rich foods. Calcium supplements in the form of calcium carbonate tablets may be used.

MAGNESIUM IMBALANCES

Magnesium is necessary for enzyme function in cells, acetylcholine release, glycolysis, stimulation of ATPases, and bone formation. Since magnesium is a component of chlorophyll, magnesium intake is aided by eating dark green leafy vegetables. Nuts and grains are also good sources of magnesium. Magnesium is absorbed primarily from the terminal ileum. Magnesium is distributed among the extracellular fluid (small amounts), the cells (larger amounts), and the bones (large amounts). Magnesium excretion occurs in urine, feces, and sweat.

Magnesium imbalances are caused by alterations in magnesium intake, distribution, or excretion; by loss of magnesium through an abnormal route; or by a combination of these factors. The plasma magnesium concentration influences the release of acetylcholine at neuromuscular junctions. Thus, magnesium imbalances are characterized by alterations in neuromuscular irritability.

Hypermagnesemia

Hypermagnesemia occurs when the plasma magnesium concentration is too high (above 2.4 mg/dL [0.99 mmol/L]). Keep in mind that the serum levels measured in the laboratory may not reflect body magnesium stores, because most of the magnesium in the body is located in the bones and inside the cells.

Clinical manifestations of hypermagnesemia include decreased muscle irritability, hypotension, bradycardia, drowsiness, lethargy, and weak or absent deep tendon reflexes. In severe hypermagnesemia, flaccid muscle paralysis, fatal respiratory depression, cardiac arrhythmias, and cardiac arrest occur.

Hypermagnesemia is caused by conditions that involve increased magnesium intake and decreased magnesium excretion. Impaired renal function leading to decreased magnesium excretion is the most common cause of hypermagnesemia in children. In both oliguric renal failure and adrenal insufficiency, magnesium ions that cannot be excreted in the urine accumulate in the extracellular fluid.

Less frequently, increased magnesium intake may cause hypermagnesemia. Magnesium sulfate ($MgSO_4$) given to treat eclampsia in the mother before delivery causes hypermagnesemia in the newborn. Abnormally high amounts may also be taken in magnesium-containing enemas, laxatives, antacids, and intravenous fluids. Aspiration of seawater, as in near-drowning, is an uncommon but potentially serious source of excessive magnesium intake. Children with Addison's disease can have abnormally high magnesium levels.

Hypermagnesemia is managed primarily by increasing the urinary excretion of magnesium. This is usually accomplished by increasing fluid intake (except in oliguric renal failure) and by the administration of diuretics. Dialysis may sometimes be necessary.

Nursing Management

Monitor serum magnesium levels. Take the child's blood pressure (to watch for hypotension), heart rate and rhythm (to monitor for bradycardia and cardiac arrhythmias), respiratory rate and depth (to watch for respiratory depression), and deep tendon reflexes (to check muscle tone and paralysis

---

NORMAL SERUM MAGNESIUM CONCENTRATION

1.5–2.4 mg/dL (0.62–0.99 mmol/L)

DRUGS THAT MAY CAUSE HYPERMAGNESEMIA

Magnesium-containing cathartics
Magnesium antacids

or movement). Keep the side rails of the bed raised. Children with hypermagnesemia or oliguria should not be given magnesium-containing medications or sea salt.

Teach parents of children with chronic renal failure that these children should never be given milk of magnesia, antacids that contain magnesium, or other sources of magnesium. When hypermagnesemia is treated with diuretics, monitor potassium levels to watch for hypokalemia.

Hypomagnesemia

Hypomagnesemia refers to a plasma magnesium concentration that is too low (below 1.5 mg/dL [0.62 mmol/L]). (Remember that the serum levels of magnesium may not reflect body stores, since most of the magnesium in the body is found in cells and bones.)

Hypomagnesemia is characterized by increased neuromuscular excitability (tetany). The clinical manifestations are hyperactive reflexes, skeletal muscle cramps, twitching, tremors, and cardiac arrhythmias. Seizures can occur with severe hypomagnesemia.

Hypomagnesemia is caused by conditions that involve decreased magnesium intake or absorption, shift of magnesium to a physiologically unavailable form, increased magnesium excretion, and loss of magnesium by an abnormal route.

Decreased magnesium intake or absorption can occur if a child who is not eating has prolonged intravenous therapy without magnesium. Chronic malnutrition is another cause of decreased magnesium intake. Magnesium absorption is decreased in chronic diarrhea, short bowel syndrome, malabsorption syndromes, and steatorrhea.

A shift of magnesium to a physiologically unavailable form may occur after transfusion of many units of citrated blood products because magnesium bound to the citrate is not physiologically active. Such transfusions cause prolonged hypomagnesemia in liver transplant patients, who have impaired citrate metabolism. Magnesium shifts rapidly into bones that have been deprived of adequate stores.

Increased magnesium excretion in the urine occurs with diuretic therapy, the diuretic phase of acute renal failure, diabetic ketoacidosis, and hyperaldosteronism. Chronic alcoholism, occasionally seen in adolescents, increases urinary magnesium excretion. Magnesium contained in gastrointestinal secretions is bound to fat and excreted in the stool.

Loss of magnesium by an abnormal route occurs with prolonged nasogastric suction and through sequestration of magnesium in acute pancreatitis. Several medications may cause hypomagnesemia.

Hypomagnesemia is managed by administering magnesium and treating the underlying cause of the imbalance.

Nursing Management

In addition to monitoring serum magnesium levels, nursing assessment of hypomagnesemia includes monitoring deep tendon reflexes, testing for Trousseau's and Chvostek's signs (see p. 320), monitoring cardiac function, and observing for muscle twitching. Children who are able to talk report muscle cramping. Because magnesium levels are not routinely measured in many settings, request the test for any child who has risk factors and early manifestations of hypomagnesemia. When intramuscular or intravenous magnesium are ordered, administer carefully as directed and monitor vital signs. Electrocardiogram and renal studies may precede drug administration. Have resuscitative drugs and equipment readily available during drug administration.

Teach parents of a child with hypomagnesemia or continuing risk factors such as chronic diarrhea to include magnesium-rich foods in the diet. Before administering magnesium supplements, verify that the child's urine output is adequate. Monitor deep tendon reflexes if intravenous magnesium is given, and observe for complications of magnesium supplementation.

► CLINICAL ASSESSMENT OF FLUID AND ELECTROLYTE IMBALANCE

How can you assess children appropriately for fluid and electrolyte imbalance without thinking through the clinical manifestations of every possible disorder one after the other? First, perform a rapid risk factor assessment on each child to see which factors are present (Tables 8–12 and 8–13).

COMPLICATIONS OF MAGNESIUM SUPPLEMENTS
Oral Magnesium
Diarrhea
Intravenous Magnesium
Flushing, warmth
Elevated serum magnesium
Cardiac arrhythmias
Decreased deep tendon reflexes

8-12	Risk Factor Assessment for Fluid Imbalances

Isotonic Fluid (Extracellular Fluid Volume Imbalances)
- Source of increased intake?
- Aldosterone secretion increased or decreased?
- Source of loss from the body?

Water
- Source of increased intake?
- Antidiuretic hormone secretion increased or decreased?
- Source of unusual loss from the body?

8-13	Risk Factor Assessment for Electrolyte Imbalances

Electrolyte Intake and Absorption
- Increased?
- Decreased?

Electrolyte Shifts
- From electrolyte pool to plasma?
- From plasma to electrolyte pool?

Electrolyte Excretion
- Increased?
- Decreased?

Electrolyte Loss by Abnormal Route
- Vomiting?
- Diarrhea?
- Nasogastric suction?
- Wound?
- Burn?
- Excessive sweating?

A risk factor assessment may be performed mentally during routine tasks. Look for factors that alter the intake, retention, and loss of isotonic fluid and water. This information is used to evaluate which fluid imbalance is most likely to occur in a particular child. Next, look for factors that alter electrolyte intake and absorption, distribution between plasma and other electrolyte pools, excretion, and abnormal routes of electrolyte loss. This information is used to evaluate which electrolyte imbalances are most likely to occur in the child. A review of pathophysiology is important to understand the role of the other electrolytes and substances, such as phosphorus, in the body.

After evaluating possible imbalances for the child, perform a clinical assessment. Assessment of fluid imbalances is performed by assessing weight changes, vascular volume, interstitial volume, and cerebral function (Table 8–14). Assessment of electrolyte imbalances is performed by assessing serum electrolyte levels, skeletal muscle strength, neuromuscular excitability, gastrointestinal tract function, and cardiac rhythm (Table 8–15). Next, check for other manifestations that are specific to a particular high-risk imbalance (eg, polyuria in hypokalemia). Evaluate any serum laboratory values available. This method of risk factor assessment followed by clinical assessment provides a rapid yet thorough approach to assessment for fluid and electrolyte imbalances.

▶ PHYSIOLOGY OF ACID–BASE BALANCE

Normal acid–base balance is necessary for proper function of the cells and the body. The number of hydrogen ions (H^+) present in a fluid determines how acidic it is. Increasing the hydrogen ion concentration makes a solution more acidic. Because the hydrogen ion concentration in body fluids is

8-14	Summary of Clinical Assessment of Fluid Imbalances	
Assessment Category	**Specific Assessments**	**Changes With Fluid Imbalances**
Rapid changes in weight	Daily weights	Weight gain—extracellular volume excess Weight loss—extracellular volume deficit; clinical dehydration
Vascular volume	Small vein filling time	Increased—extracellular volume deficit; clinical dehydration
	Capillary refill time	Increased—extracellular volume deficit; clinical dehydration
	Character of pulse	Bounding—extracellular volume excess Thready—extracellular volume deficit; clinical dehydration
	Postural blood pressure measurements	Postural drop—extracellular volume deficit; clinical dehydration
	Lung sounds in dependent portions	Crackles—extracellular volume excess
	Central venous pressure	Increased—extracellular volume excess Decreased—extracellular volume deficit; clinical dehydration
	Tenseness of fontanel (infants)	Bulging—extracellular volume excess Sunken—extracellular volume deficit; clinical dehydration
	Neck vein filling (older children)	Full with upright—extracellular volume excess Flat when supine—extracellular volume deficit; clinical dehydration
Interstitial volume	Skin turgor	Skin tents—extracellular volume deficit; clinical dehydration
	Presence or absence of edema	Edema—extracellular volume excess
Cerebral function	Level of consciousness	Decreased—clinical dehydration

8-15	Summary of Clinical Assessment of Electrolyte Imbalances	
Assessment Category	**Specific Assessments**	**Changes With Electrolyte Imbalances**
Skeletal muscle function	Muscle strength	Weakness, flaccid paralysis—hyperkalemia; hypokalemia
Neuromuscular excitability	Deep tendon reflexes	Depressed—hypercalcemia; hypermagnesemia
		Hyperactive—hypocalcemia; hypomagnesemia
	Chvostek's sign (not infants)	Positive—hypocalcemia; hypomagnesemia
	Trousseau's sign	Positive—hypocalcemia; hypomagnesemia
	Paresthesias	Digital or perioral—hypocalcemia
	Muscle cramping or twitching	Present—hypocalcemia; hypomagnesemia
Gastrointestinal tract function	Bowel sounds	Decreased or absent—hypokalemia
	Elimination pattern	Constipation—hypokalemia; hypercalcemia
		Diarrhea—hyperkalemia
Cardiac rhythm	Arrhythmia	Irregular—hyperkalemia; hypokalemia; hypercalcemia; hypocalcemia; hypermagnesemia; hypomagnesemia
	Electrocardiogram	Abnormal—hyperkalemia; hypokalemia; hypercalcemia; hypocalcemia; hypermagnesemia; hypomagnesemia
Cerebral function	Level of consciousness	Decreased—hyponatremia; hypernatremia

very small, acidity is expressed as **pH** (the negative logarithm of the hydrogen ion concentration) rather than as the hydrogen ion concentration itself. The range of possible pH values is 1 to 14. A pH of 7 is neutral. The lower the pH, the more acidic the solution. A pH above 7 is basic. The higher the pH, the more basic the solution. Body fluids are normally slightly basic.

The pH of body fluids is regulated carefully to provide a suitable environment for cell function. The pH of the blood influences the pH inside the cells. **Acidemia** is a term that refers to a decreased blood pH below normal levels, while **alkalemia** is an increased blood pH. In order for the enzymes outside the cells to function optimally, the pH must be in the normal range. If the pH inside the cells becomes too high or too low, then the speed of chemical reactions becomes inappropriate for proper cell function. Cell protein function relies on the correct level of hydrogen ions. Thus acid–base imbalances result in clinical signs and symptoms, and, in severe cases, they may cause death.

In the course of their normal function, all cells in the body produce acids. Cells produce two kinds of acids: carbonic acid (H_2CO_3) and metabolic (noncarbonic) acids. These acids are released into the extracellular fluid and must be neutralized or excreted from the body to prevent dangerous accumulation. They can be neutralized to some degree by the buffers in body fluids. Carbonic acid is excreted by the lungs in the form of carbon dioxide and water. Metabolic acids are excreted by the kidneys.

Buffers

The maintenance of hydrogen ions within normal range relies heavily on buffers. A **buffer** is a compound that binds hydrogen ions when their concentration rises and releases them when the concentration falls[17] (Figs. 8–16A and B). Several kinds of buffers are present in the body (Table 8–16). Various body fluids have buffers to meet their special needs. The bi-

NORMAL VALUES OF ARTERIAL BLOOD pH

Infants: 7.36–7.42
Children: 7.37–7.43
Adolescents: 7.35–7.41

EXAMPLES OF METABOLIC ACIDS

Pyruvic acid
Sulfuric acid
Acetoacetic acid
Lactic acid
Hydrochloric acid
Beta-hydroxybutyric acid

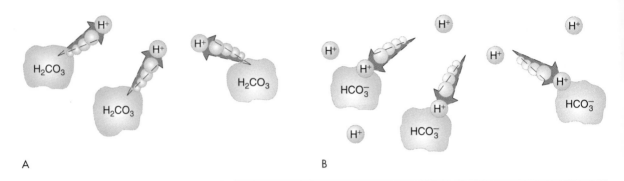

FIGURE 8–16. **A,** How buffers respond to an excess of base. If the blood has too much base, the acid portion of a buffer pair (eg, H_2CO_3 of the bicarbonate buffer system) releases hydrogen ions (H^+) to help return the pH to normal. **B,** How buffers respond to an excess of acid. If the blood has too much acid, the base portion of a buffer pair (eg, HCO_3^- of the bicarbonate buffer system) takes up hydrogen ions (H^+) to help return the pH to normal.

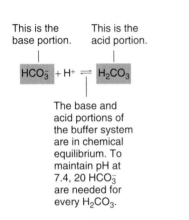

This is the base portion.   This is the acid portion.

$$HCO_3^- + H^+ \rightleftharpoons H_2CO_3$$

The base and acid portions of the buffer system are in chemical equilibrium. To maintain pH at 7.4, 20 HCO_3^- are needed for every H_2CO_3.

FIGURE 8–17. The bicarbonate buffer system.

8-16	Important Buffers	
Buffer	**Major Locations in the Body**	
Bicarbonate	Plasma; interstitial fluid	
Protein	Plasma; inside cells	
Hemoglobin	Inside red blood cells	
Phosphate	Inside cells; urine	

carbonate buffer system neutralizes metabolic acids (Fig. 8–17); however, it cannot neutralize carbonic acid.

All buffer systems have limits. For example, if there are too many metabolic acids, the bicarbonate buffers become depleted. The acids then accumulate in the body until they are excreted by the kidneys. Clinically, this is seen as a decreased serum bicarbonate concentration and decreased blood pH.

Role of the Lungs

The lungs are responsible for excreting excess carbonic acid from the body. A child breathes out carbon dioxide and water, the components of carbonic acid, with each breath. With faster and deeper breaths, more carbonic acid is excreted. Since carbonic acid is converted in the body to carbon dioxide and water by the enzyme carbonic anhydrase, an indirect laboratory measurement of carbonic acid is P_{CO_2}.

Although a child can voluntarily increase or decrease the rate and depth of respirations, they are usually involuntarily controlled. The P_{CO_2} and pH of the blood are monitored by chemoreceptors in the hypothalamus of the brain and in the aorta and carotid arteries. These arteries also monitor the P_{O_2} of the blood. The input from the chemoreceptors is combined with other neural input to change breathing according to needs. Rate and depth increase or decrease according to the amount of carbonic acid that needs to be excreted.

CARBONIC ACID

Carbonic acid = carbon dioxide + water
$$H_2CO_3 = CO_2 + H_2O$$

P_{CO_2} NORMAL ARTERIAL BLOOD VALUES

Infants: 30–34 mm Hg
Children: 35–41 mm Hg
Adolescents: 38–44 mm Hg

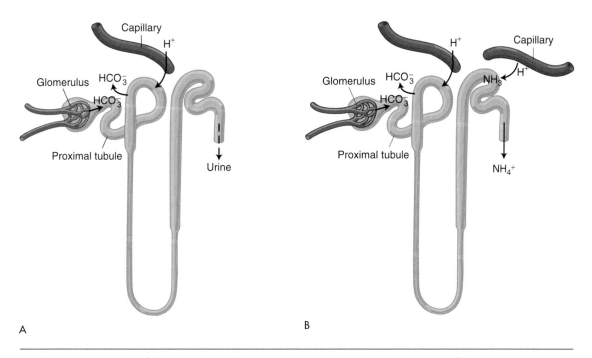

FIGURE 8–18. A, Recycling of bicarbonate by the kidneys. Bicarbonate ions that are in the blood are filtered into the renal tubules at the glomerulus. In the proximal tubules, bicarbonate ions are reabsorbed into the blood at the same time that hydrogen ions are transported from the blood into the renal tubular fluid. **B,** Secretion and buffering of hydrogen ions in the kidneys. If the urine is too acidic, the cells that line the urinary tract could be damaged. To prevent this problem, hydrogen ions secreted into the distal tubules are neutralized by phosphate buffers or bound to ammonia and excreted in the form of ammonium ions.

If a child has a condition that decreases the excretion of carbonic acid or causes breathing to be too slow or shallow (such as overmedication following surgery), carbonic acid accumulates in the blood. Clinically, this is seen as an increased blood P_{CO_2}. The reverse will also be true.

Role of the Kidneys

The kidneys excrete metabolic acids from the body in two ways. They reabsorb filtered bicarbonate and form bicarbonate when needed to restore balance. Bicarbonate is formed when acids and ammonium combine with extra ions.[18] The blood bicarbonate concentration is an indicator of the amount of metabolic acids present, since bicarbonate is used in buffering the acids. When the concentration is normal, metabolic acids are present in usual amounts (Figs. 8–18A and B).

In a healthy child, the result of these renal processes is excretion of metabolic acids and maintenance of blood bicarbonate concentration within normal limits. However, a child whose kidneys are not producing enough urine may be unable to excrete metabolic acids effectively. Accumulation of these acids uses up many of the available bicarbonate buffers, resulting in a decreased serum bicarbonate concentration.

Role of the Liver

The liver also plays a role in maintaining acid–base balance by metabolizing protein, which produces hydrogen ions. It also synthesizes proteins needed to maintain osmotic pressures in the fluid compartments.

> **NORMAL CONCENTRATIONS OF ARTERIAL BLOOD BICARBONATE**
>
> Infants: 17.2–23.6 mmol/L
> Children: 18–25 mmol/L
> Adolescents: 23–25 mmol/L

► ACID–BASE IMBALANCES

There are four acid–base imbalances. Two are the result of processes that cause too much acid in the body and are referred to as **acidosis.** The other two imbalances are the result of processes that cause too little acid in the body and are called **alkalosis.** An acid–base disorder caused by too much or too little carbonic acid is called a *respiratory* acid–base imbalance. A disorder caused by too much or too little metabolic acid is called a *metabolic* acid–base imbalance.

Arterial blood gas measurements (ABGs) provide a laboratory evaluation of a child's current acid–base status. Table 8–17 provides a method that can help you interpret the pH, PCO_2, and bicarbonate concentrations, which are the most important acid–base measures. End-tidal CO_2 can provide a continuous noninvasive measurement. (Remember that PCO_2 reflects carbonic acid status and bicarbonate concentration reflects the metabolic acid status.)

Respiratory Acidosis

Respiratory acidosis is caused by the accumulation of carbon dioxide in the blood. Since carbon dioxide and water can be combined into carbonic acid, respiratory acidosis is sometimes called carbonic acid excess. The condition can be acute or chronic. It is controlled by the lungs.

Clinical Manifestations

Acidosis in the brain cells causes central nervous system depression, manifested by confusion, lethargy, headache, increased intracranial pressure, and even coma.[19] Acute respiratory acidosis can lead to tachycardia and cardiac arrhythmias. The child's arterial blood gases always show an increased PCO_2, the laboratory sign of increased carbonic acid. Serum pH can be decreased or normal.

8-17   How to Interpret Arterial Blood Gas Measurements

Ask the following questions to analyze blood gas results.
1. **What is the pH?** If the pH is normal, the child has no imbalance or has compensated for an imbalance. If the pH is below normal, the child has acidosis. If the pH is above normal, the child has alkalosis.
2. **What is the PCO_2?** If the PCO_2 is normal, the child does not have an acid–base imbalance. If the PCO_2 is above normal, the child has respiratory acidosis. This may be the primary disorder or may be a compensatory response to metabolic alkalosis. Looking at the bicarbonate concentration helps you decide. If the PCO_2 is below normal, the child has respiratory alkalosis. Again, this can be the primary disorder or may be a compensatory response to metabolic acidosis.
3. **What is the bicarbonate concentration?** If the bicarbonate concentration is within normal range, the child does not have a metabolic acid–base imbalance. If the bicarbonate is above normal, the child has metabolic alkalosis. This can be a primary disorder or can be compensatory in respiratory acidosis. When bicarbonate is below normal, the child has metabolic acidosis, either as a direct disorder or as a compensatory response to respiratory alkalosis.
4. **What do the results together tell you?** If the pH is abnormal and either the PCO_2 or bicarbonate concentration is normal, there is an uncompensated acid–base disorder. If all three values are abnormal, the child has a partially compensated disorder and the pH will provide the definitive answer. If PCO_2, pH, and bicarbonate are all decreased, then partially compensated metabolic acidosis is most likely. If pH is normal and PCO_2 and bicarbonate are abnormal, there is a fully compensated acid–base disorder.
5. **What are the child's history and clinical signs?** Does your interpretation fit with what you know about the child's medical condition and with assessments you are making? This last step helps you to integrate laboratory data with the clinical picture to strengthen your nursing care of the child with an acid–base imbalance.

8-18	Causes of Respiratory Acidosis		
Factors Affecting the Lungs	**Factors Affecting the Neuromuscular Pump**		**Factors Affecting Central Control of Respiration**
Aspiration	Flail chest		Sedative overdose
Spasm of the airways	Pneumothorax or hemothorax		General anesthesia
Laryngeal edema	Mechanical underventilation		Head injury
Epiglottitis	Hypokalemic muscle weakness		Brain tumor
Croup	High cervical spinal cord injury		Central sleep apnea
Pulmonary edema	Botulism		
Atelectasis	Tetanus		
Severe pneumonia	Kyphoscoliosis		
Cystic fibrosis	Poliomyelitis		
Bronchopulmonary dysplasia	Muscular dystrophy		
Pulmonary embolism	Congenital diaphragmatic hernia		
	Guillain-Barré syndrome		

Etiology and Pathophysiology

Any factor that interferes with the ability of the lungs to excrete carbon dioxide can cause respiratory acidosis. These factors may interfere with the gaseous exchange within the lungs, may impair the neuromuscular pump that moves air in and out of the lungs, or may depress the respiratory rate (Table 8–18; Fig. 8–19).

As the P_{CO_2} begins to increase, the pH of the blood begins to decrease. Compensatory mechanisms begin to act in the form of nonbicarbonate

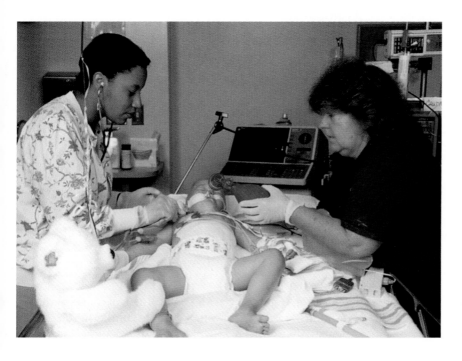

FIGURE 8–19. This child may develop respiratory acidosis or respiratory alkalosis. If the tidal volume is set too low during mechanical ventilation, carbon dioxide (carbonic acid) will accumulate in the body (respiratory acidosis) because it is not being excreted by the lungs. If the tidal volume is set too high, carbon dioxide will be depleted in the body (respiratory alkalosis) because it is being excreted in great quantities.

8-19	Laboratory Values in Uncompensated and Compensated Respiratory Acidosis		
	PCO$_2$	pH	HCO$_3^-$
Uncompensated	Increased	Decreased	Normal
Partially compensated	Increased	Decreasing but moving toward normal	Increasing
Fully compensated	Increased	Normal	Increased

buffers, additional hydrogen ion excretion by the kidneys, and formation and decreased bicarbonate excretion by the kidneys. These compensatory mechanisms take several days to become active so the child manifests a changing clinical situation, depending on the underlying cause and the amount of compensation occurring (Table 8–19).

Medical Management

Treatment of respiratory acidosis requires correction of the underlying cause. For example, treatment may include bronchodilators for bronchospasm, mechanical ventilation for neuromuscular defects, decreasing sedative use, or surgery for kyphoscoliosis.

Nursing Assessment

Nursing assessment plays a pivotal role in decisions about interventions for respiratory acidosis. This is especially true in chronic conditions such as cystic fibrosis and kyphoscoliosis. Assess respiratory rate, rhythm, and depth carefully. Take the apical pulse and be alert for tachycardia or arrhythmia. A cardiac monitor may be used. Obtain serial arterial blood gas measurements in acute conditions to evaluate changing status. Assess the level of consciousness and energy. Observe for chronic fatigue, headache, or decreased level of consciousness.

Nursing Diagnosis

Several nursing diagnoses may apply to the child with respiratory acidosis. The most important of these addresses the child's Risk for Injury. Other nursing diagnoses depend on the specific clinical manifestation and the particular cause of the acidosis. Examples include:

- Risk for Injury related to decreased level of consciousness
- Risk for Decreased Cardiac Output related to cardiac arrhythmias
- Ineffective Breathing Pattern (hypoventilation) related to inadequate neuromuscular activity
- Pain (headache) related to cerebral vasodilation
- Ineffective Management of Therapeutic Regimen related to prescribed bronchodilator therapy

Nursing Management

Teach children at risk for respiratory acidosis and their parents preventive measures to use at home. For the child with a chronic condition such as cystic fibrosis, muscular dystrophy, or kyphoscoliosis, demonstrate deep

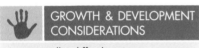
GROWTH & DEVELOPMENT CONSIDERATIONS

It is usually difficult to get a young child to do deep breathing or to use the "blow bottle" that is often given to older children and adults. To make deep breathing fun, use a pinwheel and have the child turn it during play. Alternatively, give a child a straw and have him or her blow bubbles in a glass of water, or have the child use the straw to blow scraps of paper across the bedside table.

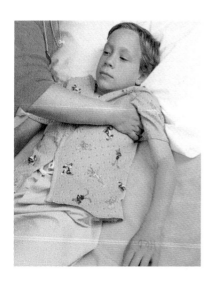

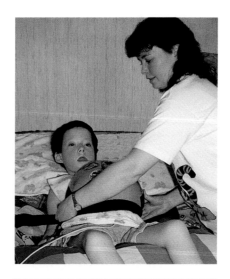

FIGURE 8–20. Positioning to facilitate chest expansion. If the child is positioned to avoid chest compression or slumping to the side, this will help correct respiratory acidosis.

FIGURE 8–21. This child, who has muscular dystrophy, uses a "turtle" respirator at home to assist with breathing. His parents required instructions from the nurse on use of the respirator. The family has a generator to provide electricity for the respirator during power outages.

breathing and encourage its use several times each day. Teach the family signs of infection—including fever, increased respiratory secretions, and discomfort with breathing—so they can be treated promptly, preventing further respiratory involvement. Position the child to facilitate chest expansion (Fig. 8–20). Teach parents about proper administration of any necessary medications. For example, the child with cystic fibrosis may receive antibiotics to prevent respiratory infections. Teach parents and older children about home respirator use (Fig. 8–21).

For the hospitalized child, the focus is on ensuring safety. Keep side rails raised, and turn and position the child frequently. Evaluate mental status and document and report any changes in alertness. When laboratory values of blood pH and P_{CO_2} are available, evaluate them promptly and report any changes or abnormalities. Administer medications as ordered. Carefully watch the doses of sedatives to avoid further respiratory depression. Provide suctioning and encourage deep breathing.

Respiratory Alkalosis

Respiratory alkalosis occurs when the blood contains too little carbon dioxide. It is sometimes called carbonic acid deficit.

Arterial blood gas measurements show a decreased P_{CO_2} in respiratory alkalosis. Blood pH is generally elevated. The lack of carbon dioxide causes neuromuscular irritability and paresthesias in the extremities and around the mouth. Muscle cramping and carpal or pedal spasms can occur. The child may be dizzy or confused.

Excess carbon dioxide loss is caused by hyperventilation, in which more air than normal is moved into and out of the lungs. Common causes of hyperventilation are listed in Table 8–20.

In many cases, respiratory alkalosis lasts for several hours only. Renal compensation does not occur, as these compensatory mechanisms take several days to begin action. An example is the hyperventilation that occurs

8-20	Causes of Hyperventilation

Hypoxemia

Anxiety

Pain

Fever

Salicylate poisoning

Meningitis

Encephalitis

Septicemia caused by gram-negative bacteria

Mechanical overventilation

8-21	Laboratory Values in Uncompensated and Compensated Respiratory Alkalosis		
	P_{CO_2}	pH	HCO_3^-
Uncompensated	Decreased	Increased	Normal
Partially compensated	Decreased	Increased but moving toward normal	Decreasing
Fully compensated	Decreased	Normal	Decreased

with acute anxiety. If the condition persists, however, the kidneys will begin to retain more acid and excrete more bicarbonate. Hydrogen ions will be released from body buffers to decrease plasma bicarbonate. While the imbalance continues, cellular function is thus protected by returning pH to normal levels (Table 8–21).

Medical management focuses on correcting the condition that caused the hyperventilation so that the body's compensatory mechanisms can return carbon dioxide levels to normal.

Nursing Management

Assess the child's level of consciousness and ask if the child feels light-headed or has tingling sensations or numbness in the fingers, toes, or around the mouth. Assess the rate and depth of respirations. Monitor the hospitalized child's P_{O_2} with serial arterial blood gas measurements to evaluate changes in status. A careful assessment is needed regarding the cause of hyperventilation. Did an occurrence cause anxiety for the child? Is pain present (see Chap. 7)? Has the child received salicylates in any form? Is the child mechanically ventilated? Is there a central nervous system infection such as meningitis?

Nursing care for the child with respiratory alkalosis centers on teaching stress management techniques, maintaining pain control, promoting respiratory function, ensuring safety, maintaining fluid status, and providing health supervision and home care.

Teach Stress Management Techniques. When anxiety is the cause of respiratory alkalosis, instruct the child to breathe slowly, in rhythm with your own breathing. Teach stress control techniques such as relaxation and imagery for situations that cause anxiety (Table 8–22).

Maintain Pain Control. Use medications, imagery, distraction, positioning, massage, and other techniques to decrease pain and maintain pain management. Chapter 7 describes these and other measures to assist with pain control.

Promote Respiratory Function. Have the child cough, or suction as needed. Be certain that mechanical ventilation systems are working properly.

Ensure Safety. Provide a safe environment for the child who has a decreased level of consciousness. Be sure the child is supervised when sitting or standing up. Keep bed rails up.

Regulate Fluid Status. Renal compensation to manage ongoing respiratory alkalosis requires adequate urinary output. Regulate fluid intake to ensure urine output unless fluids are restricted due to medical condition.

NURSING ALERT

The P_{O_2} must be checked before any therapy for respiratory alkalosis is started, because it is dangerous to stop hyperventilation if oxygenation is poor.

<table>
<tr><td>8-22</td><td>Techniques for Reducing Anxiety in Children With Parethesias</td></tr>
</table>

Infant
Calming touch, quiet voice, swaddling, holding quietly

Toddler or Preschooler
Stuffed toy to hug, singing familiar quiet nursery songs, acknowledging the child's feelings, holding calmly

Young School-age Child
Talking quietly about a happy event, telling a familiar story, reading a familiar book together, explaining that the tingling will go away, use of simple guided imagery, supportive listening

Older School-age Child or Adolescent
Explaining the reason for the tingling and that it will go away, use of guided imagery, familiar music on tape or radio, asking what the child does when anxious or "scared," and talking about coping strategies

Care in the Community. Teach parents to keep aspirin and other salicylate products out of reach of children, preferably in a locked medicine box. Instruct parents to keep syrup of ipecac in their homes and how to use it. Provide stickers with the number of the Poison Control Center.

Metabolic Acidosis

Metabolic acidosis is a condition in which there is an excess of any acid other than carbonic acid. For this reason, it is sometimes called noncarbonic acid excess.

Clinical Manifestations

Laboratory values show decreased blood pH and decreased HCO_3 and Pco_2. An attempt at respiratory compensation causes one of the most important signs of metabolic acidosis, increased rate and depth of respirations (hyperventilation) or *Kussmaul respirations.* Severe acidosis can cause decreased peripheral vascular resistance and resultant cardiac arrhythmias, hypotension, pulmonary edema, and tissue hypoxia.[19] Confusion or drowsiness may result, as well as headache or abdominal pain.

Etiology and Pathophysiology

Metabolic acidosis is caused by an imbalance in production and excretion of acid or by excess loss of bicarbonate (Table 8–23). Excess accumulation occurs by one of two mechanisms. First, a child can eat or drink acids or substances that are converted to acid in the body. Examples include aspirin, boric acid, and antifreeze. Second, cells can make abnormally high amounts of acid that cannot be excreted. This is the case in ketoacidosis of untreated diabetes mellitus or the starvation that can occur in anorexia or bulimia. A disorder of excretion occurs in conditions such as oliguric renal failure (Fig. 8–22).

Bicarbonate can be lost from the body through the urine or through excessive loss of intestinal fluid. Diarrhea, fistulas, and ileal drainage are all possible sources. Carbonic anhydrase inhibitors can cause loss of excess bicarbonate in the urine.[17]

When the pH of the blood decreases below normal, the chemoreceptors in the brain and arteries are stimulated and respiratory compensation begins.

<table>
<tr><td>8-23</td><td>Causes of Metabolic Acidosis</td></tr>
</table>

Gain of Metabolic Acid
Ingestion of acids (eg, aspirin)
Ingestion of acid precursors (eg, antifreeze)
Oliguria (eg, renal failure)
Distal renal tubular acidosis
Hyperalimentation
Diabetic ketoacidosis
Starvation ketoacidosis
Some inborn errors of metabolism (eg, maple syrup urine disease)
Tissue hypoxia (lactic acidosis)

Loss of Bicarbonate
Diarrhea
Intestinal or pancreatic fistula
Proximal renal tubular acidosis

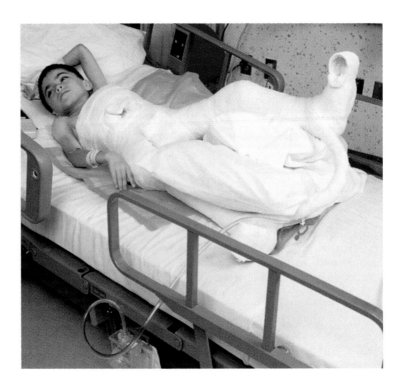

FIGURE 8–22. With any postoperative or immobilized child, it is important to monitor urine output to detect oliguria. If the kidneys do not produce very much urine, the metabolic acids accumulate in the body and cause metabolic acidosis. Inadequate fluid intake in the postoperative or immobilized child can lead to oliguria and, potentially, metabolic acidosis.

The child's rate and depth of breathing increase and carbonic acid is removed from the body. The blood pH shifts to a more normal range even though the cause is not corrected. The underlying condition and the degree of compensation will alter the clinical laboratory values observed (Table 8–24).

Medical Management

Treatment of metabolic acidosis depends on identification and treatment of the underlying cause. In severe metabolic acidosis, intravenous sodium bicarbonate may be used to increase the pH and to prevent cardiac arrhythmias. This treatment is difficult to manage, because renal excretion can cause excess retention of bicarbonate; therefore, intravenous sodium bicarbonate is used only in severe situations, such as prolonged cardiac arrest.[20]

Nursing Assessment

Assess the rate and depth of respirations. Evaluate the child's level of consciousness frequently. Be alert for signs or complaints of headache and abdominal pain. Serial arterial blood gas measurements will usually be obtained to evaluate changes in status.

8-24	Laboratory Values in Uncompensated and Compensated Metabolic Acidosis		
	HCO_3^-	pH	PCO_2
Uncompensated	Decreased	Decreased	Normal
Partially compensated	Decreased	Decreased but moving toward normal	Decreasing
Fully compensated	Decreased	Normal	Decreased

Nursing Diagnosis

Several nursing diagnoses can apply to the child with metabolic acidosis, including:

- Risk for Injury related to confusion/drowsiness or decreased responsiveness
- Risk for Decreased Cardiac Output related to cardiac arrhythmias
- Altered Tissue Perfusion: Cerebral related to tissue hypoxia
- Ineffective Breathing Pattern related to compensatory mechanisms
- Knowledge Deficit related to effective control of ketone production in diabetes mellitus

Nursing Management

Ensure safety, taking into account the child's level of consciousness and alertness. Turn the child and change his or her position to prevent pressure on the skin. Limit the child's activities to decrease cardiac workload.

Position the child to facilitate chest expansion. Provide oral care during rapid respirations since the mouth may become dry.

Monitor intravenous solutions and laboratory values indicating acid–base balance. Report changes promptly.

Once the child is stabilized, provide teaching to compensate for knowledge deficits. Teach parents of young children to keep medications and acids locked up and out of reach to prevent poisoning (Fig. 8–23). This includes medicines with aspirin as well as substances commonly kept in the garage for car maintenance. Teach about home management of diabetes and about early identification and treatment to avoid diabetic ketoacidosis.

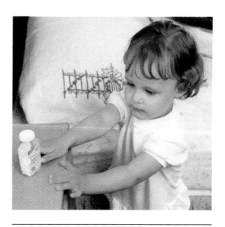

FIGURE 8–23. The parents of this child need teaching by a nurse! Teaching parents to use safety latches on cabinets to keep aspirin away from small children can help prevent metabolic acidosis.

Metabolic Alkalosis

Metabolic alkalosis occurs when there are too few metabolic acids. It is sometimes called noncarbonic acid deficit.

Blood pH, bicarbonate, and P_{CO_2} are usually elevated in metabolic alkalosis (Table 8–25). Hypokalemia often occurs simultaneously (refer to p. 313 to review signs of hypokalemia). Respiratory rate and depth usually decrease. Increased neuromuscular irritability, cramping, paresthesia, tetany, seizures, and excitation can occur. Finally, this state can progress to weakness, confusion, lethargy, and coma.

A gain in bicarbonate or a loss of metabolic acid can cause metabolic alkalosis (see Table 8–26). Bicarbonate is gained through excessive intake of bicarbonate antacids or baking soda or through metabolism of bicarbonate

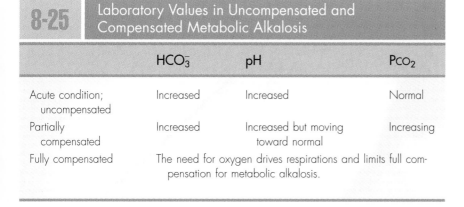

8-25	Laboratory Values in Uncompensated and Compensated Metabolic Alkalosis		
	HCO₃⁻	pH	P$_{CO_2}$
Acute condition; uncompensated	Increased	Increased	Normal
Partially compensated	Increased	Increased but moving toward normal	Increasing
Fully compensated	The need for oxygen drives respirations and limits full compensation for metabolic alkalosis.		

8-26 Causes of Metabolic Alkalosis

Gain of Bicarbonate
Ingestion of baking soda
Ingestion of large quantities of bicarbonate antacids
Exchange transfusion or massive transfusion (citrate is metabolized to bicarbonate)
Increased renal absorption of bicarbonate

Loss of Metabolic Acid
Prolonged vomiting (eg, pyloric stenosis)
Nasogastric suction
Cystic fibrosis
Hypokalemia
Diuretic therapy
Hyperaldosteronism
Adrenogenital syndrome
Cushing's syndrome

precursors such as the citrate contained in blood transfusions. Increased renal absorption of bicarbonate can occur in profound hypokalemia, primary hyperaldosteronism, or extreme deficit in extracellular fluid volume. Acid can be lost through severe vomiting, such as that seen in infants with pyloric stenosis and in continued removal of gastric contents through suction.

When the chemoreceptors in the brain and arteries detect the rising pH of metabolic alkalosis and respirations decrease, carbonic acid is retained in the body. This carbonic acid can neutralize the bicarbonate and return pH toward normal.

Medical management is directed at treating the underlying cause of the condition. Increasing the extracellular fluid volume with intravenous normal saline is used to facilitate renal excretion of bicarbonate.

Nursing Management

Assess the child's level of consciousness frequently. Alertness may decrease after an initial period of excitement, so regular assessments are needed. Monitor neuromuscular irritability. Observe for nausea and vomiting. Assess the rate and depth of respirations carefully. Obtain serial arterial blood gas measurements as ordered.

Facilitate ease of respirations. Ensure safety by keeping bed rails elevated and by turning the child frequently. Position the child on the side to avoid aspiration of vomitus.

If antacids were the cause of the alkalosis, teach the child and parents about correct use of these medications.

Mixed Acid–Base Imbalances

It is possible for two acid–base imbalances to occur at the same time. For example, a child with cystic fibrosis can develop respiratory acidosis from lung problems and concurrent metabolic alkalosis from vomiting during an illness. Treatment with diuretics may cause concurrent metabolic alkalosis resulting from extracellular volume depletion and hypokalemia in a child with congestive heart failure and chronic respiratory acidosis. In these cases, all of the underlying causes must be identified and treated. Care of children with mixed acid–base imbalances is often complicated, requiring hospitalization and careful management. Upon discharge, the nurse can teach parents about signs of imbalance that need to be reported and treated in order to prevent further complications.

REFERENCES

1. Trachtman, H. (1995). Sodium and water homeostasis. *Pediatric Clinics of North America, 42*(6), 1343–1364.

2. Davenport, M. (1996). Pediatric fluid balance. *Care of the Chronically Ill Child, 12*(1), 26–28, 30–31.

3. Seaman, S.L. (1995). Renal physiology part II: Fluid and electrolyte regulation. *Neonatal Network, 14*(5), 5–11.

4. Dabbagh, S., Ellis, D., & Gruskin, A.B. (1996). In E.K. Motoyama & P.J. Davis (Eds.), *Smith's anesthesia for infants and children* (6th ed., pp. 105–137). St. Louis: Mosby–Year Book.

5. UNICEF. (1990). *State of the world's children*. Oxford, England: University Press for UNICEF.

6. Gavin, N., Merrick, N., & Davidson, B. (1996). Efficacy of glucose-based oral rehydration therapy. *Pediatrics, 98*(1), 45–51.

7. Avery, E.A., & Snyder, J.D. (1990). Oral rehydration for acute diarrhea: The underused simple solution. *New England Journal of Medicine, 323*, 891–894.

8. Rice, K.H. (1994). Oral rehydration therapy: A simple, effective solution. *Journal of Pediatric Nursing, 9*(6), 349–356.

9. Duggan, C. (1992). The management of acute diarrhea in children: Oral rehydration, maintenance, and nutritional therapy. *Morbidity and Mortality Weekly Reports, 41*(RR-16), 1–20.

10. Travis, L.B. (1997). Disorders of water, electrolyte, and acid–base physiology. In A.M. Rudolph, J.I.E. Hoffman, & C.D. Rudolph (Eds.), *Rudolph's pediatrics* (20th ed., pp. 1319–1331). Stamford, CT: Appleton & Lange.

11. Farrar, H.C., Chande, V.T., Fitzpatrick, D.F., & Shema, S.J. (1995). Hyponatremia as the cause of seizures in infants: A retrospective analysis of incidence, severity, and clinical predictors. *Annals of Emergency Medicine, 26*(1), 42–48.

12. White, V.M. (1997). Hyperkalemia. *American Journal of Nursing, 97*(6), 35.

13. Nativ, A., Agostini, R., Drinkwater, B., & Yeager, K.K. (1994). The female athlete triad: The interrelatedness of disordered eating, amenorrhea, and osteoporosis. *Clinics in Sports Medicine, 13*(2), 405–418.

14. Sommerauer, J., Gayle, C., Jenner, M., & Stiller, C. (1988). Intensive care course following liver transplantation in children. *Journal of Pediatric Surgery, 23*, 705–708.

15. Johnson, M.D. (1994). Disordered eating in active and athletic women. *Clinics in Sports Medicine, 13*(2), 355–369.

16. Snow-Harter, C.M. (1994). Bone health and prevention of osteoporosis in active and athletic women. *Clinics in Sports Medicine, 13*(2), 389–404.

17. Halperin, M.L., & Goldstein, M.B. (1994). *Fluid, electrolyte, and acid–base physiology* (2nd ed., pp. 69–144). Philadelphia: Saunders.

18. Hanna, J.D., Scheinman, J.I., & Chan, J.C.M. (1995). The kidney in acid–base balance. *Pediatric Clinics of North America, 42*(6), 1365–1396.

19. Adelman, R.D., & Solhung, M.J. (1996). Pathophysiology of body fluids and fluid therapy. In R.E. Behrman, R.M. Kliegman, & A.M. Arvin (Eds.), *Nelson textbook of pediatrics* (15th ed., pp. 185–214). Philadelphia: Saunders.

20. Lustig, J.V. (1997). Fluid and electrolyte therapy. In W.W. Hay, J.R. Groothuis, A.R. Hayward, & M.J. Levin (Eds.), *Current pediatric diagnosis and treatment* (13th ed., pp. 1106–1115). Stamford, CT: Appleton & Lange.

ADDITIONAL RESOURCES

American Academy of Pediatrics, Provisional Committee on Quality Improvement, Subcommittee on Acute Gastroenteritis. (1996). Practice parameter: The management of acute gastroenteritis in young children. *Pediatrics, 97*(3), 424–431.

Bindler, R., & Howry, L. (1997). *Pediatric drugs and nursing implications* (2nd ed.). Stamford, CT: Appleton & Lange.

Corbett, J.V. (1996). *Laboratory tests and diagnostic procedures* (4th ed.). Stamford, CT: Appleton & Lange.

Cullen, L. (1992). Interventions related to fluid and electrolyte balance. *Nursing Clinics of North America, 27*(2), 569–597.

Gaylord, M.S., Lorch, S., Lorch, V., & Wright, P. (1995). The novel use of sterile water gastric drips for management of fluid and electrolyte abnormalities in extremely low birth weight infants. *Neonatal Intensive Care, 8*(3), 44–48, 64.

Goldberg, G., & Greene, C. (1992). Update on inborn errors of metabolism: Primary lactic acidemia. *Journal of Pediatric Health Care, 6*, 176–181.

Maguire, D., & Doyle, P. (1994). Sodium balance in very-low-birth-weight infants. *Critical Care Nurse, 14*(5), 61–66.

Merenstein, G.B., Kaplan, D.W., & Rosenberg, A.A. (1997). *Handbook of pediatrics* (18th ed.). Stamford, CT: Appleton & Lange.

O'Donnell, D., & Lathrop, J. (1989). *Pediatric fluids and electrolytes: A self-study text.* Milwaukee: Maxishare.

Poulson, N. (1995). Fluid and electrolyte management of the very-low-birth-weight infant. *Journal of Perinatal and Neonatal Nursing, 8*(4), 59–70.

Reid, S.R., & Bonadio, W.A. (1996). Outpatient rapid intravenous rehydration to correct dehydration and resolve vomiting in children with acute gastroenteritis. *Annals of Emergency Medicine, 28*(3), 318–323.

Weizman, Z., Houri, S., & Gradus, D. (1992). Type of acidosis and clinical outcome in infantile gastroenteritis. *Journal of Pediatric Gastroenterology and Nutrition, 14*, 187–191.

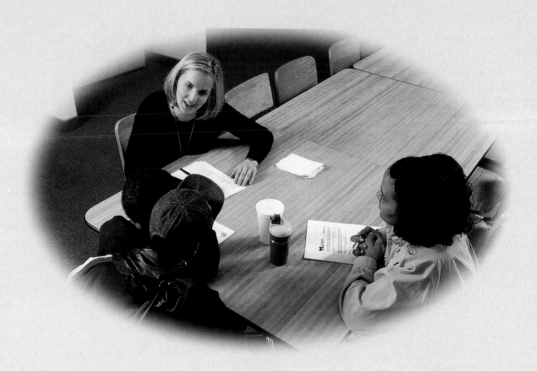

Raymond, a 2-year-old child, has had recurrent infections since he was born. In the last 3 months he has had bronchitis twice, otitis media three times, and several colds. Raymond has had a slight fever, vomiting, and diarrhea for several days. His mother brings him to a walk-in clinic to find out what is wrong.

Blood tests are performed to assess Raymond's immune function. On the basis of a thorough evaluation of Raymond's clinical symptoms and the results of the laboratory tests, he is diagnosed with acquired immunodeficiency syndrome (AIDS). Raymond is admitted to a special unit of the hospital for children with AIDS where special precautions are taken to prevent infection. Like many of the other children, Raymond is often irritable and difficult to console. Because he vomits frequently, the nurses pay particular attention to Raymond's nutritional problems, giving him frequent small feedings.

Raymond is diagnosed as having failure to thrive, a common sequela of AIDS. Broad-spectrum antibiotics are given, and he is assessed frequently for the development of new infections. A multidisciplinary team, including nurses, physicians, nutritionists, and social services professionals, are involved in planning Raymond's care.

ALTERATIONS IN IMMUNE FUNCTION 9

"Raymond's family is learning to deal with the reality of AIDS. All of us on the team are trying to give them the support they need now and to prepare them for the future."

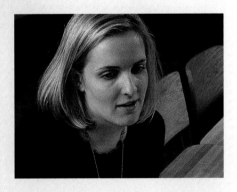

TERMINOLOGY

- **allergen** An antigen capable of inducing hypersensitivity.
- **antibody** A protein capable of reacting to a specific antigen.
- **antigen** A foreign substance that triggers an immune system response.
- **graft-versus-host disease** A series of immunologic responses mounted by the host of a transplanted organ with the purpose of destroying the transplant cells.
- **hypersensitivity response** An overreaction of the immune system, responsible for allergic reactions.
- **immunodeficiency** A state of the immune system in which it cannot cope effectively with foreign antigens.

- **immunoglobulin** A protein that functions as an antibody. Immunoglobulins are responsible for humoral immunity.
- **opportunistic infection** An infection that is often caused by normally nonpathogenic organisms in persons who lack normal immunity.
- **primary immune response** The process in which B lymphocytes produce antibodies specific to a particular antigen on first exposure.

What are the signs and symptoms of immunologic disorders in children? Many times they are nonspecific. Raymond's admitting signs and symptoms, described in the opening scenario, are characteristic of several different immunodeficiency disorders. The immune system is one of the few body systems that regulates, either directly or indirectly, all other body functions. Thus, a problem with the immune system can have multisystem consequences and may be life threatening. Allergic reactions to food or frequent episodes of otitis media may indicate a disorder of immune function. Congenital abnormalities sometimes signal a defect in cellular immunity. In this chapter, we will examine some of the more common disorders of immune function and discuss nursing care of children who have these diseases and their families.

▶ ANATOMY AND PHYSIOLOGY OF PEDIATRIC DIFFERENCES

The function of the immune system is to recognize any foreign substances within the body—in simple terms, to distinguish "nonself" from "self"—and to eliminate those foreign substances as efficiently as possible. Whenever the body recognizes the presence of a substance that it cannot identify as part of itself, the body protects itself through the immune response. Normally, the immune system responds to an invasion of foreign substances, or **antigens,** in numerous ways. It produces **antibodies,** or proteins that work against antigens. There are many types of antibodies, which are described later in this section. The immune system also produces other types of cells, such as T lymphocytes and natural killer (NK) cells.

Immunity is either natural or acquired. Natural immune defenses are those an infant is born with, such as intact skin, body pH, natural antibodies from the mother, and inflammatory and phagocytic properties. Acquired immunity is composed of humoral (antibody-mediated) and cell-mediated immunity and is not fully developed until a child is about 6 years of age.

Humoral immunity is responsible for destroying bacterial antigens. B lymphocytes, produced in the bone marrow, develop into plasma cells that produce antibodies. Antibodies are a type of protein called **immunoglobulins.** There are five types of immunoglobulins: IgM, IgG, IgA, IgD, and IgE (Table 9–1). IgM, IgG, and IgA act to control a number of body infections, whereas IgE is useful in combating parasitic infections and is part of the allergic response. The role of IgD is not known.

Antibodies are found in serum, body fluids, and certain tissues. When a child is first exposed to an antigen, the B lymphocyte system begins to

9-1	Classes of Immunoglobulins
IgM	Present in intravascular spaces
IgG	Present in all body fluids
IgA	Present in secretions of gastrointestinal, respiratory, and genitourinary tracts
IgD	Presence and function not yet described
IgE	Present in internal and external body fluids

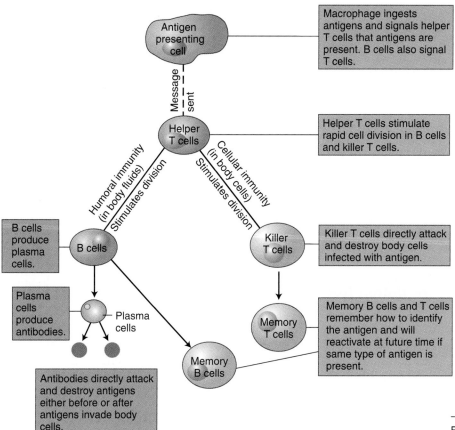

FIGURE 9-1. Primary immune response.

produce antibodies that react specifically to that antigen (Fig. 9–1). It takes approximately 3 days for this process, known as **primary immune response,** to occur. Subsequent encounters with the antigen trigger memory cells, resulting in an immune response within 24 hours.

Infants and children have differing amounts of some immunoglobulins. IgG is the only immunoglobulin that crosses the placenta; as a result, a newborn's levels are similar to those of his or her mother. This maternal IgG disappears by 6–8 months of age. The infant's IgG then increases gradually until mature levels are reached at 7–8 years. IgM levels are low at birth, rise markedly at 1 week of age, and continue to increase until adult levels are reached at about 1 year. IgA and IgE are not present at birth. Manufacture of these immunoglobulins begins by 2 weeks of age; however, normal values are not achieved until 6–7 years. It is thus easy to see why children under 6 years of age become ill so often—they do not have a full complement of immunoglobulins.

In contrast, *cell-mediated immunity* achieves full function early in life. T lymphocytes, produced in the thymus, provide cellular immunity and protect against most viruses, fungi, slowly developing bacterial infections such as tuberculosis, and tumors. In addition, they control the timing of the response in delayed hypersensitivity reactions, such as the purified protein derivative (PPD) test, and they are responsible for the rejection of foreign grafts, such as transplants. For this reason, the blood infused into newborns is generally irradiated to prevent **graft-versus-host disease** (a series of immunologic reactions in response to transplanted cells) from transfused lymphocytes.[1] Specialized types of T lymphocytes include killer T cells, suppressor T cells, and helper T cells. Suppressor T cells inhibit B lymphocytes from differentiating into plasma cells. Helper T cells aid this process.

Natural killer (NK) cells (also known as non-B/non-T lymphocytes) originate in the bone marrow and thymus and migrate to the blood and spleen. They play a role in control of viral infection, tumors, and autoimmune disease. Newborns have somewhat lower numbers of NK cells than older children and adults, decreasing their ability to respond to certain antigens.

Complement is a component of blood serum consisting of 11 protein compounds. It is an inactive enzyme that activates in response to antigen–antibody functions, resulting in a generalized inflammatory reaction that kills foreign cells. It also plays a role in causing some autoimmune diseases. The levels of some of the complement proteins is lower in newborns than in older children and adults, thus delaying and hampering response to certain infections.

► IMMUNODEFICIENCY DISORDERS

Immunodeficiency, a state of decreased responsiveness of the immune system, can occur to varying degrees in response to any number of events. Children with congenital immunodeficiency, or primary immune deficiency, are born with a failure of humoral antibody formation (B-cell disorder), a deficient cellular immune system (T-cell disorder), or a combination of both defects. In congenital disorders, the immune deficiency is not caused by another condition. However, immunodeficiency may also be acquired, as in human immunodeficiency virus (HIV) infection.

B-CELL AND T-CELL DISORDERS

In B-cell disorders, immunoglobulins may be present in inadequate numbers or nearly absent. X-linked hypogammaglobulinemia, selective IgA deficiency, and common variable immunodeficiency are examples of such disorders. Because newborns are protected from infection by maternal antibodies in the first months after birth, symptoms of B-cell disorders usually become apparent after 3 months of age. Infants with these disorders have frequent recurrent bacterial infections and failure to thrive. With treatment, consisting of intravenous immunoglobulins and antibiotics, most children survive into adulthood. Prognosis depends on the degree of antibody deficiency.

T-cell disorders are characterized by inadequate numbers of T lymphocytes or absence of T-cell functions. Isolated T-cell disorders are rare and may be associated with congenital abnormalities (as in DiGeorge syndrome) or of unknown cause. DiGeorge syndrome has only recently been recognized as a genetic disease, with most cases demonstrating characteristic chromosomal deletions. The syndrome is characterized by the absence of parathyroid or thymus glands, cardiac and ear defects, tetany 48 hours after birth, and viral and fungal infections in the neonatal period (Fig. 9–2). Children with the disorder are treated with antibiotics, oral calcium, thymus transplantation, and HLA-identical bone marrow transplantation. Without thymus transplantation, few children survive beyond 5 years. X-linked immunodeficiency with hyper-IgM is a T-cell disorder that affects mainly males and causes decreased T-cell function, variable abnormal levels of immunoglobulins, and high titers of some antibodies.

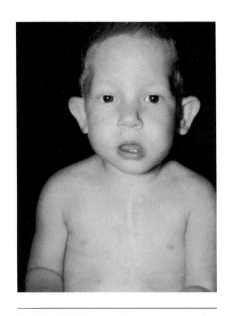

FIGURE 9–2. This infant has characteristic features of DiGeorge syndrome. Note the low-set and malformed ears.
From Stites, D.P., & Terr, A.I. (1997). Basic & clinical immunology (7th ed., p. 346). Stamford, CT: Appleton & Lange.

9-2 Selected Congenital Immunodeficiency Disorders

Disorders	Laboratory Findings
B cell	
X-linked hypogammaglobulinemia	Reduced IgA, IgM, IgE, IgG (<100 mg/dL), absence of B cells in peripheral blood, normal T cells
Selective IgA deficiency	IgA < 10 mg/dL
Common variable immunodeficiency	IgA, IgM reduced; IgG < 250 mg/dL
T cell	
DiGeorge syndrome	Lymphopenia; absent T-cell functions, decreased T cells, normal B cells
X-linked immunodeficiency with hyper-IgG	Reduced IgG, IgA; normal or elevated IgM; mutations in T-cell surface proteins
Combined	
Severe combined immunodeficiency syndrome (SCID)	Complete absence of both T- and B-cell immunity
Wiskott–Aldrich syndrome	Thrombocytopenia, normal IgG, decreased IgM, increased IgA, increased IgE; inability to respond to polysaccharide antigens

Refer to Table 9–2, which compares laboratory values for selected congenital immunodeficiency disorders.

SEVERE COMBINED IMMUNODEFICIENCY DISEASE

Severe combined immunodeficiency disease (SCID) is a congenital condition characterized by absence of both humoral and cellular immunity. SCID occurs in X-linked recessive, autosomal recessive, and sporadic forms. Without appropriate treatment, children born with SCID usually die within the first 2 years of life.

Clinical Manifestations

Symptoms in a child born with SCID develop early in life. The neonate often demonstrates a susceptibility to infection by 3 months of age. The disorder is characterized by chronic infection, failure to completely recover from infection, frequent reinfection, and infection with viruses such as cytomegalovirus and the bacterium *Pneumocystis carinii*. Often the first infection seen is a resistant oral candidiasis. Children are also highly susceptible to sepsis and pneumonia. Failure to thrive is a consequence of persistent illness.

Some infants experience graft-versus-host disease as a result of placental transfer of maternal T lymphocytes. If the child receives foreign tissue, for example, in a blood transfusion, signs such as skin rash, fever, hepatosplenomegaly, and diarrhea may occur.

Etiology and Pathophysiology

The exact cause of SCID is unknown. Defective stem cells, thymus dysfunction, and enzymatic disorder have been proposed as possible etiologies.

9-3   Cells Evaluated in Laboratory Studies for Immune Conditions

Test and Type of Cell Evaluated	Action	Implication of Increased or Decreased Levels
White blood cell (WBC) count		
Neutrophil	Phagocytic cell that defends against bacteria	Increased in bacterial infection, inflammatory processes, and some malignancies
Eosinophil	Associated with antigen–antibody reaction	Increased in allergic reaction; decreased in children receiving corticosteroids
Lymphocytes (T, B, non-B/non-T [NK])	Major components of immune system	Increased in many infections; decreased in children with immune deficiency
Immunoglobulins		
(IgM, IgG, IgA, IgD, IgE)	Many roles in a number of immunologic reactions	Increased in presence of infection or allergic response; decreased in children with immune deficiency

Diagnostic Tests and Medical Management

A marked reduction in lymphocyte counts is indicative of SCID. B and T lymphocytes are generally few in number or absent from the peripheral blood and lymphoid tissues. In some cases, the B-lymphocyte count may be elevated, although these cells do not function. NK cells are few in number. Immunoglobulin levels are significantly reduced. Refer to Table 9–2 for laboratory findings in SCID. Diagnosis is usually made only after extensive laboratory testing. In addition to a complete blood count, erythrocyte sedimentation rate, and B and T-cell lymphocyte counts, other studies including IgA, IgG, and IgM antibody titers to immunizations received and neutrophil count may be performed (see Table 9–3).

The goal of medical management is to restore immune function. Thymic hormones have been given to some children with limited success. Intravenous immune globulin (IVIG) may be administered. Bone marrow transplantation offers hope for children with SCID (see Chap.13). However, the donor must be a histocompatible donor, such as a sibling. T-cell function is corrected with the marrow transplantation, and new cells appear 3–4 months after infusion of the donor marrow.

Prognosis is poor without aggressive therapy. Some children have survived 10 years after a successful bone marrow transplant.[2]

Nursing Assessment

Obtain a thorough history of infections, including age of onset, type of causal organism, frequency, and severity. Take a family history, and find out if the child has had any unusual reactions to vaccines, medications, or foods. Measure the child's height and weight accurately to identify failure to thrive. Look for any evidence of infections involving the skin, subcutaneous tissues, respiratory system, and mucous membranes. Palpate the abdomen for hepatomegaly and the lymph nodes for lymphadenopathy.

Assess family support systems and coping mechanisms.

Nursing Diagnosis

The primary nursing diagnosis for a child with SCID is Risk for Infection related to immunodeficiency. Other nursing diagnoses may include:

- Risk for Altered Nutrition: Less Than Body Requirements related to chronic diarrhea and infections
- Risk for Impaired Skin Integrity related to chronic infections
- Risk for Caregiver Role Strain related to a child with a chronic, life-threatening disease
- Risk for Altered Growth and Development related to restricted activities and chronic illness

Nursing Management

Nursing care of the immunodeficient child focuses on preventing infection. However, even with the use of environmental controls, such as keeping children inside bubbles to maintain a sterile environment, these children are prone to **opportunistic infections** (infections caused by normally nonpathogenic organisms in persons who lack normal immunity).

Prevent Systemic Infection

Frequent and thorough handwashing is important. Standard precautions are always used, with transmission-based precautions when needed. Use sterile aseptic technique when caring for all sites where needles, catheters, central lines, endotracheal tubes, pressure-monitoring lines, and peripheral intravenous lines enter the child's body. Food and other items entering the hospital room may need special treatment. The child should be placed in a private room, and contact with infectious individuals should be minimized.

Promote Skin Integrity

The skin is the only intact defense that many immunodeficient children have. Provide good skin care, and observe all possible pressure areas closely for signs of breakdown or infection. Turn the child frequently. Encourage range of motion exercises. Avoid any skin trauma.

Manage Medication Therapy

Many of the medications used long term in the treatment of children with SCID have numerous side effects. Monitor closely for side effects of antibiotics, such as overgrowth of resistant organisms (eg, thrush infections in the mouth, *Clostridium difficile* infections of the gastrointestinal tract) and administer IVIG safely (see Table 9–4).

Provide Emotional Support and Referral to Appropriate Support Groups and Services

SCID is a life-threatening and devastating disease. Even with aggressive therapy, the prognosis is poor. Evaluate the family's knowledge about the disease. The parents may be experiencing guilt because of the genetic nature of the disease and the difficulties of treatment. Listen closely to their concerns and encourage them to discuss their fears. Refer them to an appropriate support group or counselor if needed. Genetic counseling should be encouraged if the parents plan to have more children.

The family of a child who undergoes bone marrow transplantation requires additional support and referrals. The transplantation procedure involves surgery for both the ill child and the donor, often another child in the family. (Refer to the discussion in Chapter 13.) After the infusion of the donor marrow, the ill child will be hospitalized for several months until T-lymphocyte levels are sufficient to provide resistance to infection. During this period, parents may need to rely on social services to help manage the

9-4	Nursing Considerations in the Administration of Intravenous Immune Globulin (IVIG)

Used in treatment of
- Immunodeficiency disease, such as severe combined immunodeficiency and acquired immunodeficiency syndrome (AIDS)
- Antibody deficiency associated with other conditions such as malignancy
- Kawasaki disease

Administration
- IVIG must be administered as stated in the package insert.
- Use separate tubing and do not mix with other medications.
- Start infusion slowly and increase to recommended rate after 30 minutes if no reaction occurs (see below).
- Monitor for hypersensitivity reaction (fever, increased pulse or respiration, decreased blood pressure, chest pain, shaking, chills).
- Schedule immunizations 14 days before or 3 months after IVIG infusion, since immune response will be altered.

Possible adverse reactions[3]
- Headache
- Fever
- Nausea, vomiting
- Arthralgia
- Anaphylaxis

Special Types available
- RespiGam (helpful in respiratory syncytial virus)
- CytoGam (enriched with antibodies to cytomegalovirus)

family situation, particularly if the child is hospitalized at a medical center far from the family's home. Assess the family's situation and make appropriate referrals to social service and to support groups. Introduce parents to other families undergoing bone marrow transplantation.

WISKOTT–ALDRICH SYNDROME

A combined congenital immunodeficiency syndrome, Wiskott–Aldrich syndrome is an X-linked disorder characterized by thrombocytopenia, eczema, hemorrhagic tendencies, and recurrent infections. Thrombocytopenia with bleeding tendencies appears during the neonatal period. Eczema appears by 1 year of age. Infections involve the middle ear and often lead to chronic otitis media. Children are particularly susceptible to infections from herpesviruses and lymphoreticular malignancies, especially of the lymphatic system.

The diagnosis is made in the early neonatal period on the basis of the thrombocytopenia (refer to Table 9–2). How and when Wiskott–Aldrich syndrome manifests itself varies, with some children maintaining normal lymphocyte levels for years. Treatment is symptomatic and includes antibiotic prophylaxis together with platelet infusions and intravenous immunoglobulin therapy. Without bone marrow transplantation, most children die within the first 5 years of life. Survival beyond adolescence is unusual. Infection, bleeding, or malignancy may be the cause of death.[4]

Nursing Management

Nursing care is similar to that for the child with SCID. Refer the parents for genetic counseling to help them understand the transmission of the disease and the probability of having another child with the same disorder. Arrange for psychologic support for those parents who may be overwhelmed with guilt from learning that the illness is inherited.

Help the parents and family cope with the knowledge that the child has a chronic and potentially fatal illness. Referral to family counseling may be appropriate.

ACQUIRED IMMUNODEFICIENCY SYNDROME

Soon after acquired immunodeficiency syndrome (AIDS) was recognized in homosexual adults and intravenous drug abusers, cases of AIDS were seen in children. Increasing numbers of children infected with the human immunodeficiency virus (HIV) have been diagnosed, making HIV infection a leading cause of immune disease in infants and children and the leading cause of death in children 1–4 years of age.

Most cases of HIV in children—and virtually all new cases—are the result of perinatal transmission.[5] Each year in the United States, approximately 1500–1750 children become infected after being born to mothers infected with HIV. It is expected and hoped that the number will decrease with new therapies for treating infected women during pregnancy and labor/delivery and their infants after birth. Because of the high rate of transfer from mother to infant, HIV counseling and voluntary testing are encouraged for all pregnant women.[6]

The virus affects multiple systems and eventually destroys the child's immune system (Fig. 9–3). An understanding of the natural history of HIV disease is still evolving, and there are several important differences in the disease progression and clinical manifestations of pediatric and adult HIV infection.

Clinical Manifestations

The interval from HIV infection to the onset of overt AIDS is shorter in children than in adults, and shorter in children infected perinatally than in those infected through transfusion.[7] Most children with AIDS have nonspecific findings, including lymphadenopathy, hepatosplenomegaly, nephropathy, oral candidiasis, failure to thrive and weight loss, diarrhea, chronic eczema and dermatitis, and fever. Raymond, described at the beginning of this chapter, had several of these findings, as well as a history of recurrent, acute infections (bronchitis, otitis media, and colds).

Bacterial and opportunistic infections, such as *Streptococcus, Haemophilus influenzae, Salmonella,* and *Pneumocystis carinii* pneumonia (PCP), as well as

NURSING ALERT

Certain infections are common in HIV-infected children, even before diagnosis. They include chronic and bilateral otitis media, thrush (oral candidiasis), and *Pneumocystis carinii* (PCP) respiratory infection. Be alert for the possibility of HIV infection in infants with such infections, especially in infants known to be at risk.

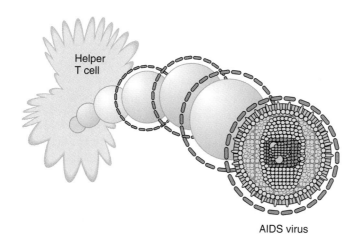

Helper T cell

AIDS virus

FIGURE 9–3. The AIDS virus selectively targets and destroys the body's T cells, eventually destroying the body's ability to combat infection.

malignancies such as lymphomas frequently occur as the disease progresses. Lymphocytic interstitial pneumonitis is a common manifestation of pediatric AIDS. Frequently children develop encephalopathy resulting in developmental delay or a deterioration of motor skills and intellectual functioning.

Etiology and Pathophysiology

Acquired immunodeficiency syndrome is caused by the human immunodeficiency virus (HIV-1). Children may acquire HIV infection from their mothers transplacentally or during delivery. Transmission can occur during birth from blood, amniotic fluid, and exposure to genital tract secretions, and after birth through breast milk from HIV-positive mothers. However, risk for perinatal transmission is significantly reduced if the infected mother receives zidovudine (ZDV) (formerly called azidothymidine [AZT]) during pregnancy.[8]

HIV has also been transmitted to children through transfusions of infected blood before mandatory screening of blood and blood products was instituted in 1985. Most of these children were infected during treatment of hemophilia. Although 30% of adolescents with AIDS also have hemophilia, with infected blood the expected etiology,[10] adolescents now most commonly acquire the virus through intravenous drug abuse or through unprotected sexual activities.

The HIV virus selectively targets and destroys T cells, thereby decreasing and eventually eliminating cellular immunity. Humoral immunity is also affected. Thus, the child is left unprotected against a myriad of bacterial, viral, fungal, and opportunistic infections, which are ultimately fatal. Every organ system can be affected.

Diagnostic Tests and Medical Management

Most children with AIDS are diagnosed early in life. Serologic tests for detection of the virus are monitored in infants born to HIV-positive mothers. These tests are performed at birth and repeated at 3 and 6 months. The preferred test is the polymerase chain reaction (PCR); other tests include p24 antigen, or HIV culture (which is not universally available). Any positive result is confirmed by retesting. When the infant has had two negative tests, testing with enzyme-linked immunosorbent assay (ELISA; HIV antibody) should be done at 12, 15, and 18 months. After two consecutive negative results with ELISA, the child is considered free of HIV. In addition, a complete blood count (CBC) and CD4+ T-cell subset is performed at 3–6 months.

The Centers for Disease Control and Prevention (CDC) considers children under 13 years of age to be infected if their symptoms meet the CDC criteria for AIDS, if they have HIV in the blood or tissues, or if they have antibodies to HIV. The CDC criteria address two issues: first, the diagnosis of HIV, and second, the clinical classification of children infected with HIV (Table 9–5).

Because of the rapidity of disease progression in perinatally transmitted HIV infection, early identification of infected infants is important to ensure the most effective treatment. HIV-infected mothers should be identified during pregnancy, and their infants should undergo periodic laboratory testing, as described above. Regardless of the results of these tests, all infants of infected mothers should start prophylaxis against PCP (a commonly serious or fatal outcome in infants) by the age of 4–6 weeks and continue to 12 months, or until two negative HIV tests have been documented (at 1 and 4 months of age). Drugs used for PCP prophylaxis in-

RESEARCH CONSIDERATIONS

An AIDS clinical trial that began in 1991 included administration of zidovudine to HIV-positive women during pregnancy, labor, and delivery, and to the infant orally after birth. The study was discontinued in 1994 when a significant drop in transmission of HIV to the baby was noted in those receiving the drug. Thus all the control group fetuses and infants born to HIV-positive mothers could be treated rather than recieve the placebo.[9]

9-5 Clinical Staging of Pediatric HIV Infection

Diagnosis of HIV infection in children
- HIV infected (two or more positive tests for HIV or demonstrates AIDS)
- Perinatally exposed (born to a mother known to be infected with HIV)
- Seroconverter (born to a mother known to be infected with HIV but has had two negative HIV tests)

When infected, the child with HIV is classified as
- Category N (not symptomatic)
- Category A (mildly symptomatic)
- Category B (moderately symptomatic)
- Category C (severely symptomatic)

clude trimethoprim-sulfamethoxazpole (Bactrim or Septra), dapsone, or aerosolized pentamidine.[11] In addition, all infected mothers should receive oral zidovudine (ZDV) after the first trimester of pregnancy and intravenous ZDV during labor and delivery; and the newborn should receive 6 weeks of oral ZDV after birth. A CBC with differential is performed at birth, 4–6 weeks, and 12 weeks to monitor for drug side effects.

Medical management is supportive, as there is no cure for AIDS. Intravenous immune globulin (IVIG; see Table 9–4) has been used to prevent bacterial infections in children under the age of 2 years. Treatment involves prompt therapy for bacterial and opportunistic infections. Children between 3 months and 12 years of age are given antiretroviral drugs, including nucleoside reverse transcriptase inhibitors such as zidovudine (ZDV), didanosine (DDI), zalcitabine (DDC), lamivudin (3TC), and stavudine (D4T). Also under investigation are protease inhibitors such as saquinivir, indinivir, ritonivir, and nelfinavir. The protease inhibitors appear to be most effective when used in combination with nucleoside reverse transcriptase inhibitors, which slow replication of the virus. Recent drug trials have demonstrated reduction of serum HIV load in infants who acquired the infection from their mothers and were treated with a combination of several antiviral drugs.[12]

The earlier the child develops AIDS, the poorer the prognosis. The average age for survival of a child after diagnosis of HIV infection is 8 years.[5]

RESEARCH CONSIDERATIONS

Researchers at the National Institutes of Health ended a study of AIDS therapy in children while it was in process because the results indicated that those children treated with combination antiviral drugs (zidovudine and either lamivudine or didanosine) had a better outcome than those treated with didanosine alone. The researchers recommend the combination drug therapy for children under 3 years of age who are HIV positive and have not received antiviral therapy.[13]

Nursing Assessment

For infants at risk of HIV infection, obtain the HIV test results of the mother if available. When these are positive, the infant will need to be screened numerous times during infancy for HIV infection, as described in the previous section. Facilitate the screening and explain the necessity to the family.

Physiologic Assessment

Assessment centers on observation and evaluation of potential sites of infection. Assess breath sounds, respiratory status, arterial blood gases, level of consciousness, and mental status. Any evidence of lymphocytic interstitial pneumonitis or neurologic abnormalities should be reported. Assess the child's height and weight frequently. Observe for signs of failure to thrive and assess for anemia. Look for *Candida* infections in the mouth and the diaper area. Note any developmental delays in motor skills or intellectual functioning, which could result from encephalopathy and poor nutrition.

Psychosocial Assessment

Assess family support systems and coping mechanisms, as the stressors of caring for a child with AIDS may overwhelm parents. Assess the family's ability to care for the child. If the mother is infected, inquire about the extended family's ability to provide daily care as well as emotional support. When assessing an adolescent with AIDS, evaluate the teen's understanding of how AIDS is transmitted and his or her response to the diagnosis.

Nursing Diagnosis

The accompanying Nursing Care Plan includes common nursing diagnoses that may apply to a child hospitalized with AIDS. Other nursing diagnoses may include:

- Diarrhea related to gastrointestinal infection, malignancy, or drug reactions
- Impaired Gas Exchange related to pulmonary disease
- Altered Growth and Development related to chronic infection and poor nutrition
- Risk for Ineffective Family Coping: Compromised related to life-threatening illness

Nursing Management

When the mother is known to be infected with HIV, ensure that the infant is followed closely through HIV testing, prophylaxis for HIV and PCP, and evaluation of general health and development.[8]

Nursing care of the child with AIDS is similar to that of a child with any serious chronic, life-threatening disease. It centers on preventing infection, managing pain, promoting respiratory and other organ function, promoting adequate nutritional intake, and providing emotional support to the parents and child, while promoting the child's development. The accompanying Nursing Care Plan summarizes nursing care for the child hospitalized with acquired immunodeficiency syndrome.

Prevent Infection

Immunosuppressed children become infected with bacteria as well as other organisms that are common in the environment. Frequent handwashing and limiting exposure of the child to individuals with upper respiratory or other infections are a few of the interventions used to protect the child with HIV from acquiring other infections.[14] A modified immunization schedule that avoids exposure to the live polio and varicella vaccines should be followed.[15] Perform annual tuberculosis (TB) testing for children infected with HIV. Teach sexually active adolescents the importance of practicing safe sex and the ramifications of high-risk sexual behaviors and intravenous drug abuse.

Promote Respiratory Function

Because many children with AIDS develop pneumonia, encourage the child to cough and deep breathe every 2–4 hours. Blowing cotton balls with a straw, blowing bubbles, or other games may engage the interest of a younger child. Reposition infants frequently so all areas of the lungs can

SAFETY PRECAUTIONS

Health care workers who come in contact with blood or other body fluids of children infected with HIV are at risk for exposure to the virus. Standard precautions should be used in caring for all children, as HIV status and presence of other infections may not be known. (Refer to the *Quick Reference to Pediatric Clinical Skills* accompanying this text.)

SAFETY PRECAUTIONS

Children with immune disorders, their siblings, or other household contacts should not be immunized with live oral polio virus or live varicella vaccine because of the risk of transmitting the virus to the immunodeficient child. Inactivated (injectable) polio vaccine can be used.

NURSING CARE PLAN
THE CHILD WITH ACQUIRED IMMUNODEFICIENCY SYNDROME

GOAL	INTERVENTION	RATIONALE	EXPECTED OUTCOME

1. Risk for Infection related to immunosuppression

The child will remain free of infection.	• Assess the child every 2–4 hours for fever; lesions in the mouth; redness, inflammation, soreness, and lesions on the skin or around intravenous lines.	• Fever is one of the few signs of infection in the immunosuppressed child who does not have a sufficient number of white blood cells.	The child has no fever and shows no other signs of infection.
	• Auscultate for changes in breath sounds every 2 hours. Perform pulmonary toilet (coughing, deep breathing, incentive spirometry) every 2–4 hours.	• Pneumonia is a likely infection in the child with AIDS.	
	• Enforce strict handwashing. Allow no fresh flowers, fruits, or vegetables in child's room. Screen visitors for colds or recent exposure to varicella. Use blood and body fluid precautions (refer to the *Quick Reference to Pediatric Clinical Skills* accompanying this text.) Practice strict asepsis for dressing changes and suctioning.	• Control of environmental factors helps prevent infection.	
	• Coordinate patient care assignments to avoid exposing the child to individuals with recent infections or immunizations.	• Planning minimizes chances for infection.	
	• Organize patient care activities to allow for adequate period of rest.	• Rest periods allow the child to regain energy.	
	• Follow recommendations of CDC and AAP for immunizing immunosuppressed children. Avoid live oral polio virus vaccine and live varcella vaccine. Perform annual TB testing.	• Special recommendations consider the child's decreased immune response and the danger of acquiring disease from certain live virus vaccines.	

Continued . . .

NURSING CARE PLAN
THE CHILD WITH ACQUIRED IMMUNODEFICIENCY SYNDROME— *Continued*

GOAL	INTERVENTION	RATIONALE	EXPECTED OUTCOME

2. Altered Nutrition: Less Than Body Requirements *related to decreased intake and absorption of nutrients*

GOAL	INTERVENTION	RATIONALE	EXPECTED OUTCOME
The child will have adequate nutritional intake to meet metabolic needs.	• Encourage frequent small meals to promote nutritional and fluid intake. • Maintain nasogastric tube feeding, if ordered. Hyperalimentation may be necessary to ensure adequate nutrition. • Eliminate unpleasant stimuli and odors from the environment during meals. • Monitor skin turgor every shift. • Involve a nutritionist in planning a diet for the child that includes favorite foods.	• Additional nutrition is required to rebuild the immune system. • Unpleasant stimuli decrease the desire for food. • Skin turgor reflects hydration status. • Including favorite foods encourages intake.	The child eats frequent meals of adequate nutritional content.

3. Risk for Impaired Skin Integrity *related to skin infection, immobility, or diarrhea*

GOAL	INTERVENTION	RATIONALE	EXPECTED OUTCOME
The child will have minimal or no skin breakdown.	• Observe all pressure areas closely for signs of infection or breakdown. • Keep skin clean and dry. Provide perineal care to minimize irritation from diarrhea.	• Skin care is important in the immunocompromised child. The skin may be the only intact defense the child has. • Prevents breaking or cracking of skin.	The child is free of preventable skin breakdown.

4. Risk for Altered Oral Mucous Membrane *related to infection*

GOAL	INTERVENTION	RATIONALE	EXPECTED OUTCOME
The child will have intact oral mucous membranes.	• Inspect mouth for sign of blistering or lesions. • Provide mouth care with normal saline solution or lemon–glycerine swabs every 2–4 hours.	• Candidal infection is frequently associated with immunodeficiency. • Provides comfort and promotes healing.	The child has intact oral mucous membranes.

NURSING CARE PLAN
THE CHILD WITH ACQUIRED IMMUNODEFICIENCY SYNDROME– *Continued*

GOAL	INTERVENTION	RATIONALE	EXPECTED OUTCOME

5. Pain related to infections

The child will be free of pain or experience only mild pain/discomfort.	• Observe for signs of pain and discomfort. • Medicate for pain as ordered and document results. • Implement general comfort measures (holding, rocking, etc).	• Pain relief adds to comfort of the child and family.	The child shows evidence of pain relief.

6. Knowledge Deficit (Parent) related to home care of child with AIDS

The parent(s) will verbalize knowledge about home care, measures to prevent infection, and signs and symptoms to report to health care providers.	• Explain the importance of optimizing the child's health status and reducing risk of complications through diet, rest, and meticulous personal hygiene. Be sure that parents and other family members understand how AIDS is spread and appropriate precautions. • Discuss with the parents and the child reasons for protective measures. • Inform the family about signs and symptoms of infection that should be reported promptly to the physician or nurse (fever, chills, cough, mild erythema).	• Knowledge about the disorder and preventive measures is necessary to provide safe and effective home care for the child. • Knowledge of rationale increases compliance. • Prompt treatment improves outcome.	The parent describes appropriate home care and preventive measures for a child with AIDS.

7. Caregiver Role Strain related to anxiety about child's condition and demands of providing care

The parent(s) will report decreased anxiety related to the child's condition and care.	• Encourage family members to express fears and concerns regarding the child's prognosis. • Advise family about support services or other resources available in the community.	• Expression of fears helps to decrease anxiety. • Provides additional support to help family cope with the child's illness and the dying process, when needed.	The parent states decreased anxiety.

aerate. Rest periods to conserve energy and lower the body's demand for oxygen are important.

Promote Adequate Nutritional Intake

Because many children with AIDS have failure to thrive, nutrition is an important part of their care. A nutritionist should be involved in planning an appropriate diet for the child that provides necessary calories, protein, and other nutrients. Vitamins may be especially lacking in the diets of infected children. Antioxidants (vitamin A, vitamin E, zinc, and selenium) are known to enhance general immune system function and should be at recommended levels. Periodic dietary analysis and teaching are needed. Adequate nutrition is sometimes provided by hyperalimentation.

Diarrhea resulting from gastrointestinal infection and lactose intolerance is a common finding in these children and complicates other nutritional disturbances. Antidiarrheal medications may be prescribed, or alternative formulas tried. Keep the child's lips and mouth moist and pay close attention to hydration status. Monitor the skin turgor and urine output, and provide careful perineal skin care to prevent infection.

The frequency of *Candida* infections leads to blisters, cracking, and discharge involving the oral mucous membranes. Mouth care with a non-alcohol-based solution such as normal saline or lemon–glycerine swabs should be done every 2–4 hours.

Provide Emotional Support

The family of the child with AIDS is under great strain. The mother and others in the family may also be infected. Integrate social services and support groups into the care of the child as soon as the diagnosis is made. Spend time talking with the family about their fears and feelings. In many parts of the United States, AIDS still carries a tremendous stigma, and the family may not be able to discuss their feelings outside of the health care environment. Safeguard the wishes of the family regarding the privacy of the diagnosis.

Clarify any misconceptions the older child with AIDS may have about the transmission of the disease. Routes of transmission and the need for safe sexual practices must be clearly discussed with adolescents. Providing support for adolescents is particularly important, as the dependence which this chronic and terminal disease brings can make it difficult to meet the developmental task of independence. Adolescents may benefit from contact with other infected peers.

Discharge Planning and Home Care Teaching

The diagnosis of AIDS is surrounded by strong emotions and fears. Be honest and direct. Education is essential. Explain that there is no evidence that casual contact among family members can spread the infection. For the child who has been hospitalized, home care needs should be identified well in advance of discharge.

School attendance guidelines for children with AIDS have been published by the American Academy of Pediatrics (AAP) and the CDC. These guidelines recommend unrestricted school attendance for children with AIDS or AIDS-related complex as long as their physician approves. Contraindications to school attendance include lack of control of body secretions, biting, and open wounds that cannot be covered. The nurse often prepares the school personnel with training related to care for children with known and unknown cases of HIV. The nurse also may be responsible for providing medicines or other care for the HIV-infected child at school.[15]

LEGAL & ETHICAL CONSIDERATIONS

Disclosure of patient information is a breach of confidentiality that may subject a nurse to legal action. Disclosure of confidential information occurs whenever a patient's condition—for example, a diagnosis of AIDS—is discussed inappropriately with any third party.

Support groups, home health care nursing services, financial assistance, and psychological counseling are usually needed at some point during the child's illness, and the family should be aware of the availability of such services. Help the family deal with guilt feelings about the child's condition.

Care in the Community

Much of the care of the child with HIV infection or AIDS takes place in the community. Discuss the family's finances as well as health insurance coverage for the child's care. Evaluate the family and community support systems. Many children with HIV infection are placed in foster homes, and these families need careful instruction to manage this multifaceted illness.

Assist the family to alter the home environment to provide standard precautions during care. Make sure the child and family understand that HIV is transmitted through blood, urine, stool, and other body secretions. Teach family members the importance of careful hygiene. Encourage careful handwashing and tell parents to use precautions when handling body fluids. Explain that they should wear gloves when changing diapers; disposing of urine, stool, and emesis; or treating the child's cuts and scrapes. Instruct parents to use a bleach solution for disinfection of objects when necessary and to avoid contact with persons with infectious illnesses. Parents will also need instruction on correct administration and side effects of any medications the child is taking.

Emphasize the importance of promoting the child's development. Frequent developmental screening should be performed. Teach the parents how to support the child in achieving developmental milestones. Encourage contact with other children and adults, provide for appropriate toys, teach parents how to encourage the child's communication, and praise the family for what the child has already accomplished. Children who manifest decreasing developmental milestones or other neurologic symptoms should be assessed for HIV-induced encephalopathy by the primary care provider. The nurse's record of development will be of great importance in this situation.

The child needs to receive regular health maintenance care, such as child health supervision visits, immunizations, and care for health conditions (asthma is a common occurrence).[17]

► AUTOIMMUNE DISORDERS

In an immune system damaged by pathologic changes, an immune response may occur to some of the body's own proteins, resulting in the production of autoantibodies. These pathologic conditions in which the body directs the immune response against itself—identifying "self" as "nonself"—are called autoimmune disorders.

The primary feature of autoimmune disorders is tissue injury caused by a probable immunologic reaction of the host with its own tissues. Structural or functional changes occur as immune cells attack other cells in the body.

The autoimmune disorders are grouped into systemic and organ-specific diseases. Systemic diseases, which largely involve more than one organ, include systemic lupus erythematosus and juvenile rheumatoid arthritis. Organ-specific diseases, which primarily affect a single organ, include insulin-dependent diabetes mellitus (IDDM; see Chap. 20) and thyroiditis.

SAFETY PRECAUTIONS

Because children with HIV or other bloodborne infections may be enrolled in child care centers, staff in these centers should use standard precautions in handling blood and body fluids. Instruct day-care center personnel in use of these precautions. Assist child-care centers in establishing procedures to notify all parents when a child with an infectious disease has been at the center. Parents of immunocompromised children can then take any necessary precautions to minimize the chances of their children becoming ill. Parents of HIV-infected children must be very cautious to limit the exposure of their children to infectious diseases.[16]

NURSING ALERT

When a child has been diagnosed with HIV, even common childhood infections are a cause for concern. Conditions such as respiratory infection, fever, chickenpox, or gastrointestinal illness can progress rapidly to a life-threatening stage. Teach families to seek prompt treatment at the first sign of illness.

SYSTEMIC LUPUS ERYTHEMATOSUS

Systemic lupus erythematosus (SLE), a generalized disorder seen mainly in females, is a chronic inflammatory disease of unknown origin that involves many organ systems. SLE is more common in African-Americans, Hispanics, and Asians than in Caucasians, affecting 4.4 per 100,000 Caucasian females from 10 to 20 years of age, 20 per 100,000 African-American females, 13 per 100,000 Hispanic females, and 31 per 100,000 Asian females.[18] The majority of cases are diagnosed in the teenage and early adult years. A genetic component is suspected as the disease is often more common in certain families.

Clinical Manifestations

Symptoms depend on the organ involved and the amount of tissue damage that has occurred. Initial symptoms include fever, chills, fatigue, malaise, and weight loss. The most common symptoms are arthritis and skin rash. A butterfly rash on the face, consisting of a pink or red rash over the bridge of the nose extending to the cheeks, is a characteristic finding. Children with SLE may have hemolytic anemia, with a low white blood cell and platelet count; bleeding disorders; hypergammaglobulinemia; and vasculitis.

Etiology and Pathophysiology

The exact etiology of SLE is unknown. It is believed that an outside environmental agent causes the body to initiate an abnormal immune system response to its own tissues. Antigen–antibody complexes are deposited in the vascular system, leading to widespread inflammation and tissue damage. The tissues most likely to be affected are the small blood vessels, glomeruli, joints, spleen, and heart valves. Because many systems can be affected at the same time, organ damage with subsequent system failure may occur.

Diagnostic Tests and Medical Management

Blood tests reveal anemia, an elevated blood urea nitrogen (BUN), abnormal plasma proteins, abnormal erythrocyte sedimentation rate (ESR), presence of antinuclear antibodies, and a positive LE (lupus erythematosus) cell reaction, which indicates nonspecific inflammation. The Coombs test is positive. Urinalysis may reveal proteinuria.

The goals of medical management are to create a remission of symptoms and to prevent complications. Corticosteroids, such as prednisone, are prescribed to control inflammation. Antimalarial preparations, such as hydroxychloroquine and chloroquine, are used to treat symptoms associated with skin lesions and renal and arthritic problems. Although the exact action of these drugs on SLE is not known, they often permit continued remission with a lowered dose of steroids. Nonsteroidal antiinflammatory drugs (aspirin, ibuprofen, naproxen) are used to relieve muscle and joint pain. Immunosuppressant drugs, such as cyclosporin and methotrexate, have been used to help control SLE. Diet may be restricted if the child has excessive weight gain or fluid retention from steroids and renal damage.

Prognosis depends on the severity of the disease. The 5-year survival rate now approaches 80%–90% because of improved treatment measures.[19]

Nursing Assessment

Physiologic Assessment

A thorough assessment is needed, as symptoms are widespread. Assess for rash, petechiae, cyanosis, skin ulcers, joint deformity, friction rub, edema, and splenomegaly.

Psychosocial Assessment

Because SLE is a chronic disease that affects primarily adolescents, psychosocial assessment is indicated. Assess family interactions, exploring stressful situations such as divorce or trauma. Treatment-related restrictions and changes in appearance can lead to withdrawal, depression, and suicidal tendencies.

Nursing Diagnosis

Several nursing diagnoses may apply to the child with SLE. These include:

- Risk for Ineffective Management of Therapeutic Regimen related to denial
- Risk for Altered Tissue Perfusion (Renal) related to inflammatory process in kidneys
- Risk for Impaired Skin Integrity related to rashes and photosensitivity
- Risk for Activity Intolerance related to chronic disease
- Risk for Body Image Disturbance related to side effects of medications
- Risk of Infection related to immunosuppressive medications
- Pain related to joint inflammation

Nursing Management

The goals of nursing care are to assist the child to manage and cope with a chronic disease, and to facilitate a remission.

Maintain Fluid Balance

Because most children with SLE have renal involvement, it is important to monitor intake and output and frequently evaluate the child's fluid and electrolyte status. Renal dysfunction can manifest itself by edema, muscle cramps, diarrhea, tetany, and convulsions.

Promote Skin Integrity

Presence of the rash on mucous membranes can cause weakening of the tissues, placing the child at increased risk for infection. Encourage the use of good hygienic measures and a mild soap. Recommend that adolescents limit their use of cosmetics. Reinforce the importance of avoiding sunlight as much as possible and the use of sun protection factor (SPF) of 15 or higher at all times when in the sun.

Promote Rest and Comfort

Because of fatigue and joint pain, the child has little energy reserve during acute episodes of the disease. Encourage frequent rest periods and a nutritious diet to maximize energy stores. A physical therapist can plan a program to encourage mobility and increase muscle strength.

Manage Side Effects of Medications

Observe for side effects of medications used for treatment, and teach the child and family about these effects. For example, immunosuppressant

NURSING ALERT

The side effects of the corticosteroids, immunosuppressants, and antimalarial drugs used in the treatment of children with SLE are significant and include hair loss, susceptibility to infection, "moon face," retinal damage, and bone loss.

drugs can promote infection anywhere in the body; and nonsteroidal antiinflammatory drugs commonly cause gastric distress and bleeding of the gastrointestinal tract. The antimalarial drug hydroxychloroquine can cause serious vision changes; thus, frequent eye examinations are needed.[20]

Provide Emotional Support

Adolescents may have an altered body image as a result of rash, alopecia, arthritic changes in the joints, and chronic disease. Referral to a lupus support group, social services, or counseling may be helpful. The American Lupus Society and the Lupus Foundation of America can provide information to help parents and children adjust to the disease (see Appendix F). The Arthritis Foundation also publishes a useful pamphlet, *Meeting the Challenge: A Young Person's Guide to Living with Lupus.*

JUVENILE RHEUMATOID ARTHRITIS

Juvenile rheumatoid arthritis (JRA) is an autoimmune inflammatory disease that occurs slightly more often in girls than in boys. It usually occurs in children between 2 and 5 or between 9 and 12 years of age, and it may disappear in adolescence[2] or occasionally continue as a chronic disease.[21]

Clinical Manifestations

JRA may be restricted to a few joints or be systemic with involvement of multiple joints. Symptoms can include fever, rash, lymphadenopathy, splenomegaly, and hepatomegaly. The child may develop a limp or obviously favor one extremity over the other. Pain, stiffness, loss of motion, and swelling occur in the large joints such as the knees. Older children may develop symmetric involvement of the small joints of the hand.

Etiology and Pathophysiology

The cause of JRA is unknown, but it is thought to have an autoimmune basis. Inflammation begins in the joint and leads to pain and swelling. Scar tissue eventually develops, resulting in limited range of motion. There are three types of JRA: pauciarticular, systemic, and polyarticular.

Diagnostic Tests and Medical Management

Diagnosis is made primarily on the basis of the history and assessment findings, in particular, arthritis having an onset before 16 years of age and persisting for at least 6 weeks, with no other identifiable cause.[22] There are no specific laboratory tests for the disease. In some children, rheumatoid factor and antinuclear antibody (ANA) tests are positive.

Medical management involves drug therapy, physical therapy, and, when necessary, surgery. The goals of treatment are to relieve pain and prevent contractures. Salicylates (aspirin) or nonsteroidal antiinflammatory drugs (tolmetin sodium, naproxen, diclofenac, ibuprofen) are prescribed to reduce inflammation. Steroids may be used with children who have moderately active disease. Children who do not respond to aspirin or nonsteroidal antiinflammatory drugs may be treated with sulfasalazine and methotrexate. Physical therapy is performed to increase strength and mobility of joints while protecting them from injury. Surgery is occasionally performed to relieve pain and maintain or improve joint function in children with joint contractures.

Seventy percent of children with JRA experience a spontaneous and permanent remission of the disease by adulthood. Rarely, the disease is unresponsive to treatment. Children with early onset have a better prognosis.[2]

Nursing Assessment

A careful history is important, as it is sometimes the primary mode of diagnosis. Assess for joint swelling and deformities, fever, nodules under the skin, and enlarged lymph nodes.

Nursing Diagnosis

Several nursing diagnoses may apply to the child with JRA. They include:

- Activity Intolerance related to joint swelling and pain
- Impaired Physical Mobility related to joint inflammation
- Anxiety related to chronic illness and uncertain prognosis
- Pain related to joint inflammation
- Body Image Disturbance related to appearance and physical immobility
- Risk of Infection related to chronic disease and aspirin therapy

Nursing Management

Nursing care focuses on promoting mobility, encouraging adequate nutrition, and teaching the parents and child about the disease and its management. Most care will occur in the community, including physical therapy, with only occasional hospitalizations at the time of an exacerbation of the disease.

Promote Improved Mobility

Physical therapists play an essential role in the child's treatment. The goals of physical therapy are to maintain joint function, strengthen muscles, increase tone, maintain body alignment, and prevent permanent deformities such as contractures. Range-of-motion exercises, stretching, hydrotherapy, and swimming exercises help to prevent deformities (Figs. 9–4 and 9–5). Encourage the child to perform activities of daily living. Medications may be given to reduce joint swelling and inflammation. Warm compresses to the involved joints are soothing.

Encourage Adequate Nutrition

Promote general health by encouraging a well-balanced diet. Children with decreased mobility may have reduced metabolic needs, and excess weight causes additional muscle strain.

Care in the Community

The child with JRA may never, or rarely, be hospitalized. Most care takes place during visits to health care offices, clinics, and physical therapy. Teach parents about the child's condition and prognosis, and answer their questions about the child's treatment. The child may need support to adjust to the diagnosis of a chronic illness. Encourage the child to maintain contact with peers and to attend school whenever possible. Explain to the child and parents that overexertion may lead to exacerbation of the disease. Inform parents about possible complications of JRA, such as altered growth related to early closure of epiphyseal plates, small joint contractures, and synovitis.

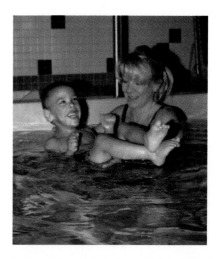

FIGURE 9–4. The physical therapist uses hydrotherapy to help maintain joint function in a child who has juvenile rheumatoid arthritis.

NURSING ALERT

Infants and children with juvenile rheumatoid arthritis who are receiving aspirin therapy are at risk of developing Reye syndrome if they contract influenza. These children should be immunized with influenza vaccine in the fall of each year.

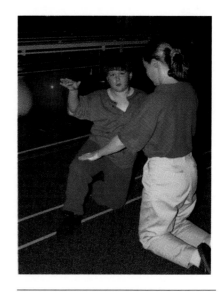

FIGURE 9–5. Stretching exercises are an important part of physical therapy for a child who has juvenile rheumatoid arthritis.

Parents and children can be referred to the Arthritis Foundation and the American Juvenile Arthritis Foundation for further information and support (see Appendix F).

▶ ALLERGIC REACTIONS

Allergy is one of the major chronic illnesses of children today. Why are some children allergic to cats, for instance, while no one else in the family has allergies? In order to answer this question, the nurse needs to have a basic understanding of the mechanisms of allergy.

Allergy is an abnormal or altered reaction to an antigen. Antigens responsible for clinical manifestations of allergy are called **allergens.** Allergens can be ingested in food or drugs or injected or absorbed through contact with unbroken skin. An allergic reaction is an antigen–antibody reaction and can manifest itself as anaphylaxis, atopic disease, serum sickness, or contact dermatitis. Characteristic findings in children with allergies are summarized in Table 9–6.

The **hypersensitivity response,** an overreaction of the immune system, is responsible for allergic reactions. Hypersensitivity reactions have been classified into four types (Table 9–7). Type I hypersensitivity reactions are immediate reactions that occur within seconds or minutes of exposure to the antigen. Symptoms can include a wheal and flare in the skin, edema, spasm of smooth muscle, wheezing, vomiting, diarrhea, or anaphylaxis. The release of chemical substances such as histamine is responsible for the signs and symptoms exhibited. The first time a child is exposed to the allergen, there is no reaction. With every exposure thereafter, however, the allergic child may have a reaction to the allergen.

Type IV reactions are delayed responses that do not appear until several hours after exposure and require 24–72 hours to develop fully. A type IV reaction, which is not confined to any specific tissue, is elicited by relatively complex antigens such as those of bacteria and viruses and by simple antigens such as drugs and metals. Symptoms include contact dermatitis, itching, and blistering.

NURSING ALERT

Anaphylaxis is an exaggerated hypersensitivity reaction that may manifest with itching; localized or generalized hives on the hands, feet, or mucosa; soft tissue swelling; cough; dyspnea; pallor; sweating; and tachycardia. Severe reactions may lead to respiratory distress or death.

9-6   Characteristic Findings in Children With Allergies

Respiratory system: Asthma, rhinitis (seasonal and perennial), serous otitis media, cough, pneumonia, croup, edema of glottis

Gastrointestinal system: Abdominal pain and colic, stomatitis, constipation, diarrhea, bloody stools, geographical tongue, vomiting

Skin: Angioedema, urticaria, eczema, atopic dermatitis, erythema multiforme, purpura, drug and food rashes, contact dermatitis

Nervous system: Headache, tension, fatigue, convulsions, Ménière syndrome, tremor

Eye: Conjunctivitis, cataract, ciliary spasm, iritis

Blood: Thrombocytopenic purpura, hemolytic anemia, leukopenia, agranulocytosis

Musculoskeletal system: Arthralgia, myalgia, rheumatoid arthritis, torticollis

Genitourinary system: Dysuria, vulvovaginitis, enuresis

Miscellaneous: Anaphylactic shock, serum sickness, autoimmune diseases

9-7   Types of Hypersensitivity Reactions

Type	Mechanism of Action	Clinical Manifestations	Examples
Type I Localized or systemic reactions (anaphylaxis)	Antibodies bind to certain cells, causing release of chemical substances that produce an inflammatory reaction.	Hypotension, wheezing, gastrointestinal or uterine spasm, stridor, urticaria	Extrinsic asthma, hay fever
Type II Tissue-specific reactions	Antibodies cause activation of complement system, which leads to tissue damage.	Variable; may include dyspnea or fever	Transfusion reaction, ABO incompatibility, hemolytic disease of the newborn
Type III Immune-complex reactions	Immune complexes are deposited in tissues, where they activate complement, which results in a generalized inflammatory reaction.	Urticaria, fever, joint pain	Acute glomerulonephritis, serum sickness
Type IV Delayed reactions	Antigens stimulate T cells that release lymphokines, which cause inflammation and tissue damage.	Variable; may include fever, erythema, itching	Contact dermatitis, tuberculin skin test, graft-versus-host disease, allograft rejection

Nursing Management

The child with allergies requires a thorough assessment, including a complete past medical history, family history, personal and social history, and review of symptoms. The history focuses on the following areas:

- What symptoms does the child experience? Encourage the child to describe the difficulty in his or her own words.

- Are the symptoms continuous or intermittent? What are the frequency and duration of episodes?

- When did the child first begin to experience symptoms? Did the child have eczema or a feeding problem in infancy or childhood? Did the infant have frequent bouts of colic or skin problems when new foods were introduced? Was there a change in symptoms at puberty? Are the symptoms becoming worse or spontaneously improving?

- What known agents in the environment cause difficulties?

- Are there seasonal variations in symptoms? At what time of the day or night do symptoms usually occur?

Assessment should also include a complete physical examination; laboratory, x-ray, and pulmonary function studies; tests of nasal function; and skin testing. Nursing care focuses on treating the symptoms, alleviating the anxiety of the child and parents, and identifying the allergens. Teaching the child and family how to minimize or avoid exposure to allergens is important. Parents of children who have had severe reactions to bee or wasp stings should be taught how to take precautions and how to provide emergency treatment if the child is stung.

Families may need instructions on allergy-proofing the home. Pets, dust, carpets, fabrics, feather pillows and bedding, and cigarette smoke can all cause allergic reactions. If families are reluctant to give up pets, frequent baths can reduce dander, which is the usual allergen.

RAST

The radioallergosorbent test (RAST) is a common laboratory test used to detect IgE antibodies. It measures circulating IgE antibodies to many allergens and generally correlates well with skin test results. It is not as sensitive as skin tests, however, so those tests are generally preferred.

 SAFETY PRECAUTIONS

If the child has had a severe or systemic reaction in the past to a bee or wasp sting, ensure that the parents know how to handle an anaphylactic reaction if the child is stung again. Kits with syringes of premeasured adrenaline are available on a prescription basis. Instruct family members how to use the kit. Make sure that the kit is properly stored without exposure to sun or high temperature. Have the family check the expiration date of the adrenaline frequently. The child should wear a medical alert bracelet. An allergy specialist should be consulted to determine whether desensitization injections would be helpful for the child.

Review any dietary restrictions for a child who has a food allergy with the child and family, and teach parents to read labels. Referral to a nutritionist is usually necessary.

LATEX ALLERGY

NURSING ALERT

In September 1997, the Food and Drug Administration (FDA) issued a labeling requirement for all medical devices containing latex. By September 1998, these products must carry a warning label that reads: "Caution: This product contains natural rubber latex, which may cause allergic reactions."

Latex allergy has been growing in incidence among both health care workers and patients. Many health care products, such as gloves, drains, catheters, and intravenous ports contain latex, a sap from the rubber tree. Latex allergy is caused by an IgE-mediated response that develops after repeated exposure to latex. In some cases, intraoperative deaths have occurred when allergic individuals were exposed to latex products during surgery.

Children most at risk for latex allergy include those with myelodysplasia and congenital urinary tract anomalies. Persons who have had repeated surgeries are also at higher risk due to high exposure to latex during surgery. Health care personnel may also be at risk for latex allergy (Table 9–8).

Children and adolescents at high risk should receive allergy skin testing for latex.[23,24] Health care personnel should use alternative products whenever possible in caring for those persons at risk.

When a positive skin test has occurred or when the person has had a reaction to latex, all latex products must be removed from the allergic individual's environment. Alternative products, such as nonlatex gloves and catheters, must be used when providing health care. These individuals should also wear a medical identification bracelet at all times. Emphasize to parents and children that many everyday products contain latex, including latex balloons and condoms (Table 9–9).

9-8   Measures to Protect Against Latex Allergy

Health care personnel are at high risk of developing latex allergy because of intense exposure to products containing latex. An estimated 8–12% of health care workers are latex sensitive. You can protect yourself by using the following measures:[22]

- Decrease exposure by using alternative products whenever available (use synthetic rubbers, polyethylene, nitrile, neoprene, vinyl gloves).
- Use powder-free gloves if using latex gloves (the powder has high amounts of latex, which are inhaled).
- Avoid use of oil-based hand creams and lotions before putting on latex gloves, as these preparations break down the latex.
- When symptoms of sensitivity to latex occur on exposure (rash, hives, nasal congestion, conjunctivitis, cough, or wheeze), contact the Employee Health Department of your facility.
- If severely allergic, avoid all contact and wear a medical identification bracelet.
- Contact the National Institute for Occupational Safety and Health (NIOSH) at 800–346–4647 or the American Nurses Association at 800–637–0323 for more information.

9-9 Latex-Free Alternatives for the Home

Frequently Contain Latex	Latex-Safe Alternatives/Manufacturers[a]
Art supplies—paint markers, paints, glue, erasers	Elmers (School Glue, Glue-All, GluColors, Carpenters Wood Glue, Sno-Drift Paste), Crayola products *(except for rubber stamps and erasers)*, Liquitex paints, Silly Putty; FarberCastle art erasers *(available through Staples catalog)*, Dick Blick art materials
Balloons	Mylar balloons (Marketing Innovations Enterprises)
Balls—Koosh, tennis, rubber, basketball	PVC (Hedstrom Sports Ball)
Bath mat	Gerry baby products (Pound Pales)
Bathroom throw rugs (nonskid latex backing)	100% cotton reversible throw rugs
Bungee cords	None or rope
Carpet backing, gym floors	Provide barrier (cloth or mat), wooden floors
Chewing gum	Warner Lambert
Cleaning/kitchen gloves	Magla
Food handled with latex gloves	Synthetic gloves for food handling
Condoms, diaphragms	Polyurethane female condom (Reality), polymer male condom (Avanti) (order through Condomania [800-926-6366] www.condomania.com)
Cosmetic applicators sponges (Buff Puffs)	Cotton balls, latex-free sponges (Rickies Beauty, Cosmetic Plus)
Crutches—axillary, hand pads	Cover with cloth or tape
Disposable diapers, rubber pants, incontinence pads	Tranquillity, First Quality, Gold Seal, Huggies Drypers, Some Attends, Confidence
Elastic on underwear, leg and waist of clothing	Cover with cloth (Decent Exposures) (Special clothes for children 508-430-5172) ARC
Erasers	FarberCastle (Castle Art erasers)
Feeding nipples	Silicone (Gerber, Evenflo, MAM, some Ross, Mead Johnson)
Feminine sanitary pads	Kimberly-Clark products
Foam rubber lining of braces	Cover with felt cloth
Infant tooth brush massager	Soft bristle brush or cloth, Gerber/NUK
Pacifiers	Plastic, silicone, and vinyl made by INFA, Gerber, MAM, binky, Kip, Soothie, and Wee Soothie (Childrens Medical Venture)
Handles—Racquet (ping-pong), golf clubs, bats, tools, ski poles	Vinyl, leather
Rain coats, rubber boots	Neoprene-coated nylon
Rubber bands	String, spring clips, Plasti Band (Baumgartens)
Socks	Buster Brown cotton socks without elastic (Vermont Country Store)
Toys, rubber ducky, teething toys	Plastic, cloth vinyl
Toys—Stretch Armstrong, old Barbies, bowling balls	Jurassic Park figures (Kenner); 1993 Barbie; Disney Dolls (Mattel); many toys by Fisher Price, Little Tykes, Playschool, and Discovery; trolls (Norfin); The First Years; Shelcore; Safety First; *(JC Penney and Toys R Us have a catalog for special needs children with product content listed for most of the toys)*
Water toys, scuba gear, snorkels, wet suits, beach thongs	PVC plastic
Wheelchair—cushions, tires	Jay, ROHO; cover seat, use gloves when handling tires
Zippered storage bags	Waxed paper, plain plastic bags, Ziploc (Dow)

[a]Last updated December 1997.
Courtesy of Debra Adkins, Latex Allergy News, Torrington, CT.

REFERENCES

1. Buckley, R.H. (1996). Allergy, immunology, and rheumatology. In A.M. Rudolph, J.I.E. Hoffman, & C.D. Rudolph (Eds.), *Rudolph's pediatrics* (20th ed., pp. 431–498). Stamford, CT: Appleton & Lange.

2. Stiehm, E.R., & Ammann, A.J. (1997). Combined antibody (B-cell) and cellular (T-cell) immunodeficiency disorders. In D.P. Stites, A.T. Terr, & T.G. Parslow (Eds.), *Basic & clinical immunology* (9th ed.). Stamford, CT: Appleton & Lange.

3. Lederman, H.M. (1996). IVIG therapy: Separating fact from wishful thinking. *Contemporary Pediatrics, 13*(6), 75–92.

4. Workman, L., Ellerhorst-Ryan, J., & Hargrave-Koertge, V. (1993). *Nursing care of the immunocompromised patient*. Philadelphia: Saunders.

5. Boland, M. (1996). Overview of perinatally transmitted HIV infection. *Nursing Clinics of North America, 31*(1), 155–164.

6. MMWR. (1996). AIDS among children—U.S. 1996. *Morbidity and Mortality Weekly Report, 45*(46), 1005–1010.

7. McClintock, L., & Corrall, J. (1994). Pediatric presentation of the immunocompromised patient. *Topics in Emergency Medicine, 16*(1), 45–67.

8. Rogers, M.F., Moseley, R.R., Simonds, R.J., Moore, J.S., Gwinn, M., Elsner, L.G., Curran, J.W., Bloom, A.S., & Peterson, H.B. (1995). U.S. Public Health Service recommendations for human immunodeficiency virus counseling and voluntary testing for pregnant women. *Morbidity and Mortality Weekly Report, 44*(RR-7), 1–15.

9. MMWR. (1994). CDC: Recommendations for the use of zidovudine to reduce perinatal transmission of human immunodeficiency virus. *Morbidity and Mortality Weekly Report, 43*, 1–20.

10. Hall, C.S. (1994). The experience of children with hemophilia and HIV infection. *Journal of School Health, 64*(1), 16–17.

11. Grubman, S. (1995). 1995 revised guidelines for prophylaxis against *Pneumocystis carinii* pneumonia for children infected with or prenatally exposed to human immunodeficiency virus. *Morbidity and Mortality Weekly Report, 44*(RR-4), 1–11.

12. Luzuriaga, K., Bryson, Y., Krogstad, P., Robinson, J., Stechenberg, B., Lamson, M., Cort, S., & Sullivan, J. (1997). Combination treatment with zidovudine, didanosine, and nevirapine in infants with human immunodeficiency virus type infection. *New England Journal of Medicine, 336*(19), 1343–1344.

13. National Institutes of Health. (1997). Combination regimens favored in symptomatic HIV children. *Clinician Reviews, 7*(9), 104.

14. Kaplan, J.E., Masur, H., & Holmes, K.K. (1997). 1997 USPHS/IDSA guidelines for the prevention of opportunistic infections in persons infected with human immunodeficiency virus. *Morbidity and Mortality Weekly Report, 46*(RR-12), 1–46.

15. Gross, E.J., & Larkin, M.H. (1996). The child with HIV in day care and school. *Nursing Clinics of North America, 31*(1), 231–242.

16. Pizzo, P.A., & Wilfert, C.M. (Eds.). (1994). Pediatric AIDS: The challenge of HIV infection in infants, children, and adolescents (2nd ed.). Baltimore: Williams & Wilkins.

17. O'Hara, M.J., & D'Orlando, D. (1996). Ambulatory care of the HIV-infected child. *Nursing Clinics of North America, 31*(1), 179–206.

18. Lehman, T.J.A. (1995). A practical guide to systemic lupus erythematosus. *Pediatric Clinics of North America, 42*(5), 1223–1238.

19. Sack, K.E., & Fye, K.H. (1997). Rheumatic diseases. In D.P. Stites, A.T. Terr, & T.G. Parslow (Eds.), *Basic & clinical immunology* (9th ed.). Stamford, CT. Appleton & Lange.

20. Kuper, B.C., & Failla, S. (1994). Shedding new light on lupus. *American Journal of Nursing, 8*(5), 26–33.

21. Dunkin, M.A. (1994). When kids get arthritis. *Arthritis Today, 94*(11), 45–49.

22. Warren, R.W., Perez, M.D., Wilking, A.P., & Myones, B.L. (1994). Pediatric rheumatic diseases. *Pediatric Clinics of North America, 41*(4), 783–818.

23. Petonsk, E.L. (1997). Nurses should take action to avoid occupational latex allergy. *Journal of Emergency Nursing, 32*(2), 91–92.

24. Wilburn, S. (1997). Latex allergy. *Journal of Emergency Nursing, 32*(2), 93–94.

ADDITIONAL RESOURCES

Barrett, D.J., & Sleasman, J.W. (1997). Pediatric AIDS: So now what do we do? *Contemporary Pediatrics, 14*(6), 111–124.

Baumeister, L.L., & Nicol, N.H. (1994). Pediatric lupus and the role of sun protection. *Pediatric Nursing, 20*(4), 371–375.

Bok, M., & Morales, J. (1997). The impact and implications of HIV on children and adolescents: Social justice and social change. *Journal of HIV/AIDS Prevention & Education for Adolescents and Children, 1*(1), 9–33.

Czarniecki, L. (1996). Advanced HIV disease in children. *Nursing Clinics of North America, 31*(1), 207–220.

Dickover, R.E., Garraty, E.M., & Herman, S.A. (1996). Identification of levels of maternal HIV-1 RNAA associated with risk of perinatal transmission, effect of maternal zidovudine treatment on viral load. *Journal of the American Medical Association, 275,* 599–605.

Emery, H.M., Bowyer, S.L., & Sisung, C.E. (1995). Rehabilitation of the child with a rheumatic disease. *Pediatric Clinics of North America, 42*(5), 1263–1284.

Fritsch, D.F., & Fredrick Pilat, D.M. (1993). Exposing latex allergies. *Nursing, 23*(8), 46–48.

Giannini, E.H., & Cawkell, G.D. (1995). Drug treatment in children with juvenile rheumatoid arthritis: Past, present, and future. *Pediatric Clinics of North America, 42*(5), 1099–1126.

Grzybowski, M., Ownby, D.R., Peyser, P.A., Johnson, C.L., & Shork, M.A. (1996). The prevalence of anti-latex IgE antibodies among registered nurses. *Journal of Allergy and Clinical Immunology, 98,* 535.

Hartley, B., & Fuller, C.C. (1997). Juvenile arthritis: A nursing perspective. *Journal of Pediatric Nursing, 12*(2), 100–109.

Hudack, C.M., & Gallo, B.M. (1997). What to expect when your patient has AIDS. *American Journal of Nursing, 97*(9), 16CC–16HH.

Hughes, C.B., & Caliandro, G. (1996). Effects of social support, stress, and level of illness on caregiving of children with AIDS. *Journal of Pediatric Nursing, 11*(6), 347–358.

Leung, D.Y.M. (1994). Mechanisms of the human allergic response: Clinical implications. *Pediatric Clinics of North America, 41*(4), 727–744.

Levinson, W., & Jawetz, E. (1996). *Medical microbiology and immunology* (14th ed). Stamford, CT: Appleton & Lange.

Lewis, S.Y., Wesley, Y., & Haiken, H.J. (1996). Pediatric and family HIV: Psychosocial concerns across the continuum of disease. *Nursing Clinics of North America, 31*(1), 221–230.

Lyons, M. (1993). Immunosuppressive therapy after cardiac transplantation: Teaching pediatric patients and their families. *Critical Care Nurse, 13*(1), 39–45.

Nicholson, J.K.A., & Hearn, T.L. (1997). 1997 revised guidelines for performing CD4 and T-cell determinations in persons infected with human immunodeficiency virus (HIV). *Morbidity and Mortality Weekly Report, 46*(RR-2), 1–29.

Schelonka, R.L., & Yoder, B.A. (1996). The WBC count and differential: Its uses and misuses. *Contemporary Pediatrics, 13*(10), 124–141.

Young, M.A., & Meyers, M. (1997). Latex allergy. *Nursing Clinics of North America, 32*(1), 169–182.

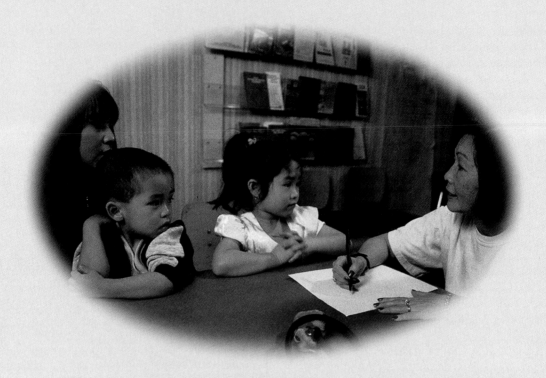

L ian, 5 years old, has accompanied her mother and 2-year-old brother Chang to the pediatric clinic. Her mother is concerned because Chang has had a fever of 38.3°C (101°F) for the past 3 days. Chang has been to this office several times in the past few months for health care, but this is the first time Lian has come along.

When the nurse asks about Lian's last visit to the doctor and the status of her immunizations, her mother says Lian has not been seen for about 2 years. She is not sure whether Lian has had all of her shots. In checking Lian's health records, the nurse notes that she is in need of several immunizations, including DPT, polio, varicella, and hepatitis B. Chang needs polio, MMR, and Hib vaccines.

Should Lian be given any of these immunizations today, even though her brother is ill? Which immunizations could be given at the same time? Should Chang also receive any immunizations today?

INFECTIOUS AND COMMUNICABLE DISEASES 10

"Both Lian and Chang need several immunizations, and we don't want to miss this opportunity to catch them up. Chang was found to have only a minor illness. Lian will be going to kindergarten in the fall, so it is very important for her to get all of the immunizations she needs now."

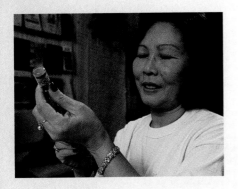

TERMINOLOGY

- **acellular vaccine** A vaccine that uses proteins from the microorganism rather than the whole cell to stimulate the process of active immunity.
- **active immunity** Stimulation of antibody production without causing clinical disease.
- **communicable disease** An illness that is transmitted directly or indirectly from one person to another.
- **direct transmission** The passage of an infectious disease through physical contact between the source of the pathogen and a new host.
- **indirect transmission** The passage of an infectious disease involving survival of pathogens outside humans before they invade a new host.
- **infectious disease** Illness, caused by a microorganism, that is commonly communicated from one host (human or otherwise) to another.

- **killed virus vaccine** A vaccine that contains a killed microorganism that is still capable of inducing the human body to produce antibodies to the disease.
- **live virus vaccine** A vaccine that contains the microorganism in a live but attenuated, or weakened, form.
- **nosocomial infection** An infection acquired in a health care agency, not present at the time of entrance to the agency.
- **passive immunity** Immunity produced through introduction of specific antibodies to the disease, which are usually obtained from the blood or serum of immune persons and animals. *Does not confer lasting immunity.*
- **toxoid** A toxin that has been treated (by heat or chemical) to weaken its toxic effects but retain its antigenicity.
- **transplacental immunity** Passive immunity that is transferred from mother to infant.

Young children such as Lian and Chang are particularly susceptible to illnesses that are transmitted among close contacts or through exposure to microorganisms in various settings. Many of these illnesses can be prevented by following a recommended schedule of childhood immunizations. Why are children more vulnerable than adults to infectious and communicable diseases? How do you recognize the common infectious and communicable diseases, and what is the medical and nursing management of these diseases? Using information in this chapter, you will be able to answer these questions.

An **infectious disease** is an illness caused by microorganisms that are commonly communicated from one host (human or otherwise) to another. A **communicable disease** is an illness that is directly or indirectly transmitted from one person to another. Communicable diseases are a major cause of morbidity in infants and children in the United States, and in some cases result in death.

For a communicable disease to occur, the following need to be present (Fig. 10–1):

- An infectious agent, or pathogen
- An effective means of transmission
- A susceptible host

An effective chain of transmission for infection requires a suitable habitat, or reservoir, for the pathogen. A reservoir may be living or nonliving. Transmission may be direct or indirect. **Direct transmission** involves physical contact between the source of the infection and the new host. **Indirect transmission** occurs when pathogens survive outside humans before causing infection and disease.

A susceptible host is also necessary for the occurrence of an infectious disease. Young children, whose immune systems are not fully developed and who have not yet developed antibodies to many agents, cannot defend themselves against disease as well as older children. Other characteristics,

CULTURAL CONSIDERATIONS

In some cultures infectious diseases are seen as punishment or the result of curses or evil spirits. For example, Native Americans traditionally view illnesses as the result of disharmony or displeasing the spirits. They may not believe in the germ theory of disease causation.

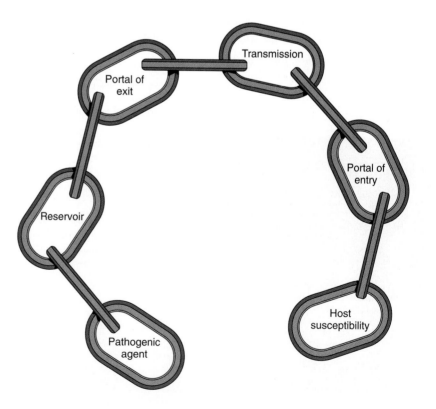

FIGURE 10–1. The chain of infection. To achieve infection control, one of the links in the chain must be broken.

such as immunodeficiency and poor health, may increase a child's risk of contracting an infectious disease.

Control of infectious diseases is usually directed at interrupting the chain of transmission or eliminating one or more of the habitats or reservoirs (eg, spraying insecticide to kill mosquitoes that carry malaria). Isolating an infected individual interferes with disease transmission, and killing the pathogen eliminates the causal agent. Public health authorities monitor patterns of disease occurrence, and health care workers are required to report cases of many infectious diseases to state health officials.

As a result of major public health programs and scientific advances such as safer drinking water, better sanitation, improved standards of living, immunizations, and advanced medical treatment, infectious and communicable diseases have decreased in occurrence but remain a significant source of morbidity and mortality in infants and children, especially in developing countries.

▶ SPECIAL VULNERABILITY OF CHILDREN

The capability and function of the immune system, especially of infants, is poorly understood. Infants are particularly vulnerable to infectious diseases for the following reasons:

- Their immune responses are immature.
- Passively acquired maternal antibodies are decreasing.
- Disease protection through immunization is as yet incomplete.

As children grow, they develop immunity through immunization or exposure to the natural disease. As children mature and become more active, they interact more frequently with other children and adults, which increases their exposure to infectious agents (Fig. 10–2). As healthy children are exposed to more infections, they develop antibodies naturally. Thus, subsequent infections with the same type of organism may be less severe or avoided. (Refer to the discussion of "Anatomy and Physiology of Pediatric Differences" in Chapter 9.)

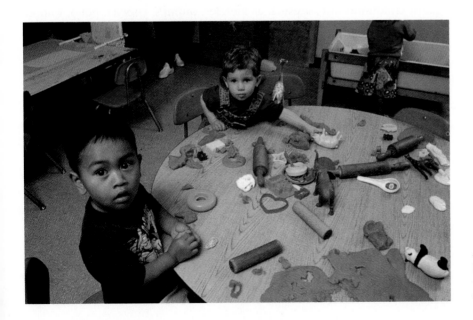

FIGURE 10–2. Infectious diseases are easily transmitted in settings such as day-care centers where children handle common objects.

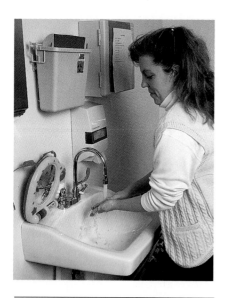

FIGURE 10–3. Proper handwashing is one of the most effective measures in preventing transmission of microorganisms.

TYPES OF VACCINES

- **killed virus vaccine** A vaccine that contains a microorganism that has been killed but is still capable of inducing the human body to produce antibodies. EXAMPLE: inactivated poliovirus vaccine.
- **toxoid** A toxin that has been treated (by heat or chemical) to weaken its toxic effects but retain its antigenicity. EXAMPLE: tetanus toxoid.
- **live virus vaccine** A vaccine that contains a microorganism in live but attenuated, or weakened, form. EXAMPLE: measles vaccine.
- *recombinant forms* An organism that has been genetically altered for use in vaccines. EXAMPLES: hepatitis B and **acellular pertussis vaccine** (a vaccine that uses proteins from pertussis rather than the whole cell to stimulate the process of active immunity).
- *conjugated forms* An altered organism that is joined with another substance to increase the immune response. EXAMPLE: *Haemophilus influenzae* type b (Hib) vaccine.

Transmission of infectious diseases in day care and other close environments is facilitated by the poor hygiene behaviors of young children. The fecal–oral and respiratory routes are the most common sources of transmission in children. Children usually do not wash their hands after toileting unless they are closely supervised. They put toys and their hands in their mouths, and then rub their nose and eyes. They often are unable to care for a runny nose without help. Diapers may leak stool and provide the fecal exposure to organisms. In addition, the staff in a day-care center or other persons caring for children may not use proper handwashing techniques (Fig. 10–3). All of these behaviors promote the transmission of infection.

► IMMUNIZATION

The development and widespread availability of immunizations has been one of the great breakthroughs of modern medicine. Immunization introduces an antigen (a foreign substance that triggers an immune system response) into the body, allowing immunity against a disease to develop naturally. The person produces antibodies, which are proteins capable of responding to specific antigens.

In **active immunity** (in which antibody production is stimulated without causing clinical disease) an antigen is given in the form of a vaccine. However, a child may need antibodies faster than the body can develop them. In this case, **passive immunity** may be induced with antibodies produced in another human or animal host and given to the child. This approach is also used with at-risk children after a single exposure to a disease to prevent the disease from occurring or to reduce its severity. For example, if a child who has never had a tetanus immunization steps on a rusty nail, the child needs immediate protection (passive immunity) from tetanus. Tetanus immune globulin injection is given to combat the tetanus toxin produced by the bacterial spores introduced by the nail. Because passive immunity does not confer lasting immunity, the process of antibody development (active immunity) is then initiated with the administration of a tetanus toxoid vaccine.

Since vaccines were first developed in the late 1800s, many diseases have decreased dramatically in incidence. The introduction of vaccines against childhood diseases such as measles, mumps, rubella, polio, whooping cough, diphtheria, *Haemophilus influenzae* type b, hepatitis B, and chickenpox has greatly improved the quality of life for children and adults. Improvements in vaccine technology continue to increase the safety and efficacy of immunization against an increasing number of diseases. Today's vaccines are often produced synthetically by means of recombinant DNA technology or genetic engineering.

Vaccines should be administered at specific ages and intervals. Timing for first immunizations is determined by the age at which **transplacental immunity** (passive immunity transferred from mother to infant) decreases or disappears, and the infant or child develops the ability to make antibodies in response to the vaccine. Scientists continue to study the duration of protection from vaccines. Some vaccines do not confer lifelong immunity. The recommended schedule for immunization is updated annually to reflect new vaccines and the need for repeat immunization. The Advisory Committee on Immunization Practices (ACIP), the American Academy of Pediatrics (AAP), and the American Academy of Family Practitioners (AAFP) have collaborated to recommend a single vaccination schedule that is updated annually. The 1998 recommendations are given in Table 10–1.

10-1 Recommended Childhood Immunization Schedule United States, January–December 1998

Vaccines[a] are listed under the routinely recommended ages. [Bars] indicate range of acceptable ages for vaccination. Shaded ovals indicate *catch-up vaccination:* at 11–12 years of age, hepatitis B vaccine should be administered to children not previously vaccinated, and varicella vaccine should be administered to children not previously vaccinated who lack a reliable history of chickenpox.

Age ▶ Vaccine ▼	Birth	1 mo	2 mo	4 mo	6 mo	12 mo	15 mo	18 mo	4–6 yr	11–12 yr	14–16 yr
Hepatitis B[b,c]	Hep B-1										
		Hep B-2			Hep B-3					Hep B[c]	
Diphtheria, tetanus, pertussis[d]		DTaP or DTP	DTaP or DTP	DTaP or DTP	DTaP or DTP		DTaP or DTP[d]		DTaP or DTP	Td	
H. influenzae type b[e]		Hib	Hib	Hib[e]		Hib[e]					
Polio[f]		Polio[f]	Polio		Polio[f]				Polio		
Measles, mumps, rubella[g]						MMR			MMR[g]	MMR[g]	
Varicella[h]						Var				Var[h]	

[a]This schedule indicates the recommended age for routine administration of currently licensed childhood vaccines. Some combination vaccines are available and may be used whenever administration of all components of the vaccine is indicated. Providers should consult the manufacturers' package inserts for detailed recommendations.

[b]*Infants born to HBsAg-negative mothers* should receive 2.5 μg of Merck vaccine (Recombivax HB) or 10 μg of SmithKline Beecham (SB) vaccine (Engerix-B). The 2nd dose should be administered ≥ 1 mo after the 1st dose. The 3rd dose should be given at least 2 months after the 2nd dose, but not before 6 mo of age.

Infants born to HBsAg-positive mothers should receive 0.5 mL hepatitis B immune globulin (HBIG) within 12 hr of birth, and either 5 μg of Merck vaccine (Recombivax HB) or 10 μg of SB vaccine (Engerix-B) at a separate site. The 2nd dose is recommended at 1–2 mo of age and the 3rd dose at 6 mo of age.

Infants born to mothers whose HBsAg status is unknown should receive either 5 μg of Merck vaccine (Recombivax HB) or 10 μg of SB vaccine (Engerix-B) within 12 hr of birth. The 2nd dose of vaccine is recommended at 1 mo of age and the 3rd dose at 6 mo of age. Blood should be drawn at the time of delivery to determine the mother's HBsAg status; if it is positive, the infant should receive HBIG as soon as possible (no later than 1 wk of age). The dosage and timing of subsequent vaccine doses should be based upon the mother's HBsAg status.

[c]Children and adolescents who have not been vaccinated against hepatitis B in infancy may begin the series during any childhood visit. Those who have not previously received 3 doses of hepatitis B vaccine should initiate or complete the series during the 11–12-year-old visit and unvaccinated older adolescents should be vaccinated whenever possible. The 2nd dose should be administered at least 1 mo after the 1st dose, and the 3rd dose should be administered at least 4 mo after the 1st dose and at least 2 mo after the 2nd dose.

[d]DTaP (diphtheria and tetanus toxoids and acellular pertussis vaccine) is the preferred vaccine for all doses in the vaccination series, including completion of the series in children who have received ≥ 1 dose of whole-cell DTP vaccine. Whole-cell DTP is an acceptable alternative to DTaP. The 4th dose of DTaP may be administered as early as 12 mo of age, provided 6 mo have elapsed since the 3rd dose, and if the child is considered unlikely to return at 15–18 mo of age. Td (tetanus and diphtheria toxoids, absorbed, for adult use) is recommended at 11–12 yr of age if at least 5 yr have elapsed since the last dose of DTP, DTaP, or DT. Subsequent routine Td boosters are recommended every 10 years.

[e]Three H. influenzae type b (Hib) conjugative vaccines are licensed for infant use. If PRP-OMP (PedvaxHIB [Merck]) is administered at 2 and 4 mo of age, a dose at 6 mo is not required. After completing the primary series, any Hib conjugate vaccine may be used as a booster.

[f]Two poliovirus vaccines are currently licensed in the United States: inactivated poliovirus vaccine (IPV) and oral poliovirus vaccine (OPV). The following schedules are all acceptable by the ACIP, the AAP, and the AAFP, and parents and providers may choose among them:

1. IPV at 2 and 4 mo; OPV at 12–18 mo and 4–6 yr
2. IPV at 2, 4, 12–18 mo, and 4–6 yr
3. OPV at 2, 4, 6–18 mo, and 4–6 yr

The ACIP routinely recommends schedule 1. IPV is the only poliovirus vaccine recommended for immunocompromised persons and their household contacts.

[g]The 2nd dose of MMR is routinely recommended at 4–6 yr of age or at 11–12 yr of age, but may be administered during any visit, provided at least 1 mo has elapsed since receipt of the 1st dose and that both doses are administered at or after 12 mo of age.

[h]Susceptible children may receive varicella vaccine (Var) at any visit after the first birthday, and those who lack a reliable history of chickenpox should be immunized during the 11–12-year-old visit. Children ≥ 13 yr of age should receive 2 doses, at least 1 mo apart.

Supplemental immunizations for influenza, meningococcal, and pneumococcal infections are recommended for certain children, as noted in Table 10–2.

The effectiveness of vaccines depends on the proper storage of vaccines and the immunization of all susceptible individuals. Lower immunization rates of children are often associated with economic factors, limited

CLINICAL TIP

The pertussis vaccine is given in combination with the diphtheria and tetanus toxoids (DTP). Pertussis immunization has been associated with neurologic events. A new acellular, highly refined pertussis vaccine is available that has less potential for causing serious side effects. It is recommended for use whenever possible in combination with diphtheria and tetanus toxoid for all doses.

10-2 Supplemental Immunizations

Vaccine	Recommendation
Influenza	For children with chronic pulmonary disease, cardiac disease, sickle cell disease or other hemoglobinopathies, diabetes, metabolic disease, human immunodeficiency virus (HIV) infection, or those undergoing immunosuppressive therapy or chronic aspirin therapy (eg, for rheumatoid arthritis or Kawasaki disease). Administered annually in autumn. Children with no history of influenza illness or vaccine need two doses 1 mo apart.[1]
Meningococcal	For children older than 2 years of age with asplenia. Vaccine duration is 5 years or longer in children older than 4 years at the time of immunization. The vaccine should be repeated after 1 year if the child is younger than 4 years at the time of initial immunization.[1]
Pneumococcal	For children older than 2 years of age with sickle cell disease, asplenia, chronic cardiovascular and pulmonary disorders, nephrotic syndrome, renal failure, HIV infection, cerebrospinal fluid leaks, or those undergoing immunosuppressive therapy. Repeat the immunization after 3–5 years if the child is younger than 10 years and at severe risk for pneumococcal infection.[1]

access to health care, the lack of available primary care at hours when working parents can get there, inadequate education regarding the importance of immunization, and religious prohibitions. Currently, efforts to initiate, complete, and monitor immunizations in children are increasing. For example, managed care organizations require that contracted health care providers comply with the pediatric immunization standards, and patient records are audited to ensure compliance.

NURSING ASSESSMENT

Nurses are responsible for reviewing a child's immunization record and determining whether the child needs immunization. Inquire about the child's preventive care as well as health problems. Make sure you use the most current guidelines for comparison with the child's record. If the child is behind in appropriate immunizations for age, determine the best combination of vaccines to give at this visit to better protect the child. Also take advantage of opportunities to give needed immunizations to siblings accompanying the family on the visit, such as Lian in the opening scenario. A minor illness should not deter the nurse from giving an immunization to a child, such as Lian's brother Chang.

Many missed opportunities to immunize children have been identified. Children (and siblings present) should have their immunization status assessed during each health care visit. To reduce the number of missed opportunities for full immunization of children, use the following guidelines.[2]

CLINICAL TIP

Make sure vaccines are stored properly in the refrigerator or freezer. An improperly stored or poorly administered vaccine may be rendered ineffective, thus preventing the child from developing immunity. Read the package inserts of vaccines to determine proper storage conditions. Some vaccines are frozen; others are refrigerated. When reconstituting vaccines, it is important to use the solution provided or follow the manufacturer's directions. Write the date and time on the bottle if it is a multidose vial. Many reconstituted vaccines (eg, varicella vaccine) have a very short shelf life.

- Several vaccines—diphtheria, tetanus, and pertussis (DTP), measles, mumps, and rubella (MMR), hepatitis B (HBV), *Haemophilus influenzae* type b (Hib), and oral or inactivated polio (OPV or IPV) vaccines—can be given at the same visit.

- Two injections can be given in different sites on the same extremity.
- Immunizations can be given when the child has a minor illness with or without a low-grade fever, and with antibiotic treatment. Recent exposure to an infectious disease is *not* a reason to defer a vaccine.
- Premature infants have the same requirements for immunizations as full-term infants.
- Immunizations can be given when there was a local reaction to a prior vaccine or a family member had an adverse response.

True contraindications for a vaccine are an anaphylactic reaction to the vaccine or one of its components and a moderate to severe acute illness. Some additional contraindications for specific vaccines may also exist, such as pregnancy and allergy to some components of the vaccine (eg, neomycin, eggs) (see Table 10–3).

Assess the child for potential contraindications to vaccines. Inquire about past reactions to vaccines as well as allergy to key vaccine components such as eggs or neomycin. Determine whether female teens could be pregnant.

Text continues on page 377.

NURSING ALERT

The inactivated poliovirus vaccine (IPV) is the only vaccine that should be used for immunocompromised persons and their household contacts. Some cases of paralytic polio in immunocompromised individuals and healthy children resulted after exclusive use of the oral polio vaccine (OPV). The new immunization guidelines permit parents and providers to choose among three options to fully immunize a child against poliomyelitis, using either vaccine exclusively or giving two doses of IPV followed by two doses of OPV.

10-3   Common Pediatric Immunizations

Immunization Type	Side Effects	Contraindications	Nursing Considerations
Diphtheria and Pertussis Vaccines and Tetanus Toxoid (DTP or DTaP)			
Route: Intramuscular *Dosage:* 0.5 mL *Age(s) Given:* 2, 4, 6, 15–18 months; 4–6 years (five doses) *Storage:* Store in body of refrigerator at 2°–8°C (35°–46°F). Do not freeze.	*Common:* Redness, pain, nodule at injection site; temperature up to 38.3°C (101°F); drowsiness; fussiness; anorexia *Serious:* Anaphylaxis; shock or collapse; residual seizure disorder; fever above 38.8°C (102°F); persistent inconsolable crying	Occurrence of a serious side effect after previous administration of DTP or DTaP, such as anaphylaxis. Administration to be delayed for 1 month after immunosuppressive therapy and until moderate to severe febrile illnesses have resolved. Administration of immune serum globulin within last 90 days.	Prior to immunization, ask about previous reactions to immunization. Ask for history of seizures or neurologic diseases. In children with a history of seizures with or without fever, give acetaminophen at the time of the vaccine and then every 4 hours for 24 hours. Shake vaccine before drawing. Solution will be cloudy. Td is used in children over 7 years of age and in adults. Acellular pertussis preparation has a lower incidence of some side effects and may be used for all doses. When required, simultaneous administration of tetanus immune globulin or diphtheria antitoxin should be given in separate sites with a new needle and syringe.

Continued . . .

10-3 Common Pediatric Immunizations (continued)

Immunization Type	Side Effects	Contraindications	Nursing Considerations
Poliovirus Vaccine Live Oral Trivalent (OPV) *Route:* Oral *Dosage:* 0.5 mL, or drops, or entire contents of single-dose dispenser *Age(s) Given:* 2, 4, 12–18 months; 4–6 years (four doses) *Storage:* Keep frozen at –10°C (14°F). Refreeze thawed container if temperature did not exceed 8°C (46°F) during thaw period. Vial can go through maximum of 10 thaw/freeze cycles. Alternatively, thawed vial can be stored in refrigerator at 2°–8°C (35°–46°F) for maximum of 30 days.	*Common:* None *Serious:* Paralytic polio disease in child or caregiver	Immunosuppression or lack of acquired immunity of infant or caregiver. If a family member is immunosuppressed, infant or child can be immunized with injectable inactivated polio vaccine rather than OPV. Pregnancy.	Prior to immunization, ask if child or family members are immunosuppressed or have been immunized. Live virus vaccine must be handled carefully. Wipe spill from surface. Instruct parents that caregivers must wash hands carefully after diaper changes for first month to avoid transmission of live virus from infant's stool to nonimmunized caregiver.
Poliovirus Vaccine Inactivated (IPV) *Route:* Subcutaneous *Dosage:* 0.5 mL *Age(s) Given:* 2, 4, 12–18 months; 4–6 years (four doses) *Storage:* Store in body of refrigerator at 2°–8°C (35°–46°F). Do not freeze.	*Common:* Swelling and tenderness, irritability, tiredness *Serious:* Anaphylaxis	Hypersensitivity to vaccine components: neomycin, streptomycin, polymyxin B. Anaphylactic response.	Prior to immunization, ask if the child has an allergy to neomycin, streptomycin, or polymyxin B. Recommended for all doses when the child or a caretaker is immunodeficient or immunosuppressed. May be used as first 2 polio vaccine doses in all children.
Measles, Mumps, Rubella Vaccines (MMR) *Route:* Subcutaneous *Dosage:* 0.5 mL *Age(s) Given:* 12–15 months; 4–6 years (two doses) *Storage:* Store in body of refrigerator at 2°–8°C (35°–46°F). When reconstituted, keep refrigerated and away from light; discard if unused within 8 hours. Diluent is stored at room temperature.	*Common:* Elevated temperature 5–12 days after immunization; redness or pain at injection site; noncontagious rash; joint pain *Serious:* Anaphylaxis; encephalopathy, residual seizure disorder	Allergy to neomycin, eggs. Impaired immune system due to malignancy, immune deficiency disease, or immunosuppressive therapy. Measles vaccine is recommended for those infected with HIV. Administration of immune serum globulin or blood products in past 3–11 months. Pregnancy.	Prior to immunization, ask if child has allergy to eggs or neomycin. Inquire about immunosuppression. Instruct adolescent girls of childbearing age to avoid pregnancy for 3 months after immunization. Giver tuberculosis (TB) test at same time as MMR or 4–6 weeks later.

10-3   Common Pediatric Immunizations (continued)

Immunization Type	Side Effects	Contraindications	Nursing Considerations
Hepatitis B Vaccine (HB) *Route:* Intramuscular *Dosage:* Engerix-B: 0.5 mL or Recombivax HB: 0.5 mL *Age(s) Given:* Birth–2 months; 1 month after first dose; 6 months after first dose; or birth–2 months, 1–4 months, and 6–18 months (three doses) *Storage:* Store in body of refrigerator at 2°–8°C (35°–46°F). Do not freeze.	*Common:* Pain or redness at injection site; headache; photophobia; altered liver enzymes *Serious:* Anaphylaxis	Prior anaphylaxis, liver abnormalities. Serious allergic reaction to past dose.	Prior to immunization, check status of mother's hepatitis B test and presence of other liver disease. *Note:* If mother has HBsAg+, vaccine must be given to infant within 12 hours of birth along with hepatitis B immune globulin at the same time in another site. Shake vaccine before withdrawing. Solution will appear cloudy. Various formulations (pediatric, adult, dialysis) are available in different strengths. Read package insert carefully to determine proper dosage for age for the particular formulation used.
***Haemophilus influenza* Type B (Hib)** *Route:* Intramuscular *Dosage:* 0.5 mL *Age(s) Given:* 2, 4, 6, 12–15 months; (four doses for HbOC[a] and PRP-T[a]); or 2, 4, 12–15 months (three doses for PRP-OMP[a]) *Storage:* Store in body of refrigerator at 2°–8°C (35°–46°F). Do not freeze.	*Common:* Pain, redness, or swelling at site *Serious:* Anaphylaxis (extremely rare)	Prior anaphylactic reaction to this vaccine.	Prior to immunizations, ask if child is immunosuppressed. Since schedules for products of different companies vary, it is important to read package insert carefully. New preparations have become available that combine DTP and Hib as well as DTaP and Hib.
Varicella Virus Vaccine *Route:* Subcutaneous *Dosage:* 0.5 mL *Age(s) Given:* 12–18 months; or any time up to 12 years of age (one dose); 13 years or older (two doses 4–8 weeks apart) *Storage:* Frozen at −15°–5°F. May be stored in refrigerator up to 72 hours before reconstitution. Once reconstituted, vaccine must be used within 30 minutes or discarded. Do not refreeze. Diluent kept at room temperature	*Common:* Pain or redness at injection site; fever up to 38.8°C (102°F) in children or up to 37.7°C (100°F) in adults; rash at injection site or generalized *Serious:* Anaphylaxis	Allergy to neomycin or gelatin. Immunodeficiency or receiving immunosuppression therapy. Active untreated TB. Pregnancy. Moderate or severe febrile illness. Recently received blood products.	Prior to immunization, ask if child is immunodeficient or on immunosuppression treatment or had an allergic reaction to a past vaccine with neomycin components. Instruct adolescent girls of child-bearing age to avoid pregnancy for 3 months after immunization.

[a]Trade names.
Data from Bindler, R.M., & Howry, L.B. (1997). Pediatric drugs and nursing implications (2nd ed.). Stamford, CT: Appleton & Lange.

NURSING CARE PLAN
THE CHILD NEEDING IMMUNIZATIONS

GOAL	INTERVENTION	RATIONALE	EXPECTED OUTCOME

1. Risk for Infection related to incomplete immunization series

GOAL	INTERVENTION	RATIONALE	EXPECTED OUTCOME
The child will become adequately protected from vaccine-preventable illnesses.	• Review the child's immunization record for needed vaccines at each health care visit. • Identify all due vaccines that can be provided simultaneously. • Identify potential contraindications to needed vaccines. Review past reactions to vaccines given.	• Assessment identifies the children who have missed needed immunizations. • Many vaccines can be given at the same visit to more adequately protect the child. This also saves health care trips for families. • Reduces the risk for the child and other caretakers to have adverse reactions to vaccines.	The child is adequately protected from vaccine-preventable illnesses.

2. Knowledge Deficit (Parent) related to potential side effects of vaccines

GOAL	INTERVENTION	RATIONALE	EXPECTED OUTCOME
Parents will sign consent for vaccines to be given.	• Educate the parents about the need for specific vaccines and the risk if not given. Obtain signed consent before giving vaccine.	• Informed consent is required for all treatments.	The parent(s) complete(s) consent form, which is placed in the child's file.
Parents will state the side effects of vaccines given	• Review past reactions to vaccines and describe common potential reactions and why they occur. • Describe serious side effects that should be reported to the health care provider.	• Parents should expect common reactions and know they indicate the child's body is building protection to the illness. • Parents need to be prepared for potential serious side effects so they can obtain care.	Parents report all serious side effects to the health care provider.
Parents will manage common side effects of vaccines.	• Teach parents general comfort measures for children's common side effects; for example: 　• Cool pack to tender leg 　• Acetaminophen for fever and discomfort 　• Rocking and holding the infant 　• Gentle movement of affected extremity	• Parents will know how to make the child more comfortable during the 24–48 hours after the vaccine is given.	The child is given comfort measures after vaccine administration.

NURSING CARE PLAN
THE CHILD NEEDING IMMUNIZATIONS– *Continued*

GOAL	INTERVENTION	RATIONALE	EXPECTED OUTCOME

3. Risk for Injury related to vaccine reaction

GOAL	INTERVENTION	RATIONALE	EXPECTED OUTCOME
The child's potential vaccine reactions will be safely managed.	• Prepare for life-threatening reactions by having resuscitation drugs and equipment immediately available.	• Anaphylactic reactions must be managed quickly and effectively.	The child has no reaction or has a severe reaction to a vaccine that is managed effectively.
	• Monitor the child for 15 minutes after the vaccine is given before letting the child go home.	• A life-threatening response will usually appear within this time frame.	
	• Assess the child for extreme anxiety and injection fearfulness.	• These are potential signs the child may have a vasovagal response to the injection.	
	• Have the fearful child sit or lie down until symptoms of vasovagal response have disappeared.	• The child who faints may sustain a head injury.	
	• Report all vaccine-related reactions to the appropriate agency using the standard form.	• Legal requirement for all health care providers.	

Inquire about recent administration of immune globulin or blood products. Antibody response to vaccines may be decreased. Follow guidelines for administration of specific live virus vaccines (eg, measles, varicella).

NURSING DIAGNOSIS

The accompanying Nursing Care Plan explores three potential nursing diagnoses that may apply to the child needing immunizations. Additional nursing diagnoses may include:

- Ineffective Breathing Pattern related to anaphylactic response to vaccine
- Risk for Impaired Skin Integrity related to response to vaccine
- Altered Health Maintenance related to incomplete immunization series for age

NURSING MANAGEMENT

Nursing management focuses on informing parents about immunizations and possible side effects, addressing their fears about possible reactions, obtaining consent, and reporting adverse reactions.

LEGAL & ETHICAL CONSIDERATIONS

Federal legislation requires consent to be obtained before administering a vaccine. In most institutions it is the nurse's responsibility to inform the parents or the child's legal guardian, supply literature, and obtain written consent before the vaccine is administered. The nurse is required to record the (1) month, day, and year of administration, (2) vaccine given, (3) manufacturer, (4) lot number and expiration date of the immunization given, (5) site and route of administration, and (6) name, title, and address of the person who administers the vaccine. In addition, the nurse is obligated to report any severe immunization reactions to the state health department.

NURSING ALERT

Be prepared for potential vaccine anaphylaxis. Keep epinephrine 1:1000 and resuscitation equipment immediately available.

LEGAL & ETHICAL CONSIDERATIONS

The National Childhood Vaccine Injury Act of 1986 provides compensation if a link between immunization and a serious adverse effect is found. This act resulted after serious neurologic adverse reactions from the pertussis immunizations were reported, creating significant liability concerns for health care professionals. The Vaccine Adverse Event Reporting System was established in 1988 to track serious vaccine reactions (see Fig. 10–5 and Table 10–4).

Nurses should be strong advocates for immunization. Being well informed about immunizations, their potential side effects, and recommended schedules assists immunization efforts (see Table 10–3).

Provide written materials about immunizations to the parents or guardian. When teaching about immunizations, explain the risks and benefits of immunization, risks of disease, and common side effects and treatments. Record the child's history carefully, specifying any previous reactions to immunizations, allergies, and immune diseases.

Some parents have fears about immunization reactions based on stories they have heard. Talk with parents to understand their concerns. Be able to explain the risks and benefits of each immunization. Parents have the right to refuse immunizations for their child on the basis of religious beliefs, but they must sign a waiver noting their decision. If there is a disease outbreak, the nonimmunized child must be kept out of school. Local, city, or state courts decide how to settle any conflicts.

Obtain written consent to give the needed vaccines from the parent or guardian. Give the appropriate immunizations to the child as efficiently as possible, while providing support to the child (Fig. 10–4). Injections are always stressful to young children, and some older children will also react with anxiety. Do not prolong the process of giving immunizations, and give the child honest answers that the needles will cause some pain. Help the child cope by having the child select the arm or leg for the injection and forms of distraction. After the injections are completed, let the parent comfort the child. Schedule the child's next appointment for a health supervision visit to complete needed immunizations for age.

Certain reactions following immunization are reportable by law to the U.S. Department of Health and Human Services (Table 10–4). Follow guidelines for reporting according to the Vaccine Adverse Event Reporting System (Fig. 10–5). Provide parents with a record of the child's immunizations, and record the vaccines given in the health care agency's official records.

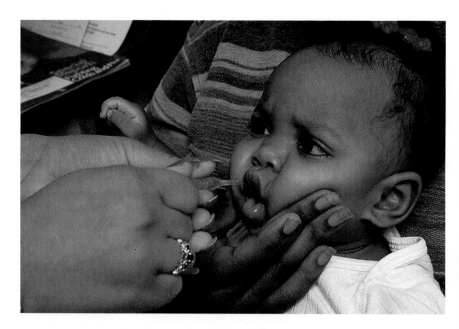

FIGURE 10–4. Give immunizations quickly and efficiently. Do not prolong the wait and let fear grow. The child will be anxious, especially if more than one injection must be given.

10-4	National Vaccine Injury Compensation Program—Vaccine Injury Table[a]	

Vaccine	Illness, Disability, Injury, or Condition Covered	Time Period for First Symptom or Manifestation of Onset or of Significant Aggravation After Vaccine Administration
I. DTP; P; DT; Td; or tetanus toxoid; or in any combination with polio; or any other vaccine containing whole cell pertussis bacteria, extracted or partial cell pertussis bacteria, or specific pertussis antigen(s)	A. Anaphylaxis or anaphylactic shock[b] B. Encephalopathy (or encephalitis) C. Any sequela (including death) of an illness, disability, injury, or condition referred to above which illness, disability, injury, or condition arose within the time period prescribed	4 hours 72 hours Not applicable
II(a). Measles, mumps, rubella, or any vaccine containing any of the foregoing as a component needed	A. Anaphylaxis or anaphylactic shock B. Encephalopathy (or encephalitis) C. Residual seizure disorder D. Any sequela (including death) of an illness, disability, injury, or condition referred to above which illness, disability, injury, or condition arose within the time period prescribed	4 hours 5–15 days (not less than 5 days and not more than 15 days) for measles, mumps, rubella, or any vaccine containing any of the foregoing as a component. 5–15 days (not less than 5 days and not more than 15 days) for measles, mumps, rubella, or any vaccine containing any of the foregoing as a component. Not applicable
II(b). In the case of measles, mumps, rubella (MMR), measles, rubella (MR), or rubella vaccines only	A. Chronic arthritis B. Any sequela (including death) of an illness, disability, injury, or condition referred to above which illness, disability, injury, or condition arose within the time period prescribed	42 days Not applicable
III. Polio vaccine (other than inactivated polio vaccine)	A. Paralytic polio —in a non-immunodeficient recipient —in an immunodeficient recipient —in a vaccine-associated community case B. Any acute complication or sequela (including death) of an illness, disability, injury, or condition referred to above which illness, disability, injury, or condition arose within the time period prescribed	 30 days 6 months Not applicable Not applicable
IV. Inactivated polio vaccine	A. Anaphylaxis or anaphylactic shock B. Any acute complication or sequela (including death) of an illness, disability, injury, or condition referred to above which illness, disability, injury, or condition arose within the time period prescribed	4 hours Not applicable

[a]Effective date: March 10, 1995.

[b]Anaphylaxis and anaphylactic shock mean an acute, severe, and potentially lethal systemic allergic reaction. Most cases resolve without sequelae. Signs and symptoms begin minutes to a few hours after exposure. Death, if it occurs, usually results from airway obstruction caused by laryngeal edema or bronchospasm and may be associated with cardiovascular collapse. Other significant clinical signs and symptoms may include the following: Cyanosis, hypotension, bradycardia, trachycardia, arrhythmia, edema of the pharynx and/or trachea and/or larynx with stridor and dyspnea.

Adapted from American Academy of Pediatrics In: Peter, G. (Ed.) (1997). Red Book: Report of the Committee on Infectious Diseases (24th ed.). Elk Grove Village, IL: AAP.

VACCINE ADVERSE EVENT REPORTING SYSTEM
24 Hour Toll-free information line 1-800-822-7967
P.O. Box 1100, Rockville, MD 20849-1100
PATIENT IDENTITY KEPT CONFIDENTIAL

VAERS

For CDC/FDA Use Only

VAERS Number _____

Date Received _____

Patient Name:	Vaccines administered by (Name):	Form completed by (Name):
Last First M.I.	_____	_____
	Responsible Physician _____	Relation ☐ Vaccine Provider ☐ Patient/Parent
Address	Facility Name/Address	to Patient ☐ Manufacturer ☐ Other
		Address *(if different from patient or provider)*
City State Zip	City State Zip	City State Zip
Telephone no. (____) _____	Telephone no. (____) _____	Telephone no. (____) _____

1. State	2. County where administered	3. Date of birth ___/___/___ mm dd yy	4. Patient age	5. Sex ☐ M ☐ F	6. Date form completed ___/___/___ mm dd yy

7. Describe adverse event(s) (symptoms, signs, time course) and treatment, if any	8. Check all appropriate:
	☐ Patient died......... (date ___/___/___ mm dd yy) ☐ Life threatening illness ☐ Required emergency room/doctor visit ☐ Required hospitalization (_____ days) ☐ Resulted in prolongation of hospitalization ☐ Resulted in permanent disability ☐ None of the above

9. Patient recovered ☐ YES ☐ NO ☐ UNKNOWN	10. Date of vaccination ___/___/___ mm dd yy	11. Adverse event onset ___/___/___ mm dd yy
12. Relevant diagnostic tests/laboratory data	Time _____ AM PM	Time _____ AM PM

13. Enter all vaccines given on date listed in no. 10

	Vaccine (type)	Manufacturer	Lot number	Route/Site	No. Previous doses
a.	_____	_____	_____	_____	_____
b.	_____	_____	_____	_____	_____
c.	_____	_____	_____	_____	_____
d.	_____	_____	_____	_____	_____

14. Any other vaccinations within 4 weeks of date listed in no. 10

	Vaccine (type)	Manufacturer	Lot number	Route/Site	No. Previous doses	Date given
a.	_____	_____	_____	_____	_____	_____
b.	_____	_____	_____	_____	_____	_____

15. Vaccinated at: ☐ Private doctor's office/hospital ☐ Military clinic/hospital ☐ Public health clinic hospital ☐ Other/unknown	16. Vaccine purchased with: ☐ Private funds ☐ Military funds ☐ Public funds ☐ Other/unknown	17. Other medications

18. Illness at time of vaccination (specify)	19. Pre-existing physician-diagnosed allergies, birth defects, medical conditions (specify)

20. Have you reported this adverse event previously?	☐ No ☐ To health department ☐ To doctor ☐ To manufacturer	*Only for children 5 and under*

		22. Birth weight _____ lb. _____ oz.	23. No. of brothers and sisters

21. Adverse event following prior vaccination (check all applicable, specify)	*Only for reports submitted by manufacter/immunization project*

	Adverse Event	Onset Age	Type Vaccine	Dose no. in series	24. Mfr./imm. proj. report no.	25. Date received by mfr. /imm. proj.
In patient	_____	_____	_____	_____		
In brother	_____	_____	_____	_____	26. 15 day report?	27. Report type
or sister	_____	_____	_____	_____	☐ Yes ☐ No	☐ Initial ☐ Follow-Up

Health care providers and manufacturers and required by law (42 USC 300aa-25) to report reactions to vaccines listed in the Vaccine Injury Table
Reports for reactions to other vaccines are voluntary except when required as a condition of immunization grant awards.

FIGURE 10–5. Vaccine Adverse Event Reporting System Reporting Form.

▶ INFECTIOUS AND COMMUNICABLE DISEASES IN CHILDREN

Infectious and communicable diseases cause acute illnesses. These diseases are caused by bacterial, viral, protozoan, or fungal organisms. As noted earlier, infants and children develop infectious and communicable diseases more frequently than adults do. They develop antibodies as they are exposed to infectious organisms, so they frequently become symptomatic after exposure. The epidemiology, clinical manifestations, treatment, prevention, and nursing care of selected infectious and communicable disease of childhood are described in detail in Table 10–5.

Text continues on page 400.

NURSING ALERT

Chickenpox can be fatal in immuno-compromised children. Children who are undergoing chemotherapy, steroid treatment, or transplant therapy should be carefully monitored after exposure to the disease. Varicella-zoster immune globulin is usually administered as soon as possible after exposure. A chickenpox vaccine is available and recommended for use in all children who have not had the disease.

10-5   Selected Infectious and Communicable Diseases in Children

Disease	Clinical Manifestations	Treatment	Nursing Management
Chickenpox (Varicella)† *Causal agent:* Varicella-zoster, human herpesvirus 3. *Epidemiology:* Peak occurrence is in the late fall, winter, and spring. Maternal antibodies disappear 2–3 months after birth. *Transmission:* Direct contact with lesions or airborne spread of secretions. *Incubation period:* 14–21 days. *Period of communicability:* As long as 5 days before the onset of the rash to a maximum of 6 days after the appearance of the first group of vesicles, when all lesions have crusted over. This period may be prolonged after passive immunization or in immunodeficient children.	The onset of symptoms is acute. Mild fever, malaise, and irritability occur before and with eruption. The rash begins as a macule on an erythematous base and progresses to a papule, then to a clear, fluid-filled vesicle, and then to a pustule. Lesions are often described as a "teardrop on a rose petal" and may erupt for 1–5 days. Lesions of all stages may be present at any one time. Crusts may remain for 1–3 weeks. Lesions in the mouth may lead to decreased fluid intake and dehydration. *Complications:* Complications are rare but can include secondary infection, encephalitis, varicella pneumonia, thrombocytopenia, arthritis, meningitis, and Reye syndrome. This disease may cause very significant illness or death to immunocompromised children.	There is no cure for chickenpox. Medical management is supportive. Acyclovir if started within 24 hours will decrease new lesion formation and the total number of lesions,[3] but this is not recommended for healthy children with uncomplicated chickenpox.[1] *Prognosis:* Most children recover fully. Children who are immunocompromised must be treated aggressively. *Prevention:* Chickenpox is a vaccine-preventable disease. The immunization may be given to susceptible children at any time after 12 months of age. Varicella-zoster immune globulin may be given to exposed immunocompromised children with no history of chickenpox.	• Use airborne and contact precautions for hospitalized children while they are contagious (usually a period before the lesions appear until all lesions are dry). Hospitalization is generally reserved for children with complications or other illnesses. Varicella history, especially recent exposure in susceptible children, should be obtained for all children entering the hospital. Children who have been exposed to varicella and require admission should be placed in isolation as a means of protecting immunocompromised patients. Nurses caring for the child should have a varicella titre done to be certain of their immune status if they have not had a documented case of chickenpox. • Most children are treated at home. While contagious, they should be isolated from all susceptible individuals, especially medically fragile or immunocompromised children or adults, and women early in pregnancy. The school or child care facility should be notified of the child's illness. • Give nonaspirin antipyretics to control fever. • Give oral antihistamines for relief of discomfort from itching. Oatmeal and Aveeno baths are soothing. Caladryl lotion applied in moderation to lesions may also provide relief.

Note: An asterisk (*) after the disease name indicates that a vaccine or antitoxin is available for use in high-risk or as-needed situations. A dagger (†) indicates that the disease currently has a safe and effective vaccine.

Continued . . .

Disease	Clinical Manifestations	Treatment	Nursing Management

Chickenpox (Varicella)[†] (continued)

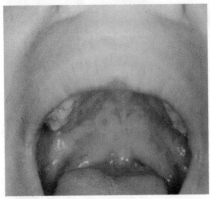

Mouth lesions of chickenpox.
Courtesy of Centers for Disease Control and Prevention, Atlanta, GA.

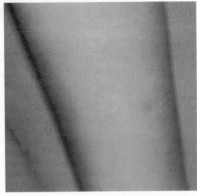

Skin lesions of chickenpox.

- Observe the child closely for drowsiness, meningeal signs, respiratory distress, and dehydration.
- Keep the child's fingernails short and clean. Young children may need to wear soft cotton mittens to prevent infections when itching cannot be controlled. Observe skin closely for evidence of secondary infection.
- Change bed linens frequently. Linen should be washed in mild soap and rinsed well.
- Watch for symptoms of complications.
- Disorientation and restlessness may indicate viral encephalitis.
- Reassure the child that the lesions are temporary and will go away. Children, especially of school age, fear disfigurement.

Coxsackievirus

Causal agent: Coxsackieviruses cause a wide group of acute diseases that range from minor and self-limiting to potentially fatal.

Epidemiology: Occurs worldwide, most commonly in summer and early fall. Sporadic outbreaks are seen, especially among children in out-of-home settings. Illnesses include the common cold; phar-yngitis; pneumonia; hand, foot, and mouth disease; and herpangina. Immunity probably occurs after clinical or subclinical infection, but duration of the immunity is unknown.

Transmission: Fecal–oral route; possibly respiratory route.

Incubation period: 3–6 days.

Period of communicability: 2 days before rash to 2 days after it disappears.

Each of the coxsackieviruses is responsible for a different set of manifestations. Herpangina is an acute, self-limiting viral disease characterized by the sudden onset of fever, sore throat, and small, discrete grayish papulovesicular ulcerative pharyngeal lesions that gradually increase in size. In hand, foot, and mouth disease the lesions are more diffuse and may occur on the buccal surfaces of the cheeks, gums, and sides of the tongue. Papulovesicular lesions occur on the hands and feet and last for 7–10 days. Children may be irritable and have a fever, anorexia, dysphagia, malaise, and a sore throat.

There is no specific treatment.

Prognosis: Recovery is generally good with supportive care.

Prevention: Avoid contact with infected persons early in the disease.

- Isolate the child while contagious. Use contact precautions if the child is hospitalized.
- Apply topical lotions and give systemic medications as ordered to lessen the pain and relieve any irritation.
- Offer cool drinks and soft, bland foods (no citrus, salty, or spicy foods). Swallowing may be painful.
- Offer warm saline mouth rinses.
- Observe for dehydration.
- Provide reassurance and support to parents.
- Give nonaspirin antipyretics for fever. Keep the child out of school or day care while the child is febrile.

Disease	Clinical Manifestations	Treatment	Nursing Management
Diphtheria†* *Causal agent:* *Corynebacterium diphtheriae,* a bacterium. *Epidemiology:* Occurs mostly during colder months in temperate zones in unimmunized, partially immunized, and immunized children with waning immunity. In tropical areas, cases of cutaneous and wound diphtheria occur sporadically. Maternal immunity lasts as long as 6 months after birth. *Transmission:* By contact with an infectious patient or carrier's nasal or eye discharge, or skin lesions; or, less commonly, indirectly by contact with contaminated articles. Unpasteurized milk has also served as a vehicle. *Incubation period:* 2–5 days, sometimes longer. *Period of communicability:* Varies but is usually 2–4 weeks or until 4 days after antibiotics were initiated.	Symptoms can be mild or severe. Low-grade fever, anorexia, malaise, rhinorrhea with a foul odor, cough, hoarseness, stridor or noisy breathing, and pharyngitis may be present. In more severe cases the membranes of the tonsils, pharynx, and larynx are affected. The characteristic membranous lesion is a thick, bluish white to grayish black patch that covers the tonsils. It can spread to cover the soft and hard palates and the posterior portion of the pharynx. Attempts to remove the membrane result in bleeding. *Complications:* Produces an endotoxin that causes myocarditis and neuropathy (diplopia, slurred speech, difficulty swallowing, or paralysis of the palate) or ascending paralysis similar to Guillain-Barré syndrome.	Administration of antitoxin and antibiotics within 3 days of the onset of symptoms. The child must be tested for sensitivity to horse serum before giving the antitoxin. When diphtheria is strongly suspected, antibiotic therapy (penicillin G or erythromycin) should be initiated without waiting for laboratory results. Removal of the membrane may be needed to treat airway obstruction. *Prognosis:* With treatment, prognosis is good. If untreated, diphtheria can cause death from airway obstruction. *Prevention:* Diphtheria is a vaccine-preventable disease. The immunization series is initiated at 2 months of age and is usually given in combination with tetanus and pertussis. Diphtheria-tetanus (Td) is administered to children over the age of 7. This is a reportable disease.	• Use droplet precautions for pharyngeal disease and contact precautions for cutaneous disease. • Monitor closely for signs of increasing respiratory distress, as well as cardiac and neurologic complications. Provide humidified oxygen as necessary. • Have emergency airway equipment readily available. • Administer antibiotics. Give no medications containing caffeine or other stimulants. • Use oral suction gently as necessary. • Allow children to use mouthwash if desired. Gargling is not permitted because it can irritate the back of the throat. • Encourage liquids as tolerated. Intravenous fluids may be necessary. • Provide emotional support to the family.

Continued . . .

10-5   Selected Infectious and Communicable Diseases in Children (continued)

Disease	Clinical Manifestations	Treatment	Nursing Management

Erythema Infectiosum (Fifth Disease)

Causal agent: Human parvovirus B19.

Epidemiology: Occurs worldwide, most often in winter and spring. The disease also occurs in epidemics, with peak activity every 6 years. The incidence is highest in children between the ages of 5 and 14 years.

Transmission: Respiratory secretions and blood.

Incubation period: 4–14 days.

Period of communicability: Believed to be the highest before the onset of the disease. Not contagious after rash appears unless in aplastic crisis.[4]

The child first manifests a flu-like illness (headache, nausea, body ache); 1 week later, a red rash appears. It begins on the cheeks as an erythematous, maculopapular rash that coalesces, giving a "slapped face" appearance. The rash is accompanied by circumoral pallor. In 2–4 days the second stage develops. A lace-like, symmetric, erythematous, maculopapular rash appears on the trunk and limbs and spreads from proximal to distal surfaces of the body. During the third stage, which lasts 1–3 weeks, the rash fades but can reappear if the skin is irritated or exposed to cold or heat. The rash may be mildly pruritic.

Complications: Children with diseases such as hemolytic condition may have transient aplastic crisis. The child has flu-like symptoms but not rash.

There is no specific treatment, and recovery is spontaneous. Children with hemolytic conditions may need blood transfusion if aplastic crisis occurs.

Prognosis: Fetal infection may occur resulting in spontaneous abortion.

Prevention: Avoid contact with infected persons early in the disease.

- Children are rarely hospitalized unless they have preexisting diseases. Isolation is needed only for children with aplastic crisis or when immunosuppressed. Use standard precautions.
- Antipyretics (acetaminophen) may be given to control fever.
- Use soothing oatmeal-based commercial bath products (Aveeno) if the rash is pruritic. Antipruritics may also help to relieve itching.
- Encourage rest and offer frequent fluids.
- Keep children out of direct sunlight if possible.
- Provide protective, light, loose clothing if exposure to sunlight cannot be avoided.
- Provide quiet diversionary activity. There is no reason to keep the child out of school or day care.
- Explain the three stages of rash development to parents.

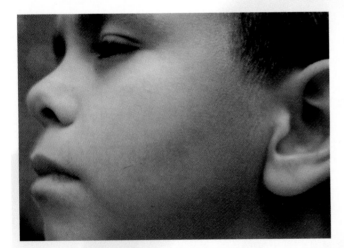

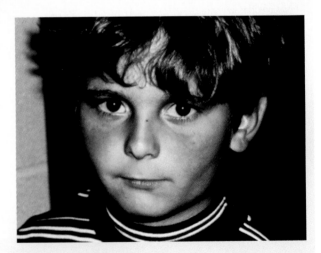

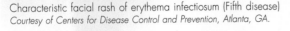

Characteristic facial rash of erythema infectiosum (Fifth disease)
Courtesy of Centers for Disease Control and Prevention, Atlanta, GA.

Disease	Clinical Manifestations	Treatment	Nursing Management

Haemophilus Influenzae Type B (H-Influenzae Type B; H-Flu Type B)†

Causal agent: Coccobacilli *H. influenzae* bacteria, which has several serotypes and can be encapsulated or nonencapsulated.

Epidemiology: Occurs most often in the spring and summer. Most commonly affected are infants and young children who are African-Americans, Native Americans, Alaskan Natives, or members of group settings such as day-care centers. Low-birth-weight children and children with chronic illnesses also have an increased susceptibility. The epidemiology is currently being altered with the introduction of the Hib vaccine.

Transmission: Direct person-to-person contact or droplet inhalation. The organism is frequently asymptomatically colonized in the respiratory tract.

Incubation period: Unknown.

Period of communicability: 3 days from onset of symptoms.

H. influenzae type B can cause several severe illnesses, including meningitis, epiglottitis, pneumonia, septic arthritis, and cellulitis. It is also a cause of sepsis in infants. Other illnesses include sinusitis, otitis media, bronchitis, and pericarditis. Each disease has very specific clinical manifestations.

Complications: Illness caused by *H. influenzae* type B responds to antibiotic therapy. Left untreated, severe sequelae and death, especially in young infants, can occur from conditions such as meningitis, epiglottitis, sinusitis, pneumonitis, and cellulitis.

Treatment consists of antibiotic therapy. Rifampin may be given to unprotected household contacts (not pregnant women) within 1 week after diagnosis.

Prognosis: With rapid diagnosis and treatment, the outlook for recovery is good but highly dependent on the disease the organism has caused. When treatment has been delayed, the prognosis for full recovery becomes much more guarded.

Prevention: Immunization is now available for *H. influenzae* type B as part of the recommended childhood immunization series beginning at 2 months of age. Although the vaccine has been available for only a few years, there have already been dramatic declines in illness caused by this organism.

- Use droplet precautions until 24 hours after the initiation of antibiotics.
- Antibiotic therapy is administered intravenously for severe infections. Infections such as otitis media can be managed at home with oral antibiotics.
- Children under the age of 4 years who have not been immunized are at increased risk for developing disease from *H. influenzae*. Specific prophylactic measures for susceptible children may be ordered by the physician.
- Administer antipyretics to help the child feel more comfortable.
- Closely monitor IV sites for patency and infiltration.
- Perform nursing care measures specific to the illness.
- Inform family members that rifampin turns urine and other body fluids orange.

Continued . . .

Disease	Clinical Manifestations	Treatment	Nursing Management
Hepatitis B[†] *Causal agent:* Hepatitis B virus (HBV), a member of the family Hepadnaviridae. *Epidemiology:* Occurs worldwide. In the United States, hepatitis B is seen in greater frequency among certain high-risk groups and among immigrants from areas of high incidence. High-risk groups include intravenous drug users; homosexual men; persons with multiple sexual partners; health care workers; funeral directors; household contacts of HBV carriers; patients on hemodialysis or who have received multiple blood transfusions, especially before blood product screening began; inmates in correctional facilities; and children in long-term care facilities.[5] *Transmission:* Primarily by body fluids, particularly blood, semen, saliva, and vaginal secretions. Exposure to blood or blood products and use of unsterilized needles. Sexual transmission is one of the most common methods of transmission.[6] Tatooing and sharing of toothbrushes. Perinatal transmission is a significant source of infection in the newborn. *Incubation period:* 45–160 days (average: 60–90 days). *Period of communicability:* During incubation period and throughout clinical course of disease.	Onset is insidious, with malaise and weakness. Muscle aches, anorexia, nausea, vomiting, diarrhea, jaundice, arthralgias, and vague abdominal discomfort may occur. Papular acrodermatitis may be seen in some children. *Complications:* Because diagnosis can be made only by serologic testing, hepatitis B may go undiagnosed and lead to chronic active hepatitis, which can severely affect the liver and eventually cause liver failure. Increased risk of liver cancer. 25–50% of children under 5 years of age become chronic carriers.[7]	There is no cure for hepatitis B. Treatment is supportive. Alfa-interferon injections may be used to treat chronic infections. Hepatitis B immune globulin may be given after exposure to unprotected persons.[8] *Prognosis:* Children may become lifelong carriers even if they have shown no signs of the illness. *Prevention:* Hepatitis B is a vaccine-preventable disease. The hepatitis B vaccine is now recommended for all children, anyone living in a household with a carrier, and all teens. All health care workers should be immunized. Blood supplies in the United States are now screened for HBV.	• Children with acute hepatitis B are usually not hospitalized. If the child is hospitalized, maintain strict isolation and use standard precautions when obtaining specimens and performing care. • Encourage the child to rest. • Observe sclera for change from white to yellow. • Observe closely for prolonged or unusual bleeding. Watch for bruising. • Provide high-calorie liquids and encourage small, frequent feedings. • Avoid medications metabolized by the liver (acetaminophen, sedatives, and tranquilizers). • Provide diversionary activities. • Educate parents about transmission. (Refer to Chapter 15 for further discussion of acute hepatitis.)

CLINICAL TIP

Hepatitis B can be transferred from mother to infant, either transplacentally during delivery or during breastfeeding if the mother has cracked nipples. Infection in the newborn often results in a chronic carrier state. An infant born to an infected mother should be immunized in separate sites with both hepatitis B immune globulin and hepatitis B vaccine within 12 hours of birth.

Disease	Clinical Manifestations	Treatment	Nursing Management

Lyme Disease

Causal agent: Borrelia burgdorferi, a spirochete, which is transmitted by ixodid ticks.

Epidemiology: Distribution in the United States correlates highly with the distribution of the various tick carriers (vectors). Animals such as dogs and cats can also have the disease. Lyme disease occurs year round, with the highest risk of infection in summer. Infection does not induce immunity.

Transmission: Tick bite. The tick transmits the infected spirochete when it draws blood. The tick must feed for 36 hours to transmit the disease.

Incubation period: 3–32 days after an infected tick bite.

The most typical early symptom is a slowly expanding red rash, called erythema migrans, at the site of the bite, often found on the groin, axilla, or thigh. The rash starts as a flat or raised red area and may progress to partial clearing, develop blisters or scabs in the center, or have a bluish discoloration. The rash has a red-ringed border and is at least 5 cm in diameter. In the first stage, symptoms include malaise, fatigue, headache, stiff neck, mild fever, and muscle and joint aches. Stage 2 occurs 1–4 months after the bite. The most common symptom of untreated disease is pain and swelling of the joints, most commonly the knee (Lyme arthritis). Stage 3 occurs months later and includes problems such as Lyme arthritis and central nervous system changes. These may become chronic problems.

Complications: Left untreated, Lyme disease can cause significant neurologic deficits, including arm and leg weakness, Bell's palsy, encephalitis, meningitis, and sometimes depression. Cardiac problems include mild congestive heart failure and AV block.

Antibiotics are the treatment of choice. Amoxicillin, cefuroxime axetil, or erythromycin are most often used in children 8 years of age or younger. Doxycycline or tetracycline is given to children over the age of 8 years. A 14–21-day course is given with required reevaluation to determine if a change in or continued use of antibiotics is needed to prevent progression to later phases because of relapse.[9] Intravenous antibiotics are often required in the later stages of the disease.

Prognosis: Lyme disease does not cause acute, life-threatening illness, but it may result in significant morbidity, especially when chronic.

Prevention: Avoid areas that are heavily tick infested, and wear protective clothing. Check for ticks (especially hidden in hair) after every outing. Check pets because they can carry home ticks that are then transferred to the child. Remove ticks as soon as possible. If symptoms develop, seek medical attention promptly for a child who has been bitten. There is no acquired immunity.

- Children with early disease are usually treated at home. Children with progressive symptoms may be hospitalized. Use standard precautions.
- Administer antibiotics. Tell parents to have the child avoid sun exposure when taking doxycycline. Nonaspirin analgesics and antipyretics may provide relief of mild fevers, headaches, and muscle and joint aches.
- Allow children to rest. Children with Lyme disease may tire easily. Vigorous activities may be difficult.
- Educate parents and children about the disease and early recognition of the symptoms. Teach them to safely remove ticks.
- Provide emotional support.

CLINICAL TIP

To remove a tick, grasp it gently but firmly with fine-point tweezers where the mouth parts are attached. Pull gently until it releases. Clean the area with soap and water. If any tick parts are left under the skin, take the child to a health care provider for removal.

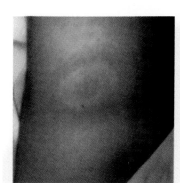
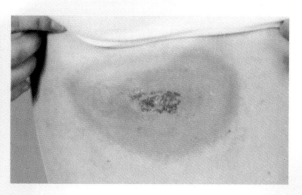

The appearance of the erythema migrans rash may vary in early Lyme disease.
From Pfizer Central Research. (1989). Lyme disease. Groton, CT: Author.

Disease	Clinical Manifestations	Treatment	Nursing Management

Measles (Rubeola)[†]

Causal agent: Morbillivirus, a member of the paramyxovirus group.

Epidemiology: Occurrence peaks in the late winter and early spring. In developed countries, measles occurs mostly in outbreaks among adolescents, which are largely the result of lack of immunization or possibly declining immunity. Maternal immunity is active in the infant until the age of approximately 12–15

Children are quite ill in the prodromal phase, with symptoms including high fever, conjunctivitis, coryza, cough, anorexia, and malaise. Small, irregular, bluish white spots on a red background, called Koplik spots, appear on the buccal mucosa about 2 days before and after the onset of the rash. The characteristic red, blotchy, maculopapular rash usually appears 2–4 days after onset of prodromal phase. The rash begins on the face and spreads to the trunk and extremities. Symptoms gradually subside in 4–7

There is no cure for measles. Treatment is supportive.

Prognosis: Recovery is generally good with supportive care.

Prevention: Measles is a vaccine-preventable disease. The measles vaccine is available alone (M), in combination with the rubella vaccine (MR), or in combination with the rubella and mumps vaccines (MMR). Immune globulin, administered up to 6 days after exposure, may be helpful in preventing the disease in susceptible persons (immunocompromised

- If the child is hospitalized, maintain airborne precautions during the contagious period (4 days after the rash appears).
- Use a cool-mist vaporizer to help clear respiratory passages.
- Suction nose and oral cavity very gently as necessary.
- Give nonaspirin antipyretics for fever and antipruritics for itching.
- Assess lungs carefully, especially in young children, in whom pneumonias are a common complication.
- Antitussives may be ordered to control coughing.
- If the child has conjunctivitis, remove crusting around eyes with tepid water.
- Keep lights dim, and cover windows if the child has photophobia.

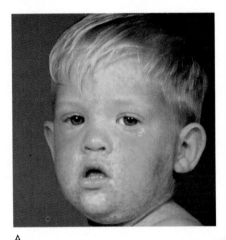 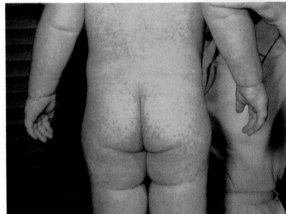

A   B

Measles, third day of rash. **A,** Facial rash. **B,** Posterior view.
Courtesy of Centers for Disease Control and Prevention, Atlanta, GA.

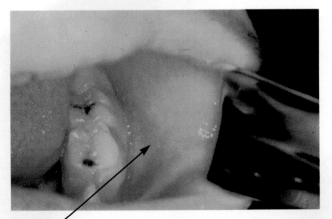

Koplik spots on oral mucosa, fifth day of rash.
Courtesy of Centers for Disease Control and Prevention, Atlanta, GA.

Disease	Clinical Manifestations	Treatment	Nursing Management

Measles (Rubeola)[†] (continued)

months. Vaccination induces lifelong immunity. In developing countries, measles remains largely an endemic problem and is a significant cause of infant and childhood morbidity and mortality.

Transmission: Airborne; respiratory droplets and contact with infected persons.

Incubation period: about 8–12 days.

Period of communicability: Begins during the prodromal phase and ends about 2–4 days after the rash appears.

days. Other symptoms include anorexia, malaise, fatigue, and generalized lymphadenopathy.

Complications: Diarrhea, otitis media, bronchopneumonia, bronchiolitis, laryngotracheitis, and encephalitis. Complications and sequelae occur most often in children who are malnourished, medically fragile, and immunosuppressed. The younger the child, the greater the risk for complications.

children, infants less than 1 year of age, pregnant women). All health care workers should have documented immunity.

This is a reportable disease.

- Elevate the head of the bed. Keep the room cool with good air circulation. Provide light, nonirritating blankets.
- Keep skin clean and dry. No soaps should be used.
- Offer cool liquids frequently in small amounts. Blended, pureed, and mashed foods are most easily tolerated.
- Maintain bed rest. Visitors should be immune to measles.
- Provide diversions such as music, stories, and favorite toys.

Mononucleosis

Causal agent: Epstein-Barr virus (EBV), a member of the herpesvirus group.

Epidemiology: Occurs worldwide. In developing countries, the disease occurs in young children and may be asymptomatic or mild. In developed countries, the disease is more common in older children and adolescents.

Transmission: Direct contact with infected oropharyngeal secretions (saliva, kissing). EBV can also be transmitted by blood transfusion.

Incubation period: 30–50 days.

Period of communicability: Virus is shed for up to 18 months after the clinical course of the disease.

In very young children mononucleosis may cause irritability, but be otherwise asymptomatic. A maculopapular rash may be seen in a few cases. In other children, the disease is characterized by malaise, headache, anorexia, abdominal pain, fatigue, and fever for 2–3 days, followed by lymphadenopathy and a sore throat. Splenomegaly may occur. Pain from swelling of the tonsils and lymph nodes may be significant.

Complications: Rare side effects include central nervous system symptoms such as encephalitis, aseptic meningitis, and Guillain-Barré syndrome. Splenic rupture, respiratory failure, and hematologic complications such as thrombocytopenia can also occur. In immunodeficient children, fatal infections or lymphomas can develop.

There is no specific treatment. Corticosteroids may be used to control tonsillar swelling and pain when there is impending airway obstruction. Antibiotics (penicillin or erythromycin) are used for secondary infections.[10]

Prognosis: After recovery, the virus remains latent in the lymphoid system. It can be reactivited during periods of immunosuppression. The child will be a virus carrier for life.

Prevention: No known prevention.

- Children are usually treated at home. Standard precautions should be used. Give antipyretics and analgesics for fever and sore throat. Offer warm salt water for gargling. Offer soft foods and encourage fluids.
- Maintain bed rest.
- Give adolescents a sense of responsibility by involving them in decisions about care whenever possible. Be sure to include parents and adolescent in discussions.
- Reassure adolescents who may be worried about keeping up with schoolwork that they can return to school when the fever is gone and swallowing is normal.
- Teens should avoid kissing until the fever has been gone for several days.
- Contact sports should be avoided until the liver and spleen are normal, usually in about 4 weeks.

Continued . . .

10-5   Selected Infectious and Communicable Diseases in Children (continued)

Disease	Clinical Manifestations	Treatment	Nursing Management

Mumps (Parotitis)†

Causal agent: A paramyxovirus.

Epidemiology: Occurs worldwide in unvaccinated children, most often in winter and spring. Infection and vaccination induce lifelong immunity. Maternal immunity begins to disappear in infants at the age of 12–15 months. Vaccine failure and lack of immunization have been implicated in cases occurring in vaccinated populations.[11]

Transmission: Saliva droplets and direct contact.

Incubation period: 12–25 days.

Period of communicability: 7 days before parotid swelling until 9 days after swelling subsides.

Malaise; low-grade fever; and earache, pain with chewing, decreased appetite and activity; followed by bilateral or unilateral parotid gland swelling. Swelling peaks around the third day. Meningeal signs (stiff neck, headache, photophobia) occur in about 15% of patients.

Complications: Orchitis (inflammation of the epidydimis, pain on testicular palpation, and scrotal swelling—most often unilateral) may occur in postpubertal males; sterility is relatively rare.[12] Oophoritis, pancreatitis, aseptic meningoencephalitis, and unilateral permanent deafness are sometimes seen.

There is no specific treatment. Therapy is supportive.

Prognosis: Mumps is usually self-limiting.

Prevention: Mumps is a vaccine-preventable disease. The vaccine is usually administered in combination with the measles and rubella vaccines (MMR) at 12–15 months of age and again at either 4–6 years or 11–12 years.

This is a reportable disease.

- Children are generally uncomfortable but are rarely very ill. They are usually treated at home.
- Use droplet precautions for hospitalized children while contagious. Avoid exposure to immunocompromised individuals or susceptible persons.
- Keep children out of school or day care until all symptoms subside. Encourage diversional activities.
- Give nonaspirin analgesics and antipyretics to control fever and pain. Give steroids if ordered. Encourage fluid intake. Swallowing and chewing may be painful. Offer soft and blended foods. Avoid foods and beverages that increase salivary flow (citrus, spices, and candies) because they cause pain.
- Talking may be painful. Provide a bell or other attention-getting device.
- Apply warm or cool compresses, whichever is preferred, to the parotid area.
- Be alert for signs of complications. Headache, stiff neck, vomiting, or photophobia may indicate meningeal irritation.
- Provide scrotal supports if testicular swelling occurs.
- Reassure children who may be upset about the facial swelling that it will go away.

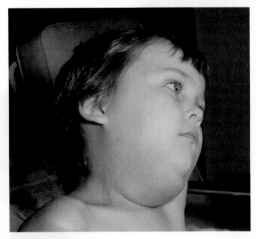

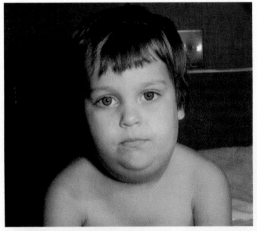

A   B

This child has mumps with diffuse lymphedema of the neck. **A,** Side view. **B,** Front view.
Courtesy Centers for Disease Control and Prevention, Atlanta, GA.

10-5 Selected Infectious and Communicable Diseases in Children (continued)

Disease	Clinical Manifestations	Treatment	Nursing Management

Pertussis (Whooping Cough)[†]

Causal agent: Bordetella pertussis.

Epidemiology: Occurs worldwide. Predominantly a childhood disease that is most common in children under 6 months of age. Pertussis also occurs in health care workers or adults who may have weakened or incomplete immunity. Adults may become only mildly ill but can spread the disease to unimmunized children.

Transmission: Respiratory droplets and direct contact with discharge from the respiratory membranes.

Incubation period: 7–21 days (commonly 7–10 days).

Period of communicability: Begins approximately 1 week after exposure. Pertussis is communicable for 5–7 days after the initiation of antibiotic therapy. The disease is most contagious before the paroxysmal cough stage.

The onset is insidious. The disease begins with a runny nose, followed by an irregular, nonproductive cough. The cough becomes more severe at night and changes into spasms of paroxysmal coughing followed by inspiration, stridor, or "whooping." (Young infants do not manifest the "whooping.") Sucking on a bottle may trigger the coughing spell. May be accompanied by flushing, cyanosis, vomiting, and dehydration from decreased oral intake. Coughing may last 1–4 weeks or more.

Complications: Pneumonia, atelectasis, otitis media, and seizures.

Treatment consists of antibiotics (erythromycin), corticosteroids, if ordered, and supportive care.

Prognosis: The disease is most severe in infants under 1 year of age, and most deaths occur in this age group.

Prevention: Pertussis is a vaccine-preventable disease. Active immunization should be given in early infancy. Health care professionals who are in close contact with infected children before diagnosis may need antibiotics to prevent transmission.

This is a reportable disease.

- Use droplet precautions until 5–7 days after the initiation of antibiotics. Most hospitalized cases occur in children under the age of 5 years.
- Closely monitor respirations and oxygen saturation. The smaller the child, the greater the risk for respiratory distress and apnea.
- Remain with the child during coughing spells, when hypoxic and apneic episodes are most likely. Give oxygen if ordered. Have emergency equipment readily available.
- Provide humidification. Gentle suctioning may be necessary.
- Give nonaspirin antipyretics as needed for fever.
- Encourage frequent rest periods.
- Allow the child to eat desired foods.
- Encourage the child to take fluids. The child may need IV hydration if oral intake is not tolerated.
- Provide emotional support to parents.
- Teach parents to watch for signs of respiratory failure and dehydration if the child is managed at home.

Continued . . .

10-5 Selected Infectious and Communicable Diseases in Children (continued)

Disease	Clinical Manifestations	Treatment	Nursing Management
Poliomyelitis[†] *Causal agent:* There are three serotypes of poliovirus. *Epidemiology:* Occurs worldwide. Polio primarily affects children, although some of the cases involve transmission to immunocompromised or non-polio-protected adults caring for infants who have received the live polio virus vaccine. The disease can be mild or severe. The vaccine induces lifelong immunity. The live poliovirus vaccine has been associated with paralytic disease (1 case/7.8 million doses) with the greatest risk occurring with the first dose.[8] *Transmission:* Primarily by the fecal–oral route, possibly respiratory. *Incubation period:* Usually 7–10 days (range 3–36 days). *Period of communicability:* Unknown. Infectious for up to several weeks before symptoms develop. The virus is shed in pharyngeal secretions for a few days and in the stool for several weeks.	Affects the central nervous system. Less severe infections may be limited to fever and stiffness in the neck or back, headache, vomiting, and sore throat. In other cases, fever, headache, stiff neck, Kernig or Brudzinski sign, decreased deep tendon reflexes, and progressive weakness occur. There may be respiratory difficulties, and an increased respiratory rate that may interfere with the ability to talk because frequent pauses are needed. Paralysis results from damage to neurons. *Complications:* Permanent motor paralysis, respiratory arrest, and post-polio syndrome.	Treatment is supportive. No chemotherapeutic agents that directly kill the polio virus are available. *Prognosis:* Respiratory complication is life threatening and involves 5–10% of all cases. Respiratory paralysis may lead to death. *Prevention:* Poliomyelitis is a vaccine-preventable disease. Children should be immunized with either the inactivated poliovirus vaccine (IPV) or the live oral poliovirus vaccine (OPV) according to the recommended schedule. OPV is excreted in the stool for about 1 month after administration. Young children should be kept away from immunocompromised, elderly, or unimmunized persons for 7–10 days after receiving OPV. This is a reportable disease.	• Use standard and droplet precautions in the hospital and keep the child on strict bedrest. • Observe closely for respiratory paralysis (ineffective cough, talking with frequent pauses, shallow and rapid respiratory rate). Have emergency equipment at bedside. Assist ventilations as needed. • Administer sedatives and nonaspirin analgesics as ordered to allow for rest and comfort. Moist hot packs may relieve discomfort. • Encourage fluids. • Position the child to promote body alignment. • Perform range-of-motion exercises to prevent contractures after the acute phase. • Provide emotional support. • Long-term orthopedic (physical therapy) support may be needed by some children.

10-5   Selected Infectious and Communicable Diseases in Children (continued)

Disease	Clinical Manifestations	Treatment	Nursing Management

Rabies (Hydrophobia)*

Causal agent: Rhabdoviridae, two types (urban, in dogs; wild, in wildlife).

Epidemiology: Occurs worldwide. Urban rabies is generally controlled by vaccination of domestic animals susceptible to the infection, especially dogs and cats. Rural rabies can occur in many wild animals, particularly bats, foxes, skunks, and raccoons.

Transmission: Infected saliva from bite of rabid animal. Virus enters the wound and travels along the nerves from point of entry to the brain where it multiplies and migrates along the efferent nerves to the salivary glands.

Incubation period: Highly variable (3–7 weeks; average, 6 weeks). This period depends on the amount of virus in the saliva, how close to the brain or major nerves the bite occurred, and how deeply the saliva penetrated the skin.

Children may be free of symptoms during the long incubation period. Initial acute symptoms include headache, fever, loss of appetite, and malaise. Painful contractures in the muscles used in swallowing lead to hydrophobia, a reflex contraction at the sight of liquid. Neurologic symptoms such as hallucinations, disorientation, periods of excitability (mania) and quiet, and seizures later occur. Usually results in death.

Animal bites should be washed thoroughly with soap and water and irrigated well. Suturing should be avoided if possible. Rabies immune globulin (RIG) or human diploid cell rabies vaccine (HDCV) should be given to all persons bitten by animals that may be rabid.[13] The vaccine is of no value once rabies symptoms are present.

Prognosis: If symptoms develop, no drug improves the prognosis. Only 7 patients with human rabies have survived with intensive care support.[1]

Prevention: Immunization with RIG and HDCV should be given as soon as possible after exposure. HDCV is repeated on days 3, 7, 14, and 28 days after the bite (5 doses). The HDCV series may be stopped if the animal is found free of rabies. Expert advice on the administration of these vaccines can be supplied by state and local health officials. Prevention also includes immunizing all domestic animals against rabies. Tell children to avoid contact with wild animals that seem friendly.

This is a reportable disease.

- Administer RIG and HDCV as ordered. Assist family with obtaining help to find and quarantine the animal for observation.
- Provide emotional support to the family while reinforcing the urgency for the vaccine and the need for a series of injections.
- If the child acquires rabies, he or she will be hospitalized.
- Institute standard precautions. The virus is transmitted primarily in the saliva and cerebrospinal fluid.
- Make the child as comfortable as possible.
- Keep liquids out of sight of the hydrophobic child.
- Use caution in the late stages of the disease when children are usually combative. Various medications, paralyzing agents, and sedatives may be used to provide relief. Coma and death occur after an exhaustive period of excitement and agitation that may last for days.
- Provide emotional support to the family.

 CLINICAL TIP

Any animal suspected of having rabies should be quarantined, if possible.[13] Rabies is diagnosed on the basis of history and clinical symptoms. The importance of history cannot be underestimated. Diagnosis is usually confirmed by fluorescent antibody staining of the dead animal's brain tissue.

Continued . . .

10-5   Selected Infectious and Communicable Diseases in Children (continued)

Disease	Clinical Manifestations	Treatment	Nursing Management

Rocky Mountain Spotted Fever (Tickborne Typhus Fever, São Paulo Typhus)

Causal agent: Rickettsia rickettsii, a bacterium that is transmitted by infected ticks.

Epidemiology: Rocky Mountain spotted fever (RMSF) occurs in most of the United States, southwestern Canada, and Mexico. In the United States most cases have been reported from the south Atlantic and south central states. Generally occurs between April and September. Most infections occur in children who are less than 15 years of age. Infection induces immunity.

Transmission: Transmitted by bites of ticks, principally dog ticks. There is no evidence of person-to-person transmission.

Incubation period: 3–14 days (most commonly 7 days) after bite of an infected tick.

RMSF is a multisystem disease that can be mild, moderate, or severe. Onset may be gradual or rapid. Children may be very ill. Sudden onset is characterized by a moderate to high fever that ordinarily lasts for 2–3 weeks, significant malaise, deep muscle pain, severe headache, chills, and conjunctival injection. The characteristic rash, which usually appears between the third and fifth days, starts on the extremities, including the palms and soles, and moves to the trunk. Initially the rash is maculopapular and blanches with pressure. It later becomes petechial and more defined; it is rarely pruritic. The child may have splenomegaly, hepatomegaly, and jaundice.

Complications: In severe cases bleeding from disseminated intravascular coagulation (DIC) can be significant. Gastrointestinal symptoms often occur early in the disease. Pulmonary complications, especially pneumonitis, are common and can become life threatening. Central nervous system involvement can cause significant encephalitis and overall severe neurologic dysfunction. Cardiac and renal complications can also occur, leading to shock in severe cases.

Treatment consists of antibiotics, such as chloramphenicol, and doxycycline.[1]

Prognosis: Without early recognition and treatment, morbidity is significant and mortality in children is usually less than 20%.[14] If the rash occurs late or not at all, the disease is likely to be more severe.

Prevention: Avoid areas that are heavily tick infested, and wear protective clothing. Check for ticks and if found remove promptly. Seek medical attention promptly for a child who has been bitten and becomes symptomatic.

- Use standard precautions.
- Children may require prolonged hospitalization, including monitoring in the intensive care unit.
- Have hemodynamic monitoring equipment and emergency supplies readily available.
- Administer antibiotics as ordered.
- Observe for any abnormal bleeding.
- Make the child as comfortable as possible. If the child is unconscious, support the extremities and keep the eyes closed and lubricated.
- Provide quiet diversional activities.
- Provide emotional support, and keep parents informed about the child's condition.

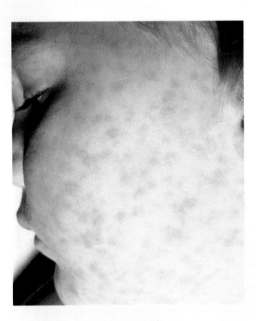

Rash of Rocky Mountain spotted fever.

10-5	Selected Infectious and Communicable Diseases in Children (continued)

Disease	Clinical Manifestations	Treatment	Nursing Management
Roseola (Exanthem Subitum) *Causal agent:* Herpesvirus type 6. *Epidemiology:* Occurs worldwide, primarily in children 6–24 months of age during the spring and summer months. *Transmission:* Unknown. *Incubation period:* Appears to be 5–15 days. *Period of communicability:* Unknown, but the child is probably contagious during the fever phase before the rash appears.	Sudden, high fever up to 40.5°C (105°F) for 3–8 days, during which the child does not appear toxic. The fever phase is followed by a characteristic erythematous, maculopapular rash, which starts on the trunk and spreads to the face, neck, and extremities. The rash can last for 1–2 days. The child's appetite is normal. *Complications:* Children may have febrile seizures.	Roseola is self-limiting, and there is no treatment other than supportive care. *Prognosis:* Roseola is benign in most cases.	• Children are rarely hospitalized, but if they are, use standard precautions. • Give nonaspirin antipyretics to control fever. • Observe closely for any seizure activity, especially during the acute febrile periods. • Encourage fluids. • Reassure parents that the rash will disappear in a few days.

Continued . . .

Disease	Clinical Manifestations	Treatment	Nursing Management

Rubella (German Measles)[†]

Causal agent: An RNA virus, member of the family Togaviridae.

Epidemiology: Occurs worldwide and is most prevalent in the winter and spring. Children are susceptible after loss of transplacentally acquired maternal antibodies about 6–9 months after birth. Natural infection or vaccination induces lifelong immunity. Congenital rubella syndrome is most likely the result of lack of immunization rather than vaccine failure.

Transmission: Droplet spread, direct contact with infected persons, or contact with articles soiled by nasal secretions.

Incubation period: 14–21 days (most commonly 16–18 days).

Period of communicability: From about 7 days before until about 4 days after the onset of the rash. Infants with congenital rubella may shed the virus for months after birth and should not be exposed to or cared for by persons who are not immune to the disease.

Rubella is generally a mild disease with a characteristic pink, nonconfluent, maculopapular rash. The rash appears on the face, progresses to the neck, trunk, and legs, and disappears in the same order. Symptoms include low-grade fever, headache, malaise, coryza, sore throat, and anorexia. Generalized lymphadenopathy involving the postauricular, suboccipital, and posterior cervical areas is common.

Treatment is supportive. Rubella is generally self-limiting in children.

Prognosis: Disease is usually mild and benign. Major risk is for the fetus if the mother is infected. Abortion, stillbirth, or death under 6 months are common (10% die after birth). Many other anomalies may be present, such as cardiac, ear, and eye deficits.

Prevention: Rubella is a vaccine-preventable disease. It is important that females of childbearing age be immunized because of the severe complications rubella poses to the fetus during the first trimester. All health care workers should have documented immunity.

- Children are usually treated at home and rarely require hospitalization. They should not attend school or day care while contagious, and they should be isolated from pregnant women. School and child care facilities should be notified of the child's illness.
- Maintain droplet precautions for contagious children. Maintain contact precautions for infants with congenital rubella until 1 year of age.[1]
- Give nonaspirin analgesics and antipyretics for any pain and fever.
- Allow children to choose what they would like to eat and drink. Encourage fluids.
- Provide quiet activities.

NURSING ALERT

Congenital rubella syndrome occurs in at least 25% of infants born to women who acquired rubella during the first trimester of pregnancy. Infants can be born with cardiac defects, ophthalmologic disturbances (blindness, cataracts), mental and physical retardation, deafness, and neurologic complications.

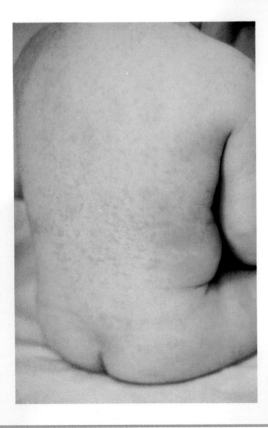

Discrete maculopapular erythematous rash of rubella.

Disease	Clinical Manifestations	Treatment	Nursing Management

Streptococcus

Causal agent: Group A streptococci (GAS).

Epidemiology: The illness is caused by various M-protein groups of group A alpha- and beta-hemolytic streptococci. In recent years severe infections have appeared, in some cases threatening life and limb. Different strains are associated with pharyngeal and pyodermal infections. Pharyngeal infections tend to occur more in late fall, winter, and spring. Pyodermal infections tend to occur in warmer seasons because of the association with minor skin trauma and insect bites.

Transmission: Airborne respiratory droplets, and direct contact.

Incubation period: Pharyngeal: usually 2–5 days.
Pyodermal: usually 7–10 days

Period of communicability: For weeks in untreated pharyngeal infections.

Pharyngeal: Onset is abrupt, with a sore throat, malaise, high fever, chills, headache, abdominal pain, anorexia, and vomiting. A beefy red pharynx with exudate (strep throat), and tender cervical nodes is seen. A characteristic erythematous rash associated with scarlet fever appears in some cases 12–48 hours after onset of symptoms, starting on the neck and spreading to the trunk and extremities. In 3–4 days, the rash begins to fade and the tips of the toes and fingers begin to peel. The classic strawberry tongue is seen on day 4–5.

Pyodermal: Lesions (impetigo) are honey-colored crusts at the site of open lesions.

Complications: If untreated, acute rheumatic fever, acute glomerulonephritis, toxic shock syndrome, bacteremia, and necrotizing fasciitis or myositis can occur. The incidence of severe, invasive GAS infections has increased in recent years.[1]

Prompt antibiotic treatment is effective. Penicillin is the drug of choice. Erythromycin is used if the child is allergic to penicillin. The fever decreases after treatment is begun. Uncomplicated impetigo is treated with bacitracin or mupirocin ointment. Invasive strains causing necrotizing fasciitis or myositis need surgical intervention (exploration and debridement of dead tissue). Clindamycin may be needed for toxic shock syndrome and necrotizing fasciitis.[15]

Prognosis: Recovery is usually good with antibiotic therapy.

Prevention: None.

- Children with uncomplicated streptococcal infections are usually cared for at home. Promote bed rest during the febrile state. Give nonaspirin antipyretics to control fever. Teach parents important signs of a worsening condition.
- For pharyngeal infections, offer warm salt water for gargling; a soft diet and nonacidic beverages. Encourage fluids. Provide cool, clear liquids. Swallowing may be difficult.
- Explain to parents the importance of the child's taking anitbiotics for the full number of days prescribed.
- Encourage other family members with sore throats to have throat cultures taken.
- For impetigo, teach the parents to wash the skin, remove crusts, and apply antibiotic ointment. If the child is hospitalized, maintain droplet precautions for pharyngeal infections and contact precautions for skin lesions for 24 hours after beginning antibiotics. Monitor vital signs, especially temperature. Administer antibiotics as ordered.
- If the child develops invasive streptococcal infection, use standard precautions. The child with toxic shock syndrome will need intensive care to manage shock and fluid and electrolyte imbalances.

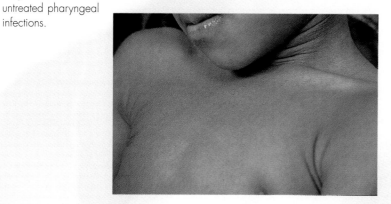

Skin rash of scarlet fever.

Continued . . .

10-5   Selected Infectious and Communicable Diseases in Children (continued)

Disease	Clinical Manifestations	Treatment	Nursing Management
Tetanus *Causal agent: Clostridium tetani* or tetanus bacillus *Epidemiology:* The bacillus is common and exists as a spore in soil, dust, and animal excretions. The organism produces an endotoxin that affects the central nervous system. *Transmission:* The organism is transmitted to humans through wounds in the skin from contact with contaminated soil or implements. Newborns can acquire tetanus via the umbilical cord if they are born in an unclean area or if a contaminated instrument is used to cut the cord. *Incubation period:* 3 days–3 weeks (average 8 days). *Period of communicability:* Not communicable to other individuals except through skin wounds.	Stiffness of the neck and jaw, with painful facial spasms over a few days. Spasms may be stimulated by noise or sudden movement. There is eventual rigidity of the abdomen and trunk. There is difficulty swallowing the increased oral secretions. Newborns have difficulty with sucking, progressing to an inability to suck, irritability, and nuchal rigidity. *Complications:* Laryngospasm, respiratory distress, death.	Tetanus immune globulin is given to unimmunized persons as soon as possible. Tetanus toxoid is given at the same time in a separate site. Medications are provided to treat muscle spasms. Intensive care is provided with cardiorespiratory monitoring, assisted ventilation, IV metronidazole or penicillin G, and supportive care. Survival beyond 4 days indicates an increased chance of recovery. Paroxysms become less frequent and complete recovery may take weeks. *Prognosis:* 30% mortality; much higher in newborns. *Prevention:* Tetanus immunizations are routinely given. They must be updated every 10 years, or, if a potentially contaminated wound occurs, in 5 years. Proper surgical debridement of wounds decreases the chance of infection.	• Prevent disease by checking immunization records and administering immunizations as necessary. • Give immune globulin to unimmunized persons. • Assist with wound debridement. • The child with tetanus is hospitalized. Use standard precautions. • Monitor the child's condition. Handle as little as possible. • Offer skin and respiratory care. The child may need an endotracheal tube for airway support. • Provide feedings via total parenteral nutrition or feeding tube. • Maintain hydration with IV fluids and electrolytes. • Try to reduce the child's anxiety, as mental status may be unaffected. • Prepare the family for a possible poor prognosis.
Tuberculosis See Chapter 11.			

10-5	Selected Infectious and Communicable Diseases in Children (continued)

Disease	Clinical Manifestations	Treatment	Nursing Management

Typhoid Fever[†] (Enteric Fever)

Causal agent: Salmonella typhi, a gram-negative bacterium.

Epidemiology: Occurs worldwide but is very rare in developed countries. Between 1% and 4% of patients who recover from typhoid fever become carriers. In underdeveloped countries, the disease is a significant source of morbidity and mortality, especially in school-age children. Clinical illness confers immunity.

Transmission: Fecal–oral route; ingestion of food and water contaminated with human waste. Transmission to the neonate from either the mother or medical personnel can occur at delivery.

Incubation period: 5–14 days.

Period of communicability: Variable. Typhoid fever is communicable as long as bacteria are excreted, usually from the first week until disease recovery.

Initial symptoms are malaise, high fever, chills, headache, cough, sore throat, anorexia, and abdominal pain. The fever ascends and after 7 days, reaches a plateau, at which point the patient is more ill. The child may have marked constipation or "pea soup" diarrhea. Older children may complain of muscle aches and headaches. Generalized lymphadenopathy, spleen and liver enlargement, bradycardia, conjunctival irritation, and abdominal distention and tenderness may occur. During the second week of the disease, discrete, rose-colored spots (caused by bacterial emboli in the skin capillaries) may appear on the trunk.

Complications: Intestinal perforation and hemorrhage, cholecystitis, urinary retention, pneumonia, and hepatitis are the most common severe complications.

Antimicrobial drugs of choice are chloramphenicol, trimethoprim/sulfamethoxazole, cephalosporins, and ampicillin.

Prognosis: With treatment the prognosis is good. Victims may become carriers who can be treated.

Prevention: Vaccines against typhoid fever are available. Immunization is advised for travelers to areas where typhoid incidence is high. Oral and injectable vaccines require boosters. Water supplies can be kept free from contamination by appropriate waste disposal.

- Use contact precautions. Wash hands after contact with excreta from the child. Proper disposal of gloves and gowns is necessary. Separate toilet facilities are necessary.
- Monitor vital signs, and examine chest and abdomen frequently. Observe for respiratory problems and intestinal perforation.
- Monitor intake and output. Encourage fluids. Administer intravenous fluids as necessary.
- Administer antibiotics.
- Maintain bed rest. Keep room quiet.
- Provide diversionary activities such as board games and videos when the child is feeling better.
- Instruct visitors not to use the child's toilet facility.
- Provide emotional support to the parents and family.
- The school or child-care facility should be notified of the child's illness.

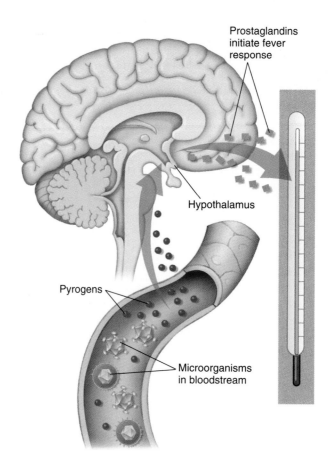

Prostaglandins
initiate fever
response

Hypothalamus

Pyrogens

Microorganisms
in bloodstream

FIGURE 10–6. The hypothalamus functions as the body's thermostat, directing the body to conserve or to dissipate heat. When microorganisms invade the body, endogenous pyrogens are released into the bloodstream. These substances travel to the hypothalamus, where they trigger the production and release of prostaglandins, which initiate the fever response.

CLINICAL MANIFESTATIONS

The child with an infectious or communicable disease will have several symptoms. Each disease has its own specific cluster of symptoms. Skin rash, poor appetite, malaise, vomiting and/or diarrhea, and body aches are some common signs and symptoms. Fever in a child is often a sign of infectious disease. Why does fever develop in response to certain illnesses and infections? What methods can be used to manage fever in children?

Physiology of Fever

The hypothalamus is the control center for the regulation of body temperature and is frequently compared to a thermostat because of its regulatory function (Fig. 10–6). As blood circulates through the hypothalamus, this brain structure regulates body temperature by directing body systems to conserve or dissipate heat, depending on the temperature of the blood.

- If body temperature is lower than normal, vasoconstriction is initiated to conserve heat. The adrenal glands produce epinephrine and norepinephrine, which cause an increase in metabolism, more vasoconstriction, and more heat production.

- Shivering or chills may occur, which in turn may increase heat production.

- When excess heat is produced, the body responds with an increase in temperature. The heart rate and respiratory rate increase.

CLINICAL TIP

One degree of temperature elevation causes an increase in respiratory rate by four breaths per minute and increases oxygen need by 7%.

- Vasodilation occurs and the skin flushes, becoming warm to the touch. As the temperature decreases, the child may start to perspire, and the heart and respiratory rates return to normal.

Endogenous pyrogens are released by macrophages in response to an invasive organism. These pyrogens travel through the circulatory system to the hypothalamus, where they trigger the production of prostaglandins. Prostaglandins are believed to raise the body's thermoregulatory set point, thus causing the fever to occur.[16]

DIAGNOSTIC TESTS AND MEDICAL MANAGEMENT

Diagnostic tests include cultures from sites where the infection may potentially be located (skin, pharynx, blood, urine, feces, cerebrospinal fluid, etc). In some cases x-rays or special imaging may be used to identify localized infection in an organ, such as the lungs.

For many infectious and communicable diseases, management is supportive. An elevated temperature can be a beneficial physiologic response, helping to eradicate organisms that thrive at lower body temperatures, and mobilizing the immune response. It may also enhance the effect of antibiotics. In addition, fever decreases the plasma iron concentration, which may limit the growth of microorganisms.[17] Fever is not inherently harmful until it reaches 41°C (105.9°F). For this reason, medical management may include postponing treatment of low-grade fevers under 38.9°C (102°F) to promote the body's natural defenses against an infection. If not managed, elevated temperatures can result in febrile seizures, which ususally have no long-term sequelae. Thus, fevers greater than 38.9°C (102°F) should be treated, especially if associated with discomfort. Persistent temperatures of 38.3–38.5°C (101–101.5°F) may also benefit from antipyretic treatment. Acetaminophen and ibuprofen are the preferred antipyretics for children. Aspirin is no longer recommended for children because of its association with Reye syndrome.

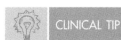

CLINICAL TIP

Antipyretics reduce fever by inhibiting prostaglandin synthesis, which results in lowering of the body's temperature set point.

Administration of antibiotics is often another component of medical management of infectious diseases. Before the introduction of antibiotics, children were often unable to fight infection and died as the result of overwhelming sepsis. Antibiotics have been responsible for decreases in morbidity and mortality from infections among children. However, strains of bacteria and viruses that are resistant to many antibiotics have developed. Children with chronic illnesses such as cystic fibrosis, sickle cell disease, and acquired immunodeficiency syndrome (AIDS) are particularly susceptible to infection by drug-resistant pathogens.

NURSING ASSESSMENT

Assess the child's hydration status and fluid intake, vital signs, comfort level, and appetite and observe for seizures and for a toxic appearance (lethargy, poor perfusion, hypoventilation, hyperventilation, and cyanosis). The child with a fever may be irritable and restless, sleep fitfully, and have nonspecific muscular pain. Identify those children who may be at higher risk for a serious illness in association with a fever,[18] in particular:

- Children having a toxic appearance
- Children less than 28 days of age with a temperature over 38°C (100.4°F)
- Children less than 4 years of age with a temperature over 41°C (105.8°F)

- Children with conditions such as a ventriculoperitoneal shunt, congenital heart disease, asplenia, and sickle cell anemia

Observe the child for other signs of infection, such as a rash, nausea and vomiting, and/or diarrhea, as well as generalized symptoms of a poor appetite and malaise.

NURSING DIAGNOSIS

The following nursing diagnoses may be appropriate for children with infectious and communicable diseases:

- Hyperthermia related to infectious disease process
- Risk for Fluid Volume Deficit related to the inability to drink adequate liquids
- Impaired Skin Integrity related to secondary infection of skin lesions associated with an infectious disease process
- Altered Oral Mucous Membranes related to infectious disease process
- Risk for Infection (Secondary) related to scratching pruritic lesions
- Fluid Volume Deficit related to repeated episodes of vomiting
- Knowledge Deficit (Parents) related to care of child with an infectious disease process

NURSING MANAGEMENT

Most children with infectious diseases are cared for at home; however, children may be evaluated in various health care settings.

Care of the Child at Home

Teach parents to care for their child at home. This includes how and when to give antipyretics and antibiotics if ordered, appropriate foods and beverages to provide, care of rashes, and other topical symptoms. Parents often fear fevers and need information and reassurance. Table 10–6 provides guidelines that parents can use in responding to fever in children. Help them to recognize the signs of the child's worsening condition in association with the child's specific disease.

Correct any misconceptions parents may have about the occurrence or cause of the infectious disease in their child. The parents may feel that they have exposed their child to certain germs or bacteria. Teach them that infection control in the home will reduce exposure of other family members to the infectious disease. Specific infection-control measures that parents can take include:

- Teaching good handwashing. This is one of the best ways to decrease the spread of infection.
- Disinfecting hard surfaces such as those touched by the child with a cold, diaper changing areas, diaper pails, and cribs.
- Telling children not to kiss pets on the mouth.
- Removing toys that the child has mouthed and disinfecting them before other children play with them.
- Making sure all children in the house are fully immunized.

CULTURAL CONSIDERATIONS

Many Latino and Asian cultures subscribe to the hot and cold theory of disease causation. Fever, a hot condition, is treated by giving the patient cold substances (foods or medicines). "Hot" and "cold" do not refer to temperature but to categories. Cold foods include vegetables, fruits, and fish. Cold medicines include orange flower water, linden, and sage.

NURSING ALERT

Make sure the family or caregiver gives the correct dose of antipyretic medication. Reinforce the following points: (1) Drops and elixir preparations do not have the same concentration. (2) Ibuprofen lasts 1–2 hours longer than acetaminophen, so it may be given less frequently. (3) Acetaminophen given in a dose of 15 mg/kg has the equivalent efficacy of 10 mg/kg of ibuprofen.

10-6   Parent Teaching: Guidelines for Evaluating Fever in Children

Call your health care provider immediately if:
- The child is under 2 months old or has a fever over 40.1°C (104.2°F).
- The child is crying inconsolably or whimpering.
- The child cries when moved or otherwise touched by the parent or other family members.
- The child is difficult to awaken.
- The child's neck is stiff.
- There are any purple spots present on the skin.
- Breathing is difficult and no better after the nose is cleared.
- The child is drooling saliva and is unable to swallow anything.
- The child has a convulsion.
- The child acts or looks very sick.

Call your health care provider within 24 hours if:
- The child is 2–4 months old (unless fever occurs within 48 hours of a DTP shot and the infant has no other serious symptoms).
- The fever is higher than 40.1°C (104.2°F) (especially if the child is under 3 years old).
- The child complains of burning or pain with urination.
- The fever has been present more than 24 hours without an obvious cause or location of infection.
- The fever went away for more than 24 hours and then returned.
- The fever has been present for more than 72 hours.

Modified from Hay, W.W., Jr., Groothuis, J.R., Hayward, A.R., & Lewin, M.J. (Eds.). (1997). Current pediatric diagnosis and treatment (13th ed.). Stamford, CT: Appleton & Lange.

Care of the Child in the Health Care Setting

Nursing care of children with infectious diseases in health care settings focuses on preventing the spread of infection. Children with suspicious rashes should be isolated from other children. When possible, hard surfaces in the examining room where the child was seen should be wiped down with antiseptic solution before another child uses the room. Linens are disposed of in appropriately marked linen bags.

Nursing care for treatment of fever includes administering antipyretics, removing unnecessary clothing, and encouraging increased fluid intake. Tepid baths or sponging may be ordered when the child's temperature is greater than 40°C (104°F) while waiting for the antipyretic to work. Use water that is about 26.6°C (80°F).

Children are often admitted to the hospital for treatment of severe infections. In addition, countless numbers of **nosocomial** (hospital-acquired) **infections** occur each year. The fecal–oral and respiratory routes are the most common sources of infections in children. All items with which the infected child comes into contact are considered contaminated (linens, toys, medical equipment, etc.). Transmission-based precautions, including isolation, must be implemented to reduce exposure of other children and staff to the infectious agent. Follow your facility's standard precautions and transmission-based precautions to reduce the spread of infectious diseases to staff and other patients. Bring any questions and concerns to your hospital's infection control nurse. (Refer to the *Quick Reference to Pediatric Clinical Skills* accompanying this text for more detailed information.)

RESEARCH CONSIDERATIONS

A recent study compared fever reduction in febrile children with temperatures of more than 38.9°C (102°F) when given acetaminophen alone or with a 15-minute tepid sponge bath. No significant differences were found in temperature between the two study groups over a 2-hour period. However, the children who were given sponge baths had significantly higher discomfort scores.[19]

Involve the parents by allowing them to assist with their child's care. Nursing care also includes treating infection, administering antibiotics on schedule, monitoring antibiotic blood levels if indicated to ensure appropriate results, and educating parents.

REFERENCES

1. Peters, G. (Ed.). (1997). *1997 red book: Report of the Committee of Infectious Diseases* (24th ed.). Elk Grove Village, IL: American Academy of Pediatrics.
2. Osguthorpe, N.C., & Morgan, E.P. (1995). An immunization update for primary care providers. *Nurse Practitioner, 20*(6), 52–65.
3. Asano, Y., Yoshikawa, T., Suga, S., Kobayashi, I., Nakashima, T., et al. (1993). Postexposure prophylaxis of varicella in family contact by oral acyclovir. *Pediatrics, 92*(2), 219–222.
4. Adams, D.M., & Ware, R.E. (1996). Parvovirus B19: How much should you worry? *Contemporary Pediatrics, 13*(4), 85–96.
5. Alter, M.J., Hadler, S.C., & Margolis, H.S. (1990). The changing epidemiology of hepatitis B in the United States: Need for alternative vaccination strategies. *Journal of the American Medical Association, 263,* 1218–1222.
6. Alter, M.J., & Margolis, H.S. (1990). The emergence of hepatitis B as a sexually transmitted disease. *Medical Clinics of North America, 74*(6), 1529–1541.
7. Ramos-Soriano, A.G., & Schwarz, K.B. (1994). Recent advances in the hepatides. *Gastroenterology Clinics of North America, 23*(4), 753–767.
8. Kline, N.E. (1997). Infectious diseases. In J.A. Fox (Ed.), *Primary health care of children.* (pp. 797–825). St. Louis: Mosby.
9. Gordon, S.L. (1994). Lyme disease in children. *Pediatric Nursing, 20*(4), 415–418.
10. Cozad, J. (1996). Infectious mononucleosis. *Nurse Practitoner, 21*(3), 14–27.
11. Briss, P.A., Fehrs, L.J., Parker, R.A., et al. (1994). Sustained transmission of mumps in a highly unvacci-

nated population: Assessment of primary vaccine failure and waning vaccine-induced immunity. *Journal of Infectious Diseases, 169,* 187–193.
12. Shulman, A., Shohat, B., Gillis, D., Yavetz, H., Homonnai, Z.T., & Paz, G. (1992). Mumps orchitis among soldiers: Frequency, effect on sperm quality, and sperm antibodies. *Fertility and Sterility, 57*(6), 1344–1346.
13. Centers for Disease Control and Prevention. (1992). Human rabies, California, 1992. *Morbidity and Mortality Weekly Reports, 41*(26), 461–463.
14. Hashmey, R., & Shandera, W.X. (1997). Infectious diseases: Viral and rickettsial. In L.M. Tierney, S.J. McPhee, & M.A. Papadakis (Eds.), *Current medical diagnosis and treatment 1997* (37th ed.). Stamford, CT: Appleton & Lange.
15. Denny, F.W., & Henderson, F.W. (1996). Group A invaders. *Contemporary Pediatrics, 13*(9), 104–115.
16. Sapir, C.B., & Breder, C.D. (1994). The neurologic basis of fever. *New England Journal of Medicine, 330,* 1880.
17. Thomas, V., Riegel, B., Andrea, J., Murray, P., Gerhart, A., and Gocka, I. (1994). National survey of pediatric fever management practices among emergency department nurses. *Journal of Emergency Nursing, 20*(6), 505.
18. Thomas, D.O. (1995). Fever in children: Friend or foe? *RN, 58*(4), 42–47.
19. Sharber, J. (1997). The efficacy of tepid sponge bathing to reduce fever in young children. *American Journal of Emergency Medicine, 15*(2), 211–213.

ADDITIONAL RESOURCES

Adcoch, L.M. (1992). A new look at measles. *Infectious Disease Clinics of North America, 6*(1), 133–147.

Advisory Committee on Immunization Practices. (1998). What's new in the 1998 immunization schedule? *Contemporary Pediatrics, 15*(2), 22–23.

Benenson, A.S. (Ed.). (1995). *Control of communicable diseases in man* (16th ed.). Washington, DC: American Public Health Association.

Broome, C.V., & Wenger, J.D. (1993). Decline of childhood *Haemophilus influenzae* type b disease in the Hib vaccine era. *Journal of the American Medical Association, 269*, 221–226.

Castiglia, P.T. (1996). Hepatitis in children. *Journal of Pediatric Health Care, 10*(6), 286–288.

Feigen, R.D., & Cherry, J.D. (1992). *Textbook of pediatric infectious diseases* (3rd ed.), Vols. 1 & 2. Philadelphia: Saunders.

Gildea, J.H. (1992). When fever becomes an enemy. *Pediatric Nursing, 18*(2), 165–167.

Groleau, G. (1992). Rabies. *Emergency Medicine Clinics of North America, 10*(2), 361–368.

Kamper, C. (1992). Treatment of Rocky Mountain spotted fever. *Journal of Pediatric Health Care, 5*, 216–222.

Kline, N.E. (1997). Infectious diseases (pp. 797–825). In Fox, J.A. (Ed.), *Primary health care of children*. St. Louis: Mosby.

Pauley, J.G., & Gaines, S.K. (1993). Preventing day care-related illnesses. *Journal of Pediatric Health Care, 7*(5), 207–211.

Salsberry, P.J., Nickel, J.T., & Mitch, R. (1995). Missed opportunities to immunize preschoolers. *Applied Nursing Research, 8*(2), 56–60.

Schmitt, B.D. (1996). When your child has hand, foot, and mouth disease. *Contemporary Pediatrics, 13*(11), 89.

Schmitt, B.D. (1996). When your child has mononucleosis. *Contemporary Pediatrics, 13*(4), 66–69.

Strebel, P.M., Sutter, R.W., Cochi, S.L., Biellik, R.J., Brink, E.W., et al. (1992). Epidemiology of poliomyelitis in the United States one decade after the last reported case of indigenous wild virus–associated disease. *Clinical Infectious Diseases, 14*, 568–579.

Torrigiani, G. (1993). Communicable diseases: A major burden of morbidity and mortality. *Vaccine, 11*(5), 570–572.

Walker, D.H. (1995). Rocky mountain spotted fever: A seasonal alert. *Clinical Infectious Diseases, 20*, 111.

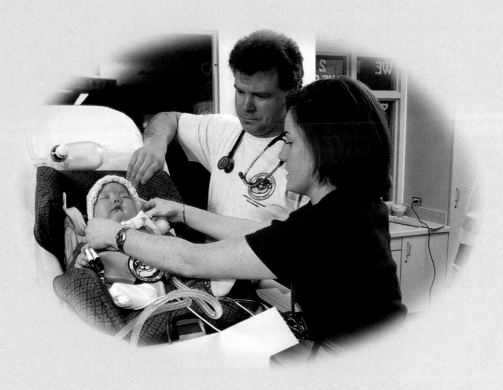

E
mily, an 8-month-old infant with bronchopulmonary dysplasia, is cared for at home by her mother. She has a tracheostomy and is hooked up to humidification. When Emily develops a fever, more secretions than usual in the tracheostomy, and labored breathing, her mother arranges for an urgent care visit to the pediatrician. Emily's mother knows how important it is to obtain prompt treatment for her daughter's respiratory problems.

When Emily is seen by the pediatrician, her temperature is 38.8°C (102°F), her respiratory rate is 50, and her heart rate is 130. Intercostal and substernal retractions are visible, and crackles can be heard over the lower right lobe. The pediatrician decides that a chest x-ray is needed. Because of the potential for Emily's respiratory difficulty to worsen, he plans to have her observed in the hospital's 23-hour unit. Intravenous antibiotics may be needed if an infection is confirmed by x-ray. The hospital's transport team is called to take Emily from the office to the hospital.

The transport team takes Emily to the hospital in a car safety seat strapped to a stretcher. This promotes safe travel and provides the proper position to assist breathing. Oxygen is administered to prevent hypoxia. Suction is available if needed. The trip by ambulance to the hospital takes only 20 minutes.

Why are infants with bronchopulmonary dysplasia at higher risk for respiratory problems? What are the signs of respiratory distress? What nursing care is required when an infant experiences respiratory distress?

ALTERATIONS IN RESPIRATORY FUNCTION 11

"During the transport, we will be monitoring Emily for signs of increased respiratory distress that could be caused by excessive secretions or a worsening condition. It is safer to transport a child with these problems with all of the treatment resources at hand, rather than let the mother take her to the hospital by car."

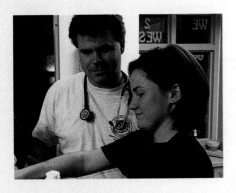

TERMINOLOGY

- **adventitious** Breath sounds that are not normally heard, such as crackles and rhonchi.
- **airway resistance** The effort or force needed to move oxygen through the trachea to the lungs.
- **alveolar hypoventilation** The condition in which the volume of air entering the alveoli during gas exchange is inadequate to meet the body's metabolic needs.
- **apnea** Cessation of respiration lasting longer than 20 seconds.
- **dysphonia** Muffled, hoarse, or absent voice sounds.
- **dyspnea** Shortness of breath; difficulty in breathing.
- **hypercapnia** Greater than normal amounts of carbon dioxide in the blood.
- **hypoxemia** Lower than normal amounts of oxygen in the blood.
- **hypoxia** Lower than normal amounts of oxygen in the tissues.
- **laryngospasm** Spasmodic vibrations of the larynx, which create sudden, violent, unpredictable, involuntary contraction of airway muscles.

- **paradoxical breathing** Severe respiratory distress in which the chest falls and the abdomen rises on inspiration.
- **periodic breathing** Pauses in respiration lasting less than 20 seconds; a normal breathing pattern in infancy and childhood.
- **retractions** A visible drawing in of the skin of the neck and chest, which occurs on inhalation in infants and young children in respiratory distress.
- **stridor** An abnormal, high-pitched musical respiratory sound caused when air moves through a narrowed larynx or trachea.
- **tachypnea** An abnormally rapid rate of respiration.
- **trigger** A stimulus that initiates an asthmatic episode; a substance or condition, including exercise, infection, allergy, irritants, weather, or emotions.

This chapter explores several special factors in the child's respiratory system that create ongoing threats to respiratory function and overall health. Most respiratory problems in children produce mild symptoms, last a short time, and can be managed at home. Nevertheless, acute respiratory problems are the most common cause of illness requiring hospitalization in infants and children under 15 years of age.[1]

Pediatric respiratory conditions may occur as a primary problem or as a complication of nonrespiratory conditions and may be life threatening or have long-term implications. Nurses must learn to assess the child's current respiratory status quickly, monitor progress, and anticipate potential complications (Table 11–1).

Respiratory problems may be a result of structural problems, functional problems, or a combination of both. Structural problems involve alterations in the size and shape of parts of the respiratory tract. Functional problems involve alterations in gas exchange and threats to this normal

---

11-1 | Assessment Guidelines for a Child in Respiratory Distress[a]

Quality of Respirations
- Inspect the rate, depth, and ease of respirations.
- Identify the signs of respiratory distress: tachypnea (abnormally rapid rate of respirations), retractions, nasal flaring, inspiratory stridor, expiratory grunting.
- Note lack of simultaneous chest and abdominal rise with inspiration (paradoxical breathing).
- Auscultate breath sounds: bilateral, diminished or absent, **adventitious** (sounds that are not normally heard, such as wheezes, crackles, rhonchi).

Quality of Pulse
- Assess the rate and rhythm: tachycardia may indicate hypoxia.
- Compare pulse sites (apical to brachial) for strength and rate.

Color
- Observe overall color: with respiratory distress, color progresses from pallor to mottled to cyanosis; central cyanosis is a late sign of respiratory distress.
- Compare peripheral and central color: assess capillary refill and nailbed color and inspect mucous membranes; central cyanosis in mucous membranes is more ominous.
- Note whether crying improves or worsens color.

Cough
- Quality: note whether dry (nonproductive), wet (productive, mucousy), brassy (noisy, musical), croupy (barking, seal-like).
- Effort: note whether forceful or weak; weak cough may indicate an airway obstruction or fatigue from prolonged respiratory effort (not valid in neonates).

Behavior Change
- Note level of consciousness: alert or lethargic
- Restlessness and irritability are associated with hypoxia.
- Watch for abrupt behavior changes (restlessness, irritability) and lowered level of consciousness, which indicate increasing hypoxia.

Signs of Dehydration
- Inspect for dry mucous membranes, lack of tears, poor skin turgor, and decreased urine output, which indicate that fluid needs are not being met.

---

[a]Refer to Chapter 3 for the actual techniques of assessment mentioned in this table.

process from irritants (such as large particles and chemicals) or invaders (such as viruses or bacteria). Alterations in other organ systems, especially the immune and neurologic systems, may also threaten respiratory function. As you read this chapter, keep the distinction between structural and functional problems in mind to help you understand what is normal and what is abnormal about the child's maturing respiratory system.

► ANATOMY AND PHYSIOLOGY OF PEDIATRIC DIFFERENCES

The child's respiratory tract constantly grows and changes until about 12 years of age. The young child's neck is shorter than an adult's, resulting in airway structures that are closer together.

UPPER AIRWAY DIFFERENCES

The child's airway is shorter and narrower than an adult's. These differences create a greater potential for obstruction (Fig. 11–1 and Table 11–2). The infant's airway is approximately 4 mm in diameter, about the width of

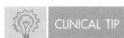

CLINICAL TIP

The diameter of a child's trachea closely approximates the diameter of the child's little finger. This "rule of finger" can be used for quick assessment of airway size.

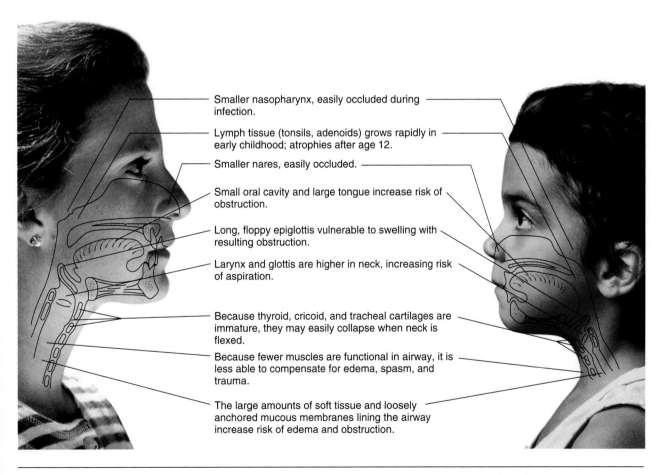

Smaller nasopharynx, easily occluded during infection.

Lymph tissue (tonsils, adenoids) grows rapidly in early childhood; atrophies after age 12.

Smaller nares, easily occluded.

Small oral cavity and large tongue increase risk of obstruction.

Long, floppy epiglottis vulnerable to swelling with resulting obstruction.

Larynx and glottis are higher in neck, increasing risk of aspiration.

Because thyroid, cricoid, and tracheal cartilages are immature, they may easily collapse when neck is flexed.

Because fewer muscles are functional in airway, it is less able to compensate for edema, spasm, and trauma.

The large amounts of soft tissue and loosely anchored mucous membranes lining the airway increase risk of edema and obstruction.

FIGURE 11–1. It is easy to see that a child's airway is smaller and less developed than an adult's airway, but why is this important? An upper respiratory tract infection, allergic reaction, positioning of the head and neck during sleep, and the small objects children play with can have serious consequences in the child.

11-2	Summary of Upper Airway Differences Between Children and Adults

Difference in Children	Significance
Small oral cavity and large tongue	Increases risk of obstruction; nasal patency is critical in infants
Rapid growth of lymph tissue (tonsils and adenoids) during early childhood, atrophy after age 12	Larger tissues in smaller pharyngeal structures; infection can easily cause obstruction of upper airway as lymph tissues swell in response
Larynx and glottis high in neck	Increases chance of aspiration
Thyroid, cricoid, and tracheal cartilages immature and incomplete	Easily collapse when neck is flexed, further narrowing airway; less protective of glottis
Large amount of soft tissue and loosely anchored mucous membranes lining length of airway	Increases likelihood of airway edema and obstruction
Long, floppy epiglottis	Vulnerable to swelling with resultant obstruction
Fewer functional muscles in the airways	Less able to compensate for edema, spasm, and trauma; may swallow more mucus than able to sneeze or cough out

GROWTH & DEVELOPMENT CONSIDERATIONS

Airway resistance in infancy is 15 times greater than in adults.[2]

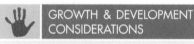

GROWTH & DEVELOPMENT CONSIDERATIONS

At birth the lung tissue contains only 25 million alveoli, which are not fully developed. The number of alveoli increases to 300 million by 8 years of age, after which these structures begin increasing in size and complexity until puberty.[2]

a drinking straw, in contrast to the adult's airway diameter of 20 mm. The upper airway primarily increases in length rather than diameter during the first 5 years of life.

The child's narrower airway causes an increase in **airway resistance,** the effort or force needed to move oxygen through the trachea to the lungs. As air moves from the child's nares down the trachea to the distal airways (alveoli), it must flow through a relatively small area. Friction and increasing resistance are generated as air passes through the airway. When edema and swelling occur in response to a virus, bacterium, or other irritant, the airway is further narrowed, increasing airway resistance even more. The trachea in a child is higher and at a different angle than the adult's (Fig. 11–2).

Physiologically the upper airway is the port for inspiration of oxygen and expiration of carbon dioxide. Infants, children, and adults can breathe through either the nose or the mouth. Until 4 weeks of age, newborns are obligatory nose breathers. The coordination of mouth breathing is controlled by maturing neurologic pathways; thus, young infants do not automatically open the mouth to breathe when the nose is obstructed. The only time a newborn breathes through the mouth is when he or she is crying. Nasal patency in newborns is therefore essential for such activities as breathing and eating.

LOWER AIRWAY DIFFERENCES

The child's lower airway is also constantly growing. The developing alveoli change size and shape, and their numbers increase until respiratory maturity is attained at 12 years of age. This alveolar growth increases the area available for gas exchange. At birth the distal (peripheral) bronchioles that extend to the alveoli are narrow and fewer in number than in an adult. The

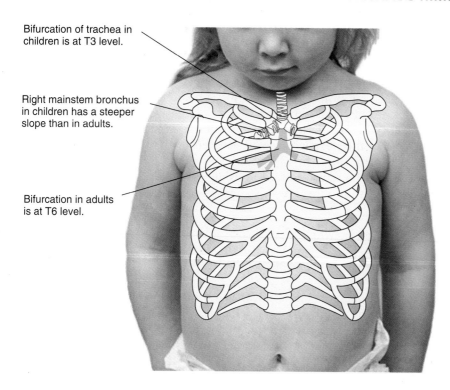

Bifurcation of trachea in children is at T3 level.

Right mainstem bronchus in children has a steeper slope than in adults.

Bifurcation in adults is at T6 level.

FIGURE 11–2. In children the trachea is shorter and the angle of the right bronchus at bifurcation is more acute than in the adult. When you are resuscitating or suctioning, you must allow for the differences. Do you think that this difference is significant in respiratory infection? Why?

child's overall growth can be correlated to the increased branching of the peripheral bronchioles as the alveoli continue to multiply. The taller the child, the greater the lung surface area.

The bronchi and bronchioles are lined with smooth muscle. The newborn does not have enough smooth muscle bundles to help trap airway invaders. By 5 months of age, however, sufficient muscles exist to react to irri-

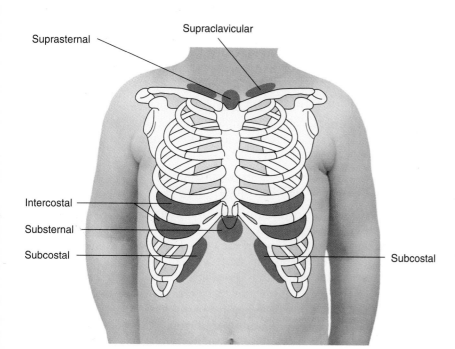

Suprasternal

Supraclavicular

Intercostal

Substernal

Subcostal

Subcostal

FIGURE 11–3. Retraction sites. Retractions may occur in the very young infant in the suprasternal area. In the older infant and child, retractions occur when the airway is severely obstructed, as in croup.

NURSING ALERT

The depth and location of retractions is associated with the severity of respiratory distress. Isolated intercostal retractions indicate mild distress. Subcostal, suprasternal, and supraclavicular retractions indicate moderate distress. These retractions accompanied by use of accessory muscles indicate severe distress.

NURSING ALERT

These signs and symptoms signal the body's response to increased metabolic demands for oxygenation as a result of stress or impending illness:
- Increasing restlessness, irritability, unexplained sudden confusion
- Rapid heart rate accompanied by rapid respiratory rate

tants by bronchospasm and muscle contraction. Smooth muscle development is complete and comparable to that of an adult by 1 year of age.[2]

The lungs, which have no muscles of their own, rely on the diaphragm and intercostal muscles to power respiration. Children up to 6 years of age are primarily diaphragmatic breathers. Because the intercostal muscles are immature and the ribs are primarily cartilage and very flexible, their efficiency in assisting ventilation is reduced. The chest wall is so flexible that the negative pressure created by the downward movement of the diaphragm draws in air, but in cases of respiratory distress causes the chest wall to be drawn inward, causing **retractions.** By 6 years of age, the child begins to use the intercostal muscles more effectively for breathing (Fig. 11–3).

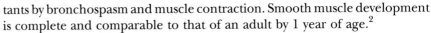

► URGENT RESPIRATORY THREATS

From the moment a child is born, airway integrity is threatened because of the immaturity of the respiratory muscles and neurologic system. Learn to recognize the early signs of respiratory compromise so that you will be able to intervene quickly to assist the infant in distress.

APNEA

Infants normally breathe with an irregular rhythm and may have pauses of up to 20 seconds between breaths. This **periodic breathing** should not be confused with apnea. **Apnea,** by definition, is cessation of respiration lasting longer than 20 seconds. Apnea may be the first major sign of respiratory dysfunction in the neonate.[3,4]

There are two types of apnea: apnea of prematurity (AOP) and an apparent life-threatening event (ALTE). AOP occurs in preterm infants, usually as a result of immaturity. ALTE (sometimes referred to as apnea of infancy) occurs in near-term or term infants. In the past, both AOP and ALTE were often called "near-miss sudden infant death" or "aborted crib death." These terms erroneously implied a close association between such episodes and sudden infant death syndrome (SIDS). SIDS should *not* be confused with apnea and is discussed later in this chapter.

Apnea of Prematurity

AOP may be caused by functional or structural problems. Functional problems involve neurologic and immunologic immaturity. Structural problems involve immature muscle development and coordination. Table 11–3 summarizes possible causes of AOP.

Apparent Life-threatening Event

ALTE is defined as an episode of apnea accompanied by a color change (cyanosis, pallor, or occasionally ruddiness), limp muscle tone, choking, or gagging occurring in a near-term or term infant who is greater than 37 weeks' gestation. These episodes may occur during sleep, wakefulness, or feeding. A variety of identifiable diseases and conditions can cause ALTE (see Table 11–3). In 50% of cases, however, no cause is ever identified. These cases are sometimes called apnea of infancy.[4]

ALTE can frighten the parent or observer, who often fears the infant has died. Emergency resuscitation is usually required.

11-3 Causes and Clinical Manifestations of Apnea of Prematurity and Apparent Life-threatening Event

Cause	Clinical Manifestations	Diagnostic Tests
Functional or structural airway problem or immaturity	Apnea of 20 sec or longer; accompanied by bradycardia or cyanosis	Cardiorespiratory monitoring, sleep study, sepsis workup
Aspiration as a result of dysfunctional swallowing or gastroesophageal reflux	Choking, coughing, cyanosis, vomiting	Barium swallow, esophageal pH probe
Cardiac problems	Tachycardia, tachypnea, dyspnea	Cardiorespiratory monitoring, electrocardiogram, echocardiogram
Drug toxicity or poisoning; maternal history of ingestion	Central nervous system depression, hypotonia	Serum magnesium level, toxicity screen
Environmental	Lethargy, tachypnea, hypothermia or hyperthermia	Cardiorespiratory and temperature monitoring, environmental temperature level (ambient air temperature)
Impaired oxygenation, respiratory disease	Cyanosis, tachypnea, respiratory distress, anemia, choking, coughing	Oximetry, chest radiograph, arterial blood gases, complete blood count, upper airway evaluation, sleep study, serum electrolytes
Acute infection	Feeding intolerance, lethargy, temperature instability	Complete blood count, cultures when appropriate
Intracranial pathology	Abnormal neurologic examination, seizures	Cranial ultrasound, computed tomography scan, electroencephalogram, magnetic resonance imaging
Metabolic disorders	Jitteriness, poor feeding, lethargy, central nervous system depression or irritability	Serum electrolytes, glucose, calcium

Modified from Eichenwald, E., & Stark, A. (1992). Apnea of prematurity: Etiology and management. Tufts University School of Medicine Reports on Neonatal Respiratory Diseases, 2(1), 1–11.

Nursing Management

After AOP or ALTE, infants are usually admitted to the hospital for 48 hours for evaluation and cardiorespiratory monitoring. Nursing care includes observing and monitoring cardiorespiratory status, providing supportive care to the infant and family, and anticipating the need for emergency resuscitation.

Monitor Cardiorespiratory Status
Cardiorespiratory monitoring records heart rate and respiratory rate while the infant is awake and asleep (Fig. 11–4). Transcutaneous PO_2 (oxygen saturation or oximetry) monitoring provides continuous evaluation of the infant's oxygenation status.

Provide Emotional Support
Establishing rapport and open communication with the parents is essential for creating a sense of trust. To obtain further information about the episode, use open-ended questions and active listening skills. Do not give parents the impression that their parenting skills are being judged or questioned. Parents experience fear and anxiety about the infant's prognosis. Explanations of tests and treatment help to decrease their anxiety and increase their understanding of the situation.

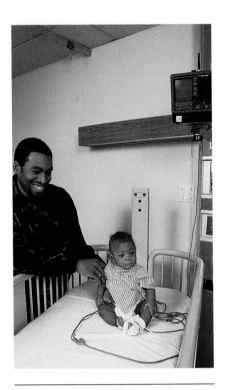

FIGURE 11-4. Infants who experience an episode of apnea are usually admitted to the hospital for cardiorespiratory monitoring.

During hospitalization the infant should be held and cuddled to provide a sense of security and well-being. Encouraging parents' participation in the infant's care helps to meet these needs and promotes family bonding. Often parents are afraid to touch the infant because they might disconnect the monitoring cable. Wrapping the cable inside the infant's blanket helps secure the wires, increasing parents' feelings of confidence in handling the infant.

Provide Tactile Stimulation

Tactile stimulation, such as rubbing the infant's back or feet, often is enough to halt an apneic episode. Continuous stimulation from an oscillating waterbed reduces the frequency of apneic episodes in some infants.[4] Both methods of stimulation remind the infant to take a breath.

Administer Medications

Methylxanthines (aminophylline, caffeine) or doxapram may be administered to stimulate the respiratory center in the brain. Infants have immature hepatic and renal systems, so the rate and efficiency of drug absorption and excretion are affected. Serum drug levels should be monitored frequently because the metabolism and distribution of the drug can be unpredictable.

Anticipate Emergency Resuscitation

Because the infant who has had AOP or ALTE continues to be at risk for cardiopulmonary arrest, emergency resuscitation equipment and drugs should be readily accessible at all times.

Discharge Planning and Home Care Teaching

Home care needs should be identified and addressed well in advance of discharge. Parents need to be taught how to operate an apnea monitor, what to do when the infant has an apneic episode (Table 11-4), and how to perform cardiopulmonary resuscitation (CPR) and choking-prevention techniques. (Refer to the *Quick Reference to Pediatric Clinical Skills* accompanying this text.)

SUDDEN INFANT DEATH SYNDROME

SIDS has been defined as the sudden death of an infant under 1 year of age that remains unexplained after a complete autopsy, a death scene investigation, and review of the history. It remains the leading cause of death in infants between 1 month and 1 year of age.[5] The peak incidence is between 2 and 4 months of age. SIDS occurs rarely in infants less than 2 weeks or older than 6 months of age. It is currently unpredictable and unpreventable. The first symptom is cardiopulmonary arrest.[6]

SIDS is referred to as a "syndrome" because of the many and varied autopsy and clinical findings that characterize most infants who die of the disorder. The autopsy typically does not identify a disease process that caused the death. Clinical findings include evidence of a struggle or change in position and the presence of frothy, blood-tinged secretions from the mouth and nares. SIDS occurs more often in the fall and winter and during periods of sleep. Most deaths are unobserved. Typically parents find the infant dead in the crib in the morning and report having heard no cries or disturbances during the night. A mild respiratory illness often precedes the death.

Although many reasons have been proposed for SIDS, including airway obstruction (as a result of anatomic, neuromuscular, and developmental factors), abnormal cardiorespiratory control, and hyperactive airway re-

11-4	Parent Teaching: Home Care Instructions for the Infant Requiring Apnea Monitoring

Apnea Equipment
- Understand monitor type, lead wires, placement of skin electrodes or chest belt, battery power, manual for troubleshooting.

Emergency Preparation
- Notify telephone company, electric company, local rescue squad, local emergency department (establishes priority status).
- Post phone numbers of rescue squad, physician, equipment company, power company, emergency number, cardiopulmonary resuscitation (CPR) guidelines, other important numbers (neighbor, parents' work numbers) in at least two places in the home; have at least one added extension phone.
- Keep the apnea monitor battery fully charged.

Safety Precautions
- Place monitor on firm surface; keep away from other appliances (television, microwave oven) and water.
- Ensure that alarms are audible from all locations.
- Double-check that monitor is *on* before going to bed.
- Thread cable and wires through lower end of infant's clothes.
- Ensure integrity of leads, monitor cable, power cord (replace if frayed).

Routine Care
- Understand reasons for apnea monitor and frequency of use.
- Be able to attach and detach infant chest leads and belt.
- Evaluate skin for irritation or breakdown from electrode placement and give skin care (no oils or lotion; move patches correctly).

Emergency Care
- Develop plan for respiratory failure and power failure.
- Demonstrate CPR and back blows and chest thrusts for airway obstruction.
- Understand how to respond to alarms for apnea, bradycardia, or loose lead.

Apnea Alarm
- Observe infant's respiratory movement.
- If respiration is absent or infant is lethargic, stimulate by calling name and gently touching, proceeding to vigorous touch if needed.
- If no response, proceed with CPR.

Bradycardia Alarm
- Stimulate infant; infant should respond quickly.

Loose Lead
- Check electrode patch. Is it loose? Dirty? Belt loose?
- Check wires from electrode or monitor cable.
- Check power supply. Is battery low? Power failure? Monitor malfunctioning?

---

flexes, the cause of the disorder remains unknown. Several infant, maternal, and familial factors appear to place infants at risk for SIDS (Table 11–5). SIDS has not been found to be associated with newborn apnea or immunizations for diphtheria, tetanus, and pertussis (DTP).

Nursing Management

The sudden, unexpected nature of the infant's death is confirmed in the emergency department. The nurse's role is to be empathetic and provide support during one of the greatest crises a family must face. The focus is on supporting the family during the acute grieving period (Table 11–6).

11-5   Risk Factors for Sudden Infant Death Syndrome

Infant
- Prematurity
- Low birth weight
- Twin or triplet birth
- Race (in decreasing order of frequency): most common in Native American infants, followed by African-American, Hispanic, white, and Asian infants
- Gender: more common in males than females
- Age: most common in infants between 2 and 4 months of age
- Time of year: more prevalent in winter months
- Exposure to passive smoke (reduces arousal to hypoxia)[7]
- History of cyanosis, respiratory distress, irritability, and poor feeding in the nursery

Maternal and Familial
- Maternal age less than 20 years
- History of smoking and illicit drug use (increases incidence 10 times)
- Anemia
- Multiple pregnancies, with short intervals between births
- History of sibling with sudden infant death syndrome (increases incidence four to five times)
- Low socioeconomic status; crowding
- Poor prenatal care, low weight gain

SAFETY PRECAUTIONS

Research shows a relationship between sudden infant death syndrome (SIDS) and sleeping on the abdomen. For this reason, the American Academy of Pediatrics now advises that infants be placed on their side or back for sleep. Over the past several years, the number of SIDS deaths has decreased. This decrease is thought to be related to the increased public awareness of this recommended sleeping position.

LABORATORY VALUES: RESPIRATORY FAILURE

Arterial blood gas levels indicative of respiratory failure are a PO_2 level less than 50 mm Hg and a PCO_2 level greater than 50 mm Hg.

Reassure the parents that they are not responsible for the infant's death and assist them in contacting other family members and mobilizing support. Older children may need reassurance that SIDS will not happen to them. They may also believe that bad thoughts or wishes about their baby brother or sister caused the death. Support groups can help parents, siblings, and other family members express these fears and work through their feelings about the infant's death. The SIDS Alliance and SHARE (see Appendix F) are organizations that can help families locate a support group in their geographic area.

Nurses can play an important role in educating the public about the link between SIDS and infant positioning during sleep.

RESPIRATORY FAILURE

Respiratory failure occurs when the body can no longer maintain effective gas exchange because of a functional or structural failure of the mechanisms of respiration. Other body systems may also contribute directly or indirectly to an increased workload, causing the respiratory system to fail. The clinical manifestations of respiratory failure are signs of respiratory distress: **hypoxemia** (lower than normal blood oxygen level) and **hypercapnia** (an excess of carbon dioxide in the blood) (Table 11–7).

The physiologic process that ends in respiratory failure begins with **alveolar hypoventilation.** Alveolar hypoventilation occurs when any of these factors exist: (1) oxygen need exceeds actual oxygen intake, (2) the airway is partially occluded, or (3) the transfer of oxygen and carbon dioxide in the alveoli is disrupted. This disruption may occur either because of a mal-

11-6 Supportive Care for the Family of an Infant with Sudden Infant Death Syndrome (SIDS)

Nursing Interventions	Rationale
1. Provide parents with a private area and a support person who reinforces that the infant's death was not their fault.	1. Parents need to be able to express their grief in their own way and know that they are not being blamed for the infant's death.
2. Prepare the family for the viewing of the infant. Describe how the infant will look and feel.	2. You can say "Paul's (use the infant's name) skin will feel cool. He will be very still and his eyes will be closed." They probably know this, but a gentle explanation demonstrates empathy. Explain that pooling of blood on the dependent areas will look like bruises.
3. Allow parents to hold, touch, and rock the infant if desired.	3. Viewing the infant allows parents a chance to say good-bye. Before bringing the infant to parents, wrap in a clean blanket, comb the hair, wash the face, swab the mouth clean, and apply Vaseline to lips.
4. Reinforce the physician's explanation about the need for an autopsy.	4. An autopsy is required for all unexplained deaths. You can say to parents, "It is the only way we can be sure of what caused your baby's death."
5. Answer parents' questions and provide them with sources for further information. Provide literature and a name of the local contact for a SIDS support group, as well as for the national foundation.	5. Parents may not be able to take in all of your answers. Many emergency departments and pediatric units have a social worker who provides ongoing contact with the family. Provide names of resource persons and phone numbers for SIDS support groups.
6. Advise parents that surviving siblings may benefit from psychologic support.	6. Siblings often require emotional support in the weeks and months after the death. Social workers can help the family obtain counseling and support for all members.
7. Provide parents with a lock of hair, footprints, and handprints, if they desire.	7. Personal items can be placed in a memory book. This reaffirms the child's existence for many parents.

function of respiratory center stimulation (the alveoli do not receive the message to diffuse) or because the alveolar membrane is defective (a structural problem).

Alveolar hypoventilation results in hypoxemia and hypercapnia. When the blood levels of oxygen and carbon dioxide reach abnormal levels, **hypoxia** (lower than normal oxygen in the tissues) occurs and respiratory failure begins. Signs of impending respiratory failure include irritability, lethargy, cyanosis, and increased respiratory effort such as **dyspnea** (difficulty breathing), **tachypnea** (increased respiratory rate), nasal flaring, and intercostal retractions.[8] Any signs of respiratory failure should be reported immediately.

11-7	Clinical Manifestations of Respiratory Failure and Imminent Respiratory Arrest

Clinical Manifestations	Physiologic Cause
Respiratory failure	
Initial signs Restlessness Tachypnea Tachycardia Diaphoresis	These signs occur because the child is attempting to compensate for oxygen deficit and airway blockage. Oxygen supply is inadequate; behavior and vital signs reflect compensation and beginning hypoxia.
Early decompensation Nasal flaring Retractions Grunting Wheezing Anxiety and irritability Mood changes Headache Hypertension Confusion	The child attempts to use accessory muscles to assist oxygen intake; hypoxia persists and efforts now waste more oxygen than is obtained.
Imminent respiratory arrest	
Severe hypoxia Dyspnea Bradycardia Cyanosis Stupor and coma	These signs occur because oxygen deficit is overwhelming and beyond spontaneous recovery. Cerebral oxygenation is dramatically affected; central nervous system changes are ominous.

Nursing Management

Early recognition of impending respiratory failure is the most important aspect of care for a child with any signs of respiratory compromise. The child who has even a slight degree of respiratory distress should immediately be placed in an upright position (by elevating the head of the bed). Assess respiratory quality and rate, followed by apical pulse rate and temperature. Oxygen administration equipment and respiratory emergency equipment should be kept at the child's bedside. Ensure that an order for oxygen is obtained or that oxygen is administered. Monitor the child for changes in vital signs, respiratory status, and level of consciousness. Be prepared to assist ventilations if respiratory status deteriorates.

Using Artificial Airways

Respiratory problems that do not respond to oxygen therapy, medications, or position changes require the insertion of an artificial airway. As the child's level of consciousness deteriorates, the ability to keep the airway open decreases. Endotracheal intubation is a short-term, emergency measure to stabilize the airway by placing a tube in the trachea. A tracheostomy is the creation of a surgical opening into the trachea through the anterior neck at the cricoid cartilage. Surgeons prefer to perform this procedure in the operating room; however, a tracheostomy may also be performed in an emergency department or other setting when the situation dictates immediate intervention. (Refer to the *Quick Reference to Pediatric Clinical Skills* ac-

NURSING ALERT

When the child has a chronic respiratory condition, development of respiratory failure may be gradual. Signs will be subtle. Be particularly alert to behavior changes in addition to respiratory signs. Serial blood gases may be needed to monitor the child.

companying this text for additional information on endotracheal and tracheostomy tubes.) These children usually require admission to the intensive care unit (ICU) for monitoring.

Because endotracheal and tracheostomy tubes prevent vocal cord vibration, intubated children cannot cry or talk. Infants and young children often express initial frustration when they realize they cannot communicate verbally. They often develop other noise-making behaviors, such as striking the mattress to gain attention. When time permits, the nurse should teach the parents and child what to expect before insertion of the endotracheal or tracheostomy tube. A communication board can be used with older children.

Many children are discharged from the hospital and cared for at home for an extended period with a tracheostomy tube in place. It is essential to teach parents how to maintain the airway, clean the tracheostomy site, and change the tube. A home health care nurse can provide follow-up care and support for the child and family.

▶ REACTIVE AIRWAY DISORDERS

Reactive airway disorders occur when airway tissue reacts to invasion by a virus, bacterium, allergen, or irritant. These invaders cause airway tissue to respond with inflammation, edema, increased mucus production, and bronchospasm. Reactive airway disorders are reversible, usually self-limiting, and generally responsive to supportive therapies. They occur in either upper or lower airways and include croup syndromes, asthma, and bronchiolitis.

CROUP SYNDROMES

Croup is a term applied to a broad classification of upper airway illnesses that result from swelling of the epiglottis and larynx. The swelling usually extends into the trachea and bronchi. Included under the classification of croup syndromes are viral syndromes, such as spasmodic laryngitis (spasmodic croup), laryngotracheitis, and laryngotracheobronchitis (LTB), and bacterial syndromes, such as bacterial tracheitis and epiglottitis (Fig. 11–5, Table 11–8).

LTB, epiglottitis, and bacterial tracheitis are referred to as the "big three" of pediatric respiratory illness because they affect the greatest number of children across all age groups in both sexes. The initial symptoms of all three conditions include inspiratory **stridor** (a high-pitched, musical sound that is created by narrowing of the airway), a "seal-like" barking cough, and hoarseness. LTB is the most common disorder, but epiglottitis and bacterial tracheitis are more serious.

Laryngitis and laryngotracheitis are mild illnesses that can be managed at home. LTB is the most serious type of viral croup, frequently necessitating an emergency department visit for infants and children under 6 years of age.

Laryngotracheobronchitis

Although the term *croup* is applied to several viral and bacterial syndromes, it is most often used to refer to LTB, a viral invasion of the upper airway that extends throughout the larynx, trachea, and bronchi. Table 11–8 compares LTB and other croup syndromes.

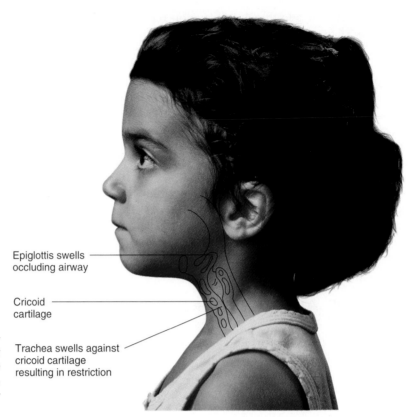

Epiglottis swells
occluding airway

Cricoid
cartilage

Trachea swells against
cricoid cartilage
resulting in restriction

FIGURE 11–5. There are two important changes in the upper airway in croup: the epiglottis swells, thereby occluding the airway, and the trachea swells against the cricoid cartilage, causing restriction.

NURSING ALERT

Throat cultures and visual inspection of the inner mouth and throat are *contraindicated* in children with LTB and epiglottitis. These procedures can cause laryngospasms (spasmodic vibrations that close the larynx) to occur as a result of the child's anxiety or of probing this reactive and already compromised area.

Clinical Manifestations

A child who is brought to the emergency department with LTB has usually been ill for several days with upper respiratory symptoms. These symptoms progress to a cough and hoarseness. Fever may or may not be present. Common presenting signs are tachypnea, inspiratory stridor, and a seal-like barking cough.

Etiology and Pathophysiology

Acute viral LTB is most common in children 3 months to 4 years of age but can occur up to 8 years of age. Boys are affected more often than girls. LTB is of greatest concern in infants and children under the age of 6 years, because of potential airway obstruction. The causative organism is usually parainfluenza virus type I or II, which appears during winter months in clustered outbreaks.[9]

Airway tissues respond to the invading virus by producing copious, tenacious secretions and swelling, which increase the child's respiratory distress. The edema causes the airway diameter to narrow in the subglottic area, the narrowest part of the airway. Even small amounts of mucus or edema can quickly obstruct the airway (see Fig. 11–5). Both the large and small airways can be affected.

Diagnostic Tests and Medical Management

Diagnosis is often made by clinical signs. Pulse oximetry is used to detect hypoxemia. If the diagnosis of LTB is in question, anteroposterior (AP) and lateral x-rays of the upper airway are taken; these may show symmetric subglottic narrowing called a "steeple sign."

11-8   Summary of Croup Syndromes

	Viral Syndromes			Bacterial Syndromes	
	Acute Spasmodic Laryngitis (Spasmodic Croup)	*Laryngotracheitis*	*Laryngotracheo-bronchitis*	*Bacterial Tracheitis*	*Epiglottitis (Supraglottitis)*
Severity	Least serious	Most common[a]	Most serious; progresses if untreated	Guarded; requires close observation	Most life threatening (medical emergency)[a]
Age affected	3 months to 3 years	3 months to 8 years	3 months to 8 years	1 month to 13 years[a]	2 years to 8 years
Onset	Abrupt onset; peaks at night, resolves by morning (recurs)[a]	Gradual onset; starts as URI, progresses to moderate respiratory difficulty	Gradual onset; starts as URI, progresses to symptoms of respiratory distress	Progressive from URI (1–2 days)	Progresses rapidly (hours)[a]
Clinical manifestations	Afebrile; mild respiratory distress; barking-seal cough	*Early:* mild fever [<39.0°C (102.2°F)]; hoarseness; barking-seal, brassy, croupy cough; rhinorrhea; sore throat; stridor; apprehension (inspiratory) *Progressing to* labored respirations	*Early:* mild fever; [<39.0°C (102.2°F)]; barking-seal, brassy, croupy cough; rhinorrhea; sore throat; stridor (inspiratory); apprehension; restless/irritable *Progressing to* retractions (progressive); increasing stridor; cyanosis	High fever [>39.0°C (102.2°F)]; URI appears as viral croupy cough; croup initially; stridor (tracheal); purulent secretions	High fever [>39.0°C (102.2°F)]; URI; intense sore throat; dysphagia[a]; drooling[a]; increased pulse and respiratory rate; prefers upright position (tripod position with chin thrust)[a]
Etiology	Unknown; suspect viral with allergic/emotional influences	Parainfluenza, types I and II, RSV, or influenza	Parainfluenza, types I and II, RSV, or influenza	*Staphylococcus*	*Haemophilus influenzae*

[a]Classic parameter or key point (distinguishes condition).

Medical management consists of maintaining and improving respiratory effort with humidification, medications, and supplemental oxygen when the saturated oxygen level is less than 92% (Table 11–9).

Children with a good response to medications are often sent home from the emergency department after an observation period. Children with moderate to severe symptoms after medications are admitted for further observation and treatment. Airway obstruction is a potential complication of LTB. The child may require intubation and transfer to the ICU to maintain airway patency if obstruction occurs. Most children, however, respond positively to the high humidity and oxygen therapy and are discharged within 48–72 hours.

Nursing Assessment

The initial and ongoing physical assessment of the child focuses on adequacy of respiratory functioning. Close monitoring is required to identify changes in airway patency. The child should be continuously monitored in

NURSING ALERT

Observe the child continuously for inability to swallow, absence of voice sounds, increasing degree of respiratory distress, and acute onset of drooling (an ominous sign of supraglottic obstruction). If *any* of these signs occur, get medical assistance *immediately.* The quieter the child, the greater the cause for concern.

11-9	Medications Used for Symptomatic Treatment of Laryngotracheobronchitis	
Medication	Action/Indication	Nursing Considerations
Beta-agonists and beta-adrenergics (eg, albuterol, racemic epinephrine): aerosolized through face mask	Rapid-acting bronchodilator, used to decrease symptoms of respiratory distress; and constriction of subglottic mucosa and submucosal capillaries	Provides only temporary relief; the child may develop tolerance quickly, increasing frequency with which drug is required; *the child may experience tachycardia* (160–200 beats/min) and hypertension; dizziness, headache, and nausea may necessitate stopping medication; does not alter the course of viral croup; reduces the need for artificial airway; tendency to return to pretreatment level of distress
Corticosteroids (eg, dexamethasone): IM, IV, PO	Antiinflammatory, used to decrease edema	The child may experience cardiovascular symptoms (hypertension): requires close observation for individual response; children less frequently need emergency airways; stridor resolves faster

the emergency department observation area or the intensive care unit. When the child's condition stabilizes, monitoring can be less frequent (Tables 11–10 and 11–11).

Particular attention should be paid to the child's respiratory effort, breath sounds, and responsiveness. Physical exhaustion can diminish the intensity of retractions and stridor. As the child uses the remaining energy reserve to maintain ventilation, breath sounds may actually diminish. Noisy breathing (audible airway congestion, coarse breath sounds) in this situation verifies adequate energy stores. Responsiveness will decrease as hypoxemia increases.

Nursing Diagnosis
The following nursing diagnoses might be appropriate for the child with acute LTB:

- Ineffective Breathing Pattern related to tracheobronchial obstruction, decreased energy, and fatigue
- Impaired Gas Exchange related to altered oxygen supply (narrowed air inlet)
- Altered Nutrition: Less Than Body Requirements related to expenditure of glycogen stores and to inadequate food and fluid intake prior to admission
- Fear/Anxiety (Parent or Child) related to acute illness, uncertainty of prognosis, unfamiliar surroundings and procedures
- Knowledge Deficit (Parent) related to diagnosis, treatment, prognosis, and home care needs

GROWTH & DEVELOPMENT CONSIDERATIONS

Infants and preverbal toddlers with laryngotracheobronchitis require constant supervision to monitor respiratory status. A means of communication (sign language or simple word cues) must be established to enable the older child to alert nursing staff to respiratory difficulty.

11-10 — Nursing Assessment of Child With a Reactive Airway Disorder

Nursing Action	Rationale
Assess heart rate and respiratory rate	Tachypnea and tachycardia indicate increasing respiratory effort
Check position of the child (sitting? prone? supine?)	Upright or semi-Fowler's promotes airway patency; the child's change to a more upright position may signal increased distress
Assess overall quality of respiratory effort: Determine inspiratory and expiratory breath sounds, ability to speak, and presence of stridor, cough, retractions, nasal flaring, cyanosis	Reflects overall adequacy of airway and respiratory function
Initiate croup score (Table 11–11) and continue scoring every 2–4 hours or more frequently if distress increases; initiate nursing actions appropriate for croup score	Provides consistent and objective assessment data with quantitative score for future comparison
Attach cardiorespiratory monitor and pulse oximeter	Provides continuous assessment data as part of ongoing physiologic monitoring

11-11 — Croup Scale to Identify the Severity of Croup

Signs	Severity Score 0	1	2	3
Stridor	None	Mild	Moderate at rest	Severe, on inspiration + expiration
Retractions	None	Mild	Suprasternal, intercostal	Severe, may see sternal retractions
Color	Normal	Normal score = 0	Normal score = 0	Dusky or cyanotic score = 0
Breath sounds	Normal	Mildly decreased	Moderately decreased	Markedly decreased
Level of consciousness	Normal	Restless when disturbed	Anxious, agitated	Lethargic

Scoring: To quantify the severity of croup, add up the individual scores for each of the sign categories. A score between 0 and 15 is possible. The rating of mild, moderate, and severe is as follows: 4–5 is mild, 6–8 is moderate, >8 or any sign in the severe category is severe.
Modified from Davis H.W., Gartner, J.C., Galvis, A.G., Michaels, R.H., and Mestad, P.H. (1981). Acute upper airway obstruction: croup and epiglottitis. Pediatric Clinics of North America, 28(4), pp. 859–880.

Nursing Management

Skillful nursing care can greatly assist children with LTB and their families to cope with the symptoms of the illness. Nursing care focuses on maintaining airway patency, promoting fluid balance, reducing stress, and teaching the family how to care for the child at home.

Maintain Airway Patency. Supplemental oxygen with high humidity may be needed for hypoxemia. High-humidity mist tents are rarely used as studies have not demonstrated any improvement in symptoms. Allow the child to assume a position of comfort.

An important developmental consideration is the child's ability to communicate reliably. The nurse must be immediately available to attend to the child's respiratory needs. The child should be roomed near the nurses' station and emergency resuscitation equipment kept at the bedside.

Meet Fluid and Nutritional Needs. The illness preceding the emergency department visit may have compromised the child's fluid status. Recognizing fluid deficit and monitoring the child's hydration and nutritional status are essential. Fluids promote liquification of secretions and provide calories for energy and metabolism. Parents can be encouraged to participate in gaining the child's cooperation in taking oral fluids. An intravenous infusion may be necessary to rehydrate the child, maintain fluid balance, or provide emergency access. The child should be observed closely for difficulty in swallowing, which may be an early sign of epiglottitis or bacterial tracheitis.

Discharge Planning and Home Care Teaching. During the child's observation period nurses should take every opportunity to assess the parents' knowledge of symptoms of LTB and discuss actions to take if symptoms recur. For example, instruct parents to call the child's physician if:

- Mild symptoms do not improve after 1 hour of humidity and cool air treatment.
- The child's breathing is rapid and labored.

Epiglottitis (Supraglottitis)

Epiglottitis (also known as supraglottitis) is an inflammation of the epiglottis, the long narrow structure that closes off the glottis during swallowing (see Fig. 11–5). Because edema in this area can rapidly (within minutes or hours) obstruct the airway by occluding the trachea, epiglottitis is considered a potentially life-threatening condition. (Table 11–8 compares epiglottitis and other croup syndromes.)

Characteristically, a previously healthy child *suddenly* becomes very ill. The child initially develops a high fever (greater than 39°C [102.2°F]), with a sore throat, **dysphonia** (muffled, hoarse, or absent voice sounds), and dysphagia (difficulty in swallowing). As the larynx becomes obstructed, inspiratory stridor develops. The child resists normal swallowing of saliva because of intense throat pain and swelling, resulting in drooling. To fully open the airway and improve air intake, the child sits up and leans forward with the jaw thrust forward in the classic "sniffing" or tripod posture and refuses to lie down.

Epiglottitis is often caused by bacterial invasion of the soft tissue of the larynx by *Haemophilus influenzae* type B (Hib), but it can also be caused by streptococcus and staphylococcus. The resulting inflammation and edema in the tissues and surrounding the epiglottis lead to airway obstruction. For-

---

CLINICAL TIP

Children with laryngotracheobronchitis usually prefer cool, noncarbonated, nonacidic drinks such as apple juice or fruit-flavored drinks. Remember that gelatin, ice, and fruit-flavored ice pops are also fluids. Oral rehydration fluids may also be used.

THE FOUR Ds OF EPIGLOTTITIS

The four classic signs of epiglottitis, in order of their appearance, are:
- **D**ysphonia
- **D**ysphagia
- **D**rooling
- **D**istressed respiratory effort

tunately, since use of the Hib vaccine has become widespread, the number of cases of epiglottitis has decreased significantly.

Diagnosis is often based on a lateral neck x-ray (Fig. 11–6), which reveals an enlarged, rounded epiglottis, seen as a mass at the base of the tongue. A narrowed airway is also visible. A blood culture may be taken after the child is stabilized. **Laryngospasm** can occur as a result of the severe irritation and hypersensitivity of the airway muscles. For this reason, visual inspection of the mouth and throat is contraindicated in children with suspected epiglottitis unless carried out by a physician in an environment where immediate intubation can be performed.[9] Obstruction is almost certain if stress or physical manipulation further irritates the fragile airway.

Immediate medical therapy consists of interventions to maintain an open airway, usually by insertion of an endotracheal tube. Antibiotics effective for *H. influenzae* and gram-positive organisms are given until blood culture sensitivities are available. Antipyretics (acetaminophen, ibuprofen) may be useful in managing fever and sore throat pain.

Nursing Management

Nursing management consists of airway management, drug therapy, hydration, and emotional and psychosocial support of the child and parents. Until the endotracheal tube is removed, the child is usually managed in the intensive care unit to ensure continual observation.

Maintain Airway Patency. Cool mist and supplemental oxygen promote better airway function. The child may be placed in a high-humidity tent to provide oxygen and cool moisture. The child should be observed closely and often. A quiet environment with as little stress as possible is essential. A quiet, undisturbed child will be less anxious and less inclined to cry. Crying stimulates the airway, increases oxygen consumption, and can precipitate laryngospasm; the calmer the child, the better the respiratory function.[10] A supine position is contraindicated because it can compromise the function of the diaphragm and make the child feel as if he or she is choking.

Administer Medications and Fluids. Antibiotics are administered to treat the infection and fluids to provide hydration. Because the child was febrile with a sore throat before admission, fluid intake may have been com-

NURSING ALERT

Because infants and preverbal toddlers cannot alert the nurse if they have respiratory distress, they must not be left alone during the acute phase of epiglottitis.

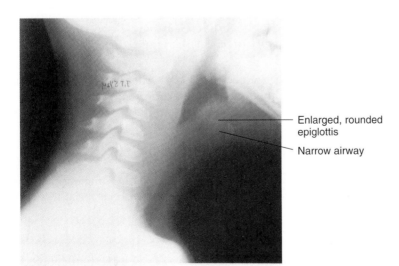

— Enlarged, rounded epiglottis
— Narrow airway

FIGURE 11–6. The phrase "thumb sign" has been used to describe this enlargement of the epiglottis. Recall the trachea's usual "little finger" size. Do you see the stiff, enlarged "thumb" above it in this lateral neck x-ray?

promised. The nurse should be alert for signs of dehydration. Careful monitoring of intake and output and specific gravity provides valuable data about hydration status.

Provide Emotional Support. The loss of voice, or even the inability to create sounds, can be frightening to a child. The unfamiliar hospital environment and strange equipment can create stress for child and parent alike. The nurse reassures the parents that the child's voice loss is temporary and explains the need for the various pieces of equipment. Twenty-four-hour visitation for parents or immediate family members is advisable. This provides reassurance for the child and allows parents to take turns so that each can have a break.

Discharge Planning and Home Care Teaching. Most children show rapid improvement once cool mist and oxygen, antibiotics, and fluid therapy are started. Usually recovery occurs quickly and the endotracheal tube can be removed within 24–36 hours.[11] Home care may involve completing the course of antibiotics. Parents need instructions on proper administration and potential problems of drug therapy.

Bacterial Tracheitis

Bacterial tracheitis is an infection of the upper trachea that is most often caused by *Staphylococcus aureus.* It is believed to start with a viral infection or preexisting anatomic lesion that develops into a bacterial superinfection. The disorder starts with croupy cough and stridor but progresses to include a high fever (greater than 39°C [102.2°F]), which persists for several days.[9] (Table 11–8 compares bacterial tracheitis and other croup syndromes.)

Because of the similarity of symptoms, bacterial tracheitis is often misdiagnosed initially as LTB. Instead of improving with therapy, however, the child's condition becomes worse. Children generally prefer lying flat to sitting up. This seems to be a position of comfort that allows the child to conserve energy. Diagnosis is often made by blood cultures after the child is found unresponsive to usual LTB management. Most children need an artificial airway and ventilatory support.

Nursing Management
Nursing management involves the following:

- Careful airway assessment and support
- Airway maintenance (artificial airway assistance is often required because of the thick tracheal secretions that pool high in the upper airway)
- Suctioning as needed (mechanical suction enables easier removal of secretions and helps maintain a patent airway)
- Administration of humidified oxygen
- Administration of antibiotics
- Preparation for resuscitation

The earlier section on epiglottitis discusses other nursing care interventions that may also be appropriate for the child with bacterial tracheitis.

ASTHMA

Asthma (also called bronchial asthma) is a chronic inflammatory disorder of the airway.[12] It has been described in medical writings since ancient times. This common chronic illness occurs in infants, children, and adolescents and accounts for a large percentage of school absenteeism.[13] Most children with asthma experience their first symptoms before the age of 5 years. Asthma occurs more frequently in boys than girls until the teen years, when the incidence equalizes.[14]

Asthma is a chronic condition with acute exacerbations or persistent symptoms. Children require continuous coordinated care to control sudden symptoms and minimize long-term airway changes. Although unusual in the past, severe persistent asthma is more common now. Mortality from asthma in children rose 31% between 1980 and 1987,[16] and continues to rise. How does this chronic condition pose a threat to children?

Clinical Manifestations

Asthma is characterized by airway inflammation, airway obstruction or narrowing, and airway hyperreactivity. The sudden appearance of breathing difficulty is often referred to as an asthma "attack" or "episode."

During an acute attack, respirations are rapid and labored and the child often appears tired because of the ongoing exertion of breathing. Nasal flaring and intercostal retractions may be visible. The child exhibits a productive cough and expiratory wheezing, use of accessory muscles, decreased air movement, and respiratory fatigue. The resulting hypoxia, as well as the cumulative effect of previously administered medications, contributes to behaviors ranging from wide-eyed agitation to lethargic irritability.

In children who have repeated acute exacerbations, a barrel chest and the use of accessory muscles of respiration are common findings (see Fig. 11–12, p. 439). The child with chronic asthma is often small according to standard growth charts but usually catches up in adolescence.

Etiology and Pathophysiology

The respiratory difficulties of an asthma attack result from inflammation that contributes to airway obstruction.[12] The inflammation causes the normal protective mechanisms of the lungs (mucus formation, mucosal swelling, and airway muscle contraction) to react excessively in response to a stimulus.

The stimulus, more correctly termed a **trigger,** that initiates an asthmatic episode can be a substance or condition. Asthmatic triggers include exercise, viral or bacterial agents, allergens (mold, dust, or pollen), food additives, pollutants, weather changes (humidity and temperature), and emotions. The role of emotions as a trigger is often misunderstood and misinterpreted. A common myth is that children with asthma have psychologic problems that precipitate acute attacks. Although psychologic problems may be present, they do not account for the acute attack. The reactive airway responses to stimuli are present *before* the trigger initiates the physiologic sequence that results in an asthma attack.

Airway narrowing results from airway swelling and production of copious amounts of mucus. Mucus clogs small airways, trapping air below the plugs (Fig. 11–7). The airways swell, creating muscle spasms that often become uncontrolled in the large airways. With time, repeated episodes of bronchospasm, mucosal edema, and mucus plugging can damage the respiratory cells that line the airway. This process leaves the airway chronically irritated and scarred and results in air trapping, called hyperinflation.

The psychologic sequence of events during an asthmatic episode starts with moderate anxiety as the episode begins. The anxiety becomes severe as the episode intensifies. Severe anxiety, in turn, intensifies physical responses and symptoms, and a vicious cycle is established. Recognizing and

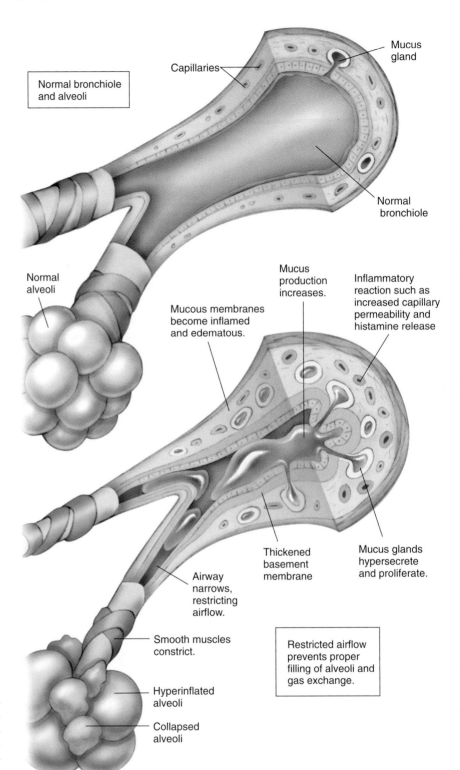

Normal bronchiole and alveoli

Capillaries

Mucus gland

Normal bronchiole

Normal alveoli

Mucous membranes become inflamed and edematous.

Mucus production increases.

Inflammatory reaction such as increased capillary permeability and histamine release

Thickened basement membrane

Mucus glands hypersecrete and proliferate.

Airway narrows, restricting airflow.

Smooth muscles constrict.

Restricted airflow prevents proper filling of alveoli and gas exchange.

Hyperinflated alveoli

Collapsed alveoli

FIGURE 11–7. What can cause an asthma attack? Some asthma triggers are exercise, infection, and allergies. Shown is how asthma obstructs airflow through constriction and narrowing of the airway.

| 11-12 | Assessing Peak Expiratory Flow Rate (PEFR)[14] | |

Zone	PEFR (Best or Predicted for Age)	Action
Green	80–100%	Continue regular management plan.
Yellow	50–80%	Implement action plan provided by physician.
Red	<50%	**Medical Alert:** Implement action plan predetermined by physician. Call provider if PEFR does not return to yellow or green zone.

The child's personal best is determined after reviewing the recorded PEFRs measured two to four times a day for 2–3 weeks. The child should be optimally treated with medications during the day so an optimal reading is obtained.[12]

addressing the child's fear and panic are essential for reestablishing normal respirations.

Diagnostic Tests and Medical Management

The diagnosis of asthma is confirmed through pulmonary function studies. A spirometer is used to measure the volume of air the lungs can move in and out. Because the test requires children to cooperate and follow instructions, it is usually administered to children over 4 or 5 years of age.[17] Findings determine the extent of airway restriction and assist in selecting the appropriate treatment. (See Tables 11–12 and 11–13.) Skin testing may be used to identify allergens (asthma triggers).

| 11-13 | Revised Asthma Severity Classification |

Classification (Steps)	Description
Step 1: Mild intermittent	Brief exacerbations with symptoms no more often than twice a week. PEFR ≥ 80% of predicted with variability < 20%
Step 2: Mild persistent	Exacerbations more than twice a week, but less than once a day. May affect activity. PEFR ≥ 80% of predicted with variability of 20–30%
Step 3: Moderate persistent	Daily symptoms. Daily use of inhaled short-acting beta-agonist. Exacerbations at least twice a week that may last for days. Affects activity. PEFR > 60% but < 80% of predicted with variability > 30%
Step 4: Severe persistent	Continuous symptoms, limited physical activity. Frequent exacerbations. PEFR ≤ 60% of predicted with variability > 30%

From National Asthma Education and Prevention Program. (1997). Expert Panel Report II: Guidelines for the diagnosis and management of asthma. (NIH Publication No. 97-4051). Bethesda, MD: National Institutes of Health.

CLINICAL TIP

To help toddlers learn to use a peak flow meter, have them practice by blowing into party favors (eg, noise-makers). To learn to use a metered-dose inhaler, let the child learn to breathe in slowly with straws. Make sure you teach the child the proper use of the inhaler first.

Medical management includes medications, support of parents and child, and education (Table 11–14). Pharmacologic treatment attempts to promote optimal respiratory function. In children as young as 4–5 years, the use of a peak expiratory flow meter can assist in the management of asthma by helping to identify when obstruction occurs.[14] This device measures the child's ability to push air forcefully out of the lungs. Medication administration can be based on peak expiratory flow rate (PEFR) readings and the effectiveness of treatment confirmed by improved PEFR numbers.

Most children with acute exacerbations respond to aggressive management in the emergency department. Children who do not respond or who are already being managed at home on corticosteroids have a greater chance of being admitted. Some children will need mechanical ventilation. Support of the parents and child should focus on helping them to cope

11-14   Medications Used to Treat Asthma

Medication	Action/Indication	Nursing Considerations
Bronchodilators		
Beta-agonists Albuterol, metaproterinal, or terbutaline: aerosol, subcutaneous, or by mouth	Relax smooth muscle in airway, resulting in rapid bronchodilation; *drugs of choice for acute or daily therapy (inhaled route)*	Have some side effects (tachycardia, nervousness, nausea and vomiting, headaches), but these are usually dose related; repetitive or excessive use can mask increasing airway inflammation and hyperresponsiveness
Methylxanthines Theophylline (related to caffeine): by mouth	Relax muscle bundles that constrict airways; dilate airway; provide continuous airway relaxation	Used for long-term control, so continuous administration needed; works best when a specific amount is maintained in the bloodstream (therapeutic serum level, 10–20 µg/L); requires serum level checks and dose adjustment; have many and varied side effects (including tachycardia, arrythmias, restlessness, tremors, seizures, insomnia, hypotension, severe headache, vomiting, and diarrhea)
Antiinflammatory Agents		
Cromolyn sodium: aerosol only Nedocromil: aerosol only	*Preventive medications*, best taken daily to stop chemicals associated with producing asthma; controls seasonal, allergic, and exercise-induced asthma	Less effective in older children; prophylactic medications, once wheezing starts, these medications are ineffective
Corticosteroids intravenous, by mouth, or aerosol Bechlomethasone, triamcinolone, prednisone	Effectively reduce mucosal edema in airways; best absorbed intravenously, but can be useful if inhaled; usually combined with other asthma medications	Side effects (such as abnormalities in glucose metabolism, increased appetite, fluid retention, weight gain, moon face, mood alteration, and hypertension) may be severe if used long term; if used on daily basis, lowest therapeutic dose should be given; growth suppression possible with long-term use
Other		
Hyposensitization (allergy shots): subcutaneous	Series of injections that can reduce sensitivity to unavoidable allergens (eg, environmental organisms—mold, pollen); gradual dose increase over time (called a "build-up") increases the child's tolerance to allergic substances; has been of help in some children	Use is controversial; some question about actual effect

with and understand the diagnosis and the need for daily management to promote near-normal respiratory function while the child continues to grow and develop normally.

Nursing Assessment

The nurse usually encounters the child and family in the emergency department or nursing unit. Acute care has become necessary because the child's level of respiratory compromise cannot be managed at home. What needs to be done first? What is the nurse's role during an acute asthmatic episode?

Physiologic Assessment

Identify the child's current respiratory status first by assessing the airway, breathing, and circulation (Table 11–15). If the child is moving air or talking, assess the quality of breathing. Is the child wheezing? Is stridor present? Are retractions visible (see Fig. 11–3)? What is the respiratory rate? What is the quality of breath sounds? Observe the child's color and assess the heart rate. Oxygen saturation is obtained via pulse oximeter. Only after no life-threatening respiratory distress is found should the assessment move on to other systems. Assess PEFR, skin turgor, intake and output, and specific gravity. Because asthma can be a symptom of another illness, a head-to-toe

NURSING ALERT

The infant or child who has had episodes of frequent coughing or frequent respiratory infections (especially pneumonia or bronchitis) should also be evaluated for asthma. The *cough* is the warning signal that the child's airway is very sensitive to stimuli; it may be the only sign in "silent" asthma.

11-15	Estimation of Severity of Acute Exacerbations of Asthma in Children

Assessment Criteria	Mild	Moderate	Severe
PEFR[a]	70–90% predicted or personal best	50–70% predicted or personal best	< 50% predicted or personal best
Respiratory rate, resting or sleeping	Normal to 30% increase above the mean	30–50% increase above mean	Increase over 50% above mean
Alertness	Normal	Normal	May be decreased
Dyspnea[b]	Absent or mild; speaks in complete sentences	Moderate; speaks in phrases or partial sentences; infant's cry softer and shorter; has difficulty sucking and feeding	Severe; speaks only in single words or short phrases; infant's cry softer and shorter; stops sucking and feeding
Pulsus paradoxus[c]	< 10 mm Hg	10–20 mm Hg	20–40 mm Hg
Accessory muscle use	No intercostal to mild retractions	Moderate intercostal retractions with tracheosternal retractions; use of sternocleidomastoid muscles; chest hyperinflation	Severe intercostal retractions, tracheosternal retractions with nasal flaring during inspiration; chest hyperinflation
Color	Good	Pale	Possibly cyanotic
Auscultation	End-expiratory wheeze only	Wheeze during entire expiration and inspiration	Breath sounds becoming inaudible
Oxygen saturation	> 95%	90–95%	< 90%
PCO$_2$	< 35	< 40	> 40

Note: Within each category, the presence of several parameters, but not necessarily all, indicate the general classification of the exacerbation.
[a]For children 5 years of age or older.
[b]Parents' or physicians' impressions of degree of children's breathlessness.
[c]Pulsus paradoxus does not correlate with phase of respiration in small children.
From National Asthma Education and Prevention Program. (1994). Acute exacerbations of asthma: Care in a hospital-based emergency department (p. 13). Bethesda, MD: National Heart, Lung, and Blood Institute, National Institutes of Health.

assessment should be performed to identify other associated problems (Tables 11–1 and 11–10).

Psychosocial Assessment

Is the child anxious? Crying? (See Table 11–16.) In an older child whose asthma was previously diagnosed, have the asthmatic episode and hospitalization created guilt about doing something the child thinks he or she should have avoided or about forgetting to take medication? The nurse should look for clues to hidden stress and self-blaming.

Nursing Diagnosis

Common nursing diagnoses for the child experiencing an acute asthmatic episode include the following:

- Ineffective Airway Clearance related to airway compromise, copious mucus secretions, and coughing
- Ineffective Breathing Pattern related to airway obstruction, possible additional respiratory illness, and poor response to medication
- Anxiety/Fear (Child or Parents) related to change in health status, difficulty breathing
- Knowledge Deficit related to medical management of chronic disease

Nursing Management

Pharmacologic and supportive therapies are used to reverse the airway obstruction and promote respiratory function. Nursing interventions center on maintaining airway patency, meeting fluid needs, promoting rest and stress reduction for the child and parents, supporting the family's participation in care, and providing the family with information to enable them to manage the child's acute asthmatic episodes and ongoing needs.

Maintain Airway Patency

If the child is exhibiting breathing difficulty, supplemental oxygen is required. Oxygen is best administered by nasal cannula or face mask. (Refer to the *Quick Reference to Pediatric Clinical Skills* accompanying this text.) Humidified oxygen

---

11-16	Psychosocial Assessment of the Child With an Acute Respiratory Illness

Child
- Assess for indications of anxiety or fear that may have an impact on respiratory status.
- For young children, inquire about security objects (such as a blanket or doll), the child's reaction to strangers, and reaction to absence of parents.
- For older children, ask whether this is the first hospital stay and what previous illness and hospital experiences have meant to the child.

Parents
- Assess parents' reactions: Are they anxious? Fearful? Verbal or quiet? Asking appropriate questions?
- Observe for nonverbal cues. Often parents have financial worries (cost of hospital stay, lost work and wages) and personal worries (siblings at home who are ill) that they may not readily share with staff.

should be used to prevent drying and thickening of mucus secretions. The child should be placed in a sitting (semi-Fowler's) or upright position to promote and ease respiratory effort. The effectiveness of positioning and oxygen administration is evaluated by transcutaneous oxygen monitoring (pulse oximeter) and by observing for improved respiratory status.

The respiratory distress and need for supplemental oxygen can be stressful for parents and child alike (Fig. 11–8). Encouraging the parents' presence can be reassuring for the child. The parents should be kept informed of procedures and results, and their input should be obtained in developing the treatment plan.

Many medications are given by the aerosol route (Fig. 11–9). The advantages of aerosol are that the medication acts quickly, enabling the pulmonary blood vessels to absorb the inhaled medication, systemic effects are minimized, and the inhaled droplets provide the added benefit of moisture. Because the medication is quickly absorbed, continuous aerosol treatments may be implemented. Monitor the child for side effects. The frequency of vital sign assessment is related to the severity of symptoms.

Meet Fluid Needs

Fluid therapy is often necessary to restore and maintain adequate fluid balance. Adequate hydration is essential to thin and break up trapped mucus plugs in the narrowed airways. An adequate oral intake may not be possible with the child's compromised respiratory status. An intravenous infusion may be needed, and this route also may be used for administering medications and providing glucose. Overhydration must be avoided to prevent pulmonary edema in severe asthma attacks.

As respiratory difficulty diminishes, oral fluids can be offered slowly. Intake and output are monitored and specific gravity is assessed frequently

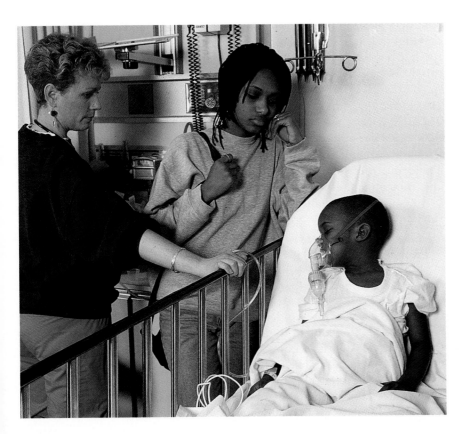

FIGURE 11–8. Acute exacerbations of asthma may require management in the emergency department. The child is positioned in a semi-sitting position to facilitate respiratory effort. Providing support to both the child and parent is an important part of nursing care during these acute episodes. This mother is exhausted after a sleepless night of caring for her son.

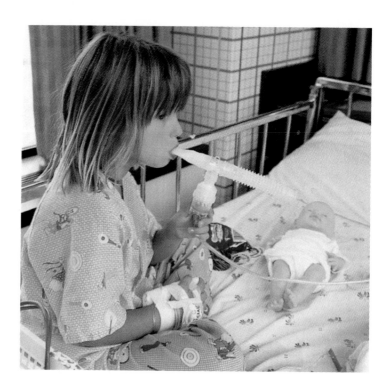

FIGURE 11-9. Medications given by aerosol therapy allow children the freedom to play and entertain themselves.

SAFETY PRECAUTIONS

Iced beverages precipitate bronchospasms in some children with asthma. It is safest to offer the asthmatic child room temperature or slightly cooled fluids without ice.

to evaluate the child's hydration status. Involving parents in feeding can help gain the child's cooperation in taking oral fluids. The child's fluid preferences should be determined and choices provided where possible.

Promote Rest and Stress Reduction

The child who has had an acute asthmatic episode is usually very tired when admitted to the nursing unit. Labored breathing and low oxygen status have left the child exhausted. The child should be placed in a quiet, private room if possible, to promote relaxation and rest. By grouping tasks, nurses can avoid repeatedly disturbing the child.

Support Family Participation

The parents may stay with the child, but may be exhausted after hours of their child's respiratory distress. Give parents the option of assisting with the child's treatments, rather than expecting them to do it in addition to comforting the child. Provide frequent updates about the child's condition and encourage the parents to take breaks as needed.

Length of hospitalization depends on the child's response to therapy. Any underlying or accompanying health problem, such as preexisting lung disease or pneumonia, can complicate and extend the child's hospital stay. Communicate with the family of the hospitalized child at least once a day about the child's condition.

Discharge Planning and Home Care Teaching

Parents need a thorough understanding of asthma—how to prevent attacks and treatment to maintain the child's health and avoid unnecessary hospitalization. The American Lung Association is an excellent resource for parents (see Appendix F). Through printed educational materials and referral to a local support group, parents gain additional knowledge and confidence that enable them to help their child lead a normal life[18] (Fig. 11–10). Special summer camps for asthmatic children are available.

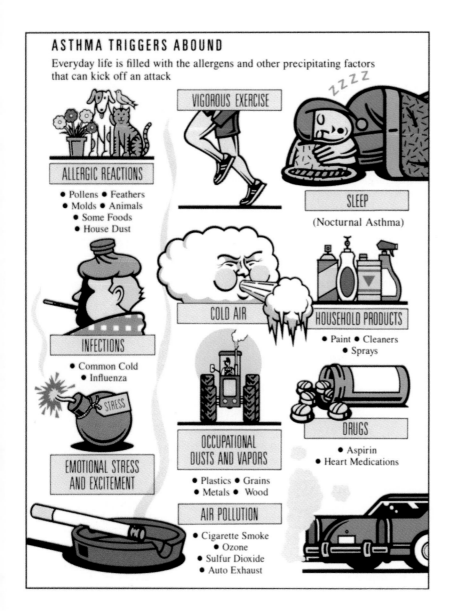

ASTHMA TRIGGERS ABOUND

Everyday life is filled with the allergens and other precipitating factors that can kick off an attack

VIGOROUS EXERCISE

SLEEP
(Nocturnal Asthma)

ALLERGIC REACTIONS
- Pollens • Feathers
- Molds • Animals
- Some Foods
- House Dust

COLD AIR

HOUSEHOLD PRODUCTS
- Paint • Cleaners
- Sprays

INFECTIONS
- Common Cold
- Influenza

EMOTIONAL STRESS AND EXCITEMENT

STRESS

OCCUPATIONAL DUSTS AND VAPORS
- Plastics • Grains
- Metals • Wood

DRUGS
- Aspirin
- Heart Medications

AIR POLLUTION
- Cigarette Smoke
- Ozone
- Sulfur Dioxide
- Auto Exhaust

FIGURE 11–10. This educational piece from the American Lung Association explains what triggers an asthma attack. The required life-style changes for the child and family will be significant, so be sensitive to the family's situation and needs. Culture sometimes plays a significant part in exposure to life-style triggers. *From American Lung Association—The "Christmas Seal" People. Copyright © 1989 American Lung Association.*

Discharge planning for the asthmatic child focuses on increasing the family's knowledge about the disease, medication therapy, and the need for follow-up care (Table 11–17). The required life-style changes may be difficult for the child and parents. The need to modify the home by removing a loved pet, for example, may create stress. The nurse can play a role in keeping lines of communication open and can facilitate discussion and clarification of ways to prevent asthmatic episodes. Teach the family how to measure peak expiratory flow and necessary medications to manage asthma attacks early on. The family should be reassured that most children with asthma can lead a normal life with some modifications.

Care in the Community

Nurses provide care to children with asthma in pediatricians' offices, specialty asthma clinics, schools, and summer camps. Once the stress of the acute episode has passed, opportunities exist to provide more extensive education (Fig 11–11).

If the child uses aerosol or oral glucocorticoids to control asthma attacks, monitor the child carefully as these medications may affect overall

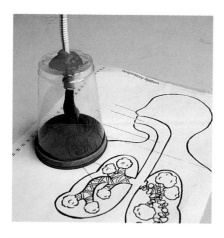

FIGURE 11–11. School-age children can be taught how the lung functions using simple activities such as this project, in which a "lung" is made using a plastic cup, a straw, and balloons. The school nurse who organized the asthma club described in Chapter 1 uses this activity to illustrate how the lung takes in air, expanding and contracting during breathing.

11-17   Parent Teaching: Home Care Instructions for the Child with Asthma

1. Identify parents' knowledge about the condition:
   a. Review why asthma occurs and evaluate parents' understanding of the physiologic process. Ask:
      - Do you understand what happens in your child's lungs during an asthma attack?
      - Do you know the early warning signs of an asthma episode in your child?
      - What are your child's symptoms and how does he or she respond to them? Does your child use the peak expiratory flow meter to evaluate symptoms?
   b. Identify asthma triggers and evaluate parents' understanding of how to prevent, avoid, or minimize their effect in a timely manner. Ask:
      - Do you know your child's personal asthma triggers? (Suggest that the parents and child keep a notebook to track episodes so they can learn more about these triggers.)
      - What steps can you take to minimize or eliminate your child's exposure (quitting smoking, environmental control, etc)?
2. Set up a schedule for parents to learn asthma management. Ask:
   - Do you know when and where to seek emergency medical help?
   - What actions can you take before seeking medical assistance?
3. Review parents' understanding of medication therapy:
   - Provide information about medications: name, type of drug, dose, method of administration, expected effect, possible side effects.
   - Evaluate the child's technique for the use of an inhaler and peak flow meter.
4. Address associated issues:
   - Do parents know how to store and properly transport medications?
   - What are the financial considerations of medication cost and life-style changes?
   - Has the child's school or teacher been notified? What arrangements have been made for the child's use of medications at school?
   - Has a medical identification bracelet or medallion been obtained for the child to facilitate assistance when away from home?
5. Identify need for follow-up care:
   - Do parents know when to see a physician? When drug levels need to be checked?
   - Does child need to see an allergist?
   - Do the child or parents have special emotional needs?
   - Would a self-help group or camp experience be helpful for the child?

growth. Review the family's daily plan for monitoring the child's respiratory status. Evaluate the child's technique for PEFR and the parent's ability to identify the timing and type of stepped-443up care needed to manage worsening symptoms. The goal is to bring asthma attacks under control with stepped-up care before a significant episode occurs. This can be achieved only with daily monitoring.

Environmental control is an important part of asthma management. When possible, pets should not be kept in the home (and never in the child's bedroom). Cockroaches and dust mites should be eliminated or controlled. Smoke from cigarettes, wood stoves, and fireplaces all have the potential to trigger an asthma attack.

Parents should communicate with school personnel regarding the child's condition, need to take medications, and ability to participate in activities.[13]

Refer to the Nursing Care Plan for the child with asthma in the community setting, in Chapter 5, for additional information.

STATUS ASTHMATICUS

Status asthmaticus is unrelenting, severe respiratory distress and bronchospasm in an asthmatic child, which persists despite pharmacologic and supportive interventions. Without immediate intervention the child with status asthmaticus may die. The child is placed in an intensive care unit and may require endotracheal intubation with assisted ventilation. The section on respiratory failure earlier in the chapter gives additional information on the nurse's role in providing emergency respiratory care.

► LOWER AIRWAY DISORDERS

The lower airway, or bronchial tree, lies below the trachea and includes the bronchi, bronchioles, and alveoli. Lower airway disorders occur because a structural or functional problem interferes with the lungs' ability to complete the respiratory cycle. Lower airway disorders include neonatal respiratory distress syndrome, bronchopulmonary dysplasia, bronchitis, bronchiolitis, pneumonia, tuberculosis, and cystic fibrosis.

NEONATAL RESPIRATORY DISTRESS SYNDROME

Neonatal respiratory distress syndrome (RDS) manifests during the first hours of life in newborn infants with severely compromised respiratory systems. It may be caused by hyaline membrane disease or meconium aspiration. RDS is the most common cause of respiratory failure during the first days after birth, but due to improved technology, 80–90% of affected infants survive.[19]

Clinical manifestations include tachypnea (70–120 breaths/min), retractions, grunting, rales, cyanosis, slow capillary refill, **paradoxical breathing** (in which the chest falls and the abdomen rises on inspiration), decreased breath sounds, and labored breathing.

RDS results from inadequate or inactivated pulmonary surfactant.[19] Surfactant is a substance that lowers the surface tension of the alveoli by keeping the alveoli inflated and preventing the interior walls from adhering. Without sufficient surfactant, the alveoli collapse and cannot reinflate.

In utero, the fetal lungs are filled with fluid. When the infant takes the first breath after birth, this fluid is expelled from the alveoli. If insufficient surfactant is present, the alveolar walls adhere together. As a result, oxygen and carbon dioxide cannot be exchanged, which creates a threat to life. The alveoli themselves become damaged and die, creating thick scar tissue (the hyaline membrane tissue) in the alveolar space. The alveoli are replaced with fibrous nonfunctional tissue that stiffens the lung.[19]

Diagnosis usually occurs in the newborn nursery. A chest x-ray showing air in the bronchial tree and decreased lung expansion confirms the diagnosis. Medical management focuses on adequate resuscitation at birth, good temperature control, and assisted ventilation to expand the alveoli and preserve respiratory function. Intravenous fluid therapy and medications (primarily theophylline and dexamethasone) are administered to support function of the respiratory and other body systems.[20] Synthetic surfactant given

CLINICAL TIP

An alveolus can be thought of as a small balloon filled with water. When the balloon is emptied, the water droplets that remain inside the balloon cause the surface tension to increase. As a result, the sides of the balloon stick together. The increased surface tension makes reinflation almost impossible.

within 24 hours of birth has decreased mortality, but it has not changed the development of chronic inflammation.[21] Blood products may be administered to expand blood volume, increasing oxygen capacity.

Nursing Management

The respiratory status of the infant with RDS is closely monitored. Nursing assessment focuses on identifying changes in respiratory status, such as quality of respirations and pulse, overall color, signs of dehydration, and changes in the infant's behavior. Pulse oximetry and blood gases are monitored to aid in assessment.

Care of the infant is organized to eliminate any unnecessary physical stimulation, as this additional stress contributes to respiratory compromise. The infant is usually placed in a warmer to reduce metabolic demands. Position the infant to facilitate breathing. Parents need clear explanations about the infant's health status and planned interventions. By remaining available to parents and answering their questions, the nurse establishes a positive relationship and facilitates essential communication.

Because of the potential for respiratory distress and ongoing respiratory problems after discharge, parents should be taught CPR. (Refer to *Quick Reference to Pediatric Clinical Skills* accompanying this text.) The infant is also monitored at home for apnea, and medical follow-up should be continuous. Parents may benefit from a referral to a support group.

BRONCHOPULMONARY DYSPLASIA

Bronchopulmonary dysplasia (BPD) is an iatrogenic (treatment-induced) condition that results in chronic respiratory dysfunction. It is the most prevalent and serious chronic respiratory disorder that begins during infancy. Premature infants are affected more often than full-term infants, and morbidity is greater in males than in females. The incidence is increasing due to advances in medical technology that permit very-low-birth-weight infants to survive.[20]

The infant with BPD has persistent signs of respiratory distress: tachypnea, cyanosis, irritability, nasal flaring, grunting, retractions, and pulmonary edema. Normal activities, such as feeding, can create increased oxygen demands that are difficult for the compromised infant to meet.

BPD is a direct result of the treatment provided to premature and term infants with such conditions as RDS, congenital heart disease, meconium aspiration, and tracheoesophageal fistula. Treating these conditions with oxygen and positive-pressure ventilation for a minimum of 3 days contributes to BPD.[21]

In BPD, the alveoli and bronchioles are damaged by an inflammatory response that leads to scarring, fibrosis, and smooth muscle hypertrophy, resulting in inefficient gas exchange and poor mucus clearing. Air trapping and small airway obstruction cause areas of overdistention; and carbon dioxide retention then causes airway collapse and more air trapping. Increased lung fluid results from damage at the alveolar–capillary membrane. This, in turn, creates chronic low oxygenation (hypoxemia). The alveoli continue to develop, but the lungs never completely heal.

The chest x-ray is the best indicator of lung changes and is the key to medical diagnosis. There may be cystic changes or fine lacy densities with or without hyperinflation.[22] The air trapping persists and in time causes the chest to assume a barrel shape (Fig. 11–12). Medical management focuses on symptomatic treatment that supports respiratory function and on good

LONG-TERM OUTCOMES OF BPD

- Developmental delays
- Growth retardation
- Continuing airway obstruction
- Persistent airway hyperactivity

nutrition, which helps to accelerate lung maturity. Supplemental oxygen, chest physiotherapy, and medication therapy are used (Table 11–18).[22]

Nursing Management

Nursing management focuses on promoting respiratory function and preparing the family for home care needs. Nursing assessment includes close monitoring of respirations, pulse, color, behavior changes, and vital signs. The infant with chronic BPD may become acutely ill at any time.

Once home, many infants need ventilation therapy, oxygen respiratory support, and drug therapy (Fig. 11–13). Frequent rehospitalization may be necessary because, although the lungs may function adequately, they remain vulnerable throughout childhood to common respiratory illnesses. Infants with BPD do not have the same respiratory reserve as healthy infants, and they can become very ill very quickly. This was illustrated by the case of Emily, described in the vignette at the beginning of this chapter. Nutritional requirements to support growth must be balanced with fluid restrictions. Electrolytes must be monitored monthly.

It is important to provide for the infant's normal development through rest, nutrition, stimulation, and family support. Including parents in the infant's care early on promotes bonding and prepares them for home care responsibilities. Some families require home nursing assistance. Referrals for needed respiratory supplies, medications, an early intervention program, and follow-up care must be carefully planned and coordinated well in advance of the infant's discharge date.

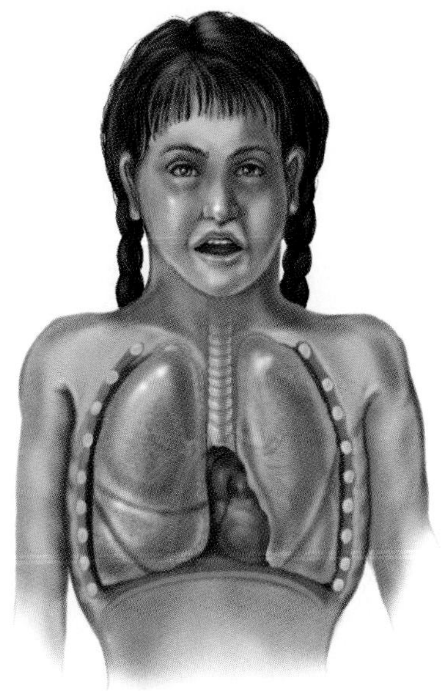

BRONCHITIS

Bronchitis, inflammation of the bronchi, rarely occurs in childhood as an isolated problem. The bronchi can be affected simultaneously with adjacent respiratory structures during a respiratory illness. Bronchitis occurs most often in children under 4 years of age, usually following a mild upper respiratory

FIGURE 11–12. A barrel chest may result from chronic respiratory conditions such as bronchopulmonary dysplasia or asthma, in which air trapping and hyperinflation of the alveoli occur.

11-18	**Medications Used to Treat Bronchopulmonary Dysplasia**
Medication	Action/Indication
Bronchodilators (beta-adrenergics, anticholinergics, theophylline)	Open the airways by relaxing smooth muscles in airway; different drugs work together for best response; improve gas exchange, decreases wheezing and coughing
Antiinflammatory agents (corticosteroids, cromolyn)	Reduce pulmonary edema and inflammation in small airways; enhance effect of bronchodilators
Diuretics (furosemide, chlorothiazide, spironoloactone)	Help remove excess fluid from lungs; decrease pulmonary resistance and increase pulmonary compliance; may cause electrolyte imbalances
Potassium chloride	Prevents electrolyte imbalances associated with diuretics
Antibiotics	Low-dose prophylactic therapy to prevent severe illness; specific treatment for identified organisms

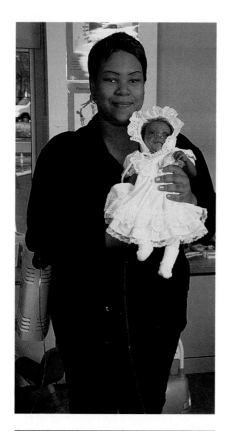

FIGURE 11-13. Many children with BPD are cared for at home, with the support of a home care program to monitor the family's ability to provide airway management, oxygen, and ventilator support. This premature infant girl, who is now 4-months old but weighs only about 5 pounds, requires respiratory support, which is provided by a portable oxygen tank.

RESPIRATORY SYNCYTIAL VIRUS

Respiratory syncytial virus (RSV) occurs in annual epidemics from October to March. By the age of 3 years, most children have been infected with RSV, and reinfection (via siblings or close family contacts) throughout life is common. RSV causes severe or fatal illness in infants with conditions such as congenital heart disease, bronchopulmonary dysplasia (BPD), prematurity, and immunosuppression.[24] Hospital personnel should follow principles of good handwashing, as the virus is easily transmitted.

tract problem.[23] Bronchitis is caused most often by a virus but may also result from invasion of bacteria or in response to an allergen or irritant.

The classic symptom of bronchitis is a coarse, hacking cough, which increases in severity at night. Children with bronchitis look tired and report that they feel awful. The chest and ribs may be sore because of the deep and frequent coughing. There is often a deep, rattling quality to breathing. Some children have audible wheezing that can be heard without a stethoscope.

Nursing Management

Nursing management includes supporting respiratory function through rest, humidification, hydration, and symptomatic treatment. Refer to the sections on asthma and pneumonia for detailed information on treatment measures.

Home care should emphasize the self-limiting nature of the disorder. Parents who smoke should be advised that quitting or refraining from smoking in the child's presence may benefit the child.

BRONCHIOLITIS

Bronchiolitis is one of the most frequent causes of hospitalization in infants[2] and poses one of the greatest threats to the respiratory system of infants and small children. Although some infants and children have mild symptoms that are easily managed at home, others become acutely ill with severe respiratory distress that can become a life-threatening emergency. What makes bronchiolitis such a potential threat?

Bronchiolitis is a lower respiratory tract illness that occurs when an infecting agent (virus or bacterium) causes inflammation and obstruction of the small airways, the bronchioles. Infection occurs most frequently in toddlers and preschoolers. Infection is most severe in infants under 6 months of age. Infants under 2 months of age are particularly vulnerable, and they are routinely hospitalized when bronchiolitis is diagnosed.

Clinical Manifestations

The infant or child with bronchiolitis may have been ill with upper respiratory symptoms such as nasal stuffiness, cough (not usually noted in infants), and fever (less than 39°C [102.2°F]) for a few days. As the illness progresses and the lower respiratory tract becomes involved, symptoms increase and include a deeper, more frequent cough and more stressful, labored breathing. Respirations are rapid, shallow, and accompanied by nasal flaring and retractions (signs of severe distress). Parents report that the infant or child is acting more ill—appearing sicker, less playful, and less interested in eating. Infants, especially, may refuse to feed or may spit up what they do eat along with thick, clear mucus.

Etiology and Pathophysiology

Bacterial, mycoplasmal, and viral organisms may cause bronchiolitis; however, infection with respiratory syncytial virus (RSV) is the most common cause. RSV is transmitted through direct or close contact with respiratory secretions of infected individuals. Viruses, acting as parasites, are able to invade the mucosal cells that line the bronchioles. The invaded cells die when the virus bursts from inside the cell to invade adjacent cells. The resulting cell debris clogs and obstructs the bronchioles and irritates the airway. In response, the airway lining swells and produces excessive mucus. Despite this protective effort by the bronchioles, the actual effect is partial airway obstruction and bronchospasms.

The cycle is repeated throughout both lungs as the airway cells are invaded by the virus. The partially obstructed airways allow air in, but the mucus and airway swelling block expulsion of the air. This creates the wheezing and crackles in the airways. Air trapped below the obstruction also interferes with normal gas exchange. The child with RSV is therefore at risk for respiratory failure as the oxygen level decreases and the carbon dioxide level increases. Apnea and pulmonary edema may occur.

As the airflow continues to decrease, breath sounds diminish. Thus the noisier the lungs, the better, as this indicates that the child is still able to move air in and out of the lungs.

Diagnostic Tests and Medical Management

The history and physical examination provide the data needed to diagnose bronchiolitis. Chest x-rays show nonspecific findings of inflammation.

Viral cultures or antigen testing of an immunofluorescence stain of respiratory secretions obtained by either a nasal swab in special culture medium or a nasopharyngeal wash confirm the presence of RSV.[24] Children who test positive for RSV are isolated, roomed together, or placed on the same ward to minimize the spread of the virus to other hospitalized children. Medical management is frequently supportive, especially when the causative agent is unknown and the condition is mild to moderate in severity (Table 11–19). Ribavirin is given by small-particle aerosol when RSV has been diagnosed.

There is evidence that bronchiolitis in infancy may increase the chances of childhood wheezing and asthma. It also may be a major risk factor for chronic obstructive pulmonary disease later in life.[2]

Nursing Assessment

Physiologic Assessment

Assess airway and respiratory function carefully. Good observation skills are important to ensure timely interventions for worsening respiratory symptoms and prevention of respiratory distress (see Tables 11–1 and 11–7).

Psychosocial Assessment

Children and their parents should be observed for signs of fear and anxiety (see Table 11–16). The unfamiliar hospital environment and procedures can increase stress. Parents' questions, as well as their nonverbal cues, help direct nursing interventions during admission and throughout hospitalization.

Developmental Assessment

Observe for signs of stranger and separation anxieties, which are common in the age group most often hospitalized for bronchiolitis (infants and small children). Involving parents in procedures and care, when appropriate, can promote emotional security.

Nursing Diagnosis

The accompanying Nursing Care Plan lists common nursing diagnoses for the child with bronchiolitis. The following diagnoses might also be appropriate:

- Ineffective Airway Clearance related to increased airway secretions, fatigue from coughing and dyspnea, and air trapping

NURSING ALERT

Ribavirin is usually administered through an endotracheal tube or double hood to reduce exposure to care providers and visitors. Although some caregivers advocate limiting ribavirin use because of its teratogenicity when given through aerosol route, efforts must be made to reduce exposure to staff, visitors, and other patients so that this lifesaving medication is not eliminated as a treatment option.[25] Pregnant health care workers should not care for children receiving this therapy.

11-19	Medical Management of Bronchiolitis

Medical Therapy	Rationale
Cardiorespiratory monitor and pulse oximetry	Enable provider to follow course and assess need for specific therapies
Humidified oxygen therapy via hood or face tent, tent, or nasal cannula	Delivery method determined by desired concentration of oxygen, degree of moisture, and child's response
Intubation and assisted ventilation	Used when the child becomes too fatigued to breathe effectively
Hydration via intravenous or oral fluids	Provider must consider insensible fluid loss, decreased intake, the child's current electrolyte and hydration status, and risk for pulmonary edema
Aerosol medications	Bronchodilators, steroids, and beta-antagonists act directly on inflamed and obstructed airways; bronchodilators help prevent apnea episodes in premature infants; ribavirin (RSV antiviral agent) reduces the severity of the illness, improves oxygenation, and decreases inflammatory injury
Pulmonary hygiene (postural drainage and chest physiotherapy)	Helps to further loosen trapped mucus
Systemic medications	Symptomatic treatment may include antipyretics (acetaminophen or ibuprofen preferred; no antibiotics are given unless evidence of secondary bacterial infection [eg, otitis media] is present)
High-Risk Infant or Child[a] Intravenous immunoglobulins	May prevent RSV bronchiolitis

[a]Defined as an infant or child with congenital heart disease, bronchopulmonary dysplasia, chronic lung problems, or cystic fibrosis or who is premature or severely ill and less than 6 weeks old.

- Ineffective Breathing Pattern related to inflamed tracheobronchial tree and progression of bronchiolitis
- Fluid Volume Deficit related to inability to meet fluid needs and increased metabolic demands (insensible loss, fever, thickened or increased respiratory secretions)

Nursing Management

Nursing management focuses on maintaining respiratory function, supporting overall physiologic function and hydration, reducing the child's and family's anxiety, and preparing the family for home care. Refer to the accompanying Nursing Care Plan, which summarizes nursing care for the child with bronchiolitis.

Maintain Respiratory Function
Close monitoring is essential to evaluate the child's improvement or to spot early signs of deterioration. Oxygen and pulmonary care therapies are administered. High humidity and supplemental oxygen may be provided with

NURSING CARE PLAN
THE CHILD WITH BRONCHIOLITIS

GOAL	INTERVENTION	RATIONALE	EXPECTED OUTCOME

1. Ineffective Breathing Pattern related to increased work of breathing and decreased energy (fatigue)

The child will return to respiratory baseline. The child will not experience respiratory failure.	• Assess respiratory status (Table 11–1) a minimum of every 2–4 hours or more often, as indicated for a decreasing respiratory rate and episodes of apnea. Cardiorespiratory monitor and pulse oximeter attached with alarms set, if ordered. Record and report changes promptly to physician.	• Changes in breathing pattern may occur quickly as the child's energy reserves are depleted. Assessment and monitoring baseline reveal rate and quality of air exchange. Frequent assessment and monitoring provides objective evidence of changes in the quality of respiratory effort, enabling prompt and effective intervention.	The child returns to respiratory baseline within 48–72 hours.

2. Altered Tissue Perfusion (Cardiopulmonary) related to partially obstructed airway

The child's oxygenation status will return to baseline.	• Administer humidified oxygen via mask, hood, or tent.	• Humidified oxygen loosens secretions and helps maintain oxygenation status and ease respiratory distressed.	The child's respiratory effort eases. Pulse oximetry reading remains > 94% oxygen saturation during treatment.
	• Note child's response to ordered medications (nebulizer treatments).	• Medications act systemically and locally (on respiratory tissue) to improve oxygenation and decrease inflammation.	The child tolerates therapeutic measures with no adverse effects.
	• Position head of bed up or place the child in position of comfort on parent's lap, if crying or struggling in crib or bed.	• Position facilitates improved aeration and promotes decrease in anxiety (especially in toddlers) and energy expenditure.	The child rests quietly in position of comfort.

3. Risk for Fluid Volume Deficit related to inability to meet body requirements and increased metabolic demand

Child's immediate fluid deficit is corrected.	• Evaluate need for intravenous fluids. Maintain IV, if ordered.	• Previous fluid loss may require immediate replacement	Child's hydration status is maintained during acute phase of illness.
Child will be adequately hydrated, be able to tolerate oral fluids, and progress to normal diet.	• Maintain strict intake and output monitoring and evaluate specific gravity at least every 8 hours.	• Monitoring provides objective evidence of fluid loss and ongoing hydration status.	Child takes adequate oral fluids after 24–48 hours to maintain hydration.

Continued . . .

NURSING CARE PLAN
THE CHILD WITH BRONCHIOLITIS– *Continued*

GOAL	INTERVENTION	RATIONALE	EXPECTED OUTCOME

3. Risk for Fluid Volume Deficit related to inability to meet body requirements and increased metabolic demand (continued)

	• Perform daily weight measurement on the same scale at the same time of day. Evaluate skin turgor.	• Further evidence of improvement of hydration status.	Child's weight stabilizes after 24–48 hours; skin turgor is supple.
	• Assess mucous membranes, and presence of tears. Report changes promptly to physician.	• Moist mucous membranes and tears provide observable evidence of hydration.	Child shows evidence of improved hydration.
	• Offer clear fluids and incorporate parent in care. Offer fluid choice when tolerated.	• Choice of fluid offered by parent gains the child's cooperation.	The child accepts beverage of choice from the parent or nursing staff.

4. Fear/Anxiety (Child and Parent) related to acute illness, hospitalization, and uncertain course of illness and treatment

Child and parents will demonstrate behaviors that indicate decrease in anxiety.	• Encourage parents to express fears and ask questions; provide direct answers and discuss care, procedures, and condition changes.	• Provides opportunity to vent feelings and receive timely, relevant information. Helps reduce parents' anxiety and increase trust in nursing staff.	Parents and child show decreasing anxiety and decreasing fear as symptoms improve and as child and parents feel more secure in hospital environment. *Parent* freely asks questions and participates in the child's care. The *child* cries less and allows staff to hold and/or touch him or her.
	• Incorporate parents in the child's care. Encourage parents to bring familiar objects from home. Ask about and incorporate in care plan the home routines for feeding and sleeping.	• Familiar people, routines, and objects decrease the child's anxiety and increase parents' sense of control over unexpected, uncertain situation.	

5. Knowledge Deficit (Child or Parent) related to diagnosis, treatment, prognosis, and home care needs

Parent will verbalize knowledge of symptoms of bronchiolitis and use of home care methods before the child's discharge from the hospital.	• Explain symptoms, treatment, and home care of bronchiolitis.	• Anticipate potential for recurrence. Assist family to be prepared should croup symptoms recur after discharge.	Parent accurately describes croup symptoms and says that a mist vaporizer is available in the child's room at home.
	• Provide written instructions for follow-up care arrangements, as needed.	• Written, as well as oral, instructions reinforce knowledge. Parents may not "hear" and remember the particulars of home care if presented only orally.	Parents take instructions home when the child is discharged.

a mist tent if the child requires only moisture and minimal oxygen. If more concentrated oxygen is required, it can be given via nasal cannula, hood, or tent. Pulse oximetry is used to evaluate oxygenation.

Patent nares are important to promote oxygen intake. A bulb syringe is a helpful tool that can quickly and easily clear the nasal passages. The head of the bed should be elevated to ease the work of breathing and drain mucus from the upper airways. Pulmonary hygiene and nebulized medications are usually administered by a respiratory therapist. Maintenance of a nebulizer for medications may be needed.

Support Physiologic Function

Grouping nursing tasks promotes the child's physiologic function by decreasing stress and promoting rest. Rest is a key component in improving the child's breathing and overall health. Medications may be administered to control temperature and promote comfort as needed. An intravenous infusion may be ordered to rehydrate and maintain fluid balance until the child is capable of taking sufficient oral fluids.

Reduce Anxiety

The need for hospitalization and assistive therapies creates anxiety and fear in the child and parents. An important part of nursing care is anticipating, recognizing, and acting to decrease the child's and parents' anxiety. Provide parents with thorough explanations and daily updates, and encourage their participation in the child's care.

The presence of parents and their ability to calm the infant or child can be helpful in the child's recovery. The parents may themselves be frightened by the child's continued respiratory difficulty and the presence of assistive equipment at the bedside. They should be reassured that holding or touching the child will not dislodge wires or tubing.

If the child has been ill for a few days before admission, the parents are likely to be tired. Acknowledging parents' physical and emotional needs facilitates a spirit of caring and enhances communication between staff and family. The parents should be encouraged to take turns at the child's bedside and to take breaks for meals and rest.

Discharge Planning and Home Care Teaching

Children are discharged once they show sufficient stability in maintaining adequate oxygenation (as evidenced by easing of respiratory effort, decreased mucus production, and absence of coughing). In most children, symptoms abate within 24–72 hours. The same supportive therapies implemented in the hospital may be needed at home:

- Use of the bulb syringe to suction the nares of an infant under 1 year of age (See *Quick Reference to Pediatric Clinical Skills.*)
- Fluid intake to thin respiratory secretions (making them easier to clear) and provide glucose for energy (since the child's appetite may not return to normal for several days)
- Rest

Children are usually capable of recognizing their own activity limits. However, parents should encourage active toddlers to nap and take rest periods. Teach the parents proper administration of medications. Acetaminophen may be prescribed for persistent low-grade fevers and general discomfort. Advise parents that RSV infection can recur; therefore, they need to know how to recognize symptoms and when to call the physician.

DISCHARGE TEACHING: BRONCHIOLITIS

Advise parents to call the physician if:
- Respiratory symptoms interfere with sleep or eating
- Breathing is rapid or difficult
- Symptoms persist in a child who is less than 1 year old, has heart or lung disease, or was premature and had lung disease after birth
- The child acts sicker—appears tired, less playful, less interested in food (parents just "feel" the child is not improving)

PNEUMONIA

Pneumonia is an inflammation or infection of the bronchioles and alveolar spaces of the lungs. It occurs most often in infants and young children. Pneumonia in children often resolves much sooner than in adults. The key is early recognition, enabling the child to be managed at home rather than in the hospital.

Pneumonia may be viral, mycoplasmal, or bacterial in origin. Common organisms causing pneumonia include RSV, parainfluenza virus, adenovirus, enterovirus, and pneumococcus. Children who are immunosuppressed are susceptible to many other bacterial, parasitic, or fungal infections. Regardless of the causative agent, symptoms include elevated temperature, cough, dyspnea, tachypnea, and abnormal breath sounds.

What physiologic process occurs to precipitate the symptoms? Bacterial and viral invaders act differently within the lungs. Bacterial invaders circulate through the bloodstream to the lungs, where they damage cells. Bacteria tend to be distributed evenly throughout one or more lobes of a single lung, a pattern termed *unilateral lobar pneumonia*. Viral or mycoplasma invaders, on the other hand, are parasites of cells. Viruses frequently enter from the upper respiratory tract, infiltrating the alveoli nearest the bronchi of one or both lungs. There they invade the cells, replicate, and burst out forcefully, killing the cells and sending out cell debris. They rapidly invade adjacent areas, distributing themselves in a scattered, patchy pattern referred to as bronchopneumonia. The end result of bacterial, viral, or mycoplasma invasion is the presence of exudate resulting from cell death, which fills the alveolar spaces, pooling and clumping in dependent areas of the lung to create areas of consolidation.

Diagnosis is made by chest x-ray, which shows an abnormal density of tissue, such as a lobar consolidation. The child's age, severity of symptoms, and presence of an underlying lung, cardiac, or immunodeficiency disease can create varying responses.

Medical management for all types of pneumonia includes symptomatic therapy (pain and fever control) and supportive care through airway management, fluids, and rest. Mycoplasma and other bacterial pneumonias are treated with organism-sensitive antibiotics; viral pneumonias usually improve independent of antibiotics.

Nursing Management

Nursing care incorporates supportive measures and medical therapies as appropriate. Nursing measures used to manage the child with bronchiolitis are generally applicable to the child with pneumonia.

In addition to ongoing respiratory assessment and supportive therapies (pulmonary care, antibiotics, hydration), the child may need relief from pain when coughing and deep breathing. Pain medication (acetaminophen or ibuprofen) can provide the added benefits of temperature control and may aid in sleep. Hospitalization is reserved for seriously ill children.

The goal of nursing care is to restore optimal respiratory function. Discharge planning should be addressed early in the hospital stay. Medications, especially antibiotics, must be taken at prescribed intervals and for the full course. Parents should be taught the proper administration of drugs and any side effects. Follow-up may include a chest x-ray to see if the lungs are clear. Symptoms of pneumonia usually disappear long before the lungs are completely healed. Some children continue to have worsening reactive airway problems or abnormal results on pulmonary function tests. Most children, however, recover uneventfully.

CLINICAL TIP

Teach the child and parent how to splint the chest, by hugging a small pillow, teddy bear, or doll, to make coughing less painful.

Preventive measures against pneumonia are limited. An immunization against pneumococcal bacteria is recommended for children over 2 years of age who are immunosuppressed or have chronic diseases.[26]

TUBERCULOSIS

Tuberculosis (TB) is caused by the organism *Mycobacterium tuberculosis*, which is transmitted through the air in infectious particles called droplet nuclei. Since 1988, the incidence of TB has been on the rise, particularly among minorities and children younger than 5 years.[27] Adults with active laryngeal or pulmonary TB may transmit the disease to children.

Clinical manifestations of TB in infants include a persistent cough, weight loss or failure to gain weight, and fever. Wheezing and decreased breath sounds may be present. Older children may be asymptomatic.

By coughing, sneezing, speaking, or singing, a person with active TB sends out tiny droplets of moisture that remain in the air. If these droplets are inhaled, the bacillus may infect the new host. Frequently, however, the organism is trapped in the upper airway, preventing infection. Infection occurs *only* when the bacillus reaches the alveoli.[28]

Once the organism reaches the alveoli, an immune response is initiated to combat the invader. The immune system sends macrophages to surround and wall off the bacillus in small hard capsules, called tubercles. There the bacillus can remain dormant (inactive) indefinitely or can progress to active TB. In young children, the disease develops as an immediate complication of the primary infection.[29] Children with HIV infection or immunosuppression may have more rapidly progressive disease. If the tubercle extends into a blood vessel, the bacillus may spread through the bloodstream to affect the liver, spleen, bone marrow, or meninges (tubercular meningitis). This systemic form of TB (called miliary tuberculosis) may lead to serious illness or death. Miliary tuberculosis is not, however, transmissible; only active pulmonary TB has the potential to infect another individual.

Several tests may be required to confirm the diagnosis (Table 11–20). Medical management focuses on diagnosis and treatment of active TB with antitubercular drug therapy. Challenges to treatment have occurred with the development of multidrug-resistant TB. Tuberculosis is a major public health problem and must be promptly reported to local health departments.

Nursing Management

Nursing care centers on administering medications and providing supportive care. Parents need to be taught about the disease process, medications, possible side effects, and the importance of long-term therapy (eg, that drug therapy may last for 6–12 months). Most children with TB are able to lead essentially normal lives. Emphasize the importance of taking medications as prescribed, and ensuring proper nutrition and rest to promote normal growth and development.

The discussion of pneumonia earlier in this chapter and the discussion of tubercular meningitis in Chapter 18 give other nursing care measures appropriate for the child with TB.

CYSTIC FIBROSIS

Cystic fibrosis is an inherited autosomal recessive disorder of the exocrine glands that results in physiologic alterations in the respiratory, gastrointestinal, integumentary, musculoskeletal, and reproductive systems. The

11-20	Diagnostic Tests for Tuberculosis
Test	**Indication**
Mantoux test (intradermal injection of purified protein derivative [PPD])	Confirms *infection* with the TB organism (2–10 weeks after exposure)
Chest x-ray examination (anteroposterior and lateral views)	Confirms presence of pulmonary tuberculosis (small, seedlike opacities may be visible)
Blood cultures for *Mycobacterium tuberculosis*	Proves diagnosis; defines specific drug sensitivity
Gastric washings (early morning after overnight fast; 3 consecutive days)	Confirms pulmonary tuberculosis (active form of tuberculosis)
Sputum cultures (expectorated or from bronchoscopic examination)	Confirms active pulmonary tuberculosis
Pleural biopsy for culture and tissue examination	Taken when pleural effusion is present
Lumbar puncture	Confirms meningeal tuberculosis (inactive form of tuberculosis)

THE FOUR Fs OF CYSTIC FIBROSIS

Stools of a child with cystic fibrosis are characteristically:
- **F**rothy (bulky and large quantity)
- **F**oul smelling
- **F**at containing (greasy)
- **F**loat

Ralph Turner's Story

My name is Ralph Turner and I am a cystic.

One day I went to the store with my mother. It was winter and it was real cold outside and when I got in the store I started coughing. And my mother started pounding on me so I could get up the mucus and I wouldn't be coughing. But then this lady said, "Look at that mother beating on that kid who has a cold." And my mother told the lady to shut up and she told her what I had. And the lady didn't say nothing else.

I know some more things about cystic fibrosis. When I play baseball, I run to the bases and start coughing sometimes and I have to rest for a little while and then I am fine. And then I can play again. I can ride my bike and—ooh!—I ride my bike and that is good for us. It helps us bring up the mucus. That's right! When we go real fast we bring up the mucus!

The mucus is the stuff that I cough up. It is called phlegm. If I told you everything I did when I cough—you'd be amazed! Like when I jump and I land real hard on my feet—I cough! I want to be like Reggie Jackson and be on the Orioles. When people grow up they don't have that much trouble. They have to cough but not that much. Like I know this man who has cystic fibrosis and he is my father's friend and he doesn't have that much trouble.

My cousin has cystic fibrosis and his name is Ralph Paul Turner. He is 14 years old. Sometimes he has trouble like me. We were born with cystic fibrosis but they didn't know I had cystic fibrosis until I was 4 months old. Now I am 7.

I hope they find a cure for us kids soon.

by Ralph Dwayne Turner. Age, 7 years old
Died, 9 years old

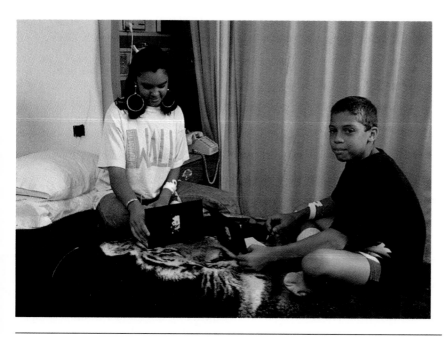

FIGURE 11–14. Cystic fibrosis is an inherited autosomal recessive disorder of the exocrine glands, so it is not uncommon to see siblings with it such as this brother and sister.

disorder occurs predominantly in white children, but other populations are also affected. Gender is not a factor in incidence (Fig. 11–14).

Clinical Manifestations

The primary symptom of cystic fibrosis is the production of thick, sticky mucus. One of the earliest signs in the newborn is meconium ileus, a small bowel obstruction that occurs during the first few days of life. In infants and toddlers, fecal impaction and intussusception ("telescoping" of the bowel) may be the first signs of the disorder. Steatorrhea (fatty stool) is one of the characteristic signs of cystic fibrosis. The sticky, thick stool is thought to create the initial obstruction. Intestinal peristalsis (controlled by the autonomic nervous system) is also adversely affected. Rectal prolapse, resulting from the large, bulky, difficult-to-pass stools, occurs in 20% of infants and children with cystic fibrosis[31] (Fig. 11–15).

Other signs and symptoms include a chronic moist, productive cough and frequent respiratory infections. Most children have difficulty maintaining and gaining weight despite a voracious appetite. Infants and children may have a delayed bone age, short stature, and delayed onset of puberty. Clubbing of the tips of the fingers and toes occurs as the disease progresses (Fig. 11–16).

Etiology and Pathophysiology

A gene isolated on chromosome 7 directs the function of the cystic fibrosis transmembrane conductance regulator (CFTR). With a defective CFTR, there is defective chloride-ion transport across the secretory epithelial cells. When the chloride ions are not permeable, water does not move across cell membranes, leading to viscous secretions. Ultimately, all body organs with mucous ducts become obstructed and damaged.[32]

Because of the blocked pancreatic ducts and resulting pancreatic damage, the natural enzymes necessary to digest fats and proteins are not secreted and essential nutrients are excreted in the stool.

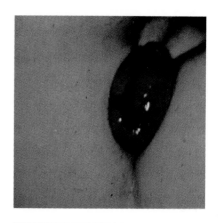

FIGURE 11–15. Rectal prolapse.

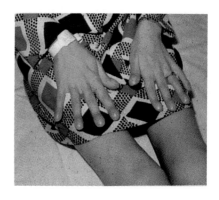

FIGURE 11–16. Digital clubbing.

The classic cough occurs because the lungs are always filled with mucus, which the respiratory cilia cannot clear. This causes air to become trapped in the small airways, resulting in atelectasis (pulmonary collapse). Secondary respiratory infections occur because secretions provide an environment conducive to bacterial growth.

Nearly all males who have cystic fibrosis are sterile because of blockage or absence of the vas deferens.[32] Females have difficulty conceiving because increased mucus secretions in the reproductive tract interfere with the passage of sperm.[32]

Metabolic function is altered as a result of the imbalances created by excessive electrolyte loss through perspiration, saliva, and mucus secretion. The "salty taste" of the skin is the result of sodium chloride that makes its way through skin pores to the skin surface.

Diagnostic Tests and Medical Management

Cystic fibrosis is usually diagnosed in infancy or early childhood with one of three major presentations: newborn meconium ileus, malabsorption or failure to thrive, or chronic recurrent respiratory infections. Some children with a milder form of the disease, however, may reach the teen or young adult years before symptoms appear.

Cystic fibrosis is diagnosed definitively by a positive sweat test and the presence of classic symptoms or a positive family history[32] (Table 11–21). Genetic testing of the child's DNA is possible if symptoms are present and the sweat test is not diagnostic.[31]

The sweat test may be performed at the child's bedside or on an outpatient basis. The parents should be present to hold and reassure the infant or small child (Fig. 11–17). They should be informed that the test will indicate whether the child has cystic fibrosis and that a second test may be ordered to confirm the diagnosis.

Medical management focuses on maintaining respiratory function, managing infection, promoting optimal nutrition and exercise, and preventing gastrointestinal blockage (Table 11–22). Improvements in medical management now enable many children with cystic fibrosis to survive into adulthood. The disease is ultimately terminal, however, because of the progressive multisystem changes and the difficulty of long-term infection management.

Care of the child with previously diagnosed cystic fibrosis is the focus of the following discussion.

DIAGNOSTIC CLUE

"I kissed my baby's cheek and tasted salt! Nothing would be the same after that."
—The mother of a 1-week-old infant with cystic fibrosis

GENETIC CONSIDERATIONS

Recent advances in localization of the cystic fibrosis gene (on chromosome 7) by genetic linkage studies have led to successful techniques for prenatal diagnosis and carrier testing. The possibility of gene therapy by transfer of the normal gene to airway epithelial cells is also being investigated.

11-21	Diagnostic Test for Cystic Fibrosis (Sweat Test)		
Test	Purpose	Normal Values	Diagnostic Values
Sweat test (pilocarpine iontophoresis)	Analysis of sodium and chloride content in sweat	Sodium: 10–30 mEq/L; Chloride: 10–35 mEq/L	Chloride: 50–60 mEq/L—suspicious; > 60 mEq/L—diagnostic with other clinical signs

11-22   Medical Management of Cystic Fibrosis

Medical Therapy	Rationale
Respiratory Therapy	
Aerosol bronchodilators	Opens large and small airways; used if reactive airway disease responds positively to use before chest physiotherapy
Aerosol Dornase alfa	Loosens, liquefies, and thins pulmonary secretions; decreases risk of developing pulmonary infections requiring parenteral treatment in some patients[33]
Antiinflammatory agents: steroids, high-dose ibuprofen	Reduces inflammatory response to chronic infection; short courses to decrease side effects of steroids; decreases progression of lung damage in preadolescents with mild disease
Chest physiotherapy for all lung segments (bilateral percussion-vibration and forceful coughing)	Mobilizes secretions to bronchi for expectoration
Infection Management (Most Susceptible to *H. influenzae, S. aureus,* and *P. aeruginosa* Bacteria and Viral Agents)	
Antibiotics (oral, IV, aerosol routes)	Treatment based on sputum-culture results; may need higher than normal doses to be effective[34]
Nutritional Needs	
Pancreatic enzyme supplements (Cotazym-S, Pancrease, Viokase) taken with meals and snacks	Assists in digestion of nutrients and decreasing fat and bulk
Diet supplies well-balanced, nutritious food with 120–150% of RDA recommended calories and 200% of RDA recommended protein, and moderate fat; nutritional counseling necessary	Promotes essential nutrient balance for health, growth, and weight maintenance; considers child, food, and cultural-socioeconomic issues
Multivitamins and vitamin E in water-soluble form; vitamins A, D, and K given when deficient; iron supplementation	Cystic fibrosis interferes with vitamin production; supplements are required in water-soluble form for better absorption (vitamins A, D, E, and K are naturally fat soluble); iron deficiency results from malabsorption syndrome

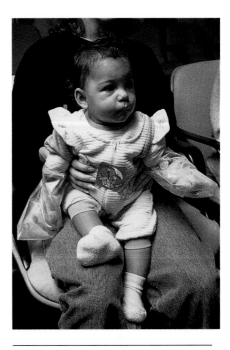

FIGURE 11–17. This 6-month-old girl is being evaluated for cystic fibrosis using the sweat test.

Nursing Assessment

Physiologic Assessment

Physical assessment of the child focuses on adequacy of respiratory function. The child with cystic fibrosis usually is admitted with symptoms of an upper respiratory infection. A set of baseline vital signs, including temperature, pulse, respirations, and blood pressure, along with a weight measurement, should be obtained on admission. Observe the child's physical appearance, noting overall body proportions and any changes characteristic of long-term cystic fibrosis.

Psychosocial Assessment

The emotional stress of this chronic disease may not be readily apparent on admission, particularly if the child's symptoms are mild and not imminently life threatening. Ongoing observation of the child's and parents' behavior helps direct nursing interventions throughout hospitalization (see Table 11–16). Sblings may also show signs of difficulty in dealing with the illness.

The nurse should ask parents how the child's illness has affected day-to-day functioning. What have parents told the child and siblings about the disease? What kind of questions have the child and siblings asked about cystic fibrosis, and how have parents answered them? Has the child ever asked about his or her life expectancy? If not, what would parents say if asked?

Developmental Assessment

Growth and development may be altered by the chronic nature of the disease. Children with cystic fibrosis are growth retarded, with 40% of them below the 5% weight for age level on a growth curve.[35] Compare the child's height and weight to age norms and observe the adolescent for the appearance of secondary sex characteristics, which are often delayed. School-age children and adolescents often are embarrassed at being viewed as different from playmates and peers. Ask how the child and adolescent feels about the need for a special diet, medications, and limitations.

Nursing Diagnosis

Common nursing diagnoses for the child with cystic fibrosis include the following:

- Ineffective Airway Clearance related to thick mucus in lungs
- Ineffective Breathing Pattern related to thick tracheobronchial secretions and airway obstruction
- Risk for Infection related to the presence of mucous secretions conducive to bacterial growth
- Altered Nutrition: Less Than Body Requirements related to inability to digest nutrients
- Fear/Anxiety (Parent or Child) related to prognosis and effect of illness on growth and development
- Knowledge Deficit (Parent or Child) related to diet, therapies, and follow-up care

Nursing Management

Nursing management involves supporting the child and family initially, when the diagnosis is made, during subsequent hospitalizations, and during visits to specialty and primary health care providers. The nurse's role begins with implementing specific medical therapies and providing nursing care to meet the child's physiologic and psychosocial needs. Respiratory therapy, medications, and diet must be coordinated to promote optimal body function. Psychosocial support and reinforcement of the child's daily care needs are important in preparation for home care.

Children with cystic fibrosis require periodic hospitalization when a severe infection occurs. Including parents in the child's routine care as much as possible helps them to maintain the child's home schedule while hospitalized. However, parents may view the hospital stay as a break from the rigorous daily pulmonary routine at home and need support in taking advantage of some "down" time. The family often becomes proficient at providing physical care to the child, but the nurse should take the opportunity provided during rehospitalization to review basic information about respiratory care, medications, and nutrition. Keeping lines of communication open and validating parents' understanding of their child's disease and care needs are important steps in preparing the family to cope with this chronic health challenge.

Provide Respiratory Therapy

Chest physiotherapy is usually performed one to three times per day before meals to clear secretions from the lungs (Fig. 11–18). Parents and other family members can learn to help with these necessary treatments. (Refer to the *Quick Reference to Pediatric Clinical Skills* accompanying this text.) Pulmonary care may involve aerosol treatments and antibiotics when indicated (see Table 11–22).

Administer Medications and Meet Nutritional Needs

Digestive problems can be eased with special medications and dietary modification (see Table 11–22). Pancreatic enzyme supplements come in powder sprinkles and capsule form and are taken orally with all meals and large snacks. The amount needed is individualized based on the child's nutritional needs and digestive response to these supplements. The goal is to achieve near-normal, well-formed stools and adequate weight gain.

Some fat-soluble vitamins (A, D, E, and K) are not completely absorbed from food; therefore they must be taken in water-soluble form. Multivitamins taken twice daily usually are sufficient to prevent deficiency. The diet should be well-balanced, with an emphasis on high caloric value. Respiratory complications necessitate additional energy expenditure, and some

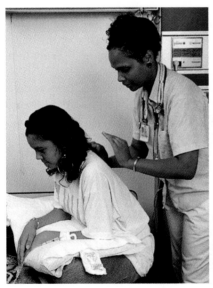 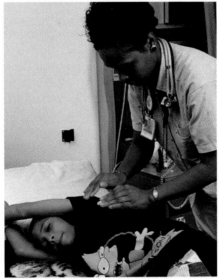

A   B

FIGURE 11–18. Postural drainage can be achieved by clapping with a cupped hand on the chest wall over the segment to be drained to create vibrations that are transmitted to the bronchi to dislodge secretions. **A,** If the obstruction is in the posterior apical segment of the lung, the nurse can do this with the child sitting up. **B,** If the obstruction is in the left posterior segment, the child should be lying on the right side. Several other positions can be used depending on the location of the obstruction.

children require special nutritional supplements, and sometimes supplemental nasogastric or gastrostomy feedings, to gain and maintain weight.

Fats and salt are both necessary in the diet. Balanced with pancreatic enzyme supplements, moderate fat intake adds an important source of extra fuel.

Provide Anticipatory Guidance

The nurse should assist the parents and child to learn what they must do to maintain health after discharge. Emotional support is essential because the diagnosis of this invariably fatal disorder creates anxiety and fear in both the parents and the child. They need assistance with emotional and psychosocial issues relating to discipline, body image (stooling and odor), frequent rehospitalization, the fatal nature of the illness, the child's feeling of being different from friends, and overall financial, social, and family concerns. Because the disorder is inherited, families may have more than one child with cystic fibrosis. Parents may have unspoken feelings of anger and guilt, blaming themselves for their children's condition.

Discharge Planning and Home Care Teaching

The financial burden of medications, supplies, and medical follow-up may not be recognized immediately by a family already overwhelmed by the diagnosis. Because of the chronicity of cystic fibrosis, home care is as important as care of the child in the hospital. Initially, parents need assistance in obtaining necessary equipment. If the family requires financial assistance, they should be referred to the appropriate social services. Home care of the child with cystic fibrosis is expensive and can be draining on the family's finances.

Parents need to learn chest physiotherapy, which the child will need as often as three or four times a day. Arranging for a visiting nurse and a respiratory therapist to visit the family frequently can provide reassurance and relief to the family. Managing the child's nutritional needs is important and takes time and energy.

Parents need to learn how to mix enzymes for young children, what vitamins need to be given daily, and what foods should be avoided or eliminated because of the child's digestive problems. Referral should be made to a nutritionist either before or at the time of discharge.

Cystic fibrosis affects all family members and disrupts activities of daily living for everyone. It is important to refer familes to family counseling and group therapy with familes of other children with cystic fibrosis if indicated. The Cystic Fibrosis Foundation (see Appendix F) is a source for information on current advances in cystic fibrosis. Local chapter activities also provide emotional support for parents and children.

Care in the Community

Nurses may encounter the child with cystic fibrosis in any of the following settings: clinics specializing in the disease, pediatricians' offices, and schools. The primary goal is to keep the disease under control by promoting optimal nutrition and assisting the family reduce the incidence of infection. Nurses may also provide home care to the child with cystic fibrosis following hospitalization for an acute exacerbation or provide hospice care.

Assessment. Assess the child's respiratory status. Inquire about the frequency and character of the child's cough and characteristics of the sputum. Compare this information with the child's baseline. Changes in the cough may be more important than its presence or absence. Auscultate the chest for breath sounds, crackles, and wheezes. Note any cyanosis or clubbing of the extremities. Oxygen saturation and spirometry readings should be obtained if changes in respiratory status are suspected.

Evaluate the child's growth, plotting the weight and height on a growth curve. Determine whether the child is maintaining an appropriate growth pattern. Inquire about the child's appetite and dietary intake. How are nutritional supplements, pancreatic enzymes, and vitamins used?

Assess the child's stooling pattern. Identify whether the child has problems with abdominal pain or bloating, and whether these problems can be related to eating, stooling, or other activities. Palpate the abdomen for liver size, fecal masses, and evidence of pain.

Inquire about the family's and child's emotional and psychosocial responses to managing the illness. These issues are very important when the child is going through major developmental stages.

Management. Review the child's use of bronchodilators and airway clearance techniques. To prevent a change in pulmonary status from progressing, short-term changes in care may be recommended. These may include antibiotics and an increase in the number of times chest physiotherapy is performed daily. Help the family select the best time to fit the additional treatment into their schedule.

Malnutrition is a major problem for children with cystic fibrosis. Parents often need to plan meals and snacks for the young child to ensure that adequate calories are consumed. Nutritional supplements may be suggested when growth is not adequate. Arrange for a consultation with a nutritionist if the family would benefit from new strategies to help meet the child's nutritional needs.

Children with cystic fibrosis lose more than normal amounts of salt in their sweat. This loss can become intensified during hot weather, strenuous exercise, and fever. Parents should allow the child to add extra salt to food and should permit some salty snacks (pretzels with salt, pickles, carbonated soda). During periods of increased sweating, the child should be encouraged to drink more fluids and increase salt intake. Teach parents to recognize early symptoms of salt depletion, including fatigue, weakness, abdominal pain, and vomiting, and to contact the child's health care provider if these symptoms occur.

Talk with the child and family to identify any assistance needed with emotional and psychosocial issues. Depending on the child's developmental stage, issues related to discipline, body image (stooling and odor), or the child's feeling of being different from friends may be major concerns. The family may also have overall financial, social, and family management concerns that can be discussed.

CLINICAL TIP

Parents often have a difficult time getting the child with cystic fibrosis to eat the extra calories needed for optimal nutrition, setting the stage for a potential mealtime battleground. To be successful, parents need guidance about managing mealtime behaviors in addition to guidelines for preparing nutritional calorie-dense foods.[36]

► INJURIES OF THE RESPIRATORY SYSTEM

Airway compromise after an unintentional injury is a major cause of death in children.[11] Why are children so vulnerable to changes in respiratory function after accidental injury?

The small size of the child's airway makes it vulnerable to obstruction. The tongue, small amounts of blood, mucus, or foreign debris or swelling in the respiratory tract or adjacent neck tissue may block the airway and lead to hypoxia and respiratory failure. If the child's neck is flexed or hyperextended, the soft laryngeal cartilage may compress and obstruct the airway.

NURSING ALERT

Never allow a child's neck to hyperextend (bend completely backward) or hyperflex (bend completely forward). Hyperextension flattens the trachea because there is no firm cartilage to provide structural support. Hyperflexion can kink and compress the trachea. Both maneuvers obstruct rather than open the airway.

Infants and young children rely on the diaphragm for air movement. They are abdominal (or "belly") breathers. Excessive crying and anxiety deplete metabolic reserves. External ventilatory support and vigorous crying may impede diaphragm function if the stomach becomes distended with air. Because the child's metabolic rate is about double that of an adult, the child has a greater need for oxygen. Respiratory distress, anxiety, and even fever can dramatically add to the child's oxygen demand.

AIRWAY OBSTRUCTION

Airway obstruction exists when air passage in the respiratory tract and lungs is slowed or blocked. If the blockage occurs above the trachea, inspiration is more affected. If the blockage occurs below the trachea, expiration is more affected. Earlier sections dealt with structural and functional problems that may lead to airway obstruction. This section addresses two common conditions of airway obstruction in children that result from unintentional injury: foreign body aspiration and near-drowning.

Foreign-Body Aspiration

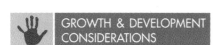

GROWTH & DEVELOPMENT CONSIDERATIONS

Foreign-body aspiration is a major health problem for infants and young toddlers because of their increasing mobility and tendency to place small objects in the mouth.

Foreign-body aspiration is the inhalation of any object (solid or liquid, food or nonfood) into the respiratory tract. Aspiration occurs most often during feeding and reaching activities, while crawling, or during playtime in children aged 6 months to 4 years of age.[9] However, aspiration may occur in children of any age.

Clinical Manifestations

Children are usually brought to the hospital after a sudden episode of coughing. Discovery of an open container with small objects may prompt parents to seek medical assistance for the child. The child may have spasmodic coughing, respiratory distress, or gagging. Sudden respiratory distress in the absence of fever or other symptoms of illness strongly suggests foreign-body aspiration.[9]

Etiology and Pathophysiology

In infants over 6 months of age and in children, aspiration may be caused by any number of small objects that make their way into the child's mouth. Foods such as nuts, popcorn, or small pieces of raw vegetables or hot dog; small, loose toy parts such as small wheels and bells; or household objects and substances such as beads, safety pins, coins, buttons, latex balloon pieces, colorful liquids (mouthwash, perfume) in enticing packages (screw top bottles) are frequent causes of airway obstruction.

The severity of the obstruction depends on the size and composition of the object or substance and its location within the respiratory tract. The majority of aspirated foreign bodies (AFBs) usually cause bronchial, not tracheal, obstruction. An object lodged high in the airway above the vocal cords is frequently coughed out easily or with some assistance (such as use of chest thrusts and back blows or the abdominal thrust). (Refer to the *Quick Reference to Pediatric Clinical Skills* accompanying this text.) An object lodged in the trachea is a life-threatening situation.

Coughing, choking, gagging, dysphonia, and wheezing may be brief or may persist for several hours if the object drops below the trachea into one of the mainstem bronchi. The right lung is the most common site of lower airway aspiration because of the sloped angle of its bronchus (see Fig. 11–2). Objects may migrate from higher to lower airway locations. An object may also move back up to the trachea, creating extreme respiratory difficulty.[9] If oxygen is depleted for an extended time, brain damage may occur.

Diagnostic Tests and Medical Management

Medical management focuses on taking a careful history to determine whether aspiration has indeed occurred. Choking associated with feeding or crawling on the floor is usually a confirming event. The physical examination often reveals decreased breath sounds, stridor, and respiratory distress in the child without a witnessed aspiration. A special radiograph, called a forced expiratory film, may be ordered. This shows local hyperinflation and mediastinal shift away from the affected side.[9] Sometimes, when the object aspirated is radiopaque, it can be seen on an x-ray film (Fig. 11–19). Fluoroscopy and fiberoptic bronchoscopy may be used to identify, locate, and extract the AFB.

The child with an AFB that is removed is usually stabilized in the emergency department and observed for a few hours. Depending on the type of object and degree of obstruction, surgical removal of the object and hospitalization may be required.

Nursing Assessment

Physiologic Assessment. If the object remains lodged, the child is observed for increasing signs of respiratory distress, especially vital signs and audible wheezing on auscultation. Changes in breath sounds, from noisy to decreasing to absent, on the affected side are noted. This can indicate that the object is moving and blocking a mainstem bronchus.

Psychosocial Assessment. The unexpected and acute nature of the event creates anxiety for both parents and child. The child and parents also may be experiencing a variety of other emotions—fear, anger, or guilt. The nurse should assess coping and level of stress. Providing a quiet environment and encouraging the presence of the parents can help to reduce the child's fear and anxiety.

Developmental Assessment. As the child's condition stabilizes, the nurse observes how well the child's abilities match the parents' understanding of age-appropriate behaviors. Providing anticipatory teaching or reinforcing information about developmental characteristics (see Chap. 2) helps parents to anticipate safety hazards in the future.

Nursing Diagnosis

Common nursing diagnoses for a child with an AFB include the following:

- Ineffective Airway Clearance related to foreign object trauma (previously removed or coughed out object)
- Ineffective Breathing Pattern related to inflamed tracheobronchial tree (object in place, or removed with traumatic edema)
- Fear/Anxiety (Parent or Child) related to uncertainty of prognosis, unfamiliar surroundings and procedures
- Knowledge Deficit (Parent) related to follow-up required after discharge, childproofing the home

Nursing Management

The first 12 hours after aspiration are critical, and subtle changes in the child's respiratory status during this period must be documented and re-

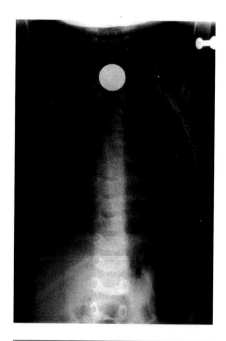

FIGURE 11–19. An aspirated foreign body (coin) is clearly visible in the child's trachea on this chest x-ray.
Courtesy of Rockwood Clinic, Spokane, WA.

CLINICAL TIP

If the child cannot say the "P" in words like Pluto or Peter Pan, the expiratory effort is noticeably diminished as a result of the foreign body.

ported promptly. The child and family should be apprised of procedures and provided with emotional support.

Discharge Planning and Home Care Teaching. Discharge planning centers on anticipatory guidance about childproofing the home (see Chap. 2) and encouraging the parents to learn CPR, choking-prevention techniques, and back blows, chest thrusts, or abdominal thrusts. (Refer to the *Quick Reference to Pediatric Clinical Skills* accompanying this text.)

NEAR-DROWNING

Near-drowning incidents and death by drowning are most prevalent in children under 5 years of age. In this age group, drowning is a leading cause of death resulting from injury.[37] Groups at high risk include toddlers, teenage boys, and children with seizure disorders. Children with seizure disorders may experience sudden and uncontrollable loss of body position that places them at risk without warning.

Near-drowning is defined as resuscitation and survival for 24 hours following a submersion injury. Near-drowning may result in complete recovery, severe brain injury, or variable neurologic deficits.[37] A key feature influencing survival is initiation of immediate resuscitation, followed, it is hoped, by spontaneous respiratory effort by the child within 5 minutes after removal from the water.[37] The mouth is cleaned of foreign matter, but time should not be wasted trying to remove water from the lungs. The sooner the child is ventilated, the better the chance of survival with normal neurologic potential. Emergency transport to a hospital should occur as soon as possible, even if spontaneous breathing is initiated.

Most drownings occur in the child's home pool or at the residence of a neighbor, friend, or relative. Usually the child is playing, is not wearing a swimsuit, and is briefly unsupervised before the immersion. Other common drowning sites for young children include bathtubs, hot tubs, toilets, and even large water-filled buckets. A child can drown in as little as 2 in. (5 cm) of water and an infant in 1 in.(2.5 cm).[37] In most immersion cases, hypoxemia begins within seconds and irreversible nervous system cell changes begin within 4–6 minutes (refer to Chap. 18). Hypoxemia is the most important consequence of near-drowning. Supportive care for any progression of pathology related to cerebral edema and aspiration of water is key. Damage to the airways from loss of surface-active material can lead to capillary leakage and pulmonary edema.[37]

Nursing Management

Nursing management focuses on observation and support of cardiopulmonary and central nervous system function (see Chap. 18). Frequent neurologic monitoring with the Glasgow Coma Scale and assessment of vital signs provide valuable baseline information. A chest x-ray may be ordered to establish baseline information about lung expansion and pulmonary integrity. Pulse oximetry will be ordered to provide ongoing data about the child's oxygenation status. The nurse should document any change in respiratory status and notify the physician promptly.

The child and family need support to work through the feelings surrounding the near-drowning incident, the unexpected hospitalization, and an uncertain prognosis that may mean the child will not return to normal functioning. Prevention is the key to avoiding a similar mishap in the future.

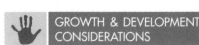

GROWTH & DEVELOPMENT CONSIDERATIONS

Toddlers have large heads, which makes them top heavy, and an unsteady gait that compromises body control and speed of movement. When propelled into a body of water, they may be unable to escape. Teenage boys may engage in risky behavior around or in a body of water, placing themselves or others at risk.

SMOKE-INHALATION INJURY

Exposure to fire conditions sets up dramatic responses in the respiratory tract of children. In every age group, inhalation injury significantly increases the child's chance of death.[38]

The severity of the smoke-inhalation injury is influenced by the type of material burned and whether the child was found in an open or closed space. The composition of materials determines how easily they ignite, how fast they burn, and how much heat they release. These factors influence the production of smoke and toxic gases. Smoke, a product of the burning process that is composed of gases and particles, is generated in varying volumes and density. The type and concentration of toxic gases, which are usually invisible, affect the severity of pulmonary damage. The duration of exposure to the smoke produced and any toxic gases contribute significantly to the child's prognosis.

Exposure to extreme heat, common in house fires, leads to surface injury and upper airway damage. The upper airway normally removes heat from inhaled gases, sparing the lower airway from thermal damage. However, this action results in marked edema, placing the small child at particular risk for airway obstruction. Edema develops rapidly over a few hours and may lead to acute respiratory distress syndrome. Burns of the face and neck, singed nasal hairs, soot around the mouth or nose, and hoarseness with stridor or voice change all indicate inhalation injury.

Carbon monoxide (CO) is a clear, colorless, odorless gas that is present in all fire conditions. The CO molecule binds more firmly to hemoglobin than does oxygen. As a result, it replaces oxygen in circulation and rapidly produces hypoxia in the child. The longer the exposure to CO, the greater the hypoxia. The brain receives inadequate oxygen, resulting in confusion. This accounts for the inability of fire victims to escape as confusion progresses to loss of consciousness. The process can be rapidly reversed, however, by timely administration of 100% oxygen.[39]

Damage to the lower airway most often results from chemicals or toxic gas inhalation. Soot is carried deep into the lungs, where it combines with water in the lungs to deposit acid-producing chemicals on the lung tissue. These acids burn the tissue, causing loss of cilia, loss of surfactant, and edema. Tissue destruction, edema, and disruption of gas exchange produce the initial insult to the lungs. Days later, the damaged tissue sloughs off, obstructing the airways. Because the cilia that normally help in removing debris have been destroyed, the lungs become a breeding ground for microorganisms. Pneumonia becomes a major health concern. The damaged alveoli heal by scar tissue formation. This can greatly reduce the future functioning of the lungs.

Nursing Management

Most children who survive smoke-inhalation injury are admitted for close observation, airway management, and ventilatory support, if indicated. Respiratory assessment and pulmonary therapy are usually required to reestablish adequate oxygenation and respiratory function.

BLUNT CHEST TRAUMA

Blunt trauma is a common injury in children, especially associated with motor vehicle crashes.[40] Chest injuries may not be obvious and can be extremely difficult to evaluate.

After sustaining severe blunt trauma, most children die from lack of oxygen caused by poor airway and ventilatory control. A child's elastic, pliable chest wall and thin abdominal muscles provide minimal protection to underlying organs. This elasticity often spares bone but not the underlying organs. The presence of a rib fracture in children under 12 years old indicates trauma of significant force. The energy from blunt trauma is transferred directly from an external force to the internal organs, often causing a pulmonary contusion or pneumothorax.

PULMONARY CONTUSION

A pulmonary contusion is defined as bruising damage to the tissues of the lung. This causes bleeding into the alveoli, which may lead to capillary rupture in the air sacs. Edema develops in the lower airways as blood and fluid from damaged tissues accumulate. Lower airway obstruction and atelectasis may result.[38]

Pulmonary contusion occurs in up to 76% of children with nonpenetrating chest trauma. Initially the child may appear asymptomatic. Careful observation is required during the first 12 hours after the injury to detect decreased perfusion related to ventilatory impairment.

Nursing Management

Nursing care centers on providing necessary physiologic support, such as oxygen therapy, positioning, and comfort measures. The child's level of consciousness is an excellent indicator of respiratory function. Agitation and lethargy can signal increasing hypoxia. The thorax should be inspected for symmetric chest wall movement and equal presence of breath sounds in both lungs. The child may initially appear well but requires careful and thorough monitoring to detect signs of deterioration. Children with significant injuries are cared for in the intensive care unit. Some children require ventilator support as the pulmonary tissues heal.

PNEUMOTHORAX

A pneumothorax occurs when air collects between the pleural layers, causing the lung to collapse. If blood collects in the pleural space, it is called a *hemothorax,* and if blood and air collect, it is called a *pneumohemothorax.* A pneumothorax is one of the more common thoracic injuries in pediatric trauma patients.

There are three types of pneumothorax: open, closed, and tension. An open pneumothorax, sometimes referred to as a sucking chest wound, results from any penetrating injury that exposes the pleural space to atmospheric pressure, thereby collapsing the lung.

A closed pneumothorax is sometimes caused by blunt chest trauma with no evidence of rib fracture (Fig. 11–20). The chest may be compressed against a closed glottis, causing a sudden increase in pressure within the thoracic cavity. The child spontaneously holds his or her breath when the thorax is struck, accounting for the involuntary closing of the glottis. The pressure increase is transferred to the alveoli, causing them to burst. A single burst alveolus may be able to seal itself off, but with the destruction of many alveoli the lung collapses. Breath sounds are decreased or absent on the injured side, and the child is in respiratory distress.[38] A thoracostomy is performed and a chest tube inserted. A closed drainage system is attached to help remove the air and reinflate the lung by reestablishing negative pressure. (Refer to the *Quick Reference to Pediatric Clinical Skills* accompanying this text.)

CLINICAL TIP

When monitoring the status of a child who has a pulmonary contusion, do not rely on the child's color as an indicator of adequate oxygenation. Cyanosis in children is often a late indicator of respiratory distress. Observe for hemoptysis (fresh blood in the emesis), dyspnea, decreased breath sounds, wheezes, crackles, and a transient temperature elevation.

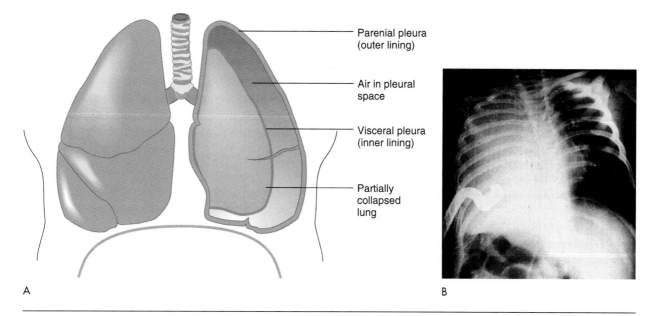

Parenial pleura
(outer lining)

Air in pleural
space

Visceral pleura
(inner lining)

Partially
collapsed
lung

A   B

FIGURE 11–20. **A,** A pneumothorax is air in the pleural space that causes a lung to collapse. Whether the air results from an open injury or from bursting of alveoli due to a blunt injury, it is important to focus on airway management and maintain lung inflation. **B,** Pneumothorax. B, copyright © 1975 MEDCOM, Inc.

A tension pneumothorax is a life-threatening emergency that results when the internal pressure from a closed pneumothorax is not vented and continues to build, compressing the chest contents and collapsing the lung. Air leaks into the chest cavity during inhalation but is trapped from escape during exhalation. Venous return to the heart is impaired as the trachea, heart, vena cava, and esophagus are compressed toward the unaffected lung when the mediastinum shifts. Signs of tension pneumothorax include increasing respiratory distress, decreased breath sounds, and paradoxic breathing.

Nursing Management

Nursing management focuses on airway management and maintaining lung inflation. The child arrives on the nursing unit with a chest tube and drainage system in place. Continued close observation for respiratory distress is essential. Vital signs are carefully monitored. Complications include hemothorax (if the thoracostomy and chest tube are improperly placed), lung tissue injury, and scarring from poor tube placement (especially if the tube is placed too near the breast in girls).

 ## REFERENCES

1. Maternal and Child Health Bureau, Health Resources and Services, Department of Health and Human Services. (1996). Causes of hospitalization by age: 1993. *Child health USA '95.* Rockville, MD: Author.

2. Webster, H., & Huether, S.E., (1998). Alterations in pulmonary function in children. In K.L. McCance & S.E. Huether (Eds.), *Pathophysiology: The biologic basis for disease in adults and children* (3rd ed., pp. 1201–1220). St. Louis: Mosby.

3. Brooks, J.G. (1992). Apparent life-threatening events and apnea of infancy, *Clinics in Perinatology. 19*(4), 809–838.

4. Eichenwald, E., & Stark, A. (1992). Apnea of prematurity: Etiology and management. *Tufts University School of Medicine Reports on Neonatal Respiratory Diseases, 2*(1), 1–11.

5. Sudden infant death syndrome—US, 1983–1994. (1996). *Morbidity and Mortality Weekly Report, 45*(40), October 11, 862.

6. National SIDS Resource Center. (1994). *Sudden infant death syndrome: Trying to understand the mystery.* McLean, VA: Author.

7. Lewis, K.W., & Bosque, E.M. (1995). Deficient hypoxia awakening response in infants of smoking mothers: Possible relationship to sudden infant death syndrome. *Journal of Pediatrics, 127,* 691–699.

8. Bechler-Karsch, A. (1994). Assessment and management of status asthmaticus, *Pediatric Nursing, 20*(3), 217–223.

9. Bank, D.E., & Krug, S.E. (1995). New approaches to upper airway disease. *Emergency Medical Clinics of North America, 13*(2), 473–487.

10. Eichelberger, M.R., Ball, J.W., Pratsch, G.S., & Clark, J.R. (1998). *Pediatric emergencies* (2nd ed.). Englewood Cliffs, NJ: Brady.

11. Hazinski, M.F. (1992). *Nursing care of the critically ill child* (2nd ed.). St. Louis: Mosby.

12. Richman, E. (1997). Asthma diagnosis and management: New severity classifications and therapy alternatives. *Clinician Reviews, 7*(8), 76–112.

13. Swanson, M.N., & Thompson, P.E. (1994). Managing asthma triggers in school. *Pediatric Nursing, 20*(2), 181–184.

14. Kieckhefer, G., & Ratcliffe, M. (1996). Asthma. In P.L. Jackson & J.A. Vessey (Eds.), *Primary care of the child with a chronic condition* (2nd ed., pp. 121–144). St. Louis: Mosby.

15. Beeber, S.J. (1996). Parental smoking and childhood asthma. *Journal of Pediatric Health Care, 10*(2), 58–62.

16. National Asthma Education Program, Expert Panel on the Management of Asthma. (1991). *Guidelines for the diagnosis and management of asthma* (DHHS Publication No. 91-3042A). Washington, DC: Government Printing Office.

17. Rachelefsky, G.S. (1995). Asthma update: New approaches and partnerships. *Journal of Pediatric Health Care, 9*(1), 12–21.

18. National Asthma Education Program. (1994). *Nurses: Partners in asthma care* (NIH Publication No. 95-3308). Bethesda, MD: National Heart, Lung, and Blood Institute.

19. Tooley, W.H. (1996). Hyaline membrane disease. In A.M. Rudolph, J.I.E. Hoffman, & C.D. Rudolph (Eds.), *Rudolph's pediatrics* (20th ed., pp. 1598–1605). Stamford, CT: Appleton & Lange.

20. Rastogi, A., Akintorin, S.M., Bez, M.L., Morales, P., & Pildes, R.S. (1996). A controlled trial of dexamethasone to prevent bronchopulmonary dysplasia in surfactant-treated infants. *Pediatrics, 98*(2), 204–210.

21. Parker, R.A., Lindstrom, D.P., & Cotton, R.B. (1992). Improved survival accounts for most, but not all, of the increase in bronchopulmonary dysplasia. *Pediatrics, 90,* 663–668.

22. Harvey, K. (1996). Bronchopulmonary dysplasia. In P.L. Jackson & J.A. Vessey (Eds.), *Primary care of the child with a chronic condition* (2nd ed., pp. 172–192). St. Louis: Mosby.

23. D'Auria, J.P. (1997). Respiratory system. In J.A. Fox (Ed.), *Primary health care of children* (pp. 415–418). St. Louis: Mosby.

24. Chiocca, E.M. (1994). RSV and the high-risk infant. *Pediatric Nursing, 20*(6), 565–568.

25. Jury, D.L. (1993). More on RSV and ribavirin. *Pediatric Nursing, 20*(1), 89–92.

26. Koslap-Petraco, M. (1997). Immunizations. In J.A. Fox (Ed.), *Primary health care of children* (p. 168). St. Louis: Mosby.

27. Starke, J. (1992). Childhood tuberculosis during the 1990s. *Pediatrics in Review, 13,* 43–53.

28. Boutette, J. (1993). T.B. The second time around . . . *Nursing, 5,* 42–50.

29. American Thoracic Society. (1994). Treatment of TB and tuberculosis infection in adults and children. *American Journal of Respiratory Critical Care Medicine, 149,* 1359–1374.

30. Doerr, C.A., & Starke, J.R. (1996). Tuberculosis: When to test. *Contemporary Pediatrics, 13*(1), 82–104.

31. Duffield, R.A. (1993). Cystic fibrosis and the gastrointestinal tract. *Journal of Pediatric Health Care, 10*(2), 51–57.

32. McMullen, A.H. (1996). Cystic fibrosis. In P.L. Jackson & J.A. Vessey (Eds.), *Primary care of the child with a chronic condition* (2nd ed., pp. 324–349). St. Louis: Mosby.

33. Gutteridge, C., & Kuhn, R.J. (1994). Pulmozyme—Dornase alfa. *Pediatric Nursing, 20*(3), 278–279.

34. Hagemann, T. (1996). Cystic fibrosis—Drug therapy. *Journal of Pediatric Health Care, 10*(3), 127–134.

35. Fitzsimmons, S.C. (1993). The changing epidemiology of cystic fibrosis. *Journal of Pediatrics, 122,* 1–9.

36. Stark, L.J., Knapp, L., Bowen, A.M., Powers, S.W., Jelalian, E., et al. (1993). Behavioral treatment of calorie consumption in children with cystic fibrosis: Replication with 2 years' follow-up. *Journal of Applied Behavior Analysis, 26*(4), 435–450.

37. Fields, A.I. (1993). Near drowning. In M.R. Eichelberger (Ed.), *Pediatric trauma: Prevention, acute care, rehabilitation* (pp. 606–615). St. Louis: Mosby.

38. Allshouse, M.J., & Eichelberger, M.R. (1993). Patterns of thoracic injury. In M.R. Eichelberger (Ed.), *Pediatric trauma: Prevention, acute care, rehabilitation* (pp. 437–448). St. Louis: Mosby.

39. Kane, T.D., & Warden, G.D. (1996). Pediatric burn injury. In A.M. Rudolph, J.I.E. Hoffman, & C.D. Rudolph (Eds.), *Rudolph's pediatrics* (20th ed., pp. 866–867). Stamford, CT: Appleton & Lange.

40. Templeton, J.M. (1993). Mechanism of injury: Biomechanics. In M.R. Eichelberger (Ed.), *Pediatric trauma: Prevention, acute care, rehabilitation* (p. 21). St. Louis: Mosby.

ADDITIONAL RESOURCES

Ahmann, E. (1996). *Home care of the high risk infant* (2nd ed.). Rockville, MD: Aspen Systems.

Allen, D.B. (1996). Growth suppression by glucocorticoid therapy. *Endocrinology and Metabolism Clinics of North America, 25*(3), 699–717.

Back, K.J. (1991). Sudden, unexpected pediatric death: Caring for the parents. *Pediatric Nursing, 17*(6), 571–575.

Berti, L.C. (1996). Childhood tuberculosis. *Journal of Pediatric Health Care, 10*(3), 106–114.

Campbell, L.S., & Thomas, D.O. (1991). Pediatric trauma: When kids get hurt. *RN, 8,* 32–39.

Castiglia, P.T. (1996). Adjusting to childhood asthma. *Journal of Pediatric Health Care, 10*(3), 82–84.

Cruz, M.N., Stewart, G., & Rosenberg, N. (1995). Use of dexamethasone in the outpatient management of acute laryngotracheitis. *Pediatrics, 96*(2), 220–223.

Cunningham, J.C., & Taussig, L.M. (1991). An introduction to cystic fibrosis for patients and families (Publication No. N8554A-4). Bethesda, MD: Cystic Fibrosis Foundation.

Coffman, S.P. (1992). Home care of the child and family after near-drowning. *Journal of Pediatric Health Care, 6,* 18–24.

Dickison, A.E. (1990). Child with upper airway obstruction: Part I. *Choices in Respiratory Management, 20*(2), 29–34.

Dickison, A.E. (1990). Child with upper airway obstruction: Part II. *Choices in Respiratory Management, 20*(3), 66–68.

Fernbach, S.D., & Thomson, E.J. (1992). Molecular genetic technology in cystic fibrosis: Implications for nursing practice. *Journal of Pediatric Nursing, 7*(1), 20–25.

Ferrante, S., & Painter, E. (1995). Continuous nebulization: A treatment modality for pediatric asthma patients, *Pediatric Nursing, 21*(4), 327–331.

Geller, G. (1995). Cystic fibrosis and the pediatric caregiver: Benefits and burdens of genetic technology. *Pediatric Nursing, 21*(1), 57–61.

Hay, W.W., Groothuis, J.R., Hayward, A.R., & Levin, M.J. (Eds.). (1997). *Current pediatric diagnosis & treatment* (12th ed.). Stamford, CT: Appleton & Lange.

Keens, T.G., & Ward, S.L.D. (1993). Apnea spells, sudden death and the role of the apnea monitor. *Pediatric Clinics of North America, 40*(5), 897–911.

McDonald, H. (1996). Mastering uncertainty: Mothering a child with asthma. *Pediatric Nursing, 22*(1), 55–59.

National Education and Prevention Program. (1997). *Expert Panel Report II: Guidelines for diagnosis and management of asthma* (NIH Publication No. 97-4051). Bethesda, MD: National Institutes of Health.

Ott, M.J., Horn, M., & McLaughlin, D. (1995). Pediatric TB in the 1990s. *American Journal of Maternal Child Nursing, 20*(1), 16–20.

Rothbaum, R.J. (1996). Improving digestion in children with cystic fibrosis. *Contemporary Pediatrics, 13*(2), 39–54.

Wagner, M.H., & Sherman, J.M. (1997). Cystic fibrosis and the general pediatrician. *Contemporary Pediatrics, 14*(2), 89–112.

Williams, J.K. (1995). Genetics and cystic fibrosis: A focus on carrier testing. *Pediatric Nursing, 21*(5), 444–448.

Wintemute, G.J. (1992). Drowning in early childhood. *Pediatric Annals, 21*(7), 417–421.

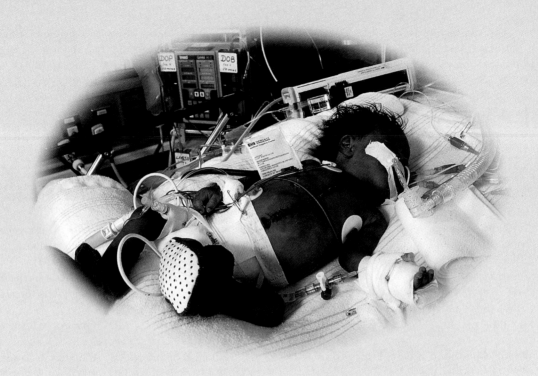

B randy, who is 1 month old, was diagnosed with a ventricular septal defect (VSD) at birth. Her parents were just beginning to accept
that she had a heart defect that might require surgical repair when
signs of respiratory distress and difficulty in feeding developed.

Brandy's mother had been alerted to watch for these signs as a possible indication of congestive heart failure. Brandy was quickly hospitalized so her
congestive heart failure could be treated with digoxin, furosemide (Lasix),
and potassium. Over the next 2 days she lost the fluid weight she had gained.

Because Brandy developed problems so soon after birth, it was decided that
she should undergo surgical correction of her heart defect. Corrective surgery
was performed to place a patch over the septal opening. Brandy was cared for
in the intensive care unit for several of days before being transferred to another unit.

What are the causes of congestive heart failure? How is this condition
treated? Is Brandy at risk to develop congestive heart failure again despite
having had corrective surgery? What teaching and support do Brandy's parents need to care for her at home after the heart surgery? Answers to these and
other questions can be found throughout this chapter.

ALTERATIONS IN CARDIOVASCULAR FUNCTION 12

"Brandy got so sick so fast. We didn't expect her to have to have surgery when she was still so small. I just want her to get stronger and have the chance to grow up to be like other kids."

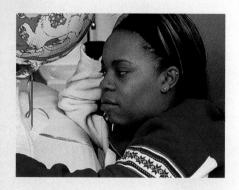

TERMINOLOGY

- **compliance** Amount of distention or expansion the ventricles can achieve to increase stroke volume.
- **desaturated blood** Blood with a lower than normal oxygen level resulting when a heart defect causes oxygenated and unoxygenated blood to mix.
- **digitalization** Process of giving a higher than normal dose of digoxin initially to speed response to the drug.
- **hemodynamics** Pressures generated by blood and passage of blood through the heart and pulmonary system.
- **palliative procedure** Intervention used to preserve life in children with a potentially fatal or lethal condition.
- **polycythemia** Above-normal increase in the number of red cells in the blood to increase the amount of hemoglobin available to carry oxygen.

- **preload** Volume of blood in the ventricle at the end of diastole that stretches the heart muscle before contraction.
- **pulmonary hypertension** Condition resulting from a chronic blood volume overload through the pulmonary arteries. It is often irreversible and leads to a life-threatening increase in pulmonary vascular resistance.
- **shunt** Movement of blood between heart chambers through an abnormal anatomic or surgically created opening.
- **syncope** Transient loss of consciousness and muscle tone.

Alterations in cardiovascular function may be a result of a congenital defect, acquired infection, or injury. Heart disease is the fourth leading cause of death in children aged 1–9 years in the United States.[1] Congenital heart defects, like Brandy's ventricular septal defect, occur in approximately 1% of all live births[2] and often require surgical correction. Rapid advances in the treatment of congenital heart defects have resulted in children having surgery at younger ages. As a result, nursing care required to identify and manage responses of infants and children with heart disease has become more challenging.

► ANATOMY AND PHYSIOLOGY OF PEDIATRIC DIFFERENCES

TRANSITION FROM FETAL TO PULMONARY CIRCULATION

After the umbilical cord has been cut, the newborn must quickly adapt to receiving oxygen from the lungs. The transition from fetal to pulmonary circulation occurs in just a few hours. During fetal circulation the constricted pulmonary vessels limit blood flow to the lungs (high pulmonary vascular resistance). Blood, however, flows easily to the extremities because systemic vascular resistance is low. The foramen ovale, an opening between the atria in the fetal heart, allows blood to flow from the right to the left atrium. Systemic vascular resistance increases after the umbilical cord is cut, causing a backup of blood flow. The pressure in the left side of the heart increases, stimulating closure of the foramen ovale. Once breathing has been initiated, the lungs expand and pulmonary vascular resistance falls. Blood that was previously shunted through the ductus arteriosus to the aorta flows to the lungs. Figure 12–1 compares fetal and pulmonary circulation.

The ductus arteriosus, responding to higher oxygen saturation, normally constricts and closes within 10–15 hours after birth. Permanent closure occurs by 10–21 days after birth, unless oxygen saturation remains low. Fetal tissues are accustomed to low oxygen saturation. This may explain why newborns with cyanotic heart disease appear relatively comfortable even when the arterial partial pressure of oxygen (PaO_2) is 20–25 mm Hg. Acidosis, cerebral anoxia, and death would occur in minutes in older children and adults with a comparable PaO_2.[3]

The ventricles are equal in size at birth, but by 2 months of age the left ventricle is twice as large as the right ventricle. The higher systemic vascular pressures force the left ventricle to develop quickly.

Infants have a greater risk of heart failure than older children because the immature heart is more sensitive to volume or pressure overload. During infancy the muscle fibers of the heart are less developed and less organized, resulting in limited functional capacity. Less **compliance** (amount of distention or expansion the ventricles can achieve to increase stroke volume) of the heart muscle means that stroke volume cannot increase substantially. The heart muscle fibers develop during early childhood so that heart function is comparable to a healthy adult's by 5 years of age.[4]

OXYGENATION

Oxygen bound to hemoglobin is transported to the tissues by the systemic circulation. Hematocrit and hemoglobin concentrations appropriate for the child's age are necessary for adequate oxygen transport (see Chap. 13).

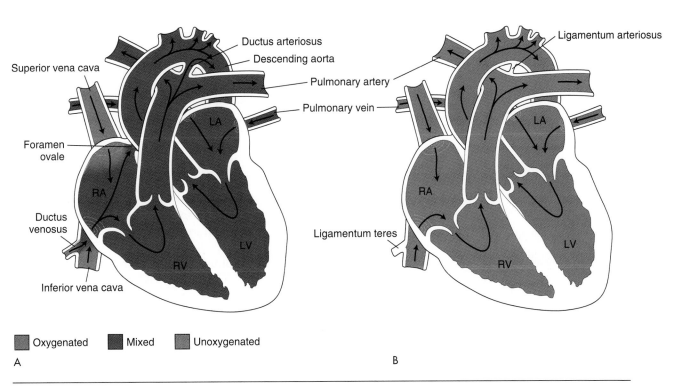

Oxygenated   Mixed   Unoxygenated

A

B

FIGURE 12–1. Normal circulation of the heart. **A,** Fetal (prenatal) circulation. **B,** Pulmonary (postnatal) circulation. *LA,* left atrium; *LV,* left ventricle; *RA,* right atrium; *RV,* right ventricle.

The oxygen arterial saturation is the amount of oxygen that can potentially be delivered to the tissues. **Desaturated blood** results when oxygenated and unoxygenated blood mix because of a congenital heart defect. Cyanosis, which indicates hypoxemia (lower than normal amounts of oxygen in the blood), results from the presence of 5 or more grams of unoxygenated hemoglobin per 100 mL of blood.[5]

The child's bone marrow responds to chronic hypoxemia by producing more red blood cells to increase the amount of hemoglobin available for oxygenation. This increase is known as **polycythemia.** A hematocrit value of 50% or higher is common in children with cyanotic heart defects.

CARDIAC FUNCTIONING

Oxygen requirements are high for the first 8 weeks of life. Normally the newborn's heart rate increases to provide adequate oxygen transport. The infant has little cardiac output reserve capacity until oxygen requirements begin to decrease. Cardiac output depends almost completely on heart rate until the heart muscle is fully developed at 5 years of age. Weight-specific cardiac output decreases during childhood. During stress, exercise, fever, or respiratory distress, infants and children have tachycardia, which increases their cardiac output.

Children respond to severe hypoxemia with bradycardia. Cardiac arrest in children generally results from prolonged hypoxemia related to respiratory failure or shock rather than from a primary cardiac insult as in adults. Bradycardia is therefore a significant warning sign of cardiac arrest. Appropriate management of hypoxemia reverses bradycardia and prevents cardiac arrest.

CLINICAL TIP

A pulse oximeter can be used to measure arterial oxygen saturation. A reading of 95–98% is normal in children. The following values indicate hypoxemia:
- Mild hypoxemia: 90–95%
- Moderate hypoxemia: 85–90%
- Severe hypoxemia: <85%

NURSING ALERT

Extreme polycythemia as determined by a hemoglobin concentration greater than 20 g/dL and a hematocrit greater than 55–60% is dangerous. Blood viscosity is increased, and the child is at risk for a thromboembolism.[5]

▶ CONGESTIVE HEART FAILURE

Congestive heart failure is a condition in which cardiac output is inadequate to support the body's circulatory and metabolic needs. It may result from a congenital heart defect that causes an obstruction or fluid overload in the heart, from problems with heart contractility, or from pathologic conditions that require high cardiac output, such as severe anemia, acidosis, or respiratory disease.

Clinical Manifestations

Congestive heart failure often develops subtly, and symptoms may not be recognized at first. The infant tires easily, especially during feeding. Weight loss or lack of normal weight gain, diaphoresis, irritability, and frequent infections may be evident.

As the disease progresses, symptoms such as tachypnea, tachycardia, nasal flaring, grunting, retractions, cough, or crackles may occur. Generalized fluid volume overload is seen more commonly in toddlers and older children. Periorbital and facial edema, jugular vein distention, and hepatomegaly are signs of fluid volume excess.

Cardiomegaly always occurs as the heart attempts to maintain cardiac output. Cyanosis, weak peripheral pulses, cool extremities, hypotension, and heart murmur are precursors of cardiogenic shock, which can occur if congestive heart failure is not adequately treated. (Cardiogenic shock is discussed later in this chapter.)

Etiology and Pathophysiology

Congenital heart defects are the most common cause of congestive heart failure in children.[7] Brandy, described in the scenario at the beginning of this chapter, developed congestive heart failure as a result of one such defect. Some defects allow blood to flow from the left side of the heart to the right so that extra blood must be pumped to the pulmonary system rather than through the aorta when the left ventricle contracts. Even though the heart rate increases to manage the extra blood volume, the pulmonary system becomes overloaded. Other congenital defects restrict the flow of blood so that normal pressures in the heart are disrupted. For example, if the aorta or pulmonary vessels are abnormally small, the heart must work harder to force blood through these structures. As a result the heart muscle hypertrophies, which increases cardiac output initially, but eventually the hypertrophied muscle becomes ineffective.[8] Initially the right or left side of the heart may fail, but eventually failure is bilateral.

When cardiac output remains insufficient, the body's sympathetic response is activated. Peripheral vasoconstriction and decreased blood flow to internal organs such as the brain and kidneys lead to fatigue and dizziness. The kidneys respond to the lowered volume by activating the renin–angiotensin mechanism, which temporarily corrects the problem. Renal vasoconstriction results when aldosterone is secreted, and salt and water are retained. This protective measure eventually fails, leading to systemic edema or pulmonary congestion.

Diagnostic Tests and Medical Management

Diagnosis is based primarily on clinical manifestations such as tachycardia, respiratory distress, and crackles. A chest x-ray study reveals cardiac enlargement and increased pulmonary vascular markings. Echocardiography may be performed to diagnose cardiac dysfunction. An electrocardiogram rarely shows abnormalities but may rule out cardiac dysrhythmias.

NURSING ALERT

When the heart rate reaches 180 beats/min in a child (220 beats/min in an infant), the time needed for blood to fill the ventricles during diastole is too short. As a result, the cardiac output and stroke volume fall. Life-threatening shock may develop if corrective action is not taken to reduce the heart rate.[6]

The goals of medical management are to make the heart work more efficiently and to remove excess fluid, thus improving peripheral circulation. Inotropic medicines and afterload-reducing agents are now sometimes used to lessen the workload of the heart and help it to work more efficiently.[9] Digoxin is the drug most commonly used to improve the heart's ability to contract and therefore increase its output. Occasionally a higher than normal dose is given initially, followed by a lower maintenance dose. This process, called **digitalization,** speeds the child's response to the drug.

Diuretics, such as furosemide, chlorothiazide, and spironolactone, are given to promote fluid excretion. Furosemide is the most commonly used medication during hospitalization; thiazides are commonly used to maintain diuresis at home (Table 12–1). Because most diuretics (except for spironolactone) cause potassium loss, serum potassium levels are monitored and potassium supplements may be ordered. Vasodilating drugs may be given to reduce pulmonary and systemic vasoconstriction and to decrease the work of the heart.

Other medical therapy is supportive. Oxygen therapy, rest, and fluid and dietary management are also part of the treatment plan (Fig. 12–2).

Most children improve rapidly after medication is administered. When congestive heart failure develops in a child with a correctable heart defect, surgery may be scheduled sooner than had been planned to prevent further deterioration and damage to the heart. This was the case with Brandy, in the opening scenario.

Nursing Assessment

Physiologic Assessment

As diagnosis of congestive heart failure depends primarily on physical symptoms, nursing observations are important. Assess the child's behavioral patterns, cardiac function, respiratory function, and fluid status (Table 12–2). Obtain a detailed history of the onset of symptoms from the parents, as congestive heart failure often develops slowly.

Psychosocial Assessment

Take a history of the child's previous hospitalizations and assess the family's knowledge about the child's condition. Families of children with congestive heart failure are anxious and fear the potential serious outcome of the problem and the need to provide ongoing care.[9] Assess the family's anxiety level and coping strategies. Evaluate the family's economic status. Medica-

NURSING ALERT

Digoxin and digitoxin are both digitalis preparations but are not the same drug. Digoxin is the drug of choice in pediatrics. Digitoxin is 10 times more powerful than digoxin, and is rarely used in children. Read labels carefully and double-check doses to ensure that the child receives the right dose of the right drug.

12-1	Drugs Used in Treatment of Congestive Heart Failure

Drug	Action
Digoxin	Increases myocardial contractility
Furosemide	Rapid diuresis
Thiazides	Maintenance diuresis
Chlorothiazide (suspension)	
Hydrochlorothiazide (tablets)	
Spironolactone	Potassium-sparing diuretic

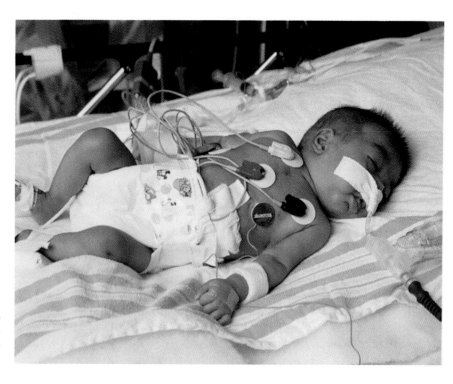

FIGURE 12–2. Jooti is receiving intravenous fluids and oxygen. Her condition is being continuously monitored for congestive heart failure.

tion is crucial to treatment, and a family's inability to afford or obtain the necessary medications jeopardizes the child's outcome.

The family is often overprotective and reluctant to leave the child with other caregivers. Find out if a knowledgeable person who can safely administer medications and watch the child is available for respite care.

12-2	Physical Assessment of a Child in Congestive Heart Failure

Behavioral Manifestations	**Respiratory Function**
Lethargy	Tachypnea
Listlessness	Nasal flaring
Tiring on feeding (infant)	Retractions
Tiring with play (child)	Crackles
Irritability	Orthopnea
Cardiac Function and Fluid Status	Cough
Tachycardia	Grunting
Cyanosis (late sign unless a cyanotic defect)	**Nonspecific Signs**
Cool extremities	Poor weight gain (infant)
Peripheral edema	Ascites
Slow capillary refill time	Hepatomegaly
Hypotension (rare; late sign)	Diaphoresis
Jugular vein distention (children)	Frequent infections (eg, otitis media, respiratory)
Heart murmur	
Oliguria	

Developmental Assessment

Since fatigue limits the activities of the child with congestive heart failure, the child does not have the opportunity to practice the skills needed to attain normal developmental milestones. Perform developmental assessment with a tool such as the Denver II (see Chap. 5). In addition, ask parents about the attainment of expected developmental milestones such as sitting, manipulating objects, standing, or walking. When congestive heart failure is well controlled, the child's energy level increases and developmental skills often improve. In infants and toddlers assessments every 2–3 months are useful to observe development and evaluate disease management.

Parents may limit the child's contact with other children because of frequent infections and exercise intolerance. Ask parents about contact and play with other children and a typical day's activity schedule.

Nursing Diagnosis

Several nursing diagnoses that may apply to the child with congestive heart failure are given in the accompanying Nursing Care Plans. The primary nursing diagnosis is Decreased Cardiac Output related to cardiac defect.

Nursing Management

Nursing care for the child with congestive heart failure focuses on administering and monitoring effects of medications, maintaining adequate oxygenation and myocardial function, promoting rest, fostering development, providing adequate nutrition, and providing emotional support to the child and family. The first of the two accompanying Nursing Care Plans summarizes nursing care for the child who is hospitalized with congestive heart failure.

Administer and Monitor Prescribed Medications

Children with congestive heart failure usually receive digoxin and furosemide. These medications are potent and must be administered correctly. Digoxin is given intravenously or orally in extremely small doses. Carefully measure and verify the doses. If a child taking digoxin orally is NPO or vomiting, seek a physician's order regarding the course of action to be taken; the drug must not be omitted. On the other hand, vomiting can be a signal that digoxin is at a toxic level. It is important to observe the child carefully for digoxin toxicity. Blood is drawn 6–8 hours after digoxin is given to monitor serum levels. A therapeutic serum level ranges from 1.1 to 1.7 ng/mL. Levels below 0.5 ng/mL are ineffective, and those over 2 ng/mL can lead to toxicity. Digoxin overdose is more common when potassium levels are low, so check serum potassium levels when a potassium-depleting diuretic is given. Serum potassium of 3.5 mmol/L or less may be a contraindication to digoxin administration; clarify this possible contraindication with the child's physician.

Measure intake and output carefully. Weigh the infant's diapers before and after changing (1 g = 1 mL urine). Observe for changes in peripheral edema and circulation. Weigh the child at the same time each day because fluid volume varies throughout the day. If ascites is present, take serial abdominal measurements to monitor changes (see Fig. 8–11). Turn the child frequently, and provide skin care when edema is present (see Fig. 8–12).

Maintain Oxygenation and Myocardial Function

Oxygen therapy may be ordered. Make sure that tubing is patent, the oxygen flow rate is correct, the oxygen delivery device is working properly, and humidification is provided. Keep the child calm and quiet. Position the

NURSING ALERT

Take an apical pulse with a stethoscope for 1 full minute before every dose of digoxin. If bradycardia is detected (< 100 beats/min for infants and toddlers, < 80 beats/min in older children, or < 60 beats/min in adolescents), call for a physician's advice before administering the drug.

NURSING ALERT

Signs of digoxin toxicity include:
- Bradycardia (pulse usually < 100 beats/min in a young child)
- Arrhythmia
- Nausea, vomiting, anorexia
- Dizziness, headache
- Weakness, fatigue

NURSING CARE PLAN
THE CHILD HOSPITALIZED WITH CONGESTIVE HEART FAILURE

GOAL	INTERVENTION	RATIONALE	EXPECTED OUTCOME

1. Decreased Cardiac Output related to congenital heart defect

The child's cardiac output will be sufficient to meet body's metabolic demands.	• Administer digoxin as ordered.	• Digoxin increases contractility of heart and force of contraction.	The child's cardiac output is sufficient as indicated by increased energy, adequate feeding intake, and decreased edema.
	• Take apical pulse and listen to heart sounds regularly, especially before each dose of digoxin. Record apical pulse with each recorded dose of digoxin.	• Digoxin may cause bradycardia. Pulse and heart sounds provide information about heart functioning.	
	• Use cardiac monitor if ordered.	• Monitor notes tachycardia and arrhythmias.	
	• Prevent injury by monitoring for digoxin side effects. Monitor serum level of digoxin and serum potassium level.	• Digoxin is a potent drug with serious side effects. Hypokalemia increases risk of digoxin toxicity.	The child maintains normal serum levels of potassium and therapeutic levels of digoxin.
	• Provide for rest periods each hour.	• Rest decreases need for high cardiac output.	The child rests hourly and has adequate energy to eat and play.

2. Altered Tissue Perfusion (Cardiopulmonary, Renal) related to sympathetic response to congestive heart failure

The child's peripheral and central edema will decrease.	• Provide skin care for edematous body parts and elevate extremities.	• Edematous skin breaks down easily. Elevation promotes return of fluid from extremities	The child shows no edema.
	• Weigh daily. Measure abdominal girth daily if ascites is present. Observe for peripheral edema.	• Evaluations demonstrate effectiveness of therapy.	
The child's urinary output will remain within normal levels. Intake and output will be balanced.	• Measure intake and output carefully. Weigh diapers to obtain output of young child.	• Adequate output is a good indicator of renal perfusion.	The child's intake and output are proportional, and electrolyte levels remain within normal ranges.
	• Maintain fluid-restricted diet if ordered.	• Fluid restriction is sometimes used to decrease cardiac fluid load.	
	• Administer diuretics as ordered.	• Diuretics mobilize fluids and facilitate excretion.	
	• Monitor electrolytes.	• Electrolyte imbalance is common when fluids are restricted and diuretics are given.	

NURSING CARE PLAN
THE CHILD HOSPITALIZED WITH CONGESTIVE HEART FAILURE– *Continued*

GOAL	INTERVENTION	RATIONALE	EXPECTED OUTCOME

3. Impaired Gas Exchange related to pulmonary congestion

GOAL	INTERVENTION	RATIONALE	EXPECTED OUTCOME
The child will manifest adequate oxygenation.	• Place child in semi-Fowler's position. • Evaluate respiratory rate and sounds. Take pulse oximetry readings to determine oxygen saturation. • Provide oxygen and humidification if ordered. Observe for diaphoresis, a sign of increased respiratory effort.	• Position facilitates lung expansion. • Absence of tachypnea and adventitious sounds and oxygen saturation above 95% indicate ease of respiration. • Supplemental oxygen decreases tachypnea, and humidification moistens secretions to keep airway clear.	The child has normal respiratory rate for age with no evidence of adventitious sounds or diaphoresis.

4. Altered Nutrition: Less Than Body Requirements related to rapid tiring while feeding

GOAL	INTERVENTION	RATIONALE	EXPECTED OUTCOME
The infant or child will demonstrate normal weight gain for age.	• Hold infant at 45 degree angle for feeding. • Record intake carefully. • Weigh child daily. • Give frequent small meals with rest periods in between. Give high-calorie snacks. • Use soothing approaches such as holding infants for feeding and having parents eat with older child.	• Position facilitates breathing while eating. • Evaluation of intake indicates whether caloric and other nutritional needs are met. • Weight gain indicates growth (in absence of edematous symptoms of congestive heart failure). • Digesting small meals requires less energy. High-calorie snacks provide calories efficiently. • Restful approach facilitates intake with minimal cardiac work.	The infant or child gains recommended weight according to growth grids. All dietary requirements are met, and mealtimes are pleasant.

5. Anxiety (Parent) related to unknown nature of child's disease

GOAL	INTERVENTION	RATIONALE	EXPECTED OUTCOME
Parents will express lessened anxiety as hospitalization proceeds.	• Encourage parents to room in or stay with child. Explain procedures and treatment. Involve parents in care as much as possible. Have parents plan child's play periods.	• Involvement in child's care lessens parental anxiety and fear of unknown.	Parents demonstrate comfort in providing care for child.

Continued . . .

NURSING CARE PLAN
THE CHILD HOSPITALIZED WITH CONGESTIVE HEART FAILURE– *Continued*

GOAL	INTERVENTION	RATIONALE	EXPECTED OUTCOME

5. Anxiety (Parent) related to unknown nature of child's disease (continued)

	• At discharge, provide clear instructions and information about whom and where to call with questions.	• Having resources available provides feeling of security.	
	• Allow parents to verbalize questions, concerns, and feelings. Refer parents to support groups or other resources as needed.	• Emotional support is needed to lessen anxiety.	

child in a semi-Fowler's or 45 degree angle position to promote maximum oxygenation. Infants are generally most comfortable eating at a 45 degree angle, which facilitates breathing while eating.

Promote Rest

Group assessments and interventions together to ensure that the child has some uninterrupted rest each hour. Feedings should last no more than 20–30 minutes. Frequent small feedings generally work best, with burping after every half ounce of intake to minimize vomiting. Rocking is restful for infants. Encourage older children to engage in quiet activities such as playing board games or watching television.

Foster Development

Encourage parents to play with the child, using toys to stimulate eye–hand coordination and fine motor movements. Such toys include rattles, blocks, and stuffed animals for infants and books, paper and pencil, and dolls for older children. Encourage sitting, standing, or walking for short periods with adequate rest afterward to promote the development of large muscles. Singing, talking, and playing music facilitate cognitive and language skills.

Provide Adequate Nutrition

Teach parents about feeding techniques. The mother who chooses to breast-feed the infant should not be discouraged. The antibodies contained in breast milk reduce infections, and the milk is naturally low in sodium. However, the sucking involved in feeding may cause dyspnea that forces the infant to rest frequently during feeding.

Infants should be burped frequently to permit rest and prevent vomiting. They may need small frequent feedings and longer feeding periods. Positioning the baby in an infant seat at a 45 degree angle decreases venous return to the heart and decreases its metabolic demand. This is a favorable position for feeding and other activities.[10]

Make sure that parents understand that changes in feeding habits (decreased intake, vomiting, sleeping through feedings, increased perspiration with feedings) may indicate deteriorating cardiac status. The American Heart Association publishes the booklet *Feeding Infants with Congenital Heart Disease* for parents (see Appendix F).

Adequate nutrition is needed to support the infant's growth. It is not unusual for infants with heart problems to develop failure to thrive as the result of feeding difficulties. When infants have significant dyspnea with feeding, special feeding techniques are needed. Some infants need a higher caloric formula (24 calories per ounce or higher) to obtain adequate nutrition. Other infants require nutritional supplementation by nasogastric or gastrostomy tube (Fig. 12–3). Parents are often advised to give the infant a chance to feed normally for a specific period. The remainder of the formula is then given by nasogastric or gastrostomy tube.

Provide Emotional Support

When a child is hospitalized with congestive heart failure, the family is often anxious about his or her condition. Give parents an opportunity to express concerns about their child's condition. Explain the child's treatment regimen, and make sure family members understand the child's need for nutrition and rest. Answer any questions about the child's prognosis and the ultimate outcome. Provide family members with information, and relay questions to the physician. Talking to other parents of children with cardiac conditions may be a source of emotional support. Refer parents to the appropriate support groups.

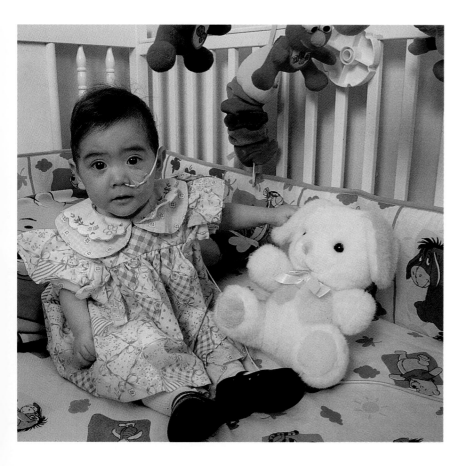

FIGURE 12–3. Infants with cardiac conditions often require supplemental feedings to provide sufficient nutrients for growth and development. The parents of this infant girl have been taught how to give her nasogastric feedings at home.

Discharge Planning and Home Care Teaching

Home care needs should be identified and addressed well in advance of discharge. While the child is hospitalized, teach the family about the administration of medications and signs of a worsening condition.

Demonstrate administration of drugs, and then supervise while the parents show how to measure and administer medications. Teach parents about the toxic effects of digoxin and other drugs. Advise them to notify the physician immediately if any of these side effects occur.

Show parents how to feed the child to maximize nutritional intake. Tell them to watch for symptoms such as increased feeding difficulty, irritability, lethargy, breathing difficulty, and puffiness around the eyes or extremities, which indicate that congestive heart failure is worsening. Parents are frequently taught to take the child's pulse and to report any significant change to the physician. An increase in pulse rate can signal congestive heart failure, and a decrease in pulse rate can indicate digoxin toxicity.

Care in the Community

The second of the two accompanying Nursing Care Plans outlines home care of the child with congestive heart failure. Parents play a critical role in the care of the child with heart disease by facilitating normal development and limiting the incidence of congestive heart failure.[10]

Evaluate family resources so that adequate child or respite care can be arranged if needed. Demonstrate to the family how to assess the child's energy level, and how to observe for feeding problems and edema. Observe medication administration and correct any errors. Watch the child feeding and provide suggestions (eg, positioning at a 45 degree angle and allowing adequate time), as necessary.

HOME CARE CONSIDERATIONS

Digitalis is a *very* dangerous drug. Encourage parents to keep it locked up at home and away from children. In case of accidental ingestion, immediate medical care is needed.

CLINICAL TIP

Evidence is emerging that the use of multivitamins by women at the time of conception may reduce the risk of certain defects (transposition of the great vessels, tetralogy of Fallot, and truncus arteriosus).[11]

► CONGENITAL HEART DISEASE

Congenital heart disease refers to a defect in the heart or great vessels, or persistence of a fetal structure after birth. Congenital heart defects are estimated to occur in 10 per 1000 live births.[2] In spontaneously aborted and stillborn fetuses the incidence is much higher.

Congenital heart defects are usually the result of a combined or interactive effect of genetic and environmental factors, such as:

- Fetal exposure to drugs such as phenytoin and lithium
- Maternal viral infections such as rubella
- Maternal metabolic disorders such as phenylketonuria and diabetes mellitus
- Maternal complications of pregnancy such as increased age and antepartal bleeding
- Genetic factors (family recurrence patterns)
- Chromosomal abnormalities such as Turner syndrome, cri du chat syndrome, Down syndrome, and trisomy syndromes 13,15, and 18[12]

Because of this genetic component, the incidence of congenital heart defects is expected to slowly rise as persons with some of these defects survive and have children of their own.[2]

A child often has more than one defect at the same time. Depending on the type of defect, signs and symptoms may be present at birth or develop later.

NURSING CARE PLAN
THE CHILD WITH CONGESTIVE HEART FAILURE BEING CARED FOR AT HOME

GOAL	INTERVENTION	RATIONALE	EXPECTED OUTCOME
1. Altered Growth and Development related to low energy level			
The child will meet developmental milestones for age group.	• Perform baseline developmental assessment.	• Assessment provides comparison for later assessments and basis for planning specific games, toys, and activities.	The child displays normal language, fine motor, and gross motor activity.
	• Plan for short play periods after rest.	• Short play periods maintain energy and facilitate play.	
	• Introduce age-appropriate toys and activities such as rattles and blocks for infants and art projects for older children.	• Play activities facilitate learning and mastery of developmental tasks.	
	• Plan for interactions with healthy children.	• Social skills are learned through contact with others.	
2. Knowledge Deficit (Parent) related to treatment regimen			
Parents will demonstrate correct administration of medications.	• Demonstrate administration of digoxin, diuretics, and other medications. Have parents administer them under supervision of nurse.	• Demonstration with return demonstration is an excellent method of learning psychomotor skills.	Parents report that child continues to demonstrate improvement and adequate cardiac output with absence of congestive failure episodes.
Parents will state side effects of medications and symptoms of congestive heart failure.	• Describe side effects of medications. Give parents handouts with telephone number to call to ask questions or report side effects.	• If side effects are understood, serious complications can be avoided.	
	• Describe subtle onset of congestive heart failure and its symptoms (increasing weakness, exhaustion, irritability, difficulty feeding, cough or difficult respirations, edema).	• Parents can evaluate child regularly and note subtle changes requiring medical management.	

Continued . . .

NURSING CARE PLAN
THE CHILD WITH CONGESTIVE HEART FAILURE BEING CARED FOR AT HOME– *Continued*

GOAL	INTERVENTION	RATIONALE	EXPECTED OUTCOME

3. Altered Nutrition: Less Than Body Requirements related to tiring while feeding

The infant or child will demonstrate normal weight gain for age.	• Teach parents methods to promote food intake related to positioning, size of feedings, food choices.	• Positioning, frequency of feedings, size of feedings, and use of high-calorie foods can enhance nutritional intake.	The infant or child shows normal weight gain.
	• Observe feeding during home visit.	• Feedback can assist parents in integrating positive feeding techniques.	Parents report and demonstrate successful feedings of child.

4. Caregiver Role Strain (Parent) related to demands of child

Parents will express ability to meet own needs.	• Assess family and community supports. Provide information related to respite care.	• Variable family and community supports are available.	Parents report some time away from the child and report renewal in caring for the child.
	• Encourage parents to seek activities to meet personal needs.	• Parents need time to meet own personal needs in order to successfully care for child.	

5. Activity Intolerance (Child) related to poor cardiac output

The child will perform all necessary activities of daily living without undue tiring.	• Help parents alternate activities and rest throughout the child's day.	• Activities to promote development must be alternated with rest due to decreased cardiac output.	The child performs necessary activities and rests frequently each day.
	• Have parents limit child's exposure to persons with contagious infections.	• When the child is ill and tired, the immune system can be compromised.	
	• Help family plan quiet surroundings to provide for child's rest.	• Home setting may need to be altered to promote rest.	

Congenital heart defects are generally divided into two categories, cyanotic and acyanotic, based on the hallmark sign of cyanosis. However, a child with an acyanotic defect may show clinical signs of cyanosis. The pathophysiology of a heart defect is related to **hemodynamics,** which refers to the pressures generated by blood and the pathways blood takes through the heart and pulmonary system.

ACYANOTIC DEFECTS

The majority of children with congenital heart defects have acyanotic conditions. There are two types of acyanotic defects: nonobstructive lesions, which do not interfere with the flow of blood, and obstructive lesions, which block the outflow of blood from the heart. Nonobstructive defects include patent ductus arteriosus (PDA), atrial septal defect (ASD), atrioventricular canal (endocardial cushion defect), and ventricular septal defect (VSD). Obstructive defects include pulmonic stenosis (PS), aortic stenosis (AS), and coarctation of the aorta. Tables 12–3 and 12–4 summarize clinical manifestations, diagnostic tests, and medical management for these defects.

Clinical Manifestations

The child with a nonobstructive acyanotic heart defect may be asymptomatic except for a heart murmur. The most important consequence of these defects is volume overload. Congestive heart failure may develop if the amount of blood passing from the left to the right side of the heart overloads the pulmonary system.[13] If this occurs, the child has hepatomegaly, dyspnea, tachypnea, intercostal retractions, poor growth, and frequent respiratory infections. The more severe and complex the heart defect, the earlier symptoms of congestive heart failure appear.

The child with an obstructive acyanotic heart defect also has a heart murmur. Obstructive defects cause pressure overload and hypertrophy of the closest ventricle. Although some children experience fatigue and exercise intolerance because of their inability to increase cardiac output, many children are asymptomatic and grow normally.

Older children with a diagnosis of congenital heart disease may have additional symptoms. Exercise-induced dizziness and **syncope** (transient loss of consciousness and muscle tone) are serious signs indicating a need for medical evaluation.

Etiology and Pathophysiology

Beginning at birth the left side of the heart normally generates higher pressures than the right side in response to increasing systemic vascular resistance and decreasing pulmonary vascular resistance. In children who have nonobstructive defects such as openings in the septal wall, a left-to-right **shunt** (movement of blood between heart chambers through an abnormal opening) occurs. Oxygenated blood mixes with unoxygenated blood, and the extra blood volume overloads the pulmonary system, causing congestive heart failure. **Pulmonary hypertension,** an often irreversible condition leading to life-threatening pulmonary vascular resistance, occurs if chronic volume overload of the pulmonary arteries is not corrected.

Diagnostic Tests and Medical Management

The presence of a heart murmur is often the first indication of an acyanotic defect. A loud murmur indicates higher pressures of blood flowing across the shunt or through the narrowed valve or vessel. Once the heart murmur is discovered, a chest x-ray study, electrocardiography, and echocardiography are performed. The echocardiogram usually clearly shows the defect, shunt, and heart pressures.

The selection of treatment for acyanotic defects depends on the severity of symptoms and whether the condition is imminently life threatening. Surgical correction is the treatment of choice for most acyanotic defects.

CLINICAL TIP

Signs and symptoms of congenital heart disease in older children include:
- Exercise intolerance
- Chest pain
- Arrhythmias
- Syncope
- Sudden death

12-3   Acyanotic Heart Defects—Nonobstructive Lesions

Patent Ductus Arteriosus (PDA)

Common congenital defect caused by persistent fetal circulation that accounts for 5–10% of all congenital heart defects. When pulmonary circulation is established and systemic vascular resistance increases at birth, pressures in aorta become greater than in the pulmonary arteries. Blood is then shunted from aorta to pulmonary arteries, increasing circulation to pulmonary system.

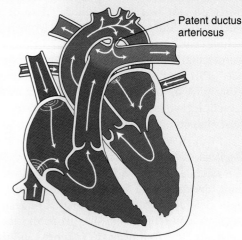

Patent ductus arteriosus

Clinical Manifestations

Dyspnea; tachypnea; full, bounding pulses; and poor development occur. Infant is at risk for frequent respiratory infections and subacute endocarditis. When a large PDA exists, congestive heart failure, intercostal retractions, hepatomegaly, and growth failure are also seen. A continuous systolic murmur is auscultated, and a thrill may be palpated in pulmonic area.

Diagnostic Tests

When murmur is detected, diagnosis is confirmed by chest x-ray study, electrocardiogram (ECG), and echocardiogram. Chest x-ray film and ECG show left ventricular hypertrophy. PDA can be visualized, and left-to-right shunt can be measured on echocardiogram.

Medical Management

Surgical ligation of PDA is the treatment of choice. Intravenous indomethacin often stimulates closure of the ductus arteriosus in premature infants. Transcatheter closure by obstructive device is sometimes attempted in children over 18 months of age.

PROGNOSIS: If PDA is not treated, child's life span is shortened because pulmonary hypertension and vascular obstructive disease develop.

Atrial Septal Defect (ASD)

An opening at any point in the atrial septum that permits left-to-right shunting of blood. The opening may be small, as when the foramen ovale fails to close, or septum may be completely absent. Of children with congenital heart defects, 30–50% have an ASD.

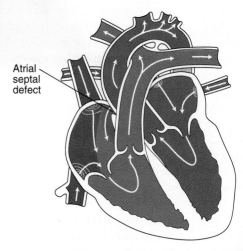

Atrial septal defect

Clinical Manifestations

Infants and young children usually have no symptoms. Small and moderate-sized ASDs are usually not diagnosed until preschool years or later. Congestive heart failure, easy tiring, and poor growth occur with a large ASD. A soft systolic murmur is usually heard in pulmonic area with wide splitting of S_2.

Diagnostic Tests

Diagnosis is made by echocardiogram that identifies right ventricular overload and shunt size. Chest x-ray film and ECG reveal little information unless ASD is large and excessive shunting is present.

Medical Management

Surgery to close or patch ASD is performed to prevent pulmonary vascular obstructive disease. Some ASDs may be closed by transcatheter device during cardiac catheterization.

PROGNOSIS: Many persons with uncorrected small and moderate-sized ASDs have lived to middle age without symptoms. Atrial arrhythmias are common late complications.

Atrioventricular Canal (Endocardial Cushion Defect)

Atrioventricular (AV) canal refers to a combination of defects in the atrial and ventricular septa and portions of tricuspid and mitral valves. Of children with congenital heart defects, 3–4% have a total or partial AV canal. This defect is associated with Down syndrome. Endocardial cushions are fetal growth centers for mitral and tricuspid valves and AV septum. The most complex AV canal malformation results in one AV valve and large septal defects between both atria and ventricles.

12-3 Acyanotic Heart Defects—Nonobstructive Lesions (continued)

Clinical Manifestations

Severity of symptoms depends on amount of mitral regurgitation. Infants have congestive heart failure, tachypnea, tachycardia, poor growth, and repeated respiratory failure, as well as systolic murmur, which is loudest at left lower sternal border.

Diagnostic Tests

On chest x-ray film, heart appears large and pulmonary vascular markings are present. Echocardiogram reveals presence of septal defects and details of valvular malformation. Cardiac catheterization is performed to evaluate pulmonary hypertension and pulmonary resistance.

Medical Management

Surgery is performed during infancy to prevent pulmonary vascular disease. Patches are placed over septal defects, and valve tissue is used to form functioning valves. Occasionally the mitral valve is replaced. Oxygen may be required until surgery.

PROGNOSIS: Information on long-term survival following successful surgery is lacking. Arrhythmias occur postoperatively. There is no difference in short-term survival rates between infants with and without Down syndrome.

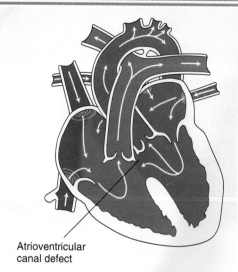

Atrioventricular canal defect

Ventricular Septal Defect (VSD)

An opening in the ventricular septum results in increased pulmonary blood flow. Blood is shunted from left ventricle directly across the open septum into the pulmonary artery. This most common congenital heart defect occurs in approximately 30–40% of all children with congenital heart disease[a]

Clinical Manifestations

Only 15% of VSDs are large enough to cause symptoms, such as tachypnea, dyspnea, poor growth, reduced fluid intake, congestive heart failure, and pulmonary hypertension. Systolic murmur is auscultated in lower left sternal border.

Diagnostic Tests

Chest x-ray film and ECG reveal few findings in cases of small VSDs. Larger VSDs with shunting are associated with enlarged heart and pulmonary vascular markings on chest x-ray film and left ventricular hypertrophy on ECG. Echocardiogram establishes diagnosis if shunting is present. Cardiac catheterization is used only in preparation for surgery.

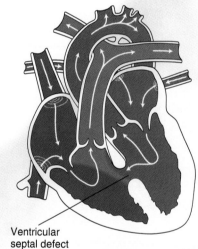

Ventricular septal defect

Medical Management

Most small VSDs close spontaneously. Treatment is conservative when no signs of congestive heart disease or pulmonary hypertension are present. Surgical patching of VSD during infancy is performed when poor growth is evident. Closure of VSD by transcatheter device during cardiac catheterization may be attempted for some defects. Prophylaxis for infective endocarditis is required.

PROGNOSIS: Highest risk associated with surgical repair is in the first few months of life. Children respond well to surgery and experience substantial "catch-up" growth. An arrhythmia, complete right bundle branch block, is a complication found in more than 30% of patients.[b]

[a]*Information from Hoffman, J.I.E. (1990). Congenital heart disease: Incidence and inheritance. Pediatric Clinics of North America, 37, 25–43.*
[b]*Information from Fyler, D.C. (1992). Ventricular septal defect. In Nadas' pediatric cardiology (pp. 453–457). Philadelphia: Hanley & Belfus.*

Table 12–5 lists the types of surgical procedures performed on children with congenital heart defects. Conservative treatment, such as waiting until the child is symptomatic or older, may be selected initially. For example, a ventricular septal defect may close spontaneously or growth of the child may increase the probability of success of surgery. Surgical correction of defects

12-4   Acyanotic Heart Defects—Obstructive Lesions

Pulmonic Stenosis

Stenosis (narrowing of valve or valve area) can be above valve, below valve, or at valve. Stenosis obstructs blood flow into pulmonary artery. This increases preload. Right ventricular hypertrophy occurs. Pulmonic stenosis is the second most frequent congenital heart defect, accounting for 8–12% of all cases.

Clinical Manifestation

Children with mild stenosis may have no symptoms and grow normally. In moderate stenosis, dyspnea and fatigue occur on exertion. Signs of heart failure are rare but may result from chronic pressure overload. A systolic murmur with a fixed split S_2 and thrill may be found in the pulmonic listening area. Heart failure and chest pain on exertion may occur in severe cases.

Diagnostic Tests

Diagnosis is usually made at birth after auscultation of murmur. The chest x-ray film may show heart enlargement, and the ECG may demonstrate right ventricular hypertrophy. Echocardiogram provides information about pressure gradient across valve and size of valve ring.

Medical Management

Dilation by balloon valvuloplasty, performed during cardiac catheterization, has been widely successful for treatment of simple pulmonic stenosis. Surgical valvotomy is still used, especially when other defects such as ASD are present. Surgical resection may be needed for narrowing above the valve area. Pulmonary regurgitation may result, but is not a significant problem.

PROGNOSIS: Pulmonic stenosis does not typically increase in severity. Lifelong infective endocarditis prophylaxis is necessary.

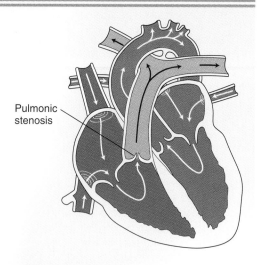

Pulmonic stenosis

Aortic Stenosis

Narrowing of the aortic valve obstructs blood flow to systemic circulation. Aortic stenosis accounts for 3–6% of all cases of congenital heart defects. This defect is often associated with bicuspid rather than normal tricuspid valve. Stenosis is usually progressive during childhood.

Clinical Manifestations

A majority of infants and young children are asymptomatic and grow and develop normally. The blood pressure is normal, but there is often a narrow pulse pressure. Occasionally the child complains of chest pain after exercise, but exercise intolerance is uncommon. Peripheral pulses may be weak. Fainting and dizziness are serious signs that require intervention. Congestive heart failure develops in symptomatic infants. A systolic heart murmur and thrill in the aortic listening area are usually detected in routine physical examination in the school-age child or adolescent.

Diagnostic Tests

Chest x-ray film and ECG are usually normal in mild cases. An echocardiogram reveals number of the valve cusps, pressure gradient across valve, and size of aorta. Stress testing may be used in asymptomatic children to determine amount of obstruction present with exercise.

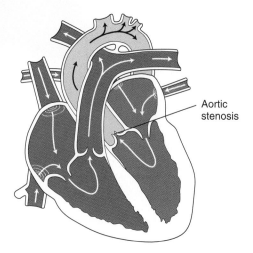

Aortic stenosis

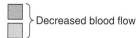

Decreased blood flow

Medical Management

The aortic valve may be successfully dilated by balloon valvuloplasty during cardiac catheterization. Surgical valvuloplasty may also be performed. Aortic valve replacement is performed when stenosis is severe or if significant regurgitation results from other interventions. Surgical treatment is palliative rather than curative.

PROGNOSIS: Chest pain, syncope, and sudden death can occur in symptomatic children, particularly during vigorous exercise. Stenosis is usually progressive during childhood as the valve calcifies. Valve replacement may ultimately be necessary. Lifelong infective endocarditis prophylaxis is required.

Coarctation of the Aorta

Narrowing or constriction in the descending aorta, often near the ductus arteriosus, obstructs systemic blood outflow. This defect is common, occurring in 8–10% of all children with congenital heart disease.

Clinical Manifestations

Many children are asymptomatic and grow normally, but constriction is progressive; 20–30% of children develop congestive heart failure by 3 months of age. Reduction in blood flow through descending aorta causes lower blood pressure in legs and higher blood pressure in arms, neck, and head. Brachial and radial pulses are full, but femoral pulses are weak or absent. Older children may complain of weakness and pain in the legs after exercise.

Diagnostic Tests

ECG shows left ventricular hypertrophy. Chest x-ray film may reveal enlargement and pulmonary venous congestion, and indentation of descending aorta. Rib notching (change in the smooth contour of the rib apparent on x-ray) is rarely seen before 10 years of age. Magnetic resonance imaging shows coarctation.

Medical Management

Balloon dilation during cardiac catheterization may provide initial relief. Surgical resection and anastomosis are palliative, since coarctation usually recurs. The subclavian artery can be used as a patch in the infant.

PROGNOSIS: Persistent hypertension in adulthood is common, especially if surgery occurs after 9 years of age.[a] Endocarditis prophylaxis is needed.

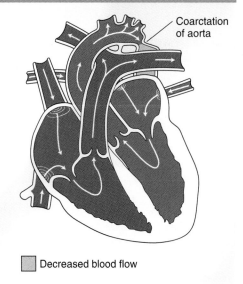

Coarctation of aorta

☐ Decreased blood flow

---

[a]Information from Ing, F.F., Starc, T.J., Griffiths, S.P., & Gersony, W.M. (1996). Early diagnosis of coarctation of the aorta in children: A continuing dilemma. Pediatrics, 98(3 Pt. 1), 378–382.

12-5 Surgical Procedures for Congenital Heart Defects

Procedure	Purpose	Therapeutic Use
Angioplasty	Dilatation of recoarctation of aorta during cardiac catheterization	Palliative
Arterial switch (Jatene)	Reattachment of great arteries with correct ventricle for transposition of great vessels	Corrective
Fontan	Creation of conduit between right atrium and pulmonary artery to increase pulmonary blood flow	Corrective
Modified Blalock–Taussig	Creation of conduit to increase pulmonary blood flow	Palliative
Mustard or Senning	Baffling blood in the atria to reestablish a proper blood flow in transposition of the great vessels	Corrective
Norwood	Creation of conduit between aorta and pulmonary artery to increase blood flow to aorta	Palliative or corrective
Patent ductus arteriosus closure	Closure of ductus arteriosus by surgery or an umbrella device during cardiac catheterization	Corrective
Pulmonary artery banding	Placement of constricting band around pulmonary artery to reduce pulmonary blood flow	Palliative
Rashkind	Creation of larger defect between atria to increase blood mixing during cardiac catheterization	Palliative
Transcatheter closure	Closure of septal defect by umbrella device during cardiac catheterization	Corrective
Transplant	Replacement of diseased heart with donor heart	Corrective
Valvuloplasty	Repair of valve to relieve stenosis by balloon dilation during cardiac catheterization or surgery	Palliative or corrective

The following tests are used in the diagnosis of congenital heart disease:

Chest x-ray study
Reveals size and contour of the heart and characteristics of pulmonary vascular markings

Electrocardiogram (ECG)
Records quality of major electrical activity in the heart, identifies arrhythmias

Echocardiogram
Identifies heart's structures, the pattern of movement, hemodynamics, and the presence of defects

Cardiac catheterization
Allows precise measurement of oxygen saturation and pressures in each chamber and heart vessel; also identifies anatomic alterations

Holter monitor
Allows 24–48 hour ECG recording

Exercise testing
Enables ECG recording with controlled increase in activity to identify significant cardiac compensation or inadequate cardiac output

that cause pulmonary hypertension is performed in infancy to prevent irreversible pulmonary vascular disease.

Surgery often results in complete repair of the acyanotic defect. Unless complications develop before surgery, the child should make a complete recovery without limitations. The major complication of acyanotic heart defects is pulmonary hypertension.

Cardiac catheterization, an invasive procedure previously used exclusively for diagnosis of some congenital heart defects, is now more often performed as a therapeutic procedure. Recently developed techniques using balloons and other transcatheter devices permit treatment of many acyanotic heart defects during cardiac catheterization.

Potential complications of cardiac catheterization include perforation of the pulmonary artery, allergic reaction to the contrast media, dysrhythmias, hypotension, stroke, vascular compromise in the leg, and bleeding.

Nursing Care of the Child Undergoing a Cardiac Catheterization

Prepare the child for cardiac catheterization with age-appropriate information. A tour of the catheterization laboratory may reduce the child's fears about the large equipment. Because the child will be sedated but arousable for the procedure, explain the sensations that he or she will experience.

Cardiac catheterization is often an outpatient procedure, but some children will be admitted for observation. The child is NPO after midnight, except for medications, and arrives at the catheterization laboratory the morning of the procedure. Before entering the laboratory, the child is asked to void and is given an oral sedative.

Nursing Assessment

Before the procedure, assess the child's vital signs, hematocrit and hemoglobin concentrations, and strength of pedal pulses for comparison with postcatheterization assessments.

For several hours after the procedure, monitor the child for potential complications such as arrhythmia, bleeding, hematoma development, thrombus formation, and infection. No bleeding should occur at the catheterization site. Assess vital signs, neurovascular status of the lower extremities, and the pressure dressing over the catheterization site every 15 minutes for 1 hour and then every 30 minutes for 1 hour. The child's temperature, heart rate, respiratory rate, and blood pressure should remain stable. Monitor intake and output because the contrast medium may cause diuresis. The child's intake and output should be balanced. Pedal pulses, capillary refill, sensation, warmth, and color of the lower extremities should match the precatheterization assessment.

Nursing Diagnosis

The following nursing diagnoses may apply to the child who undergoes cardiac catheterization:

- Knowledge Deficit (Child and Parent) related to cardiac catheterization procedure
- Risk for Infection related to invasive procedure
- Risk for Fluid Volume Deficit related to blood loss, period of time NPO, and diuretic effect of contrast medium
- Altered Tissue Perfusion (Cardiopulmonary) related to potential thrombus formation and hemorrhage

• Risk for Decreased Cardiac Output related to obstruction by balloon catheter

Nursing Management

Nursing care during a cardiac catheterization focuses on monitoring the child's vital signs, reassuring the child, and providing emergency care if necessary. After the catheters and guidewires are removed at the end of the procedure, direct pressure must be applied for 15 minutes. A pressure dressing is then placed over the site for 6 hours.

The child is kept on bedrest for 6 hours. Activity is then limited for 24 hours. Provide quiet diversional activities to keep the child occupied.

Encourage the intake of small amounts of clear liquids initially, and then progress to other fluids and food as the child tolerates them. Maintaining hydration is important because the contrast medium used during the procedure has a diuretic effect. Monitor intake and output.

Discharge Planning and Home Care Teaching. Routinely children are discharged several hours after the cardiac catheterization. Teach the parents to watch the child for signs of complications and make sure they know when to notify the physician. An elevated temperature may indicate infection. It is essential that parents specifically check the catheterization site for bleeding or a hematoma for the first 24 hours after catheterization. Emphasize that quiet play, *only*, is allowed for 24 hours.

Children whose heart defect is corrected by cardiac catheterization have the same risks for infective endocarditis as children with surgical correction. Use the information provided in Table 12–8, later in this chapter, to teach parents about antibiotic prophylaxis.

Nursing Care of the Child Undergoing Surgery for an Acyanotic Defect

Children with acyanotic heart defects are hospitalized either because of complications, such as congestive heart failure, or for surgery. Refer to the earlier discussion of nursing management in congestive heart failure for care of children with this condition.

Nursing Assessment

Assess the ability of the parents to cope with the diagnosis of their child's congenital heart defect. Initially parents may be in shock and feel guilty and anxious. The child often looks healthy and has few symptoms.

Parents need an opportunity to express their feelings and to begin learning to cope with their child's illness. They need special support if their infant has a life-threatening heart defect. Members of the cardiology team, including nurses, must provide counseling for the family. Counseling information may include the following:

• General information about the congenital heart disease, including a description of the heart's anatomy and physiology and the defect
• Specific information about the multiple interactive factors associated with congenital heart disease; this information can often help reduce parents' guilt about the child's defect
• Sample case histories with good and poor prognoses
• Overview of the child's prognosis and timing of medical and surgical interventions

12-6 Fetal Development of Specific Heart Defects	
Defect	Critical Time (Weeks of Gestation)
Patent ductus arteriosus	3–8
Coarctation of the aorta	4–28
Ventricular septal defect	4–7
Transposition of the great vessels	3–4
Tricuspid or mitral atresia	3–6
Truncus arteriosus	6–7
Total anomalous pulmonary venous return	3–8

From Keith, J.D., Rowe, R.D., & Vlad, P. (Eds.). (1978). Heart disease in infancy and childhood (3rd ed.). New York: Macmillan.

CLINICAL TIP

Parents are at higher risk of having a child with a congenital heart defect if any of the following factors are present:[14]

- Family history of congenital heart disease
- Maternal age > 35 years
- Coexisting maternal disease (diabetes mellitus, collagen vascular disease, phenylketonuria)
- Exposure to teratogens or rubella infection

Parents may need genetic counseling if planning a future pregnancy. Fetal echocardiography can identify structural heart defects as early as 18–20 weeks of gestation (Table 12–6).

The American Heart Association publishes the booklet *If Your Child Has a Congenital Heart Defect.* See Appendix F for information about contacting the national headquarters.

Following surgical correction of the heart defect, the child is usually cared for in an intensive care unit until stable. The child may be intubated and ventilated for a few hours. In the immediate postoperative period, assess the child's vital signs, level of consciousness, pain level, heart functioning, and arrhythmias. Monitor intake and output. Monitor for hemorrhage, adequate ventilation and tissue perfusion, and acid–base and electrolyte imbalances.

After the child's return to the general nursing unit, nursing assessment focuses on signs of surgical complications such as infection, arrhythmias, and impaired tissue perfusion. Monitor the child's temperature, and inspect the surgical incision site. Fever, excessive incisional pain, spreading erythema around the incision, and wound drainage beginning 3–4 days postoperatively may be early signs of infection. Assess the respiratory system for breath sounds, respiratory effort, and signs of distress that may indicate pneumonia or fluid in the pleural space.

Because the child may no longer be on a cardiac monitor, auscultation of the apical pulse to detect an irregular heart rate or bradycardia is essential. Either condition is an indication of reduced cardiac output that requires intervention. To assess for impaired tissue perfusion, check capillary refill, extremity warmth, pedal pulses, level of consciousness, and urine output. Reduced urine output is a sign of decreased cardiac output. Continue to assess the child's pain.

Nursing Diagnosis

Several nursing diagnoses may be associated with acyanotic heart defects and their complications. They include:

- Fluid Volume Excess related to pulmonary vasculature overload
- Decreased Cardiac Output related to an obstructed outflow tract
- Ineffective Breathing Pattern related to pulmonary vasculature overload

- Altered Nutrition: Less Than Body Requirements related to ineffective feeding pattern
- Ineffective Infant Feeding Pattern related to shortness of breath and fatigue
- Risk for Infection related to altered immune function, surgery, or pulmonary overload
- Risk for Activity Intolerance related to chronic pulmonary vasculature overload
- Altered Family Processes related to guilt and grieving over lack of perfect infant
- Risk for Caregiver Role Strain related to child with chronic health condition
- Knowledge Deficit (Parents) related to special care for chronic condition

Nursing Management

Children are often managed at home until surgery is scheduled. See Table 12–7 for parent education guidelines.

Nursing care following surgery focuses on promoting the child's recuperation. Pain management should be provided for several days postoperatively. Follow the guidelines given in Chapter 7.

Encourage the child to perform spirometry exercises regularly to promote full lung expansion. Chest physiotherapy may be performed in children under 3 years of age. Inspect the child's incision regularly and cleanse it with hydrogen peroxide if ordered (Fig. 12–4).

Administer antibiotics as ordered. Intravenous lines are often converted to heparin or saline locks to continue antibiotic administration once the child's oral intake is normal. Although oral fluids are rarely limited, intake and output should be assessed carefully.

Encourage the child to increase activity gradually with longer periods out of bed every day. Provide opportunities for therapeutic play so the child can better manage the stresses associated with pain and frightening procedures.

Discharge Planning and Home Care Teaching. Infants and children may be discharged from the hospital within a few days of surgery.

12-7   Home Care of Children with Congenital Heart Defects Before Surgery

Routine Health Care
Provide well-child care and all immunizations, including pneumovaccine and influenza vaccine.
Provide preventive dental care with fluoride treatment beginning at 2 years of age.

Administration of Medications
Give medications safely with a dosage schedule that fits the family's routine.

Signs of Illness
Notify physician if the child has the following signs: fever, vomiting, diarrhea, or is feeding poorly.

Activity
Allow the child to set his or her own activity level. Children with congenital heart defects usually do not overexert themselves.

From Stinson, J., & McKeever, P. (1995). Mother's information needs related to caring for infants at home following cardiac surgery. Journal of Pediatric Nursing, 10(1), 48–57.

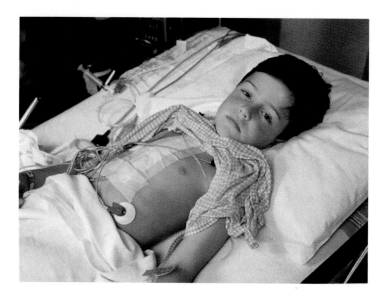

FIGURE 12–4. A child with atrial septal defect repair. Surgery is performed with this type of defect to prevent pulmonary vascular obstructive disease.

Parents need discharge teaching in preparation for continuing care of the child at home.[15] Instructions should include the following:

- Allow the child to increase activity gradually as tolerated. Report any changes in activity level to the physician.

- Observe for signs of wound infection, fever, flu-like symptoms, or an increased respiratory rate or respiratory distress. Report these signs to the physician.

- Allow the child to return to school in approximately 3 weeks. Physical activities such as rough play, bike riding, or climbing should be postponed for 6 weeks until the incision has healed completely.

Reassure parents by telling them that the child with a repaired cardiac defect should have no further cardiovascular problems. Encourage them to allow the child to live a normal and active life.

Children are at risk for infective endocarditis, especially within the first 6 months after surgery. The child should receive prophylactic antibiotics according to the American Heart Association recommendations (Table 12–8). Any unexplained fever or malaise seen in the 2 months following repair or after dental work may be a sign of infection. The child should be examined for petechiae and splenomegaly. Blood cultures, blood cell count, and urinalysis should be performed.

CYANOTIC DEFECTS

Cyanotic heart disease is generally caused by a valvular or vascular malformation. The most common malformations are tetralogy of Fallot and transposition of the great vessels (Fig. 12–5). Table 12–9 summarizes clinical manifestations, diagnostic tests, and medical management for these defects.

Other less common congenital heart defects include hypoplastic left heart syndrome, tricuspid atresia, pulmonary atresia, truncus arteriosus, and total anomalous pulmonary venous return (Table 12–10). Not all of these defects cause cyanosis.

Clinical Manifestations

Cyanosis often occurs when the ductus arteriosus closes, causing hypoxemia. Signs and symptoms of chronic hypoxemia include fatigue, clubbing of the

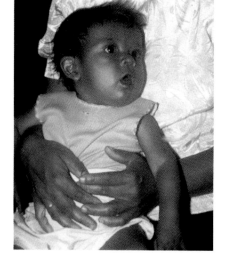

FIGURE 12–5. This infant has a cyanotic heart defect. What is the prognosis for an infant who has either of the most common malformations—tetralogy of Fallot or transposition of the great vessels?

12-8 | Antibiotic Recommendations for Endocarditis Prophylaxis in Children[a]

For Dental, Oral, or Upper Respiratory Tract Procedures
Amoxicillin

For Children Allergic to Penicillin
Clindamycin, cephalexin, cefadroxil, azithromycin, clarithromycin

For Genitourinary and Gastrointestinal Procedures
Ampicillin, gentamicin, amoxicillin

For Children Allergic to Penicillin
Vancomycin, gentamicin

[a]*Routine dosage:* Large dose is given 1 hour before procedure. Smaller dose is given 6 hours after procedure. Modified from Dajani, A.S., Taubert, K.A., Wilson, W., Bolger, A.F., Bayer, A. et.al. (1997). Prevention of bacterial endocarditis: Recommendations of the American Heart Association. *Journal of the American Medical Association, 277* (22), 1794–1801.

fingers and toes, exertional dyspnea, and delayed developmental milestones. Because infants tire easily with feeding, they receive fewer calories, and do not grow normally. Congestive heart failure develops in some children.

The skin may have a ruddy or mottled appearance before cyanosis is observed. When pulmonary circulation is impaired, hemoglobin may not become reoxygenated. The appearance of cyanosis is related to the hemoglobin level and the oxygen saturation level.

Cyanotic (hypoxic) spells, the most significant problem to develop in infants and toddlers with heart defects, usually appear between 2 months and 2 years of age. Cyanotic spells can develop suddenly. Signs include:

- Increased rate and depth of respirations
- Increased cyanosis
- Increased heart rate
- Pallor and poor tissue perfusion
- Agitation or irritability

Children with uncorrected cyanotic heart disease often squat to relieve dyspnea (Fig. 12–6). The knee–chest position reduces the cardiac output by decreasing the venous return from the lower extremities and by increasing the systemic vascular resistance.

Etiology and Pathophysiology

Cyanotic defects are generally caused by a malformation or combination of defects that prevents adequate oxygenation of the blood. When the defect is associated with decreased pulmonary blood flow, pressures from obstructed blood in the right side of the heart exceed those in the left. Unoxygenated blood is shunted to the left side of the heart. Oxygenated blood destined for the systemic circulation is diluted, resulting in chronic hypoxemia and cyanosis.

When children with cyanosis rise in the morning, they may experience an abrupt decrease in pulmonary blood flow. A cyanotic spell may be triggered by this decrease when combined with a sudden increase in cardiac output and venous return caused by crying, feeding, exercise, and straining with defecation. The partial pressure of oxygen (Po_2) is lowered, and the partial pressure of carbon dioxide (Pco_2) rises. The hypoxemia becomes progressively worse as the respiratory center in the brain overreacts, in-

 CLINICAL TIP

Cyanosis is seen at a higher oxygen saturation level when the child's hemoglobin level is normal or polycythemia exists.[5]

Hemoglobin Level	Oxygen Saturation Level
6 g% (anemia)	45–50%
15 g% (normal)	75–80%
20 g% (polycythemia)	80–85%

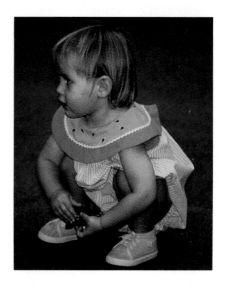

FIGURE 12–6. A child with a cyanotic heart defect squats (assumes a knee–chest position) to relieve cyanotic spells.

12-9   Cyanotic Heart Defects

Tetralogy of Fallot

Combination of four defects: pulmonic stenosis, right ventricular hypertrophy, ventricular septal defect (VSD), and overriding of aorta. Some children have a fifth defect: open foramen ovale or atrial septal defect (ASD). About 10% of children with congenital heart defects have tetralogy of Fallot. This defect is characterized by elevated pressures in right side of heart, causing right-to-left shunt.

Clinical Manifestations

As ductus arteriosus closes, infant becomes hypoxic and cyanotic. The degree of pulmonary stenosis determines severity of symptoms. Polycythemia, hypoxic spells, metabolic acidosis, poor growth, clubbing, and exercise intolerance may develop. Infants have a systolic murmur heard in pulmonic area that is transmitted to suprasternal notch.

Diagnostic Tests

Chest x-ray film shows a boot-shaped heart due to the large right ventricle with decreased pulmonary vascular markings. Electrocardiogram (ECG) shows right ventricular hypertrophy. Echocardiogram demonstrates VSD, obstruction of pulmonary outflow, and overriding aorta. Cardiac catheterization is required before surgical correction to completely identify the location of all anatomic structures and any additional defects.

Medical Management

Cyanotic spells are managed according to guidelines given in section on nursing management of cyanotic defects. Monitoring child for metabolic acidosis or prolonged unconsciousness is critical. Palliative surgery may be performed before corrective surgery. Corrective surgery may be attempted in symptomatic children by 6 months of age.

PROGNOSIS: Arrhythmias and myocardial dysfunction are believed to be related to surgical intervention. A pacemaker may be needed for some children. Sudden death from ventricular arrhythmias occurs in 2–7% of patients several years after surgery.[a] Lifelong infective endocarditis prophylaxis is required.

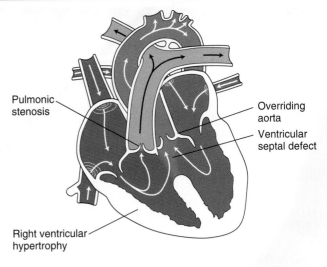

Pulmonic stenosis

Overriding aorta

Ventricular septal defect

Right ventricular hypertrophy

■ Decreased blood flow

creasing the respiratory effort. The additional respiratory effort further increases the cardiac output and contributes to a life-threatening decline unless rapid intervention is successful.

Children with cyanotic defects are at increased risk for thromboembolism. The chronic hypoxemia leads to polycythemia in an attempt to increase the hemoglobin available to carry oxygen. Brain abscesses are more common in children with cyanotic heart defects. Bacteria in the blood returning from the systemic circulation are usually filtered out by the capillaries in the lungs. However, when unoxygenated blood enters the systemic circulation through the right-to-left shunt, bacteria can travel directly to the brain.

Diagnostic Tests and Medical Management

A systolic heart murmur may be apparent after cyanosis develops. A chest x-ray study, electrocardiogram, and echocardiogram are obtained. Usually

12-9 Cyanotic Heart Defects (continued)

Transposition of the Great Vessels (TGV)

Pulmonary artery is the outflow for left ventricle, and aorta is outflow for right ventricle. This condition is life threatening at birth, and survival initially depends on open ductus arteriosus and foramen ovale. This condition occurs in about 5% of children with congenital heart disease. ASD or VSD may also be present with TGV.

Clinical Manifestations

Cyanosis, apparent soon after birth, progresses to hypoxia and acidosis. Cyanosis does not improve with oxygen administration. However, cyanosis may be less apparent when a large VSD is also present. Congestive heart failure may develop over days or weeks. Tachypnea (60 respirations/min) is often present without retractions or other signs of dyspnea. Infants take a long time to feed and need frequent rest periods because of rapid respiratory rate and fatigue. Growth failure may be evident as early as 2 weeks of age if corrective surgery is not performed.

Diagnostic Tests

Chest x-ray study may reveal a classic egg-shaped heart with a narrow superior mediastinum. Diagnosis is made by echocardiogram when position of arteries arising from ventricles is visible.

Medical Management

Prostaglandin E_1 is initially ordered to maintain patent ductus arteriosus until palliative procedure can be performed. Corrective surgery is usually performed before 1 week of age. Large opening between atria is created with balloon during cardiac catheterization in newborns. This may also be corrected surgically.

PROGNOSIS: Survival without surgery is impossible. Arrhythmias occur in many patients after a Mustard or Senning procedure. Infective endocarditis prophylaxis may be necessary.

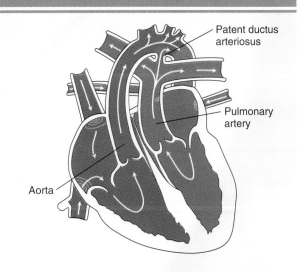

Labels: Patent ductus arteriosus; Pulmonary artery; Aorta

aFyler, D.C. (1992). Tetralogy of Fallot. In Nadas' pediatric cardiology (pp. 471–491). Philadelphia: Hanley & Belfus.

the echocardiogram clearly shows the defect, shunt, and heart pressures. Cardiac catheterization is often used to obtain detailed anatomic information before surgery.

Early management of cyanotic heart defects is important to prevent secondary damage to the heart, lungs, and brain, including the adverse effects of hypoxemia on the child's cognitive and psychomotor development.[16] For this reason, corrective surgery is being performed at younger ages, often in infancy. A **palliative procedure** may be performed to preserve life in children with potentially lethal heart defects and complications (see Table 12–5). With many defects, the success of corrective surgery is better after the infant has had an opportunity to grow.

If closure of the ductus arteriosus causes life-threatening cyanosis in newborns, prostaglandin E_1 (PGE_1) is prescribed to reopen the ductus arteriosus. These infants depend on a patent ductus arteriosus for survival or improvement in pulmonary or systemic blood flow. Treatment with PGE_1 provides time for the newborn to be transferred to a cardiac center for surgical intervention. Response time to PGE_1 varies depending on the type of defect. Cyanotic infants respond within 30 minutes, but infants with acyan-

12-10	Less Common Congenital Heart Defects		
Condition	**Clinical Manifestations**	**Diagnostic Tests**	**Medical Management**
Hypoplastic Left Heart Syndrome Absence or stenosis of mitral and aortic valves associated with an abnormally small left ventricle and aortic arch. Signs are initiated with closure of ductus arteriosus.	Signs include tachypnea, retractions, decreased peripheral pulses, poor peripheral perfusion, pulmonary edema, and congestive heart failure eventually leading to shock, acidosis, and death.	Echocardiogram is used for initial diagnosis.	Prostaglandin E_1 given to maintain patent ductus arteriosus. Palliative Norwood procedure, and then a modified Fontan procedure or transplantation may be performed. Survival rate is low.
Tricuspid Atresia/Pulmonary Atresia Absence of tricuspid or pulmonary valve. A ventricular septal defect (VSD) or transposition of the great vessels (TGV) is also often present.	Early cyanosis, dyspnea, congestive heart failure, hepatomegaly, acidosis, hypoxic spells, clubbing, polycythemia, and growth delays occur. Continuous murmur is heard in aortic area.	Chest x-ray study and echocardiogram are used for initial diagnosis.	Prostaglandin E_1 is given to maintain patent ductus arteriosus. Digoxin and diuretics are also used. Palliative surgery increases pulmonary blood flow. The Rashkind procedure is used. The modified Fontan procedure results in improved survival.
Truncus Arteriosus A single large vessel empties both ventricles. VSD is usually present.	Cyanosis develops soon after birth. Severe congestive heart failure, dyspnea, retractions, fatigue, poor feeding, polycythemia, clubbing, increased pulse pressure, bounding peripheral pulses, increased respiratory infections, and cardiomegaly also occur.	Chest x-ray study and echocardiogram give initial diagnosis. Cardiac catheterization is done before surgery.	Surgery is performed to close VSD and create a passage to pulmonary arteries. Digoxin and diuretics are given. Repeated surgery is necessary to enlarge pulmonary artery conduit. Survival is improved, but long-term prognosis is unknown.
Total Anomalous Pulmonary Venous Return Pulmonary veins empty into right atrium or veins leading to the right atrium.	Increased right ventricular impulse may occur. With severe pulmonary overload, tachycardia, dyspnea, pulmonary edema, retractions, cyanosis, hepatomegaly, poor feedings, irritability, and failure to thrive are seen.	Chest x-ray study, echocardiogram, and cardiac catheterization are used for diagnosis.	Surgery to reconnect or baffle the pulmonary veins to the left atrium is performed. Survivors have lived more than 20 years after correction.

otic lesions such as coarctation of the aorta may take up to 3 hours to respond.[17]

The child's hemoglobin level and hematocrit values must be monitored to ensure that the blood does not become too viscous. Polycythemia may be managed by red blood cell pheresis if the blood viscosity becomes too high.

Cyanotic spells are treated aggressively. To decrease the pulmonary vascular resistance, the initial treatment involves calming the child, giving oxygen, and administering intravenous morphine and intravenous propranolol. All unpleasant procedures must be postponed. To increase the systemic vascular resistance, the child is placed in knee–chest position and given intravenous fluids to expand circulatory volume. Dopamine or phenylephrine (Neosynephrine) are also given. Once a cyanotic spell has occurred, immediate palliative or corrective surgery is often scheduled. Oral propranolol is administered to decrease the frequency of cyanotic spells because of its action to minimize spasms of the pulmonary outflow tract.[18]

Antibiotic prophylaxis for infective endocarditis is needed before and after surgical correction for all cyanotic conditions. See Table 12–8 for a list of recommended antibiotics.

Nursing Assessment

Frequently monitor the cardiovascular status of infants receiving PGE_1 therapy. Assess vital signs, heart rhythm, skin color, peripheral pulses, and capillary refill time. Observe for signs of improvement in vital signs and color as the oxygen saturation increases and acidosis decreases following the initial treatment. In addition, watch for tachycardia, tachypnea, crackles, frothy secretions, low urine output, and edema because these infants are at risk for congestive heart failure.

Observe the child carefully for signs of increased cyanosis in the morning or at other high-risk times. Watch for neurologic signs of thromboembolitic complications from polycythemia such as headache, dizziness, excessive irritability, and paralysis. Older children with cyanotic defects may have clubbing of the fingers (Fig. 12–7).

Nursing Diagnosis

Among the nursing diagnoses that might apply to a child with cyanotic heart disease are:

- Altered Tissue Perfusion (Cardiopulmonary) related to reduced pulmonary blood flow
- Decreased Cardiac Output related to development of congestive heart failure
- Risk for Infection related to unfiltered bacteria in the blood and sites of blood shunting that promote bacterial growth
- Altered Nutrition: Less Than Body Requirements related to dyspnea and fatigue with feeding
- Ineffective Infant Feeding Pattern related to dyspnea and fatigue
- Risk for Caregiver Role Strain related to care of a child with chronic illness
- Activity Intolerance related to cyanosis and dyspnea on exertion
- Altered Growth and Development related to hypoxemia
- Risk for Ineffective Management of Therapeutic Regimen related to prophylactic antibiotics for dental care procedures
- Knowledge Deficit (Parents) related to assessment and management of cyanotic spells, which are unpredictable events

Nursing Management

Children with tetralogy of Fallot are often managed at home until surgery is scheduled. Home care involves reducing parental anxiety, providing adequate nutrition, helping parents recognize signs of illness, and formulating a plan for emergency treatment. Nursing care of the hospitalized child focuses

 CLINICAL TIP

Crying may improve cyanosis caused by lung disease or disorders of the central nervous system. In children with cyanotic heart disease, crying usually makes cyanosis worse.

 NURSING ALERT

Cyanotic spells become life threatening if not treated immediately. The child becomes progressively more hypoxic and limp, loses consciousness, is likely to have a seizure or cerebrovascular accident, and may die.

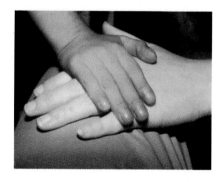

FIGURE 12–7. Clubbing of the fingers is one manifestation of a cyanotic defect in an older child. What neurologic signs may be associated with such a defect?

 CLINICAL TIP

To calm and reassure the infant while simultaneously positioning him or her in knee–chest position, hold the infant facing your chest. Place one arm under the knees and fold the legs upward toward the infant's chest. Use the other arm to support the infant's back.

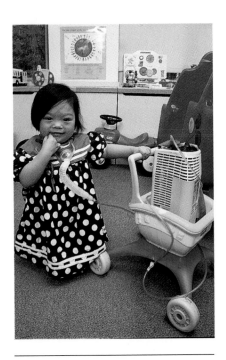

FIGURE 12–8. By pushing her oxygen cannister in a toy shopping cart, this toddler is able to move around in her environment. This strategy meets both her physiologic need for supplemental oxygen and her developmental need for independence.

NURSING ALERT

Common side effects of PGE₁ therapy include cutaneous vasodilation, bradycardia, tachycardia, hypotension, seizure activity, fever, and apnea.

on monitoring PGE₁ therapy (for newborns only; used until palliative surgery is performed), treating cyanotic spells, and providing postsurgical care.

Home Care of the Child Before Surgery

Parents are usually anxious because of the need to wait before surgery can be performed. They often fear that the infant will not survive until surgery or that they will be unable to manage any problems the infant may have. Provide parents with information and teach them how to care for the child at home. Some infants have such special home care needs that home health nursing and other community services are required. Many of these children require supplemental oxygen and nutrition, either for emergencies or for regular use (Fig. 12–8).

Cyanosis with or without congestive heart failure often results in delayed gross motor skills. Developmental specialists can help parents set realistic developmental goals for the child. Make referrals to community-based early-intervention programs to promote the child's development.

Encourage parents to treat the infant as normally as possible. The child should be able to tolerate crying for a few minutes without difficulty. Prolonged crying should not be permitted because it causes fatigue and further hypoxia.

Vomiting and diarrhea may lead to dehydration, and parents must notify the physician whenever the infant or child has these symptoms. Dehydration is a particular risk in children with polycythemia because the blood can become even more viscous. Fever and dehydration may increase cyanosis. The systemic vascular resistance is decreased, resulting in a further decrease in blood flow to the pulmonary system. Aggressive management with antipyretic medication and fluid volume replacement is necessary.[18]

Teach parents to observe the child for signs of infective endocarditis, including low-grade fever, fatigue, and malaise. They need to notify the physician if these symptoms occur within 2 months of surgery or a high-risk procedure. Parents must learn to request antibiotic prophylaxis for the child (see Table 12–8). Children also need preventive dental care to reduce the risk of endocarditis.

Parents may want to formulate an emergency plan in case the infant develops acute problems such as a cyanotic spell or respiratory distress. Cardiopulmonary resuscitation should be taught to the parents. Ask parents to notify the local rescue squad about the infant's problem. Prepare a card or brief history form with information about the child's condition, medications, and necessary emergency care and the physician's name for parents to keep at home[19] (Fig. 12–9). When an acute problem occurs, this form gives important information to the emergency medical technicians and emergency department staff.

Although parents may travel with cyanotic children, they should not take these children to areas of high altitude without consulting with the physician first. Arrangements for supplemental oxygen when traveling on an airplane may be necessary.

Care of the Infant and Child Undergoing Surgery

Monitor and carefully maintain the central, umbilical, or peripheral intravenous lines in the infant receiving continuous infusion of PGE₁. Observe the infant for side effects of prostaglandin treatment. Have intubation equipment and a bag and mask at the bedside in case apnea occurs. Have intravenous fluids available to control hypotension.

If a cyanotic spell occurs, immediately place the child in the knee–chest position and administer oxygen. Administer morphine as ordered. Immedi-

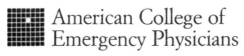

American College of Emergency Physicians

Emergency Data Set for Children with Special Needs

Date form completed _____ Initials

Revised _____ Initials

Revised _____ Initials

Name: _____ Birth date: _____

Home address: _____ Home Phone: _____

_____

Emergency Contacts: Names & Relationship 1: _____ # _____

2: _____ # _____

Physicians: Primary care physician: _____ Phone: _____

Fax: _____

Specialty physician: _____ Phone: _____

Fax: _____

Specialty physician: _____ Phone: _____

Anticipated Primary ED: _____ Fax: _____

Diagnoses:

1. _____

2. _____

3. _____

4. _____

Synopsis:

_____

_____

_____

_____

Medications:

1. _____   2. _____   3. _____

4. _____   5. _____   6. _____

Significant baseline physical findings: _____

Significant baseline ancillary findings (lab, x-ray, ECG): _____

_____

_____

MANAGEMENT DATA:

Medications to be avoided   and why:

1. _____   _____

2. _____   _____

3. _____   _____

Procedures to be avoided   and why:

1. _____   _____

2. _____   _____

3. _____   _____

Antibiotic prophylaxis

Indications: _____   Medication and dose: _____

COMMON PRESENTING PROBLEMS/FINDINGS WITH SPECIFIC SUGGESTED MANAGEMENT

Problem   Suggested Diagnostic Studies   Suggested Treatment

_____

_____

Comments on child, family, or other specific medical issues:

_____

_____

FIGURE 12-9. An emergency care form should be kept in the home to provide essential medical information to rescue personnel.
Copyright © the American College of Physicians, 1997.

ately notify the physician for further orders if these procedures are ineffective and the spell continues. Avoid any unpleasant or anxiety-provoking procedures.

Children are admitted to the intensive care unit following surgery. Refer to the section on nursing assessment in the discussion of nursing care of the child undergoing surgery on page 485. Postoperative bleeding is a potential risk in children with polycythemia because bleeding times are prolonged and platelet counts are low. Chest tube output is monitored carefully for bright red blood or excessive volume. Bright red blood in the chest tube is a significant sign of hemorrhage. Fluids and diuretics are used to maintain **preload** (the volume of blood in the ventricle at the end of diastole that stretches the heart muscle before contraction) in the right ventricle whereas inotropic drugs are used to support cardiac output. Children are transferred to the general nursing unit once heart function has stabilized.

Monitor the heart functioning of children following surgery. Assess vital signs, skin color, perfusion of the skin by capillary refill, and distal pulses. A sudden sustained increase in pulse and respirations and a decrease in peripheral perfusion may be early signs of hemorrhage. Monitoring fluid intake and output following surgery is critical. Note any signs of respiratory distress that may indicate the development of a pneumothorax or congestive heart failure.

► ACQUIRED HEART DISEASES

RHEUMATIC FEVER

COMMUNITY CARE CONSIDERATIONS

A virulent strain of group A streptococci may be causing the increase in cases of rheumatic fever that have been reported in the United States. Often, the sore throat that precedes the child's illness is mild and goes untreated. Nurses must carefully evaluate pharyngitis, especially when cases of group A streptococcal infection have been identified in the family or community.

Rheumatic fever is an inflammatory disease that follows an initial infection by some strains of group A beta-hemolytic streptococci. This disorder causes changes in the heart, joints, skin, and, less often, the central nervous system. As a result of effective treatment of streptococcal infections, the incidence of rheumatic fever reached a low in the United States in the 1970s. However, the disease has occurred more frequently in recent years, probably because of an increase in number and severity of group A streptococcal infections.[20] The exact cause of the disease is unknown. Possible causes include a bacterial toxin or an altered immune response.

Several weeks after an untreated streptococcal infection, the hallmark signs of rheumatic fever may occur. Aschoff bodies (hemorrhagic bullous lesions) develop in the connective tissue of the heart. Endocarditis may lead to permanent heart valve damage. The child's joints become inflamed and painful (migratory polyarthritis), although this condition improves in several weeks. Subcutaneous nodules may be palpable near joints. A skin rash called erythema marginatum, with pink macules and blanching in the middle of the lesions, is frequently seen. Spiking fever often occurs. A condition known as Sydenham chorea (St. Vitus dance), which is characterized by aimless movements of the extremities and facial grimacing, may be seen if the central nervous system is involved. Mild anemia may also occur.

Diagnosis is based on clinical signs (Jones criteria; Table 12–11) and laboratory testing for antistreptolysin-O (ASO). An elevated ASO antibody titer indicates a recent streptococcal infection.

Medical treatment includes antibiotics (penicillin or erythromycin) to eradicate the streptococcal infection. Aspirin may be given to control joint inflammation and reduce fever. Children should be monitored carefully for potential heart involvement. Most children recover fully.

12-11	Guidelines for Diagnosis of Initial Attack of Rheumatic Fever (Jones Criteria, updated 1992)[a]

Major Manifestations	Minor Manifestations
Carditis	**Clinical findings**
Polyarthritis	Arthralgia
Chorea	Fever
Erythema marginatum	**Laboratory findings**
Subcutaneous nodules	Elevated acute-phase reactants
	Erythrocyte sedimentation rate
	C-reactive protein
	Prolonged PR interval

Supporting evidence of antecedent group A streptococcal infection: (1) positive throat culture or rapid streptococcal antigen test; (2) elevated or rising streptococcal antibody titer.

[a]If supported by evidence of preceding group A streptococcal infection, the presence of two major manifestations or of one major and two minor manifestations indicates a high probability of acute rheumatic fever.
Data from Special Writing Group of the Committee on Rheumatic Fever, Endocarditis, and Kawasaki Disease of the Council on Cardiovascular Disease in the Young of the American Heart Association. (1992). Guidelines for the diagnosis of rheumatic fever. Jones Criteria, 1992 update. Journal of the American Medical Association, 268(15), 2069–2073.

Nursing Management

The most important role of the nurse is prevention of rheumatic fever. Nurses in clinics, offices, and schools need to ensure that all children with possible streptococcal infections have a throat culture taken. Even if the sore throat is mild, a culture is needed if family members or other contacts have had a streptococcal infection. (Refer to the *Quick Reference to Pediatric Clinical Skills* accompanying this text for throat culture technique.) Nurses can organize culture clinics in a variety of settings.[21] Emphasize to the family the importance of giving the entire 10-day course of antibiotics when a culture is positive.

In a case of severe rheumatic fever, the child will be hospitalized for a period of time. Nursing care focuses on assessing the child's condition, promoting recovery, and ensuring compliance with the treatment regimen.

During the acute inflammatory phase, take the child's temperature at least every 4 hours and monitor vital signs. Auscultate the child's heart and note any unusual sounds. Observe the child for changes in skin, joints, or behavior. Family members should have throat cultures done to identify possible asymptomatic streptococcal carriers.

Administer penicillin and aspirin as ordered. The child is usually lethargic and often has joint pain. Position the child's joints and handle them carefully. Tepid sponge baths and cool compresses may be ordered to control spiking fevers. The child is usually placed in isolation. Provide quiet activities, as the child is often confined to bed. Encourage visits or telephone calls from family members and friends. For the child with chorea, provide emotional support because the purposeless involuntary movements can be disturbing. Encourage the family to participate in the child's hospital care.

During the recovery phase, the child will generally be cared for at home. Activities may be limited, especially if heart damage is suspected. Help parents plan quiet activities, such as playing board games, working with computers, or reading, and arrange rest periods after the child returns to school. Reassure the child and parents that the effects of chorea will eventually subside.

On discharge, a daily oral low-dose antibiotic is prescribed or monthly long-acting antibiotic injection is given. Make sure the child and parents understand the importance of taking prescribed medication indefinitely to prevent future infection and possible heart damage from recurrent rheumatic fever. Stress the importance of telling future health care providers, including dentists and surgeons, about the child's rheumatic fever history so prophylactic antibiotics can be given to prevent infective endocarditis during invasive procedures.

Make sure the parents understand that the child's future sore throats may be streptococcal and that a throat culture should be taken even when the child is taking daily antibiotics. The child may need additional antibiotics for the infection. Emphasize the importance of follow-up care to prevent new infections and to monitor heart function.

INFECTIVE ENDOCARDITIS

Endocarditis is an inflammation of the lining, valves, and arterial vessels of the heart. Infective endocarditis, also known as subacute bacterial endocarditis, is the most common type of this infection.

Symptoms can be mild and develop slowly, or they can be severe and develop rapidly. Common symptoms are fever (often with elevations in the afternoon), fatigue, joint and muscle aches, headache, and gastrointestinal discomfort. Other signs include chest pain, dyspnea, weight loss, splenomegaly, hepatomegaly, and arrhythmias or murmurs.[6]

Most infections are caused by *Streptococcus* or *Staphylococcus*. Children who have a congenital heart defect, rheumatic heart disease, or a central venous catheter or who have had heart surgery are at risk for infective endocarditis. Infections frequently occur after the causal organism enters the bloodstream during dental work or surgery.

Infective endocarditis is diagnosed primarily by blood culture; however, urine and cerebrospinal fluid also may be cultured. Elevated erythrocyte sedimentation rate, anemia, elevated C-reactive protein level, increased white blood cell count, alterations in the electrocardiogram, and changes in heart sounds and murmurs are indicators of the condition. Echocardiography may be used to identify the presence of infective lesions in the heart.

Treatment consists of administering antibiotics such as penicillin G, ampicillin, vancomycin, nafcillin, or gentamicin. Intravenous administration is preferred, with therapy continuing for 2–8 weeks. Serum levels of antibiotics are monitored to maintain a therapeutic range. Occasionally surgery is necessary to drain an abscess or because of heart valve failure. If congestive heart failure occurs, bedrest and medications such as digoxin and furosemide are prescribed. Although treatment is effective in the majority of children, 20% die because of heart damage.[6]

Nursing Management

Nursing care focuses on assessing the child's condition, administering medications, and teaching the parents about the child's care. Take the child's vital signs and assess gastrointestinal discomfort. Administer medications as ordered and monitor serum antibiotic levels. Monitor for side effects of antibiotics and for infiltration or extravasation at the infusion site. Keep invasive procedures to a minimum. Use careful aseptic technique in performing venipunctures, urinary catheterizations, and other procedures.

The child is often lethargic and on bedrest. Encourage parents to assist with the child's care and plan quiet age-appropriate activities. At discharge, instruct parents about administration of oral antibiotics at home and reinforce the need for follow-up visits. Explain the importance of informing physicians and dentists about the child's history of endocarditis so that care is taken to prevent infection before invasive procedures.

CARDIAC ARRHYTHMIAS

Cardiac arrhythmias (abnormal rhythms) are not uncommon in children. Most abnormal rhythms are not harmful and do not require intervention. These include tachyarrhythmias (sinus tachycardia) and bradyarrhythmias (sinus bradycardia) that occur with acute conditions and resolve once the condition is treated. Other abnormal rates and rhythms should be evaluated by a cardiologist. Supraventricular tachycardia (SVT) is the most common abnormal arrhythmia. Other arrhythmias, which are usually associated with congenital heart disease, include atrial fibrillation, atrial flutter, ventricular fibrillation, and heart block.

Supraventricular tachycardia is the abrupt onset of a rapid, regular heart rate, often too fast to count. Neonates and young children may be predisposed to the condition because of a congenital heart defect or Wolff–Parkinson–White syndrome. Short periods of arrhythmia (several seconds), which may be caused by paroxysmal atrial tachycardia, are rarely dangerous. However, prolonged episodes of continuous SVT for more than 24 hours may lead to congestive heart failure. Recurrent attacks are common. Electrocardiography is used to confirm the diagnosis.

Prolonged episodes of SVT are life threatening and can progress to congestive heart failure or cardiogenic shock if untreated. Cardiac output is affected because diastolic filling cannot occur with such a rapid heart rate.

Vagal stimulation such as application of ice or iced saline solution to the face may reduce the heart rate. An older child can perform the Valsalva maneuver (holding the breath and straining, or blowing forcefully on the thumb) to increase intrathoracic and venous pressures and thus slow the heart rate. Adenosine is the recommended emergency medication when vagal stimulation does not work. Cardioversion may be used for life-threatening episodes if other treatments are not effective. Digoxin and propranolol may be given to reduce the frequency of episodes.[22,23]

Nursing Management

Nursing care focuses on assessing the child's condition, administering medications, and providing emotional support to the child and parents. Children are treated in the emergency department or intensive care unit. The child is placed on a cardiac monitor, and frequent assessment is critical. Report continued abnormal rates or rhythms to the physician. Carefully observe and record changes in level of consciousness, color, weakness, irritability, and feeding pattern. Administer medications as ordered. Have emergency drugs and resuscitation equipment available at the bedside. Provide for rest and adequate nutrition.

Episodes of arrhythmia are frightening for both the child and parents. Carefully explain the treatment plan and home care. Teach parents to take the child's apical pulse. Provide telephone numbers of emergency medical facilities and help parents plan how to seek emergency care. Emphasize that digoxin and propranolol help reduce the frequency of the episodes.

GROWTH & DEVELOPMENT CONSIDERATIONS

The presenting heart rate in infants with supraventricular tachycardia (SVT) may be up to 260 beats/min. In older children, a heart rate between 150 and 240 beats/min may be seen. A heart rate of 230 beats/min is seen in 60% of children under 18 years of age.[22]

NURSING ALERT

The child with supraventricular tachycardia (SVT) should avoid subsequent use of cardiac stimulant drugs such as decongestants. These drugs might trigger another episode of SVT.

► VASCULAR DISEASES

KAWASAKI DISEASE

Kawasaki disease, also known as mucocutaneous lymph node syndrome, is an acute systemic inflammatory illness. Although this disorder is most commonly found in Japanese children, it is seen in all races. The disorder occurs primarily in toddlers. In the United States, Kawasaki disease is the most common cause of acquired heart disease in children, and its incidence is increasing.[24]

There are three stages of the disease: acute, subacute, and convalescent. The acute stage of the disease is characterized by fever, conjunctival hyperemia, red throat, swollen hands and feet, rash, and enlargement of the cervical lymph nodes (Fig. 12–10). The subacute stage is characterized by cracking lips and fissures, desquamation of the skin on the tips of the fingers and toes, joint pain, cardiac disease, and thrombocytosis. In the convalescent stage, the child appears normal but lingering signs of inflammation may be present.

The etiology of Kawasaki disease is unknown, but the primary cause is theorized to be an infection with an organism or toxin. The disease occurs most often in late summer and early spring. It is not spread by person-to-person contact.

Diagnosis is based on clinical signs using the criteria given in Table 12–12. Blood studies show some abnormalities such as elevated erythrocyte sedimentation rate, elevated white blood cell count, mild anemia, elevated platelet count, and elevated C-reactive protein level. An echocardiogram may reveal some heart changes.

Medical management of Kawasaki disease involves the use of aspirin and immune globulin. High doses of aspirin (80–100 mg/kg/day) are given while the fever is high. The dose is decreased to 10 mg/kg/day or less once the fever has dropped. Aspirin is taken until the platelet count is normal and may be continued on a long-term basis if cardiac abnormalities occur. Immune globulin given early in the disease has been shown to reduce the incidence of coronary artery lesions and aneurysms, and to decrease fever, inflammation, and leukocyte and granulocyte counts, although the mechanism by which this occurs is unknown.[25, 26]

Children are usually hospitalized as long as fever persists. Most children recover fully. Careful monitoring for cardiac disease continues for sev-

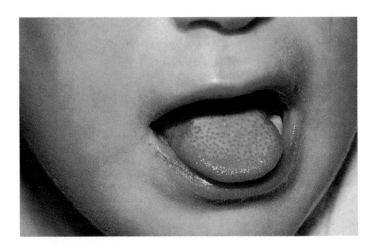

FIGURE 12-10. This child shows many of the signs of the acute stage of Kawasaki disease.

12-12	Diagnostic Criteria for Kawasaki Disease

Kawasaki disease is diagnosed when five of the following six criteria are present:
- Fever, generally ≥ 40°C (104.5°F), for 5 days or longer
- Bilateral conjunctivitis, typically with distinctly visible vessels early in the disease
- Intense erythema of the buccal and pharyngeal surfaces with dry, swollen, cracked, and fissuring lips and a strawberry tongue
- Dermatitis of the extremities, intense palmar and plantar erythema, induration of the hands and feet, and then desquamation after 2 or more weeks of symptoms
- Dermatitis of the trunk with a polymorphic erythematous maculopapular rash
- Acute cervical lymphadenopathy, frequently unilateral, with a node over 1.5 cm in diameter found early in the disease

Modified from Harville, T.O. (1996). Autoimmune vasculitides. In A.M. Rudolph, J.I.E. Hoffman, & C.D. Rudolph (Eds.),. Rudolph's pediatrics (20th ed., p. 496). Stamford, CT: Appleton & Lange.

eral weeks or months. Cardiac involvement is the most serious complication. Aneurysms and other vessel changes lead to arrhythmias, congestive heart failure, myocardial infarction, and, potentially, death.

Nursing Management

Nursing care focuses on promoting comfort, monitoring for early signs of complications or disease progression, and supporting the family.

Assessment is important in identifying signs of Kawasaki disease, as the acute phase of this disorder is commonly confused with other diseases. The nurse in the community must be alert to early signs and symptoms. When the child is hospitalized, take the temperature every 4 hours and before each dose of aspirin. Carefully assess the extremities for edema, redness, and desquamation every 8 hours. Examine the eyes for conjunctivitis and the mucous membranes for inflammation. Monitor the child's dietary and fluid intake and weigh the child daily. Carefully assess heart sounds and rhythm.

Administer aspirin and immune globulin as ordered. Monitor for side effects of aspirin such as bleeding and gastrointestinal upset. Administer intravenous immune globulin as a blood product, carefully regulating the infusion rate to run slowly according to the physician's orders, and watching for any reactions to the infusion. The infusion rate should not be over 1 mL/min. If symptoms of reaction are noted, *stop* the infusion immediately (see Chap. 9, Alterations in Immune Function).

Promote the child's comfort. Keep the child's skin clean and dry, and lubricate the lips. Use cool compresses and tepid sponges to make the feverish child more comfortable. Change the child's clothes and bed linens frequently. Give the child frequent small feedings of soft foods and liquids that are neither too hot nor too cold.

Use passive range-of-motion exercises to facilitate joint movement. Because the child with Kawasaki disease is frequently lethargic and irritable, plan rest periods and quiet age-appropriate activities. Encourage the parents to participate in their child's care. This comforts and reassures the child. Provide the parents with information about the disease and the child's treatment.

Before the child is discharged, teach the parents to administer aspirin as ordered and to watch for side effects. Advise the parents that the child may need to avoid contact sports or other activities that could cause bleeding.

NURSING ALERT

Inform the parents of a child with Kawasaki disease to postpone any scheduled immunizations for 5 months after immune globulin administration, as immune response to the vaccine may not be fully effective.[27]

12-13	Risk Factors for Hyperlipidemia

Family history of coronary heart disease before age 55

Cigarette smoking

Hypertension

Diabetes

Lack of exercise

High fat intake

Obesity

RECOMMENDED LIPID/LIPOPROTEIN LEVELS FOR CHILDREN

Total cholesterol
Recommended: < 170 mg/dL
Borderline high: 170–199 mg/dL
High: > 200 mg/dL

LDL-C
Recommended: < 110 mg/dL
Borderline high: 110–129 mg/dL
High: > 130 mg/dL

Triglyceride
Recommended: < 100 mg/dL
Borderline: 100–130 mg/dL
High: > 130 mg/dL

HDL-C
Recommended: > 35 mg/dL

Have them take the child's temperature daily and report any fever above 100°F (37.8°C) to the physician. Emphasize the need for follow-up care to monitor for cardiac complications.

HYPERLIPIDEMIA

Hyperlipidemia is a condition of excessive fat in the blood that may eventually lead to atherosclerosis. Although children do not usually die of atherosclerotic heart disease, coronary heart disease, the major cause of death in the United States, begins in childhood and progresses through the adult years.[28] It is important to identify children who have a genetic history or life-style that makes them more susceptible to future coronary heart disease (Table 12–13).

As the excessive fat circulates, it causes changes in blood vessels. The fatty streaks that appear in childhood become fibrous plaques in adolescence. These atherosclerotic plaques continue to grow in adulthood and may cause hemorrhage, thrombi, and occlusion of vessels.[29]

Hyperlipidemia is identified by a blood test. Cholesterol, including total cholesterol (TC), high-density lipoprotein cholesterol (HDL-C), and triglycerides are measured. The low-density lipoprotein cholesterol (LDL-C) level is calculated using an equation based on the triglyceride, HDL, and total cholesterol levels. It is recommended that all children who have a family history of cardiovascular disease before age 55 years (parents or grandparents) or who have a parent with elevated total serum cholesterol (240 mg/dL) be screened.[28] Some clinicians choose to screen all children, especially those with an unknown family history, during childhood or sometime after the age of 2 years. This helps to identify children who have no risk factors but demonstrate hyperlipidemia.[30] Based on total cholesterol value, children are placed in a low-, moderate-, or high-risk category. The LDL cholesterol level is examined carefully in children with elevated total cholesterol (200 mg/dL). LDL cholesterol should be less than 110 mg/dL. High HDL and low LDL cholesterol levels provide protection against heart disease.

Some children have hereditary disorders of lipid metabolism characterized by high levels of cholesterol, triglycerides, or both.[31] Children with familial hypercholesterolemia, for example, have cholesterol levels as high as 600–1000 mg/dL, resulting in lipid deposits in their corneas and tendons. These uncommon conditions require treatment by a lipid specialist.

Hyperlipidemia in most children can be managed by dietary modifications and other changes in life-style. The child's diet is carefully analyzed and changes are made to satisfy the dietary guidelines given in Table 12–14. If the child continues to have high serum lipid levels, a lipid specialist should be consulted. Cholestyramine or colestipol, which bind bile acid in the intestine, are occasionally prescribed for children over 10 years of age.

Long-term studies of the effect of childhood lipid levels on life span have not yet been concluded. It is hoped that careful monitoring and management of lipid levels in childhood will decrease the incidence of cardiovascular disease.

Nursing Management

Nursing care focuses on identifying children at risk for hyperlipidemia, providing education about diet and exercise, and monitoring eating patterns. Identification and management of hyperlipidemia takes place in a variety of community agencies. Office and clinic nurses identify children who need to have serum lipid measured. Nurses in schools provide education on ways to

12-14	Recommended Nutrient Intake in Children and Adolescents With Hyperlipidemia	
Nutrient	**Recommended Intake**	
Saturated fatty acid	Less than 10% of calories	
Total fat	No more than 30% of calories	
Polyunsaturated fat	Up to 10% of calories	
Monounsaturated fat	10–15% of calories	
Cholesterol	Less than 300 mg/day	

Modified from National Cholesterol Education Program Coordinating Committee. (1991). Report of the Expert Panel on Blood Cholesterol Levels in Children and Adolescents. Washington, DC: U.S. Department of Health and Human Services.

reduce risk factors.[32] The child's history of exercise patterns, weight percentile, and dietary intake provides important information. Obtain information on familial heart disease, hypertension, diabetes, and smoking to determine risk factors. Tell parents that the child will need to fast for 12 hours before blood is drawn to evaluate serum lipid levels.

Work with nutritionists to provide dietary teaching and monitor family eating patterns. Emphasize the importance of exercise in keeping the heart and blood vessels free from atherosclerotic changes. Help the child select an aerobic activity and encourage participation at least three times weekly.

Smoking by the child or the parents should be discouraged. Secondhand smoke may affect blood pressure and increase the risk for the development of cardiovascular disease.[32]

Include the entire family in the treatment plan, as changing eating and exercise patterns is difficult for a single family member.[33] The family of a child with hyperlipidemia requires continual teaching and reinforcement. Nutrition assessments and evaluation of family diet should be performed periodically.

HYPERTENSION

Hypertension is uncommon in children. Most cases are caused by underlying conditions such as kidney disease or heart defects. However, a genetic predisposition to hypertension may be manifested in some children by high normal or slightly elevated blood pressures. Mildly elevated blood pressure in adolescents may precede adult hypertension.[34,35] High blood pressure in adolescents is correlated with obesity and high serum lipid level.[36] All children with blood pressures in the 90th percentile for age are significantly more likely to develop hypertension as adults.[35]

Take a complete history for the child with borderline hypertension and no other associated diseases. Are parents or siblings hypertensive? Is the child obese? What is the child's daily salt intake? What are the child's daily exercise routines? Serum lipid studies should be performed to determine whether hyperlipidemia exists.

Teach both the child and the parents how to improve the diet and develop exercise routines. Emphasize the importance of avoiding smoking. Teaching that involves the entire family is usually the most effective. Take the child's blood pressure regularly to monitor changes. Compare readings to normal blood pressure for age and gender (see Chap. 3). Occasionally medications may be used to lower an elevated blood pressure that is resistant to

AEROBIC ACTIVITIES

Running	Biking
Jogging	Soccer
Fast walking	Aerobic dancing
Hiking	Rollerblading
Swimming	

CULTURAL CONSIDERATIONS

African-American children may be particularly susceptible to increased blood pressure caused by dietary intake of sodium. Encouraging these children to follow a low-salt diet is important.

other treatment approaches. Instruct the family on correct administration of prescribed medications.

PERSISTENT PULMONARY HYPERTENSION

Persistent pulmonary hypertension is a disease of newborns, especially premature infants, resulting from pulmonary artery constriction. The increased pressure leads to a right-to-left shunt. In some children with congenital heart defects, excessive pulmonary blood flow leads to pulmonary vascular resistance.

Hypoxemia results from pulmonary hypertension, and the infant displays tachypnea, cyanosis, retractions, and fatigue. Feeding is difficult, and weight loss with fluid and electrolyte imbalance is likely.

The pulmonary hypertension may be caused by hyaline membrane disease, polycythemia, meconium aspiration, a respiratory infection, or a congenital heart defect.[37] After the cause is determined, the infant is treated with oxygen, ventilation, and medications.

Nursing care focuses on promoting rest for oxygen conservation, monitoring fluid intake and output carefully, and administering medications and oxygen. Newborns often require mechanical ventilation. Give parents needed support and information about their infant. Encourage them to visit but to avoid any stimulation of the newborn.

► INJURIES OF THE CARDIOVASCULAR SYSTEM

SHOCK

Shock is an acute, complex state of circulatory dysfunction resulting in failure to deliver sufficient oxygen and other nutrients to meet tissue demands. It can be caused by a variety of conditions such as hemorrhage, dehydration, sepsis, obstruction of blood flow, and cardiac pump failure.

Hypovolemic Shock

Hypovolemic shock is a clinical state of inadequate tissue and organ perfusion resulting from the movement of blood or plasma out of the intravascular compartment[38] (Fig. 12–11). The blood or plasma in the vascular space may be decreased because of hemorrhage or fluid movement into the interstitial spaces. Hypovolemia is the most common cause of shock in infants and children.[39]

Clinical Manifestations

Signs of early hypovolemic shock in children are nonspecific but need to be recognized before hypotension occurs. Signs indicating that the child is compensating for a decreased blood volume are tachycardia, usually sustained at a rate greater than 130 beats per minute, increased respiratory effort, delayed capillary refill (> 2 seconds), weak peripheral pulses, pallor, and cold extremities (signs of decreased perfusion). Although the child's body attempts to compensate by preserving circulation to vital organs, a decreased level of consciousness ultimately results from reduced cerebral blood flow. Urine output decreases when renal blood flow drops.

If treatment is not initiated in the early stages of hypovolemic shock, the condition progresses until the child can no longer compensate. At that

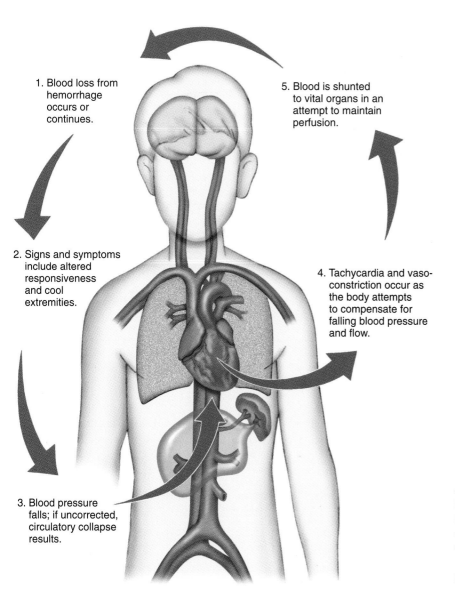

1. Blood loss from hemorrhage occurs or continues.

2. Signs and symptoms include altered responsiveness and cool extremities.

3. Blood pressure falls; if uncorrected, circulatory collapse results.

4. Tachycardia and vasoconstriction occur as the body attempts to compensate for falling blood pressure and flow.

5. Blood is shunted to vital organs in an attempt to maintain perfusion.

FIGURE 12-11. If hemorrhage reduces the circulating blood volume sufficiently, vasoconstriction occurs, shifting blood to maintain the perfusion of vital organs. When the blood loss exceeds 20–25%, the child's body can no longer compensate and hypovolemic shock ensues.

time the systolic blood pressure drops and the pulse pressure decreases. In cases of dehydration, dry mucous membranes and poor skin turgor are also present. Table 12–15 compares the signs associated with early, uncompensated, and profound shock.

Etiology and Pathophysiology

Major causes of decreased intravascular blood volume include:

- Hemorrhage from significant injury
- Plasma loss from burns, nephrotic syndrome, and sepsis
- Fluid and electrolyte loss associated with dehydration, diabetic ketoacidosis, and diabetes insipidus
- Vasodilating drugs

Shock results in inadequate delivery of oxygen and nutrients to cells and accumulation of toxic wastes in the capillaries. This reduction in circulating blood volume causes a decrease in cardiac output and mean arte-

12-15	Signs of Hypovolemic Shock		
System	Early Shock	Uncompensated Shock	Profound Shock
Cardiac	Tachycardia, weak distal pulses	Tachycardia, absent distal pulses, decreasing systolic blood pressure	Frank hypotension, bradycardia, weak central pulses
Neurologic	Normal, anxious, irritable, or combative behavior	Confusion, lethargy, decreased pain response	Comatose state
Skin	Mottled appearance; capillary refill time > 2 seconds; cool, clammy extremities	Cyanosis, capillary refill time > 3 seconds, cold extremities	Pale, cold skin
Renal	Decreased urine output, increased specific gravity	Oliguria, increased specific gravity	No urine output

Modified from Waisman, H., & Eichelberger, M.R. (1993). Hypovolemic shock. In M.R. Eichelberger (Ed.), Pediatric trauma: Prevention, acute care, rehabilitation (p. 182). St. Louis: Mosby–Year Book.

rial pressure. Cellular hypoxia and acidosis develop simultaneously. The accumulation of toxins and inadequate tissue oxygenation cause cellular damage.

The child's body attempts to compensate by the following measures:

- The heart rate and myocardial contractility increase to improve cardiac output.
- The respiratory rate increases to improve oxygenation and decrease waste accumulation in the cells.
- The hydrostatic pressure falls, permitting fluid to shift into the vascular space and increasing the circulating blood volume.
- The peripheral vasculature constricts to maintain the systemic vascular resistance as long as possible.

The child is able to compensate until 20%–25% of volume loss occurs, and then life-threatening hypotension results.

Diagnostic Tests and Medical Management

No laboratory values can be used to evaluate the volume deficit rapidly enough to diagnose hypovolemic shock. The child is examined for characteristic signs to confirm the diagnosis. Laboratory tests commonly performed after hypovolemic shock is diagnosed include hematocrit and hemoglobin, arterial blood gases, serum electrolytes, glucose, osmolality, blood urea nitrogen, and urinalysis.

Emergency care focuses on improving tissue perfusion. An open airway is established, oxygen is administered, and ventilation is assisted if necessary. Bleeding is controlled, and an intravenous line is started to provide large volumes of crystalloid fluids (Ringer's lactate).

Ringer's lactate solution is the preferred fluid for initial resuscitation. A fluid volume of 20 mL/kg is administered rapidly over 5 minutes. The same amount of fluid is given in 5 minutes if the child's physiologic condi-

CLINICAL TIP

Signs that a child is responding to fluid resuscitation include:
- Improved color
- Improved responsiveness
- Lower heart rate
- Improved capillary refill time

tion does not improve after fluid is first administered. If no improvement is seen after the second fluid bolus, blood or albumin is usually ordered.

Once the child's physiologic condition is stabilized, the cause of the hypovolemic shock becomes the focus of examination and treatment.

Nursing Assessment

Ask the parent (or child, if appropriate) about possible injuries or the duration and severity of acute illnesses. If no external bleeding is evident, determine whether an injury may be causing internal bleeding. For example, the liver and spleen are highly vascular organs that have little protection from direct blunt forces. Significant bleeding from injury to one of these organs can cause hypovolemic shock without evidence of bleeding. An acute illness such as gastroenteritis with prolonged vomiting and diarrhea can also result in dehydration and hypovolemic shock.

If external bleeding is apparent, determine the amount of blood lost. Although children lose the same amount of blood from a laceration as adults, the total volume of blood lost is proportional to their weight.

When an injured child is admitted to the hospital for a problem such as a liver or spleen laceration, assess the child's circulatory status frequently. Current medical treatment for these injuries is conservative. Surgeons give the liver or spleen a chance to heal spontaneously rather than perform immediate surgery to control bleeding and repair the laceration. Even if the child's circulatory condition was stabilized during emergency care, shock can develop again if bleeding continues.

Frequently assess the child's heart rate, respiratory rate, blood pressure, capillary refill time, level of consciousness (with the Glasgow Coma Scale; see Chap. 18), color, and skin temperature to identify any changes that indicate improvement or deterioration in the child's condition. Monitor urine output and specific gravity hourly. Signs of the child's improved status include:

- A decrease in heart rate, respiratory rate, and capillary refill time
- An increase in systolic blood pressure and urine output
- Improved color, level of consciousness, and skin temperature
- Regaining of lost weight

Nursing Diagnosis

Several nursing diagnoses may apply to the child with hypovolemic shock. They include:

- Decreased Cardiac Output related to blood loss or dehydration
- Fluid Volume Deficit related to dehydration
- Altered Tissue Perfusion (Cardiopulmonary, Renal, and Cerebral) related to decreased circulating blood volume
- Ineffective Airway Clearance related to altered level of consciousness
- Ineffective Family Coping: Compromised related to life-threatening condition of the child
- Anxiety related to unexpected hospitalization for an emergency condition

Nursing Management

Nurses in the emergency department and intensive care unit participate in the resuscitation of the child in hypovolemic shock. Assist with the child's assessment and the establishment of intravenous access. Calculate and pre-

 GROWTH & DEVELOPMENT CONSIDERATIONS

The child's total blood volume varies by weight. The child has approximately 80 mL of blood for every kilogram of body weight.[39]
- Newborn: 3 kg × 80 mL = 240 mL (1 cup)
- 5-year-old child: 25 kg × 80 mL = 2000 mL (2 quarts)
- 13-year-old child: 50 kg × 80 mL = 4000 mL (1 gallon)

pare the amount of intravenous fluid needed for administration according to the child's weight (20 mL/kg). Ensure rapid fluid administration by intravenous push or pressure bag. Monitor the child's physiologic response to the fluid bolus within 5 minutes. Prepare a second and third fluid bolus.

Use warmed intravenous fluids for resuscitation because hypothermia may interfere with the child's response to treatment. Keep the child covered or use heat lamps to reduce body-heat loss.

When packed red blood cells are administered, verify that the correct blood has been obtained for the child. Change the intravenous fluid to normal saline solution to prevent clotting during blood administration. Assess the child carefully for a transfusion reaction (see Chap. 13). Monitor the child's physiologic circulatory responses for improvement or deterioration in status. Notify the physician of any deterioration.

Provide support to the child and family during the acute phase of treatment. Parents and children with hypovolemic shock resulting from injury are usually apprehensive. The child may be fearful because of the sudden hospitalization or agitated because of an altered level of consciousness. Determine the causes of the child's anxiety. The parents often fear for the child's life in cases of injury. Update the parents about the child's condition frequently. Explain the care being provided and how it helps the child. Listen to their concerns and correct any misconceptions.

Distributive Shock

Distributive (septic) shock is an abnormal pooling of blood in the extremities that may be caused by anaphylaxis, sepsis, or spinal cord injury. Immunodeficient children are at high risk for septic shock. The blood accumulates in the extremities because of vasodilation. Less blood is returned to the heart, so preload drops and cardiac output falls.

Septic shock begins as an infection and progresses to sepsis. Once a bacterial toxin enters the circulatory system, the body's inflammatory processes go out of control. White blood cells multiply throughout the body and macrophages produce cytokines, which dilate the blood vessels and increase permeability. Neutrophils cluster and obstruct the capillaries[40] (Fig. 12–12).

Septic shock has two phases: hyperdynamic and hypodynamic. During the hyperdynamic phase, the child has a fever, tachycardia, tachypnea, warm extremities, bounding pulses, and brisk capillary refill. Perfusion appears adequate; however, because of infection and fever, oxygen demand in the tissues is much higher and perfusion is really inadequate.

Cardiac output is high but systemic vascular resistance is low, leading to an uneven flow and pooling in the extremities. Blood moves sluggishly, and anaerobic metabolism and lactic acidosis occur in tissue beds where oxygen no longer circulates. As the syndrome progresses, the hypodynamic phase develops. Cardiac output is low, and systemic vascular resistance is high. Blood has already pooled in the extremities. During the hypodynamic phase the child is cool, hypotensive, pale, and oliguric. Blood is shunted away from the kidneys, muscles, and skin to the heart and brain. Multisystem organ failure occurs if treatment does not improve regional perfusion.

Treatment for septic shock is initiated even before the diagnosis is confirmed. Fluid resuscitation is used in early septic shock to stabilize the circulation and ensure adequate tissue perfusion. Antibiotics effective against the suspected organism are given. Vasopressors are given during the hypodynamic phase. Morbidity and mortality are high even when treatment is initiated early. Complications include disseminated intravascular coagulation and adult respiratory distress syndrome.

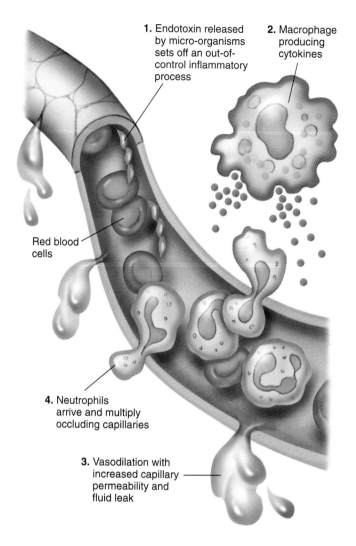

1. Endotoxin released by micro-organisms sets off an out-of-control inflammatory process

2. Macrophage producing cytokines

Red blood cells

4. Neutrophils arrive and multiply occluding capillaries

3. Vasodilation with increased capillary permeability and fluid leak

FIGURE 12-12. In septic shock, blood pools in the extremities. Blood flow is sluggish and amounts of oxygen inadequate for cell metabolism are received by the tissues.

Obstructive Shock

Obstructive shock occurs when a blockage of the main bloodstream interferes with tissue perfusion (Fig. 12–13). Causes in children include compression of the vena cava, pericardial tamponade, pulmonary embolism, tension pneumothorax, pleural effusion, and congenital heart defects with outflow obstruction (eg, coarctation of the aorta). Management is focused on treatment of the underlying condition.

Cardiogenic Shock

Cardiogenic shock is an abnormality of myocardial function in which the heart fails to maintain adequate cardiac output and tissue perfusion (Fig. 12–14). Causes of cardiogenic shock in children may include congestive heart failure, congenital heart disease, and arrhythmias such as bradycardia and supraventricular tachycardia. Cardiogenic shock may also be an end stage for other acute and chronic conditions such as sepsis, prolonged shock, hypoglycemia, and muscular dystrophy. Heart failure may result from obstructed outflow in congenital heart defects such as coarctation of the aorta.

Clinically, cardiogenic shock resembles hypovolemic shock. Tachycardia, tachypnea, decreased oxygen saturation, hypotension, and cool, pale

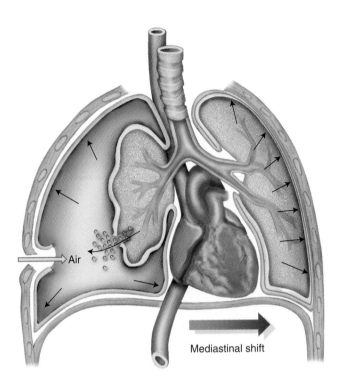

FIGURE 12-13. Obstructive shock can occur when a tension pneumothorax obstructs blood flow to and from the heart. Here, the great vessels are compressed during the mediastinal shift.

Air

Mediastinal shift

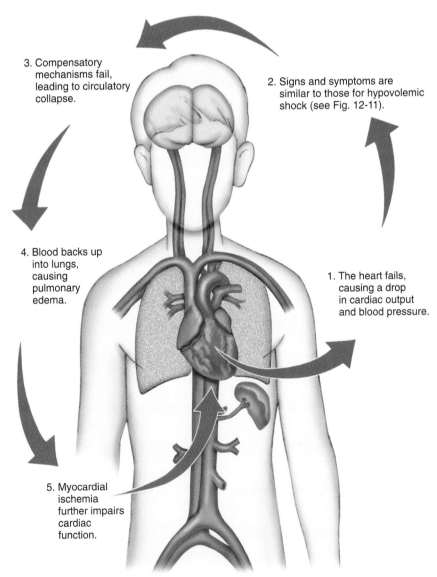

3. Compensatory mechanisms fail, leading to circulatory collapse.

2. Signs and symptoms are similar to those for hypovolemic shock (see Fig. 12-11).

4. Blood backs up into lungs, causing pulmonary edema.

1. The heart fails, causing a drop in cardiac output and blood pressure.

5. Myocardial ischemia further impairs cardiac function.

FIGURE 12-14. When the heart fails, cardiac output and blood pressure decrease. Blood backs up into the lungs, causing pulmonary edema. Inadequate amounts of oxygen reach the myocardium, further impairing the heart's pumping action. The result is cardiogenic shock.

extremities are common signs. Disorientation and restlessness occur as the compensatory mechanisms fail. Increased systemic vascular resistance puts more stress on the failing heart. Each contraction causes more blood to accumulate in the heart and pulmonary vessels, eventually leading to congestive heart failure, metabolic acidosis, and circulatory collapse.

The goal of medical treatment is restoration of myocardial function with adequate ventilation, correction of arrhythmias, fluid management, and administration of diuretics and inotropic drugs.

MYOCARDIAL CONTUSION

Myocardial contusion, a rare injury in children, results from a strong, blunt force against the chest wall that injures the heart muscle. Blood flow to areas of the heart muscle is disrupted, or myocardial cells are directly destroyed. This potentially life-threatening condition is often associated with a motor vehicle–related injury. It most often occurs in adolescents who have struck the steering wheel of a motor vehicle during a crash or children who have been struck in the chest with a baseball.

A myocardial contusion should be suspected in cases of injury to the anterior chest. This condition is often overlooked during the initial emergency assessment. The child has chest discomfort because of fractured ribs or chest wall contusion. An electrocardiogram reveals arrhythmias or signs of myocardial infarct. An echocardiogram may show an abnormality in heart wall movement. Cardiac isoenzyme concentrations are elevated. Because of the risk of sudden arrhythmias, the child is admitted to the intensive care unit for cardiac monitoring.

REFERENCES

1. National Center for Health Statistics. (1995). *National vital statistics system*, unpublished data.
2. Hoffman, J.I.E. (1995). Incidence of congenital heart disease: I. Postnatal incidence. *Pediatric Cardiology, 16*(3), 103–113.
3. Freed, M.D. (1992). Fetal and transitional circulation. In D.C. Fyler (Ed.), *Nadas' pediatric cardiology* (p. 59). Philadelphia: Hanley & Belfus.
4. Ludwig, S., & Loiselle, J. (1993). Anatomy, growth, and development: Impact on injury. In M.R. Eichelberger (Ed.), *Pediatric trauma: Prevention, acute care, rehabilitation* (pp. 39–58). St. Louis: Mosby–Year Book.
5. Park, M.K. (1996). *Pediatric cardiology for practitioners* (3rd ed.). St. Louis: Mosby–Year Book.
6. Eichelberger, M.R., Ball, J.W., Pratsch, G.S., & Clark, J.R. (1998). *Pediatric emergencies* (2nd ed.). Englewood Cliffs, NJ: Brady.
7. Wolfe, R.R., Boucek, M., Schaffer, M.S., & Wiggins, J.W. (1997). Cardiovascular diseases. In W.W. Hay, J.R. Groothius, A.R. Hayward, & M.J. Levin (Eds.), *Current pediatric diagnosis and treatment* (13th ed, pp. 474–536). Stamford, CT: Appleton & Lange.
8. Katz, A. (1990). Cardiomyopathy of overload. *New England Journal of Medicine, 322*(2), 100–110.
9. Kohr, L.M., & O'Brien, P. (1995). Current management of congestive heart failure in infants and children. *Nursing Clinics of North America, 30*(2), 261–290.
10. Werner, N.P. (1993). Congestive heart failure: Pathophysiology and management throughout infancy. *Journal of Perinatology and Neonatal Nursing, 7*(3), 59–76.
11. Botto, L.D., Khoury, M.J., Mulinare, J., & Erickson, J.D. (1996). Periconceptional multivitamin use and the occurrence of contruncal heart defects: Results from a population-based, case-control study. *Pediatrics, 98*(5), 911–917.
12. Sims, S.L. (1994). Alterations in cardiovascular function in children. In K.L. McCance, & S.E. Huether (Eds.), *Pathophysiology: The biologic basis for disease in adults and children* (2nd ed.). St. Louis: Mosby.
13. Nouri, S. (1997). Congenital heart defects: Cyanotic and acyanotic. *Pediatric Annals, 26*(2), 94–98.
14. Stumpflen, I., Stumpflen, A., Wimmer, M., & Bernaschek, G. (1996). Effects of detailed fetal echocardiography as part of routine prenatal ultrasonographic screening on detection of congenital heart disease. *Lancet, 348*(Sept. 28), 854–857.
15. Stinson, J., & McKeever, P. (1995). Mother's information needs related to caring for infants at home fol-

lowing cardiac surgery. *Journal of Pediatric Nursing, 10*(1), 48–57.

16. Castaneda, A.R. (1990). Classical repair of tetralogy of Fallot: Timing, technique, and results. *Seminars in Thoracic and Cardiovascular Surgery, 2,* 70–75.

17. Rikard, D.H. (1993). Nursing care of the neonate receiving prostaglandin E_1 therapy. *Neonatal Network, 12,* 17–22.

18. DeBoer, S. (1996). The care of the blue baby: Emergency department management of tetralogy of Fallot. *Journal of Emergency Nursing, 22*(2), 73–76.

19. Sacchetti, A., Gerardi, M., Barkin, R., et al. (1996). Emergency data set for children with special needs. *Annals of Emergency Medicine, 28,* 324–327.

20. Denny, F. (1993). New developments: Group A streptococcal infections, 1993. *Current Problems in Pediatrics, 23*(5), 179–185.

21. Freund, B.D., Scacco-Neumann, A., Pisanelli, A.S., & Benchot, R. (1993). Acute rheumatic fever revisited. *Journal of Pediatric Nursing, 8*(3), 167–176.

22. Robinson, B., Anisman, P., & Eshaghpour, E. (1996). Is that fast heart beat dangerous (and what should you do about it)? *Contemporary Pediatrics, 13*(9), 52–85.

23. Ros, S., Fisher, E., & Bell, T. (1991). Adenosine in the emergency management of supraventricular tachycardia. *Pediatric Emergency Care, 7*(4), 222–223.

24. Lux, K. (1991). New hope for children with Kawasaki disease. *Journal of Pediatric Nursing, 6*(3), 159—165.

25. Peterson-Sweeney, K.L. (1995). Systemically induced vasculitis in children. *AACN Clinical Issues, 6*(4), 657–669.

26. American Academy of Pediatrics. (1997). *1997 Redbook: Report of the Committee on Infectious Diseases.* Elk Grove Village, IL: Author.

27. Dajani, A.S., Taubert, K.A., Gerber, M.A., Shulman, S.T., Ferrieri, P., et al. (1993). Diagnosis and therapy of Kawasaki disease in children. *Circulation, 87*(5), 1776–1780.

28. National Cholesterol Education Program. (1991). *Report of the Expert Panel on Blood Cholesterol Levels in Children and Adolescents.* Washington, DC: U.S. Department of Health and Human Services.

29. Williams, C.L., & Bollella, M. (1995). Guideline for screening, evaluating, and treating children with hypercholesterolemia. *Journal of Pediatric Health Care, 9*(4), 153–161.

30. Purath, J, Lansinger, T., & Ragheb, C. (1995). Cardiac risk evaluation for elementary school children. *Public Health Nursing, 12*(3), 189–195.

31. Kwiterovich, P.O. (1989). *Beyond cholesterol.* Baltimore: Johns Hopkins University Press.

32. Howard, J.K., Bindler, R.M., Synoground, G., & Van Gemert, F.C. (1996). A cardiovascular risk reduction program for the classroom. *Journal of School Nursing, 12*(4), 5–11.

33. McCabe, E. (1993). Monitoring the fat and cholesterol intake of children and adolescents. *Journal of Pediatric Health Care, 7*(2), 61–70.

34. National High Blood Pressure Education Program Working Group on Hypertension Control in Children and Adolescents. (1996). Update on the 1987 task force report on high blood pressure in children and adolescents: A working group report from the National High Blood Pressure Education Program. *Pediatrics, 98*(4), 649–658.

35. Lauer, R., Clarke, W., Mahoney, L., & Witt, J. (1993). Childhood predictors for high adult blood pressure: The Muscatine study. *Pediatric Clinics of North America, 40*(1), 23–40.

36. Rocchini, A.P. (1993). Adolescent obesity and hypertension. *Pediatric Clinics of North America, 40*(1), 81–92.

37. Rosenberg, A.A., & Thilo, E.H. (1997) The newborn infant. In W.W. Hay, J.R. Groothius, A.R. Hayword, & M.J. Levin (Eds.), *Current pediatric diagnosis and treatment* (13th ed., pp. 20–76). Stamford, CT: Appleton & Lange.

38. Waisman, Y., & Eichelberger, M.R. (1993). Hypovolemic shock. In M.R. Eichelberger (Ed.), *Pediatric trauma: Prevention, acute care, rehabilitation* (pp. 178–185). St. Louis: Mosby–Year Book.

39. DiMaio, A.M., & Singh, J. (1992) The infant with cyanosis in the emergency room. *Pediatric Clinics of North America, 39,* 987–1006.

40. Brown, K.K. (1994). Septic shock: How to stop the deadly cascade. *American Journal of Nursing, 94*(9), 20–26.

ADDITIONAL RESOURCES

Baker, A.L., Roberts, C., & Gothing, C. (1995). Dyslipidemias in childhood: An overview. *Nursing Clinics of North America, 30*(2), 243–260.

Beaver, B.L., & Laschinger, J.C. (1992). Pediatric thoracic trauma. *Seminars in Thoracic and Cardiovascular Surgery, 4,* 255–262.

Berro, E.A., & Bechler-Karsch, A. (1993). A closer look at septic shock. *Pediatric Nursing, 19,* 289–297, 314.

Boisvert, J., Reidy, S., & Lulu, J. (1995). Overview of pediatric arrhythmias. *Nursing Clinics of North America, 29*(2), 365–380.

Caire, J.B., & Erickson, S. (1986). Reducing distress in pediatric patients undergoing cardiac catheterization. *Children's Health Care, 14,* 146–152.

Castiglia, P.T. (1993). Kawasaki disease. *Journal of Pediatric Health Care, 10*(3), 124–126.

Cowell, J., Montgomery, A., & Talashek, M. (1992). Cardiovascular risk stability: From grade school to high school. *Journal of Pediatric Health Care, 6*(6), 349–354.

DeBruin, W.J., Greenwald, B.M., & Notterman, A. (1992). Fluid resuscitation in pediatrics. *Critical Care Clinics, 8,* 423–438.

Grimes, D., & Woolbert, L. (1990). Facts and fallacies about streptococcal infection and rheumatic fever. *Journal of Pediatric Health Care, 4*(4), 186–192.

Hayden, R.A. (1992). What keeps oxygen on track? *American Journal of Nursing, 92,* 32–40.

Ing, F.F., Starc, T.J., Griffiths, S.P., & Gersony, W.M. (1996). Early diagnosis of coarctation of the aorta in children: A continuing dilemma. *Pediatrics, 98*(3), 378–382.

Jensen, C.A. (1992). Nursing care of a child following an arterial switch procedure for transposition of the great arteries. *Critical Care Nurse, 12,* 51–57.

Klein, D.M. (1991). Shock: Physiology, signs, and symptoms. *Nursing 91, 21,* 74–76.

Matthews, D. (1994). The prevention and diagnosis of infective endocarditis: The primary care provider's role. *Nurse Practitioner, 19*(8), 53–60.

McCubbin, H., Thompson, E., Thompson, A., McCubbin, M., & Kaston, A. (1993). Culture, ethnicity, and the family: Critical factors in childhood chronic illnesses and disabilities. *Pediatrics, 91*(5), 1063–1070.

Mistretta, E., & Strond, S. (1990). Hypercholesterolemia in children: Risk and management. *Pediatric Nursing, 16*(2), 152–154.

Nicklaus, T., Farris, R., Srinivasan, S., Webber, L., &

Berenson, G. (1989). Nutritional studies in children and implications for change: The Bogalusa heart study. *Journal of Advancement in Medicine, 2*(3), 451–473.

Ohler, L., Fleagle, D.J., & Lee, B.I. (1989). Aortic valvuloplasty: Medical and critical care nursing perspectives. *Focus on Critical Care, 16,* 275–287.

Pederson, C. (1995). Children's and adolescents' experiences while undergoing cardiac catheterization. *Maternal and Child Nursing Journal, 23*(1), 15–25.

Radtke, W., & Lock, J. (1990). Balloon dilation. *Pediatric Clinics of North America, 37,* 193–209.

Rowley, A., & Gonzalez-Crussi, F. (1991). Kawasaki syndrome. *Current Problems in Pediatrics, 21*(9), 380–405.

Sade, R.M., & Fyfe, D.A. (1990). Tricuspid atresia: Current concepts in diagnosis and treatment. *Pediatric Clinics of North America, 37,* 151–169.

Shulman, S.T., De Inocencio, J., & Hirsch, R. (1995). Kawasaki disease. *Pediatric Clinics of North America, 42*(5), 1205–1222.

Stewart, K.J., Lipis, P.H., Seemans, C.M., McFarland, L.D., Weinhofer, J.J., & Brown, C.S. (1995). Heart healthy knowledge, food patterns, fatness, and cardiac risk factors in children receiving nutrition education. *Journal of Health Education, 26*(6), 381–387.

Swanson, L.T. (1995). Treatment options for hypoplastic left heart syndrome: A mother's perspective. *Critical Care Nurse, 15*(6), 70–79.

Tong, E., & Sparacino, P. (1994). Special management issues for adolescents and young adults with congenital heart disease. *Critical Care Clinics of North America, 9*(2), 199–214.

Uzark, K., VonBargen-Mazza, P., & Messiter, E. (1989). Health education needs of adolescents with congenital heart disease. *Journal of Pediatric Health Care, 3,* 137–143.

Warshaw, M.P., & Winn, C.W. (1988). Pulmonary valvuloplasty as an alternative to surgery in the pediatric patient: Implications for nursing. *Heart & Lung, 15,* 521–527.

Zales, V.R., & Wright, K.L. (1997). Endocarditis, pericarditis, and myocarditis. *Pediatric Annals, 26*(2), 116–121.

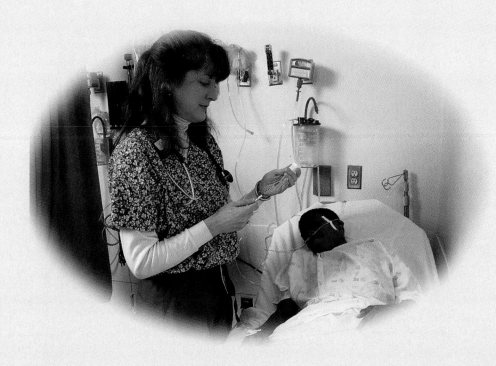

Michael is a 12-year-old African-American child who is admitted to the hospital with severe abdominal pain. He was diagnosed with sickle cell anemia at 1 year of age and has been in fairly good health. He has, however, been hospitalized on two previous occasions with complications of the disease. Recently, Michael has had several viral illnesses, leading his physician to suspect that his spleen is filled with abnormal cells, which are impairing his immune function.

Michael is small for his age and has several bruises on his lower legs. His respirations are rapid and he appears anxious. Michael's parents are knowledgeable about sickle cell anemia, as his uncle also has the disease. They know that Michael is experiencing an episode of sickle cell crisis.

An intravenous infusion is started, and Michael is medicated for pain. The nurse attempts to perform tests and procedures in groups to allow Michael time to rest in between. Michael is receiving oxygen by nasal cannula to increase his oxygen saturation to normal levels.

What immediate and long-term care does Michael require? What do Michael and his parents need to know about this crisis? How could you help them manage the challenges of this condition? This chapter will assist you in planning care for children like Michael who have disorders of the hematologic system.

ALTERATIONS IN HEMATOLOGIC FUNCTION 13

"My major concern is helping Michael to be comfortable. His pain was intense when he was admitted, and he was very anxious and breathing rapidly. Once his pain is controlled, and the results of testing show what other treatment he needs, we will begin to manage the specific complications of his condition."

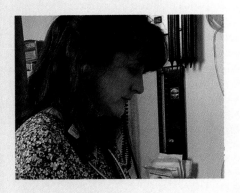

TERMINOLOGY

- **anemia** Reduction in the number of red blood cells, the quantity of hemoglobin, and the volume of packed red cells per 100 mL of blood to below-normal levels.
- **ecchymosis** A bruise.
- **erythropoiesis** Formation of red blood cells.
- **hemarthrosis** Bleeding into joint spaces.
- **hematopoiesis** Blood cell production.
- **hemoglobinopathy** Disease characterized by abnormal hemoglobin.
- **hemosiderosis** Increased storage of iron in body tissues; associated with diseases involving the destruction of red blood cells.
- **leukopenia** A lower than normal white blood cell count.

- **menorrhagia** Increased menstrual bleeding.
- **pancytopenia** A decreased number of blood cell components.
- **petechiae** Pinpoint red lesions.
- **polycythemia** Above-normal increase in the number of red cells in the blood to increase the amount of hemoglobin available to carry oxygen.
- **purpura** Bleeding into the tissues, particularly beneath the skin and mucous membranes, causing lesions that vary from red to purple.
- **thrombocytopenia** A low platelet count.
- **vaso-occlusion** Blockage of a blood vessel.

The hematologic system is one of a few body systems that regulate, directly or indirectly, all other body functions. Because blood is involved in the function of all tissues and organs, changes in the blood may result in altered functioning of many body organs and structures. Are you aware that a tendency toward easy bruising is a characteristic sign of many bleeding disorders? Other signs include nosebleeds, pallor, frequent infections, and lethargy. This chapter discusses the most common disorders of the blood and blood-forming organs in children. (See Chap. 14 for a discussion of leukemia.)

▶ ANATOMY AND PHYSIOLOGY OF PEDIATRIC DIFFERENCES

Blood has two components: a fluid portion called plasma and a cellular portion known as the formed elements of the blood. The cellular elements are red blood cells (erythrocytes), white blood cells (leukocytes), and platelets (thrombocytes) (Fig. 13–1). Table 13–1 gives normal values for these blood components in children.

Production of red blood cells occurs in the fetus by the second week of gestation, with white blood cell and platelet production beginning at 8 weeks. Most of this early production occurs in the liver; however, by 5 months' gestation, the bone marrow takes over production of these elements.[1]

At birth, **hematopoiesis,** or blood cell production, occurs in the marrow of almost every bone. The flat bones, such as the sternum, ribs, pelvic and shoulder girdles, vertebrae, and hips, retain most of their hematopoietic activity throughout life.

RED BLOOD CELLS

Red blood cells, or erythrocytes, are the most abundant of the cellular elements of blood. They are formed through a process called **erythropoiesis.** The primary function of red blood cells is to transport oxygen from the lungs to the tissues. These cells also help to carry carbon dioxide back to the lungs. Hemoglobin, a red pigment composed of protein and iron, is essential to this function.

Polycythemia is an above-average increase in the number of red cells in the blood. Any condition that causes the quantity of oxygen transported to the tissues to decrease ordinarily increases the rate of red blood cell production. When a child becomes anemic secondary to hemorrhage, for instance, the bone marrow immediately begins to produce large quantities of red cells.

At birth, the newborn has a naturally occurring elevation in red blood cells due to a high level of erythropoietin, which stimulates red cell production. Once the newborn breathes and the oxygen level in the blood increases, this production slows. Low levels of red blood cells are reached at about 2 months of age; then, by 3–4 months, values begin increasing toward childhood levels. For these reasons, the red blood cell count, hemoglobin, and hematocrit of the newborn are high (see Table 13–1). Levels are stable during childhood with an increase in hemoglobin for teenage males and a stable or slightly lower level for teenage females.[1]

WHITE BLOOD CELLS

White blood cells, or leukocytes, are the mobile units of the body's protective system. They are formed in bone marrow and lymph tissue. The white blood cell count is highest at birth, although levels vary greatly among in-

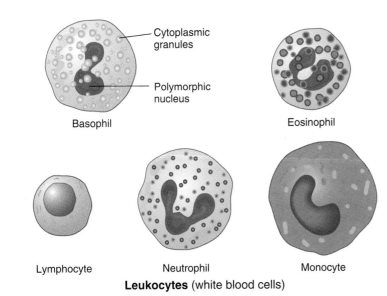

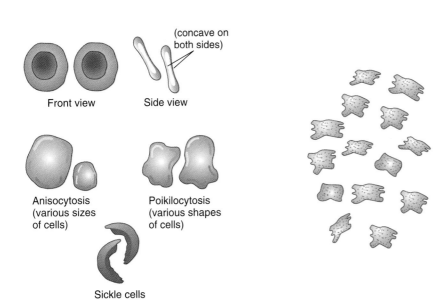

Erythrocytes (red blood cells)

Platelets

FIGURE 13-1. Types of blood cells.

	Newborn	1 Year	5 Years	8–12 Years
13-1 Normal Blood Values in Children				
Red blood cells (RBCs) (millions/μL)	5.9 (4.1–7.5)	4.6 (4.1–5.1)	4.7 (4.2–5.2)	5 (4.5–5.4)
Hemoglobin (Hgb) (g/dL)	19 (14–24)	12 (11–15)	13.5 (12.5–15)	14 (13–15.5)
White blood cells (WBCs) (per μL)	17,000 8–38	10,000 5–15	8000 5–13	8000 5–12
Platelets (per μL)	200,000	260,000	260,000	260,000
Hematocrit (Hct) (%)	54	36	38	40

Adapted from Merenstein, G.B., Kaplan, D.W., & Rosenberg, A.A. (1997).Handbook of pediatrics (18th ed., pp. 986–989). Stamford, CT: Appleton & Lange.

13-2	White Blood Cells and Their Functions
Type	**Function**
Neutrophils	Phagocytosis
Eosinophils	Allergic reactions
Basophils	Inflammatory reactions
Monocytes (macrophages)	Phagocytosis, antigen processing
Lymphocytes	Humoral immunity (B cell), cellular immunity (T cell)

TYPES OF ANEMIA IN CHILDREN

- Iron deficiency
- β-Thalassemia
- Aplastic
- Normocytic
- Sickle cell

CULTURAL CONSIDERATIONS

A number of genetic abnormalities of red blood cells that are rare in the United States are found among Southeast Asian immigrants. Many of these conditions can be confused with iron deficiency; however, most do not cause serious illness. Nurses who work with these cultural groups should seek out more specific information about such conditions.[6]

fants. By 1 week of age, white blood cell values stabilize. Throughout childhood, there is a very slow decrease in white blood cell count. [2]

There are five types of white blood cells, each with a distinct function (Table 13–2). A differential blood count indicates the percentages of the different types of white cells present in the blood and is sometimes useful in identifying the cause of an illness. For example, infections cause an increase in neutrophils; and allergies are related to an increase in eosinophils. The role of lymphocytes is discussed with acquired immunodeficiency syndrome in Chapter 9.

PLATELETS

Platelets, or thrombocytes, are cell fragments that can form hemostatic plugs to stop bleeding. They are synthesized from components in the red bone marrow and are stored in the spleen. Platelet levels in newborns are lower than in older children and adults. Levels of many clotting factors, particularly those requiring vitamin K for activation, are also lower in infants. For this reason, all newborns receive a prophylactic injection of vitamin K at birth. Values of platelets and other coagulation products soon reach normal childhood levels.[3]

► ANEMIAS

Anemia is defined as a reduction in the number of red blood cells, the quantity of hemoglobin, and the volume of packed red cells to below-normal levels. This condition can be caused by loss or destruction of existing red blood cells or by an impaired or decreased rate of red cell production. Anemia also can be a clinical manifestation of an underlying disorder, such as lead poisoning or hypersplenism (a syndrome characterized by splenomegaly and blood cell deficiencies).

IRON DEFICIENCY ANEMIA

Iron deficiency anemia is the most common type of anemia and the most common nutritional deficiency in children. It can occur secondary to blood loss, or as a result of increased internal demands (rapid growth) for blood production, or due to poor nutritional intake.

Clinical manifestations depend on the severity of the anemia. Pallor, fatigue, and irritability are characteristic findings. With prolonged anemia, nailbed deformities, growth retardation, developmental delay, tachycardia, and systolic heart murmur can occur.

Rapidly growing adolescents whose diets are high in fat and low in vitamins and minerals are particularly susceptible to iron deficiency anemia. Infants who do not take in adequate solid foods after 6 months of age and are fed only breast milk or formula that is not fortified with iron are also at risk because neonatal iron stores have been depleted by this time and their iron needs are not being met. Similarly, among mothers whose nutritional status during pregnancy was inadequate, and infants who were born prematurely or are products of multiple births, insufficient iron may have been stored in the latter part of pregnancy, placing the infant at higher risk for anemia in the first months of life.

Chronic blood loss is always a potential cause of iron deficiency anemia. The infant who has had bleeding in the neonatal period, the child who loses blood as a result of conditions such as hemophilia or parasitic gastrointestinal illness, and the adolescent girl who has **menorrhagia** (heavy menstrual bleeding), may all be at risk of anemia.

Diagnosis is made on the basis of laboratory studies, including hemoglobin level, mean corpuscular volume, microscopic analysis (Fig. 13–2), and serum iron-binding capacity. The red blood cells are microcytic (small) in size and hypochromic (pale) in appearance.[4] A diet history and analysis can provide information related to food intake.

Treatment involves correction of the iron deficiency with oral elemental iron preparations and a diet high in iron. Because oral iron preparations cause several side effects such as constipation and gastrointestinal discomfort, the child may receive iron supplements (to restore blood levels of iron) while the iron content of the diet is increased above the recommended dietary allowances (RDAs). Oral supplements can then be tapered off once the child's food intake can supply the needed iron. If the anemia is a result of bleeding, the cause is identified and treated to prevent future excess blood loss.

Nursing Management

The child with iron deficiency anemia is usually not hospitalized unless he or she has another serious illness. Nursing care focuses on screening for the disorder and educating the parents and child about the causes of iron deficiency anemia, dietary management, and the importance of complying with the medication regimen.

The American Academy of Pediatrics recommends that children be screened for anemia at 9 months of age and again at adolescence (see Chap. 5).[5] A hematocrit or hemoglobin level is obtained. More detailed tests are performed if the blood test is abnormal. Children at high risk for nutritional deficiencies, such as those in low-income groups and WIC programs, may require additional tests (Fig. 13–3). Most children in Head Start are screened annually by nurses. In addition, children showing signs of ane-

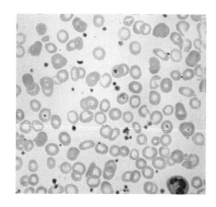

FIGURE 13–2. In iron deficiency anemia, red blood cells appear hypochromic as a result of decreased hemoglobin synthesis.
Courtesy of the Department of Hematology/Oncology, Children's National Medical Center, Washington, DC.

CULTURAL CONSIDERATIONS

According to traditional Chinese beliefs, a person who does not feel well is lacking in *chi* (inner energy) and blood. Chinese-Americans who follow traditional practices may be hesitant to have blood drawn for laboratory studies for fear of causing bodily weakness.

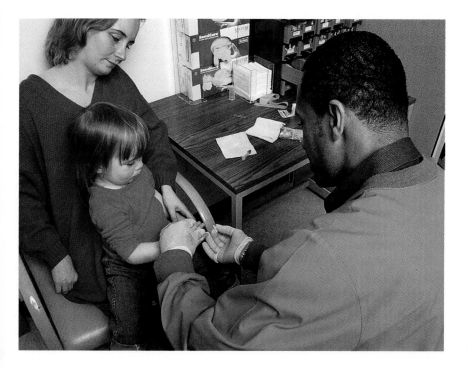

FIGURE 13–3. Most Head Start centers participate in screening programs to identify children at risk for anemia.

mia should be screened. Height and weight measurements should be obtained at each health care visit, plotted on growth charts, and compared to percentiles obtained at previous visits. Slow downward trends in percentiles are of concern and require further nutritional analysis. Developmental screening tests should be performed to assess for developmental delays (see Chap. 5).

Dietary management is the preferred long-term treatment for iron deficiency anemia. Teach the family and child about foods that are rich in iron. If the infant is anemic, encourage the parents to integrate iron-fortified formula and baby cereals into the diet. Older infants and toddlers can be provided with finger foods such as thinly sliced meats. Adolescents can be encouraged to eat foods with a high iron content, such as hamburgers and dried fruits.

Oral iron preparations are given to correct anemia. Teach the child and family that the liquid iron preparation should be taken through a straw because it stains the teeth. Instruct about side effects such as black stools, constipation, and a foul aftertaste. Emphasize the importance of drinking fluids and eating foods high in dietary fiber to minimize these side effects.

NORMOCYTIC ANEMIA

In normocytic anemia, the red blood cells, although decreased in number, are of normal size with a pale center.[4] This type of anemia may occur as a result of hemorrhage, disease-induced inflammation, disseminated intravascular coagulation (DIC; see the discussion later in this chapter), G6PD deficiency, hemolytic–uremic syndrome (see Chap. 16), or several other conditions. When one of these conditions exists in a child diagnosed with anemia, the infectious or inflammatory condition should be suspected as the cause of the identified anemia and treated first. The anemia will often then correct itself if ample time is provided.[7] Some of the infectious and inflammatory causes of anemia are listed in Table 13–3.

Clinical manifestations are similar to those seen in iron-deficiency anemia, with the possible occurrence of hepatomegaly and splenomegaly, as well. The etiology of normocytic anemia associated with chronic inflammation or infection is related to increased red blood cell destruction, decreased iron release from storage sites, and ineffective bone marrow response.[8] In hemorrhage, anemia is a direct result of loss of blood.

Treatment of normocytic anemia depends on the underlying cause. When the anemia is associated with inflammation or infection, the underlying condition is treated. For anemia caused by renal failure, recombinant human erythropoietin is administered. When hemorrhage is the underly-

CLINICAL TIP

Foods such as iron-fortified cereal, spinach, eggs, meat, kidney beans, and raisins are good sources of iron.

13-3	Infectious and Inflammatory Causes of Anemia

Infections	Inflammations
Haemophilus influenzae type b	Arthritis
HIV/AIDS	Cancers
Orbital cellulitis	Chronic heart or liver disease
Meningitis	
Septic arthritis	

ing cause, the source of the bleeding is identified and treated. In acute emergencies, blood products are infused to make up for some of the losses.

Nursing management of normocytic anemia depends on the cause of the decreased red blood cells. Children with inflammatory or infectious diseases require careful assessment and management of medication and other treatment regimens. Administer blood products and other intravenous fluids as ordered to restore blood volume. Follow-up and home visits are used to assess hematocrit, hemoglobin, and dietary intake. (Refer to the discussion later in this chapter for managment of DIC; to Chapter 15 for management of intestinal infections; and to Chapter 16 for management of hemolytic–uremic syndrome).

SICKLE CELL ANEMIA

Sickle cell anemia is a hereditary **hemoglobinopathy,** characterized by the partial or complete replacement of normal hemoglobin with abnormal hemoglobin S (Hgb S) (Table 13–4). Sickle cell anemia occurs primarily in African-Americans, although occasionally it affects people of Mediterranean descent. Sickle cell anemia occurs in about 1 in 600 African-American infants born in the United States, and 1 in 12 African-Americans have sickle cell trait (ie, they carry one gene for the disease).[9]

Clinical Manifestations

Affected children are usually asymptomatic until 4–6 months of age because sickling is inhibited by high levels of fetal hemoglobin. Clinical manifestations are directly related to the shortened life span of blood cells (hemolytic anemia) and tissue destruction resulting from **vaso-occlusion** (blockage of a blood vessel). Pathologic changes occur in most body systems and result in multiple signs and symptoms (Fig. 13–4).

13-4 | Sickle Cell Disorders

Sickle Cell Trait (Hgb SA)
Most common form of sickle cell disease in the United States

Heterozygous condition (child has one sickle cell hemoglobin gene and one normal hemoglobin gene)

Child is carrier of sickle cell anemia and rarely has symptoms of the disease

Sickle Cell Anemia (Hgb SS)
Homozygous condition (child has two sickle hemoglobin genes)

Child is subject to sickle cell crises

Sickle Cell Syndromes

Sickle cell–Hgb C disease (Hgb SC)
Second most frequent form of sickle cell disease in African-Americans

Different from sickle cell anemia only in that the sickle cell assumes a **C** shape instead of an **S** shape

Sickle Cell–β-Thalassemia Disease (Hgb SB)
Rarely occurs

Combination of sickle cell trait and thalassemia trait most often seen in people of Mediterranean descent

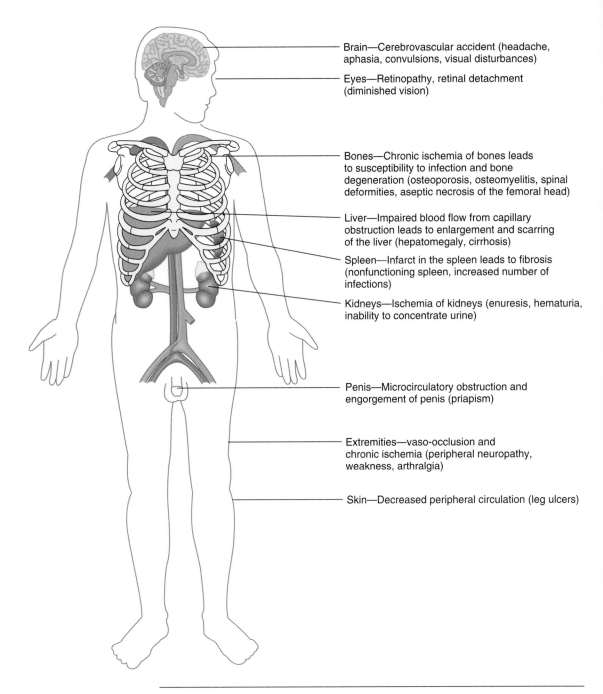

FIGURE 13–4. The clinical manifestations of sickle cell anemia result from pathologic changes to structures and systems throughout the body.

Illness results from recurrent vaso-occlusive events that involve painful crises and chronic organ damage.[10] Sickle cell crises are acute exacerbations of the disease that vary markedly in severity and frequency. Table 13–5 outlines the most common types of crises affecting children with sickle cell disease. These crises may occur individually or in combination. Michael, the boy described at the beginning of this chapter, was in sickle cell crisis.

Children with sickle cell trait rarely have such crises. However, because they have some abnormal hemoglobin, they may develop symptoms of the disease under conditions of abnormally low oxygen such as flying in an un-

13-5 Types of Sickle Cell Crises

Vaso-occlusive Crises (Thrombotic)
Most common type of crisis; painful
Caused by stasis of blood with clumping of cells in the microcirculation, ischemia, and infarction
Signs include fever, pain, tissue engorgement

Splenic Sequestration
Life-threatening crisis; death can occur within hours
Caused by pooling of blood in the spleen
Signs include profound anemia, hypovolemia, and shock

Aplastic Crises
Diminished production and increased destruction of red blood cells
Triggered by viral infection or depletion of folic acid
Signs include profound anemia, pallor

pressurized airplane over 7000 feet, or during anesthesia. The most common symptoms experienced by those with sickle cell trait are splenic infarction and hematuria. However, most persons who carry the trait never have symptoms, even with low oxygen concentrations.

Etiology and Pathophysiology

Sickle cell anemia is an autosomal recessive disorder. If both parents have the trait, with each pregnancy the risk of having a child with the disease is 25%. (See Chapter 2 for a discussion of recessive gene transmittal.)

In sickle cell anemia, the hemoglobin in the red blood cell acquires an elongated crescent or sickle shape (Fig. 13–5). The sickled cells are rigid and obstruct capillary blood flow. Microscopic obstructions lead to engorgement and tissue ischemia. This local tissue hypoxia causes further sickling and ultimately large infarctions. Damaged tissues in organs throughout the body become scarred, resulting in impaired function. For example, children with sickle cell anemia can suffer from splenic sequestration when blood is trapped in the spleen, a life-threatening complication. Many children must undergo splenectomy in early childhood, leading to severely compromised immunity.[9]

Sickling may be triggered by fever and emotional or physical stress. Precipitating factors for sickle cell crisis include increased blood viscosity (such as from a low fluid intake or fever) and hypoxia or low oxygen tension. Potential causes of hypoxia or low oxygen tension include high altitudes, poorly pressurized airplanes, hypoventilation, vasoconstriction when cold, or an emotionally stressful event. Any condition that increases the body's need for oxygen or alters the transport of oxygen (such as infection, trauma, or dehydration) may result in sickle cell crisis.

Sickled cells can resume a normal shape when rehydrated and reoxygenated. The membrane of these cells becomes more fragile, however, and cell life is shortened to 10–20 days rather than the usual 120 days. In response, bone marrow spaces enlarge to produce more red blood cells. Continuous formation and destruction of the child's red blood cells contributes to the severe hemolytic anemia that is characteristic of sickle cell anemia.

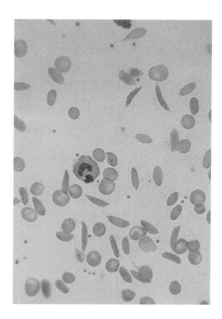

FIGURE 13–5. Many of these red blood cells show an elongated crescent shape characteristic of sickle cell anemia.
Courtesy of the American Society of Hematology, Brookline, MA.

Diagnostic Tests and Medical Management

The initial diagnosis of sickle cell anemia in newborns is often made by testing cord blood using hemoglobin electrophoresis. The sickle-turbidity test (Sickledex) may be used for quick screening purposes in children over 6 months of age, once the fetal hemoglobin levels have fallen. Hemoglobin electrophoresis is performed to verify positive Sickledex test results. Newborn screening of high-risk infants occurs in several states. However, it is recommended that all newborns be screened as the disease can occur in several groups in addition to African-Americans, such as Mediterranean, South American, Arabian, and East Indian.[11] A child's heritage should not be predicted from appearance or name alone.

No cure for sickle cell anemia exists. Supportive care is aimed at the prevention and treatment of sickling episodes. Preventing exposure to infections and maintaining normal hydration are important steps in avoiding crises. Aggressive treatment of infection with antibiotics and use of daily prophylactic penicillin in children from 2 months to 5 years of age is effective.[13] The reticulocyte count is monitored regularly to make sure that the bone marrow is still functioning.

Treatment of crises involves hydration, oxygen, pain management, and bedrest to reduce energy expenditure. Cultures (blood, urine, and throat) are taken to identify sources of infection. Other therapeutic measures include blood transfusions to treat the anemia and to make the sickled blood less viscous. If given early in the crisis, blood transfusions may sometimes relieve the ischemia in major organs and body parts (spleen, lung, kidney, brain, and penis) caused by the vaso-occlusion. Antibiotics are administered for infection control.

Children who have suffered a cerebrovascular accident (stroke) as a complication of the disease may be treated with blood transfusions on a regular basis. However, frequent transfusions may result in an overload of iron in the body. The iron is stored in tissues and organs (**hemosiderosis**) because the body has no way of excreting it. For this reason, an iron-chelating drug such as deferoxamine may be given along with vitamin C to promote iron excretion.[15]

Neonatal screening, early intervention, prophylactic antibiotics, and parent education have allowed children with sickle cell disease to live into adulthood. Prognosis depends on the severity of the child's disease. The major cause of death is from infection because the nonfunctional spleen results in an immunocompromised state.

Nursing Assessment

The nurse may be involved in sickle cell gene testing to identify carriers and children who have the disease. Once a child is diagnosed with the disease, a comprehensive physical assessment is essential because sickle cell anemia can affect any body system.

Physiologic Assessment

In children who are known to have sickle cell anemia, obtain a detailed history from the parents or child about past crises, precipitating events, medical treatment, and home management. Measure the child's height and weight accurately and compare to past measurements, since failure to thrive is common. Ask about chronic or acute pain that the child is experiencing. Pain may occur in nearly any body part, but most commonly manifests as headache, extremity pain, or abdominal discomfort.

The ill child with sickle cell disease should receive a careful multisystem assessment. Fever is an emergency necessitating prompt treatment.[16]

When the child is in crisis, assess pain and note the presence of any signs of inflammation or infection. Carefully monitor the child for signs of shock (see Chap. 12).

Psychosocial Assessment

The family of a child with sickle cell disease requires a thorough psychosocial assessment. If the child is newly diagnosed with the disorder, the family will need assistance to deal with feelings related to the serious, life-threatening nature of the disease. Assess parents' understanding of the disease transmission and ask whether genetic counseling has been obtained. Determine whether the family has adequate health care coverage to pay for the child's medical expenses. Ask older children about their knowledge of the disease, and explore their feelings related to the management of a chronic condition.

Nursing Diagnosis

Several nursing diagnoses that might apply to the child with sickle cell anemia are presented in the accompanying Nursing Care Plan. Other nursing diagnoses might include:

- Altered Family Processes related to having a child with a chronic illness
- Risk for Altered Parenting related to having a child with a genetically transmitted disease
- Altered Growth and Development related to tissue hypoxia and slow growth
- Impaired Physical Mobility related to pain in extremities

Nursing Management

The accompanying Nursing Care Plan summarizes nursing care for the child with sickle cell anemia. Nursing management for the child in crisis focuses on increasing tissue perfusion, promoting hydration, controlling pain, preventing infection, ensuring adequate nutrition, preventing complications, and providing emotional support to the child and family.

Increase Tissue Perfusion

Administer blood transfusions and oxygen as ordered. To prevent hemolysis, the intravenous fluid used before and after a blood transfusion must be saline rather than D$_5$W. In small children, the blood is usually infused without saline because the child cannot manage the extra volume. Monitor for transfusion reactions (Table 13–6). Encourage the child to rest. Work with the child and family to avoid emotional stress. Any activities that increase cellular metabolism also result in tissue hypoxia. Schedule caregiving activities and play to allow for optimal rest.

Promote Hydration

The child with sickle cell anemia is adversely affected by dehydration. Calculate the child's fluid maintenance requirements (minimum daily fluid intake) (see Chap. 8) and monitor the child's oral fluid intake. Administer intravenous fluids as ordered. Adjust oral intake as necessary to keep the child well hydrated.

Control Pain

Give prescribed analgesics around the clock during crises. If patient controlled analgesia is used, be sure that the constant infusions run as ordered

SAFETY PRECAUTIONS

It is important for all health facilities to have current guidelines for transfusion protocols. Become familiar with the policies and procedures where you work. For example, does the child's blood type and patient identification need to be checked by two nurses before starting the infusion?

CLINICAL TIP

When giving a transfusion, never infuse cold blood since it may increase sickling. Use a blood-warming coil to bring blood to room temperature.

NURSING ALERT

Blood reactions can occur as soon as the blood transfusion begins. Administer the first 20 mL of blood slowly and observe the child carefully for a reaction. Repeatedly assess the child according to hospital policy.

CLINICAL TIP

To encourage fluid intake in a small child:
- Use a favorite cup or glass
- Use straws
- Take advantage of times the child is thirsty, such as on awakening or after play
- Leave a cup within easy reach of the child
- Offer frozen juice pops, crushed ice drinks, and flavored ice chips

NURSING CARE PLAN
THE CHILD WITH SICKLE CELL ANEMIA

GOAL	INTERVENTION	RATIONALE	EXPECTED OUTCOME

1. Risk for Altered Tissue Perfusion related to sickle cell crises

GOAL	INTERVENTION	RATIONALE	EXPECTED OUTCOME
The child will show few signs and symptoms of tissue hypoxia.	• Instruct child to avoid physical exertion, emotional stress, low-oxygen environments (eg, airplanes, high altitudes), and known sources of infection.	• Decreased activity and exposure reduce body's need for oxygen.	The child has no shortness of breath and shows no signs of hypoxia.
	• Administer blood transfusions as ordered.	• Packed cells increase number of red blood cells available to carry oxygen to tissue cells. Transfusions promote circulation.	
	• Perform several caregiving activities together whenever possible.	• Grouping activities allows for optimum rest.	
	• Give oxygen as ordered.	• High concentration of oxygen in alveoli increases diffusion of gas across membranes.	
Repeated cerebrovascular accidents will be avoided.	• Administer and teach the family to administer prophylactic transfusions for the child who has had a cerebrovascular accident.	• Lowers potential for a future cerebrovascular accident.	The child does not suffer a cerebrovascular accident.

2. Risk for Fluid Volume Deficit related to sickle cell crises

GOAL	INTERVENTION	RATIONALE	EXPECTED OUTCOME
The child will maintain or be restored to adequate hydration.	• Calculate the child's daily fluid requirements. Monitor the child's usual fluid consumption and make necessary adjustments. Encourage the child to take fluids. Observe for signs of dehydration.	• Optimizing fluid intake ensures that the child gets needed fluid. Dehydration exacerbates crises.	The child shows signs of adequate hydration.
	• Record intake and output.	• Recording enables you to monitor daily fluid intake and spacing throughout the day.	

NURSING CARE PLAN
THE CHILD WITH SICKLE CELL ANEMIA— *Continued*

GOAL	INTERVENTION	RATIONALE	EXPECTED OUTCOME

3. *Pain related to sickle cell crises*

GOAL	INTERVENTION	RATIONALE	EXPECTED OUTCOME
The child will verbalize that pain is controlled.	• Administer analgesics, such as morphine or hydromorphine (Dilaudid), as ordered. Continuous intravenous infusion is used for the duration of a painful crisis.	• Pain of sickle cell crises is excruciating.	The child is pain-free or pain control is significantly improved.
	• Position carefully.	• Joints and extremities can be extremely painful.	

4. *Risk for Infection related to chronic disease and splenic malfunction*

GOAL	INTERVENTION	RATIONALE	EXPECTED OUTCOME
The child will not develop infection.	• Ensure adequate nutrition by providing high-calorie, high-protein diet. Make sure that the child's immunizations are up to date. Report any signs of infection to physician immediately.	• Chronically ill children are at greater risk of infection.	The child is free of infection.
	• Isolate the child from possible sources of infection. Instruct parents about signs of infection and encourage them to seek prompt health care.	• Restriction of persons with infection decreases the child's contact with infectious agents. Prompt care for infection reduces the chance of sickle cell crisis.	

5. *Knowledge Deficit (Child and Parents) related to cause and treatment of sickle cell anemia*

GOAL	INTERVENTION	RATIONALE	EXPECTED OUTCOME
The child and family will verbalize understanding of risk factors for sickle cell crises and how to minimize them.	• Review basics of sickle cell disease. Teach the child and family about signs and symptoms of crises.	• Knowledge of disease helps ensure compliance with treatment regimen and adherence to preventive measures.	The child and parent can verbalize precipitating events of crises.
	• Arrange for genetic counseling and testing for sickle cell trait for family members if desired.	• Questions and concerns regarding future pregnancies can be allayed through knowledge of disease and transmission.	

13-6	Nursing Considerations for Blood Transfusion Reactions		
Type of Reaction	Cause	Clinical Manifestations	Nursing Interventions
Allergic reaction	Immune response	Urticaria, itching, respiratory distress	Stop the transfusion; call physician; give antihistamines as ordered; monitor vital signs; maintain intravenous infusion of normal saline; keep intravenous line open; check urine for hematuria
Hemolytic reaction	Mismatched blood, history of multiple transfusions	Fever, chills, hematuria, headache, chest pain; can progress to shock	

NURSING ALERT

Neither hot nor cold compresses should be used for pain management in the child who has sickle cell anemia. Ischemic tissue is fragile and has reduced sensation, increasing the risk of burn injury. Cold compresses promote sickling.

COMPLICATIONS OF SICKLE CELL ANEMIA

- Poor growth
- Delayed maturation
- Nonfunctional spleen
- Infection
- Crisis

and that the parent or child understands the use of bolus infusions, when needed (see Chap. 7). Assist the child to assume a comfortable position. Avoid putting stress on painful joints.

Prevent Infection

Infection makes the child more susceptible to a crisis, and the crisis, in turn, increases susceptibility to infection. Teach the parents how to administer antibiotics for prophylaxis or treatment of infection. Be sure they have the finances and other resources to obtain and give daily antibiotics. Because pneumococcal infections are particularly virulent and can cause death in these children, parents should be instructed to obtain immediate care when the child is ill. Encourage the use of the pneumococcal vaccine in children over 2 years of age. The *Haemophilus influenzae* type b (Hib) vaccine series should be started at 2 months of age and continued at recommended ages to prevent another common source of infection.[16]

Ensure Adequate Nutrition

Emphasize the importance of adequate nutrition to promote growth. Encourage the child to eat a high-protein, high-calorie diet. Emphasize the importance of folic acid supplements as ordered.

Prevent Complications of Crises

Observe the child for signs of increasing anemia and shock (mental status change, pallor, vital sign changes). Assess the child's neurologic status for evidence of altered cerebral function. If ordered, assess for an enlarged spleen by gentle palpation. Administer blood transfusions and watch the child for any adverse reaction.

Provide Emotional Support

Sickle cell anemia is a chronic disease that is accompanied by life-threatening episodic crises. Family members often need support to help them deal with their feelings about the diagnosis and its implications. Explore resources in the home and community to see if parents will be able to administer medications and fluids and to provide adequate nutrition. Assess their knowledge of signs of infection and of sickle cell crisis and when to seek medical care for the child. Refer the parents for genetic counseling, particularly if they plan to have more children. Encourage adolescents and young adults in the family to receive genetic counseling and testing, as well. Referrals to support groups and contact with others with the disease can be helpful (see Appendix F).

Discharge Planning and Home Care Teaching

Home care needs should be identified and addressed well in advance of discharge. Provide parents with information about sickle cell disease and the child's treatment. Even parents of a child previously diagnosed with the disorder may benefit from information about the disease process and its management. Explain the basic effect of tissue hypoxia and the effects of sickling on circulation. Refer parents to support groups such as the National Association of Sickle Cell Disease for further information (see Appendix F).

Teach parents to look for signs of dehydration, such as dry mucous membranes, weight loss, and sunken fontanels in infants. Give specific instructions about how many ounces of liquid the child needs to drink each day. Emphasize that increased fluid intake is needed to replace the fluids lost from overheating or exposure to hot weather. Make sure both the child and family understand the triggers and precipitating factors for sickle cell crises. Encourage them to avoid situations that cause crises. Instruct the child and parents about signs and symptoms of crises that should be reported to their health care provider (see Table 13–5).

Provide the family with careful instructions if the child is to receive subcutaneous infusion of deferoxamine for iron overload while at home. Prompt recognition of side effects and careful management of the lengthy infusion process are important.[15] The medicine is mixed with sterile water and infused subcutaneously over several hours. The child needs to be monitored for skin reactions and allergic responses. Have parents demonstrate the infusion technique and state what to do in case of reactions.

Tell parents that it is important to inform all treating physicians and dentists of the child's medical condition. The child should also wear some type of medical identification (eg, medical identification bracelet). Special precautions are necessary when the child undergoes surgery of any kind, as hypoxia resulting from anesthesia is a major surgical risk.

Encourage older children with sickle cell anemia to participate in activities with other children between crises but to avoid strenuous physical exertion and contact sports. Play and social interactions that promote learning and development are important.

β-THALASSEMIA

The thalassemias are a group of inherited blood disorders of hemoglobin synthesis characterized by anemia that can be mild or severe. β-Thalassemia, also known as Cooley anemia, is the most common type. These disorders most often occur in people of Mediterranean descent but are also found among Middle Eastern, Asian, and African populations.[17] If both parents carry the abnormal gene, with each pregnancy there is a 25% chance of passing the disorder on to the child.

There are three types of β-thalassemia: thalassemia minor, or thalassemia trait (produces mild anemia); thalassemia intermedia (produces severe anemia); and thalassemia major (produces anemia requiring transfusion). The clinical manifestations listed in Table 13–7 are caused by the

13-7	Clinical Manifestations of β-Thalassemia

Anemia
Hypochromic and microcytic changes
Folic acid deficiency
Frequent epistaxis

Skeletal Changes
Osteoporosis
Delayed growth
Susceptibility to pathologic fractures
Facial deformities: enlarged head, prominent forehead due to frontal and parietal bossing, prominent cheek bones, broadened and depressed bridge of nose, enlarged maxilla with protruding front teeth, eyes with mongolian slant and epicanthal fold

Heart
Chronic congestive heart failure
Myocardial fibrosis
Murmurs

Liver/Gallbladder
Hepatomegaly
Hepatic insufficiency

Spleen
Splenomegaly

Endocrine System
Delayed sexual maturation
Fibrotic pancreas, resulting in diabetes mellitus

Skin
Darkening of skin

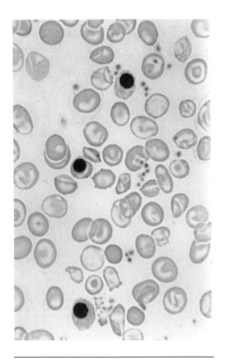

FIGURE 13-6. Red blood cell appearance in β-thalassemia. What characteristic abnormalities can be seen on this microscopic view? *Copyright © MEDCOM, Inc., Garden Grove, CA.*

defective synthesis of hemoglobin, structurally impaired red blood cells (Fig. 13–6), and the shortened life span of the red blood cells. β-Thalassemia can be detected early in infancy. The infant with β-thalassemia manifests pallor, failure to thrive, hepatosplenomegaly, and severe anemia (hemoglobin < 6 g/dL).[16] Diagnosis is made by hemoglobin electrophoresis, which shows a decreased production of one of the globin chains in hemoglobin. Characteristic erythrocyte cell changes often can be recognized in infants by 6 weeks of age.

Treatment is supportive. The goal of medical management is to maintain normal hemoglobin levels. Blood transfusion is the conventional therapy used to treat children with severe disease. Since iron overload is a side effect of this treatment, children may need to receive an iron-chelating drug such as deferoxamine, which binds excess iron so it can be excreted by the kidneys.[15] Other potential complications of long-term transfusion therapy are transfusion reactions and alloimmunization (antibody formation). Bone marrow transplantation may be offered as an alternative therapy for children newly diagnosed with the disorder.[17]

Nursing Management

Nursing care focuses on observing for complications of transfusion therapy, providing emotional support, and referring the family for genetic counseling. Transfusions of packed cells are often given (see Table 13–6). Teach parents the technique for subcutaneous infusion of deferoxamine if that route is to be used for therapy at home. Give parents information about thalassemia and its treatment, and encourage them to obtain genetic counseling. Provide emotional support and encourage parents to take an active role in the child's treatment regimen.

Compliance with transfusion therapy often becomes an issue as children reach adolescence. Offering the adolescent treatment options, such as when to undergo transfusion, can help to improve compliance.[17] Adolescents with β-thalassemia and parents of newly diagnosed children can be referred to the Thalassemia Action Group, a national organization for patients, or to the Cooley's Anemia Foundation (see Appendix F).

APLASTIC ANEMIA

Aplastic anemia is a deficiency of the blood cells that results from failure of the bone marrow to produce adequate numbers of circulating blood cells. The condition may be congenital or acquired.

Congenital aplastic anemia (Fanconi anemia) is a rare autosomal recessive syndrome consisting of multiple congenital anomalies. Symptoms can include **purpura** (bleeding into the tissues) (Fig. 13–7), **petechiae** (pinpoint lesions), bleeding, fatigue, and pallor. Laboratory findings include neutropenia or anemia and **thrombocytopenia** (low platelet count) that progresses to **pancytopenia** (decreased number of blood cell components).

Children with congenital aplastic anemia are at risk for developing malignancies such as acute nonlymphocytic leukemia.[2] The treatment of choice is bone marrow transplantation. However, the prognosis is poor, and death usually results from overwhelming infection, hemorrhage, or malignancy.

Acquired aplastic anemia in children is either idiopathic or occurs from a drug reaction. It can develop after exposure to ionizing radiation or insecticides or after ingestion of drugs such as sulfonamides, chloramphenicol, quinacrine, benzene solvents in model airplane glue, or lead.[2] This type of anemia can also be a result of an infectious process such as viral hepatitis or mononucleosis.

Symptoms are related to the degree of bone marrow failure and can include petechiae, purpura, bleeding, pallor, weakness, tachycardia, and fatigue. Diagnosis is made by blood studies, which reveal **leukopenia** (low white blood cell count) with marked neutropenia, thrombocytopenia, and pancytopenia; and by bone marrow aspiration, which reveals yellow, fatty bone marrow instead of red bone marrow.

Supportive treatment includes transfusions of packed cells and/or platelets. Immunosuppressive drug therapy is effective for many children. The treatment of choice is bone marrow transplantation from a compatible sibling or family member donor.

Nursing Management

Nursing care is similar to care provided for the child with leukemia (see Chap. 14). Nursing actions focus on preventing bleeding, administering and monitoring blood transfusions, preventing infection, encouraging mobility as tolerated, educating the parents and child about the disorder, and providing emotional support. Families need support in dealing with a child who has a life-threatening disease. Refer them to support groups for counseling, if indicated, and to social services.

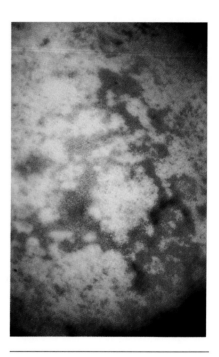

FIGURE 13–7. Nonpalpable purpura with bleeding into the tissues below the skin. *Courtesy of the Department of Hematology/Oncology, Children's National Medical Center, Washington, DC.*

► CLOTTING DISORDERS

HEMOPHILIA

Hemophilia refers to a group of hereditary bleeding disorders that result from a deficiency in specific clotting factors. Hemophilia A, or classic hemophilia, is caused by a deficiency of factor VIII in the blood and accounts for 80% of persons with hemophilia. About 1 in 5000 male births result in hemophilia A.[18] Hemophilia B, known as Christmas disease, is caused by a deficiency of factor IX. Of persons with hemophilia, 15% have hemophilia B.

Clinical Manifestations

Hemophilia is manifested in different children by bleeding tendencies that range from mild to moderate or severe. Children with hemophilia often do not manifest symptoms until after 6 months of age as they become more mobile and incur injuries and bleeding from falls or from tooth eruption. Spontaneous bleeding, **hemarthrosis** (bleeding into a joint space), and deep tissue hemorrhage occur. Affected children frequently experience bleeding into the joint spaces of the knees, ankles, and elbows. Bleeding into joint spaces or bursae causes the child to have limited motion because of pain, tenderness, and swelling.[3] Bone changes, contractures, and disabling deformities can result from immobility and from the effects of blood in the joint structures.

Children may have bleeding after circumcision, easy bruising (**ecchymosis**), nosebleeds, hematuria, and bleeding after tooth extraction, minor trauma, or minor surgical procedures. Large subcutaneous and intramuscular hemorrhages sometimes occur. Bleeding into the tissues of the neck, mouth, or chest is particularly serious because of the potential for airway obstruction. Retroperitoneal and intracranial bleeding may also occur and can be life threatening.

Females who carry the trait for hemophilia do not usually manifest symptoms of the disease. However, they may have prolonged bleeding during dental work, surgery, or trauma.

Etiology and Pathophysiology

Hemophilia is an X-linked recessive trait, which manifests almost exclusively as affected males and carrier females. A daughter who inherits the trait from her father has a 50% chance at each pregnancy of transmitting it to her sons (see Chapter 2 for a description of genetic transmission). However, as many as one third of hemophiliacs have no family members with a history of clotting disorders. In these cases, the disorder is caused by a new mutation. The degree of bleeding is related to the amount of clotting factor and the severity of the injury.

Diagnostic Tests and Medical Management

Diagnosis of affected individuals and carriers can be done before birth through chorionic villus sampling or amniocentesis. Genetic testing of family members is increasingly being used to identify carriers.[18] Diagnosis can also be made on the basis of the history, physical examination, and laboratory data. Laboratory tests will show low levels of factor VIII or IX, and prolonged activated partial prothrombin time (APPT). Prothrombin time (PT), thrombin time (TT), fibrinogen, and platelet count are normal.

The goal of medical management is to control bleeding by replacing the missing clotting factor. Replacement therapy is indicated when the child experiences a mild or major hemorrhage or faces a life-threatening situation. Prompt and adequate treatment is needed to prevent serious bleeding episodes and their sequelae.

The outlook for children with hemophilia has been greatly improved by the availability of transfusion therapy. Transfusions started at home and early interventions prevent many disease complications. In the past, many children with factor VIII deficiency died in the first 5 years of life. Today, children with moderate or mild hemophilia can lead normal lives.

A synthetic drug that is effective against mild hemophilia is desmopressin acetate (DDAVP). An analog of vasopressin, DDAVP is administered intravenously and causes a two- to fourfold increase in factor VIII activity.

Nursing Assessment

Physiologic Assessment

Obtain a complete medical history from the parents or child. In particular, ask about previous episodes of bleeding and the occurrence of hemophilia or any other bleeding disorders in family members. The history of bleeding will vary, depending on the severity of the disease.

Assess the child for any joint pain, swelling, or permanent deformity, particularly around the knees, elbows, ankles, and shoulders. Note the presence of hematuria and mild flank pain. A neurologic assessment should be conducted, as the risk for intracranial hemorrhage and bleeding can lead to peripheral neuropathies.

The adolescent with hemophilia should be screened for human immunodeficiency virus (HIV). Present testing methods make transmission of HIV to individuals with hemophilia very unusual. However, before universal testing of the blood supply began in 1985, significant numbers of hemophiliacs acquired HIV from infusions (see Chap. 9).

Psychologic Assessment

It is difficult for families to manage care of the hemophiliac child, especially if the disease is severe. Assess the family's coping mechanisms and support systems. Ask whether the family's health insurance covers the child's medical expenses; the factor concentrates and infusion equipment are costly. Find out if the parents have respite care that enables them to take time for themselves while knowing that the child is cared for safely. Assess older children's understanding of the disease and their adaptation to it.

Developmental Assessment

Because the child with hemophilia may have physical activity restrictions, physical skills may be delayed. Perform frequent developmental assessments, being particularly attentive to fine and gross motor skills.

Nursing Diagnosis

The most important nursing diagnosis for the child with hemophilia is Risk for Injury related to bleeding disorder. Some of the other nursing diagnoses that might apply include:

- Pain related to bleeding episodes
- Impaired Physical Mobility related to hemarthrosis
- Knowledge Deficit (Child and Parent) related to treatment plan
- Altered Family Processes related to care of a child with a chronic illness
- Altered Growth and Development related to bleeding and impaired mobility

Nursing Management

Nursing care focuses on preventing and controlling bleeding episodes, limiting joint involvement and managing pain, and providing emotional support. Both short-term interventions and long-term management are necessary.

Prevent and Control Bleeding Episodes

Bleeding problems are rare in infants with hemophilia. As children learn to walk and develop other motor skills, however, they often fall and suffer cuts and bruises. The risk of injury can be reduced by emphasizing to parents the need for close supervision and a safe environment. Parents should encourage children to play with toys that are safe and age appropriate.

If dental surgery or tooth extraction is necessary, it should be performed in a controlled environment by experienced staff. Use of a dental irrigation device is often recommended if the child has excess bleeding from gums. Advise adolescents to shave only with an electric razor.

Control any superficial bleeding by applying pressure to the area for at least 15 minutes. Immobilize and elevate the affected area, and apply ice packs to promote vasoconstriction.

If significant bleeding does occur, offer supportive measures and assist with factor replacement therapy. Carefully monitor the child's condition for any side effects when factor replacement therapy is administered.

Limit Joint Involvement and Manage Pain

During bleeding episodes, hemarthrosis is managed by elevating and immobilizing the joint and applying ice packs. Administer analgesics as ordered. Once bleeding has been controlled, range-of-motion exercises are performed to strengthen muscles and joints and to prevent flexion contractures. Physical therapy may be needed. Because excessive weight can place an added stress on joints, encourage the child to maintain an appropriate weight.

Provide Emotional Support

The needs of families with hemophiliac children are best met through a comprehensive team approach. Refer the parents for genetic counseling as soon as possible after diagnosis. It is important to identify family members who carry the trait, as they may suffer excessive bleeding during surgery.

Encourage the parents to verbalize their feelings. Be understanding and sensitive to their needs. Teach the parents about hemophilia and explain how the disorder affects both the child and other family members. Refer the parents and child to organizations such as the National Hemophilia Foundation for further information (see Appendix F).

Discharge Planning and Home Care Teaching

The child may be hospitalized briefly during the first manifestation of bleeding or diagnosis and management. Most care will subsequently take place in the home. Home care needs should be identified and addressed well in advance of discharge. Advise parents to have the child wear a medical identification bracelet. Explain the cause of bleeding so both the child and parents understand the disease process. Teach the child and family how to identify internal bleeding. Signs and symptoms such as joint pain, abdominal pain, and obvious bleeding are indicators for immediate factor infusion. Make sure the child and parents know what situations could cause bleeding to occur. Teach parents to give acetaminophen instead of aspirin to relieve pain.

Instruct the parents and the child, when appropriate, in the preparation and administration of factor concentrate. If infusion of the missing fac-

CLINICAL TIP

Take the following precautions when caring for children with bleeding disorders:
- Avoid taking temperatures rectally or giving suppositories.
- Check blood pressure by cuff as infrequently as possible.
- Avoid intramuscular or subcutaneous injections.
- Use only paper or silk tape for dressings.
- When indicated, perform mouth care every 3 hours with a glycerin swab.
- Except for factor replacement therapy, avoid all venipunctures.
- Use a peripheral fingerstick to obtain blood samples.
- Do not give aspirin.

tor is scheduled on a regular basis, bleeding episodes can be controlled or avoided. Have the parents demonstrate the procedure and make sure they can administer the product correctly. The parents need to be familiar with properties of the factor concentrate to prepare the mixture correctly.

The child will need an Individual School Health Plan (see Chap. 5). Members of the school staff should be instructed in management of emergencies, and infusion equipment should be readily available.

Help the family and school to plan an appropriate schedule of activities without overprotecting the child. Children with hemophilia should not engage in contact sports such as football and soccer, which may result in injury and trauma. Instead, sports such as swimming, hiking, and bicycling should be encouraged.

Explain how the parents can coordinate their child's care with a number of health professionals. Provide ongoing case management, assisting the family to take on this task if able.

Hemophilia is not only a debilitating disorder for the child. It also can be financially draining for the family. Frequent outpatient visits, emergency department visits, hospital admissions, and the cost of factor concentrate can exhaust a family's resources. If indicated, referral should be made to appropriate social services (eg, the state's maternal and child health program for children with special health care needs) and organizations such as the National Hemophilia Foundation (see Appendix F). Sharing experiences with other families of children with hemophilia can provide support.

VON WILLEBRAND DISEASE

Like hemophilia, von Willebrand disease is a hereditary bleeding disorder. There are about 20 different disorders involving a deficiency of von Willebrand factor, which is a plasma protein and the carrier for clotting factor VIII, thereby playing a necessary role in platelet adhesion.[19] The most common form of the disorder is transmitted as an autosomal dominant trait, and it can occur in both males and females. The gene for the disease is located on chromosome 12.

The characteristic manifestations are easy bruising and epistaxis. Children with von Willebrand disease frequently have gingival bleeding and increased bleeding with lacerations or during surgery. Affected teenage girls may have **menorrhagia** (increased menstrual bleeding).

Diagnosis of von Willebrand disease is made after laboratory studies reveal decreased von Willebrand factor levels, von Willebrand factor antigen levels, and factor VIII activity; reduced platelet agglutination; prolonged bleeding time; and prolonged or normal activated partial thromboplastin time (APPT). Treatment is similar to that for the child with hemophilia and involves infusion of von Willebrand protein concentrate. For bleeding episodes or prior to surgery, DDAVP is infused. Locally administered medications such as aminocaproic acid are sometimes used to manage bleeding in the mucous membranes.

Nursing Management

Teach parents about the disorder and instruct them not to give the child any aspirin or drugs that can cause bleeding or inhibit platelet function. Teach management of bleeding episodes and intravenous infusion techniques, as for hemophilia. The prognosis is good, and children with von Willebrand disease usually have a normal life expectancy.

DISSEMINATED INTRAVASCULAR COAGULATION

Disseminated intravascular coagulation (DIC) is a life-threatening, acquired pathologic process in which the clotting system is abnormally activated, resulting in widespread clot formation in the small vessels throughout the body. Excess thrombin is generated, followed by deposition of fibrin strands in body tissues. These changes cause tissue hypoxia, resulting in eventual tissue necrosis. The circulating fibrin fragments later begin to interfere with platelet aggregation and other aspects of the clotting mechanism, resulting in bleeding or hemorrhage.

DIC is a complication of other serious illnesses in infants and children, such as hypoxia, shock, cancer, and viruses. Symptoms can include diffuse bleeding manifested by hematuria, petechiae, or purpura; an injection site that continues to ooze; circulatory collapse; and major vessel thrombosis.[10] The prothrombin time and partial thromboplastin time are prolonged, platelet count and fibrinogen levels are increased, and levels of fibrin–fibrinogen split products are high.

Medical management is supportive and includes identification and treatment of the underlying disorder; replacement of depleted coagulation factors, fibrinogen, and platelets; and anticoagulant therapy (heparin).

Nursing Management

DIC is a complex disorder that is managed by a critical care team.[20] Nursing care focuses on assessing the bleeding, preventing further injury, and administering prescribed therapies. Observe for petechiae, ecchymoses, and oozing every 1–2 hours. Be sure to check dependent areas, as blood will pool in these areas. Intravenous sites are particularly prone to oozing and should be assessed every 15 minutes. Examine stool for the presence of blood, and measure blood loss as accurately as possible. Measure intake and output.

Because all body systems can be involved, careful assessment of all systems is needed on a continual basis. Institute bleeding control precautions, monitor prescribed therapy (transfusion, anticoagulant therapy), and report any signs of complications.

IDIOPATHIC THROMBOCYTOPENIC PURPURA

Idiopathic thrombocytopenic purpura (ITP), also known as autoimmune thrombocytopenic purpura, is a disorder characterized by increased destruction of platelets, even though platelet production in the bone marrow is normal. When the rate of platelet destruction exceeds the rate of platelet production, the number of circulating platelets decreases and blood clotting slows.

ITP is the most common bleeding disorder in children. It occurs most frequently in children 2–5 years of age and usually follows a viral infection such as measles, chickenpox, or rubella. Symptoms include multiple ecchymoses and petechiae. Diagnosis is made by history and through physical and laboratory findings, which show a decreased platelet count and antiplatelet antibodies in the peripheral blood. Treatment includes administering corticosteroids and intravenous immunoglobulins. For those children who do not respond to drug therapy over a period of 6 months to 1 year, splenectomy may be the treatment of choice. Spontaneous remission is seen in 90% of children with ITP.[10]

Nursing Management

Nursing care focuses on controlling and reducing the number of bleeding episodes. Preventive measures are similar to those for the child with hemophilia. Teach parents to use acetaminophen, rather than aspirin, to control pain. Provide emotional support.

MENINGOCOCCEMIA

Meningococcemia is a disease process that follows infection with *Neisseria meningitidis* or, occasionally, other microorganisms such as *H. influenzae* or *Streptococcus pneumoniae*. The disorder is thought to be an immune response to the endotoxins of the organism.

Onset is sudden: A respiratory infection is followed by high fever, rash, massive skin and mucosal hemorrhage, and shock. The child, usually under 2 years of age, is critically ill and demonstrates multisystem disease. Disseminated intravascular coagulation occurs (see previous discussion). Commonly the skin turns pink and then black as the tissues are damaged from reduced oxygen delivery. Limbs may need to be amputated as a result of impaired circulation.

Treatment consists of antibiotics, removal from sources of infection, and multisystem shock management. Prompt administration of antibiotics to the child who manifests fever with purpura can decrease the severity of outcome. Depending on the child's condition, total parenteral nutrition, sedation and pain relief, dialysis, or amputation may be required.[21]

Nursing Management

Nursing care of the child with meningococcemia is complex. The child generally has a lengthy hospitalization in a pediatric intensive care unit. Thorough assessments of all body systems are performed. Intravenous infusions must be administered when ordered to ensure correct and timely administration of antibiotics and other therapies. Urinary output is measured to evaluate kidney function. Meticulous skin care is necessary to preserve the integrity of tissues. Care is taken to prevent further infections. Nutritional support in the form of total parenteral nutrition is common. The family needs support to deal with the changing critical nature of the child's illness and the possibility that permanent deformities will result. When the child improves, continuing care in the hospital and then in the community is needed to manage growth, development, nutrition, amputations, and prosthetics.

▶ BONE MARROW TRANSPLANTATION

Bone marrow transplantation is a treatment that is used for diseases such as severe combined immunodeficiency disease, severe and unresponsive aplastic anemia, and leukemia (see Chap. 14).

There are three types of bone marrow transplant: autologous, isogeneic (or syngeneic), and allogeneic. In autologous transplantation, the child's own marrow is taken, stored, and reinfused after the child has received chemotherapy. In isogeneic transplantation, the marrow is taken from an identical twin. In allogeneic transplantation, the donor, usually a sibling, has a compatible human leukocyte antigen (HLA). When no relative is found to match the child, a histocompatible donor may be sought from the National Bone Marrow Registry.

The transplantation procedure begins with chemotherapy and, sometimes, total body irradiation directed at destroying circulating blood cells and the diseased bone marrow in the ill child. Following this treatment, the child is transfused with the donor marrow. If the transplantation is successful, the donor marrow implants itself in the bone and begins to grow. Healthy bone marrow, capable of making blood cells, is the result.

The chemotherapy program for destruction of bone marrow takes 4–12 days. During this time, the child is cared for in strict isolation in a special unit that provides a germ-free environment (Fig. 13–8). Side effects of chemotherapy provide challenges for care in addition to those of preventing infection (see Chap. 14). The child is without any immunity for a minimum of 10 days after transplantation. It takes 2–4 weeks for the donor cells to begin proliferation and maturation.[22] Medications to stimulate the production of red and white blood cells are administered during this period.

Once the bone marrow begins to produce new cells, graft-versus-host disease (rejection) is the major threat. Refer to Chapter 9 for a discussion of graft-versus-host disease.

Monitor for this multisystem disorder by assessing the skin, mucous membranes, gastrointestinal function, respiratory function, cardiac function, and hydration status. Because graft-versus-host disease may occur at any time, even after the child returns home, frequent thorough assessments are necessary after discharge.

Supportive care after the transplantation procedure focuses on preventing infection, controlling bleeding, maintaining adequate nutrition and hydration, monitoring for signs of rejection, and providing psychosocial support. The treatment is lengthy, the child is often critically ill, and parents may have traveled to a medical center many miles from home for the procedure. Ask parents about other family members and how they are managing. Provide information about inexpensive housing available near the medical center, such as in a Ronald McDonald house. Encourage parents to discuss their feelings with other parents of children receiving bone marrow transplantation. Appendix F provides listings of organizations such as the Bone Marrow Transplant Family Support Network that may serve as resources for families.

When the child is ready for discharge, be sure the family is prepared to administer medications, recognize signs of graft-versus-host disease, provide adequate nutrition for the child, and perform other necessary care. Arrange for follow-up visits and provide the names of local health care contact persons who can offer support and provide information. The child may need tutors or other educational assistance to promote integration back into the school setting.

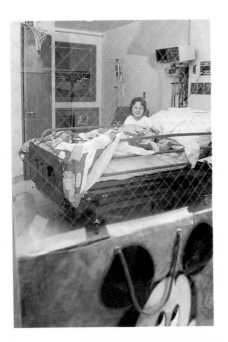

FIGURE 13–8. The child undergoing bone marrow transplantation is hospitalized in a special unit while receiving chemotherapy before the transfusion. The child remains in the unit for several weeks afterward until the new marrow produces enough cells to maintain health.

 GROWTH & DEVELOPMENT CONSIDERATIONS

Hospitalizations of children undergoing bone marrow transplantation are usually lengthy. Evaluate the child's age and developmental stage and establish developmental goals to be met during the hospitalization. Implement nursing plans to meet the child's developmental needs and encourage further growth.

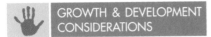 **REFERENCES**

1. Dallman, P.R., & Shannon, K. (1996). Developmental changes in red blood cell production and function. In A.M. Rudolph, J.I.E. Hoffman, & C.D. Rudolph (Eds.), *Rudolph's pediatrics* (20th ed., pp. 1167–1172). Stamford, CT: Appleton & Lange.

2. Cairo, M.S. (1996). White blood cells. In A.M. Rudolph, J.I.E. Hoffman, & C.D. Rudolph (Eds.), *Rudolph's pediatrics* (20th ed., pp. 1221–1223). Stamford, CT: Appleton & Lange.

3. Manco-Johnson, M.J. (1996). Hemostasis and bleeding disorders. In A.M. Rudolph, J.I.E. Hoffman, & C.D. Rudolph (Eds.), *Rudolph's pediatrics* (20th ed., pp. 1236–1251). Stamford, CT: Appleton & Lange.

4. Kline, N.E. (1996). A practical approach to the child with anemia. *Journal of Pediatric Health Care, 10*(3), 99–105.

5. American Academy of Pediatrics. (1997). *Guidelines for health supervision III.* Elk Grove Village, IL: American Academy of Pediatrics.

6. Glader, B.E., & Look, K.A. (1996). Hematologic disorders in children from Southeast Asia. *Pediatric Clinics of North America, 43*(3), 665–682.

7. Abshire, T.C. (1996). The anemia of inflammation: A common cause of childhood anemia. *Pediatric Clinics of North America, 43*(3), 623–638.

8. Hays, T. (1997). Hematologic disorders. In G.B. Merenstein, D.W. Kaplan, & A.A. Rosenberg (Eds.), *Handbook of pediatrics* (18th ed., pp. 601–630). Stamford, CT: Appleton & Lange.

9. Mentzer, W.C. (1996). Sickle cell disease. In A.M. Rudolph, J.I.E. Hoffman, & C.D. Rudolph (Eds.), *Rudolph's pediatrics* (20th ed., pp. 1203–1207). Stamford, CT: Appleton & Lange.

10. Lane, P.A., Nuss, R., & Ambruso, D.R. (1996). Hematologic disorders. In W.W. Hay, J.R. Groothius, A.R. Hayward, & M.J. Levin (Eds.), *Current pediatric diagnosis and treatment* (13th ed., pp. 732–780). Stamford, CT: Appleton & Lange.

11. Selekman, J. (1993). Update: New guidelines for the treatment of infants with sickle cell disease. *Pediatric Nursing, 19*(6), 600–605.

12. Rennie, J. (1994). Grading the gene tests. *Scientific American, 270*(6), 88–97.

13. Davis, H., Schoendorf, K.C., Gergen, P.J., & Moore, R.M. (1997). National trends in the mortality of children with sickle cell disease, 1968 through 1992. *American Journal of Public Health, 87*(8), 1317–1322.

14. National Heart, Lung, and Blood Institute. (1997). Periodic transfusions lower stroke risk in children with sickle cell anemia. Washington, DC: U.S. National Library of Medicine, http://www.nlm.nih.gov/

15. Day, S., Dancy, R., Kelly, K., & Wang, W. (1993). Iron overload? In sickle cell disease? *American Journal of Maternal-Child Nursing, 18*(6), 330–335.

16. Agency for Health Care Policy and Research. (1993). *Sickle cell disease: Screening, diagnosis, management, and counseling in newborns and infants.* Washington, DC: Author.

17. Martin, M.B., & Butler, R.B. (1993). Understanding the basics of ß thalassemia major. *Pediatric Nursing, 19*(2), 143–145.

18. DiMichele, D. (1996). Hemophilia 1996: New approach to an old disease. *Pediatric Clinics of North America, 43*(3), 709–736.

19. Werner, E.J. (1996). von Willebrand disease in children and adolescents. *Pediatric Clinics of North America, 43*(3), 683–708.

20. Bell, T.N. (1993). Disseminated intravascular coagulation: Clinical complexities of aberrant coagulation. *Critical Care Nursing Clinics of North America, 5*(5), 389–410.

21. Holland, J.A., Bryan, S., & Huff-Slandard, J. (1993). Nursing care of a child with meningococcemia. *Journal of Pediatric Nursing, 8*(4), 211–216.

22. Abramovitz, L.Z., & Senner, A.M. (1995). Pediatric bone marrow transplantation update. *Oncology Nursing Forum, 22*(1), 107–115.

ADDITIONAL RESOURCES

Agency for Health Care Policy and Research. (1993). *Sickle cell disease: Comprehensive screening and management in newborns and infants. Quick reference guide for clinicians.* Washington, DC: Author.

American Academy of Pediatrics. (1994). Health supervision for children with sickle cell diseases and their families. *Pediatrics, 98,* 467.

Ballas, S.K., & Mohandas, N. (1996). Pathophysiology of vaso-occlusion. *Hematology/Oncology Clinics of North America 10*(6), 1221–1239.

Coffland, F.I., & Shelton, D.M. (1993). Blood component replacement therapy. *Critical Care Nursing Clinics of North America, 5*(3), 543–556.

Kuntz, N., Adams, J.A., Zahr, L., Killen, R., Cameron, K., & Wasson, H. (1996). Therapeutic play and bone marrow transplantation. *Journal of Pediatric Nursing, 11*(6), 359–367.

Lane, P.A. (1996). Sickle cell disease. *Pediatric Clinics of North America, 43*(3), 639–664.

Manno, C.S. (1996). What's new in transfusion medicine? *Pediatric Clinics of North America, 43*(3), 793–808.

Medeiros, D., & Buchanan, G.R. (1996). Current controversies in the management of idiopathic thrombocytic purpura during childhood. *Pediatric Clinics of North America, 43*(3), 757–772.

National Heart, Lung, and Blood Institute. (1995). *Management and therapy of sickle cell disease.* (Publication No. 95-2117). Bethesda, MD: National Institutes of Health.

Ringwals-Smith, K., Krance, R., & Stricklin, L. (1995). Enteral nutrition support in a child after bone marrow transplantation. *Nutrition in Clinical Practice, 10*(4), 140–143.

Srnec, P. (1993). Congenital coagulopathies in the pediatric population. *Critical Care Nursing Clinics of North America, 5*(3), 445–452.

Sormanti, M., Dungan, S., & Rieker, P.P. (1994). Pediatric bone marrow transplantation: Psychosocial issues for parents after a child's hospitalization. *Journal of Psychosocial Oncology, 12*(4), 23–42.

Tesno, B. (1995). A comprehensive pediatric bone marrow transplant documentation tool. *Oncology Nursing Forum, 22*(5), 841–847.

Walters, M.C., & Abelson, H.T. (1996). Interpretation of the complete blood count. *Pediatric Clinics of North America, 43*(3), 599–622.

Zimmerman, S.A., Ware, R.E., & Kinney, T.R. (1997). Gaining ground in the fight against sickle cell disease. *Contemporary Pediatrics, 14*(10), 154–177.

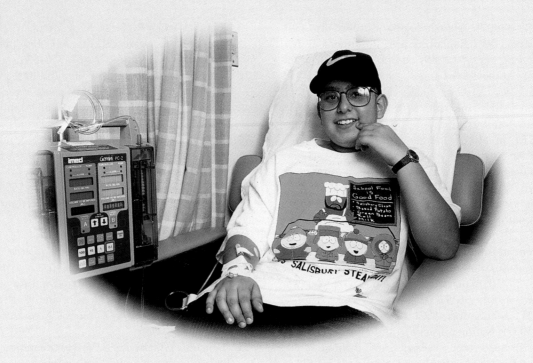

Twelve-year-old Rasheed is admitted to the hospital with fever and explosive diarrhea. He is diagnosed with enterocolitis, an invasive infection of the small intestine and colon that has occurred several months into his therapy for acute myelogenous leukemia. As Rasheed's condition worsens day by day, his anxiety grows. His mother, who took a 3-month leave from work during the early phases of his treatment, is unable to take additional time off from work to be with him. At last, with aggressive antibiotic therapy and supportive nursing care, Rasheed conquers the complication and returns home.

Rasheed and his parents feel they have met another challenge in his treatment for leukemia. When he was first diagnosed, 7 months earlier, Rasheed was severely anemic and bruised easily. He was hospitalized for a short time after diagnosis for implantation of a medication port and the first chemotherapy treatments. Soon, however, he was discharged home, returning for outpatient visits to receive chemotherapy and monitor his condition.

Rasheed has maintained a positive attitude throughout his treatment. He studied at home for a short period of time but has now returned to school. Keeping up with his school work has been made easier by the gift of a computer from the Make-a-Wish Foundation.

ALTERATIONS IN CELLULAR GROWTH 14

"The news that Rasheed had enterocolitis was a blow to him and his family, but that setback seemed to make Rasheed even more determined to fight his disease."

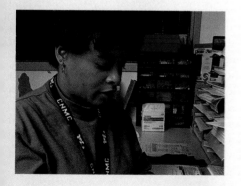

TERMINOLOGY

- **benign** A growth that does not endanger life or health.
- **biotherapy** Use of biologic response modifiers to treat cancer.
- **carcinogens** Chemicals or processes that, when combined with genetic traits and in interaction with one another, cause cancer.
- **chemotherapy** Treatment to combat cancer that involves drugs taken orally, intravenously, intrathecally, or by injection, which kill both normal and cancerous cells.
- **extravasation** Damage that occurs when a chemotherapeutic drug leaks into the soft tissue surrounding the infusion site.
- **leukocytosis** A higher than normal leukocyte count.
- **leukopenia** A lower than normal white cell count.
- **malignant** The progressive growth of a tumor that will, if not checked by treatment, result in death.
- **metastasis** The spread of cancer cells to other sites in the body.
- **myelosuppression** A decreased production of blood cells in the bone marrow.

- **neoplasms** Cancerous growths.
- **oncogene** A portion of the DNA that is altered and, when duplicated, causes uncontrolled cellular division.
- **polypharmacy** The use of many drugs at one time to treat multiple health conditions.
- **protocol** A plan of action for chemotherapy that is based on the type of cancer, its stage, and the particular cell type.
- **protooncogene** A gene that regulates cellular growth and development but can become an oncogene, capable of causing cancerous growth.
- **radiation** Cancer treatment using unstable isotopes that release varying levels of energy to cause breaks in the DNA molecule and thereby destroy cells.
- **thrombocytopenia** A low platelet count.
- **tumor suppressor genes** Genetic material that controls the growth of cells, decreasing the effects of oncogenes.

Why do children like Rasheed develop different types of cancers than adults? Cancer in adults is often the result of dietary practices or habits such as smoking. Some adult-onset cancers are the result of oncogenic responses to stimuli; that is, responses that stimulate cancerous changes in cells. Other cancers that occur in adults result from prolonged exposure to toxins such as coal dust and asbestos. Some cancers are known to be related to genetic causes. In adults, prevention through general life-style changes is a major focus of interventions. However, in children, cancer is usually embryonic (occurring during development of the fetus) or oncogenic in origin. Thus, life-style changes have little effect on the incidence of childhood cancer. Occasionally, an environmental exposure is linked to the incidence of cancer in children.

Abnormal cellular growth can occur in any area of the body. Why are some growths called cancer and others not? Changes in cellular growth within the body are called **neoplasms** (meaning new growth). A neoplasm is further classified as benign or malignant. **Benign** means that a growth does not endanger life or health. **Malignant** means that progressive growth of the tumor will, if not checked by treatment, result in spread to other sites in the body **(metastasis),** ending in death. The common term for this type of cellular growth is cancer.

▶ ANATOMY AND PHYSIOLOGY OF PEDIATRIC DIFFERENCES

The major physiologic difference between adults and children that affects cellular growth involves the immune system and how well it functions in the defense of the body. The rate of cell growth in children also can play a role in the rapidity with which some childhood cancers progress.

The immune system defends the body against foreign organisms and substances through two responses: nonspecific and specific. In a nonspecific response the components of the immune system attack a variety of targets. Nonspecific components include phagocytic (cell-destroying) cells such as mononuclear leukocytes, polymorphonuclear (PMN) leukocytes, natural killer (NK) cells, and complements (noncellular proteins) that work together to destroy invading cells and substances. During the first month of a child's life the nonspecific response is immature, so phagocytic cells have little ability to move toward cancer cells and fulfill their function. The nonspecific response is also impaired in premature and small-for-gestational-age (SGA) infants.

In a specific response, T lymphocytes and immunoglobulin (Ig) attack only one type of invader. The specific response capability also is immature in infants. B-cell production of various proteins called immunoglobins (IgM, IgG, and IgA) is below adult levels, so that the infant is vulnerable to bacterial and viral infections. (For a discussion of immune function, see Chapter 9.)

In children, many cells are growing quickly; this fast growth can lead to the proliferation of cancerous as well as normal cells.

▶ CHILDHOOD CANCER

The care of children who have cancer is a challenging specialty in pediatric nursing. For several years, the child undergoes aggressive treatments that may be life threatening and cause temporary illness. Sometimes the diagnosis is quite hopeful; at other times, a terminal result may be expected. The child is cared for at home with outpatient visits for treatment and occasional hospitalization when needed. The periods of hospitalization are times of intense physical vulnerability for the child and intense emotional vulnerability for both the child and the family. To monitor the child closely, nurses need a sound knowledge of physiologic and psychologic responses, medical interventions, and nursing care. Effective communication skills are necessary to support the child and family and promote realistic hope.

Incidence

During 1997, in the United States, cancer was diagnosed in approximately 8800 children. In children under 15 years of age, cancer is the leading cause of disease-related death.[1] In 1997, about 1700 U.S. children died of cancer, one third of these from leukemia.[2] Mortality rates have declined by over 60% since 1960. The most common forms of chilhood cancers among children in different age groups are shown in Figure 14–1.[3]

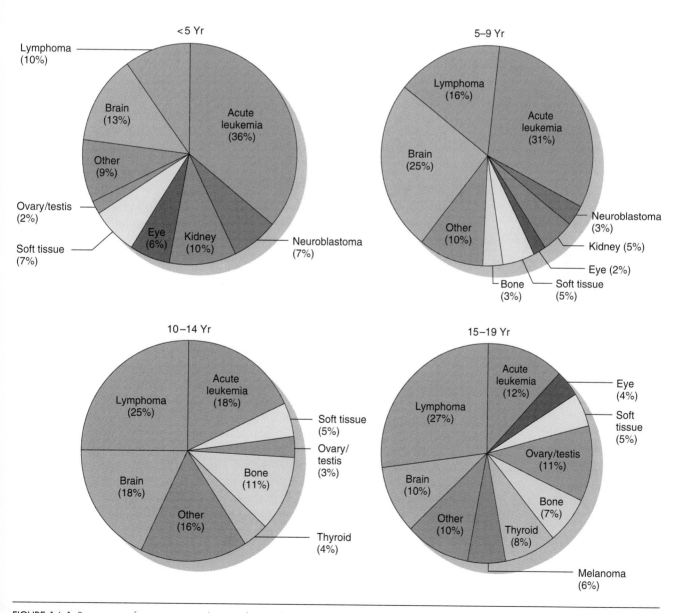

FIGURE 14–1. Percentage of primary tumors by site of origin for different age groups.
From Crist, W.M. (1995). Neoplastic diseases and tumors. In R.E. Behrman, R.M. Kliegman, & A.M. Arvin (Eds.), Nelson textbook of pediatrics (15th ed., p. 1442). Philadelphia: Saunders.

COMMON SIGNS OF CHILDHOOD
CANCER

Pain
Cachexia
Anemia
Infection
Bruising

Clinical Manifestations

Each type of childhood cancer signals its presence differently. Because many of the presenting signs and symptoms of cancer are typical of common childhood illnesses, a delay in diagnosis can occur. In some cases, no symptoms are noted until the cancer is advanced. Some of the common presenting symptoms of cancer follow.

- *Pain* may be the result of a neoplasm either directly or indirectly affecting nerve receptors through obstruction, inflammation, tissue damage, stretching of visceral tissue, or invasion of susceptible tissue.
- *Cachexia* is a syndrome characterized by anorexia, weight loss, anemia, asthenia (weakness), and early satiety (feeling of being full).
- *Anemia* may be experienced during times of chronic bleeding or iron deficiency. In chronic illness the body uses iron poorly. Anemia is also present in cancers of the bone marrow when the number of red blood cells (RBCs) is reduced, in part because of the presence of large numbers of other bone marrow products.
- *Infection* is usually a result of an altered or immature immune system. In addition, infection occurs when bone marrow cancers inhibit maturation of normal immune system cells. Infection may also occur in children who are treated with corticosteroids. Because their immune response is altered, the normal signs of infection may not appear.
- *Bruising* can occur if the bone marrow cannot produce enough platelets and bleeding occurs after minor trauma.

Etiology and Pathophysiology

Alterations in cellular growth occur in response to external and internal stimuli. Neoplasms are caused by one or a combination of three factors: (1) external stimuli that cause genetic mutations, (2) immune system and gene abnormalities, and (3) chromosomal abnormalities.

External Stimuli

External stimuli may affect the child's general health and cause mutations in body cells. **Carcinogens** are chemicals or industrial processes that, when combined with genetic traits and in interaction with one another, result in cancer. Several carcinogens cause cancers that are diagnosed during childhood. Others cause cancers that begin in childhood but are not identified until adulthood. Some chemicals suspected of causing childhood cancer include diethylstilbestrol (maternal use of therapeutic estrogen hormones), anabolic androgenic steroids, alkylating chemotherapy agents, and immunosuppressants used for organ transplantation.[3] Radiation exposure has been known to cause cancers such as leukemia and thyroid tumors in children exposed to atomic bombs and excessive radiation during diagnostic medical procedures. Secondary cancers can result when the child is treated for a primary cancer with high doses of radiation. Excessive exposure to ultraviolet radiation from the sun predisposes children to development of skin cancer in adulthood.

Immune System and Gene Abnormalities

One critical function of a normal immune system is immune surveillance, in which phagocytic cells circulate throughout the body, detecting and destroying abnormal and cancerous cells. Children with congenital immune deficiencies, such as Wiskott–Aldrich syndrome, in which immune surveillance may fail, are at high risk for cancer. A form of non-Hodgkin's lymphoma develops in some children treated with immune system–suppressing drugs.

Viruses and other substances may act in the body to alter the immune system, thereby allowing cancer to occur (Fig. 14–2). Their action is based on changing certain genes that normally regulate cellular growth and development (called **protooncogenes**) to related genes that allow unregulated cell division and cancerous growth (called **oncogenes**). Among the cancers thought to be linked to virus action and the change of protooncogenes to oncogenes are certain leukemias, rhabdomyosarcoma, Burkitt's lymphoma, and some forms of Hodgkin's disease.

Tumor suppressor genes counteract the effect of oncogenes, keeping cellular growth within normal limits. When tumor suppressor genes are missing, unstemmed cellular growth can occur. These genes are commonly missing in children with retinoblastoma and Wilms' tumor.

Chromosomal Abnormalities

Normal chromosomes undergo change as a part of the genetic process. Most of the changes are not harmful. However, some changes result in chromosomal abnormalities such as hyperploidy (more than the normal number of chromosomes), deletion, translocation, and breakage.

Some of these chromosomal abnormalities have been linked to an increased incidence of cancer. Children with Down syndrome have a 200 times higher incidence of leukemia than nonaffected children. Children who are missing a band of genetic material on chromosome 13 often have retinoblastoma. Similarly, a Wilms' tumor often develops in children missing part of the genetic material from chromosome 11.[4]

Regardless of the location of abnormal cellular growth, the pathophysiologic process is similar. The altered cell begins to multiply as directed by the altered genetic structure of its DNA and the absence or inactivation of tumor suppressor genes. Each new cell transmits the new or altered pattern to the next generation. As the abnormal cells replicate, the neoplastic mass grows. Normal cells usually die as the increased metabolic rate of the neoplastic cells depletes available nutrition. The altered DNA in the tumor cells may also cause the abnormal cells to invade adjoining tissue. Through continued growth the mass expands until it enters and disrupts a major vessel or a vital organ.

Diagnostic Tests and Medical Management

The most common diagnostic tests performed on children with cancer are complete blood counts, bone marrow aspiration, lumbar puncture (Table 14–1), peripheral blood studies, radiographic examination, magnetic resonance imaging (MRI), computed tomography (CT; Fig 14–3), ultrasound, and biopsy.

Cancer is treated with one or a combination of therapies: surgery, chemotherapy, radiation, biotherapy, and bone marrow transplantation. The choice of treatment is determined by the type of cancer, its location, and the degree of metastasis (spread to other sites in the body).

The goal of treatment may be curative, supportive, or palliative. Curative treatment rids the child's body of the cancer. Supportive treatment includes transfusions, pain management, antibiotics, and other interventions to assist the body's defenses and increase the child's comfort. Palliative treatment is designed to make the child as comfortable as possible.

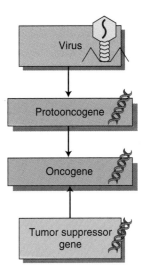

FIGURE 14–2. A protooncogene normally regulates cellular growth and development. When altered by a virus or other external cause, it can change to an oncogene, which allows unregulated genetic activity and tumor growth. Tumor-suppressor genes regulate the effects of oncogenes to decrease wildly proliferating cellular growth.

NURSING ALERT

The American Academy of Pediatrics Subcommittee on Cancer Pain in Children recommends that children be given some type of sedation before lumbar puncture is performed.

NURSING ALERT

Any child who has an implanted metallic object in his or her body should not undergo MRI scanning because of the strong magnetic field generated. Metallic objects include orthodontic braces, metal dental bridgework, surgical clips or plates, and orthopedic rods. Remove all jewelry and clothes with metal snaps from the child before the test.

14-1	Selected Diagnostic Tests for Childhood Cancer		
Test	Purpose	Normal Laboratory Values	Diagnostic Values
Bone marrow aspiration	Examines bone marrow	<5% blast cells (immature)	>25% blast cells in acute lymphoblastic leukemia, most with hypercellular marrow
Lumbar puncture	Examines cerebrospinal fluid	Cell count (mm^3) Polymorphonuclear leukocytes 0 Monocytes 0–5 RBCs 0–5	Presence of malignant cells indicates central nervous system involvement
Complete blood count and differential	Examines cellular components of blood	WBC <10,000/mm^3 Platelets 150,000– 400,000/mm^3 Hemoglobin 12–16 g/dL	WBC >10,000/mm^3 Platelets 20,000– 100,000/mm^3 Hemoglobin 7–10 g/dL

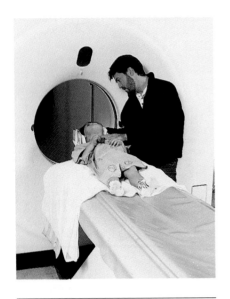

FIGURE 14–3. Computed tomography (CT) can be a frightening procedure for children. This 2-year-old boy is comforted by his father before the procedure.

COLONY-STIMULATING FACTORS

Filgrastin (Neupogen): Stimulates neutrophil production
Erythropoietin: Stimulates red blood cell production

Surgery

Surgery is used to remove or debulk (reduce the size of) a solid tumor. An example of a cancer that is commonly treated with surgery is a Wilms' tumor. Surgery is also used to determine the stage and type of cancer.

Chemotherapy

Chemotherapy is the administration of specific drugs that kill both normal and cancerous cells. The administration of various chemotherapeutic drugs (Table 14–2) is timed to achieve the greatest cellular destruction. The schedule is determined by the cell's cycle of replication (Fig. 14–4). Several chemotherapeutic drugs are administered simultaneously to maximize their lethal impact on cells at all stages of activity. Table 14–3 provides examples of some commonly used chemotherapy drug combinations.[5] Whereas DNA in a normal cell can repair itself after chemotherapy, the DNA in a neoplastic cell cannot. The particular chemotherapy treatment protocol used is based on research into different types of cancer cells. A **protocol** is a plan of action for chemotherapy that is based on the type of cancer, its stage, and the particular cell type (Fig. 14–5).

Other drugs used in the treatment of children with cancer include colony-stimulating factors, antiemetics, and nutritional supplements. Colony-stimulating factors are hormonelike glycoproteins that enhance blood cell production and counteract the myelosuppressive effects of chemotherapy drugs. Antiemetics can be used to treat the nausea and vomiting that are common side effects of therapy. Nutritional supplements can be given to maintain nutritional status.

Radiation

Radiation therapy involves the use of unstable isotopes that release varying levels of energy to cause breaks in the DNA molecule and thereby destroy cells. Radiation has been used as a treatment method since the

14-2	Chemotherapeutic Drugs and Their Actions

Cell cycle specific agents (active in specific phases of the cell cycle) (see Fig. 14–4)

Antimetabolites	Work at synthesis phase; interfere with function of nucleic acid, inhibiting DNA or RNA synthesis
	5-Azacytidine
	5-Fluorouracil
	6-Mercaptopurine
	6-Thioguanine
	Cytosine arabinoside
	Methotrexate
Vinca alkaloids	Work at mitosis phase; bind with cell proteins to inhibit nucleic acid and protein synthesis
	Etoposide
	Teniposide
	Vinblastine
	Vincristine
Miscellaneous	Work at G_1 phase; cause depletion of asparagine, needed by cancer cells and cause lysis of lymphoid cells; make cell in G phase vulnerable to other agents; interfere with prosynthesis
	L-Asparaginase
	Prednisone
Miscellaneous	Work at G_2 phase; bind cellular proteins to cause metaphase arrest
	Bleomycin
	Etoposide

Cell cycle nonspecific agents (active in all stages of the cell cycle) (see Fig. 14–5)

Alkylating agents	Substitute an alkyl group for a hydrogen atom, leading to DNA replication
	Cyclophosphamide
	Cisplatin
	Busulfan
	Chlorambucil
	Thiotepa
	Mechlorethamine
Antibiotics	Interfere with nucleic acid, inhibiting DNA or RNA synthesis
	Doxorubicin
	Mitomycin-C
	Dactinomycin
	Bleomycin
	Daunorubicin
Nitrosureas	Cause breakage in DNA; cross blood–brain barrier
	Carmustine
	Lomustine
Miscellaneous	Affect DNA and RNA synthesis
	Dacarbazine
	Procarbazine

early 1900s, shortly after its discovery. It is often used for the local and regional control of cancer, and in combination with surgery and chemotherapy.

The area to be irradiated (treatment field) includes the tumor site and sometimes other involved areas, such as lymph glands. The goal is to irra-

 SAFETY PRECAUTIONS

Nurses who care for a child receiving implant radiation need to wear a dosimeter film badge at all times.

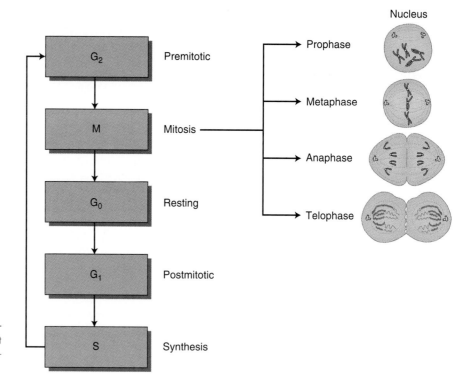

FIGURE 14-4. Chemotherapy drugs either act at specific parts of the cell cycle or are non-specific for action (act throughout all phases).

diate the tumor but not healthy adjacent tissue. The total dose of radiation is divided (or fractionated) and given over several weeks. A common course of radiation treatment might be once daily 4 or 5 days per week for a period of 2–6 weeks.

Tumors that are highly sensitive to radiation include Hodgkin's disease, Wilms' tumor, retinoblastoma, and rhabdomyosarcoma. Tumors that have a low sensitivity to radiation, such as osteosarcoma and soft tissue sarcomas require higher doses of radiation.

Biotherapy

Biotherapy is the use of biologic response modifiers, such as interleukins, interferons, or radiolabeled monoclonal antibodies, to treat cancer.[6] There are three major classes of biologic response modifiers: (1) agents that restore, augment, or modulate the host's immunologic mechanisms, (2) agents that have direct antitumor activity, and (3) agents that have other biologic effects. The actions of many of these agents are not completely understood, and some agents have more than one effect. For example, interferon has both antiviral and antiproliferative effects on some malignant cells. Interferon and tumor necrosis factor are undergoing clinical trials to study their effectiveness and to develop protocols for their safe use against selected cancers.

Bone Marrow Transplantation

Bone marrow transplantation is used to treat leukemia, neuroblastoma, and some noncancerous conditions, such as aplastic anemia. The goal of therapy is to administer a lethal dose of chemotherapy and radiation that will kill the cancer, and then to resupply the body with bone marrow stem cells either from the child's own marrow previously removed and stored or from a compatible donor.

⚖ LEGAL & ETHICAL CONSIDERATIONS

Consent by parents is mandatory if a child is to be started on a medication that is considered a clinical trial drug. Children who are cognitively able should give assent verbally or in writing. This consent can usually be obtained from children by the age of 7–9 years, depending on the child's level of understanding.

14-3   Some Commonly Used Chemotherapy Drug Combinations

Acronym	Drug Combination
A-COPP	doxorubicin + cyclophosphamide + vincristine (oncovin) + procarbazine + prednisone
ABVD	doxorubicin + bleomycin + vinblastine + dacarbazine
ACE	doxorubicin + cyclophosphamide + etoposide
APE	doxorubicin + procarbazine + etoposide
CAF	cyclophosphamide + doxorubicin + fluorouracil
CAMP	cyclophosphamide + doxorubicin + methotrexate + procarbazine
CAVe	lomustine + doxorubicin + vinblastine
CAVE or ECHO or CAPO or EVAC or VOCA	etoposide + cyclophosphamide + doxorubicin + vincristine
CHOP	cyclophosphamide + doxorubicin + vincristine + prednisone
CHOR	cyclophosphamide + doxorubicin + vincristine
CISCA	cisplatin + cyclophosphamide
CMF	cyclophosphamide + methotrexate + fluorouracil
COPP	cyclophosphamide + vincristine + procarbazine + prednisone
CY-VA-DIC	cyclophosphamide + vincristine + doxorubicin + dacarbazine
FAC	fluorouracil + doxorubicin + cyclophosphamide
MACC	methotrexate + doxorubicin + cyclophosphamide + lomustine
MOPP	mechlorethamine + vincristine + procarbazine + prednisone
MTX + MP + CTX	methotrexate + mercaptopurine + cyclophosphamide
PVB or VBP	vinblastine + bleomycin + cisplatin
T-2	dactinomycin + doxorubicin + vincristine + cyclophosphamide
VAP	vincristine + dactinomycin + cyclophosphamide
VP-L-asparaginase	vincristine + prednisone + L-asparaginase

From Bindler, R.M., & Howry, L.B. (1997). Pediatric drugs and nursing implications (2nd ed., pp. 579–580). Stamford, CT: Appleton & Lange.

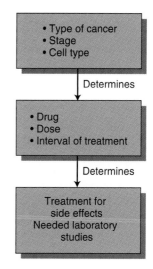

Protocol = Map or plan of action

- Type of cancer
- Stage
- Cell type

Determines

- Drug
- Dose
- Interval of treatment

Determines

Treatment for side effects
Needed laboratory studies

FIGURE 14–5. Chemotherapy protocol. A protocol is a map or plan of action that directs therapy by identifying the drug and its accompanying treatment.

Bone marrow transplantation is the treatment of choice when a relapse occurs while the child is receiving another form of cancer therapy. First, a histocompatible donor must be located. The child then receives intensive chemotherapy, often followed by total body irradiation. This treatment kills all circulating blood cells and bone marrow contents. Following this treatment, the child is transfused with the donor bone marrow. New blood cells usually form within 6–8 weeks. (See Chapter 13 for a description of care for the child undergoing bone marrow transplantation.)

Oncologic Emergencies
Oncologic emergencies can be organized into three groups: metabolic, hematologic, and those involving space-occupying lesions.

Metabolic Emergencies. Metabolic emergencies result from the lysis (dissolving or decomposing) of tumor cells, a process called tumor lysis syndrome. This cell destruction releases high levels of uric acid, potassium,

TYPES OF BONE MARROW TRANSPLANT

Allogenic: Donor and recipient are of same species
Autologous: Donor and recipient are the same person
Isogenic or syngeneic: Donor and recipient are genetically the same

 LEGAL & ETHICAL CONSIDERATIONS

A child advocate whose role is to objectively safeguard the rights and needs of a minor child involved in decisions about bone marrow harvest is frequently a part of the bone marrow transplant team.

14-4	Tumor Lysis Syndrome

Laboratory Evaluation

CBC

Serum sodium, potassium, chloride, bicarbonate, calcium, phosphorus, uric acid, BUN, creatinine, magnesium

Urinalysis

ECG if potassium is > 7 mEq/L

Management

Hydration to maintain urine specific gravity < 1.010

Alkalinization with drugs and intravenous fluids to keep urine pH between 7 and 7.5

Diuretics

Phosphate reduction with aluminum hydroxide

NURSING ALERT

Watch for signs of septic shock: hyperthermia or hypothermia, tachycardia, tachypnea, hypotension, mental changes, and peripheral cyanosis or coolness.

---

phosphates, and calcium into the blood and can lower serum sodium levels. This syndrome is seen most commonly in children with Burkitt's lymphoma and acute lymphocytic leukemia.[7] Table 14–4 presents laboratory tests and management of tumor lysis syndrome.

A second type of metabolic emergency is septic shock. Have you seen that term used in reference to oncologic emergencies? During periods of immune suppression the child is vulnerable to overwhelming infection, resulting in circulatory failure, inadequate tissue perfusion, and hypotension. Septic shock can be fatal (see Chapter 12 for a description of septic shock). Factors contributing to massive infection include inadequate neutrophil production, abnormal granulocytes (not able to be actively phagocytic), erosions through normal barriers such as blood vessels and mucous membranes, and altered bone marrow production caused by chemotherapy and some forms of radiation. Such infections must be vigorously treated with antimicrobial therapy and hydration management.

A third type of metabolic emergency occurs when large amounts of bone are destroyed by treatment, resulting in hypercalcemia (elevated calcium in the serum). Hypercalcemia is most common in children with acute lymphocytic leukemia and rhabdomyosarcoma. Treatment includes hydration and adequate intake of phosphate by oral supplement.

Hematologic Emergencies. Hematologic emergencies result from bone marrow suppression or infiltration of brain and respiratory tissue with high numbers of leukemic blast cells (hyperleukocytosis). Bone marrow suppression results in anemia and thrombocytopenia with resultant hemmorhage. Gastrointestinal and central nervous system bleeding (strokes) are common.

Treatment involves infusion of packed red blood cells for anemia; and platelet transfusion, vitamin K, and fresh frozen plasma for thrombocytopenia and hemorrhage. Hyperleukocytosis is treated by hydration, bicarbonate infusion, and allopurinol.[7]

Space-occupying Lesions. Extensive tumor growth may result in spinal cord compression, increased intracranial pressure, brain herniation, seizures, massive hepatomegaly, and superior vena cava syndrome (obstruction of the superior vena cava by tumor). These emergencies are often caused by neuroblastoma, medulloblastoma, astrocytoma, Hodgkin's disease, or lymphoma. After biopsy of the mass, treatment involves radiation therapy, chemotherapy, and corticosteroids.

Nursing Assessment

Physiologic Assessment

Physiologic assessment focuses on identifying the signs and symptoms of cancer and ongoing assessment of the side effects of treatment (see the discussion of side effects under Nursing Managment). Assessment of children with the most significant types of childhood cancers is presented later in the chapter.

Height and weight of any child who has had cancer should be carefully measured. Observe gait and coordination. Periodic laboratory studies will be performed.

Psychosocial Assessment

Assessment of body image, stress and coping abilities, knowledge of the condition and cognitive level, support systems, and developmental level provides data that helps determine the appropriate nursing interventions for the child with cancer and the family.

Body Image. Hair loss, surgical scars, and cushingoid changes are three common treatment-induced threats to body image. Most children being treated for cancer experience hair loss (Fig. 14–6). Children who have cranial surgery lose hair as part of the surgical preparation. Chemotherapy frequently results in some degree of hair loss. The speed of hair loss is unique to the child and can be as rapid as overnight or slower, evidenced by hair left on the pillow and in the hairbrush.

A second challenge to the child's body image is surgery. The scars of cranial and neck surgery are obvious, as are amputation and limb salvaging. Abdominal surgery for lymphoma is more easily concealed but is still a threat to the child's body image.

A third source of altered body image is the cushingoid features such as round and flushed face, prominent cheeks, double chin, and generalized obesity (Fig. 14–7) that result from the use of corticosteroids. As the

GROWTH & DEVELOPMENT CONSIDERATIONS

Children of different ages experience differing threats to body image as a result of cancer treatment. A preschool girl may be most upset at hair loss, since she now looks like a boy. A school-age child has the most difficult time with changes that interfere with the developmental task of industry. Amputation, which decreases the child's ability to participate in activities such as sports, dancing, and school work, can be a major challenge during the school-age years. Teenagers are often most worried about changes like hair loss and cushingoid features, which cause them to look different from peers.

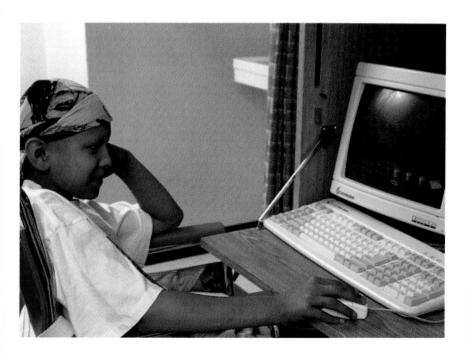

FIGURE 14–6. One of the most common threats to a child's body image at any age is hair loss induced by chemotherapy.

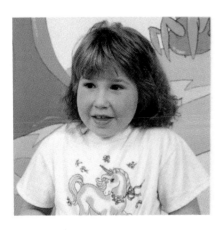

FIGURE 14–7. The child with cushingoid changes frequently has a rounded face and prominent cheeks.

child's weight increases, stretch marks similar txo those of pregnancy may occur. These stretch marks often remain after the corticosteroids are decreased.

Body image disturbances occur when a child cannot integrate changes and continues to cling to old images despite their inconsistency with reality. Common means for assessing body image are drawings, colored pictures cut out by the child to form a collage, discussion, and observation. See Chapter 4 for further discussion of these and other assessment techniques that can be used with children.

Stress and Coping. The diagnosis of cancer is a major stressor for both the child and the family. Although each child's prognosis and each family's coping mechanisms are unique, most families deal with the diagnosis in a manner similar to that of other families who have a child with a life-threatening illness (see Chap. 6). Assess the family (and child if old enough) for their understanding and acceptance of the diagnosis. Assess the level of anxiety during health care visits and scheduled treatments (Fig. 14–8). Evaluate the family's methods of coping, such as the ability to integrate relaxing and meaningful activities into family life, the use of support systems in the community and extended family, and the ability to alter expectations to take into account the child's health status. Concurrent stressors increase the family's difficulty in coping with childhood cancer. Evaluate the family for stressors such as illness or death of another family member, occupational changes, financial problems, relocation, and change in vacation plans.

Knowledge and Cognition. People who are anxious tend to narrow their scope of attention and may read unintended messages into the behaviors of health care personnel. Anxiety also limits a person's ability to retain information.[8]

The child's knowledge of cancer and its treatment should be assessed throughout the treatment period. As the child matures cognitively, new evaluations of knowledge are needed. Cancer and its treatment are complex topics and parents are exposed to information in various forms, including written material, news reports, and Internet web sites and re-

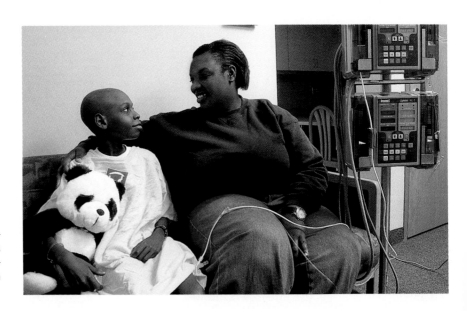

FIGURE 14–8. The child with cancer depends on parents and family members to provide support. Nurses can assist families to draw upon their strengths to help the child.

sources. Evaluate their knowledge and provide an opportunity for them to ask questions.

Children who have received cranial radiation need regular scholastic evaluations. Memory deficits and selective attention deficits as well as decreased intelligence quotients may occur as long-term effects of treatment.[9]

Support Systems. Cancer treatment generally occurs over a long period of time. The extended family is crucial in providing necessary support to the child, parents, and siblings. Identify key persons in the family. They may be the parents, grandparents, or aunts and uncles. Thoroughly assess the coping strategies used by the family to meet the various challenges posed by the child's illness. This information helps to predict the success of interventions, such as home care with intravenous medications, and to decide when referrals for other supportive therapies are needed.

Assess family resources to identify support systems available to help the family during crises.[10] Extended supports include friends, jobs, insurance coverage, religious affiliations, cultural support systems, and the school system. Parents commonly lose contact with close friends following the diagnosis of cancer in a child. This is an additional stressor for the family. Jobs are often a source of support because co-workers may have gone through the same experience. It may also be comforting for a parent to return to a job where he or she can feel a sense of security in tangible accomplishments. However, jobs can also be a source of stress if employers are unsympathetic to the demands of the child's hospitalization and clinic or office visits.

Religious affiliations can be an important source of support. Evaluate whether such affiliations are meaningful for the family and, if so, plan for visits from the appropriate clergy. In some cultures, spiritual leaders are an important part of the family's support.

The return to school may pose difficulties for the child with cancer or it may be a source of support to be connected again to peers. The child is encouraged to go to school, even if only for half a day per week, to stay connected to peers. Evaluate the ability of the school to accept a medically vulnerable child into the classroom. Assess whether the other children and teachers have been prepared for the appearance and needs of the child with cancer. Arrangements can be made for tutors to help the child keep up with schoolwork if he or she cannot attend school.

Developmental Assessment

Developmental assessment of children under 6 years of age should be performed regularly during treatment for cancer. Assessment of the child's physical and neurologic development helps in determining the progress made during treatment and provides a baseline for evaluating the long-term effects of treatment. Children under 6 years of age who have cancer should receive regular developmental assessment (see Chap. 5).

Nursing Diagnosis

Children with cancer have a variety of common psychologic and physiologic problems, regardless of their specific type of cancer. They and their families are dealing with a complex illness that influences their lives for years. The impact of this experience extends into all areas of function.

The accompanying Nursing Care Plans include several diagnoses that may be appropriate for the child with cancer who is receiving care in the

COMMUNITY CARE CONSIDERATIONS

The child who is returning to school with a changed appearance from cancer treatment needs support and assistance. Discuss and role-play how the child can tell friends about the changes. A nurse or child life specialist can visit the child's class to explain what the child is experiencing. Offer to talk with the teacher to devise a plan for preparing classmates.

RESEARCH CONSIDERATIONS

The death of a child from cancer is a major traumatic event. Research shows that during the palliative care phase, when no further treatment is possible, the family's needs are to:
- Have the child recognized as special
- Experience care and connectedness with health care professionals
- Retain responsibility for the dying child[10]

hospital or at home. Among the many other diagnoses that may be appropriate for a child with cancer are the following:

- Diarrhea related to effects of medications and radiation
- Altered Urinary Elimination related to hydration status and elimination of products of cell death
- Altered Oral Mucous Membrane related to effects of chemotherapy and radiation
- Impaired Skin Integrity related to altered nutritional state, effects of medication, radiation, and immobility
- Ineffective Individual Coping related to effects of chronic or acute illness
- Sleep Pattern Disturbance related to diarrhea, nausea, stress, anxiety, and an unfamiliar environment
- Diversional Activity Deficit related to effects of chronic illness, frequent lengthy treatments, and isolation from peers
- Body Image Disturbance related to loss of body parts or change in appearance or function
- Knowledge Deficit (Child or Parents) related to disease or treatments
- Anticipatory Grieving related to actual or potential loss of significant other

Nursing Management

The nursing care of children newly diagnosed with cancer and their families includes immediate physiologic and psychologic support, along with anticipatory guidance about imminent and future medical interventions.

Nursing care of the hospitalized child with cancer and the child receiving ongoing therapy at home is summarized in the accompanying Nursing Care Plans. These care plans are designed for the child who is beyond the cancer diagnosis phase and is receiving chemotherapy.

Physiologic care of the hospitalized child focuses on providing support during treatment. This includes ensuring optimal nutritional intake, administering medications, managing the multiple side effects of chemotherapy and radiation, ensuring adequate hydration, preventing infection, and managing pain.

Ensure Optimal Nutritional Intake

The high metabolic rate of cancer growth depletes the child's nutritional stores. Added to this is the catabolic effect of chemotherapy and radiation on normal cells, necessitating additional cellular replacement. The child needs increased nutritional intake at a time when nausea and vomiting are occurring as drug side effects, and when decreased activity and general health status result in diminished appetite.

Administer antiemetic drugs to lessen nausea from chemotherapy. Offer frequent, small meals. It may be helpful to offer the child's favorite foods at times when nausea and vomiting are decreased. Perform 24-hour dietary recalls to assess the child's intake, and evaluate height and weight regularly. Special nutritional products may be given orally, nasogastric or nasoduodenal tube feedings may be given, or total parenteral nutrition may be necessary.

Administer Medications

One of the most important interventions of the oncology nurse is administering medications safely. Most chemotherapeutic drugs are prescribed and

NURSING CARE PLAN
HOSPITAL CARE OF THE CHILD WITH CANCER

GOAL	INTERVENTION	RATIONALE	EXPECTED OUTCOME

1. Pain related to disease process

The child will report reduced pain that is manageable.	• Give analgesics as ordered. • Teach relaxation techniques, deep breathing, and distraction.	• Adequate medications can reduce pain. • Nonpharmacologic methods work with the medication to reduce pain.	The child experiences pain reduced to the level that allows child to interact appropriately and gain rest.

2. Sleep Pattern Disturbance related to physical discomfort, stress, environmental changes, or inactivity

The child will sleep for hours appropriate to age. The child will report feeling rested.	• Alter the environment to allow designated rest periods. • Plan care to reduce frequency of interruptions during normal rest and sleep times.	• A quiet environment encourages relaxation needed for resting. • Reduced interruptions allow continuous sleep and rest.	The child rests and sleeps for an age-appropriate amount of time per day.

3. Altered Nutrition: Less Than Body Requirements related to oral cavity discomfort, altered taste sensation, anorexia, or emotional stress

The child will maintain adequate nutritional intake.	• Offer small feedings. Encourage favorite foods. Refer to dietitian for special meals. Weigh daily.	• Measures can increase caloric intake. Taste changes and mouth sores alter desire for food.	The child maintains admission weight.
The child will experience reduced effects of chemotherapy (ie, nausea and vomiting).	• Teach the child distraction and relaxation techniques. Give antiemetics according to orders.	• Pharmacologic and nonpharmacologic methods are effective in helping to reduce nausea.	The child has minimal side effects of nausea and vomiting.

4. Constipation related to low-roughage diet, low fluid intake, decreased activity level, or absence of routine

The child will reestablish normal bowel pattern.	• Record all output by size and description. Administer stool softeners. Test stool for guaiac. Report changes in stool to physician. Encourage adequate fluid intake.	• Chemotherapy or tumor may create constipation, diarrhea, or blood in stool.	The child has normal bowel pattern.

Continued . . .

NURSING CARE PLAN
HOSPITAL CARE OF THE CHILD WITH CANCER– *Continued*

GOAL	INTERVENTION	RATIONALE	EXPECTED OUTCOME

5. Fluid Volume Excess or Deficit related to dietary alterations, and chemotherapy effects

The child will be adequately hydrated.	• Record all intake. Monitor intravenous rate and solution as appropriate.	• Some drugs (eg, cyclophosphamide) necessitate a high level of fluid intake to prevent complications.	The child demonstrates adequate hydration. Mucous membranes are hydrated.
	• Test specific gravity of urine daily.	• Renal function may be affected by chemotherapy.	Specific gravity remains within normal range.

6. Risk for Infection related to immunosuppression, invasive procedures, malnutrition, or pharmaceutical agents

The child will remain free of infection.	• Wash hands often. Maintain in isolation if needed.	• Handwashing is effective in killing organisms.	The child remains infection free.
	• Monitor temperature. Report elevation to physician.	• Elevated temperature is a sign of infection.	
The child will return to normal, uninfected state.	• Administer intravenous antibiotics as ordered. Monitor temperature. Use cooling mattress as ordered. Report elevations over 38°C (101°F) to physician.	• Multiple antibiotics are needed to deal with bacterial and fungal infections during neutropenia. Blood cultures may be taken to identify organism.	The child with an infection is effectively treated.

7. Impaired Physical Mobility related to neuromuscular impairment

The child experiences minimal neuromuscular complications.	• Observe for changes in level of consciousness, seizure activity, and changes in gait.	• Tumors and chemotherapy can create changes in neurologic status.	The child maintains neuromuscular capabilities.

8. Ineffective Individual Coping related to changes in body integrity, disruption of emotional bonds, or inadequate support systems

The child will demonstrate normal adaptive coping methods.	• Encourage drawings and other therapeutic play for expression of feelings. Allow for expression of angry feelings, such as hitting dolls and throwing sponge balls. Discuss how to behave during treatments.	• Expression of feelings helps identify avoidance coping for further intervention. Play is a normal way for child to express self and ideas. Misinterpretations can be corrected. Knowledge of appropriate and helpful behaviors supports self-esteem.	The child continues to use usual coping strategies expected for developmental stage.

NURSING CARE PLAN

HOSPITAL CARE OF THE CHILD WITH CANCER– *Continued*

GOAL	INTERVENTION	RATIONALE	EXPECTED OUTCOME
9. Altered Health Maintenance related to new or complex treatment, misinterpretation of information, or lack of education			
The child will state understanding of treatments and procedures.	• Use age-appropriate teaching methods. Content areas include child's cancer, medications (actions and side effects), how to deal with body changes, and how to deal with response of others to those changes. Correct misinterpretations. Anticipate upcoming events and teach the child and family about them.	• Education helps by increasing understanding, removing fantasy, and clarifying fears. Education promotes the use of new learning in all areas of life.	The child demonstrates age-appropriate knowledge of the cancer, its treatments, and medications. The child has age-appropriate understanding of how to deal with changes in the body.

NURSING CARE PLAN

HOME CARE OF THE CHILD WITH CANCER

GOAL	INTERVENTION	RATIONALE	EXPECTED OUTCOME
1. Risk for Infection related to immunosuppression, chemotherapy, and presence of invasive lines			
The child will remain infection free.	• Educate the child and parents about meaning of blood counts.	• Knowledgeable parents and child can protect themselves.	The child remains infection free.
	• Encourage parents/family members to use masks when they are ill.	• Masks help decrease airborne infection if used properly.	
	• Encourage good handwashing at all times.	• Handwashing is best prevention.	
	• Advise the child's teacher to tell parents if the child is exposed to communicable illness at school.	• Exposure can be reported to physician for possible use of acyclovir or admission for treatment.	All exposures are reported to physician immediately.
	• Clean vascular access site and inject heparin per protocol. Observe for signs of infection. Report infection to physician.	• Use of heparin maintains an open access route by preventing clotting.	

Continued . . .

NURSING CARE PLAN
HOME CARE OF THE CHILD WITH CANCER– *Continued*

GOAL	INTERVENTION	RATIONALE	EXPECTED OUTCOME

2. Altered Nutrition: Less Than Body Requirements related to hypermetabolic state and stomatitis

The child will maintain adequate nutritional intake.	• Encourage small and frequent meals. Encourage small bites of a variety of foods. • Promote good oral hygiene and use of nonalcohol mouth washes.	• Measures to increase caloric intake. Taste changes and favorite foods may no longer be preferred. • Mouth sores interrupt eating. Alcohol stings open sores.	The child maintains normal weight for height.

3. Pain related to cancer, diagnostic tests, trauma

The child will have reduced pain.	• Teach methods of distraction, relaxation, hypnotic trance, nonpharmacologic measures.	• Alteration of interpretation of pain signals allows rest.	The child's pain level is reduced to level that allows participation in activities of daily living and play.

4. Ineffective Management of Therapeutic Regimen related to increasing symptoms, side effects of therapy, complex therapy, knowledge deficit, concurrent stressors, and poor self-esteem

The child will comply with oral medication regimen.	• Educate parents and child about the importance of taking medication as prescribed. • Set up calendar with dates, times, and medications clearly labeled. • Reward the child for taking medications.	• Understanding can assist parents and child in placing importance on medication intake. • Visual reminders can help them recall instructions. • Reinforcing desired behaviors through rewards is effective with children.	The child takes all medications according to prescription.

5. Altered Growth and Development related to illness, pain, and hospitalizations

The child will demonstrate normal physical, emotional, and cognitive development.	• Encourage play appropriate to age. • Encourage the child to attend school. • Encourage seeing peers when unable to attend school. • Work with teachers to support reentry to school. Use puppets, videotape, and discussion with classmates.	• Normal activities support self-esteem and self-knowledge. • School is the work of the child and promotes cognitive and social growth. • Peer contacts help the child in normal developmental tasks. • Classmates need to understand what has happened to their friend without asking the child directly.	The child continues to develop physically, emotionally, and cognitively at a normal pace.

NURSING CARE PLAN
HOME CARE OF THE CHILD WITH CANCER– *Continued*

GOAL	INTERVENTION	RATIONALE	EXPECTED OUTCOME

6. Fatigue related to fever, anemia, and chemotherapy

The child will maintain energy levels necessary for normal activities.	• Problem-solve ways to save energy for play and school. • Plan with child for quiet activities during low-energy times.	• The child and parents are assisted to see school and play as important. • Child is empowered to select and plan own activities.	The child plans use of time effectively to maintain energy for school and play. The child conserves energy during times of increased fatigue.

7. Altered Family Processes related to illness of family member, time-consuming treatments, and separation

The child and family will demonstrate healthy adaptation.	• Encourage open communication. • Suggest that all family members develop support networks. • Parents should be proactive with siblings about their feelings and needs. • Encourage attendance of all family members at oncology camps.	• Open discussion allows problem solving and ego support. • Networks expand support systems. • Siblings feel valued and problems are confronted early. • Oncology camps promote open discussion between peers for further support and fun.	Parents report better communication between themselves and the children. Family members report an increase in friends with whom they can share feelings. Family reports attending oncology camp and describes benefit of sharing with other families in same situation.

calculated as dose per meter squared (dose/m^2), with m^2 calculated from the child's height and weight. (Refer to the section on administering medications in the *Quick Reference to Pediatric Clinical Skills* accompanying this text.)

A number of chemotherapeutic drugs are commonly used in combinations (see Table 14–3). These drugs are prepared with special techniques under laminar flow devices to minimize potential toxic effects on health care providers. Gloves and other hazardous drug protocols are used. Care must be taken to avoid **extravasation** of intravenous drugs (leakage into the soft tissue around the infusion site), as permanent tissue damage can result (Fig. 14–9).

In addition to chemotherapy drugs, the nurse administers other medications, such as antiemetics to control nausea, vitamin supplements, and antibiotics. These medications must be safely administered and the child monitored for side effects. **Polypharmacy** (the use of several drugs at one time to treat multiple health conditions) can lead to multiple side effects and can challenge the body's ability to metabolize and excrete drugs.

 SAFETY PRECAUTIONS

Health care professionals who have contact with chemotherapy drugs must follow careful guidelines. The Occupational Safety and Health Administration (OSHA) publishes an instruction manual entitled *Controlling Occupational Exposure to Hazardous Drugs*, which outlines general guidelines, protective equipment, and procedures (OSHA Instruction TED 1.15, Office of Science and Technology Assessment, Washington, DC, 1995).

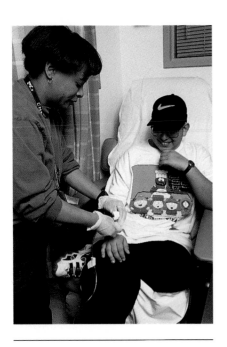

FIGURE 14–9. Chemotherapeutic drugs are given through intravenous infusion. Care should be taken to prevent leakage at the infusion site, since many drugs can cause blistering (extravasation).

NURSING ALERT

A treatment known as *leukovorin rescue* is used in conjunction with high-dose methotrexate chemotherapy. Leukovorin is a form of folic acid that helps to protect normal cells from the destructive action of methotrexate. It is started within 4 hours of methotrexate administration and is given along with hydration therapy.

Manage Treatment Side Effects

All cancer treatments affect some normal body cells as well as cancer cells, causing a wide variety of side effects (Table 14–5). A frequent occurrence is **myelosuppression,** or suppression of blood cell production in the bone marrow. Be alert for signs of a decreased white blood cell count, such as infections. Take the child's temperature, isolate the child from others with infections, and perform serum laboratory studies as ordered. A colony-stimulating factor for white cell production may be administered, if necessary.

Protect the child from bruises and be alert for signs of bleeding such as petechiae, an effect of decreased platelets. When thrombocytopenia occurs, minimize needle sticks and other intrusive procedures. Be ready to deal with nosebleeds and watch for bleeding gums. Report any bleeding episodes to the physician.

Inadequate red blood cell production can result in anemia. Encourage the child to eat iron-rich foods and administer nutritional supplements, as needed.

Chemotherapy affects all rapidly growing cells in the body, but especially those of the mucous membranes. Provide good oral hygiene with a soft toothbrush, foam wand, or water irrigation device. Report oral breakdown promptly. Be alert for blood in vomitus and stool, which can be indicators of bleeding in the gastrointestinal tract. Evaluate the effects of hair loss on the child.

Radiation can cause burns to the skin. Examine the skin daily during hospitalization or weekly when making home visits. Leave the marks on the skin that outline the radiation target area. Avoid use of lotions, powders, and soaps on the target skin area. Some children may need to be anesthetized to ensure correct positioning for radiation; post-anesthesia care will then be needed.

Ensure Adequate Hydration

Hydration management can be a challenge as the child may not be thirsty but is excreting large numbers of cell fragments and other substances as a result of treatment. Offer frequent small amounts of fluid. Include frozen ice pops or other fluid-containing foods such as Jell-O. Measure intake and output. To ensure adequate excretion, a number of chemotherapy drugs are given with intravenous fluids. It is important to administer fluids as ordered and ensure that the recommended urinary output excretion rate is maintained after drug administration.

Prevent Infection

Children with cancer have an altered immune system, both from the disease and from the effects of immunosuppressant drugs, and must be kept away from persons with known infections. Teach parents to avoid taking the child to places that attract large gatherings of people, such as department stores, once the child returns home. Emphasize the need to report any exposure to contagious diseases, especially chickenpox. Signs of infection may be masked by some drugs, so be alert for any signs of mild infection. Fever, malaise, and mild respiratory infection must all be reported promptly. Follow recommendations for the immunization of children with cancer as published by the Centers for Disease Control and Prevention and the American Academy of Pediatrics. Usually, no immunizations are given to the child until 6 months after he or she has stopped receiving chemotherapy.

Manage Pain

The child with cancer may experience pain from the disease itself and from the medical interventions, such as lumbar puncture, bone marrow aspiration, and frequent intravenous infusions and blood draws. Use all possible

14-5	Management of Common Side Effects of Chemotherapy

Side Effect	Medical Management	Nursing Interventions
Bone marrow suppression	Evidence of suppression usually appears 7–10 days after administration of chemotherapy; recovery is usually complete within 3–4 weeks Blood transfusions are administered when anemia is severe (Hgb < 7 g/dL) or platelets are < 30 Some institutions use a low-microbial diet to decrease the possibility that infectious organisms will colonize the intestine Septra is used for *Pneumocystis carinii* pneumonia prophylaxis; nystatin and oral vancomycin for antifungal and antibacterial prophylaxis	Instruct the family and child about the importance of protecting the body from bruising during periods of mild to moderate thrombocytopenia (platelet count < 5000/mm^3) Careful handwashing is essential Encourage use of masks if family or staff have nasopharyngeal infections
Nausea and vomiting	Symptoms may occur immediately or 5–6 hours after administration of chemotherapy and may last 48 hours Antiemetics, such as ondansetron, Kytril, Reglan, and Benadryl are used to treat this side effect	Teach relaxation techniques, hypnosis, and systematic desensitization (a hypnotic process that progressively reduces reactions to objects that cause strong emotional or physical responses) to help to decrease the child's symptoms Encourage mild exercise and change of diet (eating only easily digestible foods) 12 hours before chemotherapy
Anorexia and weight loss	May occur at any time; hyperalimentation is necessary if dietary changes are unsuccessful in halting the child's weight loss	Pay careful attention to changes in taste that affect food preferences Referral to a dietician may be helpful to achieve successful modification of the child's diet
Mouth sores	The oral mucositis resulting from chemotherapy usually occurs within 3–4 days and is often a contributing factor in anorexia Antifungal agents, such as nystatin or clotrimazole, lessen the possibility of candidal infection	Promote good oral hygiene, use soft foam wand or water irrigation to clean teeth; commercial mouth washes are not recommended because they contain alcohol and increase drying of the oral cavity
Constipation	Stool softeners and laxatives are used to treat this side effect	Advise parents to increase fluids and fibrous foods in the child's diet
Pain	Acetaminophen, morphine, steroids, nonsteroidal antiinflammatory drugs, and antidepressants may be used to manage pain	Careful pain assessment is important; the location of the pain may provide a clue to its cause, for example, metastasis to the skull, infiltration of joints, or damage to soft tissue; pain associated with chemotherapy may also be related to oral mucositis, myalgia, or tumor embolization; painful polyneuropathy can follow treatment with vincristine or cisplatin Acetaminophen for pain can mask the presence of fever, which signals infection; careful and complete physical assessment is needed to identify infection Pharmacologic, nonhypnotic (deep breathing, self-control), and hypnotic methods of pain control may be used; the nonpharmacologic methods often prove helpful to children with pain from multiple etiologies

pain management techniques to keep the child comfortable, as this will assist with comfort and encourage cooperation throughout the long treatment period. (See Chapter 7 for suggestions on methods of pain management.)

Conscious sedation (see Chap. 7) may be used for some procedures. Administer sedation as ordered for young children who are undergoing ra-

CLINICAL TIP

EMLA (eutectic mixture of local anesthetic) cream is a combination of lidocaine 2.5% and prilocaine 2.5% in an emulsion. Apply a thick layer of the cream to intact skin and cover with an occlusive dressing. Leave in place 1 hour for minor procedures and 2 hours for major procedures.

RESEARCH
CONSIDERATIONS

The most common unmet needs for parents when their child has cancer are:
• Financial assistance
• Time
• Rest
These needs were identified in a survey of parents of children with cancer who were receiving treatment both at a medical center and at home.[12]

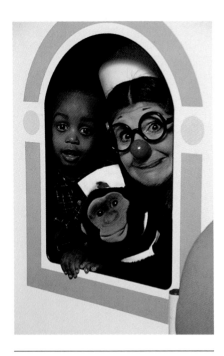

FIGURE 14–10. Clowns from the Big Apple Clown Care Unit can help to ease the stress of hospitalization for seriously ill children and their families. Here, a clown doctor and her puppet distract a toddler who is waiting for his clinic appointment.

diation. Coordinate other painful or intrusive tests so they can be done while the child is sedated for radiation.

Topical anesthetics such as EMLA cream may be used to numb the skin before an intravenous start, lumbar puncture, or bone marrow aspiration. Whenever possible, include the parents in comforting the child after painful procedures.

Provide Psychosocial Support

A diagnosis of cancer brings with it many emotions for the family. Initially parents experience shock and anger. They need basic information about the disease and the purpose of the tests that will be performed. Instructions often need to be repeated as parents may not process information the first time it is presented due to their increased stress levels. Assist the parents to plan how and when to tell the child the diagnosis. What the child needs to know is based on his or her developmental level and understanding.

Once the family has progressed from their initial state of shock about the diagnosis, they need to learn more about the disease. They may be interested in the pathophysiology, treatment, and expected outcome or the prognosis. Clarify their understanding of these areas and ask what questions they have. Provide verbal explanations and written material. Parents may talk with friends, purchase books, or search the Internet for information. Find out where they are getting information and provide additional resources when appropriate. Correct misconceptions and misinformation.

The family needs many strategies to deal with the challenge of long-term treatment for cancer. As the child experiences remissions and exacerbations or complications, the family feels alternately hopeful and discouraged. This was the case with Rasheed's family at the beginning of the chapter. Identify the family's support systems and intervene as needed to enhance these systems. Ask about extended family members who might be of help, religious or spiritual connections that can be facilitated, financial concerns, and use of social service agencies.

The child undergoing treatment for cancer needs support appropriate to his or her developmental stage and cognitive level (Fig. 14–10). (See Chapters 2 and 4 for developmental levels and effective support strategies for children of different ages.) Younger children primarily need support during painful procedures and separation from parents. Older children need intervention strategies to assist in working through feelings related to treatments (Fig 14–11). A major developmental task of adolescence is to attain independence and control, but cancer often interferes with adolescents' ability to achieve this task. Therefore, plan nursing strategies that empower adolescents as much as possible.

Talk with the child's teachers before the return to school after treatment to explain the child's condition. Arrange for tutors if necessary to assist the child with school work during hospitalization and home care. Explore the option of summer camp for children with cancer. The Make-a-Wish Foundation strives to make dreams come true for ill children by sponsoring them for a desired activity or outing (see Appendix F). Refer the child to this foundation if appropriate.

The siblings of a child who has cancer can be stressed by the changes in the family. They may grieve over the ill brother or sister and may feel sad and depressed. They also can experience anger, guilt, or resentment and may have a lack of knowledge about the disease and treatment. Inquire about siblings and ask what they know about the child's condition. Find out who is caring for siblings and whether their teachers have been informed about the family situation. Include siblings in care when possible. Invite

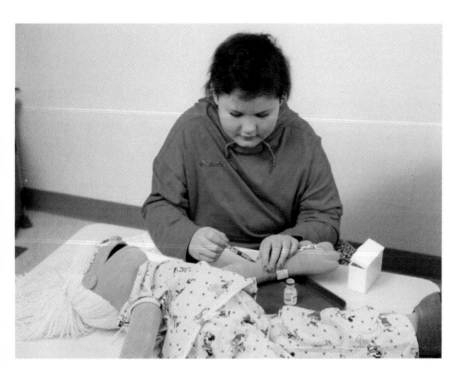

FIGURE 14–11. A child in a pediatric oncology clinic giving injections to a doll. This type of play therapy helps the child deal with fear and thus lowers his or her stress level.

them to visit and to participate both during hospitalization and at home care visits. They can be involved in play therapy sessions and recreational activities with the ill child. Ask the parents if the siblings are demonstrating symptoms such as depression, behavioral changes, or decrease in school performance and suggest interventions as appropriate. They may benefit from speaking with a school counselor or can be referred to a support group for siblings of children with cancer. Some cancer summer camps welcome siblings as well as children with cancer.

The family of a child with cancer is faced with a life-threatening illness. Refer to Chapter 6 for strategies to assist the family in coping with this stressor. For some types of cancer, the child may experience a remission with treatment, but a recurrence of disease later as cancer cells grow again. The family may become angry or depressed about the relapse. Repeated treatments challenge the family's support systems. Waiting for the outcome of diagnostic tests can be an especially challenging time. Provide information as soon as possible. If the child's illness progresses, refer the family to hospice to assist them in caring for the terminally ill child and in working through the grieving process. See Appendix F for support groups and information related to cancer.

Discharge Planning and Home Care Teaching

Preparation for home care centers on creating a normal environment while supporting the child's physiologic and psychosocial responses to the cancer and treatments. Education is the primary focus of discharge planning. Teach the parents how to ensure adequate nutritional intake, to be alert for signs of infection, to protect the child from exposure to communicable diseases during times of neutropenia, to administer medications at home, as well as methods to handle vomiting and pain. Assist the parents and child to deal with any obstacles to normal development and functioning. Teach the parents and family about symptoms that need to be treated immediately (Table 14–6).

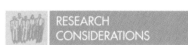

RESEARCH CONSIDERATIONS

Research has shown that two of the worst stressors for adolescents with cancer are (1) waiting for care and (2) dependence on parents. Nurses can devise interventions to minimize waiting for chemotherapy and other treatments or provide options such as meetings with other teens and computer use while waiting. Whenever possible, enable the adolescent to make choices independently of parents.[11]

14-6	Parent and Family Teaching: Reportable Events for Children Receiving Chemotherapy

Report the following events to your child's oncologist if they occur while the child is receiving chemotherapy:

- Temperature above 38°C (101°F)
- Any bleeding, such as nosebleeds, blood in stool or urine, petechiae, bruising
- Pain or discomfort with urination or defecation
- Sores in the mouth
- Vomiting or diarrhea
- Persistent pain anywhere, including headache
- Signs of infection, such as cough, fever, runny nose, tugging at ears
- Signs of infection in central lines, such as redness, drainage, or tenderness
- Exposure to communicable diseases, especially varicella (chickenpox)

Inform dentists and other health care providers that the child is receiving chemotherapy prior to procedures. Prophylactic antibiotics should be given before and after dental care.

Adapted from Bindler, R.M., & Howry, L.B. (1997). Pediatric drugs and nursing implications (2nd ed., p. 587). Stamford, CT: Appleton & Lange.

GROWTH & DEVELOPMENT CONSIDERATIONS

An adolescent can decide which type of medication port would be best (eg, an implantable port under the skin or a venous access device with tubing outside the body). This enables the teen to feel more in control of the disease and treatment.

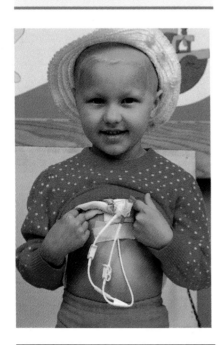

FIGURE 14–12. A vascular access device allows chemotherapeutic agents to be administered without the need for repeated "sticks" to the child.

Home management of a vascular access device or central line, such as a Broviac catheter (refer to the *Quick Reference to Pediatric Clinical Skills* accompanying this text), is an initial challenge for parents (Fig. 14–12). An implanted port may be used and allows the child freedom to swim and engage in other activities. Parents will need information about whatever device the child has received. Details about cleaning the site, instilling heparin in the line or reservoir, and other needed care are demonstrated. After teaching the parents, observe them performing the procedure before the child is discharged.

Emphasize the need for the child and family to have fun and be as normal as possible. Play distracts the child and is essential in reducing fears. Children, parents, and siblings often benefit from participation in cancer support groups and cancer summer camps. These activities create additional support systems, build the child's self-esteem, and enhance coping skills through role modeling.

Make home visits to evaluate the family's strengths and needs. Be sure that the family has adequate support from a hospice when the child's condition is terminal.

► BRAIN TUMORS

Central nervous system or brain tumors are the most commonly occurring solid tumors in children and the second most common malignancies in children, after leukemia. Each year approximately 2000 children under the age of 15 years are diagnosed with tumors of the brain and central nervous system, accounting for one in five childhood cancers.[13] Brain tumors in children usually occur below the roof of the cerebellum and involve the cerebellum, midbrain, and brainstem (Fig. 14–13). In contrast, brain tumors in adults are usually located above the areas between the cerebrum and cerebellum.

The most common brain tumors in children are medulloblastoma, cerebral and cerebellar astrocytoma, ependymoma, and brainstem glioma.

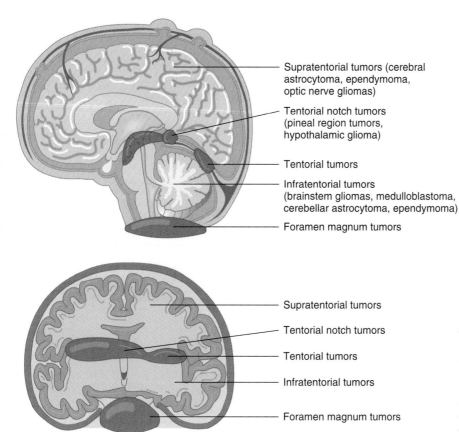

Supratentorial tumors (cerebral astrocytoma, ependymoma, optic nerve gliomas)

Tentorial notch tumors (pineal region tumors, hypothalamic glioma)

Tentorial tumors

Infratentorial tumors (brainstem gliomas, medulloblastoma, cerebellar astrocytoma, ependymoma)

Foramen magnum tumors

Supratentorial tumors

Tentorial notch tumors

Tentorial tumors

Infratentorial tumors

Foramen magnum tumors

FIGURE 14–13. Sites of brain tumors in children. Approximately 2000 children under the age of 15 years are diagnosed annually as having tumors of the brain and central nervous system. The four most common brain tumors in children are medulloblastoma, cerebral astrocytoma, ependymoma, and brainstem glioma.

Less common are supratentorial embryonal tumors and craniopharyngioma.

Clinical Manifestations and Pathophysiology

Medulloblastomas are brain tumors in the external layer of the cerebellum. They account for 20% of childhood brain tumors, and commonly occur in children aged 5–6 years.[13] Common presenting symptoms are headache, vomiting, and ataxia.

Astrocytomas arise from glial cells and can be either above or below the area between the cerebrum and cerebellum. They comprise 40% of childhood brain tumors.[13] The symptoms include seizures, visual disturbances, or symptoms of increased intracranial pressure.

Ependymomas commonly occur in the fourth ventricle of the posterior fossa and comprise 8% of childhood brain tumors. They may obstruct cerebrospinal fluid flow and cause hydrocephalus.

Brainstem gliomas are located in the pons and typically spread into the surrounding tissue. They account for 8% of childhood brain tumors.[13] Children with brainstem gliomas have symptoms of cranial nerve and long tract (motor nerve) compression. Symptoms may include ataxia, unilateral paralysis of cranial nerves VI and VII, and vertical nystagmus.

Diagnostic Tests and Medical Management

Brain tumors are commonly diagnosed by means of computed tomography (CT; Fig. 14–14A), magnetic resonance imaging (MRI; Fig. 14–14B), myelography, and angiography. Neurophysiologic tests (electroencephalography and brainstem evoked potentials) are used to assess sensory pathway

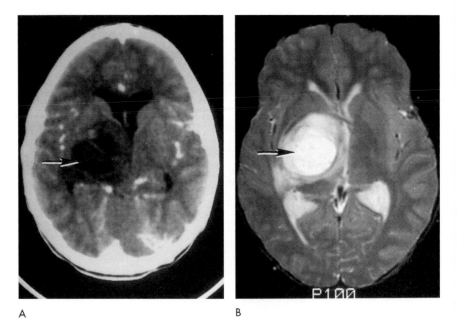

FIGURE 14–14. Radiologic imaging of a child with a brain tumor. **A,** CT scan. **B,** MRI. *Courtesy of Carlos Sivit, M.D., Children's National Medical Center, Washington, DC.*

A   B

integrity and disease- or drug-related sensory dysfunction. Other tests that may be performed are use of tumor markers and cerebrospinal fluid cytology. Lumbar puncture is used to identify abnormal cells in the cerebrospinal fluid. Bone marrow aspiration identifies any extracranial primary neoplastic growth, since cancers in other sites can metastasize to the brain.

Treatment depends on the type of brain tumor (Table 14–7). Surgery is a common treatment for brain tumors. Surgery may be performed to ob-

14-7	Comparison of Brain Tumors		
Tumor	Site	Presenting Symptoms	Medical Management
Medullo-blastoma	External layer of cerebellum	Headache, vomiting ataxia	Surgery; chemotherapy with lomustine, vincristine, prednisone, cisplatin, radiation
Astrocytomas	Glial cells, supra-tentorial or infra-tentorial	Seizures, visual disturbances, increased intracranial pressure, vomiting	Surgery; chemotherapy with vincristine, dactinomycin; radiation
Ependymoma	Fourth ventricle, posterior fossa	Hydrocephalus	Surgery, radiation
Brainstem gliomas	Pons	Cranial nerve tract signs	Surgery, radiation

tain a biopsy specimen, to debulk (reduce the tumor by partial removal) or excise the tumor, or to treat any hydrocephalus that may be present. During surgery, radiology images allow the neurosurgeon to see computerized images of the brain while at the same time stimulating nerves to determine their functioning. These techniques provide rapid feedback to the neurosurgeon. Laser surgery, which has delicate precise control and accuracy, is used when tumors are close to sensitive neural or vascular structures.

Use of radiation following surgery and chemotherapy has improved the survival of children with medulloblastoma and ependymoma. High-dose chemotherapy is often used, and this modality is improving the survival of children with central nervous system tumors.[14] Intrathecal administration of chemotherapy is useful in some cases. However, the blood–brain barrier is a factor in the effectiveness of chemotherapy for children with brain tumors. For example, when methotrexate is administered intrathecally (in the spinal canal), only a small amount crosses normal brain capillaries. Radiation is not used in children under 3 years because of resultant damage to brain cells. Bone marrow transplantation is a treatment option for some children.

Complications of treatment for children with brain tumors are significant. They include severe infections (associated with high-dose chemotherapy), seizure activity, sensorimotor defects, hydrocephalus, and growth problems. Care is taken to treat infections early and aggressively. Anticonvulsants are commonly given prophylactically following surgery.[14] Endocrine problems, such as growth hormone changes, hypothyroidism, and panhypopituitarism, may occur when the tumor is in the hypothalamic–pituitary area.[15] Treatment may also lead to a decrease in the intelligence quotient and frank mental retardation in some children. Memory deficits and selective attention deficits are the most common problems. Up to 68% of children younger than 6 years of age have intellectual deterioration.

Diabetes insipidus is a special consideration in children with midline brain tumors, such as those that compress the hypothalamus, pituitary stalk, or posterior pituitary gland. Manifestations of diabetes insipidus include voiding of large amounts of dilute urine with a specific gravity of less than 1.005.

Nursing Assessment

The focus of physiologic assessment of the child with a brain tumor is determined by the clinical manifestations (Table 14–8). Presenting signs can be categorized as follows:

- Nonspecific signs related to increasing intracranial pressure
- Secondary signs related to displacement of intracranial structures
- Focal signs suggesting direct involvement of the brain and cranial nerves

Thorough neurologic examination before surgery is essential to provide a record of baseline functioning. The neurologic examination also allows the evaluation of the child's changing physiologic status before surgery. Ask if the child has manifested slow changes over time or has had quickly developing symptoms. Measurement of head circumference and assessment of the anterior fontanel are necessary in children under the age of 18 months.[15]

Perform developmental screening on young children using the Denver II or other developmental test (see Chap. 5). Ask about the child's social interactions, school performance, and any behavior changes that have occurred.

NURSING ALERT

Some children with brain tumors have nonspecific signs. They may have a slight behavior change, perform poorly at school, or show some incoordination. Be alert to such signs and to the parents' report that they notice a change in the child. Report such findings so appropriate assessments can be made.

14-8	Physiologic Assessment of Brain Tumors

Clinical Manifestations	Assessment
Nonspecific signs: headache, morning vomiting, somnolence, irritability	Level of consciousness, pupil response, pupil shape and size
Secondary signs: disturbances of cranial nerves; other signs depend on site of tumor	All cranial nerves
Focal signs: truncal ataxia (midline brain tumors), general nystagmus, head tilting	Motor ability, head positions when watching television or looking at people (double vision, sixth cranial nerve involvement)

Nursing Diagnosis

Several nursing diagnoses can be identified for the child with a brain tumor, depending on the type and location of the tumor. Some common examples are:

- Altered Nutrition: Less Than Body Requirements related to disturbed appetite
- Impaired Physical Mobility related to tumor pressure on coordination centers
- Altered Growth and Development related to interference with normal developmental milestones
- Impaired Memory related to tumor pressure on brain memory sites
- Pain related to tumor pressure on nerve endings

Nursing Management

The child with a brain tumor requires multidisciplinary care by, among others, neurologist, neurosurgeon, pediatrician, dietician, and social worker. Other specialists are also often needed. The nurse can act as a case manager to coordinate the complex care needed by the child.[16]

For the nursing care of children immediately following surgery, refer to Chapter 4. In addition, close monitoring of neurologic status is needed postoperatively (refer to Chap. 18). Be especially alert for signs of increased intracranial pressure and infection. Observe for seizure activity. Administer drugs such as antibiotics and anticonvulsants as ordered.

Signs and symptoms of diabetes insipidus may occur following brain surgery (see Chap. 16 for a description of diabetes insipidus). Nursing care includes hourly measurement of intake and output, measurement of serum sodium levels every 4–6 hours, accurate fluid replacement, and frequent assessment of neurologic status. An indwelling urinary catheter is useful for accurate measurement of urinary output.

NURSING ALERT

Report abnormally high or low urinary output in the child after brain surgery. Either can be indicative of problems with management of urinary output.

Discharge Planning and Home Care Teaching

Teach the parents to watch for an increase in voiding of dilute urine. Be sure they can recognize the signs of infection and changes in the child's neurologic status. Once the child is ready for discharge, chemotherapy or radiation may begin; inform parents of the reason and potential side effects of these treatments. Assist the family in obtaining any special equipment they may need to care for the child at home, such as a wheelchair, bed rails, or dressings. The American Cancer Society is a potential resource for assistance with these needs (see Appendix F).

Children with brain tumors, especially those who have received radiation, are likely to have some permanent sequelae. They may have slowed development, incoordination, learning disabilities, or other effects. These sequelae are most common in children who are 3 years of age or younger at the time of radiation therapy. Perform accurate height and weight measures at each health care visit. Assess developmental milestones. Ask about progress in school and any special services that might be needed. Peform thorough neurologic assessments.

► NEUROBLASTOMA

Neuroblastoma is the solid tumor most commonly occurring outside the cranium of children. It is responsible for 8% of childhood cancers and 15% of cancer deaths in children. The average age at onset is 22 months. Prognosis varies, depending on the staging of the tumor (Table 14–9) and the age of the child, with more favorable outcomes in infants under 1 year of age.[17]

Neuroblastoma is commonly a smooth, hard, nontender mass that can occur anywhere along the sympathetic nervous system chain. A frequent

14-9	International Neuroblastoma Staging System

Stage	Description
1	Localized tumor confined to the area of origin; complete gross excision, with or without microscopic residual disease; identifiable ipsilateral and contralateral lymph nodes negative microscopically
2A	Unilateral tumor with incomplete gross excision; identifiable ipsilateral and contralateral lymph nodes negative microscopically
2B	Unilateral tumor with complete or incomplete gross excision; with positive ipsilateral regional lymph nodes; identifiable contralateral lymph nodes negative microscopically
3	Tumor infiltrating across the midline with or without regional lymph node involvement; or unilateral tumor with contralateral regional lymph node involvement; or midline tumor with bilateral regional lymph node involvement
4	Dissemination of tumor to distant lymph nodes, bone, bone marrow, liver, and/or other organs (except as defined in stage 4S)
4S	Localized primary tumor as defined for stage 1 or 2 with dissemination limited to liver, skin, and/or bone marrow

From Castleberry, R.P. (1997). Biology and treatment of neuroblastoma. Pediatric Clinics of North America, 44(4), 926; Brodeur, F.M., Pritchard, J., & Berthold, F. (1993). Revisions in the international criteria for neuroblastoma diagnosis, staging, and response to treatment. Journal of Clinical Oncology, 11, 1466; and Brodeur, G.M., Seeger, R.C., & Barrett, A. (1988). International criteria for diagnosis, staging and response to treatment in patients with neuroblastoma. Journal of Clinical Oncology, 6, 1874.

location is the abdomen, although other sites are the adrenal, thoracic, and cervical areas. It is usually diagnosed in children under 5 years of age, with the median age at diagnosis being 2 years.

Clinical Manifestations

The location of the mass determines the symptoms. Altered bowel and bladder function occur when the mass is retroperitoneal; characteristic signs are weight loss, abdominal fullness, irritability, fatigue, and fever. Dyspnea or infection may occur when the tumor is mediastinal. Neck and facial edema may result from vena cava syndrome if the tumor is mediastinal and large. Malaise, fever, and a limp can occur if there has been metastasis to the bone.[17]

Etiology and Pathophysiology

Neuroblastoma originates in primitive neurocrest cells that form the adrenal medulla, paraganglia, and sympathetic nervous system of the cervical sympathetic chain and the thoracic chain. Fifty percent of neuroblastomas develop in the adrenal medulla, 20% develop in the thorax, and the remaining 30% are elsewhere along the sympathetic chain.[18] Lymph node metastasis is common.

The cause of neuroblastoma is unknown. Theories that have been proposed center on the possible effects of environmental factors such as prenatal drug exposure from the mother and disturbed cellular nerve growth factors. Oncogenes are present in neuroblastoma cells in a DNA sequence known as N-*myc*. High levels of the N-*myc* oncogene are associated with rapid disease progression and a poorer prognosis.

Diagnostic Tests and Medical Management

The International Neuroblastoma Staging System (INSS) recommends different diagnostic and laboratory evaluations for diagnosis of the primary disease and of metastases (Table 14–10).

Vanillylmandelic acid (VMA) and homovanillic acid (HVA) levels are usually elevated in the urine and blood. They are used initially to diagnose the disease and later to follow its progress. Areas of necrosis and calcifica-

---

14-10	Diagnostic Tests for Neuroblastoma

Tests for initial diagnosis
Tumor tissue diagnosis by light microscopy, or
Biopsy of tumor cells plus laboratory evaluation showing increased urine or serum catecholamines (two separate measures each more than 3 standard deviations above the norm for age)

Tests for metastases
Bone marrow biopsy
Radiolabeled scanning with metaiodobenzylguanidine (MIBG)
Skeletal x-ray
CT or MRI of abdomen and liver
Chest x-ray, with added CT or MRI if x-ray shows lesions

tion are readily identifiable with radiologic tests. These tests also help in the staging of the disease by identifying metastases.

Routine blood cell counts may reveal anemia and thrombocytopenia (low platelet levels). There is no classic WBC response, although thrombocytopenia may occur in association with disseminated intravascular coagulation. **Leukocytosis** (higher than normal leukocyte count) and **leukopenia** (lower than normal leukocyte count) have been observed with bone marrow involvement.

The stage of the tumor (Table 14–9) determines the treatment protocol. Surgical excision of the mass is performed, followed by chemotherapy with a combination of drugs. Radiation was frequently used in the past but is now used only in certain stages of disease.[19] Bone marrow transplantation may be performed for advanced disease. Neuroblastoma is most responsive to treatment in children under 1 year of age.

Nursing Assessment

The presenting site of the tumor, such as the neck or abdomen, is assessed by observation and inspection. Palpation is contraindicated. Carefully document related functioning, such as bowel and bladder function. Take vital signs to watch for elevated temperature and vital sign changes caused by a thoracic mass. Observe gait and coordination. Take weight and height and compare to earlier percentiles for the child. Specific assessments during treatment will depend on the treatment methods used (refer to the earlier discussions of chemotherapy and radiation treatment). Psychosocial assessment and emotional assessment of the family are needed.

Nursing Diagnosis

A variety of nursing diagnoses may be appropriate for the child with neuroblastoma, depending on the location and extent of the presenting disease. Some common diagnoses might include:

- Impaired Gas Exchange related to tumor effects on respiratory system
- Impaired Physical Mobility related to tumor pressure on spine
- Sensory/Perceptual Alteration (Visual) related to ptosis and random eye movements caused by tumor presence
- Pain related to tumor pressure on nerve endings
- Anticipatory Grieving (Family) related to poor prognosis of a child with metastases

Nursing Management

The nursing management of the child with neuroblastoma can encompass the three phases of medical treatment: chemotherapy, surgery, and radiation. Specific postsurgical care depends on the size and site of the tumor. Normal postoperative care includes providing fluid support and respiratory care and preventing infection.

Nursing care during the chemotherapy phase includes minimizing side effects, preventing infection, teaching parents about the medications their child is receiving, and monitoring physical and emotional growth and development of the young child. When radiation is part of the treatment, use common nursing measures described earlier in the chapter.

Topics for parent and family teaching and discharge planning are presented in Table 14–11.

NEUROBLASTOMA: CHEMOTHERAPY DRUGS

Cyclophosphamide
Doxorubicin
Cisplatin
Ifosfamide
Teniposide
Etoposide
Carboplatin

CLINICAL TIP

Many centers give notebooks with information on chemotherapy and other relevant treatment methods to families shortly after diagnosis. Information that is pertinent to the child is highlighted during the teaching sessions. Blank pages are included to encourage parents to use the notebook for recording information, tests and results, and questions.

14-11	Parent and Family Teaching: The Child With a Neuroblastoma

Surgery Phase
- Teach the parents to observe for signs of infection at the wound site and to take the child's temperature, if necessary.
- Advise parents to note bowel movements and report a lack of one for 3 days to the physician.
- Continue with progression to a regular diet.

Chemotherapy Phase
- The child frequently has a central line placed early in the chemotherapy phase. The central line greatly reduces the emotional trauma associated with chemotherapy and blood tests.
  Teach the child how to help the parents with cleaning of the central line.
  Teach the child how to protect the central line.
  Teach the parents how to clean and dress the site of the central line.
  Have the parents practice central line care with a model and then on the child before discharge to increase the parents' confidence.
  Give the parents written and illustrated information about care of a central line.
  Arrange for home care dressing supplies before discharge.
- Give the parents detailed chemotherapy information.
- Refer the family to the American Cancer Society for coloring books for children receiving chemotherapy.
- Recommend the American Cancer Society as a resource for educational materials for the child.

▶ WILMS' TUMOR (NEPHROBLASTOMA)

Nephroblastoma, an intrarenal tumor that is called Wilms' tumor, is a common abdominal tumor of childhood and accounts for 6–7% of all childhood tumors.[20] Each year the incidence is 8.1 cases per million children. Wilms' tumor occurs most frequently between 2 and 5 years of age, but may also occur in adolescents and adults.

Clinical Manifestations

Wilms' tumor is usually an asymptomatic, firm, lobulated mass located to one side of the midline in the abdomen. Often a parent discovers the mass during the child's bath. Hypertension caused by increased renin activity related to renal damage is reported in 25% of cases. Hematuria is sometimes present. Bilateral Wilms' tumors occur in 5–10% of cases.[20]

Etiology and Pathophysiology

Wilms' tumor is associated with several congenital anomalies: aniridia (absence of the iris), hemihypertrophy (abnormal growth of one half of the body or a body structure), genitourinary anomalies, nevi, and hamartomas (benign, nodulelike growths). This connection suggests a genetic link. However, most children with Wilms' tumor have no other abnormalities. A tumor suppressor gene has been identified that acts to promote normal kidney development. This gene and others may be missing in children with Wilms' tumor.[20]

Diagnostic Tests and Medical Management

The diagnosis of Wilms' tumor is based on an ultrasound study of the abdomen and an intravenous pyelogram. CT scanning or MRI of the lungs, liver, spleen, and brain may be performed to identify any metastasis. This information is used in staging the tumor (Table 14–12). A complete blood count is obtained, as well as BUN and creatinine levels. Liver function tests are performed.

Treatment is multifaceted. Surgery is performed to remove the affected kidney, to examine the opposite kidney, and to look for other sites of metastasis. Chemotherapy or radiation therapy, alone or in combination, is sometimes used before surgery to reduce the size of the tumor. Radiation and/or chemotherapy may also follow surgery. Children whose tumors are almost completely excised and who have a favorable prognosis do not require irradiation of the tumor bed.

Long-term complications of treatment include liver damage, portal hypertension, and mild cirrhosis, which may occur in children treated for

WILMS' TUMOR: CHEMOTHERAPY DRUGS
Vincristine
Actinomycin D
Doxorubicin
Cyclophosphamide

14-12	National Wilms' Tumor Study Staging System

Stage	Description
I	The tumor is limited to the kidney and completely excised. The surface of the renal capsule is intact. The tumor is not ruptured before or during removal. No residual tumor is apparent beyond the margins of the excision.
II	The tumor extends beyond the kidney but is completely excised. Regional extension of the tumor is present, ie, penetration through the outer surface of the renal capsule into the perirenal soft tissues. Vessels outside the kidney substance are infiltrated or contain tumor thrombus. Biopsy may have been performed on the tumor, or local spillage of tumor confined to the flank has occurred. No residual tumor is apparent at or beyond the margin of excision.
III	Residual nonhematogenous tumor is confined to the abdomen. Any of the following may occur: Lymph nodes on biopsy are found to be involved in the hilus, the periaortic chains, or beyond. Diffuse peritoneal contamination by the tumor has occurred, such as by spillage of tumor beyond the flank before or during surgery, or by tumor growth that has penetrated through the peritoneal surface. Implants are found on peritoneal surfaces. The tumor extends beyond the surgical margins either microscopically or grossly. The tumor is not completely resectable because of local infiltration into vital structures.
IV	Hematogenous metastasis: deposits are present beyond stage III, eg, lung, liver, bone, and/or brain.
V	Bilateral renal involvement is present at diagnosis. An attempt should be made to stage each side according to the above criteria on the basis of extent of disease before biopsy.

From Green, G.M., D'Angio, G.L., Beckwith, J.B., et al. (1996). Wilms' tumor. CA: A Cancer Journal for Clinicians, 46 (1), 49.

right-sided Wilms' tumor. Radiation damage (such as thinning or weakening) of the skeleton, pelvis, and thorax has been reported. Kyphosis and scoliosis may occur from irradiation of vertebral bodies and the pelvis. Glomerular damage to the remaining kidney may also occur. Second malignancies in the original radiation field have occurred with orthovoltage radiation, but recent changes in radiation therapy have reduced this risk.

Nursing Assessment

Perform a thorough baseline assessment of the child. Do not palpate the abdomen because of the potential for spreading the cancerous cells. Monitor the child's blood pressure carefully as hypertension is a common finding that may require treatment.

Nursing Diagnosis

Nursing diagnoses for a child with Wilms' tumor will differ depending on the phase of treatment. Some common nursing diagnoses might include:

- Risk for Infection related to surgery
- Altered Urinary Elimination related to hematuria from tumor
- Altered Cardiopulmonary Tissue Perfusion related to hypertension caused by renin mechanism disruption
- Risk for Caregiver Role Strain related to child's immediate need for surgery
- Risk for Impaired Home Maintenance Management related to post-surgical chemotherapy or radiation

Nursing Management

Nursing management can be divided into two phases: the postrenal surgery phase and the chemotherapy phase. (See Chapter 4 for general care of the child after surgery.) Drawings and special teaching dolls with removable kidneys can be used to teach young children about the surgery. Although chemotherapy may occur at two different times, before and after surgery, nursing management considerations remain the same.

Nursing care during the postrenal surgery phase focuses on pain management and close monitoring of fluid levels. A large incision is necessary to remove the kidney, and the resultant postoperative shift of organs and fluid in the abdominal cavity may create discomfort for the child. Frequently reposition the child and use noninvasive and pharmacologic pain interventions to improve the child's comfort. Gentle handling is important. Monitor fluids closely following surgery to prevent hypovolemia and to assess the shift of fluids out of the third space and out of the body. Assess daily weight, intake and output (I&O), and urine specific gravity. Monitor the function of the remaining kidney. Take blood pressure measurements frequently to watch for signs of shock and to assess the functioning of the remaining kidney.

During the chemotherapy phase, monitor the child for side effects of drugs, the potential for infection from the central line site, and the function of the remaining kidney.

NURSING ALERT

If a mass is felt during palpation of a child's abdomen, *stop palpating immediately* and report the finding to the physician. *Never* palpate the liver or abdomen of a child with Wilms' tumor as this could cause a piece of the tumor to dislodge. Place a sign on the child's bed and in the chart alerting health providers not to palpate the abdomen.

► BONE TUMORS

OSTEOSARCOMA

Osteosarcoma is a rare, malignant bone tumor that occurs predominantly in adolescent boys. Its peak incidence is during the rapid growth years. The tumor is usually located at the metaphysis of the distal femur, proximal tibia, or proximal humerus.[21]

Clinical Manifestations

The common initial symptoms are pain and swelling. The pain can be referred to the hip or back, which can delay diagnosis. Pulmonary metastasis occurs in 20% of cases.

Etiology and Pathophysiology

Bone tissue produced by osteosarcoma never matures into compact bone. Although the cause of osteosarcoma is unknown, radiation exposure (either environmental or treatment related) is associated with its development. Survivors of retinoblastoma have a greatly increased incidence of osteosarcoma. An abnormality of gene p53 has been noted in some cases of this cancer, leading to oncogene malformations and possibly to an absence of tumor suppressor genes.[21]

Diagnostic Tests and Medical Management

Diagnosis is made through radiographic tests (radiographic studies of the affected area, bone scan, CT or MRI scans of involved bone), blood test for serum alkaline phosphatase (level may be elevated), and tumor biopsy (to confirm the diagnosis). Arteriography may be performed if limb-sparing surgery is contemplated.

Treatment involves both surgery and chemotherapy. The surgery is either a limb-sparing procedure or limb amputation. In limb-sparing procedures the tumor is removed and an internal prosthesis is inserted. A limb-sparing procedure is possible if bone growth has taken place and a neurobundle (area where several nerves converge) is not involved in the tumor. If these two criteria are not met, limb amputation is necessary. Aggressive chemotherapy following surgery has improved the survival rate. At the time of diagnosis, most children have metastases (even though they may not be identifiable), so chemotherapy is needed. Chemotherapy may be started before surgery, especially in cases where limb-sparing surgery is performed.

Research is being carried out to test the benefit of drugs to stimulate the immune system in the treatment for osteosarcoma. In addition, muramyl-tripeptide (MTP), a derivative of the tuberculosis vaccine BCG, is showing promise in reducing the risk of recurrence.[21]

OSTEOSARCOMA: CHEMOTHERAPY DRUGS
Methotrexate
Doxorubicin
Cisplatin
Cyclophosphamide
Bleomycin
Dactinomycin
Ifosfamide

EWING'S SARCOMA

Ewing's sarcoma is a malignant, small, round cell tumor usually involving the diaphyseal (shaft) portion of the long bones. The most common sites are the femur, pelvis, tibia, fibula, ribs, humerus, scapula, and clavicle, but any bone may be involved. Ewing's sarcoma occurs in 2 children per million, is most common in whites and Hispanics, and is rare in African-

American and Asian children. The incidence is highest in children between the ages of 10 and 20 years.[22]

The symptoms are similar to those of osteosarcoma and may include pain, swelling, fever, an elevated WBC count, and elevated erythrocyte sedimentation rate.

Although full mechanisms have not been described, abnormalities on chromosomes 11 and 22 have been identified in children with Ewing's sarcoma. A translocation of genetic material is apparent. In addition, these tumors express a protooncogene, c-*myc*.

A tumor biopsy is necessary for diagnosis. Diagnostic tests are the same as those for osteosarcoma.

Initial treatment for Ewing's sarcoma is chemotherapy to reduce the tumor, followed by surgical removal of the entire bone or intensive high-dose irradiation of the entire bone. Surgery is preferred because of the possibility of a secondary cancer from radiation. Chemotherapy is always used following initial treatment, as nondetectable metastases are nearly always present.[22]

EWING'S SARCOMA: CHEMOTHERAPY DRUGS

Vincristine
Cyclophosphamide
Dactinomycin
Doxorubicin
Ifosfamide
Etoposide
Adriamycin

NURSING ASSESSMENT OF BONE TUMORS

Physiologic assessment of the child with a bone tumor includes assessment of the site before surgery. Assess the child's pain or discomfort, mobility, and gait. Take careful vital signs, especially noting temperature and respirations. Psychologic assessment of the child and family are needed, especially if amputation is planned. Body image disturbances occur when a limb is lost, particularly with school-age children and adolescents. Assess the child's understanding of the treatment and of care after surgery. Find out what support systems are available for assistance.

Observe the wound postoperatively for infection and hemorrhage. Assess circulation above and below the operative site. If edema is found, elevate the limb. If a limb salvage procedure is performed, the child's extremity will be intact but it will not function as before because muscle insertion sites and mass have been removed with the tumor during surgery. Detailed charting of the condition of the surgical site and limb function is important.

If the limb has been amputated, assess the child for the following signs indicating a disturbed body image:

- Refusal to look at or touch the altered or missing body part
- Preoccupation with loss or change
- Feelings of shame or embarrassment, either verbalized or demonstrated
- Distorted perception of normal body (easily seen in the child's drawings of the body)
- Fears of rejection or unwanted attention from others
- Overexposure or hiding of the affected body part
- Actual or perceived change in the structure and function of the body or body parts

Psychosocial assessment of the child and family is discussed in more detail earlier in the general section on Childhood Cancer (see pp. 551–553).

NURSING DIAGNOSIS OF BONE TUMORS

Nursing diagnoses for the child with a bone tumor are based on the treatment and needs of each child. Among the nursing diagnoses that might be appropriate are:

- Risk for Infection related to surgery
- Impaired Skin Integrity related to use of prosthesis after surgery
- Impaired Physical Mobility related to gait disturbance
- Impaired Adjustment related to challenges in returning to normal activities after loss of a body part
- Body Image Disturbance related to visible disability
- Pain related to presence of tumor

NURSING MANAGEMENT OF BONE TUMORS

Care of the child after surgery involves general postoperative care (see Chap. 4). The child who has had an amputation has special needs regarding skin care and rehabilitation. Inspect the tissue at the surgical site, using sterile technique, and turn the child at least every 2 hours. The site needs to heal completely before chemotherapy can begin and a prosthesis can be made.

Discuss insurance and other financial arrangements with the parents, as prosthetics can be costly. Referral to a Shriners Hospital is an option for some families.

Implement plans to help the child deal with body image disturbance. Plan for a visit from another child who is well adjusted to a prosthesis. Help the child to gradually learn how to care for the stump. Slow progress may be made as the child first looks briefly, then for longer periods, and finally is willing to touch the stump. Show the child how it is possible to continue with sports such as baseball, skiing, or biking with a prosthesis. A discussion group with others can be very useful for adolescents. Plan with the child how to tell friends about the surgery and what issues he or she may face upon return to school. Make plans for elevator access if needed and emergency evacuation procedures. Some children or adolescents may need referral for counseling to assist in dealing with body image disturbance.

The child will be receiving physical rehabilitation while hospitalized and after discharge. When the child is discharged, explain to the family the importance of bringing the child for outpatient chemotherapy and physical rehabilitation visits. Special arrangements may be needed at the child's school to facilitate a wheelchair, crutches, or ambulation with a new prosthesis. Call or visit the school to evaluate the presence of buttons to open doors, wide doorways to facilitate passage, and any limitations of the building. Contact school personnel to plan the child's return.

▶ LEUKEMIA

Leukemia is the most commonly diagnosed pediatric malignancy. A cancer of the blood-forming organs, leukemia is characterized by a proliferation of abnormal white blood cells in the body. Several types of leukemia are differentiated, depending on the blood cells affected. The main types are acute lymphoblastic leukemia, acute myelogenous leukemia, and the rare chronic leukemias of childhood.

The most common type of childhood leukemia is acute lymphoblastic leukemia (ALL), which accounts for 25% of all childhood cancer and 75% of leukemias in children. The peak age at onset is 4 years. ALL is more common in Caucasians and in boys (Fig 14–15).[23]

Acute myelogeous leukemia (AML) affects all ethnic groups equally, and there is no peak age at onset.[24] Rasheed, the boy described at the beginning of the chapter, has AML.

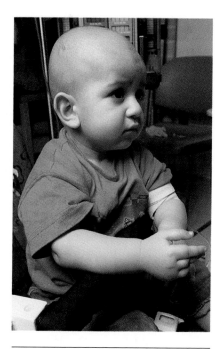

FIGURE 14–15. Acute lymphoblastic leukemia is the most common type of leukemia in children and the most common cancer affecting children under 5 years of age.

Because chronic leukemias such as chronic myelocytic, chronic myelomonocytic, and chronic lymphocytic leukemia are rare in children, the following discussion will focus on ALL and AML.

Clinical Manifestations

Children with ALL and AML usually have fever, pallor, overt signs of bleeding, lethargy, malaise, anorexia, and large joint or bone pain. Petechiae, frank bleeding, and joint pain are cardinal signs of bone marrow failure. Enlargement of the liver and spleen (hepatosplenomegaly) and changes in the lymph nodes (lymphadenopathy) are common. If the leukemia has infiltrated the central nervous system (entered it by means of the circulatory or lymphoid system), the child will have signs such as headache, vomiting, papilledema, and sixth cranial nerve palsy (inability to move the eye laterally). These findings are caused by the leukemic cells massing and putting pressure on nerves. The testicles, spinal cord, and bone marrow are common sites for infiltration. The leukemic cells in the testicle become a mass that causes the testicle to enlarge, often painlessly.

Etiology and Pathophysiology

The causes of leukemia are not well understood. Genetic factors are believed to play a role in some types of the disease. For instance, children with chromosomal defects such as Down syndrome have an increased incidence of ALL. Ionizing radiation and chemical agents such as treatment with chemotherapy for other cancers are thought to play some role in the development of AML. Children with immune deficiency states, such as ataxia-telangiectasia, congenital hypogammaglobulinemia, and Wiskott–Aldrich syndrome have an increased risk of ALL. Some investigators theorize that exposure to viruses—before or after birth—can predispose children to leukemia.[23]

Leukemia occurs when the stem cells in the bone marrow produce immature WBCs that cannot function normally. These cells proliferate rapidly by cloning instead of normal mitosis, causing the bone marrow to fill with abnormal WBCs. The abnormal cells then spill out into the circulatory system where they steadily replace the normally functioning WBCs. As this occurs, the protective lymphocytic functions such as cellular and humeral immunity are reduced, leaving the body vulnerable to infections.

The malignant WBCs rapidly fill the bone marrow, replacing stem cells that produce erythrocytes (red blood cells) and other blood products such as platelets, thereby decreasing the amount of these products in circulation. The stem cells are replaced by leukemic clones, eventually resulting in anemia. Children with leukemia commonly experience abnormal bleeding because of the reduced amounts of platelets.

Diagnostic Tests and Medical Management

Diagnosis is based initially on blood counts and bone marrow aspiration. Blood counts reveal anemia, thrombocytopenia, and neutropenia. Bone marrow aspiration reveals immature and abnormal lymphoblasts and hypercellular marrow. Bone marrow aspiration is the differential test. Neutropenia, **thrombocytopenia,** and anemia are commonly noted. Other abnormal laboratory findings include elevated serum uric acid and elevated calcium, potassium, and phosphorus levels.

Treatment of ALL involves radiation and chemotherapy. Radiation is used for central nervous system prophylaxis and involvement and for testic-

BLOOD CELL VALUES IN LEUKEMIA

	Usual	Common values in leukemia
Leukocytes	<10,000/mm^3	>10,000/mm^3
Platelets	150,000–400,000/mm^3	20,000–100,000/mm^3
Hemoglobin	12–16g/dL	7–11g/dL

ular involvement. Chemotherapy is organized into four phases: (1) induction, (2) consolidation, (3) delayed intensification, and (4) maintenance of remission. Additional drugs may be used for treatment of central nervous system involvement. Treatment of AML involves use of a wide variety of drugs during the induction and consolidation phases.

Maximum cell death occurs during the induction phase. The cells that remain after this period are more resistant to treatment. After 3–4 weeks, when a remission has occurred, central nervous system prophylaxis begins. Drugs are used in combination with cranial irradiation. During the consolidation phase, chemotherapy with L-asparaginase and doxorubicin is administered. Delayed intensification uses additional drugs to target the leukemic cells that have survived. Treatment during the maintenance phase is aimed at destroying the remaining leukemic cells. Combinations of active drugs are used to prevent resistance. Occasionally other drugs are added to the regimen, such as vincristine, prednisone, cyclophosphamide, intravenous methotrexate, cytosine arabinoside, or anthracyclines.

The prognosis for children with leukemia is much improved with current therapy. However, several risk factors affect the long-term outcome. The most favorable findings are:

- Age at onset between 2 and 10 years
- Initial hemoglobin level less than 10 g/dL
- Low initial WBC count
- Lack of B- or T-cell antigens
- Absence of extramedullary (outside bone marrow or spinal cord) involvement
- Rapid response to chemotherapy

The most important factor is the initial leukocyte count. The higher the leukocyte count (over 50,000/mm^3) at diagnosis, the worse the prognosis. For children in the low-risk group, the probability of prolonged survival is as high as 90%. Infants under 12 months of age have a poor prognosis. Treatment methods and duration are adjusted for each child, depending on that child's risk factors. More aggressive treatment is undertaken for those in the higher risk groups.

Approximately 10% of children have a relapse within a year after completing treatment. Treatment for relapse consists of additional chemotherapy drugs. The prognosis is best if the the relapse occurs late after the initial diagnosis and after the initial treatment is completed.[24] Bone marrow transplantation is a treatment option for the child who has a relapse with ALL or who is in remission from AML. Chemotherapy itself can create numerous complications, affecting all body organs. Secondary malignancies sometimes occur later in life.

Nursing Assessment

Gentle physical assessment is mandatory. Perform assessments every 8 hours or more often depending on the chemotherapy regimen. Observe carefully for bruising and other new sites of bleeding. Once chemotherapy has begun, closely monitor renal functioning through specific gravity, intake and output (I&O), and daily weight measurement. Monitor dietary intake, nausea, vomiting, and constipation. Observe for mucosal sores in the mouth. Ask the parents about any behavioral changes. Central nervous system infiltration can affect the child's level of consciousness, causing irri-

---

ACUTE LYMPHOBLASTIC LEUKEMIA: CHEMOTHERAPY DRUGS

Induction phase
  Prednisone
  Vincristine
  L-Asparaginase
  Daunorubicin
Central nervous system prophylaxis
  Intrathecal methotrexate
Consolidation phase
  L-Asparaginase
  Doxorubicin
Delayed intensification
  Vincristine
  Ara-C
  Cyclophosphamide
Maintenance phase
  6-Mercaptopurine or 6-thioguanine
  Methotrexate

ACUTE MYELOGENOUS LEUKEMIA: CHEMOTHERAPY DRUGS

Induction phase
  Daunorubicin
  Doxorubicin
  Mitoxantrone
  Cytarabin
Consolidation phase
  Etoposide
  Teniposide

COMPLICATIONS OF LEUKEMIA THERAPY

- Central nervous system toxicity or damage
- Potential damage to the pituitary, liver, kidneys, gastrointestinal tract, heart, lungs, gonads, and hematopoietic and immune systems
- Secondary malignancies

tability, vomiting, and lethargy. However, these nonspecific signs can also be induced by chemotherapeutic drugs and antiemetics.

Nursing Diagnosis

Leukemia causes many changes in the body and confirmation of the disease is difficult for families to face. Among the many nursing diagnoses that might be appropriate for the child with leukemia are:

- Altered Nutrition: Less Than Body Requirements related to anorexia from disease and treatment
- Risk for Infection related to altered immune system functioning
- Risk for Injury related to bleeding tendency
- Activity Intolerance related to fatigue from anemia and treatment
- Pain related to bone involvement and diagnostic tests
- Anxiety (Child and Parent) related to diagnosis and treatment

Nursing Management

Bone marrow suppression may necessitate transmission-based precautions. (Refer to the *Quick Reference to Pediatric Clinical Skills* accompanying this text.) Instruct parents in the prevention of infection. Care of mouth sores and other side effects of chemotherapy is presented in the Nursing Care Plan for Hospital Care of the Child With Cancer, earlier in this chapter.

Special attention to renal function is needed when the child receives cyclophosphamide. Gross hematuria is a side effect of this drug. Hydration with intravenous fluids to attain a specific gravity of less than 1.010 prevents or reduces the severity of hematuria. To achieve this specific gravity, the child receives intravenous fluids at 1½ times maintenance volume for at least 6–8 hours before and at least 1½ hours after administration of the drug. Careful monitoring of I&O is required to record the intravenous fluids and assess kidney functioning. Monitor specific gravity every 8 hours, as well as before and during administration of the drug, and when the intravenous fluids are reduced to maintenance volume levels. Daily weight measurements are important to assist in planning adequate hydration during chemotherapy, as well as to measure nutritional status.

Many children are treated in an oncology clinic, staying in the hospital only on the day of intravenous drug administration, and receiving oral medications at home. Careful teaching for the family is needed to ensure safe drug administration and identification of symptoms requiring care.

Nurses play a key role in the long-term multidisciplinary treatment of children with leukemia.[25] The impact of a diagnosis of leukemia and the long-term nature of treatment can severely stress the coping abilities of both the child and the family. Ongoing psychosocial assessment and emotional support are essential (see the general discussion of Psychosocial Assessment in the section on Childhood Cancer, pp. 551–553). Referral to support groups and social services may be beneficial.

► SOFT TISSUE TUMORS

HODGKIN'S DISEASE

Hodgkin's disease is a disorder of the lymphoid system. It usually arises in a single lymph node or an anatomic group of lymph nodes (Fig. 14–16).

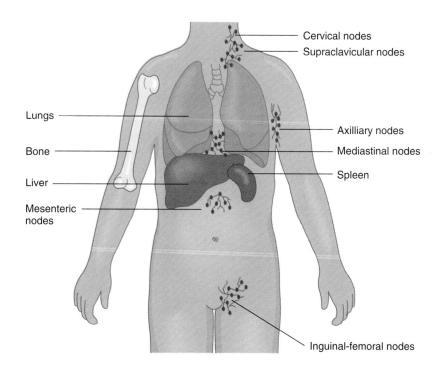

Cervical nodes
Supraclavicular nodes
Lungs
Axilliary nodes
Mediastinal nodes
Bone
Spleen
Liver
Mesenteric
nodes
Inguinal-femoral nodes

FIGURE 14–16. lymph nodes and organs affected in Hodgkin's disease in children.

There are approximately 5.7 cases per million people, with the peak occurrence in adolescent boys. Hodgkin's disease has a childhood form but is rare in those under 14 years. Most cases involve a young adult form that affects those between 15 and 35 years of age, and an older adult form, usually seen in persons over 55 years of age.[26]

Clinical Manifestations

The main symptom of Hodgkin's disease is nontender, firm lymphadenopathy, usually in the supraclavicular and cervical nodes but occasionally in the mediastinal area. A mediastinal growth can cause respiratory difficulty because of pressure on the trachea or bronchi. Fever, night sweats, and weight loss occur in one third of children with Hodgkin's disease and are associated with a more aggressive form of the disease. The leukocyte count and erythrocyte sedimentation rate (ESR) may be elevated.

Etiology and Pathophysiology

Hodgkin's disease occurs in clusters and has been reported in families. This suggests a possible genetic link as well as an infectious agent.

Diagnostic Tests and Medical Management

Diagnosis is based on lymph node biopsy. Staging is done using the Ann Arbor staging classification (Table 14–13). The basis for staging is data obtained from the history, physical examination, chest x-ray study (for metastasis), chest CT scan, CT or MRI scans of the retroperitoneal nodes, lymphangiogram, laboratory studies (complete blood count, erythrocyte sedimentation rate, serum copper level, liver function tests), and a radionuclide scan with gallium. Bone marrow biopsy, bone scan, or a staging laparotomy may be performed in certain situations when advanced disease is suspected.

RESEARCH CONSIDERATIONS

The role of an infectious agent in Hodgkin's disease is being investigated. Infectious agents associated with Hodgkin's disease include a herpesvirus, cytomegalovirus, and Epstein-Barr virus (EBV). High EBV titers and EBV-associated antigens are commonly found in individuals with Hodgkin's disease.

CLINICAL TIP

An oral contrast medium is often given to children having CT scanning of the abdomen and pelvis. Mixing this contrast medium with fruit juice or punch makes it more palatable. Mix it in a small amount so the child can easily drink it all.

14-13	Ann Arbor Staging System for Hodgkin's Disease

Stage	Description
I	Disease within a single lymph node region
IE	Disease within a single extralymphatic organ
II	Disease within two or more lymph node regions on same side of diaphragm
IIE	Disease within extralymphatic organ, and of one or more lymph node regions on same side of diaphragm
III	Disease of lymph node regions on both sides of diaphragm
IIIE	Disease of lymph node regions on both sides of the diaphragm with involvement of extralymphatic organ
IIIS	As in III, plus disease within spleen
IIISE	As in III, plus disease in extralymphatic organs and spleen
IV	Disseminated disease within one or more lymphatic organs with or without lymph node involvement

From Hudson, M.M., & Donaldson, S.S. (1997). Hodgkin's disease. In P.A. Pizzo, & D.G. Poplack (Eds.), Principles and practices of pediatric oncology (3rd ed., p. 529). Philadelphia: Lippincott–Raven.

HODGKIN'S DISEASE: CHEMOTHERAPY DRUGS

MOPP (mechlorethamine, Oncovin [vincristine], procarbazine, prednisone)

COPP (cyclophosphamide, Oncovin, procarbazine, prednisone)

COMP (cyclophosphamide, Oncovin, methotrexate, prednisone)

OPPA (Oncovin, procarbazine, prednisone, adriamycin)

ABVD (adriamycin, bleomycin, vinblastine, dacarbazine)

NON-HODGKIN'S LYMPHOMA: CHEMOTHERAPY DRUGS

Cyclophosphamide
Ifosfamide
Prednisone
Methotrexate
Ara-C
VM-26
Adriamycin
Vincristine

Chemotherapy using a four-drug combination has been found to be the most effective drug treatment. Radiation is commonly added, with low doses for children who are still growing, and larger doses for those who are physically mature or those whose disease is more advanced at diagnosis. The 5-year survival rate is approximately 80–90%, depending on the stage of the disease at diagnosis.

Bone marrow transplantation is a treatment option in children with advanced disease or relapse.

NON-HODGKIN'S LYMPHOMA

Non-Hodgkin's lymphoma includes all lymphomas that are not classified as Hodgkin's disease (about 60% of pediatric lymphomas). There are three types of pediatric non-Hodgkin's lymphoma: (1) lymphoblastic lymphoma, (2) small noncleaved cell (Burkitt's) lymphoma, and (3) large cell lymphoma. Lymphomas of all types are the third most common group of malignancies in children, following leukemia and brain tumors.[27] Non-Hodgkin's lymphomas are malignant tumors of lymphoreticular (internal framework of the lymph system) origin. The peak incidence for lymphomas occurs between the ages of 7 and 11 years, and they are three times more common in boys than in girls.

Children with non-Hodgkin's lymphoma frequently present with fever and weight loss. The lymph glands are usually enlarged or nodular, with the most frequent sites being the cervical, axillary, inguinal, and femoral nodes. However, the disease may be diffuse, without nodular glands. The anterior mediastinum is the primary site for T-cell lymphomas. Tumors that occur in this area may compress the airway (causing breathing difficulty) or superior vena cava (leading to swelling of the face, neck, or arms), and can cause pain. Jaw involvement is common in Burkitt's lymphoma.

Fifty percent of non-Hodgkin's lymphomas are caused by T-cell abnormalities. These abnormal T cells are diffuse, highly malignant, and very aggressive and do not mature. T-cell lymphomas produced by these cells often occur in children with congenital or acquired immunodeficiency states, chronic immune stimulation, or autoimmune disease. Some lymphomas are observed with B-cell abnormalities. The incidence of lymphomas shows geographic variability. For example, a high incidence of Burkitt's lymphoma is found in equatorial Africa, where it causes 50% of childhood cancer.

Diagnosis is confirmed by tissue biopsy. There are several staging systems that relate to the tumor mass and extension to other body areas. Because systemic disease is present in 80% of children with non-Hodgkin's lymphoma, the treatment is aggressive chemotherapy similar to that used for ALL. The induction phase of chemotherapy results in a 90% remission rate. Treatment also includes localized radiation and surgery to remove the tumor mass. Between 50% and 75% of children with non-Hodgkin's lymphoma have a good outcome. Children with localized diseases have a more favorable prognosis.

RHABDOMYOSARCOMA

Rhabdomyosarcoma is a soft tissue cancer that is common in children. It occurs most often in the muscles around the eyes (extraorbital), in the neck, and less commonly in the abdomen and genitourinary tract. Among children under 15 years of age, rhabdomyosarcoma occurs more often in caucasians than in African-Americans or Asians.[28] Most cases are diagnosed in children under 5 years of age.

Tumors occurring close to the eye produce swelling, ptosis, visual disturbances, and eye movement abnormalities (Fig. 14–17). When the tumor occurs in the genitourinary tract, the result can be obstruction, hematuria, dysuria, vaginal discharge, and a protruding vaginal mass. Rhabdomyosarcoma occurring in the abdomen may be asymptomatic. There is rapid metastasis to the lungs, bones, bone marrow, and distant lymph nodes.

Diagnosis is confirmed by CT, MRI, bone marrow aspiration, and biopsy. A useful biologic marker, Desmin, allows differentiation of rhabdomyosarcoma from other round cell tumors. Because 20% of children have metastatic disease at the time of diagnosis, chest and lung CT scans are performed.

Treatment includes surgical removal of the tumor followed by widefield radiation and chemotherapy with a combination of drugs. Prognosis depends on the site, staging (Table 14–14), and histologic findings. Children with stage II or IV disease or abdominal tumors have a poor prognosis.

RETINOBLASTOMA

Retinoblastoma is an intraocular malignancy of the retina. It may be bilateral (20–30%) or unilateral. In 40% of children, the disease is inherited by an autosomal dominant gene.[29]

The first sign of retinoblastoma is a white pupil, termed leukokoria or cat's-eye reflex (Fig. 14–18). Other symptoms may include a fixed strabismus (a constant deviation of one eye from the other), orbital inflammation, glaucoma, and heterochromia (irises of different colors).

Retinoblastoma is usually diagnosed when the child is between 1 and 2 years of age. The overall tumor-free survival rate is 90%, 5–10 years after diagnosis. Diagnostic tests include full ocular examination and CT or MRI scans of the eye orbit. All children with a history of retinoblastoma in the family should be examined by an ophthalmologist after birth and on a regular basis to aid in early diagnosis. Tumors are classified according to a

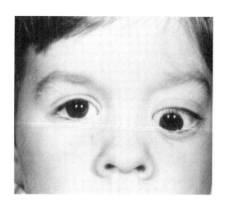

FIGURE 14–17. Rhabdomyosarcoma is characterized by ptosis and swelling.
From Vaughan, D., Asbury, T., & Riordan-Eva, P. (1995). General ophthalmology (14th ed.). Norwalk, CT: Appleton & Lange.

RHABDOMYOSARCOMA: CHEMOTHERAPY DRUGS

Dactinomycin
Cyclophosphamide
Vincristine
Doxorubicin
Cisplatin
Etoposide
Dacarbazine

14-14 Classification of Rhabdomyosarcoma

Group	Description
I	Localized, completely resected disease
II	Total gross resection with regional microscopic spread
III	Incomplete gross resection or biopsy
IV	Distant metastatic disease present

From Wexler, L.H., & Helman, L.J. (1997). Rhabdomyosarcoma and the undifferentiated sarcomas. In P.A. Pizzo, & D.G. Poplack (Eds.), Principles and practices of pediatric oncology (3rd ed., p. 808). Philadelphia: Lippincott–Raven.

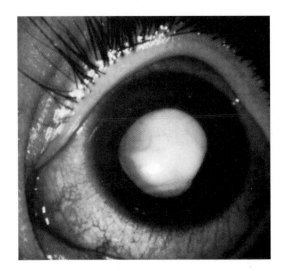

FIGURE 14–18. Retinoblastoma is characterized by leukokoria, a white reflection in the pupil.
From Hathaway, W.E., Hay, W.W., Jr., Groothuis, J.R., & Paisley, J.W. (1993). Current pediatric diagnosis and treatment (11th ed.). Norwalk, CT: Appleton & Lange.

staging system, from a very small localized tumor (group I) to tumors involving more than half the retina and with seeding into the vitreous (group V).

Treatment for retinblastoma may include removal of the eye. Other surgical treatments involve cyrotherapy or photocoagulation (argon laser therapy). Radiation is nearly always used, either as the sole treatment or before surgery to shrink the tumor. Chemotherapy is occasionally used but is generally ineffective as the drugs often fail to penetrate sufficiently into the eye. Unfortunately, children with retinoblastoma are at increased risk of developing a secondary tumor, including another retinoblastoma or a sarcoma, most commonly osteogenic sarcoma.

NURSING ASSESSMENT OF SOFT TISSUE TUMORS

Physiologic Assessment

Physiologic assessment of the child with a soft tissue tumor, such as Hodgkin's disease, non-Hodgkin's lymphoma, rhabdomyosarcoma, and other lymphomas, focuses on the child's general condition. Accurate height and weight measurements are essential to provide a baseline against which to measure the child's growth during treatment, as well as for calculation of chemotherapeutic drug dosages.

Observe the area of the tumor, such as the face, neck, and abdomen, and describe any changes. Monitor respiratory status if the tumor is in the face or neck. Report any changes in respiratory pattern to the physician. Avoid palpation of any tumor site or enlarged area; metastasis can be influenced by injudicious palpation and manipulation of a tumor site. Notify the physician of a change in any lymph node or any other area of the body.

Gastrointestinal and genitourinary function can be altered by the presence of a tumor and by treatment such as chemotherapy and radiation. Careful monitoring of the child's intake and output measurement is essential. Abdominal tumors may affect defecation, so charting of all bowel movements is important. Explain to the family and child why keeping accurate records is necessary.

Observe wounds closely for lack of healing as a result of chemotherapy or radiation. Examine the mouth and extremities for wounds or ulcers. Nutritional changes caused by treatment will affect the body's ability to support healthy cells and heal wounds.

A thorough eye examination is warranted for any child who has a family history of retinoblastoma or has undergone treatment for a prior tumor. Assess color and position of the iris, eye movements, cover–uncover test, and other eye tests described in Chapter 3. Ask whether the child has been evaluated by an ophthalmologist.

Psychosocial Assessment

Assessment of the family's psychosocial status and coping mechanisms is an essential component of nursing care. Refer to the general discussion of Psychosocial Assessment under Childhood Cancer, earlier in this chapter. Assessment of body image is needed when the child has a soft tissue tumor affecting appearance of the head and neck.

NURSING DIAGNOSIS OF SOFT TISSUE TUMORS

The location and type of soft tissue tumor determine the specific nursing diagnoses for a particular child. Common nursing diagnoses might include:

- Altered Tissue Perfusion (Peripheral) related to facial and neck edema
- Ineffective Breathing Pattern related to tumor compression in chest or neck
- Impaired Swallowing related to tumor compression on esophagus
- Altered Growth and Development related to effects of treatment
- Body Image Disturbance related to visible changes caused by tumor
- Sensory/Perceptual Alteration (Visual) related to tumor in eye

NURSING MANAGEMENT OF SOFT TISSUE TUMORS

Nursing management of children with soft tissue tumors varies depending on the specific tumor. Children with lymphoma affecting the mediastinum may need respiratory support. Position the child so that the head is elevated. Administer chemotherapy drugs as ordered, maintaining adequate fluids to facilitate excretion of the resultant breakdown products. Monitor the central line used for chemotherapy administration, and teach parents care of the central line when the child is at home.

For the child with a rhabdomyosarcoma involving the bladder, monitor urinary output carefully. Report hematuria and painful urination. Monitor the changes that occur during therapy. For example, in children with eye tumors, observe for a decrease in ptosis, which may indicate successful treatment. Administer pain medications as needed and use distraction and other techniques to decrease the child's discomfort. Emphasize to parents the need for follow-up CT and MRI scans after completion of treatment.

When the child with retinoblastoma undergoes removal of the eye, the parents and child will need detailed instructions on postsurgical care. Demonstrate to the parents care of the socket and use of a conformer to maintain the eye socket shape. When healing is complete and the child receives a prosthetic eye, instruct parents about its insertion and care. The child can gradually be taught to take over this care when old

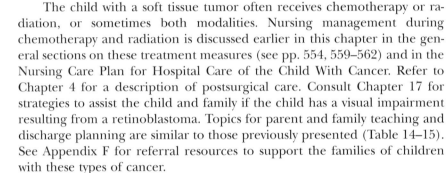

| 14-15 | Parent and Family Teaching: The Child With a Soft Tissue Tumor |

- Teach the family about the chemotherapy drugs and their side effects.
- Teach about the care of venous access devices surgically placed.
- Provide written and illustrated information about the chemotherapy protocol(s).
- Provide radiation and surgery education specific to the tumor treatment.
- Refer the family to nutrition resources such as dietitians to improve the child's nutritional status.

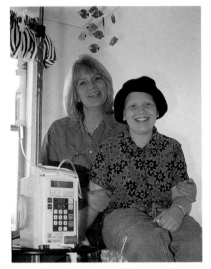

A, Nicole, 11 years old, is undergoing chemotherapy for Ewing's sarcoma. Her mother emphasizes, "It's our faith that has gotten us through this. The hardest part is how busy you are coming to treatments all the time. Nicole's younger brother sometimes feels neglected."

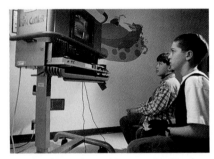

B, According to Jesse, 10 years old, "the thing that has helped me most [in dealing with acute lymphoblastic leukemia] is all the mail I got from my friends." His mother adds, "We're just really positive and think that everything will turn out alright."

enough. Encourage periodic health care visits to monitor for signs of a tumor in the other eye.

The child with a soft tissue tumor often receives chemotherapy or radiation, or sometimes both modalities. Nursing management during chemotherapy and radiation is discussed earlier in this chapter in the general sections on these treatment measures (see pp. 554, 559–562) and in the Nursing Care Plan for Hospital Care of the Child With Cancer. Refer to Chapter 4 for a description of postsurgical care. Consult Chapter 17 for strategies to assist the child and family if the child has a visual impairment resulting from a retinoblastoma. Topics for parent and family teaching and discharge planning are similar to those previously presented (Table 14–15). See Appendix F for referral resources to support the families of children with these types of cancer.

▶ IMPACT OF CANCER SURVIVAL

Over the past two to three decades, treatment for childhood cancers has been increasingly successful. About 1 in 1000 young adults is a survivor of childhood cancer.[30] The success of new modalities and treatment combinations has, however, created special health care needs for many survivors (see Figs. 14–19A, B, and C).

Surgery can have many results. Body organs may be removed and manipulated, leading to adhesions, intestinal obstruction, visual impairment, neurologic disruption, and even sterility. Removal of the spleen can lead to serious infections. Amputation necessitates the need for prosthetic devices and physical rehabilitation.

Radiation has several long-term effects. It can impair the growth of bones and teeth, leading to conditions such as scoliosis, leg length discrepancy, or poor dental health. Cardiotoxicity and pulmonary toxicity can result from mediastinal radiation. Delayed puberty and sterility can result from radiation effects to the cranium and spinal regions. Neural damage can occur. Secondary cancers, most commonly solid tumors, occur in some survivors.

Chemotherapy can cause a wide variety of effects, both during its administration and for years afterward. Cardiomyopathy can occur with some drugs, especially the anthracyclines. Pulmonary toxicity and renal complications can develop. Neurologic effects of some drugs can lead to hearing loss (eg, cisplatin and ifosfamide), cataracts, and paraplegia (eg, intrathecal methotrexate for leukemia). Learning disabilities and change in intelligence quotient (IQ) occur in some children.[31] Although radiation is responsible for most secondary tumors, some chemotherapy drugs have also been implicated.

The diagnosis and stress of treatment along with the risk of recurrence are significant stressors for the child with cancer. See Chapter 6 for a discussion of the stresses that are experienced by families when a child has a life-threatening illness. Families may find it difficult to obtain full insurance coverage for the child who has had a prior cancer. Employment can be a potential problem for cancer survivors if employers have concerns about the earlier cancer diagnosis.[32] Most people with cancer report fear of recurrence of the disease, which is a stressor. On the other hand, hopefulness and the sense of having an added purpose in life can be positive outcomes for many cancer survivors.[33]

Nurses are involved with families when a diagnosis of cancer is made, during the therapy process, and in the years that follow. For a child who survives cancer, ongoing care is essential. Evaluate the child regularly with thorough physical, psychosocial, developmental, and cognitive assessments. Carefully monitor all body systems (eg, cardiovascular; respiratory; musculoskeletal; eye, ear, nose, and throat; genitourinary). Record height and weight and general growth patterns. Ask about the child's interactions with peers and performance at school. Be alert for signs and symptoms that could indicate a secondary tumor. Ask the parents about insurance coverage and other financial difficulties with ongoing care.

Plan care to assist the family to manage any long-term effects of cancer treatment. This may involve physical rehabilitation, support related to visual impairment, or treatment for cardiac or musculoskeletal abnormalities. Provide resources for information and support (see Appendix F). Facilitate periodic evaluations in a health care agency so that serious outcomes of treatment can be identified early.

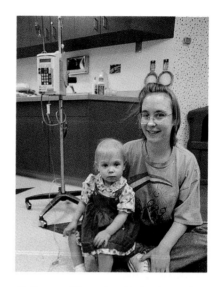

C, Cassie, 19 months old, has been diagnosed with neuroblastoma. At this age, it is hard for her to understand what is happening. Her mother has stayed with her each time she has come to the hospital, which has helped Cassie adjust to therapy. Her caregivers are confident that she will respond well to treatment.

FIGURE 14–19. Survivors of Childhood Cancer

REFERENCES

1. Wright, P.S. (1995). An overview of childhood cancer. *Nurse Practitioner Forum, 6*(4), 186–193.

2. http://www.cancer.o...97cff/97childr.

3. Crist, W.M. (1995). Neoplastic diseases and tumors: Epidemiology. In R.E. Behrman, R.M. Kliegman, & A.M. Arvin (Eds.), *Nelson textbook of pediatrics* (15th ed., pp. 1442–1444). Philadelphia: Saunders.

4. Solomon, E., Borrow, J., & Goddard, A. (1991). Chromosome aberrations and cancer. *Science, 254,* 1153–1159.

5. Bindler, R.M., & Howry, L.B. (1997). *Pediatric drugs and nursing implications* (2nd ed., pp. 579–580, 587). Stamford, CT: Appleton & Lange.

6. Bertolone, K. (1997). Pediatric oncology: Past, present, and new modalities of treatment. *Journal of Intravenous Nursing, 20*(3), 136–140.

7. Kelly, K.M., & Lange, B. (1997). Oncologic emergencies. *Pediatric Clinics of North America, 44*(4), 809–830.

8. Whitman, N., Graham, B., Gleit, C., & Boyd, M. (1992). *Teaching in nursing practice: A professional model.* Stamford, CT: Appleton & Lange.

9. Moore, I.M., Packer, R.J., Karl, D., & Bleyer, W.A. (1994). Adverse effects of cancer treatment on the central nervous system. In C.L. Schwartz, W.L. Hobbie, L.S. Constine, & K.S. Ruccione (Eds.), *Survivors of childhood cancer* (pp. 81–95). St. Louis: Mosby–Year Book.

10. James, L., & Johnson, B. (1997). The needs of parents of pediatric oncology patients during the palliative care phase. *Journal of Pediatric Oncology Nursing, 14*(2). 83–95.

11. Enskar, K., Carlsson, M., Golsater, M., & Hamrin, E. (1997). Symptom distress and life situation in adolescents with cancer. *Cancer Nursing, 20*(1), 23–33.

12. Mercer, M., & Ritchie, J.A. (1997). Home community care: Parents' perspectives. *Journal of Pediatric Nursing, 12*(13), 133–141.

13. Kun, L.E. (1997). Brain tumors: Challenges and directions. *Pediatric Clinics of North America, 44*(4), 907–918.

14. Cullen, P.M. (1995). Pharmacologic supportive care of children with central nervous system tumors. *Journal of Pediatric Oncology Nursing, 12*(4), 230–232.

15. Vernon-Levett, P., & Geller. M. (1997). Posterior fossa tumors in children: A case study. *AACN Critical Issues, 8*(2), 214–226.

16. Shiminski-Maher, T., & Wisoff, J.H. (1995). Pediatric brain tumors. *Critical Care Nursing Clinics of North America, 7*(1), 159–169.

17. Castleberry, R.P. (1997). Biology and treatment of neuroblastoma. *Pediatric Clinics of North America, 44*(4), 919–938.

18. Santana, V.M. (1995). Neuroblastoma. In R.E. Behrman, R.M. Kliegman, & A.M. Arvin (Eds.), *Nelson textbook of pediatrics* (15th ed., pp. 1460–1463). Philadelphia: Saunders.

19. Brodeur, G.M., Pritchard, J., & Berthold, F. (1993). Revisions in the international criteria for neuroblastoma diagnosis, staging, and response to treatment. *Journal of Clinical Oncology, 11*, 1466.

20. Petruzzi, M.J., & Green, D.M. (1997). Wilms' tumor. *Pediatric Clinics of North America, 44*(4), 939–952.

21. Meyers, P.A., & Gorlick, R. (1997). Osteosarcoma. *Pediatric Clinics of North America, 44*(4), 973–990.

22. Grier, H.E. (1997). The Ewing family of tumors: Ewing's sarcoma and primitive neuroectodermal tumors. *Pediatric Clinics of North America, 44*(4), 991–1004.

23. Margolin, J.F., & Poplack, D.G. (1997). Acute lymphoblastic leukemia. In P.A. Pizzo, & D.G. Poplack (Eds.), *Principles and practice of pediatric oncology* (3rd ed., pp. 409–462). Philadelphia: Lippincott–Raven.

24. Golub, T.R., Weinstein, H.J., & Grier, H.E. (1997). Acute myelogenous leukemia. In P.A. Pizzo, & D.G. Poplack (Eds.), *Principles and practice of pediatric oncology* (3rd ed., pp. 463–482). Philadelphia: Lippincott–Raven.

25. Chaney, C.N., & Jassak, P. (1997). Leukemia. In C. Varricchio (Ed.), *A cancer source book for nurses* (pp. 478–389). Atlanta: American Cancer Society.

26. Hudson, M.M., & Donaldson, S.S. (1997). Hodgkin's disease. *Pediatric Clinics of North America, 44*(4), 891–906.

27. Shad, A., & Magrath, I. (1997). Non-Hodgkin's lymphoma. *Pediatric Clinics of North America, 44*(4), 863–890.

28. Wexler, L.H., & Helman, L.J. (1997). Rhabdomyosarcoma and the undifferentiated sarcomas. In P.A. Pizzo, & D.G. Poplack (Eds.), *Principles and practice of pediatric oncology* (3rd ed., pp. 799–830). Philadelphia: Lippincott–Raven.

29. Donaldson, S.S., Egbert, P.R., Newsham, I., & Cavenee, W.K. (1997). Retinoblastoma. In P.A. Pizzo, & D.G. Poplack (Eds.), *Principles and practice of pediatric oncology* (3rd ed., pp. 699–716). Philadelphia: Lippincott–Raven.

30. Schwartz, C.L., Constine, L.S., & Hobbie, W.L. (1994). Overview. In C.L. Schwartz, W.L. Hobbie, L.S. Constine, & K.S. Ruccione (Eds.), *Survivors of childhood cancer* (pp. 5–6). St. Louis: Mosby–Year Book.

31. Blatt, J., Copeland, D.R., & Bleyer, W.A. (1997). Late effects of childhood cancer and its treatment. In P.A. Pizzo, & D.G. Poplack (Eds.), *Principles and practice of childhood oncology* (3rd ed., pp. 1301–1330). Philadelphia: Lippincott–Raven.

32. Monaco, G.P., Fiduccia, D., & Smith, G. (1997). Legal and societal issues facing survivors of childhood cancer. *Pediatric Clinics of North America, 44*(4), 1043–1058.

33. Ferrell, B.R., Dow, K., Leigh, S., Ly, J., & Gulasekaram, P. (1995). Quality of life in long-term cancer survivors. *Oncology Nursing Forums, 22*(6), 915–922.

ADDITIONAL RESOURCES

Ablin, A.R. (1993). *Supportive care of children with cancer.* Baltimore: The Johns Hopkins University Press.

Baron, M.C. (1991). Advances in the care of children with brain tumors. *Journal of Neuroscience Nursing, 23*(1), 39–43.

Bucholtz, J.D. (1992). Issues concerning the sedation of children for radiation therapy. *Oncology Nursing Forum, 19*(4), 649–655.

Buschel, P.C., & Yarbro, C.H. (1993). *Oncology nursing in the ambulatory setting.* Boston: Jones & Bartlett Publishers.

Castiglia, P.T. (1995). Lymphomas in children. *Journal of Pediatric Health Care, 9*(5), 225–226.

Close, P., Burkey, E., Kazak, A., Danz, P., & Lange. B. (1995). A prospective, controlled evaluation of home chemotherapy for children with cancer. *Pediatrics, 95*(6), 896–900.

Delbecque-Boussard, L., Gottrand, F., Ategbo, S., Nelken, B., Mazingue, P., Vic, P., Farriaux, J.P., & Turck, D. (1997). Nutritional status of children with acute lymphoblastic leukemia: A longitudinal study. *American Journal of Clinical Nutrition, 65*(1), 95–100.

Derengowski, S., & O'Brien, E. (1996). Critical care of the pediatric oncology patient. *AACN Clinical Issues, 7*(1), 109–119.

DiJulio, J. (1991). Hematopoiesis: An overview. *Oncology Nursing Forum, 18*(2), 3–6.

Fochtman, D. (1995). Follow-up care for survivors of childhood cancer. *Nurse Practitioner Forum, 6*(4), 194–200.

Foley, G.V., Fochtman, D., & Mooney, K.H. (1993). *Nursing care of the child with cancer* (2nd ed.). Philadelphia: Saunders.

Haeuber, D. (1991). Future strategies in the control of myelosuppression: The use of colony stimulating factors. *Oncology Nursing Forum, 18*(2), 16–21.

Henderson, R.C., Madsen, C.D., Davis, C., & Gold, S.H. (1996). Bone density in survivors of childhood malignancies. *Journal of Pediatric Hematology/Oncology, 18*(4), 376–371.

Hillman, K.A. (1997). Comparing child-rearing practices in parents of children with cancer and parents of healthy children. *Journal of Pediatric Oncology Nursing, 14*(2), 53–67.

Lamb, S.A. (1995). Radiation therapy options for management of the brain tumor patient. *Critical Care Nursing Clinics of North America, 7*(1), 103–114.

Lawton, K.H., Meyers, M., & Donahue, E.M. (1997). Current practices and advances in pediatric neurosurgery. *Nursing Clinics of North America, 32*(1), 73–96.

Lundquist, D.M., & Stewart, F.M. (1994). An update on non-Hodgkin's lymphomas. *Nurse Practitioner, 19*(10), 41–53.

Neville, K. (1996). Psychological distress in adolescents with cancer. *Journal of Pediatric Nursing, 11*(4), 243–251.

Papadakis, V., Tan, C., Heller, G., & Sklar, C. (1996). Growth and final height after treatment for childhood Hodgkin disease. *Journal of Pediatric Hematology/Oncology, 18*(3), 272–276.

Shelton, B.K., Baker, L., & Stecker, S. (1996). Critical care of the patient with hematologic malignancy. *AACN Clinical Issues, 7*(1), 65–78.

Stewart, E.S. (1995). Family-centered care for the bereaved. *Pediatric Nursing, 21*(2), 181–187.

Thompson, D.G., & Cohen, D.G. (1996). Nursing management of the infant with a congenital malignancy. *Journal of Obstetric, Gynecologic, and Neonatal Nursing, 25*(1), 32–38.

Varricchio, C. (Ed.). (1997). *A cancer source book for nurses* (7th ed.). Atlanta: American Cancer Society.

Wilkes, G.M., Ingwersen, K., & Burke, M.B. (1994). *Oncology nursing drug reference*. Boston: Jones & Bartlett Publishers.

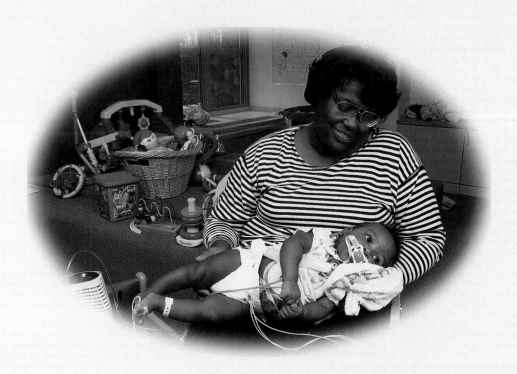

Jerome was born 2 weeks prematurely after a normal pregnancy. Soon after birth, he was diagnosed with multiple gastrointestinal anomalies, the most severe of which were an imperforate anus and esophageal atresia (an incomplete esophagus leading to a blind pouch). He underwent two major surgeries in the immediate newborn period and has been hospitalized several times since birth to treat infections and electrolyte imbalance, provide nutritional support, and evaluate his condition.

Jerome is now 8 months old and weighs 15 pounds. Although he still receives most of his nutrition through enteral feedings, he is learning to suck more vigorously and is given a bottle every few hours. The muscle development facilitated by sucking will promote his intake of foods and formation of speech later.

Jerome has a colostomy that was placed during surgery on his imperforate anus. It is hoped that this can be closed at about 2 years of age and that he will be able to develop normal bowel function. An ostomy nurse visits Jerome both at home and when he is in the hospital to evaluate his care.

Jerome's mother has been devoted to his care, providing nearly all of his tube feedings and other care at home. A home health nurse visits frequently and helps arrange occasional respite care for her. Jerome's mother has received materials and talks on the phone with members of an ostomy support group. She finds this contact very helpful in providing additional ideas about colostomy care and the opportunity to discuss her feelings and concerns about Jerome.

ALTERATIONS IN GASTROINTESTINAL FUNCTION 15

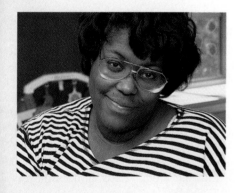

"I was so worried when Jerome was born. He had so many problems. Now he's growing and doing pretty well, and I'm so happy to see him starting to smile. I can't wait until he is able to eat on his own."

TERMINOLOGY

- **cholestasis** Disruption of bile flow.
- **constipation** Difficult and infrequent defecation with passage of hard, dry stool.
- **deamination** Removal of an amino group from an amino compound.
- **diarrhea** Frequent passage of abnormally watery stool.
- **gluconeogenesis** Formation of glycogen from noncarbohydrate sources such as protein or fat.
- **hernia** Protrusion or projection of a body part or structure through the muscle wall of the cavity that normally contains it.

- **occult blood** Blood that is present in minute quantities and can be seen only on microscopic examination or through chemical testing.
- **ostomy** An artificial abdominal opening into the urinary or gastrointestinal canal that provides an outlet for the diversion of urine or fecal matter.
- **peristalsis** A progressive, wavelike muscular movement that occurs involuntarily throughout the gastrointestinal tract.
- **projectile vomiting** Vomiting in which the stomach contents are ejected with great force.

What causes structural defects such as esophageal atresia and imperforate anus? What special care will Jerome require to promote his growth and development while he undergoes treatment for his anomalies? This chapter discusses the care of infants, like Jerome, who have structural defects and those with other common disorders of gastrointestinal functioning.

Through the gastrointestinal (GI) tract, a child ingests and absorbs the foods and fluids necessary to sustain life and promote growth. Most GI disturbances produce symptoms that are short term and interfere with nutrition and fluid balance for only a brief period. Some disorders or severe defects lead to complications that prevent optimal nutrition and adequate growth. This chapter explores some of the common GI disorders in children. (See Chapter 8 for a discussion of specific fluid imbalances that may accompany GI disorders.)

GI disorders can result from a congenital defect, acquired disease, infection, or injury. Structural problems may occur when development is altered or ceases in the first trimester of gestation. Because various parts of the gastrointestinal system are developing at this point in gestation, it is not unusual for infants to have more than one structural defect of the gastrointestinal system. This was the case with Jerome in the opening vignette. Infections can cause an increase or decrease in motility and prevent proper absorption of nutrients. Interruption or destruction of the GI system can also result from trauma or ingestion of caustic substances. As you read this chapter, remember that any interruption or alteration in the GI system will decrease the body's ability to obtain nutrients, thus impairing growth.

► ANATOMY AND PHYSIOLOGY OF PEDIATRIC DIFFERENCES

Although the fetus makes sucking and swallowing movements in utero and ingests amniotic fluid, the GI system is immature at birth. The processes of absorption and excretion do not begin until after birth because the placenta is responsible for providing nutrients and removing waste. Sucking is a primitive reflex that occurs whenever the lips or cheeks are stroked. The infant does not have voluntary control over swallowing until about 6 weeks of age.

The stomach capacity of the newborn is quite small, and intestinal motility (**peristalsis**) is greater than in older children. These characteristics explain the newborn's need for small, frequent feedings and the increased frequency and liquid consistency of bowel movements. Because of the relaxed cardiac sphincter, infants frequently regurgitate small amounts of feedings.

Digestion takes place in the duodenum. Infants have a deficiency of several enzymes: amylase (which digests carbohydrates), lipase (which enhances fat absorption), and trypsin (which catabolizes protein into polypeptides and some amino acids). Enzymes are usually not present in sufficient quantities to aid digestion until 4–6 months of age. Thus, abdominal distention from gas is common.

Liver function is also immature. After the first few weeks of life the liver is able to conjugate bilirubin and excrete bile. The processes of **gluconeogenesis** (formation of glycogen from noncarbohydrates), plasma protein and ketone formation, vitamin storage, and **deamination** (removal of amino group from amino compound) remain immature during the first year of life.

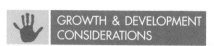

GROWTH & DEVELOPMENT CONSIDERATIONS

Stomach capacity increases throughout early childhood:

Age	Capacity (mL)
Newborn	10–20
1 week	30–90
2–3 weeks	75–100
1 month	90–150
3 months	150–200
1 year	210–360
2 years	500

By the second year of life, digestive processes are fairly complete. Stomach capacity increases to accommodate a three-meals-per-day feeding schedule. At about the same time, myelination of the spinal cord becomes complete and voluntary control over excretory functions can be achieved.

▶ STRUCTURAL DEFECTS

Structural defects can involve one or more areas of the GI tract. These defects occur when growth and development of fetal structures are interrupted during the first trimester. This can leave the structure incomplete, resulting in atresia (absence or closure of a normal body orifice), malposition, nonclosure, or other abnormalities.

CLEFT LIP AND CLEFT PALATE

Cleft lip and cleft palate are two distinct facial defects that can occur singly or in combination (Fig. 15–1). Incomplete fusion of the lip occurs in approximately 1 in 800 births.[1] It is more common in Asians and American Indians and less common in African-Americans. Incomplete fusion of the palate occurs in approximately 1 in 2000 births.[1] There are various degrees of severity with each defect.

Clinical Manifestations

A cleft that involves the lip is apparent at birth. It may be a simple dimple in the vermilion border of the lip or a complete separation extending to the floor of the nose. The defect may be unilateral or bilateral and may occur alone or in combination with a cleft palate defect. Varying degrees of nasal deformity may also be present.

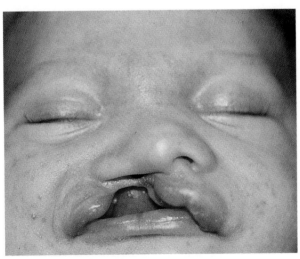

A

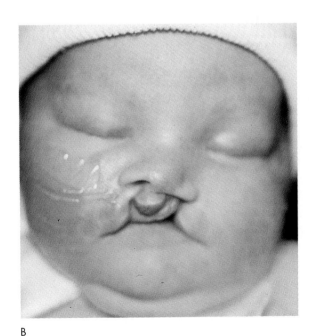

B

FIGURE 15–1. A, Unilateral cleft lip. B, Bilateral cleft lip.
Courtesy of Dr. Elizabeth Peterson.

Cleft palate defects are less obvious when they occur without a cleft lip and may not be detected at birth. Clefts of the hard palate form a continuous opening between the mouth and nasal cavity and may be unilateral or bilateral, involving just the soft palate or both the soft and hard palate.

Etiology and Pathophysiology

Cleft lip with or without cleft palate results from a failure of the maxillary processes to fuse with the elevations on the frontal prominence during the sixth week of gestation. Normally union of the upper lip is complete by the seventh week. Fusion of the secondary palate occurs between 7 and 12 weeks of gestation. Failure of the tongue to move downward at the correct time will prevent the palatine processes from fusing.

The intrauterine development of the hard and soft palates is completed in the first trimester. It is during this time that other major organ systems develop. Congenital defects such as tracheoesophageal fistula, omphalocele, trisomy 13, and skeletal dysplasias are associated with cleft lip and palate defects in 20–30% of cases. There is an increased incidence in families with a prior history of cleft lip or palate. The cause is believed to be multifactorial, involving a combination of environmental and genetic influences.[1]

Diagnostic Tests and Medical Management

Cleft lip and palate are usually diagnosed at birth or during the newborn assessment. Medical management requires the combined efforts of a multidisciplinary team. Because speech, hearing, and dentition may be affected, coordinated care by specialists in plastic surgery, hearing, speech, and dentistry is necessary.[1]

The cleft lip is usually repaired by about 2–3 months of age (Fig. 15–2). The lip is sutured together, and a Logan bow or other stabilizing device or

RESEARCH CONSIDERATIONS

Folic acid supplementation during pregnancy has been shown to decrease the incidence of neural tube defects. The benefits of folic acid supplementation for women who are planning a pregnancy appear to be supported by a recent study of 891 infants and mothers in California. Researchers found that women who took multivitamins with folic acid around the time of conception had a 25–50% lower risk of having children with orofacial clefts.[2]

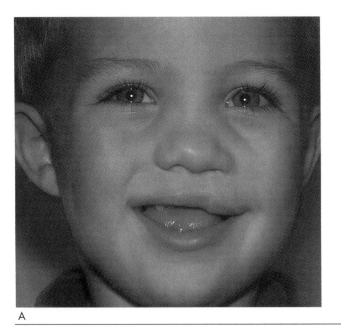
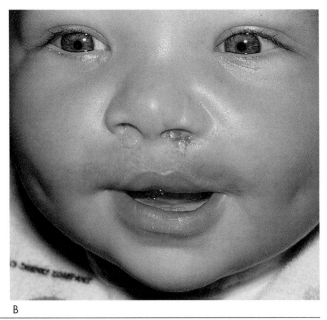

A   B

FIGURE 15–2. A, Repaired unilateral cleft lip (see Fig. 15–1A). B, Repaired bilateral cleft lip (see Fig. 15–1B).
Courtesy of Dr. Elizabeth Peterson.

dressing is put in place to prevent tension on the suture line. After surgery, the infant's elbows are restrained to prevent flexion (refer to the *Quick Reference to Pediatric Clinical Skills* accompanying this text). To prevent injury to the suture line, crying is minimized by use of medication.

Early closure of the lip enables the infant to form a better seal around the nipple for feeding. The sucking motion strengthens the muscles necessary for speech. Special feeding devices such as longer nipples with enlarged holes are available to help meet the infant's nutritional needs before surgical correction.

Timing of the cleft palate repair is controversial and depends on the size and severity of the cleft. Most surgeons perform closure operations when the infant is about 18 months old. This protects the formation of tooth buds and allows the infant to develop more normal speech patterns.

Infants with cleft lip and cleft palate are prone to recurrent otitis media, which can lead to tympanic membrane scarring and hearing loss. Antibiotic therapy is prescribed to treat any infections that might lead to an ear infection. Because infants with chronic otitis media often have difficulty hearing, speech patterns may be altered. These infants require early and continuous intervention to prevent complications. (Refer to Chapter 17 for care of the child with chronic otitis media.) The child who has had cleft palate repair will require orthodontic care. Early visits will permit assessment of tooth eruption and the need for future orthodontic work.

Nursing Assessment

Physiologic Assessment

A cleft lip defect is observable at birth. A cleft palate defect is usually noted during the newborn assessment by palpation of the hard palate with the finger. A description of the location and extent of the defect will assist the nurse in determining the correct method of feeding.

Psychosocial Assessment

Assessment of the family's reactions is an integral part of the overall nursing assessment. Physical deformities, especially of the face, can be devastating to parents. A poorly corrected defect can lead to the development of low self-esteem in the older child. Assess the child's developmental level and social interactions with peers.

Nursing Diagnosis

The accompanying Nursing Care Plan lists common nursing diagnoses for the infant with a cleft lip and/or palate. Other diagnoses that might be appropriate include:

- Anxiety (Parent) related to surgical correction of cleft lip during infancy, long-term management, and financial concerns
- Ineffective Infant Feeding Pattern related to ineffective suck and anatomic abnormality
- Risk for Caregiver Role Strain related to child with a chronic condition
- Risk for Impaired Home Maintenance Management related to infant's defect(s) and inadequate family support

NURSING CARE PLAN
THE INFANT WITH A CLEFT LIP AND/OR PALATE

GOAL	INTERVENTION	RATIONALE	EXPECTED OUTCOME

Preoperative Care

1. Risk for Aspiration (Breast Milk, Formula, or Mucus) related to anatomic defect

GOAL	INTERVENTION	RATIONALE	EXPECTED OUTCOME
The infant will have no episodes of gagging or aspiration.	• Assess respiratory status and monitor vital signs at least every 2 hours. • Position on side after feedings. • Feed slowly and use adaptive equipment as needed. • Burp frequently (after every 15–30 mL of fluid). • Position upright for feedings. • Keep suction equipment and bulb syringe at bedside.	• Allows for early identification of problems. • Prevents aspiration of feedings. • Facilitates intake while minimizing risk of aspiration. • Helps to prevent regurgitation and aspiration. • Minimizes passage of feedings through cleft. • Suctioning may be necessary to remove milk or mucus.	The infant exhibits no signs of respiratory distress.

2. Ineffective Family Coping related to birth of a child with a visible and/or structural defect

GOAL	INTERVENTION	RATIONALE	EXPECTED OUTCOME
Parents will begin bonding process with the infant.	• Help parents to hold the infant and facilitate feeding process. • Point out positive attributes of infant (hair, eyes, alertness, etc). • Explain surgical procedure and expected outcome. Show pictures of other children's cleft lip repair.	• Contact is essential for bonding. • Helps parents see the child as a whole, rather than concentrating on the defect. • Eliminating unknown factors helps to decrease anxiety.	Parents hold, comfort, and show concern for the infant.
The family's coping ability will be maximized. Parents will verbalize the nature and sequelae of the defect.	• Assess parents' knowledge of the defect, their degree of anxiety and level of discomfort, and the interpersonal relationships among family members.	• Helps to determine the appropriate timing and amount of information to be given regarding the child's defect.	The family demonstrates improved coping ability before discharge.

NURSING CARE PLAN
THE INFANT WITH A CLEFT LIP AND/OR PALATE– *Continued*

GOAL	INTERVENTION	RATIONALE	EXPECTED OUTCOME

2. Ineffective Family Coping related to birth of a child with a visible and/or structural defect (continued)

GOAL	INTERVENTION	RATIONALE	EXPECTED OUTCOME
	• Explore the reactions of extended family members.	• Extended family is an important source of support for most parents of a newborn. Family members can often help promote acceptance and compliance with the treatment plan.	
	• Support open visitation.	• Allows parents to continue the bonding process.	
	• Encourage parents to participate in caretaking activities (holding, diapering, feeding).	• Participation in infant care decreases anxiety and provides parents with a sense of purpose.	
	• Provide information about the etiology of cleft lip and palate defects and the special needs of these infants. Encourage questions.	• Concrete information allows parents time to understand the defect and reduces guilt.	
	• Refer to parent support groups.	• Support groups allow parents to express their feelings and concerns, to find people with concerns similar to their own, and to seek additional information.	

3. Altered Nutrition: Less Than Body Requirements related to the infant's inability to form an adequate seal for sucking

GOAL	INTERVENTION	RATIONALE	EXPECTED OUTCOME
The infant will gain weight steadily.	• Assess fluid and calorie intake daily. Assess weight daily (same scale, same time, with infant completely undressed).	• Provides an objective measurement of whether the infant is receiving sufficient caloric intake to promote growth. Using the same scale and procedure when weighing the infant provides for comparability between daily weights.	The infant maintains adequate nutritional intake and gains weight appropriately.

Continued . . .

NURSING CARE PLAN
THE INFANT WITH A CLEFT LIP AND/OR PALATE– *Continued*

GOAL	INTERVENTION	RATIONALE	EXPECTED OUTCOME

3. Altered Nutrition: Less Than Body Requirements related to the infant's inability to form an adequate seal for sucking (continued)

GOAL	INTERVENTION	RATIONALE	EXPECTED OUTCOME
	• Observe for any respiratory impairment.	• Any symptoms of respiratory compromise will interfere with the infant's ability to suck. Feedings should be initiated only if there are no signs of respiratory distress.	
	• Provide 100–150 cal/kg/day and 100–130 mL/kg/day of feedings and fluid. If the infant needs an increased number of calories to grow, referral to a nutritionist should be made. Formulas with higher calorie concentrations per ounce are available without increasing total fluids.	• Provides optimal calories and fluids for growth and hydration.	
	• Facilitate breast-feeding.	• Breast milk is recommended as the best food for an infant. The process of breast-feeding helps to promote bonding between mother and infant.	
	• Hold the infant in a semisitting position.	• Makes swallowing easier and reduces the amount of fluid return from the nose.	
	• Give the mother information on breast-feeding the infant with a cleft lip and/or palate such as plugging the cleft lip and eliciting a let-down reflex before nursing.	• Information and specific suggestions may encourage the mother to persist with breast-feeding.	
	• Contact the LaLeche League for the name of a support person (see Appendix F).	• The LaLeche League promotes breast-feeding for all infants. It can provide support people with experience who will aid the mother.	

NURSING CARE PLAN
THE INFANT WITH A CLEFT LIP AND/OR PALATE– *Continued*

GOAL	INTERVENTION	RATIONALE	EXPECTED OUTCOME

3. Altered Nutrition: Less Than Body Requirements related to the infant's inability to form an adequate seal for sucking (continued)

GOAL	INTERVENTION	RATIONALE	EXPECTED OUTCOME
	• If the mother is unable to breast-feed (or prefers not to), initiate bottle feeding:		
	• Hold infant in an upright or semisitting position for feeding.	• Facilitates swallowing and minimizes the amount of fluid return from the nose.	
	• Place nipple against the inside cheek toward the back of the tongue. May need to use a premature nipple (slightly longer and softer than regular nipple with a larger opening) or a Brecht feeder (an oval bottle with a long, soft nipple).	• Use of longer, softer nipples makes it easier for the infant to suck. A Brecht feeder decreases the amount of pressure in the bottle and makes the formula flow more easily.	
	• Feed small amounts slowly.	• Small amounts and allow feeding do not tire the infant as quickly as do larger amounts given at a faster rate. They also decrease the calories used during feeding.	
	• Burp frequently, after 15–30 mL of formula has been given.	• Frequent burping prevents the accumulation of air in stomach, which can cause regurgitation or vomiting.	
	• Initiate nasogastric feedings if the infant is unable to ingest sufficient calories by mouth.	• Adequate nutrition must be maintained. Use of a feeding tube allows the infant who has difficulty with oral feeding to receive adequate nutrition for growth.	

Postoperative Care

1. Risk for Infection related to surgical procedure and accumulation of formula and secretions in the oral cavity

GOAL	INTERVENTION	RATIONALE	EXPECTED OUTCOME
The infant's mucosal tissue will heal without infection.	• Assess vital signs every 2 hours.	• Elevated temperature may indicate infection.	The infant remains free of infection in the oral cavity. Tissues remain intact and pink.

Continued . . .

NURSING CARE PLAN
THE INFANT WITH A CLEFT LIP AND/OR PALATE– *Continued*

GOAL	INTERVENTION	RATIONALE	EXPECTED OUTCOME

1. Risk for Infection related to surgical procedure and accumulation of formula and secretions in the oral cavity (continued)

GOAL	INTERVENTION	RATIONALE	EXPECTED OUTCOME
	• Assess oral cavity every 2 hours or as needed for tenderness, reddened areas, lesions, or presence of secretions.	• Aids in identifying infection.	
	• Cleanse suture line with normal saline or sterile water if ordered.	• Helps decrease the presence of bacteria.	
	• Cleanse the cleft areas by giving 5–15 mL of water after each feeding.	• Prevents accumulation of carbohydrates, which encourage bacterial growth.	
	• If a crust has formed, use a cotton swab to apply a half-strength peroxide solution.	• Helps loosen the crust, aiding in removal.	
	• Apply antibiotic cream to suture line as ordered.	• Counteracts the growth of bacteria.	
	• Use careful handwashing and sterile technique when working with suture line.	• Prevents the spread of microorganisms from other sources.	

2. Ineffective Breathing Pattern related to anesthesia and increased secretions

GOAL	INTERVENTION	RATIONALE	EXPECTED OUTCOME
The infant will maintain an effective breathing pattern.	• Assess respiratory status and monitor vital signs at least every 2 hours.	• Allows for early identification of problems.	The infant shows no signs of respiratory infection or compromise.
	• Apply a cardiorespiratory monitor.	• Enables early detection of abnormal respirations, facilitating prompt intervention.	
	• Keep suction equipment and bulb syringe at bedside. Gently suction oropharynx and nasopharynx as needed.	• Gentle suctioning will keep the airway clear. Suctioning that is too vigorous can irritate the mucosa.	
	• Provide cool mist for first 24 hours postoperatively if ordered.	• Moisturizes secretions to reduce pooling in lungs. Moisturizes oral cavity.	
	• Reposition every 2 hours.	• Ensures expansion of all lung fields.	

NURSING CARE PLAN
THE INFANT WITH A CLEFT LIP AND/OR PALATE– *Continued*

GOAL	INTERVENTION	RATIONALE	EXPECTED OUTCOME

3. Impaired Tissue Integrity related to surgical correction of cleft

Lip and/or palate will heal with minimal scarring or disruption.	• Position the infant with cleft lip repair on side or back only.	• Prone position could cause rubbing on suture line.	Lip/palate heals without complications.
	• Use soft elbow restraints. Remove every 2 hours and replace. Do not leave the infant unattended when restraints are removed.	• Prevents the infant's hands from rubbing surgical site. Regular removal allows for skin and neurovascular checks.	
	• Maintain metal bar (Logan bow) or Steri-Strips placed over cleft lip repair.	• Maintaining suture line will minimize scarring.	
	• Avoid metal utensils or straws after cleft palate repair.	• These devices may disrupt suture line.	
	• Keep the infant well medicated for pain in initial postoperative period. Have parents hold and comfort the infant.	• Good pain management minimizes crying, which can cause stress on suture line. Increases bonding and soothes the child to decrease crying.	
	• Provide developmentally appropriate activities (ie, mobiles, music).	• Soothes and keeps the infant calm.	

4. Knowledge Deficit (Parent) related to diagnosis, treatment, prognosis, and home care needs

Before discharge, parents will verbalize home care methods for care of the infant with cleft lip and palate defect.	• Explain care and treatment (both short-term and long-term). Discuss potential complications.	• Assists the family to deal with the physical and psychosocial aspects of a child with a congenital defect.	Parents accurately describe and demonstrate feeding techniques to facilitate optimal growth of the infant; describe interventions if respiratory distress occurs; and take the written instructions home with them on discharge.
	• Demonstrate feeding techniques and alternatives. Allow parents to demonstrate before discharge.	• Provides visual instructions. Redemonstration confirms learning.	
	• Provide written instructions for follow-up care arrangements.	• Written instructions reinforce verbal instruction and provide a reference after discharge.	
	• Introduce the parents (if possible) to a primary care provider in the setting where the infant will receive follow-up care after discharge.	• Continuity of care is important. Since the infant will require long-term follow-up, a contact with the new provider is helpful.	

Continued . . .

NURSING CARE PLAN
THE INFANT WITH A CLEFT LIP AND/OR PALATE– *Continued*

GOAL	INTERVENTION	RATIONALE	EXPECTED OUTCOME

5. Altered Nutrition: Less Than Body Requirements related to surgery and feeding difficulties

GOAL	INTERVENTION	RATIONALE	EXPECTED OUTCOME
The infant will receive adequate nutritional intake.	• Maintain intravenous infusion as ordered.	• Provides fluid when NPO.	The infant receives adequate nutritional intake. Infant resumes usual feeding patterns and gains weight appropriately.
	• Begin with clear liquids, then give half-strength formula or breast milk as ordered.	• Ensures adequate fluids and nutrients.	
	• Use Asepto syringe or dropper in side of mouth.	• Avoids suture line and resultant accumulation of formula in that area.	
	• Do not allow pacifiers.	• Sucking can disrupt suture line.	
	• Give high-calorie soft foods after cleft palate repair.	• Rough foods, utensils, and straws could disrupt the surgical site.	

Nursing Management

Nursing care involves providing emotional support, performing postsurgical care, helping parents to coordinate care and maintain a healthy home environment, and making appropriate referrals. The accompanying Nursing Care Plan summarizes nursing care for the infant with a cleft lip and/or cleft palate.

Provide Emotional Support

Parents may need assistance to view their infant as a whole person, rather than focusing solely on the physical defect. Nurses can promote parent–infant bonding by explaining the cause of the structural defect and the procedure for correction. Interact and speak to the infant in the parents' presence and point out positive attributes such as alertness, soft skin, or active movements. Self-blame is common among parents. Parents can also be referred to the American Cleft Palate Association for information about the disorder (see Appendix F).

Parental anxiety is usual when children undergo surgery. This anxiety is heightened when the surgery involves an infant. To minimize anxiety, explanations to parents should be clear and concise. Allow sufficient time for parents to ask questions. Encourage parents to hold and cuddle the infant before surgery.

Provide Postoperative Care

Provide general postoperative care for the infant. (See the accompanying Nursing Care Plan for the Infant with a Cleft Lip and/or Palate and the Nursing Care Plan for the Child Undergoing Surgery in Chapter 4.) Assess vital signs frequently and maintain the infant's airway. Measure intake and output. When oral fluids with clear liquids are started, they are usually given through a dropper or an Asepto syringe. Position the infant in a sitting position for the feedings to avoid aspiration. The infant then progresses to half-strength formula or breast milk. After each feeding clean the suture line with water or normal saline to avoid accumulation of feedings.

It is important to maintain the suture line to ensure healing. Position the infant in a supine or a side-lying position to avoid rubbing the suture line on the bedding. Keep elbows in soft restraints. Maintain the metal device or Steri-Strips placed over the incision. Place antibiotic cream on the incision site. Medicate the infant regularly to control pain and to minimize crying and stress on the suture line. After cleft palate surgery, avoid the use of metal utensils or straws, which may disrupt the surgical site.

Discharge Planning and Home Care Teaching

Home care needs should be identified and addressed well in advance of discharge. Discuss all aspects of the infant's care with the parents throughout hospitalization and after surgery. Involve parents in the infant's care to increase their comfort level before discharge and to promote bonding. Teach them feeding techniques, how to recognize signs of infection, how to position the infant, and how to care for the suture line. Breast-feeding is usually possible with some assistance from a lactation specialist. Some infants may need a device placed in the mouth to enable them to establish suction.

Management, especially in the first few months of life, involves many different health care professionals. The parents are the best coordinators of the child's care. Encourage them to keep a diary listing the professionals with whom they talk and the content of the discussions.

Discuss with the parents the financial implications of long-term care. Private insurance does not always cover all the costs of care necessary for the child. Refer parents to social services familiar with programs and financial aid for which the parents and child may be eligible. Relief of financial worries enables parents to concentrate on caring for the child.

Teach parents how to care for the child after discharge. If the child has siblings, emphasize that they will need preparation to accept the child. Sibling rivalry can be heightened when one child receives more attention within the home. Remind parents of the importance of setting limits and of spending time with each child. Determine whether additional family supports are necessary. Provide parents with information on support groups, physicians, social workers, and local services that can help maintain family continuity.

Discuss ways to prevent the infant from touching the suture line. Teach parents how to bundle an infant in a blanket with arms tucked inside the blanket. A front-sling baby carrier may also be used to immobilize the arms. Front-sling carriers provide the additional benefits of comforting the infant through contact with the parent and of holding the infant upright, which aids in positioning during feeding.

After surgical repair, parents need to be taught how to feed the infant and how to identify signs of complications (fever, vomiting, respiratory distress). Referral to a home health care agency for support may be helpful. Encourage follow-up visits with health care professionals. The child may need further evaluation of speech development, ear infections, or a recommendation for plastic surgery.

GROWTH & DEVELOPMENT CONSIDERATIONS

An infant who has had a cleft lip repair needs stimulation to provide distraction. This approach will minimize crying, which can damage the suture line. Soft, colorful toys, mobiles, and other visual objects are helpful. Music also can be used to soothe the infant.

ESOPHAGEAL ATRESIA AND TRACHEOESOPHAGEAL FISTULA

Esophageal atresia is a malformation that results from failure of the esophagus to develop as a continuous tube during the fourth and fifth weeks of gestation. Esophageal atresia with tracheoesophageal fistula occurs in 1 in 3000 to 4000 births.[3]

Symptoms in the newborn include excessive salivation and drooling, often accompanied by cyanosis, choking, coughing, and sneezing. During feeding, the infant returns fluid through the nose and mouth. Aspiration places the infant at risk for pneumonia. Depending on the type of defect, the abdomen may become distended because of air trapping.

In esophageal atresia, the foregut fails to lengthen, separate, and fuse into two parallel tubes (the esophagus and trachea) during fetal development. Instead the esophagus may end in a blind pouch or develop as a pouch connected to the trachea by a fistula (tracheoesophageal fistula) (Fig. 15–3). Esophageal atresia is often associated with a maternal history of polyhydramnios. Associated anomalies may occur, including congenital heart defects, gastrointestinal or urinary tract anomalies, and musculoskeletal abnormalities. Jerome, described at the beginning of the chapter, had esophageal atresia as well as an imperforate anus.

Diagnosis is usually confirmed by attempting to pass a 5 or 8 French nasogastric tube into the stomach. In most cases, the tube meets resistance and can be advanced only minimally. Specific defects and associated anomalies are determined by x-ray examination. Echocardiogram and abdominal ultrasound are performed. Careful examination of the lungs is needed. A delay in diagnosis can be fatal because ingested fluid or secretions may enter the lungs.

A tube is inserted to suction the upper pouch. Intravenous antibiotics and fluids are begun. Surgery is performed as soon as possible. Surgical correction may be accomplished in several stages. The first stage usually involves ligation of the fistula and insertion of a gastrostomy tube. In the second stage, the two ends of the esophagus are reconnected, if possible. When surgical closure (anastomosis) is not possible, a gastrostomy tube must remain in place for use in feeding. Potential postoperative complications include gastroesophageal reflux, aspiration, and stricture formation.[1] The prognosis is usually good with surgery.

Nursing Management

Esophageal atresia is a surgical emergency. Preoperatively the infant requires close observation and intervention to maintain a patent airway.

CLINICAL TIP

When using a small-bore nasogastric tube, gurgling can occur when the tube is in the esophagus or lung. To confirm placement, aspiration of stomach contents and pH testing are required.

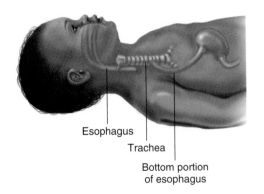

FIGURE 15–3. In the most common type of esophageal atresia and tracheoesophageal fistula, the upper segment of the esophagus ends in a blind pouch connected to the trachea; a fistula connects the lower segment to the trachea.

Esophagus

Trachea

Bottom portion of esophagus

Suction should be readily available to remove any secretions that accumulate in the nasopharyngeal airway. Place the infant with the head of the bed slightly lowered to minimize aspiration of secretions into the trachea. Continuous or low intermittent suction is used to remove secretions from the blind pouch. Oral fluids are withheld, and the infant is maintained with intravenous fluids administered through an umbilical artery catheter.

After surgery, gastrostomy drainage is maintained, and intravenous fluids and antibiotics are administered. Total parenteral nutrition may be needed until gastrostomy or oral feedings are tolerated.

The parents require emotional support throughout the infant's hospitalization. All procedures should be clearly explained. Encourage parents to bond with the infant by stroking and talking to the infant. Eliciting questions and allowing parents to participate in the infant's care, especially feeding (when permitted), can facilitate bonding and help to prepare parents for care of the infant after discharge.

Once enteral feedings have been established, the infant may be discharged from the hospital with a gastrostomy tube in place (Fig. 15–4). (Refer to the *Quick Reference to Pediatric Clinical Skills* accompanying this text for care of the child with a gastrostomy tube.) Teach the parents about gastrostomy tube care and feeding, signs of infection, and how to prevent postoperative complications (Table 15–1).

PYLORIC STENOSIS

Pyloric stenosis is a hypertrophic obstruction of the circular muscle of the pyloric canal. It is a common problem that most often affects first-born male infants.

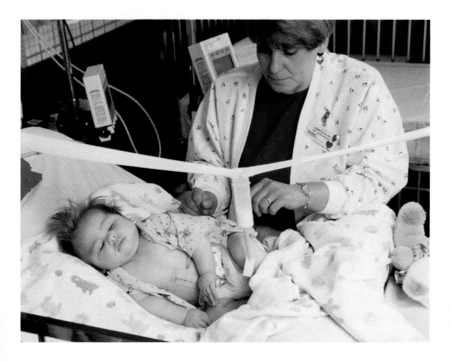

FIGURE 15–4. A gastrostomy tube is used to feed the child with a gastrointestinal disorder such as esophageal atresia.

15-1   Parent Teaching: Home Care Instructions for the Child Requiring Gastrostomy Tube Feedings and Care

Equipment
Prepared, prescribed feeding; enteral feeding pump; long-nosed syringe

Procedure
1. Wash hands.
2. Warm prescribed formula to room temperature.
3. Pour formula to run through the feeding bag.
4. Allow formula to run through the tubing to remove air. Close clamp.
5. Attach syringe to the end of the gastrostomy tube. Unclamp the gastrostomy tube.
6. Pull plunger back until resistance is felt. Check amount of formula in syringe. If more than half of the prescribed amount is withdrawn, refer to the section on problem solving (below). If less than the prescribed amount is withdrawn, push the formula gently back through the syringe.
7. Instill water through the tube.
8. Attach the feeding bag to the gastrostomy tube. Infuse at the prescribed rate.
9. Burp or bubble the infant throughout the feeding.
10. After feeding, flush the gastrostomy tube with water and clamp the tube.
11. Position the infant prone or side lying for ½–1 hour after feedings.

Psychosocial Needs
Hold and rock the infant or child during feedings.
Give a pacifier to an infant or a bottle or cup to a child to meet developmental needs.

Medication Administration
Use liquid medication whenever possible.
Crush only uncoated tablets.
Crush tablets to a find powder and mix with water or juice.
Flush tubing before and after medication administration.

Stoma Care
Wash the area around the stoma twice a day with soap and water.
Use half-strength hydrogen peroxide to remove any crusting.
Look for signs of infection, such as redness, swelling, and discharge.
Notify the physician if any signs of infection or leakage are present.

Problem Solving

Problem	Cause	Action
Formula will not flow	Blocked tube (clamping, foreign material)	Check clamp. Reposition. Pull back on syringe. Instill water. Notify physician.
	Viscous formula	
	Pump malfunction	Check plug. Call company. Give feeding by gravity.
Large volume of undigested formula removed before feeding	Delayed absorption	Reinfuse remaining formula. If more than half of feeding, subtract from the next feeding. Do not discard the residual.
	Constipation	Check for last bowel movement. Notify physician.
Constipation	Decreased free fluids	Give water and juice between feedings as tolerated. Report bowel problems or hard stools to physician.
Diarrhea	Hyperosmolar formula	Dilute formula.
	Rapid rate of flow	Feed at a slower rate.
	Cold formula	Warm formula to room temperature before feeding.
	Bacterial contamination	Treat with antibiotics.

Data from Gulanick, M., Knoll-Puzas, M., & Wilson, C. (Eds.). (1992). Nursing care plans for newborns and children: Acute and critical care. St. Louis: Mosby–Year Book; Skale, N. (1992). Manual of pediatric nursing procedures. Philadelphia: Lippincott; and Young, C., & White, S. (1992). Preparing patients for tube feeding at home. American Journal of Nursing, 92, 46–53.

Clinical Manifestations

Symptoms usually become evident 2–4 weeks after birth, although onset may vary. Initially the infant appears well or regurgitates slightly after feedings. The parents may describe the infant as a "good eater" who vomits occasionally. As the obstruction progresses, the vomiting becomes projectile. In **projectile vomiting,** the contents of the stomach may be ejected up to 3 feet from the infant. The vomitus is nonbilious and may become blood tinged because of repeated irritation to the esophagus. The infant is always hungry, appears irritable, fails to gain weight, and has fewer and smaller stools. Dehydration, alkalosis, and hyperbilirubinemia can occur.[4]

Etiology and Pathophysiology

The exact cause of pyloric stenosis is unknown, although frequently there is a family history of the disorder. It is relatively common, with about 4–5 cases in 1000 births.[5] Hypertrophy of the circular pylorus muscle results in stenosis of the passage between the stomach and the duodenum, partially obstructing the lumen of the stomach (Fig. 15–5). The lumen becomes inflamed and edematous, which narrows the opening until the obstruction becomes complete. At this time vomiting becomes more projectile. As the obstruction progresses, the infant becomes dehydrated and electrolytes are depleted, resulting in metabolic imbalances.

Diagnostic Tests and Medical Management

On physical examination, visible peristaltic waves across the abdomen and an olive-sized mass in the left upper quadrant are often found. A sonogram is usually performed to confirm the diagnosis, and an upper GI series may be performed as well. Blood tests are used to determine the degree of dehydration, electrolyte imbalance, and anemia (see Chap. 8).

Surgical correction is the treatment of choice. Preoperatively the infant's condition is stabilized with intravenous fluids and electrolytes. A na-

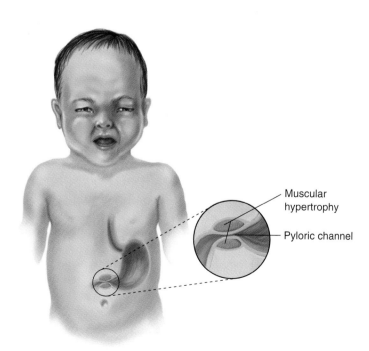

Muscular
hypertrophy

Pyloric channel

FIGURE 15–5. In pyloric stenosis, the hypertrophied pyloric muscle causes symptoms of projectile vomiting and visible peristalsis.

sogastric tube is inserted to decompress the stomach. Surgery is performed as soon as possible after the infant's condition is stabilized. During surgery the circular muscle fibers are released to allow the passage of food and fluid (pyloromyotomy). The prognosis is good. The infant is usually taking fluids in 2 days and discharged within 72 hours of surgery.

Nursing Assessment

Observe the infant's abdomen for the presence of peristaltic waves. Bowel sounds are hyperactive on auscultation. Palpation reveals an olive-shaped mass in the right upper quadrant of the abdomen.

Assess skin turgor, fontanels, urinary output, and mucous membranes to determine whether hydration is adequate. Measure vomitus and describe vomiting episodes. Be alert for signs of an electrolyte imbalance, particularly low levels of serum chloride, sodium, and potassium, and an elevated pH. (See Chapter 8 for a discussion of these electrolyte imbalances.)

Assess the parents' level of anxiety related to the child's condition.

Nursing Diagnosis

Among the nursing diagnoses that might be appropriate for the child with pyloric stenosis are:

- Fluid Volume Deficit related to frequent vomiting
- Altered Nutrition: Less Than Body Requirements related to vomiting and lack of absorption of nutrients
- Sleep Pattern Disturbance related to constant hunger, vomiting, and esophageal irritation or pain
- Risk for Infection related to surgical incision
- Altered Family Processes related to seriously ill infant requiring hospitalization and surgery

Nursing Management

Nursing care centers on meeting the infant's fluid needs, minimizing weight loss, promoting rest and comfort, preventing infection, and providing supportive care for parents.

Meet Fluid Needs

Because projectile vomiting will continue until the obstruction is relieved surgically, oral feedings are withheld. Intravenous fluid therapy is administered to correct fluid and electrolyte imbalances and to maintain adequate hydration. Monitor intake and output (including vomitus) and urine specific gravity. Inform parents that all diapers will be weighed to measure the infant's output of urine and stool.

Minimize Weight Loss

The infant loses weight because of frequent vomiting. Monitor weight daily both preoperatively and postoperatively. Small, frequent feedings consisting of clear liquids are begun within 4–6 hours postoperatively. If clear liquids are tolerated, the infant is advanced to formula feedings.

Promote Rest and Comfort

During the preoperative period the infant is hungry and cries often. The infant is swaddled to maintain warmth and provide comfort. Encourage the

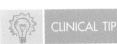
CLINICAL TIP

Auscultate for bowel sounds before palpating the abdomen because bowel patterns may change in response to the examiner's touch.

parents to hold and cuddle the infant. Provide a pacifier to meet the infant's need to suck.

Postoperatively the infant is uncomfortable because of the surgical incision. Instruct parents to avoid pressure on the incision. When diapering the infant, slide the diaper gently under the buttocks rather than lifting the legs. Swaddling, rocking, and use of a pacifier help to relax the infant. Acetaminophen or other analgesics can be administered to relieve discomfort as ordered. (See Chapter 7 for a discussion of pain management.)

Prevent Infection

Postoperatively the incision is covered with collodion or Steri-Strips and should be kept clean and dry. Check the incision site for redness, swelling, or discharge. Monitor the infant's temperature every 4 hours.

Provide Supportive Care

The need for hospitalization and surgery creates anxiety for parents. Encourage them to participate in the infant's care and to discuss their fears and concerns. Provide simple and clear explanations about the infant's condition and care. Advise parents that occasional vomiting after surgery may occur.

Discharge Planning and Home Care Teaching

Instruct parents to observe the incision for redness, swelling, or discharge and to notify the physician immediately if these occur or if the infant's temperature is higher than 38.5°C (101°F). To reduce the possibility of infection, advise parents to fold the infant's diaper so that it does not touch the incision.

GASTROESOPHAGEAL REFLUX

Gastroesophageal reflux, the return of gastric contents into the esophagus, is the result of relaxation of the lower esophageal sphincter. It may occur at any time and is not necessarily related to having a full stomach.

Children with gastroesophageal reflux are frequently hungry and irritable. They eat often but still lose weight. They have a history of vomiting and frequent upper respiratory infections. Reflux of stomach contents can lead to aspiration, resulting in frequent bouts of pneumonia, reactive airway disease, or apnea.

Some "spitting up" after feedings is considered normal in newborn infants, because of the weak cardiac sphincter of the stomach. However, regurgitation that continues and increases in frequency, resulting in delayed growth, requires further investigation. Gastroesophageal reflux is more common in premature infants and in children with neurologic impairments. It often resolves without surgical intervention by 12–18 months of age.[6]

Diagnosis is confirmed by a thorough history of the child's feeding patterns and by diagnostic evaluation using barium swallow, upper gastrointestinal endoscopy, pH probe monitoring (insertion of a small catheter into the esophagus through the nose that is left in place for 18–24 hours to measure pH and thus determine number of reflux episodes), or gastroesophageal scintigraphy (radionuclide scanning to evaluate gastric emptying).[7]

Treatment depends on the severity of the condition. Mild cases may require only a modification of feeding habits. The use of rice cereal in the infant's bottle to thicken feedings is often used. Fatty foods and citrus juices

CLINICAL TIP

To thicken formula add 1 tablespoon of rice cereal to 6 ounces of formula. Cut a slightly larger hole in the infant's nipple to accommodate the thicker feeding.

are avoided. Medications (cholinergics, antacids, and histamine antagonists) may be prescribed to reduce the amount of stomach acid and lessen the child's discomfort (Table 15–2). The child should be positioned with the upper body raised 30 degrees after feedings.

Treatment for severe cases may include surgery to create a valve mechanism by wrapping the greater curvature of the stomach (fundus) around the distal esophagus (Nissen fundoplication). A gastrostomy tube is usually inserted during surgery and left in place for 6 weeks.[8] Both infants with mild conditions and those undergoing surgical correction usually have decreased incidence of reflux. They may have episodes of mild reflux throughout life and may occasionally require medication for treatment.

Nursing Management

Nursing management focuses on obtaining a thorough history of the child's feeding patterns. Observe vomiting episodes and document amount, color, and consistency of emesis.

Monitor the infant's weight daily and plot on a growth chart to note progress. Observe for any signs of respiratory distress, and keep the infant's nose and mouth clear of vomitus.

Adequate nutrition must be maintained. Infants receiving oral feedings should be given small, frequent feedings. Place the infant in a prone position with the head of the bed elevated to prevent aspiration if vomiting should occur. If the child has difficulty maintaining this position, a Tracy harness or reflux board may be used. The harness, which is pinned to the mattress, supports the infant in an upright position. If the child has a gastrostomy tube, it is important to maintain skin integrity around the stoma site. Secure the tube so the infant cannot dislodge or pull on it.

Discharge planning focuses on instructing parents in how to feed and position the infant (eg, avoid use of infant seat), as well as providing comfort and emotional support. Encourage parents to hold and cuddle the infant during all feedings. Providing the infant with a pacifier helps to meet nonnutritive sucking needs. Teach parents how to suction the nose and mouth if vomiting occurs.

CLINICAL TIP

Measure and record the length of the gastrostomy tube daily to be sure it remains properly placed. Coil the tube that is outside the body, tape in place, and put a shirt on the infant to cover it. Frequently clean any drainage around the tube as the acidic gastric contents are harmful to the skin.

NURSING ALERT

Do not place an infant with gastroesophageal reflux in an infant seat. The infant's position in this type of seat increases intraabdominal pressure and will actually worsen the condition.

15-2	Medications Used to Treat Gastroesophageal Reflux	
Drug	**Action**
Antacid (aluminum hydroxide, aluminum carbonate)	Neutralize refluxed material and decrease resultant discomfort
Histamine blockers Ranitidine Cimetidine	Decrease gastric acid production
Metoclopramide	Increases esophageal motility and tone
Cisapride	Increases esophageal motility and tone
Acetaminophen	Controls pain

OMPHALOCELE

Omphaloceles are congenital malformations in which intraabdominal contents herniate through the umbilical cord (Fig. 15–6). They result from failure of the abdominal contents to return to the abdomen when the abdominal wall begins to close by the tenth week of gestation. The protrusion is covered by a translucent sac into which the umbilical cord inserts. Omphalocele is often associated with other congenital anomalies such as cardiac defects, genitourinary anomalies, chromosomal defects, craniofacial abnormalities, and diaphragmatic abnormalities. It occurs in 1 in 3,000–10,000 births.[3]

The size of the sac varies depending on the extent of the protrusion. Rupture of the sac results in evisceration of the abdominal contents. Treatment involves protecting the sac from injury, providing fluids and warmth, and surgical repair to replace the abdominal contents and close the abdominal wall. For smaller defects, primary closure is accomplished with one surgery. If the defect is severe, surgical correction may be performed in several steps.[3] If an omphalocele occurs without associated defects, the child usually recovers from the surgery without incident and leads a normal life.

Nursing Management

Be alert for signs of associated congenital anomalies. (Refer to the discussions of tracheoesophageal fistula earlier in this chapter; to genitourinary anomalies in Chapter 16; and to congenital heart defects in Chapter 12.)

Immediately after birth, the sac is covered with sterile gauze soaked in normal saline solution to prevent drying of the abdominal contents. A layer of plastic wrap is placed over the gauze to provide additional protection against heat and moisture loss. Monitor vital signs every 2–4 hours, paying close attention to temperature, as the infant can lose heat through the sac. Inspect the area for signs of infection.

Because the infant is NPO preoperatively, fluid and electrolyte balance is maintained by administering intravenous fluids. Postoperative care includes measures to control pain, prevent infection, maintain fluid and electrolyte balance, and ensure adequate nutritional intake.

Throughout the infant's hospitalization, parents need clear, accurate explanations about the infant's condition. To help the parents deal with the crisis of an acutely ill newborn, provide emotional support and encourage

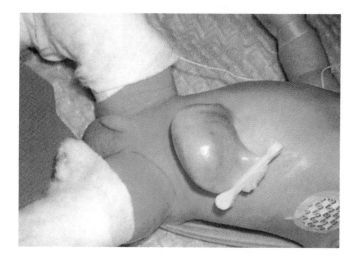

FIGURE 15–6. In omphalocele, the size of the sack depends on the extent of the protrusion of abdominal contents through the umbilical cord. *From Rudolph, A.M., Hoffman, J.I.E, & Rudolph, C.D. (Eds.). (1991). Rudolph's pediatrics (19th ed., p. 1040). Stamford, CT: Appleton & Lange.*

parents to express their feelings. When the child has multiple anomalies, parents need ongoing support for the lengthy treatment, numerous hospitalizations, and management of nutritional intake.

INTUSSUSCEPTION

Intussusception occurs when one portion of the intestine invaginates or telescopes into another. It is one of the most frequent causes of intestinal obstruction during infancy, with an incidence of 1–4 in 1000 births.[9] Most cases occur in boys between the ages of 2 months and 5 years.

The onset is usually abrupt. A previously healthy infant or child suddenly experiences acute abdominal pain with vomiting and passage of brown stool. There may be periods of comfort between acute episodes of pain. As the condition worsens, painful episodes increase. The stools become red and resemble currant jelly because of the mix of blood and mucus. A palpable mass may be present in the upper right quadrant or mid-upper abdomen.

The most common site of intussusception is the ileocecal valve (Fig. 15–7). Telescoping of the intestine obstructs the passage of stool. The walls of the intestine rub together, causing inflammation, edema, and decreased blood flow. This can lead to necrosis, perforation, hemorrhage, and peritonitis.

Diagnosis is made on the basis of the history and confirmed by radiographs of the abdomen and by a barium enema. In some cases the hydrostatic pressure from the barium moves the bowel back into place. If this does not occur, surgical intervention to reduce the invaginated bowel and remove any necrotic tissue is necessary. Surgery is usually successful in correcting the problem.

Nursing Management

Nursing management focuses on maintaining or restoring fluid and electrolyte balance. Intravenous fluids are started immediately. Serum electrolyte monitoring is essential to correct imbalances.

Postoperative care focuses on monitoring for early signs of infection, managing the child's pain, and maintaining nasogastric tube patency. Assess

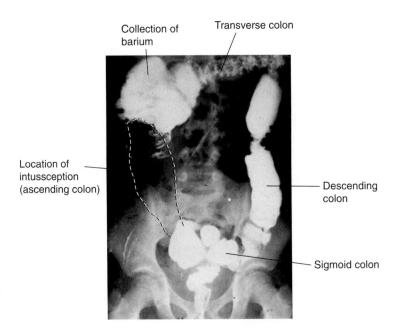

FIGURE 15–7. In infants, intussusception is commonly associated with measles, viral diseases, and gastroenteritis syndromes. *Copyright © MEDCOM, Inc., Garden Grove, CA.*

vital signs, check for abdominal distention, and listen for bowel sounds every 4 hours. After normal bowel function returns, clear liquid feedings are begun. Feedings are advanced to half-strength milk and other foods as the infant or child tolerates it.

Discharge usually occurs shortly after the infant or child begins taking full feedings. Instruct parents to watch for infection and to call the physician if symptoms recur, a fever develops, or appetite decreases.

HIRSCHSPRUNG'S DISEASE

Hirschsprung's disease, also known as congenital aganglionic megacolon, is a congenital anomaly in which inadequate motility causes mechanical obstruction of the intestine. The absence of autonomic parasympathetic ganglion cells in the colon prevents peristalsis at that portion of the intestine, resulting in the accumulation of intestinal contents and abdominal distention. Hirschsprung's disease is more common in boys and can occur in combination with congenital heart defects, Down syndrome, and some other syndromes such as Smith-Lemli-Opitz syndrome and Waarendenburg's syndrome. It can be acute or chronic and occurs in 1 in 5000 births.[11]

RESEARCH CONSIDERATIONS

Hirschprung's disease is now believed to be inherited in a recessive manner by mutations of the net oncogene.[10]

Clinical manifestations vary depending on the child's age at onset. In newborns symptoms include failure to pass meconium, refusal to suck, abdominal distention, and bile-stained emesis. If Hirschsprung's disease is not treated, the condition can lead to complete obstruction, respiratory distress, and shock.

In the older child, symptoms may include failure to gain weight and delayed growth. The child may have a history of abdominal distention, severe constipation alternating with diarrhea, and vomiting. The stool may be normal or have a ribbonlike appearance.[12]

Diagnosis is made on the basis of the history, bowel patterns, and radiographic contrast studies. The rectum is small in size on palpation and does not contain stool. Treatment in infancy involves surgical removal of the aganglionic bowel. A temporary colostomy is created to rest the bowel. Closure of the colostomy and reanastomosis are performed when the child reaches a weight of approximately 8–10 kg (17.6–22 lb).

For the child with a milder defect, management may involve dietary modification, stool softeners, and isotonic irrigations to prevent impaction until the child is toilet trained.

The return of normal bowel function depends on the amount of bowel involved. Some fecal incontinence and constipation may persist following closure of the colostomy. A serious complication is enterocolitis, which can lead to severe illness or death. Symptoms of enterocolitis include gastrointestinal bleeding and diarrhea. Enterocolitis can occur before or after surgery, resulting in ischemia and ulceration of the bowel wall. Treatment may include total parenteral nutrition and a lactose-free diet.[13]

Nursing Management

Nursing assessment in the newborn period includes careful observation for the passage of meconium. When the disease is diagnosed later in infancy or in childhood, obtain a thorough history of weight gain, nutritional intake, and bowel habits.

Nursing management consists of carefully monitoring fluid and electrolyte balance and maintaining nutrition. Teach parents how to ensure regular bowel movements. Daily rectal irrigations with normal saline solution are necessary to promote adequate elimination and prevent obstruction.

NURSING ALERT

Because newborns are often discharged within 24 hours of birth, it is important to describe to parents the characteristics of infants' first bowel movements. Parents should be instructed to notify the physician if no stool is passed or if the abdomen becomes distended.

Teach parents how to prevent skin breakdown in the rectal area by changing diapers frequently, cleansing the area carefully, and applying protective ointment at each diaper change.

If surgical correction is necessary, nursing care will include monitoring for infection, managing pain, maintaining hydration, measuring abdominal circumference to detect any distention, and providing support to the child and family. Parents will need instruction in ostomy care (refer to the discussion later in this chapter). Provide appropriate referrals to an ostomy support group and enterostomal nurse specialist. Teach parents to be alert for and immediately report signs of complications. These include diarrhea and pelvic abscess from leakage of intestinal contents at the surgical site (characterized by fever and pain). Children occasionally develop constipation, and parents may need guidance to adapt the diet and fluid intake to manage this complication. Because some children develop malabsorption, be alert for signs of poor growth or malnutrition.

ANORECTAL MALFORMATIONS

Malformations of the anus and rectum are common congenital anomalies. Minor anomalies occur in 1 in 4000–5000 births. They are often associated with anomalies of the urinary tract, esophagus, and duodenum.[12] Table 15–3 describes the most common anorectal anomalies.

Diagnosis is usually made at birth or during the newborn assessment of anorectal structures and rectal patency. Failure to pass meconium may indicate a malformation high in the colon. Stool in the urine is indicative of a fistula between the colon and urinary tract. Ribbonlike stools may occur with some malformations. Ultrasound and lower GI radiographic studies are used to confirm the diagnosis and demonstrate the extent of the anomaly.

15-3	Management of Anorectal Malformations

Condition	Management
Males	
Cutaneous fistula	
Anal stenosis	No colostomy required
Anal membrane	
Rectourethral fistula	
Bulbar	
Prostatic	
Rectovesical fistula	Colostomy required
Anorectal agenesis without fistula	
Rectal atresia	
Females	
Cutaneous perineal fistula	No colostomy required
Vestibular fistula	
Vaginal fistula	
Anorectal agenesis without fistula	Colostomy required
Rectal atresia	
Persistent cloaca	

From anomalies of the anorectum. *Warner, B.W. Classification of congenital disorders of the anorectum. In Rudolph A. M., et al (1996). Rudolph's Pediatrics (29th ed., p. 1112). Stamford, CT: Appleton & Lange.*

Medical management depends on the extent of the malformation. Some stenosed anal openings can be treated with dilation alone. An imperforate anal membrane (Fig. 15–8) is excised surgically, followed by daily manual dilations. More severe defects require reconstructive surgery. A temporary colostomy is sometimes performed to rest the bowel after reconstruction. Closure of the colostomy is generally performed between the age of 6 months and 1 year.

Nursing Management

During the initial newborn assessment, the perineal area is inspected for a poorly developed anal dimple or sacral anomalies. A rectal thermometer is lubricated and inserted a short distance into the rectum to determine patency. Observation and recording of passage of meconium are essential.

Once the diagnosis has been made, intravenous fluids are initiated and a nasogastric tube is inserted to decompress the stomach. Monitor the child's intake and output and cardiorespiratory functioning. Provide emotional support to the parents and give them information about the upcoming surgery.

Postoperative care centers on preventing infection and respiratory complications from surgery, as well as maintaining hydration. Observe the incision for signs of infection, and provide careful wound care. Assess vital signs at least every 4 hours. Once the child's condition is stable, clear fluid oral intake is allowed, advancing to half- and full-strength formula or breast milk as tolerated. The infant will have a colostomy after surgery, and careful skin care around the stoma is essential to prevent breakdown of the fragile area. Colostomy care was a particular focus of nursing management for Jerome, described at the beginning of this chapter.

Discharge Planning and Home Care Teaching

Infants are increasingly discharged shortly after birth. Give mothers clear instructions about normal newborn stools and what abnormalities to report.

After surgery, teach parents how to take the infant's temperature using the axillary route. Have them demonstrate the proper technique before discharge. Explain the signs and symptoms of infection. Discuss feeding regimens and bowel habits necessary to maintain adequate nutrition for growth and development. Advise parents that children with anorectal malformations may have difficulty achieving bowel control. Patience in toilet training is important. When the child reaches an age appropriate for toilet training, encourage the family to speak with a health care provider to discuss the child's progress.

If a colostomy is performed, teach parents how to care for the ostomy site (see discussion of ostomies later in this chapter). Reassure parents that the colostomy will be closed in the future, and assist them in planning for that hospitalization. Discuss follow-up care and long-term management. Arrange follow-up visits and home care visits to evaluate the child's ostomy site and monitor growth.

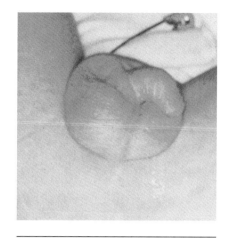

FIGURE 15–8. Imperforate anus, which is usually obvious at birth, can range from mild stenosis to a complex syndrome that includes associated congenital anomalies.

► HERNIAS

A **hernia** is the protrusion or projection of an organ or a part of an organ through the muscle wall of the cavity that normally contains it. This protrusion may result from the failure of normal openings to close during fetal development or from weakness in the supporting musculature. When intra-abdominal pressure increases (as when the infant cries or strains to pass stool), the weakened area separates, causing a protrusion of underlying organs. Inguinal hernias are the most common type of hernia occurring in children (see Chap. 16). Other hernias that occur frequently in children are diaphragmatic and umbilical.

DIAPHRAGMATIC HERNIA

In a diaphragmatic hernia, abdominal contents protrude into the thoracic cavity through an opening in the diaphragm. Sites of herniation include the substernal space, posterolateral region, and the esophageal hiatus. The posterolateral site (foramen of Bochdalek) is the most common location.[14] The cause is a delay or failure in closure of the pleuroperitoneal musculature. The overall incidence of diaphragmatic hernia is 1 in 3000–5000 live births.[15] Associated anomalies, particularly cardiac defects, occur in some infants.

A diaphragmatic hernia is a life-threatening condition. Severe respiratory distress occurs shortly after birth. As the infant cries, abdominal organs extend into the thorax, decreasing the size of the thoracic cavity. The infant becomes dyspneic and cyanotic. Characteristic findings include a barrel-shaped chest and sunken abdomen.

Some cases of congenital diaphragmatic hernia are diagnosed in utero by ultrasound. Postnatal diagnosis is confirmed by chest x-ray examination. Immediate respiratory support is essential. The infant is positioned with the head and thorax higher than the abdomen to facilitate downward movement of abdominal organs. A nasogastric tube is inserted to decompress the stomach. Ventilator support is necessary to manage respiratory compromise. Intravenous fluids are administered through an umbilical artery catheter.

Once the infant's condition is stabilized, surgery is performed to correct the defect. Extracorporeal membrane oxygenation (ECMO) may be used to provide cardiopulmonary bypass to rest the lungs. The prognosis is poor. Only 50% of infants survive, with death usually resulting from pulmonary hypoplasia. Even after surgery the infant may do well initially and then manifest severe respiratory decompensation.[14]

Nursing Management

The infant with a diaphragmatic hernia is admitted to the NICU and requires continuous monitoring. Preoperative management centers on providing supportive care to the infant and parents. Note the infant's vital signs every 30 minutes on the cardiorespiratory monitor. Observe for worsening of respiratory compromise. Maintain intravenous fluid administration. Promote decreased stimulation to keep the infant calm and thus maintain low abdominal pressure. Keep parents informed about the infant's condition, and provide emotional support both before and after surgery.

Postoperative care includes positioning the infant on the affected side to facilitate expansion of the lung on the unaffected side, observing closely for signs of infection, maintaining respiratory support, and carefully monitoring fluid and electrolyte balance.

Before discharge, instruct parents in wound care, prevention of infection, and feeding techniques.

UMBILICAL HERNIA

An umbilical hernia results from imperfect closure or weakness of the umbilical ring (Fig. 15–9). The condition is often associated with diastasis recti (lateral separation of the abdominal muscles). It is more common in African-American children and in girls.[16]

The hernia appears as a soft swelling covered by skin. The herniated area protrudes with coughing, crying, or straining during a bowel move-

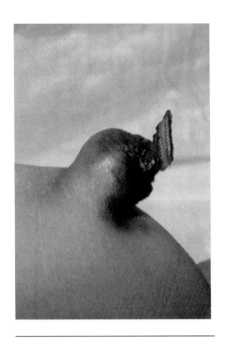

FIGURE 15–9. The umbilical hernia of the newborn usually closes as the muscles strengthen in later infancy and childhood.

From Zitelli, B., & Davis, H. (Eds.). (1994). Atlas of pediatric physical diagnosis (2nd ed.). London: Mosby–Wolfe Publishing.

ment. It is easily reduced by pushing the bowel back through the fibrous ring. The size of the defect may vary among individuals. Contents of the hernia include omentum or portions of the small intestine.

Most defects resolve spontaneously by 3–4 years of age. Surgery is indicated in cases of strangulation (closure of the umbilical ring around a portion of the bowel, preventing it from moving back into the abdomen), increased protrusion of the hernia after the age of 2 years, or little or no improvement in a large defect after the age of 4 years.

Nursing management is generally supportive. Instruct parents not to apply tape, straps, or coins to reduce the hernia. This can cause strangulation of the hernia, necessitating immediate surgery. If surgery is required, it is usually performed in a short-stay unit. Postoperatively, teach parents how to care for the surgical site, to watch for bleeding, and to recognize signs of infection. Reinforce the importance of returning for follow-up evaluation.

▶ INFLAMMATORY DISORDERS

Inflammatory disorders are reactions of specific tissues of the GI tract to trauma caused by injuries, foreign bodies, chemicals, microorganisms, or surgery. These disorders may be acute or chronic and may involve various segments of the GI tract.

APPENDICITIS

Appendicitis is an inflammation of the vermiform appendix, the small sac near the end of the cecum. The condition occurs most often in adolescent boys (10–15 years of age). It is rarely seen before 2 years of age.

Clinical Manifestations

At onset, symptoms include periumbilical cramps, abdominal tenderness, and fever. In adolescent and young adult females, symptoms must be differentiated from those associated with ovulation (mittelschmerz), ruptured ectopic pregnancy, and pelvic inflammatory disease.[17] As the inflammation progresses, pain in the right lower abdomen becomes constant. Pain is often most intense halfway between the anterior superior iliac crest and the umbilicus (Fig. 15–10). In 30% of children, however, the appendix is in a different location, so the pain may occur elsewhere. Symptoms progress to include rigidity and rebound tenderness following palpation over the right lower quadrant.

Vomiting, diarrhea, or constipation may be present. As appendicitis progresses, the child remains motionless, usually in a side-lying position with knees flexed. Sudden relief of pain usually means that the appendix has ruptured.

NURSING ALERT

Signs and symptoms of a ruptured appendix include:
- Fever
- Sudden relief from abdominal pain
- Guarding
- Abdominal distention
- Rapid shallow breathing
- Pallor
- Chills
- Irritability or restlessness

Etiology and Pathophysiology

Appendicitis almost always results from an obstruction in the appendiceal lumen. It can be caused by a fecalith (hard fecal mass), parasitic infestations, stenosis, hyperplasia of lymphoid tissue, or a tumor. Continued secretion of mucus following acute obstruction of the lumen increases pressure, causing ischemia, cellular death, and ulceration.

Perforation or rupture of the appendix may occur, resulting in fecal and bacterial contamination of the peritoneum. Peritonitis spreads quickly and if untreated can result in small bowel obstruction, electrolyte imbalances, septicemia, and hypovolemic shock.

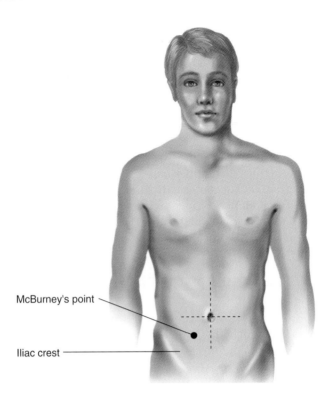

McBurney's point

Iliac crest

FIGURE 15–10. Common location of pain in children and adolescents with appendicitis.

Diagnostic Tests and Medical Management

Diagnosis of appendicitis in young children can be difficult because their pain may be less localized and their symptoms more diffuse than in the older child. Continuing evaluations over several hours are often needed to establish the diagnosis.

An elevated white blood cell count (above 15,000/μL) may occur. This leukocytosis occurs less often in young children than in teenagers. A history of abdominal pain, presence of a fecalith in the right lower abdomen on x-ray, and abdominal ultrasound help to confirm the diagnosis.

Treatment involves immediate surgical removal (appendectomy). Preoperatively the child is kept NPO. Intravenous fluids, electrolytes, and antibiotics are administered. A nasogastric tube may be inserted before or after surgery. Postoperatively the child has an abdominal incision, and intravenous antibiotics are administered to prevent infection. If the appendix has ruptured before surgery, a Penrose drain is inserted and the wound may not be completely sutured. Wound irrigations may be needed to assist with cleansing of the peritoneum. Recovery is usually complete following uncomplicated removal of the appendix.

Nursing Assessment

Physiologic Assessment

A detailed assessment of the child's pain is necessary to differentiate appendicitis from other illnesses (see Chap. 7). Ask the child to point to the painful area and to describe the pain. Note onset, location, and intensity of pain; precipitating factors; and relief measures tried. During abdominal assessment, perform palpation last to avoid causing additional pain. Assess vital signs to determine baseline values, and monitor every 4 hours thereafter.

Psychosocial Assessment

Because appendicitis usually occurs in school-age children and adolescents, assessment of the child's coping skills is important. Adolescents, because of their preoccupation with body image, may be concerned about the surgical scar. Assess the parents' and child's anxiety about the sudden hospitalization and need for emergency surgery.

Nursing Diagnosis

Among the nursing diagnoses that might be appropriate for the child with appendicitis before surgery are:

- Pain related to inflammatory process
- Risk for Fluid Volume Deficit related to vomiting
- Anxiety/Fear related to hospitalization, multiple painful procedures, and potential surgery

Postoperative nursing diagnoses might include:

- Pain related to abdominal incision
- Risk for Infection related to incision, compromised skin integrity, and bowel manipulation
- Risk for Ineffective Airway Clearance related to general anesthesia and avoidance of lung expansion due to incisional pain
- Anxiety (Parent and Child) related to child's sudden hospitalization and surgery

Nursing Management

Nursing management focuses on promoting comfort, maintaining hydration, providing emotional support, supporting respiratory function, providing care of the surgical site, and monitoring for symptoms of infection.

Promote Comfort

A side-lying position with knees bent is usually the most comfortable. Administer analgesics as ordered, and note relief from pain. Postoperative pain is managed in a similar manner. The child should be placed in a semi-Fowler or side-lying position on the right side. If the appendix has ruptured, lying on the right side facilitates drainage from the peritoneal cavity. Administer pain medication as ordered.

Maintain Hydration

Assess fluid volume status every 2 hours. Assess skin turgor, eyes, and mucous membranes for signs of dehydration. Monitor intake and output, and assess vital signs. An intravenous infusion is initiated preoperatively and continued until bowel function returns after surgery. Once bowel sounds return, offer water in small amounts and then other clear fluids.

Provide Emotional Support

For many children, this may be their first hospitalization and their first experience with health care personnel beyond their usual provider. The nurse must elicit a history, perform a physical examination, coordinate diagnostic tests, and prepare the child for surgery in a short period of time. Emotional support is essential for both child and parents. Good preoperative education can reduce anxiety. Answer any questions the child or parents may have.

NURSING ALERT

Use of a heating pad is contraindicated in children with appendicitis. Heat will only increase the inflammation and may contribute to rupture of the appendix.

Support Respiratory Function

General anesthesia during surgery compromises respiratory function. It is important for the child to turn, cough, and breathe deeply to prevent atelectasis. Encourage the child to splint the incision area with a pillow during coughing to decrease pain.

Recognize Symptoms of Infection

Assess vital signs and observe the abdominal incision every 4 hours for redness, edema, or drainage. If a drain is present, assess drainage for color, consistency, and amount. After the initial dressing has been changed, perform dressing changes frequently and keep the incision area clean and dry. Administer antibiotics as prescribed.

Discharge Planning and Home Care Teaching

The child is discharged once bowel function returns and he or she has a bowel movement. Give parents instructions on reestablishing a nutritious diet slowly and as tolerated. Teach parents to recognize the signs and symptoms of infection and to seek early treatment.

Normal activities can be resumed fairly quickly, but strenuous activities and contact sports should be avoided in the immediate postoperative period. Parents should check with the child's physician before allowing the child to resume sports activities. Home tutoring may be needed for a short time so the child can keep up with schoolwork.

NECROTIZING ENTEROCOLITIS

Necrotizing enterocolitis is a potentially life-threatening inflammatory disease of the intestinal tract that occurs primarily in premature infants. It can be caused by several factors, among them intestinal ischemia, bacterial or viral infection (a result of the premature infant's decreased immune response and greater risk for infection), and immaturity of the gut (a result of the premature infant's decreased amount of gastric acid and proteolytic enzymes and underdeveloped protective intestinal mucin layer). The disease occurs most often in the terminal ileum and colon.[18]

The infant may initially show signs of feeding intolerance (increased gastric residuals, vomiting, irritability, and abdominal distention). These signs are caused by inflammation and dilation of the bowel and accumulation of gas in the intestine. Bloody diarrhea may be present because of the hemorrhagic bowel. Signs of sepsis usually follow, and the infant's condition rapidly deteriorates. A system for staging of necrotizing enterocolitis is available (modified Bell staging), ranging from stage IA (temperature instability, apnea, bradycardia, and lethargy) to stage IIIB (respiratory and metabolic acidosis, disseminated intravascular coagulation, severe apnea, hypotension, and bradycardia).[18]

Diagnosis is made on the basis of characteristic clinical findings and the presence of free peritoneal gas, dilated bowel loops, bowel distention, and bowel wall thickening on abdominal x-rays. Necrotizing enterocolitis requires prompt intervention. Management begins with discontinuation of all enteral feedings. An orogastric tube is inserted to prevent gastric distention, and intravenous fluids are started. Total parenteral nutrition may be initiated through a central line. Antibiotics are administered prophylactically or to treat sepsis. Perforation or necrosis of the bowel necessitates surgical resection of the bowel. An ileostomy or colostomy may be performed.

All cases of necrotizing enterocolitis are treated with strict enteric precautions to prevent the spread of infection to other premature infants on

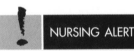

NURSING ALERT

Signs of sepsis include:
- Hypothermia or hyperthermia
- Jaundice
- Respiratory distress
- Hepatomegaly
- Abdominal distention
- Anorexia
- Vomiting
- Lethargy

the unit. Early aggressive enteral formula feedings of premature infants is avoided because of the increased incidence of the disease in these cases. Human milk has been shown to be protective against the disease; thus, breast-feeding or feeding the mother's expressed milk is the feeding method of choice for premature infants.[18]

Long-term complications of necrotizing enterocolitis include short bowel syndrome, strictures, cholestasis, impaired nutrition and growth, and delayed developmental performance.[19]

Nursing Management

Nursing care centers on early detection of necrotizing enterocolitis to minimize bowel loss and providing postoperative care. Measure abdominal circumference in the premature or high-risk infant every 4–8 hours (see Fig. 8–11). Even minimal changes in circumference can indicate necrotizing enterocolitis and should be reported to the physician. Watch for feeding intolerance by aspirating gastric residual (if the infant is receiving enteral feedings).

Maintaining fluid and electrolyte balance is essential. Provide comfort by holding and cuddling an infant who is NPO, and offer a pacifier to meet nonnutritive sucking needs. Careful assessment for infection and maintenance of skin integrity are essential. Feedings are gradually reestablished once bowel function returns.

Parents need emotional support and reassurance and help in bonding with their infant. They are coping with the birth of an infant who is critically ill. Because the symptoms of necrotizing enterocolitis do not appear until approximately 5–7 days after feedings are begun, parents may not be prepared for the infant's decline. The recovery of a premature infant is slow and can be complicated. Give clear explanations and encourage parents to ask questions and express their fears and concerns.

Once the child is discharged, frequent follow-up is needed. Encourage regular health care visits. Schedule home visits to help the family manage health care and normal developmental issues. If total parenteral nutrition is administered at home, the parents will need to know how to administer it correctly and how to care for the central line. Oral and enteral nutritional intake is carefully assessed. Growth of the child is monitored and compared to previous findings. Several medications are likely to be used, and correct administration techniques must be reinforced. The infant requires regular and thorough physical assessments to identify any complications. Parents need to learn care of the ostomy if the child has one in place. Developmental progress is assessed by regular administration of a developmental test such as the Denver II (see Chap. 5).

MECKEL'S DIVERTICULUM

Meckel's diverticulum results when the omphalomesenteric duct, which connects the midgut to the yolk sac during embryonic development, fails to atrophy. Instead, an outpouching of the ileum remains, usually located near the ileocecal valve. The pouch contains gastric or pancreatic tissue, which secretes acid, causing irritation and ulceration. Meckel's diverticulum is the most common gastrointestinal malformation and occurs in 1–2% of the population, although many individuals are asymptomatic and do not know they have the disorder.[20] It is more common in males.

Clinical manifestations usually appear by 2 years of age. The most common sign is painless dark or bright red rectal bleeding, which results from

---

CHOLESTASIS

Cholestasis is a disruption of bile flow. This is the most common problem in survivors of necrotizing enterocolitis. It is a complication of total parenteral nutrition (TPN) and commonly occurs 2 weeks after TPN therapy has been initiated. It is characterized by an elevated bilirubin (>2 mg/dL), hepatomegaly, and elevated serum transaminase.

the obstruction or ulceration. Often blood is passed without stool. Abdominal pain is uncommon, but when it occurs, it may resemble the pain of appendicitis. The child may have symptoms of intussusception, incarcerated hernia, volvulus, or intestinal obstruction. If untreated, diverticulitis may progress to perforation and peritonitis.

Diagnosis is based on the history. Contrast studies are usually not helpful because the diverticulum is often too small to visualize and may not fill with barium. Radionuclide imaging and scanning can usually detect the gastric tissue, confirming the diagnosis.

Treatment is surgical excision of the diverticulum and removal of any involved bowel. The prognosis is good following surgical excision.

Nursing Management

Preoperatively an intravenous infusion is initiated to correct fluid and electrolyte imbalances. Monitor intake and output. Observe for rectal bleeding, and test stools for occult blood. The child should be kept on bedrest. Assess vital signs every 2 hours, and monitor for signs of shock. Postoperative care is similar to that for an infant or child undergoing abdominal surgery. (See the earlier discussion of postsurgical nursing management of appendicitis and the Nursing Care Plan for the Child Undergoing Surgery in Chapter 4.)

At the time of discharge, parents need instructions on caring for the surgical site, preventing infection, providing an adequate diet, and administering prescribed medications.

INFLAMMATORY BOWEL DISEASE

Inflammatory bowel disease encompasses two distinct chronic disorders, Crohn's disease and ulcerative colitis, that have similar symptoms and treatment. Both diseases involve faulty regulation of the immune response of the intestinal mucosa.

Crohn's disease is a chronic, inflammatory process. It can occur randomly throughout the GI tract, with the ileum, colon, and rectum the most common sites. A distinct feature of Crohn's disease is the development of enteric fistulas between loops of bowel or nearby organs. Mucosal ulcers begin in small locations, and then grow in size and depth into the mucosal wall. Submucosal inflammation can be severe. The etiology is unknown. There is strong evidence to support a genetic association. Crohn's disease is more common in whites and three to six times more prevalent in individuals of Jewish descent. It most often develops between 15 and 25 years of age.

The onset of Crohn's disease is subtle. Crampy abdominal pain is usually reported first, followed by diarrhea. Other symptoms include fever, anorexia, growth failure, general malaise, and joint pain. Diagnosis is based on laboratory evaluation (anemia is common; an elevated erythrocyte sedimentation rate, hypoalbuminemia, and thrombocytosis are other possible findings) and radiologic and biopsy examinations.[21]

Ulcerative colitis is a chronic recurrent disease of the colon and rectal mucosa of unknown etiology. Inflammation is limited to the mucosa and can involve the entire length of the bowel with varying degrees of ulceration, hemorrhage, and edema. Emotional and other psychosocial factors may influence the presentation and course of the disease. It is more prevalent among persons of Jewish heritage. The disease develops before 20 years of age with peak onset at about 12 years.[22]

The first symptom of ulcerative colitis is usually diarrhea. Lower abdominal pain and cramping are present before and during a bowel move-

15-4 Comparison of Ulcerative Colitis and Crohn's Disease

	Ulcerative Colitis	Crohn's Disease
Type of lesions	Continuous, superficial involvement	Segmental, transmural (through the wall) involvement
Clinical manifestations		
Anal or perianal lesions	Rare	Common
Anorexia	Mild to moderate	Can be severe
Diarrhea	Often severe	Moderate
Growth retardation	Mild	Significant
Pain	Present	Common
Rectal bleeding	Present	Absent
Weight loss	Moderate	Severe
Risk of cancer	Slightly increased	Greatly increased

ment and are relieved by the passage of stool and flatus. The stool is often mixed with blood and mucus. Weight loss or delayed growth, nutritional deficiencies, and arthralgias often occur as effects of the disease.[23]

Diagnosis centers on evaluating the cause and identifying the extent of involved bowel and differentiating an infectious process (organisms such as *Shigella* and *Salmonella*) from ulcerative colitis. Endoscopy with biopsy is helpful to determine the extent and severity of the inflammatory process. Laboratory studies help to identify related nutritional, growth, and blood abnormalities.

Table 15–4 presents a comparison of the features of Crohn's disease and ulcerative colitis. Both diseases have periods of remission and exacerbation. Treatment for both diseases includes pharmacologic interventions (administration of antibiotic, antiinflammatory, immunosuppressive, and antidiarrheal medications), nutrition therapy, and surgery. Corticosteroids are given orally and in the form of enemas to children with more severe disease. For children with milder disease, sulfasalazine has been shown to decrease the number of relapses (Table 15–5).

A nutritionist is part of the team treating the child. The goal of nutrition therapy is to provide adequate caloric intake and nutrients necessary

15-5 Drugs Used in Treatment of Inflammatory Bowel Disease

Aminosalicylates
  Sulfasalazine
  Mesalamine

Corticosteroids
  Prednisone
  Methylprednisone
  Hydrocortisone enema

Immunosuppressants
  6-Mercaptopurine
  Azothioprine
  Cyclosporine
  Methotrexate

Antibacterial
  Metronidazole

for growth. Vitamin, iron, zinc, and folic acid supplementation is frequently required. Total parenteral nutrition (TPN) is often given to treat nutritional deficiencies and malnutrition, which accompany inflammatory bowel disease. A high-protein, high-carbohydrate, low-fiber diet with normal amounts of fat is recommended.

If other treatment measures fail to reduce inflammation, surgery is indicated. A temporary colostomy or ileostomy is performed to allow the bowel to rest. In Crohn's disease, however, ulcerations tend to recur elsewhere in the GI tract. In ulcerative colitis, removal of the diseased bowel provides a permanent cure.

Nursing Management

Nursing management occurs mainly in the community and home and focuses on helping the child and family adjust to the emotional impact of a chronic disease, administering medications and diet therapy, monitoring nutritional status, and providing appropriate referrals. Provide emotional support and counseling to help the child adjust to feeling "different" from peers. Inability to compete with peers and frequent absences from school can affect the child's self-esteem. Have the parents contact the school district to arrange for tutoring in case extended absences from school become necessary. Encourage the child who is not attending school regularly to maintain contact with friends through telephone calls, cards, and visits.

If the child is unable to eat or the intake of calories is insufficient to meet basic nutritional and metabolic needs, TPN will be ordered. If the child is able to eat, offer small, frequent, high-calorie meals or snacks. High-fiber foods should be avoided because they irritate the already inflamed bowel. Frequent growth measurements and nutritional evaluations must be carried out.

Body image is a major concern for children and adolescents with inflammatory bowel disease. Corticosteroid therapy causes growth retardation and delayed sexual maturation. Encourage the child to discuss feelings about these side effects. If a permanent colostomy or ileostomy is required, the nurse can assist the child and family to understand the need for surgical treatment. (See the discussion of ostomies that follows.) Introduce the child and family to other children who have stomas.

Teach parents about medication administration and diet therapy. Reinforce to both the parents and child the importance of adhering to a strict medication regimen. Emphasize that medications should be continued even when the child is asymptomatic. Discuss the side effects of the drugs and what to do if any of these symptoms occur.

Parents also will need instructions for TPN and care of a central venous catheter, including dressing changes, sterile and nonsterile techniques, signs of infection, how to handle infusion pumps and tubing, and how to measure the child's intake and output. Assist parents in obtaining equipment and supplies necessary for the child's care. Have parents demonstrate their mastery of care for the central venous catheter and their understanding of TPN techniques during home visits and appointments for health care.

Refer parents to social services, the visiting nurse association, and home health care agencies, if they are not receiving any of these services. For information about inflammatory bowel disease, refer families to the Crohn's Colitis Foundation (see Appendix F).

CLINICAL TIP

If lactose is tolerated, the child can be offered high-calorie foods such as cream soups, milkshakes, puddings, and custards.

CLINICAL TIP

Instruct parents to continue to provide frequent small meals and avoid a three-meals-a-day pattern with the child at home.

NURSING ALERT

Corticosteroids can decrease a child's immune response and alter growth. Immunizations (especially for polio and varicella) are contraindicated when steroids are being administered.

PEPTIC ULCER

A peptic ulcer is an erosion of the mucosal tissue in the lower end of the esophagus, in the stomach (usually along the lesser curvature), or in the duodenum. Boys are more likely to have peptic ulcers than girls. However, peptic ulcers are much less common in children than in adults.

Clinical manifestations vary according to the age of the child and location of the ulcer. The most common symptom is abdominal pain (burning) associated with an empty stomach, which may awaken the child at night. Vomiting and pain after meals, anemia, **occult blood** in stools, and abdominal distention may also be present.

Ulcers are classified as primary or secondary, depending on their etiology. Primary peptic ulcers occur in healthy children. Secondary (stress) ulcers occur in children with a preexisting illness or injury (often a burn) and in children receiving medications such as salicylates, corticosteroids, and nonsteroidal antiinflammatory drugs. Diet usually is not a major factor in the development of peptic ulcers in children, although caffeine and alcohol consumption in adolescents may exacerbate the disease. It is now known that many cases of ulcer, in both adults and children, is caused by *Helicobacter pylori*, a gram-negative rod.[24] This organism is transmitted by the fecal–oral or oral–oral routes. Infections often occur in several members of a family, especially when the family's water supply is contaminated.

Diagnosis is based on the history and radiologic studies. *H. pylori* can be diagnosed by culture of the organism taken via gastroscopy, and by measuring urea in the urine and on the breath, since the organism hydrolyzes urea.[25] The goals of medical management are to relieve discomfort and promote healing. When *H. pylori* is the causative agent, antimicrobial agents such as bismuth salts, tetracycline, and metronidazole combination are given. Other drugs combinations, such as a combination of antacids in liquid form (Maalox, Mylanta) and histamine antagonists (ranitidine, cimetidine, and famotidine), are also used. Antibody titers are measured several times over 6 months to evaluate the effectiveness of therapy. The prognosis is usually good with early intervention.

Nursing Management

Nursing care centers on interventions to promote adequate nutritional intake, promote healing, and prevent recurrences. A nutritionally sound, age-appropriate diet is provided. Foods should be omitted only if they exacerbate the disorder.

Antibiotics must be given as scheduled. Emphasize the importance of continuing drug therapy. The family needs encouragement to continue the medications as ordered and to return for follow-up visits. Children who attend school may prefer to take antacids in the form of tablets, which are easier to carry than liquid preparations. A permission form to take medications at school will need to be filled out by the prescriber. Parents should check with the child's physician before giving any additional medication. Caution parents to avoid aspirin products, which irritate the gastric mucosa. If an antipyretic or pain medication is needed, acetaminophen should be given. Advise parents to read medication labels if they are unsure of product contents.

Because psychologic stress can contribute to peptic ulcer disease, the parents and child should be assisted to identify sources of stress in the child's life. Assess coping mechanisms and provide referral for psychologic counseling, if appropriate.

► OSTOMIES

An **ostomy** is an opening into the small or large intestine or urinary canal that diverts fecal matter or urine to provide an outlet when a distal surgical anastomosis, obstruction, or nonfunctioning structures prevent normal elimination. Depending on the integrity and function of anatomic structures, the ostomy may be temporary or permanent. Infants and small children with necrotizing enterocolitis, Hirschsprung's disease, volvulus, or intussusception may require a temporary colostomy or ileostomy. Ostomies may also be indicated for children with inflammatory bowel disease, intestinal tumors, or abdominal trauma.

An ostomy may be elective or a surgical emergency. In all cases it affects a child's life-style, alters body image, causes anxiety, and increases the risk for alterations in physiologic processes (electrolyte imbalance, increased nutritional requirements). For adolescents, it may also result in dependence at a time when autonomy is a major developmental need (Fig. 15–11).

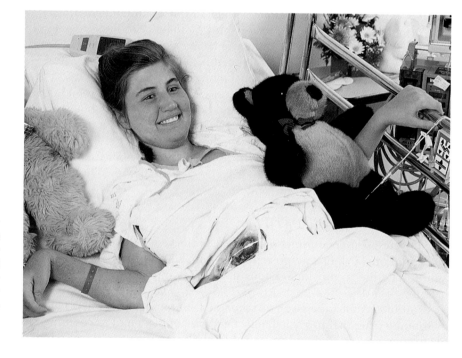

FIGURE 15–11. Nursing strategies to address altered perceptions of body image and increased feelings of dependence are important when working with adolescents who have ostomies. Support groups or a visit from another teenager who has had an ostomy can facilitate positive coping, as demonstrated by this teenage girl.

In assessing the family and child approaching ostomy surgery, it is important to determine their ability to understand and accept the physical changes that will occur.[26] Parents may feel guilt and anger about the ostomy surgery when the child has a genetically transmitted disease, has sustained an injury, or has developed an obstruction from necrosis of the bowel. Encourage the parents and child to express their feelings, and correct any misunderstandings. Parents and older children may be referred for counseling and to support groups to help them deal with their feelings. Adolescents often benefit from a visit with an adolescent ostomate (someone who has an ostomy) who can answer questions about living with an ostomy.

PREOPERATIVE CARE

Preoperative education focuses on educating the child and family and preparing them for postoperative management. Discuss how the appliance will look, and explain the purpose of the pouch in developmentally appropriate terms. Encourage the parents and child to touch and manipulate all equipment. A younger child can be shown how to place a pouch on a doll. Older children can practice placing a pouch on their skin. These measures help relieve anxiety by providing information and increasing familiarity with the appliance.

In addition to discussion of the appliance, preoperative education should include discussion of pain control and measures that will be used to prevent postoperative complications (turning, coughing, and breathing deeply). Instructions should be geared to the child's developmental level. Encourage parental participation to promote compliance.

POSTOPERATIVE CARE

Postoperative care of a child with an ostomy is similar to that for any child who undergoes abdominal surgery. (See the earlier discussion of nursing management for appendicitis and the Nursing Care Plan for the Child Undergoing Surgery in Chapter 4.)

Home care needs should be identified and addressed well in advance of discharge. Instructions include skin care, care of the stoma, appliance removal and application, and frequency of appliance changes. Teaching should begin immediately after surgery with responsibility for care transferred gradually to the parents and child as they are ready. (For information on caring for an ostomy, refer to the section on elimination in the *Quick Reference to Pediatric Clinical Skills* that accompanies this text.) Discuss diet, activity level, hygiene, clothing, equipment, and financial considerations. Arrange for home visits to check periodically on the home management program.

Parents and children can be referred to the United Ostomy Association (see Appendix F) or a local ostomy group for information and support. Referrals should be made to social service, counseling, and a home health agency, if appropriate.

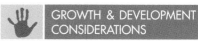

GROWTH & DEVELOPMENT CONSIDERATIONS

The preschooler has some manual dexterity and can help with some parts of the procedure for changing an ostomy appliance and cleaning the stoma. Teach the child using a doll or stuffed animal. Many school-age children are able to care for their ostomy independently. Teach them how to avoid leakage around the bag, which could be embarrassing. Adolescents are generally totally independent in their self-care of ostomies. However, they may need support to deal with the fact that they are different from their peers.[26]

CLINICAL TIP

Avoid adhesive enhancers on the skin of newborns and premature infants. Their skin layers are so thin that removal of the appliance can strip off the skin.

▶ DISORDERS OF MOTILITY

Fluids are produced in large quantities as part of normal GI functioning. As food passes through the intestines, fluids are reabsorbed and moderately soft stool is formed and evacuated. In disorders such as diarrhea and constipation, fluid production is altered, causing either more or less fluid to be reabsorbed. This can severely alter the characteristics of the stool. Reabsorption of too little water produces watery stools (**diarrhea**) and can lead to fluid and electrolyte alterations. Reabsorption of too much fluid can cause **constipation,** which if untreated can lead to bowel obstruction.

GASTROENTERITIS (ACUTE DIARRHEA)

Gastroenteritis is an inflammation of the stomach and intestines that may be accompanied by vomiting and diarrhea. It can affect any part of the GI tract. Diarrhea is a common problem in children. It may be an acute problem, caused by viral, bacterial, or parasitic infections, or a chronic problem. Children under age 5 years average approximately two episodes of gastroenteritis each year.[27] Infants and small children with gastroenteritis or diarrhea can quickly become dehydrated and are at risk for hypovolemic shock if fluid and electrolyte losses are not replaced (see Chap. 8).

Clinical Manifestations

Diarrhea may be mild, moderate, or severe. In mild diarrhea, stools are slightly increased in number and have a more liquid consistency. In moderate diarrhea the child has several loose or watery stools. Other symptoms include irritability, anorexia, nausea, and vomiting. Moderate diarrhea is usually self-limiting, resolving without treatment within 1 or 2 days. In severe diarrhea, watery stools are continuous. The child exhibits symptoms of fluid and electrolyte imbalance (see Chap. 8), has cramping, and is extremely irritable and difficult to console.

Etiology and Pathophysiology

Diarrhea in children can have many different causes (Table 15–6). The specific etiology is not always identified. The common mechanism is a decrease in the absorptive capacity of the bowel through inflammation, decrease in surface area for absorption, or alteration of parasympathetic innervation. Children in day-care centers and those living in substandard housing with improper sanitation are at increased risk.

Diagnostic Tests and Medical Management

Diagnosis is based on the history, physical examination, and laboratory findings. A thorough history may help in identifying the causative factor.

15-6   Causes of Diarrhea in Children

Causative Factor	Effect on Bowel Function
Emotional stress (anxiety, fatigue)	Increased motility
Intestinal infection (bacteria [*E. coli, Salmonella, Shigella*], viral [human rotavirus, enteric adenovirus], fungal overgrowth)	Inflammation of mucosa; increased mucus secretion in colon
Food sensitivity (gluten, cow's milk)	Decreased digestion of food
Food intolerance (lactose, introduction of new foods, overfeeding)	Increased motility; increased mucus secretion in colon
Medications (iron, antibiotics)	Irritation and suprainfection
Colon disease (colitis, necrotizing enterocolitis, enterocolitis)	Inflammation and ulceration of intestinal walls; reduced absorption of fluid; increased intestinal motility
Surgical alterations (short bowel syndrome)	Reduced size of colon; decreased absorption surface

Ask parents about recent exposure to illnesses, use of antibiotics, travel, food and formula preparation, food sensitivities or allergies, and whether the child attends day care.[28] Physical examination provides a guide to the severity of dehydration (see Chap. 8). The stool can be examined for the presence of ova, parasites, infectious organisms, viruses, fat, and undigested sugars. Laboratory evaluation of serum and urine helps in identification of electrolyte imbalances and other deficiencies.

Medical management depends on the severity of the diarrhea and fluid and electrolyte imbalances (Table 15–7). The goal of treatment is to correct the fluid and electrolyte imbalances. For mild to moderate dehydration the child is rehydrated by means of oral rehydration therapy (see Chap. 8). This may be accomplished at home or in the short-stay observation unit in a hospital with solutions such as Pedialyte, Ricelyte, or Lytren.

15-7 Treatment of Diarrhea

Degree of Dehydration	Oral Rehydration Solution[a]	Feeding
None	May not be needed if appropriate early feeding is used 10mL/kg/stool for ongoing losses	Age-appropriate diet of breast milk or regular formula, complex carbohydrates, and meats (especially chicken)
Mild (3–5%)	50mL/kg for 4–6 hours or until rehydrated 10mL/kg/stool for ongoing losses and replacement of estimated emesis volume	Same as above after rehydration is complete
Moderate (6–9%)	100 mL/kg plus replacement of continuing losses during a 4-hour period Reassess ongoing losses every hour and replace volume for volume	Same as above after rehydration is complete
Severe (≥ 10%)	True emergency which causes shock or near-shock condition Bolus intravenous therapy with normal saline or Ringer's lactate, 20–40 mL/kg/hr Begin oral rehydration solution when level of consciousness improves	Same as above after rehydration is complete

[a]If child does not tolerate oral rehydration solution, start intravenous therapy.
From Snyder, John (1997). Feeding during diarrhea: New AAP guidelines and innovations in oral rehydration solutions. Contemporary Pediatrics Meeting Reporter. July, 1997, p. 6.

Carbonated beverages and those containing high amounts of sugar should not be given. Fermentation of sugar in the GI tract causes increased gas, abdominal distention, and an increased frequency of diarrhea.

For severe dehydration, rehydration is accomplished by intravenous infusion with a solution chosen to correct the specific imbalances. Normal saline with glucose or Ringer's lactate are commonly used solutions (see Chapter 8 for further information about solutions to correct dehydration). The child is kept NPO to allow the bowel to rest. Once the dehydration has been corrected and the diarrhea has resolved, clear liquids are introduced. The child gradually progresses to a regular diet.

If the diarrhea is caused by bacteria or parasites, antimicrobial therapy may be prescribed. Absorbents such as Donnagel and Kaopectate will alter the appearance of stool but will not reduce the amount of fluid loss and are generally not recommended for children.

Nursing Assessment

The nurse may encounter the child and family in the emergency department, urgent care center, clinic, or office. If the child is hospitalized, it is important to assess onset, frequency, color, amount, and consistency of stools. If the child is also vomiting, monitor the amount and type of vomitus. Initial and ongoing physical assessment of the child focuses on observing for signs and symptoms of dehydration, which reflect underlying fluid and electrolyte status. Evaluate urinary output and specific gravity. Weigh the infant or child on admission and daily thereafter. Monitor vital signs every 2–4 hours. If the child is febrile, water loss will be increased, contributing to the dehydration. Assess skin integrity, especially in the perineal and rectal areas, and note any breakdown or rashes.

Nursing Diagnosis

The accompanying Nursing Care Plan lists common nursing diagnoses for a child with gastroenteritis. Other diagnoses that might also be appropriate include:

- Anxiety (Child and Parent) related to hospitalization
- Sleep Pattern Disturbance related to abdominal cramping and frequent bowel movements
- Altered Nutrition: Less Than Body Requirements related to inability to ingest sufficient nutrients and increased intestinal motility

Nursing Management

Nursing care focuses on providing emotional support, promoting rest and comfort, and ensuring adequate nutrition. The accompanying Nursing Care Plan summarizes nursing care for the child with gastroenteritis.

Provide Emotional Support

The child may have been ill for several days or become suddenly ill a short time before seeking health care. The child and parents are usually anxious, so it is important to allow them to talk and ask questions. The child may require blood tests to help direct rehydration therapy. Using therapeutic play techniques, such as allowing the child to manipulate equipment, can

NURSING CARE PLAN
THE CHILD WITH GASTROENTERITIS

GOAL	INTERVENTION	RATIONALE	EXPECTED OUTCOME

1. Diarrhea related to altered gastrointestinal motility

GOAL	INTERVENTION	RATIONALE	EXPECTED OUTCOME
The child's bowel function will be restored to normal.	• Obtain baseline vital signs and monitor every 2–4 hours. • Observe stools for amount, color, consistency, odor, and frequency. • Test stools for occult blood. • Monitor results of stool culture and sample for ova and parasites. • Wash hands well before and after contact with the child. • Isolate the child until the cause of the diarrhea is determined. • Assist the child with toileting and hygiene. • Administer prescribed oral rehydration and intravenous solutions. Limit solid food intake. • Notify the physician if diarrhea persists or characteristics change.	• Fluid and electrolyte imbalances can alter vital body functions. • Aids in the diagnosis and in monitoring the child's status. • Frequent defecation and some infectious organisms can cause bleeding. • Rapid notification of the physician will facilitate treatment. • Helps prevent transmission of microorganisms. • Prevents exposure of other patients and staff. • The child may be weak, incontinent, physically impaired, or anxious and require assistance to use the bathroom. • Provides necessary fluids and nutrients while allowing the bowel to rest. • Ensures early intervention.	The child's bowel function returns to normal.

2. Fluid Volume Deficit related to diarrhea and vomiting

GOAL	INTERVENTION	RATIONALE	EXPECTED OUTCOME
The child will remain hydrated and will begin to drink fluids within 24 hours of admission.	• Monitor intake and output. Be sure to document time of each voiding. • Compare admission weight to preadmission weight. Assess weight daily.	• Will determine if output exceeds input. Long periods of time without urine output can be an early indicator of poor renal function. A child should produce 1 mL of urine/kg/hr. • The degree of dehydration can be determined by the percentage of weight loss. Daily weights aid in determining progress toward rehydration.	The child has normal fluid and electrolyte balance as indicated by laboratory evaluation and physical examination.

Continued . . .

GOAL	INTERVENTION	RATIONALE	EXPECTED OUTCOME

2. *Fluid Volume Deficit related to diarrhea and vomiting (continued)*

GOAL	INTERVENTION	RATIONALE	EXPECTED OUTCOME
	• Assess level of consciousness, skin turgor, mucous membranes, skin color and temperature, capillary refill, eyes, and fontanels every 4 hours.	• Will determine degree of hydration and adequacy of interventions.	
	• Assess for vomiting.	• Vomiting frequently accompanies diarrhea and contributes to the child's fluid loss.	
	• Provide oral fluid and electrolyte replacement solution if able to tolerate.	• Less invasive than IV fluids. Provides for replacement of essential fluids and electrolytes.	
	• Provide and maintain IV replacement therapy, as ordered.	• Use of IV replacement is based on the degree of dehydration, ongoing losses, insensible water losses and electrolyte results.	

3. *Risk for Impaired Skin Integrity related to contact of skin with feces and frequent cleansing of skin*

GOAL	INTERVENTION	RATIONALE	EXPECTED OUTCOME
The child will remain free of skin breakdown and rashes.	• Assess skin of perineum and rectum for signs of skin breakdown or irritation. • Provide prevention or restorative care for infants as follows:	• Early assessment and intervention can prevent worsening of the condition.	The child's perianal and rectal tissue remains pink and intact.

Preventive care:

GOAL	INTERVENTION	RATIONALE	EXPECTED OUTCOME
	• Change diapers every 2 hours or as needed.	• Minimizes skin contact with chemical irritants from stool and urine.	
	• Use cloth diapers rather than disposable.	• Minimizes the mechanical and chemical irritation from disposables.	
	• Wash diaper area after each soiling.	• Removes traces of stool if present.	
	• Apply A & D ointment.	• Provides a barrier and protects intact or reddened skin from becoming excoriated.	

NURSING CARE PLAN
THE CHILD WITH GASTROENTERITIS– *Continued*

GOAL	INTERVENTION	RATIONALE	EXPECTED OUTCOME

3. Risk for Impaired Skin Integrity related to contact of skin with feces and frequent cleansing of skin (continued)

Restorative care:

	INTERVENTION	RATIONALE	
	• Place the infant prone and leave the buttocks open to air.	• Promotes air circulation to the area.	
	• Notify the physician if the skin is severely broken or peeling or if a rash is present.		
	• For toddlers and older children:		
	• Tub bathe at least daily (if condition allows) in tepid water. Pat the area dry.	• Helps loosen any fecal matter without scrubbing, which can cause additional irritation to the skin.	
	• Discourage the wearing of underwear if possible.	• Allows air to circulate and prevents accumulation of moisture.	
	• Apply A & D ointment at least four times daily.	• Provides a barrier and protects intact or reddened skin from becoming excoriated.	

reduce anxiety (see Chap. 4). To promote a trusting relationship, be honest if a procedure will hurt. Encourage the child to express anger, fear, and pain.

Promote Rest and Comfort

Most children with gastroenteritis are quite ill and awaken frequently with periods of vomiting and diarrhea. Provide a quiet, restful environment. Darken the room and keep interruptions to a minimum. To reduce the child's anxiety, encourage parents to room-in. Place the child's favorite toys and comfort objects within reach. Keep the child's mouth moistened with a glycerine swab, a wet washcloth, or an occasional ice chip.

Ensure Adequate Nutrition

Once the dehydration has been corrected, clear liquids are offered. If tolerated, the CRAM diet can be started. Infants are breast-fed or given formula. After about 1 week, a normal diet for the child's age is slowly reintroduced.

 CLINICAL TIP

An effective way to treat diarrhea is the CRAM diet:
Complex carbohydrates (eg, cereals, toast, pasta)
Rice
and
Milk

Discharge Planning and Care in the Community

Discharge teaching should begin on arrival at the health care facility. Instruct parents on what to expect as the child's GI system returns to normal function. Teach the parents about the symptoms of dehydration and what to do if diarrhea recurs. Be sure that parents understand the recommended diet progression. Refer them to a nutritionist, if necessary. Emphasize the necessity of good hygiene practices to prevent the spread of microorganisms that can cause gastroenteritis. If the child attends day care, have the parent inform the day-care center about the infection so the staff can be alerted to watch for other cases and can take steps to prevent the spread of infection.

Constipation

Constipation is characterized by a decrease in the frequency or passage of stools; the formation of hard, dry stools; or the oozing of liquid stool past a collection of hard, dry stool. Because stooling patterns vary among children, identification of an abnormal pattern is sometimes difficult. Infants usually have several bowel movements a day. For a young child, one bowel movement a day may be normal. As the child grows, however, three to four bowel movements a week may be a normal pattern.

Constipation may be caused by an underlying disease, diet, or psychologic factor. It may result from defects in filling, or more commonly emptying, of the rectum. Pathologic causes of defective filling include ineffective colonic propulsive activity, caused by hypothyroidism or use of medication, and obstruction, caused by a structural anomaly (stricture or stenosis) or by an aganglionic segment (Hirschsprung's disease). If the rectum fails to fill, stasis leads to excessive drying of the stools. Emptying of the rectum depends on the defecation reflex. Lesions of the spinal cord, weakness of the abdominal muscles, and local lesions blocking sphincter relaxation all may impede attempts to defecate.

Constipation during infancy is rare and is most often caused by mismanagement of diet. The transition from formula to cow's milk may cause a transient constipation because the bowel must adjust to the increased protein content of cow's milk. Constipation in young infants can usually be corrected by increasing the amount of fluids and juices given or by adding corn syrup to the formula. In older infants, increasing the intake of cereals, fruits, and vegetables in the diet should correct the problem.

Constipation occurs most frequently in the toddler and preschool age groups. This increased incidence is often associated with learning to control bodily functions. Many children do not like the sensations of a bowel movement and may begin withholding stool, which accumulates in the rectum until the next urge to defecate. The increasingly painful bowel movement reinforces the child's behavior, and a self-perpetuating pattern develops.[29] Removing constipating foods (bananas, rice, and cheese) from the child's diet often decreases the constipation. Increasing the child's intake of high-fiber foods (whole grain breads, raw fruits and vegetables) and increasing fluids also promote defecation.

In the school-age child, constipation may occur because time for toileting is limited. Busy school-age children may delay going to the bathroom. Children may also be hesitant to use an unfamiliar bathroom. Encouragement from parents and relaxation of bathroom privileges at school promote regularity and return of usual bowel patterns within a short time.

Diagnosis is based on a thorough history and physical examination. When constipation occurs along with growth failure, vomiting, or abdominal pain, further investigation is necessary to rule out other disorders. Dietary management is the treatment of choice for constipation that has no underlying pathologic cause. A single glycerin suppository or enema may be needed to remove hard stool, followed by dietary and fluid management.

Constipation may follow surgery, especially in children who are immobilized, such as by traction or a body cast. Stool softeners and a diet high in roughage and fluids are given to prevent and treat constipation.

Nursing Management

Take a diet history and obtain a description of bowel patterns from parents. Assessment of the child's food likes and dislikes may provide a clue to the cause of constipation. Nursing care focuses on teaching parents what constitutes normal bowel patterns in children and the importance of diet in maintaining normal bowel patterns. Regular bowel habits are encouraged by placing the child on the toilet 30 minutes after a meal or around the time defecation usually occurs. Providing positive reinforcement during toilet training helps to prevent a withholding pattern.

Teach parents dietary measures to promote regularity of bowel movements. Children can be given a high-fiber diet that includes fruits and vegetables. Cut-up fresh fruits, dried fruits, and fruit juice can be offered as snacks. A glycerine suppository can be used periodically. This is a natural stimulant and lubricant of the bowel. Caution parents to avoid frequent use of laxatives, stool softeners, and enemas, since overuse can cause bowel dependency.

► INTESTINAL PARASITIC DISORDERS

Intestinal parasitic disorders occur most frequently in tropical regions. Outbreaks take place in areas where water is not treated, food is incorrectly prepared, or people live in crowded conditions with poor sanitation. In the United States, outbreaks of diseases caused by protozoa or helminths (worms) are increasing. Young children, especially those in day care, are most at risk of infection. Young children often lack good hygiene practices and are more likely to put objects and their hands into their mouths. The most common intestinal parasitic disorders are summarized in Table 15–8.

Laboratory examination of stool specimens identifies the causative organism (protozoa, worms, larvae, or ova). Treatment usually involves an anthelmintic. Nursing care centers on preventive teaching. Emphasize the importance of good hygiene practices, especially careful handwashing, after toileting and when handling food. Instruct parents to give prescribed medications as directed even if the child's condition seems to be improved.

15-8 Common Intestinal Parasitic Disorders

Parasitic Infection	Transmission, Life Cycle, Pathogenesis	Clinical Manifestations	Treatment	Comments
Giardiasis Organism: protozoan *Giardia lamblia*	Transmission is through person-to-person contact, unfiltered water, improperly prepared infected food, and contact with animals. Cysts are ingested and passed into the duodenum and proximal jejunum, where they begin actively feeding. They are excreted in the stool.	May be asymptomatic. *Infants:* diarrhea, vomiting, anorexia, failure to thrive *Older children:* abdominal cramps; intermittent loose, foul-smelling, watery, pale, and greasy stools	Available medications include furazolidone and quinacrine. Furazolidone has fewer side effects than quinacrine but is more expensive. Metronidazole is also effective but is not licensed in the United States for treatment of giardiasis.	Most common intestinal parasitic organism in the United States. Infection may resolve spontaneously in 4–6 weeks without treatment. Parents or caregivers should wear gloves when handling diapers or stool of parasite-infected infant or child.
Enterobiasis (Pinworm) Organism: nematode *Enterobius vermicularis*	Transmission is from discharged eggs inhaled or carried from hand to mouth. Eggs hatch in the upper intestine and mature in 15–28 days. Larvae then migrate to the cecum. After mating, the female migrates out of the anus and lays up to 17,000 eggs. Movement of worms causes intense itching. Scratching deposits eggs on the hands and under the nails.	Intense perianal itching, irritability, restlessness, and short attention span; in females, can migrate to the vagina and urethra to cause infection. Itching intensifies at night when the female comes to the anal opening to lay eggs.	Available medications include mebendazole, pyrantel pamoate, and piperazine citrate. The child and all household members should be treated at the same time. Treatment may be repeated in 2–3 weeks.	Most common helminthic infection in United States. Transmission is increased in crowded conditions such as housing developments, schools, and day-care centers.

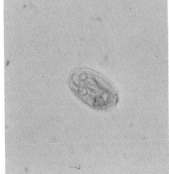

Giardia lamblia

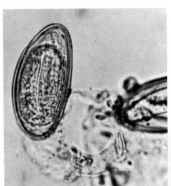

Pinworm

Giardia lamblia *courtesy of the Centers for Disease Control and Prevention, Atlanta, GA; pinworm (p. 718), roundworm (p. 714), hookworm (p. 719); and thread-worm (p. 721) from Rudolph, A.M., Hoffman, J.I.E., Rudolph, C.D. (1996). Rudolph's pediatrics (20th ed.). Stamford, CT: Appleton & Lange.*

15-8 Common Intestinal Parasitic Disorders (continued)

Parasitic Infection	Transmission, Life Cycle, Pathogenesis	Clinical Manifestations	Treatment	Comments
Ascariasis (Roundworm) Organism: nematode *Ascaris lumbricoides*	Transmission is from discharged eggs carried from hand to mouth. Adult lays eggs in small intestine. Eggs are excreted in stool, where they incubate for 2–3 weeks. Swallowed eggs hatch in the small intestine. Larvae may penetrate intestinal villi, entering the portal vein and liver, then moving to the lung. Larvae that ascend to upper respiratory tract are swallowed and proceed to the small intestine, where they repeat the cycle.	Mild infection may be asymptomatic. Severe infection may result in intestinal obstruction, peritonitis, obstructive jaundice, and lung involvement.	Available anthelmintic medications include mebendazole, pyrantel pamoate, or piperazine citrate. Stools should be examined 2 weeks after treatment and monthly for 3 months. Family members and contacts of the child should be treated if indicated. If the child has intestinal obstruction, treatment may include administering piperazine through a nasogastric tube and duodenal suction. Obstructing worms sometimes have to be surgically removed.	Most common in warm climates. Primarily affects children 1–4 years of age.
Hookworm disease Organism: nematode *Necator americanus*	Transmission is through direct contact with infected soil containing larvae. Worms live in the small intestine and feed on villi, causing bleeding. Eggs are deposited in the bowel and excreted in feces. Eggs hatch in damp shaded soil. Larvae attach to and penetrate the skin then enter the bloodstream, migrating to the lungs. Larvae then migrate to the upper respiratory passages and are swallowed.	In healthy individuals mild infection seldom causes problems. More severe infection may result in anemia and malnutrition. Presence of larvae on the skin may cause burning and itching, followed by redness and papular eruption.	Available medications include mebendazole and pyrantel pamoate. Stools should be examined 2 weeks after treatment and monthly for 3 months. Family members and contacts of the child should be treated if indicated.	Children should wear shoes when outdoors, although other unprotected areas of the skin may still come in contact with larvae.

Roundworm

Hookworm

Continued . . .

15-8 Common Intestinal Parasitic Disorders (continued)

Parasitic Infection	Transmission, Life Cycle, Pathogenesis	Clinical Manifestations	Treatment	Comments
Strongyloidiasis (Threadworm) Organism: nematode *Strongyloides stercoralis*	Transmission is from the ingestion of discharged larvae in the soil. Life cycle is similar to that of the hookworm, except the threadworm does not attach to the intestinal mucosa and feeding larvae (rather than eggs) may be deposited in the soil.	Mild infection may be asymptomatic. Severe infection may result in abdominal pain and distention, nausea, vomiting, and diarrhea. Stools may be large and pale, with mucus. Severe infection may lead to a nutritional deficiency.	Available medications include thiabendazole or mebendazole. Treatment may need to be repeated if symptoms recur after treatment. Family members and contacts of the child should be examined and treated if indicated.	Most common in older children and adolescents.

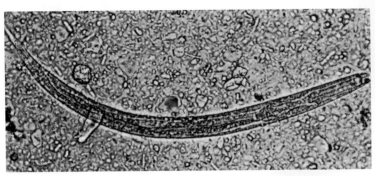

Threadworm

Parasitic Infection	Transmission, Life Cycle, Pathogenesis	Clinical Manifestations	Treatment	Comments
Visceral larva migrans (Toxocariasis) Organism: nematode *Toxocara canis* or *T. catis*, commonly found in dogs and cats	Transmission is through the ingestion of eggs in the soil. Ingested eggs hatch in the intestine. Mobile larvae then migrate to the liver and eventually to all major organs (including the brain). Once migration is complete, they encapsulate in dense fibrous tissue.	Most cases are asymptomatic. Affected children may have a low-grade fever and recurrent upper airway diseases. Severe symptoms include hepatomegaly, pulmonary infiltration, and neurologic disturbances. In all cases there is a hypereosinophilia of the blood.	There is no specific treatment. Corticosteroids have been used in severe cases. Thiabendazole has been recommended but efficacy is not established (infection usually resolves spontaneously).	Most common in toddlers. Deworm household pets monthly if indicated. Keep children away from areas contaminated with animal droppings.

▶ FEEDING DISORDERS

Feeding problems that interfere with a child's ability to ingest or tolerate formulas and foods usually become apparent during the first year of life. To prevent complications of poor nutrition, feeding methods or diet may need to be altered. The following discussion focuses on three common disorders: colic, food sensitivity and allergy, and rumination.

COLIC

Colic is a feeding disorder characterized by paroxysmal abdominal pain of intestinal origin and severe crying. It usually occurs in infants under 3 months of age.

Characteristically the infant cries loudly and continuously, often for several hours. The infant's face may become flushed. The abdomen is distended and tense. Often the infant draws up the legs and clenches the hands. Episodes occur at the same time each day, usually in the late afternoon or early evening. Crying may stop only when the child is completely exhausted or after passage of flatus or stool. Carrying the child in the upright position is often helpful.

The etiology of colic is unknown. Proposed causes include feeding too rapidly and swallowing large amounts of air. Symptoms initially may resemble intestinal obstruction or peritoneal infection. These conditions must be ruled out along with sensitivity to formula. Treatment is supportive. Usually by 3 months of age the severity and frequency of symptoms decrease.

Nursing Management

Nursing care requires a thorough history of the infant's diet and daily schedule and the events surrounding episodes of colicky behavior. Assessment of the infant's feeding patterns and diet includes type, frequency, and amount of feeding (if breast-feeding, maternal diet history) and frequency of burping. Episodes of colic are assessed for onset, duration, and characteristics of cry. What measures are used to relieve crying? How effective are they? When possible, the feeding method should be observed. Parents of infants with colic are often tired and frustrated. They require frequent reassurance that they are not to blame for the infant's condition. Suggest ways of alleviating some of the infant's symptoms and discomfort (Table 15–9).

FOOD SENSITIVITY AND ALLERGY

Food sensitivity encompasses any adverse reaction to foods or substances ingested in foods. The foods that most commonly cause a reaction are fish, shellfish, nuts, eggs, soy, wheat, corn, strawberries, and cow's milk products. Food antigens, chemical additives, antibiotics, preservatives, and food colorings also can cause food sensitivity reactions.

Allergic (IgE-mediated) reactions, on the other hand, are potentially systemic, characteristically rapid in onset, and may be manifest as swelling of the lips, mouth, uvula, or glottis, generalized urticaria, and, in severe reactions, shock. Food allergies are more prevalent in children with a family history of allergic reactions to various substances and foods (atopy). Caution parents to be aware of "hidden" substances in prepared foods. For example, the child who is allergic to nuts will experience a reaction to a food if nut extracts are used in its preparation.

15-9	Parent Teaching: Suggestions for Alleviating Colic

Provide Rhythmic Movement
Front-carrying sling carriers.
Infant swing (battery-operated swing provides continuous motion).
Car ride.

Alternate Positions
Swaddle infant in a soft, stretchy blanket with knees flexed up against abdomen or with legs straight.
Place infant prone on parent's arm, supporting the body with one hand under the abdomen and cradling the head in the crook of the other arm.

Reduce Environmental Stimuli
Respond to crying.
Provide quiet, soothing music.
Prevent sudden loud noises.
Avoid smoking.

Provide Various Tactile Stimuli
Offer a pacifier.
Provide a warm bath.
Massage abdomen.

Alter Intake
Feed smaller amount and burp frequently.
Use a bottle with a collapsible bag to prevent sucking air.
Breast-feeding mothers: eliminate milk products and spicy or gas-producing foods.
Hold upright for ½ hour after feeding.

Delayed hypersensitivity reactions are attributed to digestive products of food and require a thorough diet history over several days to identify the offending food. These reactions are more difficult to diagnose, since the reaction can occur up to 24 hours after ingestion of the food.

Cow's milk may cause an allergy or a sensitivity reaction. In allergy, an IgE-mediated systemic reaction occurs. In sensitivity reaction, there is a gastrointestinal response to milk proteins (diarrhea, vomiting, abdominal pain). Infants often have vomiting and watery, blood-streaked, mucoid diarrhea.

Diagnostic tests to identify suspected food allergies include measurement of serum IgE levels, scratch tests, and the radioallergosorbent test (RAST), in which radioimmunoassay is used to measure IgE antibodies to specific allergens (see Chap. 9). A diet diary is kept, noting date, type of foods eaten, and reaction, if any. Foods should be eaten singly for several days to determine whether they cause a reaction.

Treatment consists of eliminating the offending foods from the child's diet. Children frequently outgrow food sensitivities. Careful reintroduction of the food after a 1–2-year absence may elicit no reaction in the previously sensitive child. Allergies are more commonly lifelong. The foods involved should *always* be avoided.

Nursing Management

Prevention is the first step. Instruct parents of infants to introduce new foods at a rate of not more than one new food every 5 days. If a sensitivity is noted, the causative food can be easily identified. Discuss any changes in diet or preparation of formula. Reassure parents that the child's symptoms will disappear when the offending foods are removed from the diet.

Nursing care of a child with food allergies is primarily supportive. Help the family identify the offending foods. Explain to parents all tests, use of a food diary, and care of the child should a reaction occur. Emphasize the importance of reading food labels for hidden foods that can trigger an allergic reaction. The child with a true food allergy should wear a medical alert bracelet. Be sure that school personnel know about the allergy and know to avoid giving the child the food product. Refer the family to the Food Allergy Network (see Appendix F).

NURSING ALERT

Someone in each of the settings where the child with an allergy commonly spends time (home, day care, school, summer camp, sports team) needs to be knowledgeable in the emergency management of an allergic response using epinephrine.

RUMINATION

Rumination is a rare and serious form of chronic regurgitation that may lead to malnutrition and growth failure in infancy. Chewing movements and mouthing of fingers often precede or accompany regurgitation. Close observation may reveal the infant actively initiating gagging with the tongue and fingers.

Rumination is most often associated with poor maternal–infant bonding. This kind of behavior is seen in infants who are deprived of tactile, visual, or auditory stimuli for long periods. The infant substitutes repetitive self-stimulation for the lack of appropriate external stimulation. (See the discussion of failure to thrive in Chapter 22.)

Diagnostic evaluation focuses on ruling out an organic cause and determining the degree and type of nutritional deficiencies. Treatment involves correcting the nutritional deficits and developing normal feeding patterns. Medical and nursing staff and social services are often involved in helping parents meet the infant's nutritional and psychologic needs (see Chapter 22).

Nursing Management

Nursing care focuses on establishing a warm, caring relationship with the infant and the parents. Making eye contact with the infant, providing food regularly, and stimulating the infant through all the senses are ways to break the pattern of rumination.

Parents need to be included in the infant's care. Discuss proper nutrition and demonstrate feeding techniques and interactions that promote development. Determine the parents' support needs and make a referral to social service agencies as appropriate. A parent who is preoccupied with financial or other problems is less likely to attend to an infant's needs, resulting in continuation or recurrence of the pattern of rumination.

▶ DISORDERS OF MALABSORPTION

Malabsorption occurs when a child is unable to digest or absorb nutrients in the diet. Disorders of malabsorption include celiac disease, lactose intolerance, and short bowel syndrome. Cystic fibrosis is a common cause of malabsorption and is discussed in Chapter 11.

CELIAC DISEASE

Celiac disease, or gluten-sensitive enteropathy, is a chronic malabsorption syndrome that is more common in Caucasian, European children and is uncommon in African-American or Asian children. Current research is being directed at locating the potential genetic abnormalities that occur in celiac disease. The disease is characterized by an intolerance for gluten, a protein found in wheat, barley, rye, and oats. Inability to digest glutenin and gliadin (protein fractions) results in the accumulation of the amino acid glutamine, which is toxic to mucosal cells in the intestine. Damage to the villi ultimately impairs the absorptive process in the small intestine.

In the early stages, celiac disease affects fat absorption, resulting in excretion of large quantities of fat in the stools (steatorrhea). Stools are greasy, foul smelling, frothy, and excessive. As changes in the villi continue, the absorption of protein, carbohydrates, calcium, iron, folate, and vitamins A, D, E, K, and B_{12} becomes impaired.[30]

Symptoms usually occur when solid foods containing gluten are introduced to the child's diet (in the first 2 years of life). The child exhibits chronic diarrhea, vomiting, irritability, and failure to grow. If diagnosis is delayed, the child begins to show evidence of protein deficiency (wasted musculature, abdominal distention), delayed dentition, and changes in bone density.

Diagnosis is confirmed through measurement of fecal fat content, jejunal biopsy, and improvement with removal of gluten products from the diet. Blood screening tests are more often being used successfully for diagnosis. Serum antigliadin antibody (AGA) and reticulin antibody levels are elevated.[31] Symptoms usually improve within a few days to weeks. The intestinal villi return to normal in about 6 months.[30] Growth should improve steadily, and height and weight should reach normal range within 1 year. Vitamin supplementation may be needed for a period of time if the child has become malnourished.

Nursing Management

Nursing care focuses on supporting the parents in maintaining a gluten-free diet for the child. The parents should receive a thorough explanation of the disease process. Emphasize the necessity of following a gluten-free diet. Help parents to understand that celiac disease requires lifelong dietary modifications that should not be discontinued when the child is symptom free. Discontinuation of the diet places the child at risk for growth retardation and the development of GI cancers in adulthood. All children with celiac disease should be seen by a dietitian several times during childhood. Nutritional assessment and continued teaching to maintain a gluten-free diet take place at these visits.

The diet of an infant or toddler is easily monitored at home. When the child enters school, however, ensuring adherence to dietary restrictions becomes more difficult. In addition to easily identified gluten-based foods, such as bread, cake, doughnuts, cookies, and crackers, the child must also avoid processed foods that contain gluten as a filler. School-age children and adolescents are often tempted to eat these foods, especially when among peers. Emphasize the need for compliance while meeting the child's developmental needs.

The child's special dietary needs can place a financial burden on the family. Parents will need to purchase prepared rice or corn flour products or make their own bread and bakery products. Advise parents that obtaining a dietary prescription will enable them to deduct the cost of these ingredients and commercially prepared products as a medical expense.

Because adaptation to the diet must be made by the entire family, support and management skills are needed by parents and siblings.[32] For information and support, parents and children can be referred to several or-

NURSING ALERT

Many prepared foods contain hidden gluten. Examples include certain types of chocolate candy, some prepared hamburgers, hot dogs, luncheon meats, milk preparations such as malts and processed ice cream, canned soups, mayonnaise, catsup, malt flavoring, vinegar (except apple cider vinegar), hydrolyzed vegetable protein, and modified food starch.

ganizations, including the American Celiac Society, the Celiac Sprue Association/United States of America, and the Gluten Intolerance Group. Written materials are also available from Children's Memorial Hospital in Chicago (see Appendix F).

LACTOSE INTOLERANCE

Lactose intolerance is the inability to digest lactose, a disaccharide found in milk and other dairy products. It results from a congenital or acquired deficiency of the enzyme lactase. Congenital lactase deficiency of infancy is a rare disorder. Abdominal pain, flatulence, and diarrhea occur shortly after birth when the infant is unable to hydrolyze lactose. The prevalence of secondary (acquired) lactase deficiency is highest (approximately 100%) among Asian and Native American children and affects approximately 70% of African-Americans after the age of 3 years. Diarrhea develops rapidly after the child ingests milk and milk products. Some children are able to tolerate small ingestions of lactose but have symptoms when larger amounts are consumed.

Diagnosis is based on a thorough history and a hydrogen breath test, which measures the amount of hydrogen left after fermentation of unabsorbed carbohydrates. Implementing a lactose-free diet for a period of time may eliminate the symptoms, confirming the diagnosis. Treatment for infants includes switching to a soy-based formula. For older children, eliminating lactose-containing foods is recommended. Enzyme tablets such as LactAid can be added to milk or sprinkled on foods to aid digestion.

Nursing Management

Nursing care is primarily supportive. Carefully explain dietary modifications to parents and discuss alternate sources of calcium (see Chap. 8). Discuss the need for supplementation of calcium and vitamin D to prevent deficiencies. Caution parents to read food labels carefully to identify hidden sources of lactose. For example, milk solids are found in breads, cakes, some candies (eg, milk chocolate, caramels, and toffee), some salad dressings, margarine, and various processed foods.

SHORT BOWEL SYNDROME

Short bowel syndrome is a decreased ability to digest and absorb a regular diet because of a shortened intestine. Loss of intestine may result from extensive bowel resection for treatment of necrotizing enterocolitis or inflammatory disorders or from a congenital bowel anomaly such as intestinal malrotation, gastroschisis, or atresia.

The extent and location of the involved bowel determine the severity of the disorder. Because specific types of absorption occur primarily in certain parts of the bowel, the section lost determines the particular vitamins and other nutrients that are inadequate.[33] Over time, the remaining bowel usually compensates for the absent intestine (adaptation period). However, the infant or young child requires nutritional support initially to provide sufficient nutrients for adequate growth and development. A combination of total parenteral nutrition via central line and oral fluids may be required. Once the bowel begins to recover, enteral feedings may be started.

Nursing Management

Nursing care focuses on meeting the child's nutritional and fluid needs and teaching parents how to care for the child at home. Establishing an adequate nutritional intake and bowel pattern is a lengthy process. Total parenteral nutrition is provided initially until a feeding regimen can be established. Oral and enteral feedings are instituted gradually to allow the bowel time to compensate. Provide support to the family and child throughout this period. Teach parents how to prepare and administer total parenteral feedings and care for the central line (see description in the *Quick Reference to Pediatric Clinical Skills* accompanying this text). Once enteral or tube feedings are begun, teach management of the feeding pump and care of the feeding tube. Ensure regular bowel function and maintain skin integrity. Arrange home visits to monitor the child's growth and development, care of the central line and tube feeding site, and any side effects such as fluid and electrolyte imbalance and diarrhea.

► HEPATIC DISORDERS

The liver is one of the most vital organs in the body. Among its essential functions are blood storage and filtration; secretion of bile and bilirubin; metabolism of fat, protein, and carbohydrates; synthesis of blood-clotting components; detoxification of hormones, drugs, and other substances; and storage of glycogen, iron, fat-soluble vitamins, and vitamin B_{12}. Thus any inflammatory, obstructive, or degenerative disorder that affects liver function can be life threatening. The following discussion focuses on three common liver disorders in children: biliary atresia, viral hepatitis, and cirrhosis.

BILIARY ATRESIA

Biliary atresia is the pathologic closure or absence of bile ducts outside the liver. It is the most common pediatric liver disease necessitating transplantation.[34]

Initially the newborn is asymptomatic. Jaundice may not be detected until 2–3 weeks after birth. At that point bilirubin levels increase, accompanied by abdominal distention and hepatomegaly. As the disease progresses, splenomegaly occurs. The infant experiences easy bruising, prolonged bleeding time, and intense itching. Stools are puttylike in consistency and white or clay colored because of the absence of bile pigments. Excretion of bilirubin and bile salts results in tea-colored urine. Failure to thrive and malnutrition occur as the destructive changes of the disease progress.

The cause of biliary atresia is unknown. Absence or blockage of the extrahepatic bile ducts results in blocked bile flow from the liver to the duodenum. This altered bile flow soon causes inflammation and fibrotic changes in the liver. Lack of bile acids also interferes with digestion of fat and absorption of fat-soluble vitamins A, D, E, and K, resulting in steatorrhea and nutritional deficiencies. Without treatment the disease is fatal.

Diagnosis is based on the history, physical examination, and laboratory evaluation. Laboratory findings reveal elevated bilirubin levels, elevated serum aminotransferase and alkaline phosphatase values, prolonged prothrombin time, and increased ammonia levels. Ultrasound is used to rule out other causes, and a liver biopsy is performed.[35] Because liver damage develops rapidly in infants with biliary atresia, early diagnosis is essential.

Treatment involves surgery to attempt correction of the obstruction (hepatoportoenterostomy) and supportive care. In the hepatoportoenterostomy (Kasai procedure), a segment of the intestine is anastomosed to the porta hepatis. In most children this is a palliative treatment to promote bile drainage, maintain as much hepatic function as possible, and prevent the complications of liver failure. Supportive treatment is directed at managing the bleeding tendencies by administering oral vitamin K; preventing rickets through vitamin D supplementation; controlling itching and irritability with cholestyramine and antihistamines; and promoting adequate nutrition.

Although the hepatoportoenterostomy improves the prognosis, complications of liver disease continue to develop and eventually necessitate liver transplantation. Advances in transplantation surgery now make it possible to perform partial liver transplants from living donor resections. This enables transplantation to be performed when the child is in optimal health, rather than waiting until an appropriate-size cadaver liver is available.

These advances, along with the development of cyclosporine and other immunosuppressants, have improved the first-year survival rate for children receiving liver transplantation to between 75% and 80%.[34]

Nursing Management

Nursing care in the initial stages of biliary atresia is the same as that for any healthy newborn. As symptoms develop, the focus of nursing care becomes long-term management and support.

Diagnosis of this potentially fatal disorder can be devastating to parents. Provide emotional support and offer frequent explanations of tests during the initial diagnostic evaluation. As the disease progresses, the infant becomes irritable because of intense itching and the accumulation of toxins. Tepid baths may help to relieve itching and provide comfort. Promote rest by grouping nursing activities while the infant is awake. Care following a hepatoportoenterostomy is similar to that for a child undergoing abdominal surgery. (See the earlier discussion of postsurgical nursing management for appendicitis and the Nursing Care Plan for the Child Undergoing Surgery in Chapter 4.) Posttransplant care includes immunosuppressant drugs and close monitoring for vascular complications (see Chap. 9).

Discharge planning focuses on teaching parents how to care for the child's skin, provide for nutritional needs, administer medications, and monitor for increasing symptoms of liver disease. For the child who has received a transplant, teach parents how to identify signs of rejection (nausea, vomiting, fever, and jaundice), as well as the administration and side effects of immunosuppressant medications. Refer parents to support groups, clergy, or social services if indicated. They will need ongoing visits from a home health care nurse to help them in managing the complex care of the child.

CLINICAL TIP

When drying the skin, pat the towel against the skin rather than rubbing and massaging. Rubbing and massaging promote vasodilation, which worsens the infant's itching and irritation.

VIRAL HEPATITIS

Hepatitis is an inflammation of the liver caused by a viral infection. It may occur as an acute or chronic disease. Acute hepatitis is rapid in onset and if untreated may develop into chronic hepatitis. The most frequently diagnosed causative organisms are hepatitis A virus (HAV), hepatitis B virus (HBV), hepatitis C virus (HCV), hepatitis D virus (HDV), and hepatitis E virus (HEV). An estimated 136,000 cases of hepatitis occur annually in the United States, and one third of these are in children.[36] Most cases are types A and B.

Clinical Manifestations

Acute hepatitis infection is characterized by two phases, the anicteric (absence of jaundice) phase and the icteric (jaundice) phase. The anicteric

15-10	Comparison of Hepatitis Types			
Type	Incubation	% Icteric	% Who Become Chronic Carriers	Clinical Features
Hepatitis A Children < 5 years	4 weeks (10–50 days)	< 5	0	More acute onset; frequently subclinical in young children
Adults		50–75		
Hepatitis B Infants	12 weeks (2–20 weeks)	< 5	> 90	Extrahepatic manifestations more common
Adults		20–60	5–10	
Hepatitis C All ages	8 weeks (1–24 weeks)	20–30	≥ 60	Frequently anicteric; predisposes to hepatocellular carcinoma
Hepatitis D Coinfection with HBV	NA (probably similar to HBV)	NA	< 5	Most common viral cause of fulminant hepatitis
Superinfection of HBV carrier			> 80	
Hepatitis E All ages	~6 weeks (15–60 days)	~10	0	Severe in pregnant women; high mortality and fetal loss

NA = not available

Modified from Weintraub, P.S. (1996). Viral hepatitis. In A.M. Rudolph, J.I.E. Hoffman, & C.D. Rudolph (Eds.), Rudolph's pediatrics (20th ed., p. 647), Stamford, CT: Appleton & Lange.

phase usually lasts 5–7 days. Signs and symptoms include nausea, vomiting, anorexia, malaise, fatigue, right upper quadrant pain, hepatosplenomegaly, and fever (Table 15–10). The child becomes irritable, looks ill, and requires rest. In the icteric phase, signs and symptoms include darkening of urine, clay-colored stools, and the characteristic yellowing of the skin and sclera. In many cases of hepatitis in children, there is no jaundice, leading to difficulty in disease diagnosis and management.[36] As the jaundice worsens, the child begins to feel better. This phase lasts approximately 4 weeks. Complete recovery with return of normal liver function and laboratory values may take 1–3 months.

In some cases hepatitis becomes chronic. The individual with chronic hepatitis carries the virus, can transfer it to others, and may develop serious liver disease after several years.

Etiology and Pathophysiology

Hepatitis A is the most common form of acute viral hepatitis. It is highly contagious and traditionally has been referred to as infectious hepatitis. Infection occurs primarily through the fecal–oral route. Transmission is by di-

15-11	Transmission, Immunization, and Prophylaxis for Hepatitis		
Type	Primary Transmission	Immunization Available	Prophylaxis
Hepatitis A	Fecal–oral	Yes	Immune serum globulin Hepatitis A vaccine
Hepatitis B	Blood products Intravenous drug use In utero Sexual activity	Yes	Hepatitis B immune globulin Hepatitis B vaccine
Hepatitis C	Blood products Sexual activity Intravenous drug use	No	None
Hepatitis D	Blood products Intravenous drug use In utero Sexual activity	No	Hepatitis B vaccine
Hepatitis E	Fecal–oral	No	None

rect person-to-person spread or through ingestion of contaminated water or food (particularly shellfish). Hepatitis A frequently occurs in children in day-care settings where hygiene practices are poor. Food handlers can spread hepatitis A if not aware of their infection. Because the virus is transmitted in the early stages of the disease when individuals are often asymptomatic or only mildly ill, large numbers of people may be exposed before the diagnosis is confirmed (Table 15–11).

Hepatitis B, which has been known traditionally as serum hepatitis, is a serious disease. Transmission is usually by the parenteral route through the exchange of blood or any bodily secretion or fluid. Other common transmission routes include sexual activity and transmission from mother to fetus in utero. Adolescents who use intravenous drugs and have unprotected sexual intercourse are at risk for contracting hepatitis B. Major sources for the spread of HBV are healthy chronic carriers. All body fluids of infected individuals are potentially contaminated with the virus.

The hepatitis C virus is transmitted primarily through blood and blood products, and blood banks now test for this virus. Its incidence is low in the United States, with most infected children being those who have had repeated transfusions (as in sickle cell disease or hemophilia). Intravenous drug use and multiple sexual partners are also risk factors.

Hepatitis D (delta virus) is a defective virus that can gain entry to a human only in connection with hepatitis B. This virus is suspected when someone who has been diagnosed with hepatitis B has diminishing liver function, increasing jaundice, and deteriorating mental status.[34]

Hepatitis E infection is primarily transmitted through contaminated water and is most common in developing countries. Outbreaks may occur in flooding and rainy seasons.

The liver's response to injury by the viruses that cause hepatitis is similar (Fig. 15–12). Initially invasion of the parenchymal cells by the virus results in local degeneration and necrosis. Subsequent infiltration of the parenchyma by lymphocytes, macrophages, plasma cells, eosinophils, and

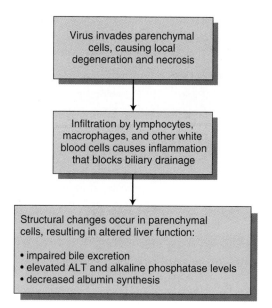

FIGURE 15–12. Pathophysiology of viral hepatitis.

NURSING ALERT

When hepatitis A is present, drug metabolism is altered and the liver's ability to detoxify drugs is decreased. As with all liver disorders, medications need to be administered carefully and the child's condition must be monitored for possible side effects.

neutrophils causes inflammation that blocks biliary drainage into the intestine. Impaired bile excretion causes a build-up of bile in the blood, urine, and skin (jaundice). Structural changes in the parenchymal cells account for other altered liver functions. Regeneration of parenchymal cells occurs within 3 months, and most children recover completely.

In some children, however, a progressive and total destruction of the hepatic parenchyma known as acute fulminating hepatitis develops. Children with this form of the disease usually die of liver failure within 2 weeks of onset unless they receive a liver transplant. Another complication, chronic active hepatitis, may lead to scarring of the liver and progressive deterioration of liver function. The prognosis depends on the degree of liver involvement. In some persons, especially those who develop chronic hepatitis, liver cancers and cirrhosis can develop.

Diagnostic Tests and Medical Management

Diagnosis is often made on the basis of a thorough history and physical examination. A history of exposure to persons with the disease is significant. Physical examination reveals a tender, enlarged liver, abdominal pain, and flu-like symptoms. Laboratory evaluation includes serologic testing (to detect the presence of antigens and antibodies to HAV, HBV, HCV, or HDV) and liver function studies. Although a test for HEV has been developed, it is not available in developing countries, so diagnosis is usually based on the history.

The three goals of medical management are early detection to prevent complications, support and monitoring during the acute phase of the disease, and prevention of the spread of the disease. Early diagnosis is essential to follow the course of the illness and identify potential complications. Management of the illness includes bedrest during the flu-like phase. If prothrombin times are increased, vitamin K is administered.

The spread of viral infections can be interrupted by elimination of the virus from the infected population, institution of proper hygiene, and passive or active immunization. To date, no antiviral agent has been developed to combat the hepatitis viruses. Prevention depends on breaking the cycle of infection. Active immunization for hepatitis A, a two-dose series, is recommended for all persons at risk of acquiring and transmitting the disease. This includes day-care staff and food handlers. Immunization for hepatitis B, a three-dose series, is recommended for many children and at-risk adults. The first dose is given within 12 hours of birth to the infant born of an infected mother. (Refer to the discussion of immunization in Chapter 10).

Passive immunity to HAV can be achieved with standard pooled immune globulin. It must be administered within 2 weeks of exposure. Passive immunity to HBV can be achieved with hepatitis B immune globulin (HBIG). It is used for one-time exposure and for infants of infected mothers and is given within 12 hours of birth.

Nursing Assessment

The nurse usually encounters the child and family in an outpatient setting. In addition to being observed for characteristic signs of hepatitis (jaundiced skin and sclera), the child is assessed for the presence of abdominal pain, anorexia, nausea and vomiting, malaise, and arthralgia. A history of the child's contacts over the past 45 days for HAV and up to 180 days for HBV is also obtained.

Nursing Diagnosis

Common nursing diagnoses for the child with acute hepatitis might include:

- Risk for Altered Nutrition: Less Than Body Requirements related to anorexia, nausea, and vomiting
- Fatigue related to flu-like symptoms and general feelings of malaise
- Risk for Diversional Activity Deficit related to change in usual daily activities
- Risk for Body Image Disturbance (Older Child) related to temporary jaundice
- Anxiety (Parent and Child) related to diagnosis and treatment measures
- Pain related to liver infection

Nursing Management

Nursing care is mainly supportive, as children with hepatitis are seldom admitted to the hospital. The hospitalized child is placed in isolation. Educating parents about necessary precautions and infection-control measures is a priority. In addition, teach parents the importance of maintaining adequate nutrition, promoting rest and comfort, and providing diversional activities.

Prevent Spread of Infection

Teach the parents and the child infection-control measures to help prevent transmission of the virus. Good hygiene practices, such as washing hands before and after toileting and proper disposal of soiled diapers, should be reinforced to parents. Siblings of a child with hepatitis B who have not already been immunized with the hepatitis B vaccine should be vaccinated immediately. Contacts of the child with hepatitis A should receive immune serum globulin and the first immunization in the hepatitis A series. Rifampin may be given in some cases.

NURSING ALERT

Health care workers who come in contact with blood or other body fluids of children infected with hepatitis B are at risk for contracting the virus. Standard precautions should be used at all times (see the *Quick Reference to Pediatric Clinical Skills* accompanying this text). Hepatitis B immunization (three doses) is recommended for nurses and other persons at high risk for exposure as well as all infants and adolescents (see Chap. 10).

CLINICAL TIP

Nurses in day-care centers can provide assessment of the center's procedures and teaching to prevent hepatitis A transmission. Help the center to set standards about:
- Handwashing after each diaper change
- Proper disposal of diapers
- Cleaning diaper-changing surfaces after each diaper change
- Never having food handlers perform diaper changes
- Instructing parents to keep children at home for at least 2 weeks after a diagnosis of hepatitis A
- Informing parents of other children when there is a case of hepatitis A and teaching them the symptoms of the condition

Maintain Adequate Nutrition

Initially the child is encouraged to eat favorite foods. Once the anorexia and nausea have resolved, a high-protein, high-carbohydrate, low-fat diet is recommended. Increased protein helps to maintain protein stores and prevent muscle wasting. Increased carbohydrates ensure adequate caloric intake and prevent protein depletion. The use of low-fat foods lessens stomach distention. Offer the child small, frequent feedings.

Promote Rest and Comfort

Bedrest is necessary only if the child has severe fatigue and malaise. However, most children voluntarily limit their activities during the initial phase of the disease. Keep the child quiet and comfortable. Offer comfort items such as favorite toys, blankets, and pillows.

Provide Diversional Activities

Hospitalized children with hepatitis are kept in isolation. Nonhospitalized children with hepatitis do not need to be isolated, but they should be kept at home for 2 weeks following the onset of symptoms. Parents who cannot arrange to take time off from work may need to arrange home sitters to stay with the child. Offer suggestions for diversional activities during this period. Young children can be provided with a new toy or favorite activities. Older children and adolescents can be provided with board games, puzzles, books or magazines, movies, or video games. Phone calls and short visits from friends help school-age children and adolescents maintain contact with peers.

CIRRHOSIS

Cirrhosis is a degenerative disease process that results in fibrotic changes and fatty infiltration in the liver. It can occur in children of any age as the end stage of several disorders. The diffuse destruction and regeneration of the hepatic parenchymal cells result in an increase in fibrous connective tissue and disorganization of the liver structure. The balance between destruction and regeneration determines the specific clinical presentation.

Clinical manifestations of cirrhosis vary. When the disease process results from obstruction, as in biliary atresia, jaundice is an initial sign that intensifies with progression of the disease. In other diseases that cause cirrhosis, jaundice may be a late sign, intermittent, or absent. Steatorrhea is frequently present and can lead to rickets, hemorrhage, and failure to gain weight. Anemia can occur as a result of chronic blood loss from the GI tract. Pruritus is common, particularly in children with biliary malformations. Clubbing of the digits and cyanosis are other common findings. Severe end-stage complications signaling hepatic failure can occur at any time and with little warning (see Table 15–12).

Diagnostic evaluation is based on the child's history of infection or disease with liver involvement. Physical examination may reveal jaundice, skin changes, ascites, and hemodynamic changes. Laboratory evaluation reveals abnormal liver function tests. A liver biopsy may help to determine the extent of the parenchymal damage.

Medical management focuses on treating the child's symptoms and achieving optimal nutritional status and growth. Table 15–12 summarizes treatment for complications of cirrhosis. Liver transplantation is the most common treatment for biliary atresia and metabolic disorders and is the only treatment for end-stage liver disease.

15-12	Treatment for Complications of Cirrhosis

Complication	Treatment
Ascites	Restrict sodium, protein, and fluids. Administer diuretics (eg, furosemide [Lasix]). Administer intravenous albumin.
Hepatic encephalopathy	Restrict protein. Administer lactulose (to control increased ammonia levels). Administer antibiotics. Correct any imbalances that can lead to coma (fluid and electrolyte imbalance).
Hemorrhage caused by esophageal varices	Administer blood and blood products. Replace fluid and electrolytes. Administer vitamin B complex and vitamin K. Insert Sengstaken-Blakemore tube in cases of severe bleeding.

Nursing Management

Nursing care focuses on monitoring physiologic and psychosocial changes to identify early signs of end-stage hepatic failure. Monitor vital signs every 2–4 hours. Daily weight measurement is performed to assess for fluid retention. Close monitoring of electrolytes and liver function test results helps determine the need for fluid replacement therapy.

Careful administration of medications and monitoring for side effects are necessary because drug metabolism is altered in liver disorders. If ascites is present, provide a low-sodium, low-protein diet and restrict fluids. Remove all water pitchers, glasses, and straws to minimize the child's desire to drink.

Parents of a child with cirrhosis are coping with a life-threatening disorder, and their anxiety and stress are high. The child may be awaiting a liver transplantation that represents the only hope for recovery. Provide support to parents and encourage them to verbalize their fears and concerns (see Chap. 6). Encourage parents to participate in the child's care. Referral to a support group or counseling may be beneficial.

▶ INJURIES TO THE GASTROINTESTINAL SYSTEM

ABDOMINAL TRAUMA

Abdominal injuries may be caused by blunt or penetrating trauma. The kind of injury determines the extent of organ damage. Low-velocity trauma, which may occur when a child strikes the handlebars of a bicycle, usually results in single-organ injury.

High-velocity blunt trauma, which may occur in motor vehicle crashes, usually results in multiple-organ involvement. Solid organs such as the liver and spleen are more vulnerable to injury than hollow organs such as the stomach, intestines, and bladder.

Motor vehicle crashes are the most common and also the most preventable unintentional injury in children.[37] On impact, small children who are held on a parent's lap or improperly restrained in a safety seat can easily become airborne, striking objects or being thrown from the car. When older children involved in severe crashes are wearing only lap

PERITONEAL LAVAGE

During peritoneal lavage, a dialysis catheter is inserted into the abdominal cavity and normal saline or lactated Ringer's solution is instilled. The fluid is then drained and analyzed for the presence of red blood cells, amylase, and bacteria, which could indicate organ damage.

belts, injury to the hollow organs may result. Bicycles are another cause of abdominal injuries in children. Such injuries commonly occur when the child strikes the handlebars during a fall or sudden stop or is struck by a car. Child abuse is another major cause of abdominal trauma.

Suspected abdominal trauma in a child necessitates a thorough history and physical examination. The description of the event should be compared with the child's signs and symptoms. Clinical manifestations of abdominal injury include pain, abdominal distention, muscle guarding, decreased or absent bowel sounds, nausea and vomiting, hypotension, and shock.

A sonogram or a CT scan is performed to assess for internal bleeding and air in the abdomen. CT scans are also used to locate areas of internal trauma. Peritoneal lavage may be performed. Baseline laboratory studies, including blood type and cross-match, are done. A urinary catheter may be inserted to check for the presence of blood and bladder rupture.

Treatment of a liver or spleen injury takes place in the ICU and focuses on preventing or managing hemorrhage and monitoring for signs of shock. An intravenous infusion is started for fluid maintenance and to provide access for blood products. The child will be kept NPO. A nasogastric tube is inserted. Blood transfusions and pharmacologic management are used to treat blood loss. Use of analgesics is minimized to avoid masking symptoms. Serial hematocrit levels are monitored during this period. Healing of the liver and spleen usually occurs without further intervention.

Exploratory laparatomy is performed to resect hollow organ injuries or to repair liver or spleen lacerations when bleeding is not controlled. The spleen is salvaged to help maintain immune function. The child is usually discharged within 5–7 days. No strenuous activity is allowed for 6–8 weeks. The prognosis is generally good.

Nursing Management

Nursing care includes initial and ongoing assessments of the child's condition. Monitor vital signs every hour as warranted. Measurement of abdominal circumference, intake and output monitoring, serial hematocrits, and auscultation of bowel sounds are also performed hourly. Notify the physician of any changes.

The child and parents are usually fearful and anxious when the child is admitted to the hospital. If the injury was preventable, parents may have feelings of guilt or anger. Provide emotional support and avoid judgmental comments or statements that assign blame.

Once the child's condition is stabilized, the focus of nursing care shifts to preventive teaching. Parents should be taught safety measures to prevent future injuries and given written materials, when available, to use as a reference when they return home.

Discuss the use of car safety restraint devices for riding in an automobile (see Chap. 2). If the child's injury was the result of a bicycle fall or crash, discuss the importance of the proper bicycle size and teach bike safety measures such as use of a helmet and knowledge and proper use of hand signals (see Chap. 2). Have the child practice safe biking habits at a bike rodeo sponsored by a local affiliate of the National SAFE KIDS Campaign (see Appendix F).

POISONING

Poisoning is a common cause of death and injury in children between 1 and 4 years of age.[38] Young children are at risk for poisoning because of their characteristic behaviors, which involve exploration of the environment (see Chap. 2). Infants and toddlers commonly place objects in their mouths. Some household items are nontoxic and cause little harm. However, items that contain caustic agents or toxic chemicals can cause irreversible damage or death.

The Poison Prevention Packaging Act of 1970 mandates child-protective devices for all potentially toxic substances, such as household cleansers and medications. Many other items commonly found in the home are less obvious sources of toxins. The leaves, stems, or flowers of many common household and garden plants are poisonous. Examples include Boston ivy, poinsettia, philodendron, lily-of-the-valley, daffodil (bulbs), azalea, and rhododendron. Table 15–13 summarizes clinical manifestations and treatment for several commonly ingested household toxins.

15-13 Commonly Ingested Toxic Agents

Type	Sources	Clinical Manifestations	Treatment
Corrosives (strong acids and alkaline products that cause chemical burns of mucosal surfaces)	Batteries, household cleaners, Clinitest tablets, denture cleaners, bleach, toilet bowl cleaners	Severe burning pain in mouth, throat, or stomach; swelling of mucous membranes; edema of lips, tongue, and pharynx (respiratory obstruction); violent vomiting; hemoptysis; drooling; inability to clear secretions; signs of shock, anxiety, and agitation	*Do not induce vomiting!* Dilute toxin with water to prevent further damage. Give activated charcoal.
Hydrocarbons (organic compounds that contain carbon and hydrogen; most are distillates of petroleum)	Gasoline, kerosene, furniture polish, lighter fluid, paint thinners	Gagging, choking, coughing, nausea, vomiting, alteration in sensorium (lethargy), weakness, respiratory symptoms of pulmonary involvement, tachypnea, cyanosis, retractions, grunting	*Do not induce vomiting!* (Aspiration of hydrocarbons places child at high risk for pneumonia.) Use gastric lavage if severe central nervous system and respiratory impairment are present. Use of activated charcoal is controversial. Provide supportive care. Decontaminate skin by removing clothing and cleansing skin.
Acetaminophen	Many over-the-counter products	Nausea, vomiting, sweating, pallor, hepatic involvement (pain in upper right quadrant, jaundice, confusion, stupor, coagulation abnormalities)	Induce vomiting or perform gastric lavage, depending on amount ingested. Administer charcoal or NAC (concentrated form of Mucomyst), which binds with the metabolite, preventing absorption and protecting the liver.
Salicylate	Products containing aspirin	Nausea, disorientation, vomiting, dehydration, diaphoresis, hyperpnea, hyperpyrexia, bleeding tendencies, oliguria, tinnitus, convulsions, coma	Depends on amount ingested. Induce vomiting. Administer intravenous sodium bicarbonate, fluids, and vitamin K.
Mercury	Broken thermometers, chemicals, paints, pesticides, fungicides	Tremors, memory loss, insomnia, weight loss, diarrhea, anorexia, gingivitis	Similar to that for lead poisoning (see text discussion).
Iron	Multiple vitamin supplements	Vomiting, hematemesis, diarrhea, bloody stools, abdominal pain, metabolic acidosis, shock, seizures, coma	Induce vomiting. Administer intravenous fluids and sodium bicarbonate. Desferoxamine chelation therapy.

CLINICAL TIP

The acronym SIRES is a useful mnemonic device for recalling the essentials of care in cases of poisoning:
Stabilize the child's condition
Identify the toxic substance
Reverse its effect
Eliminate the substance from the child's body
Support the child physically and psychologically

Most poisonings occur in the home (see Chap. 2). Parents who suspect that their child has ingested a poison should immediately call the Poison Control Center (PCC). The PCC will advise parents whether to begin treatment at home or to bring the child to the emergency department. If the child has vomited, the vomitus should be brought to the emergency department. With older children, the possibility of intentional ingestion needs to be considered.

In the emergency department the child's vital signs and level of consciousness are assessed and specific information about the poison is obtained from the parent. The goal of treatment is to prevent further absorp-

---

15-14   Emergency Management for Poisoning

1. Stabilize the child. Assess ABCs (airway, breathing, circulation). Provide ventilatory and oxygen support.
2. Perform a rapid physical examination, start an IV infusion, draw blood for toxicology screen, and apply a cardiac monitor.
3. Obtain a history of the ingestion, including substance ingested, where child was found, by whom, position, when, how long unsupervised, history of depression or suicide, allergies, and any other medical problems.
4. Reverse or eliminate the toxic substance using the appropriate method:

Syrup of ipecac[a]
- Assess level of consciousness before administering. Recommended doses are:
  - 6–12 months: 10 mL; do not repeat
  - 1–12 years: 15 mL; may repeat one time if vomiting does not occur
  - Over 12 years: 30 mL; may repeat one time if vomiting does not occur
- Administer clear fluids, 10–20 mL/kg, after giving ipecac.

Apomorphine
- Assess level of consciousness before administering.
- Given IM or SQ; has rapid onset.
- Give plenty of oral fluids.

Gastric lavage
- Insert a gastric tube through the mouth (use the largest size possible for the size of the child).
- Instill and aspirate normal saline solution until the return is clear. Considered a less effective method of removing ingested substances from the stomach than vomiting. Reserved for children with central nervous system depression, diminished or absent gag reflex, or unwillingness to cooperate with other measures.
- *Contraindicated* in children who have ingested alkaline corrosive substances, since insertion of the tube might cause esophageal perforation. Used in children who have ingested acids to decrease continued damage and potential perforation of stomach and intestines.

Activated charcoal
- Given to absorb and remove any remaining particles of toxic substances.
- Give a commercial preparation of activated charcoal orally or through a gastric tube. It is available as a ready-to-drink solution in an opaque container. Use a covered cup and straw when giving orally, to prevent the child from seeing the black liquid and to minimize spillage. Give activated charcoal only after the child has stopped vomiting, since aspiration of charcoal is damaging to lung tissue.

Cathartics
- Hasten excretion of a toxic substance and minimize absorption. The most commonly used cathartic is magnesium sulfate.

Antidotes and antagonists
There are a few of these agents. The most common is Narcan, for opiate ingestion.
5. Other measures will depend on the child's condition, the nature of the ingested substance, and the time since ingestion. May include diuresis, fluid loading, cooling or warming measures, anticonvulsive measures, antiarrhythmic therapy, hemodialysis, or exchange transfusions.
6. Remember always to treat the child first, not the poison. Maintain airway, breathing, and circulation.

---

[a]The use of ipecac is no longer widely promoted, especially in the emergency department. Activated charcoal is considered by many to be more effective in the treatment of poisoning.

tion of the poison and to reverse or eliminate its effects. Table 15–14 summarizes emergency management for poisoning.

Nursing Management

Once immediate care has been provided, the focus of nursing care shifts to providing emotional support and preventing recurrence.

Provide Emotional Support

Wait until the child is out of immediate danger before questioning parents in detail about the incident. Encourage parents to express feelings of anger, guilt, or fear about the incident.

Prevent Recurrence

Discuss with parents the need to supervise infants and young children at all times. Ask parents how medicines and cleaning agents are stored and whether the house contains any plants. Teach parents proper methods of childproofing the home. Instruct parents to keep two bottles of syrup of ipecac available for each child in the home and to be familiar with its use and proper dosage. Suggest the following measures for preventing recurrence:

- Put PCC phone number by every phone in the house.
- Place household cleaners, medications, vitamins, and other potentially poisonous substances out of the reach of children or in locked cabinets. Use warning stickers such as Mr. Yuk on all containers.
- Buy products with childproof caps.
- Store products in their original containers. *Never* place household cleansers or other products in food or beverage containers.
- Remove all house plants from the child's play areas.
- Use caution when visiting other settings that are not childproofed (eg, grandparents' homes). Remember that visitors may have pills in their purses or pockets that are easily accessible.

Lead Poisoning

Lead poisoning has been successfully prevented in many areas of the United States, with a substantial decline in lead levels from the mid 1970s. The average serum lead level for children is now 0.6 μg/dL, down from 15 μg/dL in 1976. There are still about 1.7 million children with elevated lead levels, a large proportion of whom are poor, African-American, and living in inner cities.[39] Lead in paint is the most common source of lead exposure for preschool children. Children are also exposed to lead when they ingest contaminated food, water, and soil or when they inhale dust contaminated with lead. Table 15–15 summarizes several sources of lead exposure.

Children are at greater risk for lead poisoning because they absorb and retain more lead in proportion to their weight than adults do. Lead is particularly harmful to children under the age of 7 years.

Lead interferes with normal cell function, primarily of the nervous system, blood cells, and kidneys, and adversely affects the metabolism of vitamin D and calcium. Clinical manifestations depend on the degree of toxicity (Table 15–16). Neurologic effects include decreased IQ scores, cognitive deficits, impaired hearing, and growth delays. Impaired mental function can occur with blood levels as low as 10 μg/dL. Lead ingestion by a woman during pregnancy can result in fetal malformations, reduced birth weight,

15-15	Sources of Lead Exposure

Lead-based paint

Soil and dust

Drinking water from coolers with lead-soldered or lead-lined tanks, from lead-soldered teapots, or from lead pipes or lead-soldered pipes

Food grown in contaminated soil, stored in lead-soldered cans or leaded crystal, or prepared in improperly fired pottery

Parental occupations and hobbies that involve exposure to lead (eg, plumbing, battery manufacture, highway construction, furniture refinishing, stained glass work, pottery-making)

Airborne lead in areas surrounding smelters and battery-manufacturing plants

and premature birth. Severe lead poisoning, which can result in encephalopathy, coma, and death, is now rare.

Once in the body, lead accumulates in the blood, soft tissues (kidney, bone marrow, liver, and brain), bones, and teeth. Lead that is absorbed by the bones and teeth is released slowly. Thus exposure to even small doses, over time, can result in dangerously high levels of lead in the body.

Although both the Centers for Disease Control and Prevention (CDC) and the American Academy of Pediatrics had previous recommended universal screening for all children, the decrease in incidence of elevated lead levels has led to reexamination of these guidelines. The CDC now recom-

15-16	Clinical Manifestations of Lead Poisoning		
Mild Toxicity (10–15 µg/dL)	**Moderate Toxicity (25–69 µg/dL)**	**Severe Toxicity (>70 µg/dL)**
Myalgia or paresthesia	Arthralgia	Paresis or paralysis
Mild fatigue	General fatigue	Encephalopathy (may lead abruptly to seizures, changes in consciousness, coma, and death)
Irritability	Difficulty concentrating	Lead line (blue-black) on gingival tissue
Lethargy		
Occasional abdominal discomfort	Muscular exhaustibility	Colic (intermittent, severe abdominal cramps)
	Tremor	
	Headache	
	Diffuse abdominal pain	
	Vomiting	
	Weight loss	
	Constipation	
	Anemia	

Adapted from Agency for Toxic Substances and Disease Registry. (1990). Lead toxicity. Case studies in environmental medicine (p. 11). Atlanta: Author.

mends screening children at high risk with reduced screening for those at low risk.[40, 41] A blood lead (Pb-B) level is the most useful screening and diagnostic test for lead exposure.

A Pb-B below 10 µg/dL is considered acceptable. An environmental history should be obtained for children with Pb-B levels between 10 and 19 µg/dL to identify removable sources of lead. Follow-up testing is required. Children with Pb-B levels between 20 and 69 µg/dL require a full medical evaluation, including a detailed environmental and behavioral history, physical examination, and tests for iron deficiency. Interventions to remove sources of lead from the child's environment are necessary. For levels above 25 µg/dL, chelation therapy is also administered. Children with Pb-B levels greater than 70 µg/dL are critically ill from lead poisoning and require immediate chelation therapy and interventions to provide a lead-free environment.

Chelation therapy involves the administration of an agent that binds with lead, increasing its rate of excretion from the body. Calcium disodium ethylenediamine tetraacetate (CaNa$_2$ EDTA), dimercaprol (BAL), D-penicillamine, or succimer (DMSA) may be used. Children with Pb-B levels between 25 and 69 µg/dL receive CaNa$_2$ EDTA for 5–7 days, followed by a rest period and then a second chelation treatment. Children with Pb-B levels greater than 70 µg/dL are given both BAL and CaNa$_2$ EDTA, followed by a rest period and a second chelation treatment using CaNa$_2$ EDTA alone. Long-term follow-up of children receiving chelation therapy is essential. The child should never be discharged unless a lead-free home environment has been ensured.

Nursing Management

Nursing care centers on screening, education, and follow-up. Nurses often work with state and local health officials to plan screening for children at high risk of lead exposure. Ask parents about the child's development and eating habits and be alert for risk of lead exposure. Educate parents about sources of lead in the environment and techniques to reduce exposure. Emphasize the importance of housekeeping interventions to reduce exposure to lead dust. These interventions include damp mopping of hard surfaces, floors, window sills, and baseboards; washing the child's hands and face before meals; and frequent washing of toys and pacifiers.

Teach parents the importance of including foods high in iron and calcium in the child's diet to counteract losses of these minerals associated with lead exposure. The child should eat meals at regular intervals, since lead is absorbed more readily on an empty stomach.

Be sure that parents understand the importance of follow-up testing of lead levels. If the child is developmentally delayed, refer the family to an infant stimulation or child development program. Referral to social services and either a visiting nurse or home health care nurse may also be appropriate.

CULTURAL CONSIDERATIONS

Traditional medicines and cosmetics may contain large amounts of lead. Examples include *azarcon* and *greta*, preparations that are used by Mexican-Americans to treat *empacho*, a coliclike illness; *chifong tokuwan*, *payloo-ah*, *ghasard*, *bali goli*, and *kandu*, used by some Asian communities; and *alkohl*, *kohl*, *surma*, *saoott*, and *cebagin*, used by some Middle Eastern communities.[42]

REFERENCES

1. Wetmore, R.F., & Willging, J.P. (1996). The oral cavity and oropharynx. In A.M. Rudolph, J.I.E. Hoffman, & C.D. Rudolph (Eds.), *Rudolph's pediatrics* (20th ed., pp. 949–969). Stamford, CT: Appleton & Lange.

2. Shaw, G.M., Lammer, E.J., Wasserman, C.R., O'Malley, C.D., & Tolarova, M.M. (1995). Risks of orofacial clefts in children born to women using multivitamins containing folic acid periconceptually. *Lancet, 346,* 393–396.

3. Dillon, P.W., & Cilley, R.E. (1993). Newborn surgical emergencies. *Pediatric Clinics of North America, 40*(6), 1289–1314.

4. Rudolph, C.D. (1996). Infantile hypertrophic pyloric stenosis. In A.M. Rudolph, J.I.E. Hoffman, & C.D.

Rudolph (Eds.), *Rudolph's pediatrics* (20th ed., p. 1068). Stamford, CT: Appleton & Lange.

5. Henderson, D.P. (1994). Nontraumatic surgical emergencies: Why won't Roberto stop vomiting? *Journal of Emergency Nursing, 20*(6), 575–582.

6. Berube, M. (1997). Gastroesophageal reflux. *Journal of the Society of Pediatric Nurses, 2*(1), 43–46.

7. Hebra, A., & Hoffman, M.A. (1993). Gastroesophageal reflux in children. *Pediatric Clinics of North America, 40*(6), 1233–1252.

8. Parrish, R.S., & Berube, M.C. (1995). Care of the infant with gastroesophageal reflux and respiratory disease: After the Nissen fundoplication. *Journal of Pediatric Health Care, 9*(5), 211–217.

9. Stevenson, R.J. (1996). Intussusception. In A.M. Rudolph, J.I.E. Hoffman, & C.D. Rudolph (Eds.), *Rudolph's pediatrics* (20th ed., pp. 1071–1072). Stamford, CT: Appleton & Lange.

10. Milla, P.J. (1996). Intestinal motility during ontogeny and intestinal pseudo-obstruction in children. *Pediatric Clinics of North America, 43*(2), 511–532.

11. Milla, P.J. (1996). Hirschsprung disease and other neuropathies. In A.M. Rudolph, J.I.E. Hoffman, & C.D. Rudolph (Eds.), *Rudolph's pediatrics* (20th ed., pp. 1115–1118). Stamford, CT: Appleton & Lange.

12. Loening-Baucke, V. (1996). Encopresis and soiling. *Pediatric Clinics of North America, 43*(1), 279–298.

13. Branski, D., Lerner, A., & Lebenthal, E. (1996). Chronic diarrhea and malabsorption. *Pediatric Clinics of North America, 43*(2), 307–332.

14. Greenholz, S.K. (1996). Congenital diaphragmatic hernia: An overivew. *Seminars in Pediatric Surgery, 5*(4), 216–223.

15 Rodriguez, M., Kanto, W.P., Howell, C.G., & Bhatia, J. (1996). Early diagnosis of diaphragmatic hernia and survival: A time for reappraisal? *Neonatal Intensive Care, 9*(2), 42–46.

16. Scherer, L.R., & Grosfeld, J.L. (1993). Inguinal hernia and umbilical anomalies. *Pediatric Clinics of North America, 40*(6), 1121–1132.

17. Stevenson, R.J. (1996). Appendicitis. In A.M. Rudolph, J.I.E. Hoffman, & C.D. Rudolph (Eds.), *Rudolph's pediatrics* (20th ed., pp 1105–1107). Stamford, CT: Appleton & Lange.

18. Neu, J. (1996). Necrotizing enterocolitis: The search for a unifying pathogenic theory leading to prevention. *Pediatric Clinics of North America, 43*(2), 409–432.

19. Simon, N.P. (1994). Follow-up for infants with necrotizing enterocolitis. *Clinics in Perinatology, 21*(2), 411–424.

20. Sondheimer, J.M. (1997). Gastroesophageal reflux and chalasia. In W.W. Hay, J.R. Groothius, A.R. Hayward, & M.J. Levin (Eds.), *Current pediatric diagnosis and treatment* (13th ed., pp. 537–567). Stamford, CT: Appleton & Lange.

21. Hyams, J.S. (1996). Crohn's disease in children. *Pediatric Clinics of North America, 43*(1), 255–278.

22. Seidman, E.J. (1996). Chronic inflammatory bowel diseases. In A.M. Rudolph, J.I.E. Hoffman, & C.D. Rudolph (Eds.), *Rudolph's pediatrics* (20th ed., pp. 1092–1100). Stamford, CT: Appleton & Lange.

23. Kirschner, B.S. (1996). Ulcerative colitits in children. *Pediatric Clinics of North America, 43*(1), 235–254.

24. Preud'Homme, D.L., & Mezoff, A.G. (1996). *Helicobactor pylori*: A pathogen for all ages. *Contemporary Pediatrics, 13*(11), 27–28, 31, 34, 39–40, 43, 46, 49.

25. Bujanover, Y., Reif, S., & Yahav, J. (1996). *Helicobacter pylori* and peptic disease in the pediatric patient. *Pediatric Clinics of North America, 43*(1), 213–234.

26. Garvin, G. (1994). Caring for children with ostomies. *Nursing Clinics of North America, 29*(4), 645–654.

27. Merrick, N., Davidson, B., & Fox, S. (1996). Treatment of acute gastroenteritis: Too much and too little care. *Clinical Pediatrics, 35*(9), 429–435.

28. Hellman, M.G. (1995). When a child's stomach hurts. *Emergency Medicine, 27*(8), 52–54, 56–62, 64, 69–70, 72.

29. Young, R.J. (1996). Pediatric constipation. *Gastroenterology Nursing, 19*(3), 88–95.

30. Kerr, E.C. (1995). Celiac disease in childhood. *Gastroenterology Nursing, 18*(2), 67–70.

31. Troncone, R., Greco, L., & Auricchio, S. (1996). Gluten-sensitive enteropathy. *Pediatric Clinics of North America, 43*(2), 355–374.

32. Huff, C. (1997). Celiac disease: Helping families adapt. *Gastroenterology Nursing, 20*(3), 79–81.

33. Collins, J.B., Georgeson, K.E., Vicente, Y., Kelly, D.R., & Figueroa, R. (1995). Short bowel syndrome. *Seminars in Pediatric Surgery, 4*(1), 60–73.

34. Bucuvalas, J.C., & Balistreri, W.F. (1996). The liver and bile ducts. In A.M. Rudolph, J.I.E. Hoffman, & C.D. Rudolph (Eds.), *Rudolph's pediatrics* (20th ed., pp. 1123–1166). Stamford, CT: Appleton & Lange.

35. Whitington, P.F. (1996). Chronic cholestasis of infancy. *Pediatric Clinics of North America, 43*(1), 1–26.

36. Fishman, L.N., Jonas, M.M., & Lavine, J.E. (1996). Update on viral hepatitis in children. *Pediatric Clinics of North America, 43*(1), 57–74.

37. National Safety Council (1997). *Accident facts.* Itasca, IL: Author.

38. Fingerhut, L.A., & Warner, M. (1997). *Injury chartbook. Health, United States, 1996–97.* Hyattsville, MD: National Center for Health Statistics.

39. Maternal and Child Health Bureau. (1996). *Child health USA '95.* Washington, DC: US Department of Health and Human Services.

40. Centers for Disease Control (1997). *Screening young children for lead poisoning: Guidance for state and local public health officials.* Atlanta: Author

41. Harvey, B. (1997). New lead screening guideline from the Centers for Disease Control and Prevention: How will they affect pediatricians? *Pediatrics, 100*(3), 384–388.

42. Agency for Toxic Substances and Disease Registry. (1990). *Lead toxicity. Case studies in environmental medicine.* Atlanta: Author.

ADDITIONAL RESOURCES

Armentrout, D. (1995). Gastroesophageal reflux in infants. *Nurse Practitioner, 20*(5), 54–63.

Barber, C., & Masiello, M. (1996). Oral rehydration therapy. *Topics in Emergency Medicine, 18*(3), 21–26.

Bauman, N.M., Sandler, A.D., & Smith, R.J.H. (1996). Respiratory manifestations of gastroesophageal relux disease in pediatric patients. *Annals of Otolarygology, Rhinology, and Laryngology, 105*, 23–32.

Blank, E., & Frantzides, C.T. (1995). Methods of assessing motility of the digestive system in children. *Seminars in Pediatric Surgery, 4*(1), 3–9.

Denk, M.J., & Magee, W.P. (1996). Cleft palate closure in the neonate: Preliminary report. *Cleft Palate-Craniofacial Journal, 33*(1), 57–66.

Fisher, R.S., & Krevsky, B. (1993). *Motor disorders of the gastrointestinal tract: What's new and what to do.* New York: Academy Professional Information Services, Inc.

Food Allergy Network. (1996). Food allergy network announces availability of comprehensive school food allergy program. *School Nurse News, 13*(1), 1, 3, 5.

Fox, D., & Bignall, S. (1996). Management of gastroesophageal reflux. *Paediatric Nursing, 8*(1), 17–20.

Kelley, S.J. (1994). *Pediatric emergency nursing* (2nd ed.). Stamford, CT: Appleton & Lange.

Khoshoo, V., Reifen, R., Neuman, M., Griffiths, A., & Pencharz, P.B. (1996). Effect of low- and high-fat, peptide-based diet on body composition and disease activity in adolescents with active Crohn's disease. *Journal of Parenteral and Enteral Nutrition, 20*(6), 401–405.

Kilgallen, I., & Gibney, M.J. (1996). Parental perception of food allergy or intolerance in children under 4 years of age. *Journal of Human Nutrition and Dietetics, 9*, 473–478.

Markowitz, J.F. (1996). Inflammatory bowel disease: The pediatrician's role. *Contemporary Pediatrics, 13*(5), 25–27, 30–32, 34, 42–43, 45–46.

Nordeman, L., & Hamilton, R. (1996). Dehydration and gastroenteritis. *Topics in Emergency Medicine, 18*(3), 11–20.

Putnam, P.E. (1997). Gastroesophageal reflux disease and dysphagia in children. *Seminars in Speech and Language, 18*(1), 25–37.

Reid, S.R., & Bonadio, W.A. (1996). Outpatient rapid intravenous rehydration to correct dehydration and resolve vomiting in children with acute gastroenteritis. *Annals of Emergency Medicine, 28*(3), 318–323.

Smitherman, C.H. (1996). Child and caretaker attributes associated with lead poisoning in young children. *Pediatric Nursing, 22*(4), 320–326.

Sullivan, G. (1996). Parental bonding in cleft lip and palate repair. *Paediatric Nursing, 8*(1), 21–24.

Vanderhoof, J.A. (1996). Short bowel syndrome in children and small intestinal transplantation. *Pediatric Clinics of North America, 43*(2), 530–550.

Walker, W., Durie, P., Hamilton, J., Walker-Smith, J., & Watkins, J. (1996). *Pediatric gastrointestinal disease: Pathophysiology, diagnosis, management* (2nd ed.). St. Louis: Mosby–Year Book.

Weintrub, P.S. (1996). Viral hepatitis. In A.M. Rudolph, J.I.E. Hoffman, & C.D. Rudolph (Eds.), *Rudolph's pediatrics* (20th ed., pp. 647–651). Stamford, CT: Appleton & Lange.

Whelan, E.A., Piacitelli, G.M., Gerwel, B., Schnorr, T.M., Mueller, C.A., Gittleman, J., & Matte, T.D. (1997). Elevated blood lead levels in children of construction workers. *American Journal of Public Health, 87*(8), 1352–1355.

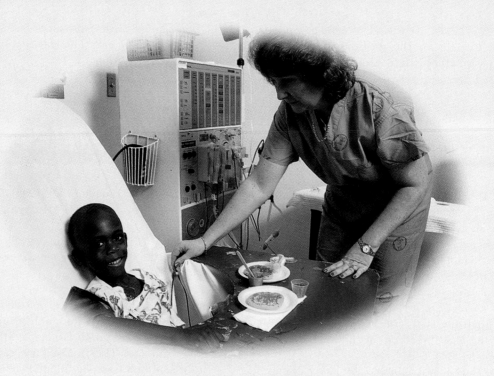

Terrell, who is now 5 years old, was born with posterior urethral valves, which caused damage to his kidneys. Despite undergoing surgery to correct the defect at 2 years of age, his kidney function continued to deteriorate. End-stage renal disease was diagnosed 2 years ago, and dialysis treatment was started 3 months later. Terrell is waiting for a kidney transplant, but no family member is able or willing to donate a kidney. As a result, Terrell has been placed on the list for a cadaver kidney.

Terrell was initially treated with peritoneal dialysis, but after having several peritoneal infections in the first year, his health care team and family decided that hemodialysis should become his recommended treatment. He comes to the dialysis center three afternoons a week for treatments that last about 3 to 4 hours. This schedule permits him to go to kindergarten classes in the morning.

What are the special concerns of the nurse in monitoring a child who is receiving hemodialysis treatment? Is Terrell at any higher risk for infection than other children? Does he need a special diet? What are the potential complications of this disease and of the hemodialysis treatments for Terrell's growth and development? If a kidney becomes available for transplant, what special teaching will the family need to receive to assure the best survival of the kidney graft? The answer to these questions and information about many other genitourinary conditions are presented in this chapter.

ALTERATIONS IN GENITOURINARY FUNCTION

16

"Providing care to children like Terrell is challenging, because the treatment often interferes with a child's regular activities. We all hope that Terrell receives a kidney transplant soon so his growth will improve and he will not have to continue to miss school during treatment."

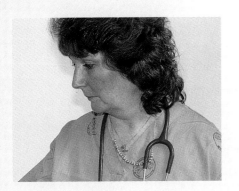

TERMINOLOGY

- **azotemia** Accumulation of nitrogenous wastes in the blood.
- **dialysate** The solution used in dialysis.
- **end-stage renal disease** Irreversible kidney failure.
- **enuresis** Involuntary micturition by a child who has reached the age at which bladder control is expected.
- **hydronephrosis** Collection of urine in the renal pelvis as a result of obstructed outflow.
- **oliguria** Diminished urine output (less than 0.5–1 mL/kg/hr).
- **osteodystrophy** Defective mineralization of bone caused by renal failure and chronic hyperphosphatemia.
- **renal insufficiency** Any degree of renal failure in which the kidneys' ability to conserve sodium and concentrate the urine decreases.
- **stent** A device used to maintain patency of the urethral canal after surgery.
- **uremia** Toxicity resulting from the buildup of urea and nitrogenous waste in the blood.
- **vesicoureteral reflux** The backflow of urine from the bladder into the ureters during voiding.

What are the consequences of urinary and renal disorders such as **end-stage renal disease,** or irreversible kidney failure, in children? What specific and nonspecific signs alert parents and health care professionals to suspect these disorders?

Many infections, structural disorders, and disease processes alter genitourinary function. Because the kidneys and other urinary system organs perform several essential body functions, including removal of waste products and maintenance of fluid and electrolyte balance, disorders that affect these organs pose a significant threat to the health of children.

Although the reproductive system is functionally immature until puberty, disorders involving these organs may also have a significant impact on the health of children. Uncorrected structural defects and sexually transmitted diseases can have both psychologic and physiologic implications on the developing child.

▶ ANATOMY AND PHYSIOLOGY OF PEDIATRIC DIFFERENCES

The genitourinary system is made up of the urinary and reproductive organs. The urinary system—kidneys, ureters, bladder, and urethra (Fig. 16–1)—functions to excrete wastes and maintain fluid and electrolyte balance. The reproductive system consists of internal and external organs that at maturity function to promote the conception and healthy development of a fetus.

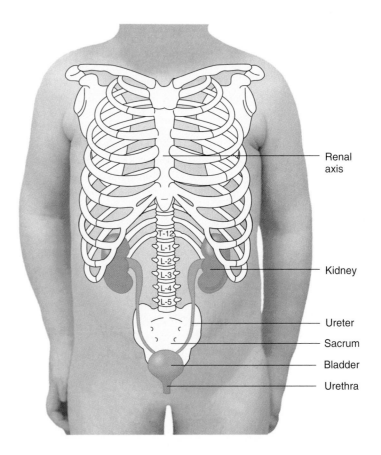

Renal axis

T-12
L-1
L-2
L-3
L-4
L-5

Kidney

Ureter

Sacrum

Bladder

Urethra

FIGURE 16–1. The kidneys are located between the twelfth thoracic (T12) and third lumbar (L3) vertebrae.

URINARY SYSTEM

All of the nephrons that will make up the mature kidney are present at birth. The kidneys grow and the tubular system matures gradually during childhood, reaching full size by adolescence. Most renal growth occurs during the first 5 years of life. This increase in size is due primarily to enlargement of the nephrons. The efficiency of the kidney also increases with age. During the first 2 years of life, the kidneys are less efficient at regulating electrolyte and acid–base balance (refer to Chap. 8) and eliminating some drugs from the body. After the age of 2 years, the kidneys' efficiency increases markedly. Because the kidney is less able to concentrate urine in infancy, urine output per kilogram of body weight is higher in infancy than in later childhood or adolescence.

Bladder capacity increases with age from 20–50 mL at birth to 700 mL in adulthood. Stimulation of "stretch receptors" within the bladder wall initiates urination. Simultaneous contraction of the bladder and relaxation of the internal and external sphincters result in emptying of the bladder. Children less than 2 years of age cannot maintain bladder control because of insufficient nerve development.

The shortness of the urethra in children may contribute to the incidence of urinary tract infection because bacteria ascend the urethra more readily than in adults.

REPRODUCTIVE SYSTEM

The reproductive system in children is functionally immature until puberty. Throughout childhood the genitalia (with the exception of the clitoris in girls) enlarge gradually. Anatomic and functional development accelerates with the hormonal changes of puberty (see Figs. 3–40 and 3–41). In girls, the mons pubis becomes more prominent and hair begins to grow. The vagina lengthens, and the epithelial layers thicken. The uterus and ovaries enlarge, and the musculature and vascularization of the uterus also increase. In boys, downy hair begins to appear at the base of the penis, and the scrotum becomes increasingly pendulous. The penis increases in length and width.

► STRUCTURAL DEFECTS OF THE URINARY SYSTEM

BLADDER EXSTROPHY

Bladder exstrophy is a rare defect in which the posterior bladder wall extrudes through the lower abdominal wall (Fig. 16–2). Failure of the abdominal wall to close during fetal development results in eversion and protuberance of the bladder wall and a wide separation of the symphysis pubis. The upper urinary tract is usually normal. The defect occurs in approximately 1 in every 30,000 live births and is more common in boys than girls by a ratio of 6 to 1.[1] The bladder mucosa appears as a mass of bright red tissue, and urine continually leaks from an open urethra. Females have a bifid clitoris. Males have a short, stubby penis, and the glans is flattened with dorsal chordee and a ventral prepuce. Epispadias and bilateral inguinal hernias are also common.

Treatment is surgical reconstruction, which is performed in several stages. The initial stage (bladder closure) is usually completed within 48

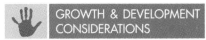

GROWTH & DEVELOPMENT CONSIDERATIONS

Urinary output per kilogram of body weight decreases as the child ages because the kidney becomes more efficient at concentrating urine. Expected output:

Infants	2 mL/kg/hr
Children	0.5–1 mL/kg/hr
Adolescents	40–80 mL/hr

CLINICAL TIP

A child's bladder capacity (in ounces) can be estimated by adding 2 to the child's age. For example, the normal bladder capacity of a 4-year-old is 6 ounces.

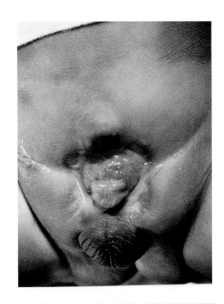

FIGURE 16–2. This child has bladder exstrophy, noted by extrusion of the posterior bladder wall through the lower abdominal wall.

hours after birth. Epispadias repair is usually begun when the infant is 9 months of age. Reconstruction of the bladder neck and ureteral reimplantation is performed when the child is 2–3 years of age. The goals of surgical reconstruction are (1) bladder and abdominal wall closure; (2) urinary continence, with preservation of renal function; and (3) creation of functional and normal-appearing genitalia. Some children require permanent urinary diversion because a functional bladder cannot be reconstructed. In some patients with a very small penis, gender reassignment may be considered.

Because the bladder epithelium is abnormal, it is prone to neoplasms. Yearly cystoscopy after the age of 20 years is recommended to evaluate for possible malignancies.[2]

Nursing Management

Preoperative nursing care centers on preventing infection and trauma to the exposed bladder. The bladder mucosa is covered in sterile plastic wrap to prevent trauma and irritation, and the surrounding area is cleaned daily and protected from leaking urine with a skin sealant.

Postoperatively the wound and pelvis are immobilized to facilitate healing. External immobilization is achieved by use of modified Bryant traction (see Chap. 19). Abduction of the infant's legs should be avoided. Nursing care includes maintaining proper alignment, monitoring peripheral circulation, and providing meticulous skin care.

Renal function is monitored by assessing the adequacy of urine output and blood and urine chemistries. Observe for any signs of obstruction in the drainage tubes such as increased intensity of bladder spasms, decreased urine output, or urine or blood draining from the urethral meatus.

Parents need emotional support to help them cope with the disfiguring nature of the infant's defect and the uncertainty of complete repair. To promote parent–infant bonding, encourage parents to participate in all aspects of the infant's care, including bathing, feeding, and wound care. Discharge teaching should include instructions about dressing changes and diapering and the need to immediately report any signs of infection or change in renal function. Emphasize the need for routine follow-up visits after surgery to assess urinary function and to ensure that the next stages of surgery are performed at the appropriate time and age in the child's development.

HYPOSPADIAS AND EPISPADIAS

Hypospadias and epispadias are congenital anomalies involving the location of the urethral meatus in males (Fig. 16–3). Both defects result from failure of the urethral folds to fuse completely over the urethral groove.

The most recent reported incidence of hypospadias is 8 in every 1000 male births, nearly double that of earlier rates.[3] The increased incidence is thought to be associated with better identification of cases and improved reporting. The urethral meatus can be located anywhere along the course of the anterior urethra on the ventral surface of the penile shaft, from the perineum to the tip of the glans. Most cases are mild, with the meatus slightly off center from the tip of the penis; in severe cases, the meatus is located on the scrotum. Hypospadias often occurs in conjunction with congenital chordee, a fibrous line of tissue that results in ventral curvature of the penile shaft.

In epispadias the meatal opening is located on the dorsal surface of the penile shaft. Epispadias often occurs in conjunction with exstrophy of the bladder.

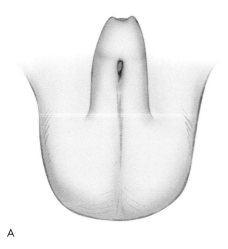
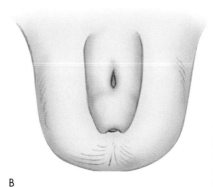

A   B

FIGURE 16–3. A, In hypospadias the urethral canal is open on the ventral surface of the penis. B, In epispadias the canal is open on the dorsal surface.

Diagnosis is made at birth. The infant should not be circumcised because the dorsal foreskin tissue will be used for surgical repair. The defects are corrected surgically, usually during the first year of life, to minimize psychologic effects when the child is older. Surgery may be performed in a single operation or as a multistage procedure. The goals of surgical repair are (1) placement of the urethral meatus at the end of the glans penis with satisfactory caliber and configuration for a urinary stream (enabling the child to void in a standing position) and (2) release of chordee to straighten the penis (enabling future sexual function).

Analgesics and muscle relaxants may be prescribed to relieve any postoperative pain.

Nursing Management

It is important for the nurse to address parents' concerns at the time of birth. Preoperative teaching can relieve some of their anxiety about the future appearance and functioning of the penis.

Postoperative care focuses on protecting the surgical site from injury (Fig. 16–4). The infant or child returns from surgery with the penis wrapped in a pressure dressing and a urethral **stent** (a device used to maintain patency of the urethral canal) in place to keep the new urethral canal open. Use of arm and leg restraints prevents inadvertent removal of the stent.

Encourage fluid intake to maintain adequate urinary output and patency of the stent. Accurate documentation of intake and output is essential. Notify the physician if there is no urine drainage for 1 hour as this may indicate kinks in the system or obstruction by sediment. Pain may be associated with bladder spasms. Anticholinergic medications such as oxybutynin or hyoscyamine may be prescribed. Acetaminophen may also be given for pain. Antibiotics are often prescribed until the urinary stent falls out.

Patients are often discharged within 1 day of surgery. Discharge teaching should include instructions for parents about care of the reconstructed area, fluid intake, medication administration, and signs and symptoms of infection (Table 16–1). Inform parents of the need to go to the physician's office for dressing removal about 4 days after surgery.

OBSTRUCTIVE UROPATHY

Obstructive uropathy refers to structural or functional abnormalities of the urinary system that interfere with urine flow. The pressure caused by urine

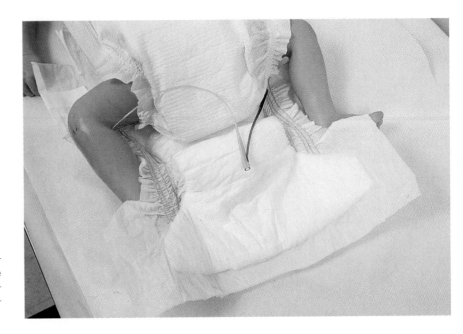

FIGURE 16–4. A double diapering technique protects the urinary stent after surgery for hypospadias or epispadias repair. The inner diaper collects stool; the outer diaper, urine.

backup compromises kidney function and often causes **hydronephrosis** (accumulation of urine in the renal pelvis as a result of obstructed outflow). Physiologic changes that may occur as a result of hydronephrosis include:

- Cessation of glomerular filtration when the pressure in the kidney pelvis equals the filtration pressure in the glomerular capillaries. In response, the blood pressure increases as the body attempts to increase the glomerular filtration pressure.
- Metabolic acidosis, which results when the distal nephrons are impaired in their ability to secrete hydrogen ions.
- Impairment of the kidney's ability to concentrate urine, resulting in polydipsia and polyuria.
- Obstruction resulting in urinary stasis, which promotes the growth of bacteria.

16-1   Parent Teaching: Hypospadias and Epispadias Repair

- Use the double-diapering technique, shown in Figure 16–4, to protect the stent (the small tube that drains the urine).
- Restrict the infant or toddler from activities (eg, playing on riding toys) that put pressure on the surgical site. Avoid holding the infant or child straddled on the hip. Limit the child's activity for 2 weeks.
- Encourage the infant or toddler to drink fluids to ensure adequate hydration. Provide fluids in a pleasant environment or using a special cup. Offer fruit juice, fruit-flavored ice pops, fruit-flavored juices, flavored ice cubes, and gelatin.
- Be sure to give the complete course of prescribed antibiotics to avoid infection.
- Watch for signs of infection: fever, swelling, redness, pain, strong-smelling urine, or change in flow of the urinary stream.
- The urine will be blood tinged for several days. Call the physician if urine is seen leaking from any area other than the penis.

- Restriction of urinary outflow, which causes progressive renal damage if left untreated. As a consequence, the growth of the kidneys may be arrested, or renal failure may occur.

Obstructive uropathy may be caused by several congenital lesions such as ureteropelvic junction (UPJ) obstruction, posterior urethral valves (PUVs), and stenosis at the ureterovesicular junction (Fig. 16–5). The ureteropelvic junction is the most common site of obstruction of the upper urinary tract in infants and children. Posterior urethral valves (abnormal folds of mucosa in the male urethra) are the most common cause of anatomic bladder outlet obstruction, occurring in approximately 1 in 5000 –8000 live male births. Other conditions that can lead to hydronephrosis include myelomeningocele, neoplasms, and prune-belly syndrome. Clinical manifestations vary, depending on the cause and location of the obstruction (Table 16–2).

PRUNE-BELLY SYNDROME

Prune-belly syndrome, also known as Eagle–Barrett syndrome, is a congenital defect characterized by failure of the abdominal musculature to develop. The skin covering the abdominal wall is thin and resembles a wrinkled prune. Other characteristics include urinary tract anomalies, poor ureteral peristalsis, enlarged bladder, high risk for recurrent urinary tract infection, and bilateral cryptorchidism. Prune-belly syndrome occurs predominantly in males (95%), with an incidence of 1 in 29,000–40,000 births.[4]

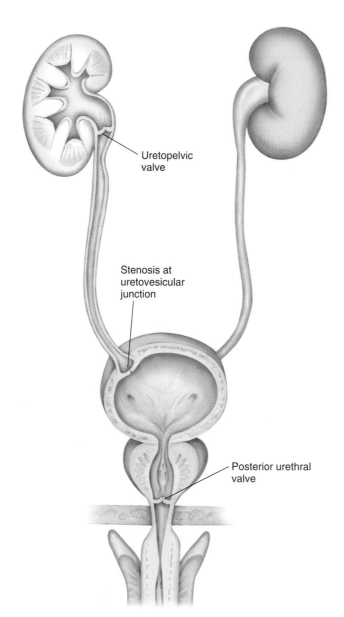

Uretopelvic valve

Stenosis at uretovesicular junction

Posterior urethral valve

FIGURE 16–5. The common sites of obstruction in the upper and lower urinary tract. Why would damage from posterior urethral valves potentially be worse than other obstructions? Upper urinary tract obstructions are often unilateral. Renal failure is most likely to occur when both kidneys are affected by hydronephrosis.

16-2	Clinical Manifestations of Obstructive Lesions of the Urinary System		
Ureteropelvic Junction Obstruction	**Posterior Urethral Valves**	**Ureterovesicular Junction Obstruction**	
In Infants Abdominal mass (enlarged kidney) Hypertension Urinary tract infection **In Children** Hematuria Pain Intermittent nausea and vomiting	**In Infants** Abdominal mass (enlarged kidney) Distended bladder Poor urinary stream Urinary tract infection, sepsis Renal concentration defect (low specific gravity, polyuria) Increased creatinine level Failure to thrive **In Children** Diurnal frequency and incontinence	Urinary tract infection, (recurrent or chronic) Hematuria Pain Abdominal mass (enlarged ureter) Enuresis	

Early diagnosis and treatment are necessary to prevent kidney damage and deterioration of renal function. Hydronephrosis may be detected by prenatal ultrasound, but milder obstructions may not become apparent until later in infancy or childhood. Table 16–3 lists diagnostic tests commonly used to identify obstructive lesions.

The goals of surgical correction or diversion are to lower the pressure within the collecting system, which prevents parenchymal damage, and to prevent stasis, which decreases the risk of infection. Surgical correction may necessitate pyeloplasty (removal of an obstructed segment of the ureter and reimplantation into the renal pelvis) or valve repair or reconstruction, depending on the cause of the obstruction. Urinary incontinence resulting from sphincter weakness is a common problem after surgery.

16-3	Diagnostic Tests for Obstructive Lesions of the Urinary System	
Test	**Use**	
Voiding cystourethrogram	Shows bladder structure and function, and detects reflux	
Renal ultrasound	Identifies scarring, masses, and hydronephrosis	
Diuretic renogram	Identifies lesions that become symptomatic during increased urine flow	
Radionucleotide scan	Differentiates hydronephrosis caused from obstructive lesions from that caused by reflux or a cyst	
Serum creatinine	Evaluates kidney function	

Nursing Management

Preoperative nursing care focuses on preparing the parents and child for the procedure and addressing parents' concerns about the postsurgical outcome. Provide parents with an opportunity to discuss concerns about the effect of the disorder on the child's long-term renal functioning.

Postoperative care involves monitoring vital signs and intake and output and observing for signs of urine retention, such as decreased output and bladder distention. Many children are discharged with stents or catheters. Teach parents how to change dressings, care for catheters, and recognize signs of possible obstruction or infection. Parents should encourage the child to participate in age-appropriate activities. However, contact sports should be avoided because of their potential to injure the bladder.

► URINARY TRACT INFECTION

A urinary tract infection (UTI) is an infection of bacterial, viral, or fungal origin that occurs in the urinary tract. Cystitis is a lower UTI that involves the urethra or bladder. Pyelonephritis is an upper UTI that involves the ureters, renal pelvis, and renal parenchyma. UTIs can be acute or chronic (the latter either recurrent or persistent).

UTIs are the second most common infections in children. What accounts for the high incidence of these infections? Among newborns most infections occur in boys. These infections are usually associated with structural defects having a higher incidence in males (eg, obstructive uropathy), which predispose the infant to infection. Among older infants and children, the incidence of UTIs is higher in girls. This is attributed to the shorter female urethra (2 cm [1 in.] in young girls) and its proximity to the anus and vagina, which increases the risk of contamination by fecal bacteria. The incidence of UTI is also increased in teenage girls who are sexually active.

Clinical Manifestations

Symptoms depend not only on the location of the infection, but also on the age of the child (Table 16–4). Symptoms in the newborn period tend to be nonspecific. Not until the toddler years are the more "classic" symptoms of

16-4	**Clinical Manifestations of Urinary Tract Infection**

Infants	Older Children (Over 2 Years of Age)
Unexplained fever	Fever
Failure to thrive	Poor appetite
Poor feeding	Dysuria
Nausea and vomiting	Urgency or hesitancy
Lethargy	Frequency
Strong-smelling urine	Enuresis or new-onset incontinence
Renal tenderness	Abdominal tenderness or lower abdominal pain
	Hematuria
	Strong-smelling urine

lower urinary tract infection—urinary frequency, dysuria, urgency, and enuresis—observed. Complicated upper urinary tract infections are characterized by high fever, abdominal pain, flank pain, persistent vomiting, and moderate to severe dehydration. About 40% of UTIs are asymptomatic.[5]

Etiology and Pathophysiology

Many first UTIs are caused by *Escherichia coli,* a common gram-negative enteric bacterium. Other causative organisms include *Staphylococcus, Klebsiella, Proteus, Pseudomonas, Enterobacter,* and *Enterococcus.*

Urinary stasis enhances the risk of UTI. Stasis may be caused by abnormal anatomic structures or abnormal function (eg, neurogenic bladder, common in children with myelomeningocele). Infrequent voiding, which is common in school-age children, also increases the risk of UTI. Children normally void four to six times a day. Some children, however, develop the habit of urinating only once or twice a day, which results in incomplete emptying of the bladder and urinary stasis.

Another cause of UTI is **vesicoureteral reflux,** the backflow of urine from the bladder into the ureters during voiding. This creates a reservoir for bacterial growth. Vesicoureteral reflux can also result from a structural anomaly in which the ureters insert in an abnormal position into the bladder.

Renal scarring and hypertension often result from vesicoureteral reflux and recurrent UTIs. The risk of kidney damage increases in the following instances:

- Children less than 1 year of age
- Delay in initiating effective antibacterial treatment for an upper UTI
- Anatomic or neurologic obstruction
- Recurrent episodes of upper UTIs

Diagnostic Tests and Medical Management

A urine specimen is examined for the presence of bacteria. A dipstick leukocyte esterase test is useful for screening, having a sensitivity and specificity rate of 80%.[6] Urine collected by midstream clean-catch void, sterile catheterization, or suprapubic aspiration is sent for culture and sensitivity to identify the specific organism and determine its sensitivity to antibiotics. Urine collection bags used on infants are reliable only when no pathogens are found. The diagnosis of infection is made from the number of colony-forming units (at least 50,000/mL) for most methods of urine collection.[7]

Radiologic studies reveal structural abnormalities in approximately 1%–2% of girls and 10% of boys with UTIs.[8] A renal ultrasound is often obtained soon after the diagnosis, and a voiding cystourethrogram (VCUG) is obtained about 3–6 weeks after the infection has cleared. These are the most commonly performed tests. Renal cortical scintigraphy and radionuclide cystography may sometimes be substituted for the renal ultrasound and VCUG.[9]

Antibiotic therapy is initiated as soon as urine samples have been collected. Sulfisoxazole, trimethoprim, or a second- or third-generation cephalosporin is commonly prescribed for uncomplicated infection. Once the culture sensitivity information is obtained, the antibiotic is changed if necessary. Follow-up cultures should be obtained 48–72 hours after drug therapy has started, at which time the urine should be sterile. Follow-up urine cultures should then be obtained monthly for 3 months, every 3 months for 6 months, and then annually.[5] Subsequent infections may be asymptomatic. For children with recurrent infections, a long-term, suppressive dose of an antibiotic may be ordered for prophylaxis.

Children with complicated UTIs are often hospitalized because of the need for rehydration, initiation of parenteral antibiotic treatment, and assessment for structural defects. Infants may develop permanent kidney damage or generalized sepsis if the UTI is not treated aggressively. If a structural defect is identified, surgical correction may be necessary to prevent recurrent infections that could lead to renal damage.

Nursing Assessment

Physiologic Assessment

A history of urinary symptoms is obtained. Assess the infant for toxic (very ill) appearance, fever, and oral fluid intake. Measure the child's height and weight and plot on a growth curve to identify any change in growth pattern associated with a chronic illness. Take the infant's or child's blood pressure. Palpate the abdomen and suprapubic and costovertebral areas for masses, tenderness, and distention. Observe the urinary stream if possible and perform a urinalysis, including specific gravity. Proper collection of the urine specimen is essential. A clean-catch urine specimen may be obtained if the child is able to cooperate. (Refer to the *Quick Reference to Pediatric Clinical Skills* accompanying this text.) If not, a catheterized sample is obtained. An early morning urine specimen is preferred because the urine is more concentrated. A blood culture may be obtained to assess for sepsis.

Psychosocial Assessment

Sexually active adolescents may deny having symptoms because they fear disclosure of their sexual activity to their parents. Careful questioning may be necessary to elicit these concerns. Be open and approachable and allow the patient and family the opportunity to address their concerns. See informed consent in *Quick Reference to Pediatric Clinical Skills*.

Nursing Diagnosis

Common nursing diagnoses for the child with a UTI include:

- Altered Urinary Elimination related to dysuria and recurrent infections
- Pain related to infection
- Altered Growth and Development related to chronic infection and renal damage
- Urinary Retention related to infrequent voiding habits
- Risk for Ineffective Management of Therapeutic Regimen related to lack of knowledge of preventive measures (adequate fluid intake, proper hygiene, signs and symptoms of recurrence)
- Risk for Fluid Volume Deficit related to fever and inadequate intake
- Knowledge Deficit (Parent) related to lack of information about diagnostic procedures and management

Nursing Management

Nursing care for the hospitalized child with a complicated UTI centers on administering prescribed medications, promoting rehydration, assessing renal function, and teaching parents and older children how to minimize the risk of future infection (see Table 16–5).

16-5	Discharge Teaching: Preventive Strategies for Urinary Tract Infections

- Teach proper perineal hygiene. Girls should always wipe the perineum from front to back after voiding.
- Encourage the child to drink plenty of fluids and avoid long periods of "holding urine."
- Caution against tight underwear; children should wear cotton rather than nylon underwear.
- Encourage the child to void more frequently and to fully empty the bladder.
- Discourage bubble baths and hot tubs, which can irritate the urethra.
- Instruct sexually active adolescent girls to void before and after sexual intercourse to prevent urinary stasis and flush out bacteria introduced during intercourse.

Administer antibiotics and antipyretics as prescribed to maintain therapeutic drug levels and reduce fever. Encourage fluid intake to dilute the urine and flush the bladder. Document intake and output. Assess renal function by comparing the child's output to the expected measure of 1 mL/kg/hr and weigh the child daily.

Frequent voiding minimizes urinary stasis. Postvoid catheterization may be needed to determine the amount of residual urine left after urinating. Palpate or percuss the bladder after voiding to evaluate bladder emptying.

Because bladder training is such an important milestone for young children, any disorder that affects voiding may have developmental implications. A toddler who has been potty trained may regress and require diapers temporarily due to incontinence related to the UTI. Reassure parents that this is normal and emphasize that they should offer the toddler support rather than disapproval. A preschooler may perceive the infection as punishment for an imagined wrong such as masturbation. Provide support and reassurance that the child is not being punished for any actions.

Care in the Community

Teach prevention through proper hygiene, especially for girls, reinforcing the importance of (1) avoiding bubble baths, (2) wearing cotton underwear, (3) avoiding tight-fitting pants, and (4) always wiping the perineum from front to back after bowel movements.

Children with UTIs are usually cared for at home. Teach parents the importance of giving antibiotics as prescribed and assist them to develop an effective schedule. Emphasize that antibiotics must be taken for the full course and that they may be continued even after the infection has cleared to prevent a recurrence.

Give parents specific guidelines for oral fluid intake. Ensure that the amount of fluids recommended for a 24–hour period equals the maintenance fluids needed plus additional fluids required because of fever and diuresis to flush out pathogens. Suggest that the parents avoid giving the child caffeinated and carbonated beverages as these may potentially irritate the bladder mucosa.[5]

Encourage the child to void more frequently even after the infection has cleared. A wristwatch with an alarm may be a helpful reminder. The child with a neurogenic bladder needs to have clean intermittent catheterization performed several times a day to reduce urinary stasis and the po-

CLINICAL TIP

Studies have documented that cranberry juice inhibits bacterial adherence to the bladder wall and alters urine pH, decreasing the risk of infection.[10]

16-6   Home Care Teaching: Clean Intermittent Catheterization

Clean intermittent catheterization (CIC) is performed to empty the bladder when nerves for bladder control are missing or damaged. This procedure must be performed every 3–4 hours during the day, but is usually not done when the child sleeps at night. The child is ready to learn self-catheterization when he or she really wants to be dry and is learning independence. Until that time, the parents usually perform CIC.

Equipment Needed
- Four or five catheters of the size and type recommended. Each catheter is used until it becomes hard and brittle (about 1 month).
- Water-soluble lubricant (not Vaseline)

How Performed
- Usually clean technique is used. Wash hands with soap and water, then spread lubricant on the tip of the catheter. Hold the catheter like a pencil in one hand, about 3 in. (8 cm) from the tip. Position the other end of the catheter over the toilet or a container.

Girls
- Spread the labia with the other hand and slide the catheter 2–3 in. (5–8 cm) into the urethra until urine begins to flow, then 1 in. (2.5 cm) further (up to 3 in. [8 cm], maximum).
- Hold the catheter in place until all urine flows out, then slowly remove it. If more urine begins to flow, let it drain before removing the catheter.

Boys
- Hold the penis outward with the other hand and slide the catheter into the penis until urine begins to flow, and then 1 in. (2.5 cm) further (up to 5–6 in. [12–15 cm], maximum). A sphincter muscle is located at the opening to the bladder, and it sometimes feels very tight. If the catheter will not slide into the bladder easily, use constant but gentle pressure on the sphincter muscle with the tip of the catheter. It will soon feel the pressure and gradually open up, allowing the catheter to slip in.
- Hold the catheter in place until all urine flows out, then slowly remove it. If more urine begins to flow, let it drain before removing the catheter.

Storage
- Wash the catheter with soap and water and shake excess water out of it. Store the catheter in a plastic bag after use.
- Keep a catheter in the car, bookbag, fanny pack, or at school. (The catheter can be carried to school in a toothbrush holder to avoid embarrassment.)

Adapted from Ball, J.B. (1998). Mosby's pediatric patient teaching guides. St. Louis: Mosby.

tential for UTI. Table 16–6 provides guidelines for teaching this procedure to families and children.

Teach parents the signs and symptoms of recurrent infection (see Table 16–4).

► ENURESIS

Enuresis is involuntary micturition by a child who has reached an age at which bladder control is expected, usually about 4–5 years of age. (See Table 16–7 for bladder control milestones.) Enuresis can occur either at night (nocturnal, 50% of cases), during the day (diurnal, 10% of cases), or

16-7	Milestones in the Development of Bladder Control

Age	Developmental Milestone
1½ years	Child passes urine at regular intervals.
2 years	Child announces when he or she is voiding.
2½ years	Child makes known need to void; can hold urine.
3 years	Child goes to the bathroom by himself or herself; holds urge if preoccupied with play.
2½–3½ years	Child achieves nighttime control.
4 years	Child shows great interest in going to bathrooms when away from home (shopping centers, movies).
5 years	Child voids approximately 7 times a day; prefers privacy; is able to initiate emptying of bladder at any degree of fullness.

16-8	Types of Enuresis

Primary enuresis: Child has never had a dry night; attributed to maturational delay and small functional bladder; not associated with stress or psychiatric cause.

Intermittent enuresis: Child has occasional nights or periods of dryness.

Secondary enuresis: Bedwetting that occurs in a child who has been reliably dry for 6–12 months; associated with stress, infections, and sleep disorders.

CLINICAL TIP

Enuretic children often have a history of constipation. Rectal pressure on the posterior bladder wall stimulates the bladder to empty.

both night and day (40% of cases).[11] Nocturnal enuresis occurs more often in boys than in girls, with 3.5:1 ratio, whereas diurnal enuresis is more common in girls. Three types of enuresis are distinguished: primary, intermittent, and secondary (Table 16–8).

Enuresis may result from neurologic or congenital structural disorders, illness, or stress. Nocturnal enuresis occurs with high frequency in children whose parents have a history of bedwetting.[11] In most children with primary enuresis, the bladder has a smaller functional capacity, and neuromuscular maturation of the inhibitory fibers is delayed. Minor abnormalities of the bladder neck and urethra are also associated with enuresis. Some children are believed to have mild developmental delays. Often children with nocturnal enuresis are harder to arouse and may fail to respond to bladder signals. The majority of cases (95%) are not associated with structural or neurologic pathology.

Diabetes mellitus or renal insufficiency should be ruled out in children with both enuresis and polyuria or oliguria. Examine the child's lower spine for fistulas or tufts of hair that could be signs of occult spina bifida. Prolonged hospitalization, family stressors, and preoccupation with school concerns also have been associated with secondary enuresis. Children with diurnal enuresis may have frequency, urgency, constant dribbling, and involuntary loss of control after voiding.

A thorough history can help identify potential causes of enuresis (Table 16–9). Asking about the child's elimination patterns and developmental milestones and the parents' methods of toilet training can provide essential information (see Table 2–19). Laboratory evaluation includes urinalysis and urine culture.

A multitreatment approach is usually most effective. Fluid restriction, bladder training, and enuresis alarms are common approaches (Table 16–10). A spontaneous cure rate occurs in 15% of children each year, regardless of intervention used or lack of intervention. Approximately one third of children with nocturnal enuresis are treated with medications. Imipramine, a tricyclic antidepressant, is often used but requires close monitoring because of its effects on mood and sleep-arousal patterns. Desmopressin, given as a nasal spray, has an antidiuretic effect but is not used long term because of its expense. Its use is usually reserved for times when the

16-9 | Questions to Ask When Taking an Enuresis History

Family History
Is there a family history of renal or urinary structural abnormalities?
Is there a family history of bedwetting?

Family Management
How serious is the problem for the family?
What happens when the child wets? (Who gets up and changes sheets?)
How is the child treated? Is the child punished or blamed for wetting?
What remedies have been tried?

Toilet Training
Did the child have a difficult time with toilet training?
What method of toilet training was used? When was toilet training initiated?
What are the child's current voiding and stooling patterns?
How long is the child's longest dry period, and when does it occur?
Does the child have a history of constipation or encopresis?

Stressors
How is the child doing in school?
Are any new or chronic stressors present in the child's life?
How does the problem interfere with play and other activities?

Risk Factors
Diabetes
- Does the child void often or have urgency?
- Is the child frequently thirsty?

Urinary Tract Infection
- Does the child experience burning on urination?
- Has the child had a urinary tract infection before?

16-10 | Treatment Approaches for Enuresis

Approach	Description
Fluid restriction	Fluid intake is limited in the evening and before the child goes to bed.
Bladder exercises	The child drinks a large amount and then holds urine as long as he or she can. The child practices stopping voiding midstream. Exercises should continue for at least 6 months.
Timed voiding	The child with diurnal enuresis is instructed to void every 2 hours and to use a double voiding pattern; this trains the bladder to empty completely and avoid overdistention.
Enuresis alarms	A detector strip is attached to the child's pants. The alarm sounds a buzzer that alerts the child when wetting occurs, so the child can get up and finish voiding in the bathroom.
Reward system	Set realistic goals for the child and reinforce dry days or nights with stars and stickers on a chart.
Medications	Desmopressin is prescribed for special situations in cases of nocturnal enuresis; oxybutynin for diurnal enuresis to relieve urgency and frequency from bladder irritability.

child is away from home for a short period (eg, sleepovers or camp). Relapse often occurs when medications are stopped. Avoidance of foods believed to contribute to enuresis may be recommended (eg, carbonated and caffeinated beverages, milk products, citrus products, sweets, vitamin C, and beverages colored with artificial dyes).[12]

Nursing Management

Enuresis is managed as an outpatient problem. Teach the child and parents about the causes and treatment of enuresis, and explore feelings of guilt or blame. Make sure the parents are aware that the child cannot control the wetting. Psychosocial support is an essential part of care since stress is an important cause of secondary enuresis. Provide emotional support to the parents and child, and encourage the child's participation in the treatment plan. Refer the child for counseling or therapy if appropriate.

Assess the parents' and child's motivation and readiness for interventions. Before parents purchase an enuresis alarm, suggest they use an alarm clock in the child's room for several nights to see if the child will arouse. Determine whether the child shares a room with others who will be disturbed by the alarm. Ask if the child and parents are willing to persist with an enuresis alarm, as the treatment may take months and the rate of success is only about 70–80%.[13]

▶ RENAL DISORDERS

NEPHROTIC SYNDROME

Nephrotic syndrome refers, not to a specific disease, but rather to a clinical state characterized by edema, massive proteinuria, hypoalbuminemia, hyperlipidemia, and altered immunity. Nephrotic syndrome is classified as congenital, primary, or secondary. Congenital nephrotic syndrome, an autosomal recessive disorder, is extremely rare. Primary nephrotic syndrome results from a disease, such as glomerulonephritis, that affects only the kidney. Secondary nephrotic syndrome results from a disease, such as diabetes, lupus, or sickle cell anemia, with multisystem effects.

Approximately 80% of children with nephrotic syndrome have a type of primary disease called minimal change nephrotic syndrome (MCNS). MCNS usually occurs in children between the ages of 2 and 7 years, with an incidence of 3 per 100,000 children,[14] and is approximately twice as common in boys as in girls.[15] MCNS derives its name from the fact that the glomeruli appear normal or show only minimal changes on light microscopic evaluation. Because MCNS is the most common form of nephrotic syndrome, it is the focus of the following discussion.

Clinical Manifestations

In most children, edema develops gradually over several weeks. Children may have a history of periorbital edema on waking that resolves during the day as fluid shifts to the abdomen and lower extremities. Other signs include hypertension, irritability, anorexia, and nonspecific malaise.[14] The child's urine may be frothy or foamy. Medical treatment often is not sought until generalized edema develops on the child's extremities, abdomen, or genitals (Fig. 16–6). Respiratory distress from pleural effusion may occur in some cases.

CLINICAL TIP

The following signs may indicate that a child has MCNS:
- Weight gain greater than expected in relation to previous pattern
- Snug fit of clothing, tight-fitting shoes
- Extreme skin pallor
- Irritability and fatigue
- Decreased urine output

Massive edema resulting in a dramatic weight gain and abdominal pain, with or without vomiting, may occur, depending on the amount of albumin lost and the amount of sodium ingested. The child becomes malnourished as a result of protein loss in the urine. The skin is pale and shiny with prominent veins, and the hair quality becomes more brittle.

Etiology and Pathophysiology

What accounts for the dramatic symptoms of altered renal functioning in children with nephrotic syndrome? Why do proteinuria, hypoalbuminemia, hyperlipidemia, and altered immunity develop in these children?

The cause of primary MCNS is unknown, and its pathophysiology is not completely understood. Normally, only a minute amount of protein is present in the urine. In MCNS, however, increased permeability of the glomerular membrane permits large, negatively charged molecules such as albumin to pass through the membrane and be excreted in the urine. Proteinuria results in decreased oncotic pressure and the development of edema, because fluid remains in the interstitial spaces instead of being pulled back into the vascular compartment. Loss of protein in the urine, as well as insufficient albumin production by the liver and a decreased albumin concentration as a result of salt and water retention by the kidney (see below) contribute to the development of hypoalbuminemia.

Because the kidney reabsorbs salt and water, edema develops. Immunoglobulins are lost, resulting in altered immunity. The liver, stimulated perhaps by hypoalbuminemia or decreased osmotic pressure, responds by increasing synthesis of lipoprotein (cholesterol), resulting in hyperlipidemia.

Diagnostic Tests and Medical Management

Diagnosis is based on the history, physical examination, presence of characteristic symptoms, and laboratory findings. Serum albumin and other blood studies may be ordered. Edema begins to develop in children when the serum albumin concentration falls below 27 g/L.[15] Urinalysis reveals massive proteinuria (50 mg/kg/day), the primary indicator of nephrotic syndrome. Microscopic hematuria may also be present. The serum creatinine or BUN are increased in some cases.

Children are often hospitalized initially, but the majority of treatment occurs on an outpatient basis. Medical management focuses on decreasing proteinuria, relieving edema, managing associated symptoms, improving nutrition, and preventing infection. Corticosteroids (such as prednisone), the drugs of choice, are prescribed to decrease proteinuria. In most children, urine protein levels fall to trace or negative values within 10–15 days of the start of corticosteroid therapy. Children who respond successfully to therapy continue to take corticosteroids daily for several weeks. The drug dosage is then gradually decreased and discontinued over a 4–6-month period.[16]

Approximately 85% of children experience complete remission with corticosteroid therapy. A relapse is commonly associated with a respiratory infection or immunizations; however, relapses become less frequent or stop during puberty.[14] Repeat therapy is administered to children who have a relapse after drug therapy is discontinued. Alkylating agents such as chlorambucil and cyclophosphamide have been effective in children with frequently recurring nephrotic syndrome, but they have serious side effects, including carcinogenesis and sterility in males. If steroid therapy is ineffective, a renal biopsy is performed to identify other causes for the child's symptoms.

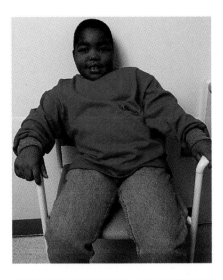

FIGURE 16–6. This boy has generalized edema, a characteristic finding in nephrotic syndrome.

To reduce massive edema, intravenous administration of albumin or oral diuretics may be ordered. Since diuretics can precipitate hypovolemia, hyponatremia, and hypokalemia, electrolyte levels should be carefully monitored. Broad-spectrum antibiotics are prescribed to treat any infections.

A diet that is normal for the child's age is recommended. No attempt should be made either to restrict or to increase protein intake. A "no added salt" diet is recommended during corticosteroid treatment.

Nursing Assessment

Physiologic Assessment

Careful assessment of the child's hydration status and edema is essential. Monitor intake and output and vital signs and record these findings accurately. Perform a careful assessment for respiratory distress associated with pleural effusion (see Chap. 11). Test urine for proteinuria and specific gravity at least once each shift.

Psychosocial Assessment

Children and parents are often fearful or anxious on admission. Because edema often develops gradually, parents may feel guilty if they did not seek medical attention immediately. School-age children with generalized edema are often concerned about their appearance. Careful questioning may be necessary to elicit these concerns. The child who is hospitalized for a recurrence of nephrotic syndrome may be frustrated or depressed. Assess individual and family coping mechanisms, support systems, and level of stress.

Nursing Diagnosis

Common nursing diagnoses for the child with MCNS include:

- Risk for Infection related to increased susceptibility and lowered resistance secondary to corticosteroid therapy
- Risk for Impaired Skin Integrity related to edema, lowered resistance to infection and injury, immobility, and malnutrition
- Fluid Volume Excess related to sodium and water retention
- Altered Nutrition: Less Than Body Requirements related to anorexia and protein loss in urine
- Fatigue related to fluid and electrolyte imbalance, albumin loss, altered nutrition, and renal failure
- Risk for Altered Family Processes related to child's hospitalization
- Knowledge Deficit (Parent) related to potential recurrence with infections and immunizations

Nursing Management

Nursing care is mainly supportive and focuses on administering medications, preventing infection, preventing skin breakdown, meeting nutritional and fluid needs, promoting rest, and providing emotional support to the parents and child.

Administer Medications

It is important to give prescribed medications at the scheduled times. Watch for side effects of corticosteroids such as moon face, increased appetite, increased hair growth, abdominal distention, and mood swings. If the child is receiving albumin intravenously, monitor closely for hypertension or signs of volume overload caused by fluid shifts. If diuretics are used, observe for shock. The child may need to have albumin infused simultaneously with diuretics.

Prevent Infection

Children with MCNS are at risk for infection because of the loss of immunoglobulins in the urine, other alterations of the immune system associated with renal failure, and corticosteroid therapy. Careful handwashing is important. Use standard precautions. Strict aseptic technique is essential during invasive procedures. Monitor vital signs carefully to detect early signs of infection that may be masked by corticosteroid therapy. Decrease the child's social contacts during immunosuppressive treatment, and caution parents and children to avoid exposure to individuals with respiratory infections and communicable diseases. Emphasize the importance of avoiding shopping malls, sporting arenas, grocery stores, game stores, and other public areas where the risk of exposure to such infections is increased.

Prevent Skin Breakdown

Meticulous skin care is essential to prevent skin breakdown and potential infection. Perform repeated skin assessments, turn the child frequently, and use therapeutic mattresses (eg, egg crate, airflow) to help prevent skin breakdown. Keep the skin clean and dry.

Meet Nutritional and Fluid Needs

Keep the child's food preferences in mind when planning menus. Encourage the child to eat by presenting attractive meals with small portions. Mealtimes should center on pleasurable socialization. Encourage the child to eat meals with other children on the unit. Fluids are not usually restricted.

Carefully monitor intake and output. Weigh the child daily using the same scale, and measure abdominal girth to monitor changes in edema and ascites (see Fig. 8–12). Monitor vital signs every 4 hours to watch for signs of respiratory distress, hypertension, or circulatory overload.

Promote Rest

Provide opportunities for quiet play as tolerated, such as drawing, playing board games, listening to tapes, and watching videos. Adjust the child's daily schedule to allow rest periods after activities. Signs of fatigue may include irritability, mood swings, or withdrawal. Inform the parents and child about the importance of rest. Limiting visitors during the acute phase of the illness may be necessary. Telephone contacts may be encouraged as an alternative to visitors. To provide a sense of control, encourage the child to set his or her own limits on activity.

Provide Emotional Support

Parents and children often need support to cope with this chronic disease. Provide parents with thorough explanations about the child's disease and treatment regimen. Parental anxiety in combination with the hospitalization may interfere with the child's independence. Assist parents to promote the child's independence by allowing the child to select food from the menu or to select the daily activity schedule. This gives the child some sense of control.

Children with MCNS may have a distorted body image because of sudden weight gain and edema. Behavioral manifestations may include refusal to look in the mirror, refusal to participate in care, and decreased interest

NURSING ALERT

Traditionally, a high-protein, low-salt diet was recommended for children with MCNS. Current data, however, suggest that the high-protein diet increases urinary protein loss and may accelerate the development of renal failure. On the other hand, low-protein diets may lead to protein deficiency. For these reasons, a regular-protein, low-salt diet is currently recommended.

in appearance. Encourage children to express their feelings. Help them maintain a normal appearance by promoting normal grooming routines. Encourage children to wear their own pajamas rather than hospital gowns. Scarves or hats may be used to lessen the child's edematous appearance.

Discharge Planning and Home Care Teaching

Home care needs should be identified and addressed well in advance of discharge. Provide parents and school-age children with explanations of the disease process, prognosis, and treatment plan. Ensure that parents know how to administer medications and can identify potential side effects. Instruct parents about the need to monitor urine daily for protein, and have them keep a diary to record results. Monitoring the child's weight each week may help identify early stages of fluid retention. This helps parents to identify signs of a relapse before edema occurs.

Tutoring may be required for a short period after discharge. However, parents should be encouraged to allow the child to return to normal activities once the acute episode has resolved. Emphasize the importance of avoiding contact with individuals who have infectious diseases, because of the child's reduced immunity. Reinforce to parents that as long as the child is receiving corticosteroid therapy or shows signs of MCNS, the "no added salt" diet should be followed. Immunizations should be withheld until 6 months after the completion of corticosteroid therapy. Although immunizations may trigger a relapse, pneumococcal vaccine and other immunizations are important to protect the child from serious preventable infections.

RENAL FAILURE

Renal failure occurs when the kidney is unable to excrete wastes and concentrate urine. There are two types of renal failure: acute and chronic. Acute renal failure occurs suddenly (over days or weeks), whereas in chronic renal failure, kidney function diminishes gradually over months or years.

Both types of renal failure are characterized by **azotemia** (accumulation of nitrogenous wastes in the blood) and sometimes **oliguria** (urine output less than 0.5–1 mL/kg/hr). The degree of renal impairment is estimated by the degree of azotemia and the increase in serum creatinine level. **Uremia** occurs when there is an excess of urea and other nitrogenous waste products in the blood.

Acute Renal Failure

Acute renal failure (ARF), which occurs when kidney function abruptly diminishes, is characterized by a rapid rise in the BUN level. The kidneys are also unable to regulate extracellular fluid volume, sodium balance, and acid–base homeostasis. ARF occurs most frequently in neonates who are critically ill with asphyxia, shock, and sepsis. It can also be a postoperative complication of cardiac surgery or may result from drug toxicity.[1]

Clinical Manifestations

Characteristically, a healthy child suddenly becomes ill with nonspecific symptoms, including nausea, vomiting, lethargy, edema, gross hematuria, and hypertension (see Table 16–11).[17] These symptoms are a result of electrolyte imbalances (Table 16–12), uremia, and fluid overload. The child appears pale and lethargic.

CLINICAL TIP

Normal renal function requires the following:
- Unimpaired renal blood flow
- Adequate glomerular ultrafiltration
- Normal tubular function
- Unobstructed urine flow

GROWTH & DEVELOPMENT CONSIDERATIONS

The following factors increase the risk of acute renal failure:

Newborn
- Critically ill neonate
- Obstructive uropathy
- Dehydration
- Hemolytic-uremic syndrome

Toddler
- Accidental poisoning (eg, acetaminophen, mushrooms)

School-age Child and Adolescent
- Trauma

16-11 Clinical Manifestations of Acute Versus Chronic Renal Failure

Acute Renal Failure	Chronic Renal Failure
Gross hematuria	Fatigue, malaise
Headache	Poor appetite
Edema	Prolonged, unexplained nausea and vomiting
Severe hypertension	Failure to thrive
Lethargy	Poor school performance
Nausea and vomiting	Complicated enuresis
	Chronic anemia
	Hypertension
	Unusual bone disease—fractures with minimal trauma, rickets, valgus deformity

From Vogt, B.A. (1997). Identifying kidney disease: Simple steps can make a difference. Contemporary Pediatrics, 14(3), 115–119.[17]

16-12 Clinical Manifestations and Causes of Electrolyte Imbalances in Acute Renal Failure

Clinical Manifestations	Cause
Hyperkalemia • Peaked T waves, widening of QRS on ECG • Arrhythmias: ventricular arrhythmias, heart block, ventricular fibrillation, cardiac arrest • Diarrhea • Muscle weakness	Results from inability to adequately excrete potassium derived from diet and catabolized cells. In metabolic acidosis, there is also movement of potassium from intracellular fluid to extracellular fluid.
Hyponatremia • Change in level of consciousness • Muscle cramps • Anorexia • Abdominal reflexes, depressed deep tendon reflexes • Cheyne–Stokes respirations • Seizures	In the acute oliguric phase, hyponatremia is related to the accumulation of fluid in excess of solute.
Hypocalcemia • Muscle tingling • Change in muscle tone • Seizures • Muscle cramps and twitching • Positive Chvostek sign (contraction of facial muscles after tapping facial nerve just anterior to parotid gland)	Phosphate retention (hyperphosphatemia) depresses the serum calcium concentration. Calcium is deposited in injured cells. Hyperkalemia and metabolic acidosis may mask the common clinical manifestations of severe hypocalcemia.

Data from Chan, J.C.M., Alon, U., & Oken, D.E. (1992). Acute renal failure. In C.M. Edelman, Jr. (Ed.), Pediatric kidney disease (2nd ed., pp. 1923–1940). Boston: Little, Brown.

Hyperkalemia is the most life-threatening electrolyte disorder associated with ARF. An increase in serum potassium adversely affects the electrical conductivity within the heart. Hyponatremia affects central nervous system function, resulting in symptoms that range from fatigue to seizures. Edema occurs as a result of sodium and water retention. (Refer to Chapter 8 for a discussion of these fluid and electrolyte alterations.) Children with ARF are also more susceptible to infection because of depressed immune functioning.

Etiology and Pathophysiology

ARF may be caused by prerenal, postrenal, or intrinsic factors. Prerenal ARF is a result of decreased perfusion to an otherwise normal kidney in association with a systemic condition. Hypovolemia (hemorrhage or dehydration), septic shock, or cardiac failure may precipitate prerenal ARF. This is the most common type of ARF in infants and young children.

Intrinsic ARF results from primary damage to the parenchymal cells of the kidneys. Damage can be caused by infection, diseases such as hemolytic-uremic syndrome or acute glomerulonephritis, cortical necrosis, nephrotoxic drugs, or accidental ingestion of drugs or poisons. The structure most susceptible to damage is the kidney tubule. Injury to the tubule resulting in acute tubular necrosis is the most frequent cause of intrinsic renal failure in children.

Postrenal ARF is caused by obstruction of the urinary flow from both kidneys, such as occurs in posterior urethral valves or a neurogenic bladder. Children may have oliguria, or normal or increased urine output. Renal failure without oliguria usually indicates a less severe renal injury. Children who recover from ARF may have residual kidney damage and compromised renal function.

NEPHROTOXIC DRUGS

- Antimicrobials: aminoglycosides, cephalosporins, tetracycline, sulfonamides
- Radiographic contrast media with iodine
- Heavy metals: lead, barium, iron
- Nonsteroidal anti-inflammatory drugs: indomethacin, aspirin

---

16-13 Diagnostic Tests for Renal Failure

Test	Normal Values	Findings in ARF
Urinalysis		
pH	4.5–8.0	Lowered
Osmolarity	50–1400 mosm/L	> 500 prerenal
		< 350 intrinsic
Specific gravity	1.001–1.030	High: prerenal ARF
		Low: intrinsic ARF
		Normal: postrenal ARF
Protein	Negative	Positive
Blood Chemistry		
Potassium	3.5–5.8 mmol/L	Elevated
Sodium	135–148 mmol/L	Normal, low, or high, depends solely on the amount of water in the body
Calcium	2.2–2.7 mmol/L	Low
Phosphorus	1.23–2.0 mmol/L	High
Urea nitrogen	3.5–7.1 mmol/L	Increased
Creatinine	0.2–0.9 mmol/L	Increased
pH	7.38–7.42	Low acidic

ARF, acute renal failure.

Diagnostic Tests and Medical Management

Diagnosis of renal failure is based primarily on urinalysis and blood chemistry results, including BUN, serum creatinine, sodium, potassium, and calcium levels (Table 16–13). The kidneys are normal in size and no signs of osteodystrophy are found on x-ray. Various imaging studies to assess kidney size, renal blood flow, and renal perfusion and function may be performed to determine whether the child has ARF or chronic renal failure.

Treatment depends on the underlying cause of the renal failure. The goal of treatment is to minimize or prevent permanent renal damage while maintaining fluid and electrolyte balance and managing complications (Table 16–14). Eliminate all potential sources of potassium intake until hyperkalemia is controlled (see Chap. 8). Initial emergency treatment of children with fluid depletion focuses on fluid replacement at 20 mL/kg of saline or lactated Ringer's solution given rapidly or over 5–10 minutes to ensure renal perfusion. Albumin may also be administered when blood loss is the cause of circulatory depletion. If oliguria persists after restoration of adequate fluid volume, intrinsic renal damage is suspected. Children with fluid overload, like those with pulmonary edema, need diuretic therapy or dialysis.

Fluid requirements are calculated to maintain zero water balance. Intake should equal output. Nutrition must be maintained with extra carbohydrate intake during the catabolic state. Antibiotics are prescribed for infection. Nephrotoxic antibiotics such as aminoglycosides are avoided.

Some children whose ARF is unresponsive to management require dialysis to correct electrolyte imbalances, manage fluid overload, and cleanse the blood of waste products. The clinical situation and age of the child will determine whether hemodialysis or peritoneal dialysis will be used. Refer to the discussion of "Renal Replacement Therapy" later in this chapter.

Prognosis depends on the cause of ARF. When renal failure results from drug toxicity or dehydration, the prognosis is generally good. However, ARF that results from diseases such as hemolytic-uremic syndrome or acute glomerulonephritis may be associated with residual kidney damage.

16-14   Medications Used to Treat Complications of Acute Renal Failure

Complication	Medication	Action or Indication	Nursing Implications
Hyperkalemia (> 5.8 mmol/L)	Kayexalate	Exchanges sodium for potassium.	May require up to 4 hours to take effect.
	Calcium gluconate 10%	Counteracts potassium-induced increased myocardial irritability.	Monitor for electrocardiographic (ECG) changes. Intravenous infiltration may result in tissue necrosis.
	Sodium bicarbonate	Helps correct metabolic acidosis by exchanging hydrogen for potassium.	Do not mix with calcium. Complications include fluid overload, hypertension, and tetany.
Hypocalcemia (< 2.2 mmol/L)	Calcium gluconate 10%	Used in presence of tetany; provides ionized calcium to restore nervous tissue function.	Administer slowly to prevent bradycardia. Monitor for ECG changes.
Malignant hypertension (blood pressure > 95% for age)	Sodium nitroprusside, nitroglycerin	Relaxes smooth muscle in peripheral arterioles.	Administer by continuous intravenous infusion; fall in blood pressure is seen within 10–20 minutes.

Nursing Assessment

A complete history and physical examination are necessary to identify progression of symptoms and possible causes for renal failure.

Physiologic Assessment. Assessment of vital signs, level of consciousness, and other neurologic indicators helps to identify clinical signs of electrolyte imbalance (see Table 16–12). Measurement of the child's weight on admission provides a baseline for evaluating changes in fluid status. Monitor urinalysis, urine culture, and blood chemistry studies. Inspect urine for color (Fig. 16–7). Cloudy urine may indicate infection; tea-colored urine suggests hematuria. Assess urine specific gravity and intake and output.

Psychosocial Assessment. The unexpected and acute nature of the child's hospitalization creates anxiety for both parents and child. Assess for feelings of anger, guilt, or fear associated with the hospitalization. Such feelings are likely if ARF developed as a result of dehydration, a preventable injury, or poisoning. Assess coping mechanisms, family support systems, and level of stress.

Nursing Diagnosis

Nursing diagnoses depend on the cause of renal failure and accompanying complications. Several nursing diagnoses may apply to the child with ARF, including:

- Altered Renal Tissue Perfusion related to hypovolemia, sepsis, or drug toxicity
- Fluid Volume Excess related to sodium and water retention
- Altered Nutrition: Less Than Body Requirements related to anorexia, nausea, vomiting, and catabolic state
- Risk for Infection related to invasive procedures and monitoring equipment, and diminished immune functioning
- Ineffective Family Coping (Compromised) related to sudden hospitalization and uncertain prognosis

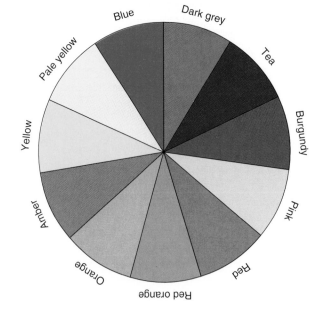

FIGURE 16–7. A color wheel, such as the one shown here, can be used as a guide in standardizing descriptions of urine color. Normal urine is pale yellow. Changes in urine color can indicate the following alterations: *yellow*—concentrated urine; *amber*—bile in urine; *orange*—alkaline or concentrated urine; *red orange*—acid pH, medications; *red*—blood, menses; *pink*—dilute blood; *burgundy*—laxatives; *tea*—melanin, hematuria; *dark gray*—medications, dyes; *blue*—dyes, medications.
From Cooper, C. (1993). What color is that urine specimen? American Journal of Nursing, 93, 37. Copyright © 1993 Connie Cooper, R.N., M.S.N.; graphics by Mike O'Grady, R.N., M.S.N.

Nursing Management

Nursing care focuses on preventing complications, maintaining fluid balance, administering medications, meeting nutritional needs, preventing infection, and providing emotional support to the child and parents.

Prevent Complications. Complications are best prevented by ensuring compliance with the treatment plan. Careful monitoring of vital signs, intake and output, serum electrolytes, and level of consciousness can alert the nurse to changes that indicate potential complications.

Maintain Fluid Balance. Estimate the child's fluid status by monitoring weight (on the same scale), intake and output, and blood pressure two or three times a day. Also monitor serum chemistry values, especially for sodium. The aim of maintaining fluid balance is to achieve a stable serum sodium concentration and a decrease in body weight by 0.5–1% a day.

If the child has oliguria, fluid intake, including parenteral nutrition, is limited to replacement of insensible fluid loss from the lungs, skin, and gastrointestinal tract (about one third the daily maintenance requirements in afebrile children). If the child is febrile, fluid administration is increased by 12% for each centigrade degree of temperature elevation.

Administer Medications. Because the kidney's ability to excrete drugs is impaired in ARF, dosages of all medications should be adjusted. The actual dosage of the drug can be reduced or the time interval between doses can be increased. Check drug levels to monitor for drug toxicity. Be aware of signs of drug toxicity for each medication the child is receiving.

Meet Nutritional Needs. Children are at risk of malnutrition because of their high metabolic rate. Parenteral alimentation or enteral feeding may be used initially to minimize protein catabolism. The diet is tailored to the individual child's need for calories, carbohydrates, fats, and amino acids or protein hydrolysates. Depending on the degree of renal failure, sodium, potassium, and phosphorus may be restricted. Oral feeding is initiated as soon as the child can tolerate it.

Prevent Infection. The child with ARF is extremely susceptible to nosocomial infections as a result of altered nutritional status, compromised immunity, and numerous invasive procedures. Thorough handwashing and standard precautions are imperative to decrease the risk of infection. Sterile technique should be used for all invasive procedures and when caring for lines. Drainage from catheter sites should be cultured to check for the presence of infectious organisms. Assess vital signs and lung sounds frequently.

Provide Emotional Support. The sudden onset of ARF presents parents with an unexpected threat to their child's life. Both the child and the parents experience anxiety because of the unexpected hospitalization and the uncertainty of the prognosis. Parents often feel guilty, regardless of the cause of renal failure. This guilt is intensified when renal failure is a result of dehydration or poisoning. Encourage parents to verbalize their fears and assist them in working through feelings of guilt. Explain procedures and treatment measures to decrease anxiety. Encouraging parents and older siblings to participate in the child's care can increase their sense of control.

Discharge Planning and Home Care Teaching. Home care needs should be identified and addressed well in advance of discharge. Encourage parental involvement early in the child's hospitalization. Be sure that parents understand the importance of administering medications correctly. Instruct family members in the proper technique for measuring

CLINICAL TIP

If serum sodium concentration rises and weight falls, insufficient fluids are being administered. If the serum sodium level falls and the weight increases, excessive fluids are being administered.

NURSING ALERT

The child with renal insufficiency has a concentrating defect. In cases of acute gastrointestinal illness, children are at greater risk for dehydration.

blood pressure so they can monitor the child's hypertension, if ordered. Have them demonstrate how to take the blood pressure.

Diet counseling is a key component of discharge planning and is usually performed by a renal dietitian. Depending on the degree of renal failure, the child's diet may include restrictions on protein, water, sodium, potassium, and phosphorus. The parents should be given written guidelines listing appropriate food choices to assist in menu planning. Ethnic and cultural preferences should be considered in listing menu options.

Continued monitoring of renal function during follow-up examinations is critical as deterioration may occur over time. Referral to support groups can be helpful for both parents and children. The National Kidney Foundation is a source of numerous publications (see Appendix F).

Chronic Renal Failure

Chronic renal failure (CRF) is a progressive, irreversible reduction in kidney function. CRF is rare in children, occurring in 3.5–6 per million.[2]

Clinical Manifestations

Children with CRF frequently have no symptoms initially. Symptoms do not appear until the child is in advanced renal failure (see Table 16–11). In the early stages, the child may appear pale and complain of headache, nausea, and fatigue. Decreased mental alertness and ability to concentrate may be seen. Anemia leading to tachycardia, tachypnea, and dyspnea on exertion may occur. As the disease progresses, the child experiences a loss of appetite and complications of renal impairment, including hypertension, pulmonary edema, growth retardation, **osteodystrophy** (defective mineralization of bone caused by renal failure and chronic hyperphosphatemia), delayed fine and gross motor development, and delayed sexual maturation.

Growth retardation is caused by disturbances in the metabolism of calcium, phosphorus, and vitamin D; decreased caloric intake; and metabolic acidosis. Osteodystrophy increases the child's risk for spontaneous fractures, rickets, and valgus deformity of the legs.

In end-stage renal disease (ESRD), the most advanced form of CRF, all body systems are adversely affected by renal failure. As the severity of the clinical and biochemical disturbances resulting from progressive renal deterioration increase, uremic symptoms develop. About 900 new cases of ESRD occur in children each year.[19]

Etiology and Pathophysiology

In children, CRF usually results from developmental abnormalities of the kidney or urinary tract. Terrell, described at the beginning of the chapter, had ESRD resulting from posterior urethral valves, which caused bilateral kidney damage. CFR may also be caused by hemolytic-uremic syndrome, glomerulonephritis, or other renal diseases. (See discussions later in the chapter.)

The gradual, progressive loss of functioning nephrons ultimately results in ESRD. ESRD is characterized by minimal renal function (less than 5% of normal), uremic syndrome, anemia, and abnormal blood values. In ESRD, the kidneys can no longer maintain homeostasis and the child requires dialysis.

The kidneys function to excrete excess acid in the body and to regulate the body's fluid and electrolyte balance. Renal failure upsets this fluid and electrolyte balance. As renal failure progresses, metabolic acidosis occurs because the kidneys cannot excrete the acids that build up in the body. Retention of excessive sodium and water is a common cause of the elevated blood pressure associated with CRF. Insufficient calcium loss, phosphorus retention, and elevated parathyroid hormone levels lead to uremic bone disease. Since the kidneys are also the site of production of erythropoietin (the growth factor responsible for the production and maturation of red cells), lack of erythropoietin and progressive renal disease are the underlying causes of the anemia of CRF.

Diagnostic Tests and Medical Management

Laboratory evaluation, including serum electrolyte, phosphate, BUN, and creatinine levels and pH, is used to confirm the diagnosis of CRF. A urine sample is collected for culture, and a 24–hour urine sample is obtained to quantify creatinine and protein excretion. From the 24–hour urine creatinine and serum creatinine levels, it is possible to calculate the remaining glomerular filtration rate. Laboratory values vary depending on the child's size and muscle mass. Age-specific normal ranges for laboratory values must be used. Tests to identify renal diseases that could be causing the renal failure are also performed if necessary. A renal biopsy is the best method for establishing or confirming the diagnosis, predicting the prognosis, and directing treatment.[18]

The goals of treatment are to slow the progression of renal disease and to prevent complications. Conservative treatment includes a combination of dietary and fluid and electrolyte management, control of hypertension, and if that fails and the child progresses to ESRD, dialysis is initiated.

Dietary management focuses on maximizing caloric intake for growth while limiting demands on the kidneys and minimizing fluid and electrolyte disturbances. Tube feedings or parenteral nutrition may be required to achieve optimal protein intake, especially in children under 1 year of age. Sodium bicarbonate (Bicitra) is used for treatment of metabolic acidosis. Restricting sodium to as little as 2 g/day may be necessary if the child is hypertensive or edematous. As renal failure progresses, potassium and phosphate restrictions become necessary. Calcium-based phosphate binders may be prescribed to remove the excess phosphate.

Diuretics are given to reduce the edema associated with renal failure. Antihypertensives are prescribed to reduce blood pressure and prevent the progression of renal disease. As in ARF, medication dosages are adjusted because of the reduced glomerular filtration rate. Supplementation of vitamins (pyridoxine and folic acid) is usually necessary to offset dietary deficiencies. Ergocalciferol and calcitriol (vitamin D) are given to increase calcium absorption. Ascorbic acid is administered to enhance iron absorption. Erythropoietin is given to stimulate increased production of red blood cells, improve energy tolerance and school performance, and reduce the need for transfusions. Human growth hormone is given during the course of renal failure, until ESRD occurs, to increase muscle mass and total body weight gain.

Children who progress to ESRD require renal replacement therapy (see the following discussion). The timetable for dialysis or renal transplantation is different from that of adults; earlier initiation can prevent some complications of ESRD. Rather than use the absolute BUN or serum creatinine as the guide, nonspecific signs such as uremic syndrome, poorly controlled hypertension, renal osteodystrophy, failure of head circumference measurement to increase normally, developmental delay, and poor growth are used in determining when to initiate therapy. (Refer to the subsequent discussion of "Renal Replacement Therapy.")

CRF is irreversible. However, the course of the disease is variable. Some children progress quickly to renal failure, necessitating dialysis. Other children are managed with a combination of medication and diet therapy for some time before significant renal impairment occurs. Frequent modifica-

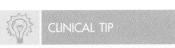

CLINICAL TIP

When CRF is present, optimal protein intake for *infants* is 2–2.5 g/kg/day; for *older children*, 1.5–2 g/kg/day.

tions in the treatment plan are often necessary to address the child's changing status.

Nursing Assessment

Physiologic Assessment. The initial and ongoing assessment of the child focuses on identifying complications of renal failure. Observe for signs of edema, poor growth and development, osteodystrophy, and anemia. Assessment of vital signs helps to identify electrolyte alterations (see Table 16–12).

Psychosocial Assessment. As renal disease progresses, the number of stressors on the child and family increases. Denial and disbelief are commonly the first reactions. A thorough family assessment can help to identify particular needs of the child and family (see Table 5–7). The development of ESRD is particularly challenging during adolescence. Noncompliance with treatments can endanger the adolescent's life.

Nursing Diagnosis

Nursing diagnoses for the child with CRF are similar to those previously listed for ARF. Additional diagnoses might include:

- Altered Growth and Development related to decreased caloric intake and metabolic disturbances
- Self-Esteem Disturbance related to perception of being "different"
- Activity Intolerance related to headaches, anemia, and fatigue
- Altered Family Processes related to a child with a life-threatening illness
- Ineffective Management of Therapeutic Regimen related to lack of knowledge of home dialysis plan and "burnout"
- Body Image Disturbance related to impaired growth and use of an external catheter for dialysis

Nursing Management

Children with CRF are usually hospitalized for initial diagnostic evaluation, to initiate dialysis treatment, to monitor problems that develop in the treatment plan, or to treat infection or another concurrent problem. Nursing care for the hospitalized child with CRF focuses on monitoring for side effects of medications, preventing infection, meeting nutritional needs, and providing emotional support and anticipatory teaching.

Monitor for Side Effects of Medications. Watch for signs of electrolyte imbalance such as weakness, muscle cramps, dizziness, headache, and nausea and vomiting in children who are taking diuretics. Supervise the child's activities closely to prevent falls resulting from dizziness, especially at the beginning of diuretic therapy. If antihypertensive medications such as hydralazine are being administered, monitor the child's weight to detect excessive gain resulting from water and sodium retention.

Prevent Infection. The child with CRF is extremely susceptible to infections. Be alert for signs of infection, such as elevated temperature; cloudy, strong-smelling urine; dysuria; changes in respiratory pattern; or productive cough. Emphasize to the child and family the importance of good handwashing practices.

Meet Nutritional Needs. Maintaining adequate nutritional intake in a child with CRF who has dietary restrictions is challenging. Provide small, frequent feedings and present meals attractively to encourage the child to eat.

Provide Emotional Support. Development of progressive CRF requires a total life-style change for the child and family. The parents and child need opportunities to express and work through their feelings related to the disease, prognosis, and treatment restrictions. Children can be assisted to express their feelings through drawings or therapeutic play.

The need for ongoing dialysis treatments and the wait for a suitable donor kidney are stressful for both parents and child. Identification of effective coping methods and family support systems is needed to promote treatment compliance. The National Kidney Foundation and local support groups for kidney disease can provide the family with information or additional support (see Appendix F).

Discharge Planning and Home Care Teaching. Home care needs should be identified and addressed well in advance of discharge. Parents need to understand the necessity of long-term treatments and follow-up care. Help the family develop a schedule for medication administration that fits with their routine. Emphasize the importance of consistency in administration times. Teach parents how to recognize side effects and complications.

Appropriate referrals should be made to the local visiting nurse association and to home care nursing agencies. Home care nurses will help the parents care for the child receiving dialysis as well as provide necessary support and reassurance. Parents of children receiving dialysis at home should be taught how to perform the treatment and how to identify complications (Table 16–15). Strict aseptic technique is necessary to prevent infection at the catheter site.

16-15   Complications of Peritoneal Dialysis

Complication	Cause
Peritonitis	
Cloudy dialysate, abdominal pain, tenderness, leukocytosis, fever (neonatal hypothermia), constipation	*Staphylococcus aureus, Staphylococcus epidermidis,* fungal infections, gram-negative rods (risk is proportional to duration of dialysis and inversely proportional to age)
Pain	
During inflow	Too rapid a rate of infusion, too large a volume of dialysate, encasement of catheter in a false passage, extremes in temperature of dialysate
During outflow at end of emptying	Omentum entering catheter at end of outflow
Leakage	
Fluid around catheter, edema of penis or scrotum secondary to leakage into abdominal subcutaneous tissue, fluid leakage to pleural spaces through diaphragm	Overfilling of abdomen, catheter that has migrated from peritoneal cavity
Respiratory symptoms	
Shortness of breath, decreased breath sounds in lower lobes, inadequate chest expansion	Abdominal fullness that compromises diaphragm movement, hole in diaphragm allowing dialysate into chest cavity

Care in the Community. Children with CRF require frequent outpatient visits to monitor the progression of signs and symptoms, and to evaluate the effectiveness of current treatments.

ASSESSMENT. Compare the child's height, weight, and head circumference to age-specific norms to identify growth retardation and to plot progress. Assess developmental progress using the Denver II or another screening tool (see Chap. 5). Assess the adolescent for signs of delayed sexual maturation and, in girls, amenorrhea. Blood and urine tests will be performed to monitor renal function. Radiographs of the bones will be taken at 6-month intervals to assess changes caused by osteodystrophy.

HEALTH SUPERVISION. Promote good dentition and oral hygiene. Regular dental visits are important to reduce infections. Make sure the family understands the need for antibiotic prophylaxis before certain invasive procedures, including dental care (see Table 12–8). If possible, all immunizations should be provided before renal transplantation, as long-term immunosuppressive therapy will then be prescribed. Live vaccines should not be given to the child taking immunosuppressive agents.

NUTRITION. Review any dietary restrictions with parents. Provide sample menus for meal planning to help parents incorporate dietary changes into daily meals. A renal dietitian usually assists the child to make food selections and to restrict fluids and sodium as necessary, taking into account the child's likes and dislikes and cultural background. School-age children may not understand the consequences of noncompliance with dietary restrictions and may perceive these restrictions as punishment. Adolescents often resent the dietary restrictions and ongoing dialysis treatments, which pose a threat to their independence and evolving sense of self. Noncooperation, depression, and hostility are common responses. Discuss possible behavioral responses to dietary restrictions and limitations imposed by the treatment plan.

EMOTIONAL SUPPORT. School-age children and adolescents are often embarrassed about being perceived as different from peers. Ask the child how he or she feels about the need to follow a special diet, take medications, and undergo dialysis treatments. To minimize the psychologic consequences of coping with a chronic disease, encourage parents to promote the child's participation in age-appropriate activities. Attendance at school and contacts with peers promote normal growth and development. Work to promote the child's self-worth and a healthy self-esteem. Prepare the child for peer conflict.

ANTICIPATORY TEACHING. Supply the parents with timely information about the disease process, dialysis treatments, and issues related to renal transplantation, as the child's renal impairment progresses.

Renal Replacement Therapy

Renal replacement therapy is the treatment for renal failure and includes both dialysis and renal transplantation. In 1994, 4000 children between birth and 19 years of age received some form of renal replacement therapy, and 1534 children received regular dialysis. Approximately 65% of children managed at home with ESRD receive peritoneal dialysis and 35% receive hemodialysis.[19] Dialysis treatment can cost up to $50,000 per year.

Peritoneal Dialysis

Peritoneal dialysis is the preferred form of dialysis for small children because continuous removal of fluids and waste products is possible. A continuous steady state of dialysis clearance occurs, decreasing the toxic effects of waste products on the child's developing body. Dietary and fluid restrictions are less severe. The timing of the treatment can be set to minimize the interruption of school, play, or other social events.

Two types of peritoneal dialysis are commonly used: continuous ambulatory peritoneal dialysis and continuous cycler-assisted peritoneal dialysis. Buretrols or graduated cylinders are used to monitor the volume of fluid exchanged.

- Continuous ambulatory peritoneal dialysis uses gravity to instill prefilled bags of **dialysate** (dialysis solution) into the peritoneal cavity four or five times a day. The fluid remains in the cavity for 4–8 hours. An attached bag is folded under the child's clothes, permitting normal activity. After the allotted time, the dialysate is drained by hanging the bag lower than the pelvis. The repeated connections and disconnections with this method are time-consuming for the child and family and increase the risk of infection.

- Continuous cycler-assisted peritoneal dialysis uses an automatic cycler to instill and drain the dialysate about five times over a 10–hour period, usually overnight. With this method, only one connection and disconnection is needed per day, which reduces demands on the family as well as the risk of infection.

In children receiving peritoneal dialysis for ARF, a catheter can be placed percutaneously that can be used for a few weeks. In children with CRF, a catheter is placed surgically for long-term use.

The primary complications of peritoneal dialysis are peritonitis and abdominal hernia (see Table 16–15). Patients average one episode of peritonitis per year.[20]

Teach the family to perform peritoneal dialysis and to use sterile technique when performing dialysis and when doing catheter care. Peritoneal dialysis is time consuming, and commitment by family members is required to manage this procedure daily. Help the family to develop home routines that minimize disruptions to daily family life. For additional information, refer to the Nursing Care Plan for the child receiving home peritoneal dialysis.

Hemodialysis

Hemodialysis is used in the critical care setting, and for those children with CRF when peritoneal dialysis is not possible for technical reasons or when the family is unable to safely provide it. In the opening scenario, Terrell's health care providers and his family decided to switch from peritoneal dialysis to hemodialysis after he developed several episodes of peritonitis in one year. Infants as small as 4 kg (8.8 lb) can be hemodialyzed with current technology. Treatment is usually performed three times a week, with each session lasting approximately 3–4 hours.

In emergency hemodialysis and for infants, a double-lumen cannula is inserted into a large vein (eg, the femoral, jugular, or subclavian vein). Children over 20 kg (44 lb) often have an artificial blood vessel, an arteriovenous shunt or fistula, created. Blood is pumped out of the body and through a dialyzer, where waste products and extra fluids diffuse out across a semipermeable membrane. Dialysate is pumped in the direction opposite blood flow to promote waste extraction. Differences in osmolarity and concentration between the child's blood and the dialysate alter the

CLINICAL TIP

Signs and symptoms of peritonitis associated with peritoneal dialysis include: fever, vomiting, diarrhea, abdominal pain, tenderness, and cloudy dialysate.

NURSING ALERT

Monitor the child receiving hemodialysis for complications that can occur suddenly.
- Hypotension—sudden nausea and vomiting, abdominal cramping, tachycardia, and dizziness
- Rapid fluid and electrolyte exchange—muscle cramping, nausea and vomiting, and dizziness
- Dysequilibrium syndrome—restlessness, headache, nausea and vomiting, blurred vision, muscle twitching, and altered level of consciousness

Text continues on page 694.

NURSING CARE PLAN
THE CHILD RECEIVING HOME PERITONEAL DIALYSIS

GOAL	INTERVENTION	RATIONALE	EXPECTED OUTCOME

1. Altered Nutrition: Less Than Body Requirements related to poor appetite and feeling of fullness after a small amount

The child will obtain adequate nutrients each day.	• With a nutritionist, develop a diet plan to identify the amounts of essential nutrients needed. • Provide small, frequent meals of needed nutrients. • Make mealtimes pleasant and avoid battles over the child's intake. • Provide supplements by tube feeding if adequate oral intake is not possible.	• Parents need concrete guidelines for food preparation. • The child will feel full with smaller amounts of food because of the dialysate. • The child will be more inclined to eat if there is less stress. • Adequate nutrition is important for growth and development, and must be supported if oral intake is inadequate.	The child's intake is adequate for an expected growth pattern to be maintained.

2. Risk for Infection related to daily invasive procedure

The child will not develop peritonitis.	• Use aseptic technique for connection and disconnection of catheters. • Perform daily catheter site care.	• Aseptic technique reduces chance of introducing bacteria into the abdomen. • Skin around the catheter site will have fewer organisms that could potentially cause infection.	The child does not develop peritonitis.
If peritonitis occurs, it will be treated appropriately.	• Observe for signs of infection (fever, abdominal pain, cloudy dialysate). • Report signs of infection to physician immediately.	• Early identification of infection will reduce complications. • Rapid intervention may reduce need for hospitalization.	Hospitalization will not be needed for peritonitis due to early identification and prompt treatment.

3. Caregiver Role Strain related to daily dialysis treatments

The family copes with daily demands for the child's dialysis treatments.	• Discuss the importance of daily, consistent dialysis treatments for the child's overall health status. • Collaborate with the family to identify strategies that could reduce the impact of dialysis on the family's life.	• If parents understand the need for consistent dialysis treatments, they are more likely to comply. • When the family participates in planning care, compliance is more likely.	The family complies with daily dialysis treatment guidelines.

NURSING CARE PLAN

THE CHILD RECEIVING HOME PERITONEAL DIALYSIS– *Continued*

GOAL	INTERVENTION	RATIONALE	EXPECTED OUTCOME

3. Caregiver Role Strain related to daily dialysis treatments (continued)

	• Refer the family to local support groups for emotional support, treatment strategies, and respite care.	• Support groups may help the family develop effective coping strategies.	

4. Body Image Disturbance related to small size and perception of being and looking different

GOAL	INTERVENTION	RATIONALE	EXPECTED OUTCOME
The child will develop a sense of self-worth and self-esteem.	• Identify and emphasize strengths the child has (eg, interaction style, skills, or cognitive abilities) despite being smaller than peers.	• Perception of personal strengths should increase self-esteem.	The child effectively interacts with peers and participates in age-appropriate activities.
	• Assist the child and family to identify popular clothing styles that hide the dialysate bag and catheter.	• Clothing that conforms to current styles, but still hides dialysate, will help the child feel less different from peers.	
	• Increase the child's participation in self-care as appropriate for developmental age.	• Ability to perform self-care increases the child's sense of control.	
	• Promote participation in safe activities with peers.	• Social interaction with peers helps reinforce similarities with others.	
	• Encourage the child to participate in support groups with other children receiving dialysis when possible.	• Interactions with other affected children provide a chance to express feelings and frustrations, and to develop successful coping strategies.	

5. Altered Health Maintenance related to chronic condition

GOAL	INTERVENTION	RATIONALE	EXPECTED OUTCOME
The child's routine health maintenance visits will be integrated with the management of the chronic condition.	• If a renal specialty team is not conveniently located and providing general health care, identify a primary care provider.	• A source of health maintenance and acute minor illness care is important, especially if the family lives a distance from the tertiary care center.	The child is fully immunized at appropriate intervals and the family has a source of regular care in the community.
	• Assess the child regularly for growth and developmental progress and signs that the chronic condition is being managed effectively.	• Routine assessments will allow potential complications to be identified earlier.	

Continued . . .

NURSING CARE PLAN
THE CHILD RECEIVING HOME PERITONEAL DIALYSIS– *Continued*

GOAL	INTERVENTION	RATIONALE	EXPECTED OUTCOME

5. Altered Health Maintenance related to chronic condition (continued)

	• Provide immunizations as recommended for the child with a chronic condition.	• Immunizations may reduce the risk of potentially life-threatening infections in a child at high risk.	
	• Provide anticipatory guidance related to safety, developmental progress, appropriate physical activities, and behavior management.	• Information will help the family support the child's health status and promote development.	

CLINICAL TIP

Carefully monitor fluid balance in the child undergoing hemodialysis. Check vital signs and blood pressure every half hour. Monitor oral intake and urinary output when on the dialysis equipment every half hour. Weigh the child before and after the dialysis to determine any fluid imbalances that must be adjusted in the next hemodialysis session.

intravascular electrolyte concentration and reduce the intravascular volume (Fig. 16–8).

Hemodialysis is more efficient than peritoneal dialysis but requires close monitoring for symptoms related to hypotension or rapid changes in fluid and electrolyte balance. Uncommonly, a disequilibrium syndrome may occur during or soon after the dialysis procedure is first performed. Other complications include access thrombosis and infection. Heparin is used to achieve an active clotting time of 150%, which reduces the risk of thrombosis.

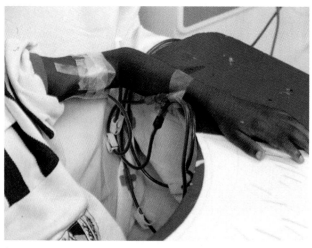

A

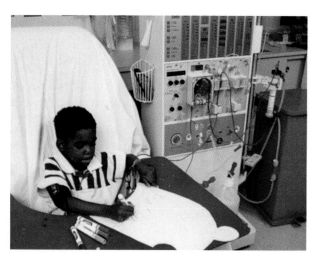

B

FIGURE 16–8. This child is undergoing hemodialysis. **A,** A surgically implanted vascular graft is being used here. One needle is placed in the arterialized end of the graft (red tubing), and one needle is placed in the venous end (blue tubing) for blood return. **B,** The child is able to draw or perform other quiet activities during dialysis treatment. Note that the child's blood pressure is monitored carefully throughout the treatment.

Nursing management focuses on teaching the child and family about the administration of heparin and the control of bleeding from minor trauma. Because dietary limitations are needed more often with hemodialysis than with peritoneal dialysis, make sure the family knows how to plan and provide for the child's daily nutritional needs. Methods to reduce the risk of infection should be reviewed, including the provision of daily care to the catheter site. Encourage showering rather than tub baths. Activities such as swimming may be discouraged.

Renal Transplantation

Renal transplantation provides the only alternative to long-term dialysis for children with ESRD. It can normalize physiology and provide a potential for normal growth. Because of the adverse effects on growth and development resulting from delaying transplantation, children are given some priority over adults awaiting transplantation. To be successful, ABO compatibility between the kidney donor and the recipient is necessary. A human leukocyte antigen (HLA) system match also improves survival of the graft. A living relative donor kidney has a higher survival rate than a cadaver kidney.

After transplantation, the child must take immunosuppressive medications such as corticosteroids, azathioprine, cyclosporine, and antilymphocyte antibodies to suppress rejection. Immunosuppression regimens use various combinations and sequences of these drugs to reduce the incidence of acute and chronic rejection. Signs of rejection include fever, increased BUN and serum creatinine levels, pain and tenderness over the abdomen, irritability, and weight gain.

Complications of immunosuppression therapy include opportunistic infection, lymphomas and skin cancer, and hypertension. Noncompliance with management is highest among families with instability, adolescents, females, and children and youth with low self-esteem.[21] Some primary kidney diseases, such as glomerulonephritis and hemolytic-uremic syndrome, can also recur in the transplanted kidney.

Nursing management includes teaching parents about the transplantation process before it occurs to help prepare them for the experience. Discuss all aspects of the child's care that will have an impact on the family's life, including follow-up appointments, medications, and general health promotion. Teach parents about the signs of acute rejection and infection, including when and how to notify the child's physician if immediate care is required.

RESEARCH CONSIDERATIONS

The kidney graft has higher survival rate when the transplant is done after the child reaches 6 years of age. It is thought that younger children have a higher immune reactivity and that the metabolism of drugs is altered, resulting in insufficient immunosuppression.[21]

POLYCYSTIC KIDNEY DISEASE

Polycystic kidney disease is a genetic disorder that has autosomal recessive and autosomal dominant forms. Liver abnormalities are associated with both forms of the disease. They each have a spectrum of severity and may be detected in the fetus or become apparent during infancy or childhood. The incidence of the autosomal recessive form is 1 per 10,000–40,000.[22] The autosomal dominant form is the most common inherited kidney disease, with a prevalence of 1 per 1000 patients.[22] The disordered gene that causes the disease has been found on chromosomes 4 and 16.

Newborns with polycystic kidney disease may have enlarged kidneys, detected at birth. Those with the most severe form of the disease die shortly after birth as a result of pulmonary hypoplasia. Clinical manifestations in infants and children include hypertension, hematuria, and proteinuria. Polyuria and polydipsia develop with progressive **renal insufficiency** (ie, as the kidneys' ability to conserve sodium and concentrate the urine decreases). As uremia develops, infants and children develop renal osteodystrophy and progressive developmental delay and growth failure.

Cellular hyperplasia of the collecting ducts causes dilation of the ducts. Fluid secreted into these ducts enables cyst sacs to form. Initially, cysts are usually less than 2 mm (1 in.) in size and do not obstruct urinary flow. As the child grows, however, the cysts become larger and fibrosis occurs. Tubular atrophy may occur in some children, whereas others have minimal changes in renal function. Polycystic kidney disease is also associated with liver abnormalities that progress to fibrosis, portal hypertension, and biliary infection, which progress in severity with age.

Diagnosis is confirmed by sonogram or renal biopsy. The disease is often diagnosed on prenatal ultrasound. If identified, other family members should be screened for subclinical cases of the disease. Liver function tests are usually normal.

Treatment is supportive. Medications such as diuretics are prescribed for hypertension. Erythropoietin is prescribed to prevent and treat anemia. Renal osteodystrophy is treated to suppress the parathyroid hormone. Chronic renal failure is managed as described earlier on pages 687–690. Surgery is performed for portal hypertension. Renal dialysis or a transplant prolong survival. However, liver problems may continue to complicate the child's health, even when the renal condition is well controlled.

Nursing Management

Nursing care is the same as that for the child with renal insufficiency and chronic renal failure. Observe the child for signs of progressive renal impairment. Ensure that follow-up appointments are scheduled to assess growth, developmental progress, and the effectiveness of the treatment plan. Family teaching for home management focuses on medications, diet, management of acute gastrointestinal illnesses, and care for the child with progressive renal insufficiency and a liver disorder.

HEMOLYTIC-UREMIC SYNDROME

Hemolytic-uremic syndrome (HUS) is a relatively rare, acute renal disease. The syndrome is characterized by a classic triad of signs: (1) hemolytic anemia, (2) thrombocytopenia, and (3) ARF. It is an important cause of CRF.[23]

HUS usually follows an episode of mild gastroenteritis with diarrhea, upper respiratory infection, or urinary tract infection. The child suddenly appears pale and develops petechiae, bruising, or bloody stools (Table 16–16). Urine output is decreased. Signs of central nervous system involvement include irritability, lethargy, gait changes, and convulsions. The child may also have edema and ascites as a result of renal failure.

The development of HUS is often linked to enterohemorrhagic *Escherichia coli*, which produces a toxin that attaches to the kidneys and other organs. Hamburger is the vector in more than half of the epidemics. Damage to the lining of the glomerular arterioles results in swelling of the endothelial cells. In response, clotting mechanisms deposit fibrin in the renal arterioles and capillaries. This partial occlusion damages the red blood cells, resulting in hemolysis and subsequent anemia. Platelet agglutination occurs in areas of vascular endothelial damage, causing thrombocytopenia. ARF develops as a consequence of blood clotting in the arterioles as well as the toxic effect of hemolyzed red blood cells on renal tubular cells leading to acute tubular necrosis.

A peripheral blood smear with fragments of red blood cells, fibrin split products, and a decreased platelet count ($< 140,000/mm^3$) confirms the diagnosis. Treatment focuses on the complications of ARF and in-

16-16   Clinical Manifestations of Hemolytic-uremic Syndrome

Prodromal Stage (1–7 days)
Upper respiratory illness
Abdominal pain with nausea, vomiting, and bloody diarrhea
Pallor
Fever
Irritability
Lymphadenopathy
Skin rash
Edema
Severe gastroenteritis with bloody diarrhea in 90% of cases

Acute Stage
Hemolytic anemia
Hypertension
Purpura
Neurologic involvement (irritability, seizures, lethargy, stupor, coma, cerebral edema)
Hematuria and proteinuria
Oliguria or anuria
Edema and ascites

cludes fluid restrictions, antihypertensive medications, and a high-calorie, high-carbohydrate diet that is low in protein, sodium, potassium, and phosphorus. Enteral nutritional support is sometimes needed. (Refer to the earlier discussion of ARF.) Dialysis may be necessary, depending on the degree of renal failure. Peritoneal dialysis is preferred unless the child has severe colitis and abdominal tenderness. Transfusions of fresh packed red blood cells may be ordered to treat severe anemia. Platelets are given if the child is bleeding or if surgery is needed. Transfusions should be administered carefully to prevent hypertension caused by hypervolemia.

Nursing Management

Nursing care is the same as that for the child with ARF, described earlier. Careful monitoring of fluid balance is essential. Observe the child carefully for signs of progressive renal impairment. Discharge planning focuses on teaching parents about medications and dietary and fluid restrictions. Follow-up visits are necessary to evaluate the effectiveness of the treatment plan.

ACUTE POSTINFECTIOUS GLOMERULONEPHRITIS

Glomerulonephritis is an inflammation of the glomeruli of the kidneys. In children, it is most often a response to a group A beta-hemolytic strepto-coccal infection of the skin or pharynx. It is also caused by other organisms including *Staphylococcus*, *Pneumococcus*, and coxsackieviruses. The incidence of acute postinfectious glomerulonephritis (APIGN) is highest in children who are 5–8 years of age, and the disorder is more common in boys than in girls. Early antibiotic therapy for streptococcal infection does not seem to prevent the development of APIGN.

Clinical Manifestations

Onset is usually abrupt. Hematuria and mild periorbital edema are usually the first clinical signs.[1] Hypertension may be severe and is the next sign to appear. As the disease progresses, the child becomes lethargic and feverish and may complain of abdominal pain, headache, and costovertebral tenderness (related to stretching of the renal capsule from edema). Gross hematuria, resulting in tea-colored urine, is a classic sign. Other signs include oliguria, anorexia, and generalized edema.

Etiology and Pathophysiology

The child with APIGN usually becomes ill after a group A beta-hemolytic streptococcal infection of the upper respiratory tract or the skin. Often the child becomes ill with strep throat, recovers, and then develops signs of APIGN after an interval of 1–3 weeks.

Glomerular damage occurs as a result of an immune complex reaction that localizes on the glomerular capillary wall. Antibody–antigen complexes become lodged in the glomeruli, leading to inflammation and obstruction. Damage to the glomerular membrane allows red blood cells and red cell casts to be excreted. Sodium and water are retained, expanding the intravascular and interstitial compartments. This process results in the characteristic finding of edema (Fig. 16–9).

Diagnostic Tests and Medical Management

Blood tests may reveal elevated BUN and creatinine concentrations. The erythrocyte sedimentation rate is increased in the acute phase, and serum

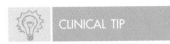

CLINICAL TIP

Encourage prompt treatment of streptococcal infections with a full course of antibiotics to prevent APIGN when possible.

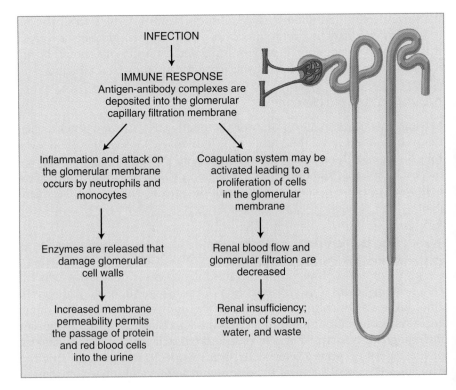

FIGURE 16–9. Pathophysiology of acute postinfectious glomerulonephritis.

lipid levels are increased in about 40% of cases. An elevated antistreptolysin O (ASO) titer reflects the presence of antibodies from a recent streptococcal respiratory infection, but the ASO level associated with a recent skin infection is low. The anti-DNAse B titer is helpful for detecting antibodies associated with recent skin infections. Anemia is common in the acute phase and is generally caused by dilution of the serum by the extracellular fluid. The hemoglobin level and hematocrit value may decrease during the late phase as a result of hematuria. The white blood cell count may be normal or slightly elevated.

Treatment focuses on relief of symptoms and supportive therapy. Bedrest is a key component of the treatment plan during the acute phase. Hypertension can be managed with a combination of an antihypertensive medication (such as hydralazine [Apresoline]) and a diuretic (such as furosemide [Lasix]). Mild to moderate hypertension should be treated with fluid and salt restriction. A course of antibiotics may be given to ensure eradication of the infectious agent.

Fluid requirements are determined by careful monitoring of urinary output, weight, blood pressure, and serum electrolytes. Initially, only insensible losses are replaced until the status of renal function is known. The degree of dietary restriction is determined by the severity of edema. Sodium and potassium intake are restricted. With severe azotemia, protein intake may have to be limited.

The prognosis for the majority of children with APIGN is good. Most children recover completely within a few weeks. Recurrences are unusual. Rarely, some children do develop CRF.

Nursing Assessment

Assess edema, which may be periorbital or dependent and shifts as the child's position is changed. Assess for circulatory congestion (crackles, dyspnea, and cough). Monitor blood pressure, which can rise as high as 200/120 mm Hg. When severe hypertension is present, assess for signs of central nervous system problems (headache, blurred vision, vomiting, decreased level of consciousness, confusion, and convulsions).

Nursing Diagnosis

The accompanying Nursing Care Plan lists several nursing diagnoses that may apply to the child with APIGN.

Nursing Management

As with other renal disorders, care of the child with APIGN requires careful monitoring of vital signs and fluid–electrolyte balance to evaluate renal functioning and identify complications. Bedrest is required during the acute phase. Immediate emergency care is needed for severe hypertension with cerebral dysfunction; diazoxide or hydralazine is administered intravenously. Nursing care focuses on monitoring fluid status, preventing infection, preventing skin breakdown, meeting nutritional needs, and providing emotional support to the child and family. The Nursing Care Plan summarizes nursing care of the child with APIGN.

Monitor Fluid Status

Monitor vital signs, fluid and electrolyte status, and intake and output. Hypovolemia can occur as a result of fluid shifting from vascular to interstitial spaces despite the outward clinical signs of excess fluid retention. Monitor

---

URINALYSIS RESULTS IN APIGN

- Acid pH
- Hematuria
- Proteinuria (trace to 2+)
- Discoloration (reddish brown to rusty color secondary to red blood cell and hemoglobin content)
- Leukocyturia

NURSING CARE PLAN
THE CHILD WITH ACUTE POSTINFECTIOUS GLOMERULONEPHRITIS

GOAL	INTERVENTION	RATIONALE	EXPECTED OUTCOME

1. Risk for Fluid Volume Excess related to decreased glomerular filtration and increased sodium retention

GOAL	INTERVENTION	RATIONALE	EXPECTED OUTCOME
The child will regain normal fluid balance.	• Assess for edema (periorbital or dependent areas). • Calculate fluid intake and plan amounts to offer throughout the day. • Limit foods with moderate to high sodium content. • Document intake and output. • Perform daily weight measurement on the same scale at the same time of day. • Administer prescribed medications (diuretics and antihypertensives).	• Sodium and water retention leads to edema. • An intake/output ratio of 1:1 reflects normal hydration and kidney function. • Further reduction in sodium intake will help balance fluid and sodium retention. • Prevents excessive fluid intake. • Weight gain is an early sign of fluid retention. Weight loss indicates improvement in condition. • Diuretics cause excretion of excess fluid by preventing reabsorption of water and sodium. Antihypertensives increase excretion of water and sodium and cause vasodilation.	The child maintains normal urine output of 0.5–1 mL/kg/hr. The child receives appropriate fluid each day.

2. Risk for Infection related to renal impairment and corticosteroid therapy

GOAL	INTERVENTION	RATIONALE	EXPECTED OUTCOME
The child will be infection free.	• Assess temperature every 4 hours. Observe for signs of infection. • Obtain throat and other cultures as ordered.	• The child is at risk for secondary infection. • Culture can identify causative microorganism in secondary infection or presence of residual streptococcal infection.	The child's temperature remains within normal limits and child is free of secondary infection.

3. Risk for Impaired Skin Integrity related to tissue edema

GOAL	INTERVENTION	RATIONALE	EXPECTED OUTCOME
The child will be free of skin breakdown.	• Assess skin for breakdown secondary to edema and bedrest. • Encourage position changes every 1–2 hours. Provide skin care. Use a therapeutic mattress.	• Ensures early identification and implementation of preventive measures. • Prolonged pressure leads to skin breakdown.	The child has unimpaired skin integrity.

NURSING CARE PLAN
THE CHILD WITH ACUTE POSTINFECTIOUS GLOMERULONEPHRITIS— *Continued*

GOAL	INTERVENTION	RATIONALE	EXPECTED OUTCOME

4. Altered Nutrition: Less Than Body Requirements *related to anorexia*

The child will maintain adequate caloric intake.	• Maintain meal schedule similar to that at home. Serve food in age-appropriate servings. Assess for food likes and dislikes. Provide favorite foods, as possible.	• Normal routine and preferred food choices help to encourage the child to eat.	Child maintains weight and tolerates daily intake that meets nutritional requirements.

5. Activity Intolerance *related to fluid and electrolyte imbalance, infectious process, and altered nutrition*

The child will progress in activity tolerance without excess fatigue as the disease process improves.	• Maintain bedrest during acute stage. Encourage gradual activity increase as the condition improves. • Provide for quiet play according to the developmental stage of the child (eg, coloring books, music, videotapes, television).	• Rest decreases the production of waste materials, which place increased stress on the kidneys. • Quiet activities minimize energy expenditures and stress on the kidneys.	The child avoids fatigue and exhibits the ability to tolerate activity for longer periods.

6. Knowledge Deficit (Parent) *related to child's medication schedule and treatment regimen after discharge*

The parents will state knowledge of the child's treatment regimen after discharge.	• Assess parents' understanding of need for compliance with medication schedule. • Describe best schedule for giving medications to match child's and family's routines. • Inform parents about potential side effects of prescribed medications and signs and symptoms of complications.	• Diuretics and antihypertensives are central to treatment plan. • Improves compliance. • Allows early intervention to prevent side effects.	The parents administer medications as prescribed.

the degree of ascites by measuring abdominal girth. Document urine specific gravity.

Prevent Infection

Impaired renal function places the child at risk for infection. Monitor for signs of infection, including fever, increased malaise, and an elevated white blood cell count. Instruct the family in good handwashing technique. Limit visitors, and screen for upper respiratory infections.

Prevent Skin Breakdown

Dependent areas or areas prone to pressure are vulnerable to skin breakdown. Turn the child frequently. Pad bony prominences or susceptible areas with sheepskin, or protect skin with a transparent dressing. Make sure the child's bed is free of crumbs or sharp toys. Keep sheets tight and free of wrinkles.

Meet Nutritional Needs

A team approach (including the nurse, renal dietitian, parents, and child) is often needed to meet the child's nutritional needs. In most cases a "no added salt" and low-protein diet is implemented. Anorexia presents the greatest challenge to meeting daily nutritional requirements during the acute phase of the disease. Encouraging parents to bring the child's favorite foods from home, to serve foods in age-appropriate quantities, and to allow the child to eat with other children or with family members may increase the child's appetite.

Provide Emotional Support

Guilt is a common reaction of parents of a child with APIGN. Parents may blame themselves for not responding more quickly to the child's initial symptoms or may believe they could have prevented the development of glomerular damage. Discuss the etiology of the disease and the child's treatment, and correct any misconceptions. Emphasize that APIGN develops in only a few children with streptococcal infection.

Discharge Planning and Home Care Teaching

Discharge planning focuses on teaching parents about the child's medication regimen, potential side effects of medications, dietary restrictions, and signs and symptoms of complications. Teach parents how to take the child's blood pressure and how to test urine for albumin, if ordered. Have them demonstrate these procedures. Emphasize that it is important to avoid exposing the child to individuals with upper respiratory tract infections. Recommend family screening for streptococcal infection if this is found to be the cause of the child's APIGN. After discharge, parents should be advised to allow the child to return to his or her normal routine and activities, with periods allowed for rest.

► STRUCTURAL DEFECTS OF THE REPRODUCTIVE SYSTEM

PHIMOSIS

In phimosis, the foreskin over the glans penis cannot be pulled back, due to adhesions or infection. Circumcision, surgical removal of the foreskin, is often performed during the newborn period to prevent phimosis, for ease of proper male hygiene, and to prevent urinary tract infections, balanitis (inflammation of the glans penis), and penile cancer. Approximately 12% of males who are not circumcised as newborns will eventually need the surgery.[24]

16-17	Discharge Teaching: Instructions Following Circumcision

- Wash hands well before and after each diaper change.
- The penis is wrapped in a bandage with petroleum jelly for the first 24 hours. To remove the bandage, soak it by dribbling water from a wet washcloth. Wet the bandage until it can be removed without disturbing the crust or clot.
- To keep the penis from sticking to the diaper, apply petroleum jelly to the head of the penis with each diaper change until the redness goes away.
- A pale yellow crust around the incision site is normal for 3–4 days after surgery.
- Call the physician if any of the following occur: bleeding that will not stop, swelling that lasts for more than 2 days, or signs of infection (tenderness after healing has started, or foul smelling drainage).

Information from Ball, J.B. (1998). Mosby's pediatric patient teaching guides. St. Louis: Mosby; and L'Archevesque, C.I., & Goldstein-Lohman, H. (1996). Ritual circumcision: Educating parents. Pediatric Nursing, 22(3), 228–234.

Nursing management involves preoperative preparation of the infant, including the advocacy for and assistance in giving the newborn local anesthesia. Teach parents to care for the surgical site, as newborns are discharged within 24–48 hours of surgery (Table 16–17).[25, 26]

CRYPTORCHIDISM

Cryptorchidism (undescended testes) occurs when one or both testes fail to descend through the inguinal canal into the scrotum. Normally, the testes descend during the seventh to ninth month of gestation.

Cryptorchidism may be the result of a testosterone deficiency, an absent or defective testis, or a structural problem such as a narrow inguinal canal, short spermatic cord, or adhesions. The disorder occurs in 3–4% of term male infants and in approximately 30% of premature infants.[27] The higher temperature in the abdomen than in the scrotum results in morphologic change to the testis, beginning after the second birthday. Lower sperm counts are the ultimate result.

Cryptorchidism is usually detected during the newborn examination when palpation of the scrotum fails to reveal one or both testes (see Fig. 3–42). It is not unusual for boys with cryptorchidism to have an inguinal hernia as well. In 75% of cases, the testes descend spontaneously by 9–12 months of age. If descent does not occur within the first year, human chorionic gonadotropin may be prescribed to induce testicular descent. An orchiopexy is performed between 1 and 2 years of age if hormone therapy is ineffective. An incision is made at the location of the testis, either in the abdomen or in the inguinal area. Blood vessels are disentangled to allow the testis to reach into the lower scrotum. A second incision is made in the scrotum at the point where the testis is stitched to the inside wall to keep it in place. If the testis is defective or undeveloped, it may be removed surgically to decrease the risk of later malignancies and a prosthesis may be placed in the scrotum.[28] The goals of surgery are repair of any hernia, enhanced fertility, and psychologic benefit. The orchiopexy also makes it easier to examine the testis for the presence of a tumor.

COMPLICATIONS OF UNCORRECTED CRYPTORCHIDISM

- Infertility
- Malignancy in undescended testis
- Torsion of the undescended testis
- Atrophy
- Psychologic effects of "empty" scrotum

Nursing Management

Preoperative nursing care includes preparing the parents and child for the procedure and addressing parents' concerns about the postsurgical outcome. Orchiopexy is often performed as an outpatient procedure. If the child is hospitalized, postoperative nursing care focuses on maintaining comfort and preventing infection. Encourage bedrest, and monitor voiding. Apply ice to the surgical area, and administer prescribed analgesics to relieve pain.

Discharge instructions should include demonstration of proper incision care. The diaper area should be cleaned well with each diaper change to decrease chances of infection. Teach parents to identify signs of infection such as redness, warmth, swelling, and discharge. All vigorous activity should be restricted for 2 weeks following surgery to promote healing and prevent injury.

INGUINAL HERNIA AND HYDROCELE

An inguinal hernia is a painless inguinal or scrotal swelling of variable size. A hydrocele is a fluid-filled mass in the scrotum. The condition is found in 1–5% of infants. Girls may have a hernia in the inguinal area, but this is uncommon.

During fetal development, a peritoneal sac precedes the testicle's descent to the scrotum. The lower sac enfolds the testis to become the tunica vaginalis, and the upper sac atrophies before birth. Fluid may become trapped in the tunica vaginalis and cause the hydrocele. When the tunica vaginalis does not atrophy, an abdominal structure may move into it.

Diagnosis is made by physical examination at the time of birth. On palpation of the scrotum, a round, smooth, nontender mass is noted. Transillumination is used to help determine whether the mass is a hernia or hydrocele (see Chap. 3, p. 154). Swelling associated with a hernia may become more apparent with straining. Some hernias reduce in size during sleep.

Outpatient surgery is performed at an early age to avoid incarceration, which is a medical emergency. The prognosis is generally excellent. Most hydroceles without inguinal hernia resolve spontaneously as the fluid reabsorbs by the time an infant is 1–2 years of age.

Nursing care for hydrocele and inguinal hernia includes explaining the disorder and its treatment and providing preoperative and postoperative teaching and care. Inform parents that the scrotum may be edematous and may appear bruised after surgery. Care of the incision involves application of a protective sealant; no dressing is applied.

NURSING ALERT

Inguinal hernias can become incarcerated when a bit of bowel becomes trapped in the inguinal opening. The child has a sudden painful swelling in the groin, increased irritability, vomiting, and abdominal distention. A bowel obstruction is seen on x-ray. Efforts are made to reduce the hernia before surgery, by placing the child in the Trendelenburg position and applying ice on the affected side.

TESTICULAR TORSION

Testicular torsion is an emergency condition in which the testis suddenly rotates, cutting off its blood supply. The arteries and veins in the spermatic cord become twisted, leading to vascular engorgement and ischemia. The incidence is highest at puberty; however, the condition may occur at any time between 3 and 20 years of age. Often the testicles are positioned horizontally in the scrotum, a situation known as a bell clapper deformity, which predisposes the boy to this condition.

Manifestations include severe pain and erythema in the scrotum, nausea and vomiting, and scrotal swelling that is not relieved by rest or scrotal support. A testicular scan or sonogram may be performed, if necessary to confirm the diagnosis.

Torsion must be reduced within 6 hours to save the testis. Manual reduction with an analgesic is sometimes attempted. More often emergency surgery is performed. During surgery, the testis is untwisted and stitched to the side of the scrotum in the correct position. The procedure is usually performed bilaterally to prevent future torsion in the other testis.

Nursing management involves psychologic support for the child and family related to the need for emergency surgery and concern about the child's future fertility. Reassure parents that as only one testis is usually affected, fertility should not be affected. The child often goes home within 8 hours of surgery; thus, the child and family need to be taught about proper care of the incision and pain management. Explain to parents that the child should not participate in strenuous activity for 2 weeks after surgery to promote healing.

► SEXUALLY TRANSMITTED DISEASES

Over the past 10 years, sexually transmitted diseases (STDs) have become a major national public health concern. There are presently more than 20 organisms of bacterial, parasitic, and viral origin, including human immunodeficiency virus (HIV), that are identified as causative agents of STDs.[29] (Refer to Chapter 9 for a discussion of acquired immunodeficiency syndrome [HIV infection].)

It is the combined responsibility of the federal, state, and local health departments to control and prevent STDs. On a national level, the Centers for Disease Control and Prevention (CDC) and the National Institutes of Health (NIH) coordinate control plans, provide surveillance, and fund basic science and clinical research. State and local health departments are responsible for controlling the spread of STDs through health-promotion programs, staff training, reporting systems, diagnosis, treatment, patient counseling, and the notification of sex partners.

Children and adolescents can become infected with sexually transmitted organisms through sexual experimentation, sexual play, molestation, and sexual abuse. Adolescents are considered an at-risk population because of their inexperience and lack of knowledge about STDs. They may disregard the importance of using barriers, may have multiple sexual partners, may have sex frequently, and often do not seek medical treatment until symptoms are well advanced.

Approximately 50% of adolescents who are 16 years of age have had sexual intercourse. This number increases to 70% by 19 years of age. More than half of the STDs reported occur in adolescents and young adults under the age of 25 years. Three million adolescents are infected with an STD each year.[30] The most frequently diagnosed STDs are chlamydia, genital herpes (herpes simplex type 2), gonorrhea, and syphilis (Table 16–18). Adolescents represent 1% of the population infected with HIV. However, there are increased numbers of individuals in the 20–29-year-old population group who may have become infected initially during their teen years.

Complications of STDs include pelvic inflammatory disease, infertility, high risk for ectopic pregnancy, and genital cancer. STDs causing an ulcerative lesion have been shown to increase the risk for HIV infection.[32] De-

LEGAL & ETHICAL CONSIDERATIONS

When a child is found to have an STD, the law requires that a report be made to social services and the local health department and that an investigation take place.

NURSING ALERT

When a child younger than 10 years of age is found to have gonorrhea, consider the possibility of sexual abuse. Whenever anorectal symptoms are found, suspect molestation.

Disease	Clinical Manifestations	Medical and Nursing Management
Chlamydia Causative organism: *Chlamydia trachomatis.* Incubation period: 5–10 days. Reportable: In most states.	*C. trachomatis* is most frequent cause of nongonococcal urethritis. Common symptoms include: Adolescent females: yellow-green mucopurulent endocervical discharge, cervicitis, salpingitis, pelvic inflammatory disease (PID). Adolescent males: urethritis, yellow-white discharge, dysuria, proctitis, epididymitis.	Recommended drug therapy includes doxycycline, tetracycline, erythromycin, or azithromycin for 7 days. Sexual partners should be treated if adolescent has had sexual contact within 30 days of onset of symptoms. Encourage use of condoms.
Genital herpes Causative organism: Herpes simplex virus (HSV-2). Incubation period: 2–12 days. Reportable: No.	Presentation can be variable and ranges from no symptoms to systemic involvement. A single lesion or a small cluster of papules appears anywhere on the genitalia, buttocks, or thighs. Papules develop into vesicles and pustules, and eventually ulcers. Ulcers can appear between vaginal folds, in posterior cervix, on glans penis or shaft of penis, in rectum, or in anus. Intense itching is followed by pain when ulcers break. Ulcers heal within 12 days. Lymph nodes closest to lesions are frequently enlarged. Disease frequently recurs.	Recommended drug therapy is acyclovir given for 7–10 days. Occasionally acyclovir is applied directly to lesions. Discourage oral sex if ulcers are present in mouth, on lips, in vagina, or on penis. Discourage anal sex when lesions are active. Encourage use of condoms.
Gonorrhea Causative organism: *Neisseria gonorrhoeae.* Incubation period: 2–7 days. Reportable: Mandatory.	Symptoms and severity vary from mild to severe and are different for males and females. In females, areas that can be infected include urethra, cervix, fallopian tubes, and Bartholin and Skene glands. In males, areas include urethra, prostate, seminal vesicles, epididymis, and Littre and Cowper glands. Classic sign is discharge from vagina or urethra; however, infections involving conjunctivae, pharynx, and anus are also seen. Prepubescent girls: heavy, thick green or creamy vaginal discharge, vulvovaginitis. Adolescent girls: purulent vaginal discharge, cervicitis, PID. Fallopian tube involvement can lead to sterility. Prepubescent and adolescent boys: yellow puslike urethral discharge, erythematous meatus, frequency, dysuria.	Recommended drug therapy includes ceftriaxone or spectinomycin IM given once and followed by 7-day course of doxycycline. For *N. gonorrhoeae* that is non-penicillin resistant, a single dose of spectinomycin is given followed by doxycycline. Sexual partners should be treated. Follow-up cultures should be obtained 4–7 days after treatment. Encourage use of condoms.
Syphilis Causative organism: *Treponema pallidum.* Incubation period: 3 weeks. Reportable: Mandatory.	Appearance of classic signs and symptoms of syphilis depends on stage of disease. *Primary stage* manifests as single lesion that appears at invasion site approximately 2 weeks to 3 months after infection. Lesion appears as ulcer that has indurated border and smooth base (chancre). It is painless and can appear on labia, within vagina, on glans penis, in anus, or on lips or tongue. Lymphadenopathy is usually present. Lesion spontaneously heals within 5 weeks. *Second stage* appears up to 10 weeks after initial infection. Child develops malaise, patchy alopecia, and diffuse rash.[1] Lesions of rash can be macular, papular, papulosquamous, or bullous. Lesions on the palms and soles are classic. Flat mucous patches called condylomata lata appear on genitals.[30,31] *Latent stage* follows beginning of second stage by about 6 weeks. Latent phase can last for several years or be lifelong.[30] *Tertiary stage* occurs more than 2 years after onset and manifests as neurosyphillis, cardiovascular disease, or congenital syphillis.	Recommended drug therapy includes single IM injection of benzathine penicillin G. For children allergic to penicillin, erythromycin is given by mouth for 15 days. Saline compresses and a topical antibiotic are often used to treat lesions on skin. Treat all sexual contacts. Encourage use of condoms plus spermicidal foams, cream, or jelly.

16-19   Patient Teaching: Preventing STDs

- Limit the number of sexual contacts.
- Always use condoms for vaginal and anal intercourse.
- Refrain from oral sex if partner has active sores in mouth, vagina, or anus or on penis.
- Reduce high-risk sexual behaviors.

spite advances in treatment, which have prolonged the survival of individuals with AIDS, HIV infection is ultimately fatal.

The nurse usually encounters the child, adolescent, and family in the emergency department, outpatient clinic, or nursing unit. Because adolescents are often afraid of the consequences of reporting symptoms, it is important for the nurse to develop good assessment skills, particularly when asking questions about sexual activity, partners, and the possibility of abuse. When a child or adolescent is diagnosed with one STD, it is important to screen for others as these diseases may coexist.

Nursing care focuses on identifying the cause and the organism, providing appropriate treatment, preventing transmission and complications, and educating the child, adolescent, and family (Table 16–19). Encourage sexually active adolescents to receive hepatitis B immunization. When counseling the adolescent, reinforce the importance of treating all sexual partners involved and modifying high-risk sexual behaviors. Be supportive and understanding—never judgmental.

REFERENCES

1. Rudolph, A.M., Hoffman, J.I.E., & Rudolph, C.D. (1996). *Rudolph's pediatrics* (20th ed.). Stamford, CT: Appleton & Lange.

2. Feeg, V., & Harbin, R.E. (1991). *Pediatric core curriculum and resource manual.* Pitman, NJ: Anthony J. Jannetti.

3. Paulozzi, L.J., Erickson, J.D., & Jackson, R.J. (1997). Hypospadias trends in two US surveillance systems. *Pediatrics, 100*(5), 831–834.

4. Becker, N., & Avner, E.D. (1995). Congenital neuropathies and uropathies. *Pediatric Clinics of North America, 42*(6), 1319–1341.

5. Miller, K.L. (1996). Urinary tract infections: Children are not small adults. *Pediatric Nursing, 22*(6), 473–480, 544.

6. Goldsmith, B.M., & Campos, J.M. (1990). Comparison of urine dipstick, microscopy, culture for detection of bacteriuria in children. *Clinical Pediatrics, 29,* 214–218.

7. Hoberman, A., & Wald, E.R. (1997). UTI in young children: New light on old questions. *Contemporary Pediatrics, 14*(11), 140–156.

8. Edelmann, C.M. (1988). Urinary tract infection and vesicoureteral reflux. *Pediatric Annals, 17,* 9.

9. Rosenfeld, D.L., Fleischer, M., Yudd, A., & Makowsky, T. (1995). Current recommendations for children with urinary tract infections. *Clinical Pediatrics, 34*(5), 261–264.

10. Sobata, A.E. (1984). Inhibition of bacterial adherence by cranberry juice, potential use for the treatment of urinary tract infections. *Journal of Urology, 131,* 1013.

11. Kelleher, R.E. (1997). Daytime and night time wetting in children: A review of management. *Journal of the Society of Pediatric Nurses, 2*(2), 73–82.

12. Maizels, M., Gandhi, K., Keating, B., & Rosenbaum, D. (1993). Diagnosis and treatment for children who cannot control urination. *Current Problems in Pediatrics, 23,* 402–450.

13. Garber, K.M. (1996). Enuresis: An update on diagnosis and management. *Journal of Pediatric Health Care, 10*(5), 202–208.

14. Gilman, C.M., & Mooney, K.H. (1994). Alterations in renal and urinary tract function in children. In K.L. McCance, & S.E. Huether (Eds.), *Pathophysiology: The biologic basis for disease in adults and children* (2nd ed., pp. 1269–1270). St. Louis: Mosby.

15. Kelsch, R.C., & Sedman, A.B. (1993). Nephrotic syndrome. *Pediatrics in Review, 14*, 33.

16. Mendoza, S.A., & Tune, B.M. (1995). Management of the difficult nephrotic patient. *Pediatric Clinics of North America, 42*(6), 1459–1468.

17. Vogt, B.A. (1997). Identifying kidney disease: Simple steps can make a difference. *Contemporary Pediatrics, 14*(3), 115–127.

18. Taylor, J.H. (1996) End stage renal disease in children: Diagnosis, management, and interventions. *Pediatric Nursing, 22*(6), 481–490.

19. National Institute of Diabetes, Digestive, and Kidney Diseases. (1995) U.S. Renal Data System 1995 annual report: Pediatric end stage renal disease (pp. 109–125). Bethesda, MD: Author.

20. Evans, E.D., Greenbaum, L.A., & Ettenger, R.B. (1995). Principles of renal replacement therapy in children. *Pediatric Clinics of North America, 42*(6), 1579–1602.

21. Bereket, G., & Fine, R.N. (1995). Pediatric renal transplantation. *Pediatric Clinics of North America, 42*(6), 1603–1628.

22. Holliday, M.A., Barratt, T.M., & Avner, E.D. (1994). *Pediatric nephrology* (3rd ed., pp. 472–485). Baltimore: Williams & Wilkins.

23. Siegel, R.L. (1995). The hemolytic uremic syndrome. *Pediatric Clinics of North America, 42*(6), 1505–1529.

24. Williamson, M.L. (1997). Circumcision anesthesia: A study of nursing implications for dorsal penile nerve blocks. *Pediatric Nursing, 23(1), 59–63.*

25. Ball, J.B. (1998). *Mosby's pediatric patient teaching guides*. St. Louis: Mosby.

26. L'Archevesque, C.I., & Goldstein-Lohman, H. (1996). Ritual circumcision: Educating parents. *Pediatric Nursing, 22*(3), 228–234.

27. Fonkalsrud, E.W. (1996). Current management of the undescended testis. *Seminars in Pediatric Surgery, 5*(1), 2–7.

28. Tanagho, E.A., & McAninch, J.W. (1995). *Smith's general urology* (14th ed.). Stamford, CT: Appleton & Lange.

29. Last, J.M., & Wallace, R.B. (1992). *Public health and preventive medicine* (13th ed.). Norwalk, CT: Appleton & Lange.

30. Coles, F.B., & Hipp, S.S. (1996). Syphilis among adolescents: The hidden epidemic. *Contemporary Pediatrics, 13*(6), 47–62.

31. Bondi, E.E., Jesothy, B.V., & Lazarus, C.S. (1991). *Dermatology: Diagnosis and therapy*. Norwalk, CT: Appleton & Lange.

32. Sieving, R., Resnick, M.D., Bearinger, L., Remafedi, G., Taylor, B.A., & Harmon, B. (1997). Cognitive and behavioral predictors of sexually transmitted disease risk behavior among sexually active adolescents. *Archives of Pediatric Medicine, 151*(3), 243–251.

ADDITIONAL RESOURCES

Castiglia, P.T. (1987). Nocturnal enuresis. *Journal of Pediatric Health Care, 1*, 280.

Druschel, C.M. (1995). A descriptive study of prune belly in New York State, 1983–1989. *Archives of Pediatrics and Adolescent Medicine, 149*(1), 70–79.

Fedewa, M.M., & Oberst, M.T. (1996). Family caregiving in a renal transplant population. *Pediatric Nursing, 22*(5), 402–407, 417.

Frauman, A.C., & Gilman, C.M. (1990). Care of the family of the child with end stage renal disease. *ANNA Journal, 17*, 383–386.

Hellerstein, S. (1995). Urinary tract infections: Old and new concepts. *Pediatric Clinics of North America, 42*(6), 1433–1457.

Koff, S.A. (1994). Obstructive uropathy: Clinical aspects. In M.A. Holliday, T.M. Barratt, & E.D. Avner (Eds.), *Pediatric nephrology* (3rd ed., pp. 1005–1017). Baltimore: Williams & Wilkins.

McNamara, E., Pike, N., Gettys, C., & Corbo-Richert, B. (1996). Organ transplants. In P.L. Jackson, & J.A. Vessey (Eds.), *Primary care of the child with a chronic condition* (2nd ed, pp. 598–622). St. Louis: Mosby.

Pan, C.G. (1997). Glomerulonephritis in childhood. *Current Opinion in Pediatrics, 9*, 154–159.

Radebough, L.C. (1986). Nursing care of the infant with bladder exstrophy. *AUAA Journal, 2*, 14–15.

Ribby, K.J., & Cox, K.R. (1997). Organization and development of a pediatric end stage renal disease teaching guide protocol for peritoneal dialysis. *Pediatric Nursing, 23*(4), 393–399.

Strupp, T.W. (1988). Post shock resuscitation of the trauma victim: Preventing and managing acute renal failure. *Critical Care Nurse Quarterly, 11,* 1–9.

Sugar, E.C., Firlit, C.F., & Reisman, M. (1993). Pediatric hypospadias surgery. *Pediatric Nursing, 19*(6), 585–588, 615.

Taylor, J.H. (1996). Renal failure, chronic. In P.A. Jackson, & J.A. Vessey (Eds.), *Primary care of the child with a chronic condition* (2nd ed., pp. 689–716). St. Louis: Mosby.

Wilson, D., & Killion, D. (1989). Urinary tract infections in the pediatric patient. *Nurse Practitioner, 14,* 38–42.

Winslow, B.H., & Devine, C.J. (1996). Principles in repair of hypospadias. *Seminars in Pediatric Surgery, 5*(1), 41–48.

Wiseman, K.C. (1991). Nephrotic syndrome: Pathophysiology and treatment. *ANNA Journal, 188,* 469–476.

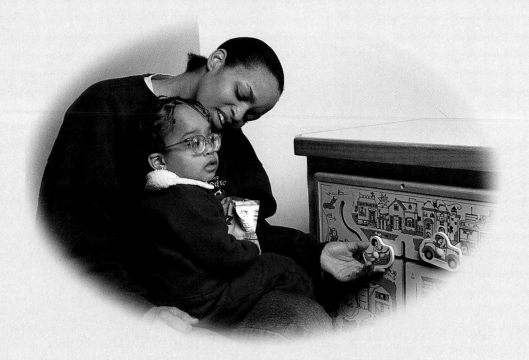

Raeanne, 3 years old, has a severe visual impairment. Born prematurely at 25 weeks of gestation, she received oxygen therapy, which damaged her retinal blood vessels. As a result, Raeanne developed retinopathy of prematurity. While in the hospital, Raeanne was given frequent ophthalmoscopic examinations. She received cryotherapy to the retinal vessels—a treatment designed to prevent detached retinae and the resulting total vision loss. Although this treatment halted progression of the disorder, Raeanne was left severely myopic (nearsighted).

For the first 3 years of life, Raeanne and her mother attended an early-intervention program, which provided stimulation for Raeanne and helped teach her mother techniques for enhancing her developmental progress. Raeanne will soon begin attending preschool. Her speech is well developed for a 3-year-old; she is socially mature, converses readily, and shows no developmental delays. However, she has had little contact with other children.

As the nurse in the preschool Raeanne will be attending, how will you assist both her parents and the preschool staff in facilitating Raeanne's adaptation to the preschool experience? Your role includes helping her parents to prepare her for this new experience. You also provide information to the other preschool staff members to help them ensure a safe environment for Raeanne, assist her in adjustment to working and playing in a group of children, and foster her development.

ALTERATIONS IN EYE, EAR, NOSE, AND THROAT FUNCTION

17

"The early-intervention program that Raeanne and I attended helped her develop the skills she'll need for preschool, but I know this will still be a big step for her. The nurse has been working with us to help prepare Raeanne to meet this new challenge."

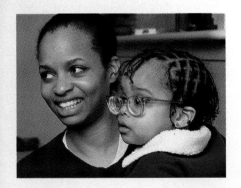

TERMINOLOGY

- **audiography** A test used to assess hearing in which sounds of various pitches and intensity are presented to children through earphones.
- **binocularity** Ability of the eyes to function together.
- **conductive hearing loss** Hearing loss caused by inadequate conduction of sound from the outer to the middle ear.
- **decibels** Units used to measure the loudness of sounds.
- **mixed hearing loss** Hearing loss having a combination of conductive and sensorineural causes.
- **myringotomy** A procedure whereby an incision is made in the tympanic membrane to drain fluid.
- **sensorineural hearing loss** Hearing loss caused by damage to the inner ear structures or the auditory nerve.

- **tympanogram** A graph showing the ability of the middle ear to transmit sound energy; measured by inserting an airtight probe into the external ear entrance and emitting a tone.
- **tympanotomy tubes** Small Teflon tubes inserted surgically into the tympanic membrane to equalize pressure, promote fluid drainage, and ventilate the middle ear.
- **visual acuity** Measurement of the ability to discriminate a letter or other object to test sight.
- **vision** A complex process of acquiring meaning from what is seen, involving the eye, brain, and related neurologic and physiologic structures.

How are conditions of the eye, ear, nose, and throat related? Which conditions have the potential to affect a child's growth, development, and behavior? In what settings do children with eye, ear, nose, and throat conditions receive care?

Because the eye, ear, nose, and throat are connected, a malformation, infection, or other condition in one of these structures may affect them all. Intact sensory structures are necessary for attainment of developmental milestones; thus alterations, especially to the eye and ear, may delay a child's development. In the preceding scenario, Raeanne's condition was diagnosed when she was very young, and she was enrolled in a program to help her develop normally. Although Raeanne received her initial diagnosis and treatment in the hospital, most children with eye, ear, nose, and throat disorders are treated at home or in the community rather than in the hospital.

▶ ANATOMY AND PHYSIOLOGY OF PEDIATRIC DIFFERENCES

EYE

How are the eyes of children different from those of adults? Chapter 3 provides a detailed discussion of the assessment of the eyes and visual acuity. The eyes of neonates differ from the eyes of adults in several ways. Visual acuity in neonates ranges between 20/100 and 20/400. The lens is more spherical and cannot accommodate to both near and far objects, which means that the neonate sees best at a distance of about 8 in. (20 cm). Since the optic nerve is not yet completely myelinated, the ability to distinguish color and other details is decreased. If the infant is preterm, especially less than 32 weeks' gestation, retinal vascularization, particularly in the periphery of the retina, may be incomplete. The rectus muscles that control binocular vision may be somewhat uncoordinated at birth. The eyes should be aligned and movement coordinated by the age of 3 months.

The eyeball of the infant and young child occupies a larger portion of the orbit than in the adult. Since the eyeball is relatively unprotected laterally, it is more easily injured. The sclera of the neonate is thin and translucent with a bluish tinge, and the iris is blue or gray. Eye color changes during the first 6 months of life. Infants produce tears to nourish and oxygenate the outer layers of the cornea. Parents do not see tears when a young infant cries because the infant's lacrimal system drains them efficiently into the nasal cavity.

As infants grow, their eyes mature and their vision improves. By the age of 2 or 3 years, most children have a visual acuity of 20/50, and by the age of 6 or 7 years, it is 20/20. **Visual acuity,** the ability to discriminate letters or other objects, is measured using standardized letter or picture charts. (See Chapter 3 and the *Quick Reference to Pediatric Clinical Skills* accompanying this text.) **Vision** refers to the complex process of acquiring meaning from what is seen, involving the eye, brain, and related neurologic and physiologic structures. Development interacts with a child's maturing physiologic system to bring increasing meaning to objects in sight (Table 17–1).[1]

EAR

Why do infants and young children have more ear problems than adults? The eustachian tube, which connects the nasopharynx to the middle ear, is proportionately shorter, wider, and more horizontal in infants than in older children or adults (Fig. 17–1). During sucking, yawning, and other move-

17-1   Visually Related Developmental Milestones

Age	Milestone
Term neonate	Demonstrates alertness to visual stimulus presented 8–12 in. (20–30 cm) from eyes
1 month	Follows an object 60 degrees horizontally and 30 degrees vertically; blinks at an approaching object
2 months	Follows a person from 6 ft (2 m) away; smiles in response to a face; raises head 30 degrees from prone
3 months	Tracks an object through 180 degrees; regards own hand; begins visual-motor coordination
4–5 months	Social smile; reaches for a cube 12 in. (30 cm) away; notices a raisin 12 in. (30 cm) away
7–8 months	Picks up a raisin by raking
8–9 months	Pokes at holes in a peg board; neat pincer grasp; crawling
12–14 months	Stacks blocks; places a peg in a round hole; stands and walks

From Scheiner, A.P. (1996). Vision problems: Impairment to blindness. In A.M. Rudolph, J.I.E. Hoffman, & C.D. Rudolph (Eds.), Rudolph's pediatrics (20th ed., p. 167). Stamford, CT: Appleton & Lange.

ments, the tube opens for milliseconds, allowing free passage of air between the nasopharynx and the middle ear.

The external ear canal is small at birth, although the internal ear and middle ear are relatively large. As a result, the tympanic membrane is close to the surface and can be easily injured.

NOSE AND THROAT

Up to the age of 6 months, infants breathe primarily through the nose and not through the mouth. Edema and nasal discharge may interfere with adequate air intake and feeding. Mucosal swelling and exudate may block the small nasal passages of young children.

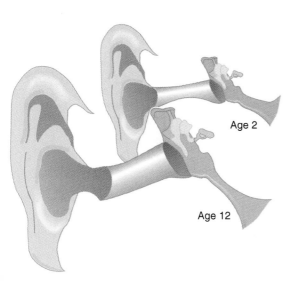

Position of eustachian tube is at a lesser angle in the young child, resulting in decreased drainage.

Age 2

End of eustachian tube in nasal pharynx opens during sucking.

Age 12

Eustachian tube equalizes air pressure between the middle ear and the outside environment and allows for drainage of secretions from middle ear mucosa.

FIGURE 17–1. Of the three anatomic differences in the eustachian tube between adults and small children (shorter, wider, more horizontal), which do you think could cause more problems for the child and why? Answer: More horizontal. Small children who are bottle-fed in a supine position have a greater probability of developing otitis media because the eustachian tube opens when the child sucks and the horizontal angle of the tube provides easy access to the middle ear. In older children the greater angle helps keep foreign substances and germs away from the middle ear.

The palatine tonsils, which are visible on oral examination, are located on each side of the oropharynx. The method for examining a child's throat is given in Chapter 3. Although tonsils vary in size considerably during childhood, they are normally large, especially in school-age children. The nasopharyngeal tonsils (adenoids) lie in the posterior wall of the nasopharynx, just above the oropharynx. In children, the adenoids may become enlarged, harboring bacteria and interfering with breathing.

▶ DISORDERS OF THE EYE

INFECTIOUS CONJUNCTIVITIS

Conjunctivitis is an inflammation of the conjunctiva, the clear membrane that lines the inside of the lid and sclera. Bacteria, viruses, allergies, trauma, or irritants cause the conjunctiva to become swollen and red with a yellow or white discharge (Fig. 17–2).

Conjunctivitis in an infant under 30 days of age is called ophthalmia neonatorum. These infections are usually acquired from the mother during vaginal delivery as a result of contact with infected vaginal discharge containing organisms such as *Chlamydia trachomatis* and *Neisseria gonorrhoeae*.[2] Prevention is of key importance; therefore, antibiotics are instilled into the eyes of all newborns soon after birth. For the infection caused by herpesvirus, prompt and vigorous treatment is needed to prevent eye injury or blindness, which can occur in children with recurrent herpesvirus infections as a result of antibody reaction to the viral antigen. Infants with herpesvirus infections of the eye are treated with intravenous acyclovir as well as topical drops.

In infants who have frequent tearing and "mattering" (eyelid discharge that has formed a crust) on awakening, a plugged lacrimal duct may mimic conjunctivitis. Treatment involves massaging the tear duct every 4 hours when the infant is awake. Lacrimal ducts that remain plugged after the age of 1 year may have to be opened surgically.

Older children with conjunctivitis complain of itching or burning, mild photophobia, and a feeling of scratching under the lids. Parents may notice increased tearing or a mucoid or mucopurulent discharge, redness and swelling of the conjunctiva, a pink sclera, and crusty eyelids, especially in the morning. There is no change in vision. Common infectious organ-

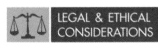

LEGAL & ETHICAL CONSIDERATIONS

By federal law, all infants born in the United States are given prophylactic eye treatment soon after delivery to help prevent ophthalmia neonatorum. It is the nurse's responsibility to administer this eye ointment. Penicillin, tetracycline, erthromycin, or povidone–iodine ointments are used.

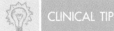

CLINICAL TIP

Sometimes an infant can develop a chemical conjunctivitis to the prophylactic eye ointment. A chemical reaction should be considered as a possible cause when conjunctivitis develops within 24–48 hours after instillation of the medication.

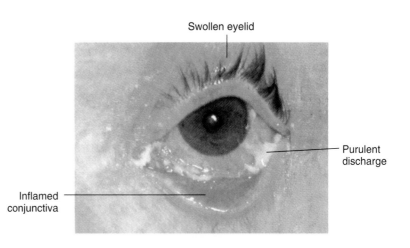

FIGURE 17–2. Acute conjunctivitis. The major difference between bacterial and viral conjunctivitis is that bacterial conjunctivitis has a purulent discharge that may result in crusting whereas discharge from viral conjunctivitis is serous (watery). Allergic conjunctivitis produces watery to thick drainage and is characterized by itching.
Adapted from Newell, F.W. (1996). Ophthalmology: Principles and concepts (8th ed.). St. Louis: Mosby–Year Book.

isms in older children include *Streptococcus pneumoniae, Haemophilus aegyptius,* and *Staphylococcus aureus.*[3]

When conjunctivitis is caused by an allergy, the child complains of intense itching. On examination, red eyes with watery discharge are observed. The eyes can also be puffy and swollen.

Antibiotic eye drops are prescribed if a bacterial infection is suspected. Instructions for instilling eye drops are given in the *Quick Reference to Pediatric Clinical Skills* accompanying this text. If an allergen is believed to be the cause, antihistamines administered orally or as drops may be prescribed. Topical steroids and vasoconstrictors may also be used.[4]

Nursing Management

Since infectious conjunctivitis is extremely contagious, tell parents that children should not return to school until they have been taking an antibiotic for 24 hours. Teach parents the importance of careful handwashing and the avoidance of shared towels. Tell parents that children should not rub their eyes. Mittens may help prevent infants from rubbing their eyes. Toddlers may be distracted by activities that keep their hands busy. Teach parents the proper techniques for instilling eye medications. Exudate may need to be removed before drops or ointment is instilled. The child's head should be elevated to reduce swelling. For children with allergies, alert parents to signs of infection so if the child gets an eye infection, prompt treatment will be obtained.

PERIORBITAL CELLULITIS

Periorbital cellulitis is an infection of the eyelid and surrounding tissues that is usually caused by bacteria (Fig. 17–3). Children present with swollen, tender, red or purple eyelids; restricted, painful movement of the area around the eye; and fever. Periorbital cellulitis should be treated promptly to prevent the spread of the infection to the posterior orbit. Management includes hospitalization for intravenous administration of antibiotics and the application of hot packs. Children usually respond favorably within 48–72 hours.

VISUAL DISORDERS

Vision, the complex process of acquiring meaning from what is seen, depends on many factors. The eyes must move quickly and in a coordinated manner. (See Chapter 3 for discussion of eye movement assessment.) They must function together in order for clear, single vision to occur. If this ability, called **binocularity,** is not present (perhaps due to strabismus or amblyopia), the child cannot make sense of the images the brain receives.

CLINICAL TIP

Place a gloved index finger on the child's nose next to the inner corner of the eye and apply gentle pressure for several seconds. If mucopurulent drainage is discharged from the eye, conjunctivitis may be present.

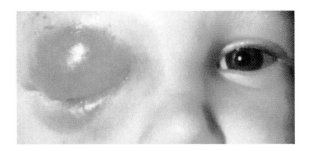

FIGURE 17–3. Periorbital cellulitis is an infection of the eyelid and surrounding tissues, not the eye itself. It is a serious bacterial infection that can spread to the optic nerve if not treated promptly with intravenous antibiotics. *From Malinow, I., & Powell, K.R. (1993). Periorbita cellulitis. Pediatric Annals, 22(4), 241–246.*

| 17-2 | Assessment Questions for Identifying Visual Disturbances in Children |

Young Child

Ask the parents:

Does your child follow you with his or her eyes as you come into a room?

Are other objects followed with ease?

Do both eyes work together or does one seem to wander off?

At what age did your baby sit, stand, walk?

Does your child have any difficulty picking up objects?

School-age Child

Ask the parents:

Does your child like to look at pictures and read?

Is he or she at grade level in all subjects?

Has your child demonstrated any learning difficulties?

Does he or she use a computer, watch television, or play computer games?

Does your child play sports and games at the same level of ability as peers?

Normally, the objects seen are integrated with other senses through eye–hand coordination, and with the brain through visual imagery and discrimination of objects seen. Although visual acuity is essential, the child's movements, mental processes, and other senses all interact to give meaning to objects that are viewed. Vision therefore, influences learning and school performance.

Visual disturbances must be diagnosed and treated promptly to prevent impairment or loss of visual acuity. Most children undergo a simple test for visual acuity during health care visits as soon as they can cooperate with the examiner. Once in school, children's visual acuity is screened every 2–3 years during the elementary years. Nurses often organize vision screening programs for children. Table 17–2 provides a series of questions that can be used to identify visual disturbances in children. A child who does not pass vision screening is referred to an ophthalmologist or optometrist for more detailed examination of near and far vision, eye structure and movement, and color discrimination.

Some of the common visual disorders in children are:

- *Hyperopia* (farsightedness): In which light rays focus posterior to the retina, resulting in an inability to focus on nearby objects. All children have some degree of hyperopia until 9–10 years of age. However, their eyes can accommodate sufficiently to enable them to see near objects clearly. Blurring of vision occurs only in children with excessive hyperopia, or a difference in accommodation between the two eyes. Amblyopia, or a weakening of the poorer eye, can occur in these children if treatment is not obtained.

- *Myopia* (nearsightedness): In which light rays focus anterior to the retina, resulting in an inability to see far-off objects. Although children of any age can manifest myopia, it most commonly develops at about 8 years of age. The child may complain of headaches and often squints to improve distance vision.

- *Astigmatism:* In which light rays are refracted differently depending on their place of entry to the eye. The curvature of the cornea or lens is distorted, causing blurred images. The child with astigmatism often holds pages very close to the face to obtain the best visual image.

The description and management of four disorders that can significantly affect vision—strabismus, amblyopia, cataracts, and glaucoma—are presented in Table 17–3.

Compensatory lenses are prescribed for most visual disorders. A significant difference in visual acuity between the eyes is often a result of amblyopia or strabismus, and further treatment may be needed (see Table 17–3). The visual acuity of a child with compensatory lenses should be reevaluated every 1–2 years. More frequent visits to an eye specialist are needed when a child is being treated for amblyopia or strabismus.

Color Blindness

Color blindness is an X-linked recessive disorder found in 8% of Caucasian and 4% of African-American males and almost never in females. The most common form affects the ability to distinguish between the colors red and green, but there are other variations. Preschool boys are often routinely tested for color blindness to identify those with the disorder. Color blindness is not treatable and management focuses on issues of safety (eg, problems in distinguishing red–green traffic signals) and techniques to improve discrimination of colors in the affected color groups.

RETINOPATHY OF PREMATURITY

Retinopathy of prematurity (ROP) occurs when immature blood vessels in the retina constrict and become necrotic. This condition, which may occur in infants of low birth weight or of short gestation, can heal completely or lead to mild myopia or retinal detachment and blindness.

Clinical Manifestations

Retinopathy of prematurity is characterized by progressive changes in the retinal blood vessels, and in severe disease, by retinal detachment. Premature and low-birth-weight infants at risk for the disease are given frequent ocular examinations to ensure early detection of these changes. For infants who do not receive ophthalmologic examinations, resulting visual impairment may be detected only later in infancy when the child progresses slowly in meeting developmental milestones, fails to reach for objects, and does not follow objects or faces with the eyes. When visual impairment is present, the child usually manifests myopia. Total loss of vision can occur in the child who suffers a retinal detachment.

Etiology and Pathophysiology

Retinopathy of prematurity results from injury to the developing capillaries of the retina.[5] Oxygen therapy is associated with the development of retinopathy of prematurity (Fig. 17–4), but other factors such as respiratory distress, artificial ventilation, apnea, bradycardia, heart disease, multiple blood transfusions, infection, hypoxia, hypercarbia, acidosis, shock, and sepsis have also been linked with the disorder. It is most common in infants born before 28 weeks of gestation and weighing under 1600 g (3 lb, 8 oz) at birth.

17-3 Visual Disorders

	Disorder	Treatment

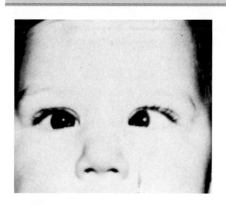

Strabismus.
From Newell, F.W., (1996). Ophthalmology: Principles and concepts (8th ed.). St. Louis: Mosby–Year Book.

Strabismus

Can be congenital or acquired.

Eyes appear misaligned to observer.

  Most common types:

    Esotropia: inward deviation of eyes ("crossed eyes")

    Exotropia: outward deviation of eyes ("wall-eyes")

May occur only when child is tired

Symptoms include: squinting and frowning when reading; closing one eye to see; having trouble picking up objects; dizziness and headache.

Corneal light reflex and cover–uncover tests confirm diagnosis.

Treatment:

Occlusion therapy (patching the fixating or good eye to force use of the weak eye)

Compensatory lenses

Surgery of the rectus muscles to correct muscle imbalance; should be performed only after eye patching

Eye drops to cause blurring of the good eye

Prisms

Vision therapy (eye exercises)

If treatment is begun before 24 months of age, amblyopia (reduced vision in one or both eyes) may be prevented.

Amblyopia ("lazy eye")

Reduced vision in one or both eyes

Amblyopia can result from untreated strabismus, with the child "tuning out" the image in deviating eye.

Symptoms are the same as for strabismus.

Vision testing can be used to diagnose condition.

Treatment:

Compensatory lenses

Occlusion therapy

Occasionally vision therapy (eye exercises) is used in an attempt to improve the weaker eye.

Treatment is discontinued when visual acuity no longer improves; 20/20 acuity rarely attained.

Treatment is most successful if done by 7–8 years of age.

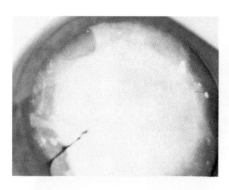

Congenital cataract.
From Vaughan, D., Asbury, T., & Riordan-Eva, P. (1992). General ophthalmology (13th ed., p. 172). Norwalk, CT: Appleton & Lange.

Cataracts

Occur when all or part of lens of eye becomes opaque, which prevents refraction of light rays onto retina

Can affect one or both eyes and may be congenital or acquired

Clouding of lens indicates presence of cataract; however, cataracts are not always visible to naked eye.

Symptoms include: distorted red reflex; symptoms of vision loss (see strabismus).

Treatment:

Specific treatment depends on whether one or both eyes are affected, extent of clouding, and presence of other ocular abnormalities.

Surgical removal of lens and corrective lenses; contact lenses frequently used; results of surgery are good; surgery before the age of 2 months is associated with the best results; visual acuity in 55% of children is 20/40 or better.

Lens implant may be used.

Eye protectors and restraints are used postoperatively to prevent injury; antibiotic or steroid drops may be used for several weeks; treatment for amblyopia may be necessary.

17-3 Visual Disorders (continued)

Disorder	Treatment

Glaucoma

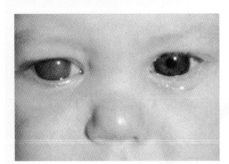

Congenital glaucoma.
From Vaughan, D., Asbury, T., & Riordan-Eva, P. (1992). General ophthalmology (13th ed., p. 172). Norwalk, CT: Appleton & Lange.

Increased intraocular pressure damages eye and impairs visual function; ciliary body of eye produces aqueous fluid that flows between iris and lens into anterior chamber; if enough fluid accumulates, blindness results.

May be congenital or acquired and affect one or both eyes

Symptoms of congenital glaucoma include: tearing, corneal clouding, eyelid spasms, and progressive enlargement of eye; photophobia (extreme sensitivity to light).

Symptoms of acquired glaucoma include: constant bumping into objects in child's periphery (painless visual field loss); seeing halos around objects.

Diagnosis is made using tonometer, which measures intraocular pressure.

Surgery to reduce intraocular pressure is treatment of choice, since medications used to combat glaucoma in adults are not effective in children.

Compensatory lenses used following surgery

Treatment is not always successful, especially if the child has congenital glaucoma, so parents' feelings regarding care of a visually handicapped child should be explored.

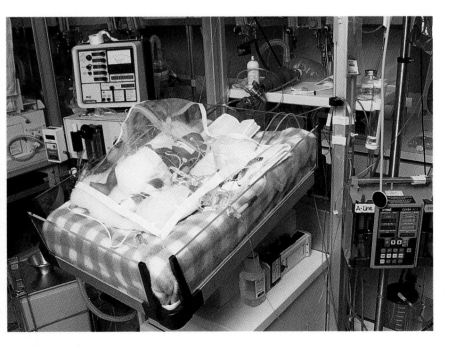

FIGURE 17–4. This premature infant in the neonatal intensive care unit is receiving artificial ventilation—a risk factor for retinopathy of prematurity. The infant will need careful management of oxygen exposure and periodic eye examinations.

The retina is normally vascularized by about 8 months' gestation. For the premature infant, however, this process must continue after birth and the environmental and other conditions listed in the preceding paragraph appear to affect its course. Arteriole constriction, followed by vascular proliferation of abnormal vessels, occurs. In most cases, the abnormal vessels gradually regress and normal vascularization occurs. Sometimes, however, the abnormal vascularization continues into the vitreous cavity, causing abnormalities of the retina, optic disc, and macula. It is not known why the disease progresses in some cases, but progression is directly linked to lower birth weight, greater prematurity, and duration (not necessarily concentration) of oxygen therapy. Raeanne, the child described in the scenario at the beginning of this chapter, developed retinopathy of prematurity after receiving oxygen therapy to aid her underdeveloped lungs.

Although the developing capillaries are lost, in up to 90% of cases, there is some degree of revascularization later.[6] The degree of visual loss, varying from slight to total, is determined by the degree of revascularization that occurs.

Diagnostic Tests and Medical Management

Diagnosis is made by ophthalmologic examination. A classification system is used to describe the location, extent, and severity of the disease.[6] All infants at risk, particularly those under 2000 g (4 lb, 3 oz) at birth or born before 33 weeks of gestation are assessed frequently by an ophthalmologist who is experienced with the condition. The disease does not manifest itself before 4–6 weeks after birth, so it is important that the infant receive regular eye examinations until the risk is discounted. If the infant shows signs of disease, eye examinations continue every 1–2 weeks. Involvement of blood vessels in the periphery of the retina rarely leads to visual impairment. With involvement in other areas of the retina, risk of visual problems is more common.

Treatment of infants with severe retinopathy of prematurity involves using cryotherapy or laser therapy to stop progression of the disease process. Other surgical procedures such as a scleral buckle procedure and vitrectomy have been used in retinal detachments. For children like Raeanne who have resulting visual impairment, it is important to treat problems such as strabismus, amblyopia, and myopia to promote maximal development.

Nursing Assessment

Assessment of the infant at risk for retinopathy of prematurity begins at birth by identifying infants who may require oxygen therapy. Look for risk factors such as prematurity and low birth weight. Assess the infant's breathing efforts and report any changes. Be certain the ventilation equipment is properly set to deliver the correct amount of oxygen. Note the cumulative risks in a particular case and suggest the need for a referral to an ophthalmologist, as necessary.

Nursing Diagnosis

The accompanying Nursing Care Plan outlines several nursing diagnoses for a child such as Raeanne with a visual impairment secondary to retinopathy of prematurity. Several other nursing diagnoses may be appropriate for an infant with the potential to develop retinopathy of prematurity or a child with resulting visual impairment. They include:

NURSING CARE PLAN
THE CHILD WITH A VISUAL IMPAIRMENT SECONDARY TO RETINOPATHY OF PREMATURITY

GOAL	INTERVENTION	RATIONALE	EXPECTED OUTCOME

1. Sensory/Perceptual Alteration related to retinopathy of prematurity

GOAL	INTERVENTION	RATIONALE	EXPECTED OUTCOME
The child will receive adequate sensory input	• Provide kinesthetic, tactile, and auditory stimulation during play and in daily care (eg, talking and playing). Provide music while bathing an infant using bells and other noises on each side of infant. Verbally describe to a child all actions being carried out by adult.	• Because visual sensory input is not present, the child needs input from all other senses to compensate and provide adequate sensory stimulation.	The child demonstrates minimal signs of sensory deprivation.

2. Risk for Injury related to impaired vision

GOAL	INTERVENTION	RATIONALE	EXPECTED OUTCOME
The child will be protected from safety hazards that can lead to injury.	• Evaluate environment for potential safety hazards based on age of child and degree of impairment. Be particularly alert to objects that give visual cues to their dangers (eg, stoves, fireplaces, candles). Eliminate safety hazards and protect the child from exposure. Take the child on a tour of new rooms, explaining safety hazards (eg, schools, hotel room, hospital room).	• The child may be at risk for injury related both to developmental stage and inability to visualize hazards.	The child will experience no injuries.

3. Risk for Altered Growth and Development related to impaired vision

GOAL	INTERVENTION	RATIONALE	EXPECTED OUTCOME
The child has experiences necessary to foster normal growth and development.	• Help parents plan early, regular social activities with other children.	• The visually impaired child benefits developmentally from contact with other children.	The child demonstrates normal growth and development milestones.

Continued . . .

- Sensory/Perceptual Alteration (Visual) related to destruction of retinal blood vessels
- Impaired Gas Exchange related to prematurity and immature lung development
- Alteration in Growth and Development related to lack of visual input to developing brain
- Altered Family Processes related to a child with a visual impairment

NURSING CARE PLAN
THE CHILD WITH A VISUAL IMPAIRMENT SECONDARY TO RETINOPATHY OF PREMATURITY– *Continued*

GOAL	INTERVENTION	RATIONALE	EXPECTED OUTCOME

3. Risk for Altered Growth and Development related to impaired vision (continued)

	INTERVENTION	RATIONALE	
	• Provide opportunities and encourage self-feeding activities.	• To obtain adequate nutrients, the child needs to feel comfortable feeding self.	
	• Provide an environment rich in sensory input.	• Sensory input is needed for normal development to occur.	
	• Assess growth and development during regular examinations to identify the child's strengths and needs.	• Regular examinations aid in early identification of growth problems or developmental delays, so that appropriate interventions can be planned.	

4. Risk for Ineffective Family Coping related to child with sensory impairment

GOAL	INTERVENTION	RATIONALE	EXPECTED OUTCOME
The family identifies methods for coping with their visually impaired child.	• Provide explanation of visual impairment as appropriate.	• The parents may feel guilt about the child's visual impairment, which can be allayed by knowledge of the cause.	The family successfully copes with the experience of having a visually impaired child.
	• Refer parents to organizations, early intervention programs, and other parents of visually impaired children.	• The parents will receive needed information and support from others.	
	• Assist parents to plan for meeting developmental, educational, and safety needs of their visually impaired child. Offer resources for changing home environment to assist visually impaired child.	• The child may require an enhanced environment in order to foster developmental progress.	

Nursing Management

The nurse plays an important role in preventing retinopathy of prematurity. Encourage early and regular prenatal care to prevent unnecessary premature births. Administer oxygen only to newborns who need it, and in the amount specified by the physician. Ensure that the proper ventilatory settings are used. Be alert for infants with multiple risk factors and refer them, when appropriate, for ophthalmologic examination. Parents of infants at risk for retinopathy of prematurity require information about the disorder, as well as support, as the long-term effects on the child's vision are often identified only after subsequent examinations as the child grows.

The accompanying Nursing Care Plan summarizes care for the child with a visual impairment resulting from retinopathy of prematurity. The nurse is instrumental in case management for such children. Reinforce to parents the importance of follow-up eye examinations. Teach methods of stimulating development for the visually impaired child (refer to the next section).

VISUAL IMPAIRMENT

Visual impairment accounts for 11% of chronic medical conditions in children. Legal blindness (defined as visual acuity of 20/200 or worse in the corrected eye or significantly reduced visual fields) occurs in 3–8 per 10,000 children. Many more children have visual impairment, or a visual acuity of between 20/70 and 20/200 in the best corrected eye.[7]

The manifestations of visual impairment depend on the cause and degree of the problem and the age of the child (Table 17–4). The child's eyes may appear crossed or watery, and the lids may be crusty. Verbal children may complain of itching, dizziness, headache, or blurred, double, or poor vision.

Many conditions discussed earlier in this chapter lead to temporary or permanent visual impairment. Infants who are premature, whose mothers were infected prenatally with rubella, toxoplasmosis, or other viruses, and who have certain congenital and hereditary conditions have a high risk of visual problems (Table 17–5). Fetal alcohol syndrome (FAS) is a major cause of visual disturbance; 90% of children with FAS have eye abnormalities.[8]

Medical management depends on the child's condition and may include surgery, medication, and supportive aids. In the case of a disorder that results in permanent visual impairment, an interdisciplinary team of specialists works with the child and family. Nurses have an important role in this team, as evidenced by the care provided to Raeanne, described at the beginning of this chapter.

NURSING ALERT

Nurses should be aware of the dangers of oxygen therapy and ventilatory support. Constant monitoring of the oxygen delivery and testing equipment is essential. Newborns in special care units should be shielded from light as much as possible, since light exposure may increase their susceptibility to retinopathy of prematurity.

NURSING ALERT

Both the Food and Drug Administration (FDA) and the American Academy of Ophthalmology have issued warnings to keep laser pointers away from infants and children. These devices can cause retinal damage if stared at for more than 10 seconds. Young children are at greater risk than adults because they fail to blink and avert their gaze in less than one-quarter of a second (the typical adult response).

17-4   Clinical Manifestations of Visual Impairment

Infants
May be unable to follow lights or objects

Do not make eye contact

Have a dull, vacant stare

Do not imitate facial expressions

Toddlers and Older Children
May rub, shut, or cover eyes

Tilt or thrust head forward

Blink frequently

Hold objects close

Bump into objects

Squint

17-5   Common Causes of Visual Impairment in Children

Congenital or Hereditary
Cataracts
Glaucoma
Tay–Sachs disease
Marfan syndrome
Down syndrome
Fetal alcohol syndrome
Prenatal infections (maternal infection)
  Rubella
  Toxoplasmosis
  Herpes simplex
Retinoblastoma

Acquired
Injury to eye or head
Infections
  Rubella
  Measles
  Chickenpox
Brain tumor
Retinopathy of prematurity
Cerebral palsy

GROWTH & DEVELOPMENT CONSIDERATIONS

Infants with visual impairment use kinesthesia, touch, and language to socialize. They will appreciate and use touch more than other children and will appreciate verbal explanations when others use nonverbal communication. Vision affects both fine and gross motor skills, so skills such as hand-to-mouth coordination and walking may be delayed in children who are visually impaired.

Nursing Assessment

Vision screening facilitates early detection and treatment of conditions that can lead to vision loss. Visual testing can be done at any age, including immediately after birth. Developmental milestones that require vision, such as following bright lights, reaching for objects, or looking at pictures in a book, can be used to assess vision. For children over the age of 3 years, visual acuity is most frequently measured by means of an age-appropriate acuity test. (See Chapter 3 and the *Quick Reference to Pediatric Clinical Skills* accompanying this text.) Visual fields and the ability to discriminate colors are tested at school age, when children can cooperate.

Children who are visually impaired may lag in development of cognitive and other skills. Sighted children learn the word "cup" using four senses—sight, touch, hearing, and taste—to obtain the information necessary to connect words with the objects they represent. In contrast, children with visual impairments rely on only three senses—touch, hearing, and taste. They learn concepts through differences in sounds, textures, and shapes.

Many visual disorders are linked with conditions that influence development. Thus, a child with cerebral palsy or fetal alcohol syndrome may need interventions to compensate for a visual disorder, as well as to meet normal developmental milestones.

Nursing Diagnosis

Nursing diagnoses for the child with impaired vision might include:

- Sensory/Perceptual Alteration (Visual) related to specific condition
- Risk for Injury related to poor vision

17-6	Strategies for Nurses Working With Visually Impaired Children

- Call the child's name and speak before touching the child.
- Tell the child when you are leaving the room.
- Describe what each procedure will feel like (eg, blood pressure cuff, otoscope).
- Let the child touch the equipment to establish familiarity.
- Describe what foods are present and their locations on the food tray.

- Risk for Altered Growth and Development related to visual impairment
- Risk for Ineffective Family Coping related to a child with a sensory impairment

Nursing Management

Table 17–6 outlines several strategies that can be used by nurses who work with visually impaired children. Nursing care focuses on encouraging the child's use of all senses, promoting socialization, helping parents to meet the child's developmental and educational needs, and providing emotional support to parents.[9] Refer the parents to an early intervention program as soon as the diagnosis is made.

Encourage Use of All Senses

Children who are partially sighted or blind use other senses to a great extent. Encouraging the use of the eyes as much as possible is important even if a child has poor vision.

- Encourage a toddler or preschooler who is visually impaired to look at pictures in well-lit settings. Have a school-age child read large-print books. Computers with large letters are also available. The Optacon (a device that raises print so it can be felt by the child) and View Scan (which magnifies print) are instruments that improve the ability to read.
- Expose the infant and child to everyday sounds.
- Suggest that the parents encourage the infant to use the sense of touch to explore people and objects. Have the parents purchase toys with sound and texture in mind. Directional concepts can be taught using games. Responding to the infant's and child's vocalizations encourages the use of speech.
- Teach specific techniques for toileting, dressing, bathing, eating, and safety.
- When the child becomes mobile, furniture and other objects in the environment should be kept in the same positions so the child can safely move around independently. Extra care must be taken to prevent injuries when a child does not see.
- Emphasize the child's abilities. Adolescents can use seeing-eye dogs or a white cane to function independently.
- If the child is in a hospital or another strange environment, orient the child to the placement of objects and do not rearrange them. Always announce your presence to the child when approaching. When walking

with a blind child, walk slightly ahead of the child so he or she can sense your movements, and let the child hold your arm rather than the reverse.

- Identify the contents of meal trays and encourage the child to feed self.
- Encourage the child to function independently within normal developmental parameters.

Promote Socialization

The child's interactions and socializations should be as normal as possible (similar to those of sighted children of the same age and development).

- Stroke, rock, and hug infants and children who are visually impaired. Sing and talk to them. These infants do not make eye contact and have rather blank expressions.

- Teach parents to read body language and vocalization as expressions of emotion. Facial expressions give a great deal of information, but infants and children with poor vision do not have the ability to learn by visual imitation. Show parents how to use tactile means to teach appropriate facial expressions. For example, a touch on the arm can be soft and stroking to indicate a smile, but firmer to indicate dismay or frown.

- Explain to parents that discipline and rewards for children with poor vision should be the same as those for other children in the family. The child should be given age-appropriate tasks.

- Encourage contact with peers as the child grows older. Teach the child to look directly at persons who are talking to him or her. Play, sports, and other activities can be modified to give the visually impaired child the same social experiences as a sighted child.

Help Parents to Meet Child's Educational Needs

Public laws require that each state provide educational and related services for children with disabilities (see Chap. 1). Parents and professionals should develop an Individualized Education Plan (as discussed in Chap. 5) that maximizes the child's learning ability. If possible, the child with a vision problem should attend day care and preschool with children who have normal visual acuity. What nursing actions are needed to help a child such as Raeanne, introduced at the beginning of this chapter, in adjusting to day care or school?

- Provide parents with information about educational options before their child reaches school age. Education should take place in a setting that allows the child to have contact with other children and to participate in social activities.

- The child may be mainstreamed with a tutor, be partially mainstreamed in a resource room, attend special classes, or be tutored at home. If the child is to attend public school, suggest to parents that they contact the school well before enrollment to ensure that school personnel understand the child's disability.

- Make sure that equipment such as large-print books, braille materials, audio equipment, or an Optacon (described earlier) is available. Ensure that frequent eye examinations are performed and assist with proper use and care of prescribed glasses or contact lenses, as necessary.

- Familiarize the child with the new environment.

Provide Emotional Support

The family often needs help to understand the child's abilities and disabilities. Support them as they learn about their child's visual problems, tell friends and family, and then adjust to supporting the child.

CLINICAL TIP

Clean the child's glasses daily with warm water and a clean, soft dry cloth. Follow the prescriber's and family's directions for care of contact lenses. General guidelines include:

- Keep the lenses in for the recommended time only.
- Store each lens in the right or left containers as labeled.
- Wash hands carefully before contact with the child's eyes or lenses.
- Use a cleaning solution on the lens after its removal.
- Rinse the lens with the recommended rinsing solution.
- Keep the lenses in the case with the disinfecting solution.
- Note on the chart that the child wears lenses.

- Encourage habilitation as soon as realistically possible. Make the adjustment easier by providing information about the child's specific type of visual impairment, available community services, and groups or associations for children with similar vision conditions. Refer to Appendix F for a list of resources for families of children with visual disorders.

- Be supportive and listen to the family's concerns regarding the child's visual deficit.

- Make sure the parents meet their own physical and emotional needs so they are better able to care for and provide support to their child.

> **GROWTH & DEVELOPMENT CONSIDERATIONS**
>
> Children with visual impairment may take longer to master self-help skills such as feeding and dressing.

17-7 Emergency Treatment of Eye Injuries

Injury	Treatment
Subconjunctival hemorrhage (caused by coughing, mild trauma, or increased physical activity)	Usually heals spontaneously; child should see ophthalmologist if most of sclera is covered or if condition does not clear up in 1–2 weeks
Periorbital ecchymosis ("black eye")	Apply ice to eye area (both eyes) for 5–15 minutes every hour for the first 1–2 days after injury (even if only one eye is affected, both eyes may discolor); then apply warm compresses
Foreign body on conjunctiva	Do not let child rub eye; remove material on surface of eye by closing upper lid over lower lid, irrigating or everting upper lid, visualizing material, and removing it with slightly damp handkerchief; patch eye and transport child to emergency department if foreign body cannot be removed
Corneal abrasion	Superficial corneal abrasions are diagnosed by touching sterile fluorescein strip to lower conjunctiva; dye remains where corneal epithelial cells are disrupted; most corneal abrasions heal spontaneously or antibiotic ointment may be prescribed and eyes patched in some children
Burns (alkaline burns readily penetrate cornea and are more serious than acid burns)	For child with chemical burn, irrigate eye for 15–30 minutes; transport child to emergency department, where irrigation should continue (see *Quick Reference to Pediatric Clinical Skills* accompanying this text); pupils are dilated to reduce pain and prevent adhesions; after irrigation is complete, eyes are patched and antibiotics are prescribed
Penetrating and perforating injuries	Obtain medical assistance immediately; *never* try to remove an object that has penetrated the child's eye; such objects should be removed by an ophthalmologist; prevent the child from rubbing injured eye; cover both eyes with shield before transportation to emergency department
Eye injuries caused by severe blows to head and eye (blunt trauma can seriously injure all eye structures, including orbit, which can be fractured)	Transport immediately to ophthalmologist's office or emergency department for evaluation and treatment

> **NURSING ALERT**
>
> Be sure to check the immunization status of the child with an eye injury. If the child has not had a tetanus booster within 5 years, this immunization should be given.

SAFETY PRECAUTIONS

Visual impairment caused by trauma is largely preventable. Dangerous chemicals and objects such as scissors and knives should be placed out of children's reach. When purchasing toys, parents should consider safety features. Protective eyewear should be encouraged during play or sports activities for children of all ages, especially in the child who already has a visual impairment.

INJURIES OF THE EYE

In the United States eye injuries are common in boys 11–15 years of age and in all children aged 9–11 years.[10, 11] Foreign bodies, blunt and sharp objects, chemical and thermal burns, physical irritants, and abuse may cause eye trauma. Recreational activities such as sports and projectile toys are common causes. Older children may be injured by chemicals in school science laboratories.

Some injuries can be treated at home, but many necessitate a trip to the emergency department or require hospitalization. A careful history of the injury is taken, assessment of the eye is performed, and visual acuity is measured.[12] Table 17–7 summarizes emergency treatment of common eye injuries. Nurses should teach children and parents methods to prevent eye injuries. This includes use of protective eye wear, especially for children who participate in athletics and have poor vision or only one functional eye.[11] (See Appendix F for educational resources focusing on protection from eye injury.)

► DISORDERS OF THE EAR

OTITIS MEDIA

Otitis media, or inflammation of the middle ear, is sometimes accompanied by infection. This condition is one of the most common childhood illnesses. Between 76% and 95% of all children have at least one episode by 6 years of age,[13] and the greatest incidence is between 6 and 36 months of age.[13, 14]

17-8	**Types of Otitis Media**	
Type	**Duration**	**Clinical Manifestations**
Acute otitis media (AOM)	Rapid onset; 1–3 weeks' duration	Tympanic membrane (TM) red, retracted or bulging, and painful; ear pulling; fever; hearing loss caused by presence of fluid; possible spontaneous TM rupture resulting in fluid drainage and reduction of pain
Recurrent otitis media (ROM)	Similar onset and duration to AOM, but repeated episodes in succession (three in 6 months or four in 12 months)	Similar to those of AOM
Otitis media with effusion (OME)	May precede or follow any stage of OM	Ear popping; feeling of pressure in middle ear; pain; hearing loss; TM retracted; fluid line or bubbles via otoscopy; symptoms of acute infection are absent
Chronic otitis media (COM)	Slow onset and persistence of 3 months of more	TM thick, immobile, retracted; if TM perforated, drainage from ear; tympanogram abnormal; hearing loss

Modified from Novak, J.C., & Novak, R.E. (1993). Small Talk, 5(2), 1, 3–7.

Otitis media occurs more frequently among boys and in children who attend day-care centers. It is most common during the winter months.

Clinical Manifestations

Otitis media is categorized according to symptoms and the length of time the condition has been present (Table 17–8). Pulling at the ear is a sign of ear pain (Fig. 17–5). Diarrhea, vomiting, and fever are typical of otitis media. Irritability and "acting out" may be signs of a related hearing impairment. Some children with otitis media are asymptomatic; therefore, an ear examination should be performed at every health care visit (see Chap. 3). A red, bulging, nonmobile tympanic membrane is a sign of otitis media (Fig. 17–6). If fluid lines and air bubbles are visible, the child has otitis media with effusion (Fig 17–7).

Etiology and Pathophysiology

The specific cause of otitis media is unknown, but it appears to be related to eustachian tube dysfunction. Often an upper respiratory infection precedes the development of otitis media. This infection causes the mucous membranes of the eustachian tube to become edematous. As a result, air that normally flows to the middle ear is blocked, and the air in the middle ear is reabsorbed into the bloodstream. Fluid is pulled from the mucosal lining into the former air space, providing a medium for the rapid growth of pathogens. The tympanic membrane and fluid behind it become infected. The most common causative organisms are *Streptococcus pneumoniae*, *Haemophilus influenzae*, and *Neisseria catarrhalis*.[15]

Conditions such as enlarged adenoids or edema from allergic rhinitis can also obstruct the eustachian tube and lead to otitis media. Since children with certain facial malformations (cleft palate) and genetic conditions (Down syndrome) usually have compromised eustachian tubes, these children are more vulnerable to the development of otitis media.[13, 14]

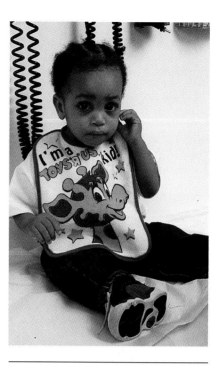

FIGURE 17–5. This young child is pulling at the ear and acting fussy, two important signs of otitis media. Ask the parents about presence of fever and night awakenings, additional signs that are often observed in children with this condition.

 GROWTH & DEVELOPMENT CONSIDERATIONS

Fluid accumulation in the middle ear prevents the efficient transmission of sound and can result in hearing loss over time, potentially delaying speech and language development. These delays may manifest as cognitive deficits or behavior problems. Motor development has been found to be impaired in children with chronic ear infections.

 CLINICAL TIP

The *Haemophilus influenzae* type B (Hib) vaccine, which is routinely given to children beginning at 2 months of age, has been influential in reducing the incidence of diseases such as otitis media that are caused by *H. influenzae* type B. Be sure to check the immunization status of each child to be sure it is up to date for Hib vaccine. (See Chapter 10 for recommended immunization schedule.)

Bulging tympanic membrane

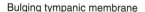

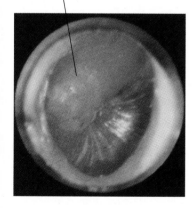

FIGURE 17–6. Acute otitis media is characterized by pain and a red, bulging, nonmobile tympanic membrane.
From Malasanos, L., Barkauskas, V., & Stoltenberg-Allen, K. (1990). Health assessment (4th ed., Plate 2). St. Louis: Mosby–Year Book. Courtesy of Richard A. Buckingham, M.D., Clinical Professor, Otolaryngology, University of Illinois College of Medicine at Chicago, Chicago, IL.

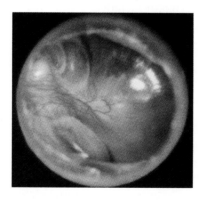

FIGURE 17–7. Otitis media with effusion is noted on otoscopy by fluid line or air bubbles.
From Malasanos, L., Barkauskas, V., & Stoltenberg-Allen, K. (1990). Health assessment (4th ed., Plate 2). St. Louis: Mosby–Year Book. Courtesy of Richard A. Buckingham, M.D., Clinical Professor, Otolaryngology, University of Illinois College of Medicine at Chicago, Chicago, IL.

Diagnostic Tests and Medical Management

Diagnosis is based on otoscopic examination. Redness, inflammation, or bulging of the tympanic membrane is usually present. A "flat" tympanogram is also suggestive of otitis media. (The tympanogram is described in the next section, on hearing impairment.) Pneumatic otoscopy can be used by a trained person to visualize movement of the tympanic membrane while a small breath of air is blown into the ear canal.[16]

Acute and recurrent otitis media are treated with antibiotic therapy for 10–14 days. The choice of antibiotic depends on the probable organism, ease of administration, cost, previous effectiveness, and any history of allergies. First-line drugs include amoxicillin and trimethoprim–sulfamethoxazole. Azithromycin and cephalosporins are used for recurrent infections.[17] Diarrhea and skin rash are the most common side effects of antibiotic therapy.[18] Treatment of recurrent or chronic otitis media may include a 6–month trial of prophylactic antibiotics (amoxicillin or sulfisoxazole).[6, 7] Prolonged otitis media may result in sensorineural or conductive hearing loss and cochlear damage, so treatment and follow-up are essential.

Neither decongestants nor antihistamines have been shown to be effective in the treatment of otitis media with or without effusion. If infection recurs despite of antibiotic treatment, **myringotomy** (surgical incision of the tympanic membrane) may be performed and **tympanotomy tubes** (pressure equalizing tubes) inserted to drain fluid from the middle ear. Tube insertion is generally recommended for children with bilateral middle ear effusion and hearing deficiency of greater than 20 **decibels** (dB) for over 3 months. Enlarged and infected adenoids may be removed at the same time.

Nursing Assessment

The tympanic membrane is assessed for color, transparency, mobility, presence of landmarks, and light reflex. Ask the parents whether the child has had a fever, been fussy, or been pulling at the ears. Observe for signs of impaired hearing.

Nursing Diagnosis

Several nursing diagnoses that may apply to the child with otitis media are included in the accompanying Nursing Care Plan. Additional nursing diagnoses might include:

- Risk for Altered Body Temperature related to infectious process
- Fatigue (Child and Parent) related to inability to obtain normal sleep
- Sensory/Perceptual Alteration (Auditory) related to chronic ear infections and loss of hearing acuity

Nursing Management

Most children with otitis media are not hospitalized; therefore, nursing management centers on care of the child in the home. The child who is having tympanotomy tubes inserted is generally treated in a day surgery setting. Occasionally, children admitted to the hospital for other problems have a concurrent ear infection that requires nursing care. The accompanying Nursing Care Plan summarizes nursing care for the child with otitis media.

Chronic otitis media can create many problems for the family. The child's waking at night with ear pain results in lack of sleep and parental fatigue. Parents often become frustrated and disillusioned because of the inability of the

NURSING CARE PLAN
THE CHILD WITH OTITIS MEDIA

GOAL	INTERVENTION	RATIONALE	EXPECTED OUTCOME

1. Pain related to inflammation and pressure on tympanic membrane

The child or parent will indicate absence of pain.	• Give analgesic such as acetaminophen. Use analgesic eardrops. • Have the child sit up, raise head on pillows, or lie on unaffected ear. • Apply heating pad or warm hot water bottle • Have the child chew gum or blow on balloon to relieve pressure in ear.	• Analgesics alter perception or response to pain. • Elevation decreases pressure from fluid. • Heat increases blood supply and reduces discomfort. • Attempts to open the eustachian tube may help aerate the middle ear.	Verbal child states that pain is relieved. Nonverbal child has improved disposition and comfort.

2. Infection related to presence of pathogens

The child will be free of infection.	• Instruct the parents to administer antibiotics exactly as directed and to complete prescribed course of medication. • Telephone the parents 2 or 3 days after initiation of antibiotic therapy. • Examine ear 3 or 4 days after completion of antibiotic treatment.	• Blood level of antibiotic must remain constant for prescribed time period to kill pathogens. • If symptoms have not improved in 36 hours, a new antibiotic may have to be prescribed. • Check-up determines whether infection has cleared up and if effusion is present.	The child's temperature is normal, symptoms have disappeared, and tympanic membrane shows no signs of infection.

3. Risk for Caregiver Role Strain related to chronic disease

The parents will manage the child's condition with minimal stress.	• Determine the parents' ability to manage condition. Provide frequent information and feedback. • Encourage parental input in managing care. • Listen carefully to parental expressions of frustration and fatigue and try to understand parents' feelings.	• Many parents can treat children at home. Knowledge of condition allows parents to make informed decisions and to manage condition effectively. • Active participation increases confidence and ability to manage condition. • Reacting empathically encourages parents to communicate.	The parents express confidence about treating the child and state that stress is reduced.

Continued . . .

NURSING CARE PLAN
THE CHILD WITH OTITIS MEDIA— *Continued*

GOAL	INTERVENTION	RATIONALE	EXPECTED OUTCOME

4. Knowledge Deficit related to common recurrence of infection in children resulting from anatomic differences in young children and frequent exposure to infectious agents

GOAL	INTERVENTION	RATIONALE	EXPECTED OUTCOME
The parents will state understanding of preventive measures.	• Teach family members to cover mouths and noses when sneezing or coughing and to wash hands frequently. Have parents isolate sick children.	• Good hygiene prevents spread of pathogens.	The child has fewer recurrences or reinfections.
	• Encourage optimal nutrition, rest, and exercise.	• Physical well-being helps the body fight disease.	
	• Position bottle-fed infants upright when feeding. Do not prop bottles.	• Elevated position prevents injection of milk and pathogens into the eustachian tube.	
	• Eliminate allergens and upper respiratory irritants such as tobacco, smoke, and dust.	• Fewer irritants and allergens may decrease susceptibility to respiratory infections. Secondhand smoke contributes to higher incidence of otitis media.	

5. Risk for Altered Growth and Development related to hearing loss

GOAL	INTERVENTION	RATIONALE	EXPECTED OUTCOME
The child will have normal hearing.	• Assess hearing ability frequently.	• Monitoring detects hearing loss early.	The child's general health and hearing improve, and incidence of condition decreases.
The child will have normal motor and language development.	• Assess motor and language development at each health care visit.	• Early detection of developmental delays can lead to appropriate intervention.	The child has language and motor development within norms for age group.

health care system to cure the child and may fear a permanent hearing impairment. Reassure parents that as the child grows older, the recurrent infections eventually cease. Exposure to secondhand smoke in the home increases the incidence of otitis media in children; therefore, parents who smoke should be encouraged to avoid smoking near the child or in the home.[6] Parents of children with tympanotomy tubes need to be taught how to care for the child and what symptoms to report (Table 17–9).

HEARING IMPAIRMENT

Approximately 1 million children in the United States have some form of hearing impairment. Hearing impairment is expressed in terms of decibels

17-9	Discharge Teaching: Care of the Child With Tympanotomy Tubes

After Surgery

Encourage the child to drink generous amounts of fluids.

Reestablish a regular diet as tolerated.

Give pain medication (acetaminophen) as ordered for discomfort and at bedtime.

Place drops in child's ears if instructed.

Restrict the child to quiet activities.

Following Postoperative Period

Follow the physician's instructions regarding swimming and water (some caution against swimming and other activities that might get water in ears; others do not).

Ear plugs can be used to prevent water from getting into ears.

Be alert for tubes becoming dislodged and falling out and alert physician (they usually fall out within 1 year).

Report purulent discharge from the ear, which may indicate a new ear infection. Contact the care provider.

(dB), which are units of loudness, and rated according to severity (Table 17–10). Children who have only a mild hearing loss (35–40 dB) may miss 50% of everyday conversation and are considered at high risk for school failure. Children with a hearing loss of more than 90 dB are considered legally deaf. From 1 to 2 children per 1000 have a bilateral hearing loss of 50 dB or more.[19]

About 50% of hearing loss is genetically caused, usually with a recessive inheritance pattern. Another 25% is due to environmental causes around the time of birth; the remainder is due to unknown causes.[20] Infants and children at risk for hearing loss include those with recurrent otitis media, congenital perinatal infections such as rubella or herpes, anatomic malformations involving the head or neck, low birth weight (less than 1500 g [3 lb, 4 oz]), hyperbilirubinemia, bacterial meningitis, and severe asphyxia at birth.[21] Parents should be aware of excessive noise at home and at school. Teenagers who use earphones at high volumes or

17-10	Severity of Hearing Loss

Type of Loss	Hearing Ability
Slight/mild	Some speech sounds are difficult to perceive, particularly unvoiced consonant sounds
Moderate	Most normal conversational speech sounds are missed
Severe	Speech sounds cannot be heard at a normal conversational level
Profound	No speech sounds can be heard; considered legally deaf
Deaf	No sound at all can be heard

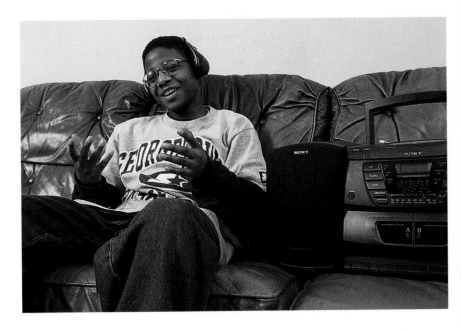

FIGURE 17–8. Listening to loud music with headphones or at rock concerts is a frequent cause of hearing loss among teenagers and young adults. This adolescent needs to be informed about the possible outcomes of this activity.

attend many rock concerts are at risk for hearing loss (Fig. 17–8). Other noise hazards include firecrackers, guns, and power and farm equipment.

Hearing disorders can be classified according to the location of the deficit. **Conductive hearing loss** occurs when conditions in the external auditory canal or tympanic membrane prevent sound from reaching the middle ear. Common causes include impacted cerumen, the most frequent reason for conductive loss; outer ear infection ("swimmer's ear"); trauma; or a foreign body. Conductive loss also occurs if the tympanic membrane does not fully vibrate, as in otitis media. The loss of acuity may be gradual or rapid and results in diminished hearing in all ranges.

Sensorineural hearing loss occurs when the hair cells in the cochlea or along the auditory nerve (cranial nerve VIII) are damaged. This leads to permanent hearing loss. Conditions leading to this type of hearing loss may be congenital (maternal rubella), genetic (Tay–Sachs disease), or acquired (from ototoxic drugs or loud noise).[21] In sensorineural hearing loss, high-frequency sounds are most affected.

A **mixed hearing loss** indicates a hearing loss having a combination of conductive and sensorineural causes.

Hearing is both an innate and a learned behavior. Infants and children who are hearing impaired exhibit a range of behaviors, depending on the child's age and the severity of the deficit. Infants who hear normally respond to sound in both obvious and subtle ways that do not occur in those who are hearing impaired (Table 17–11). As children with hearing impairments mature, language skills are affected. Hearing loss is often manifest as a cognitive deficit, a behavioral problem, or both.

Nursing Assessment

Detection of hearing loss in infants is important to ensure optimal development. Universal screening of all infants and children is recommended with rescreening and monitoring of those at risk.[22]

The child's hearing should be assessed at every well child visit. The best judges of hearing are parents; they should be asked if they have any concerns about their child's hearing. An infant's reaction to rattles, bells, or

GROWTH & DEVELOPMENT CONSIDERATIONS

Infants and young children respond automatically with a blink or the startle reflex to unexpected or loud noises. As they mature, they localize the sound source, then understand speech, and then communicate verbally.

17-11 Behaviors Suggestive of Hearing Impairment

Age	Behavior
Infant	Has a diminished or absent startle reflex to loud sound
	Does not awaken when environment is very noisy
	Awakens only to touch
	Does not turn head to sound at 3–4 months
	Does not localize sound at 6–10 months
	Babbles little or not at all
Toddler and preschooler	Speaks unintelligibly, in a monotone, or not at all
	Communicates needs through gestures
	Appears developmentally delayed
	Appears emotionally immature, yells inappropriately
	Does not respond to doorbell or telephone
	Appears more interested in objects than people and prefers to play alone
	Focuses on facial expressions rather than verbal communications
School-age child and adolescent	Asks to have statements repeated
	Answers questions inappropriately, except when able to view speaker's face
	Daydreams and is inattentive
	Performs poorly at school or is truant
	Has speech abnormalities or speaks in a monotone
	Sits close to or turns television or radio up loudly
	Prefers to play alone

handclapping (about 12 in. [30 cm] from the ear) is an important observation. Language milestones should be evaluated when the older infant and child are examined. Language development is a major area of focus in deaf children.[23] Deaf infants begin to babble at about 5–6 months of age, the same age as hearing infants. However, this babbling ceases several months later in the hearing-impaired child.

An otoscopic examination with a tympanogram can be performed on an older infant to determine conductive hearing loss. The **tympanogram** is a test that provides a graph of the ability of the middle ear to transmit sound. An airtight probe is inserted into the external ear canal and a tone is emitted. The pressure is measured by the probe and plotted on a graph. A "flat" tympanogram suggests conductive hearing loss (Fig. 17–9A and B). **Audiography** can be used with cooperative children over 3 years of age. Sounds of various frequencies and intensities are presented to the child through earphones, and the child is instructed to raise his or her hand when the sound is heard. Audiography cannot detect hearing loss caused by middle ear effusion but can indicate sensorineural loss.

The hearing of preschool and school-age children is tested by asking them to repeat whispered words or to indicate whether or not they hear a ticking watch. Hearing of school-age children and adolescents also is assessed with the Weber and Rinne tests (see Chap. 3).

If a hearing loss is uncorrectable, a team composed of physician, audiologist, speech–language pathologist, psychologist, nurse, teacher, and social worker should work with the child and family. A hearing aid may be

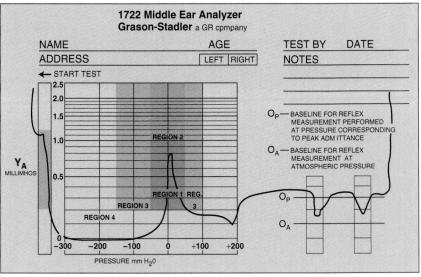

A

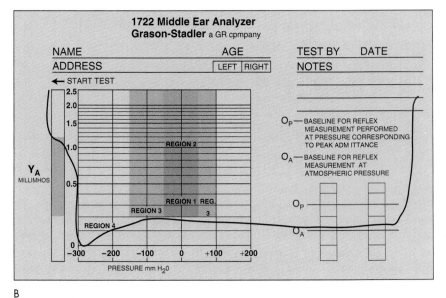

FIGURE 17–9. A, This tympanogram demonstrates normal hearing as evidenced by the curve showing the tympanic membrane's movement when a sound wave is emitted into the ear canal. Mobility is between 0.2 mL and 1.0 mL, the normal range. B, In contrast, note the flat pattern in the second tympanogram, which shows very restricted mobility of the tympanic membrane in response to sound.

B

prescribed for a conductive loss. A sensorineural loss is more difficult to treat, but cochlear implants and bone conduction hearing aids have been used in some children. For children with both types of hearing loss, several approaches are used to enhance communication (Table 17–12). Children with hearing impairment may receive speech therapy and instructions in lipreading, signing, cuing, and fingerspelling.

Nursing Diagnosis

Common nursing diagnoses for the child with impaired hearing include:

- Sensory/Perceptual Alteration (Auditory) related to a specific condition
- Risk for Impaired Verbal Communication related to hearing loss
- Risk for Altered Growth and Development related to communication impairment

17-12	Communication Techniques for Children Who Are Hearing Impaired

Technique	Description
Cued speech	Supplement to lipreading; eight hand shapes represent groups of consonant sounds and four positions about the face represent groups of vowel sounds; based on the sounds the letters make, not the letters themselves; child can "see-hear" every spoken syllable a hearing person hears
Oral approach	Uses only spoken language for face-to-face communication; avoids use of formal signs; uses hearing aids and residual hearing
Total communication	Uses speech and sign, fingerspelling, lipreading, and residual hearing simultaneously; child selects communication technique depending on the situation

From Schwartz, S. (1996). Choices in deafness: A parent's guide (2nd ed.). Rockville, MD: Woodbine House. Reprinted with permission.
For publications related to hearing-impaired children, contact Woodbine House (see Appendix F).

- Risk for Ineffective Family Coping related to a child with a hearing impairment

Nursing Management

Nurses can encourage prevention of hearing loss from exposure to loud noises such as loud music and power and farm equipment. Music should be turned down and ear protection worn for other activities.[24] Early identification of hearing loss in infants and children is facilitated by developmental assessment and hearing screening.

Nursing care of the child with a hearing impairment focuses on facilitating the child's ability to receive spoken language and to send information, helping parents to meet the child's schooling needs, and providing emotional support to parents. Refer the parents to an early intervention program as soon as the diagnosis of hearing impairment is made, in order to foster the child's development.

Facilitate Ability to Receive Spoken Language

Be aware of how the child compensates for hearing loss and use these strategies in communication.

- If hearing loss is mild or temporary or if the child reads lips, first obtain the child's visual attention by lightly touching the child or saying the child's name.

- Position your face 3–6 ft (1–2 m) from the child's face and make sure that the child's eyes are focused on your face and lips. Make sure the room is well lit, with no backlighting. Speak at a normal rate and tone, and use facial expressions that show caring or concern. If the child does not understand, rephrase the information in shorter, simpler sentences. Use specific, concrete explanations, and give the child time to comprehend. Watch for subtle signs of misinterpretations and give consistent and immediate feedback since only 30% of the English language is visible on the lips.

CLINICAL TIP

There are three types of hearing aids: those that fit totally in the ear canal, those that fit in the external ear canal, and those that fit behind the ear. The hearing aid should be cleaned each day with a damp cloth. Change the batteries as needed, usually about once a week. Disconnect the battery when not in use. Place the hearing aid in the ear with the volume off, then slowly turn up to half volume. Adjust as needed. Be sure the hearing aid fit is checked yearly, as the child's growth may necessitate a new fitting.

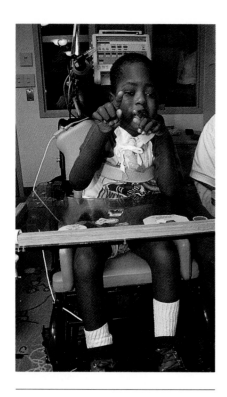

FIGURE 17–10. This child with a hearing impairment, is communicating by means of American Sign Language.

- Be familiar with the different types of hearing aids. Hearing aids, which are microphones that amplify all sounds, can be worn in or behind the ear, in the frame of glasses, or on the body with a wire attached to the ear. When talking to a child with a hearing aid, speak slowly within 6–18 in. (15–45 cm) from the microphone using a normal conversational tone. Talk to the child even if the child is not looking at you. Make sure the batteries are fresh for the best reception. Since all sound is amplified, reduce background noise as much as possible.

Acoustic feedback, an audible whistling sound that cannot always be heard by the child, is one of the most common problems with hearing aids. To eliminate this sound, readjust the hearing aid to make sure that it is inserted properly and that no hair or ear wax is caught between the ear mold and canal. Turning down the volume may also help.

A remote microphone system is another type of device designed to improve hearing. This is often used in the classroom situation because background noise is eliminated. The speaker wears a transmitter that picks up the voice and transmits it to a receiver worn by the child.

Facilitate Ability to Send Information

Maintain the child's hearing aid in proper condition. Many children with impaired hearing communicate using speech, which is enhanced through speech therapy. In addition, they are taught to sign, fingerspell, or use cued speech (Fig. 17–10). Articulation may be difficult, and understanding what the child is trying to say may be frustrating for both the nurse and the child. Taking time to listen carefully is important.

Ask the parents to explain the child's communication techniques and to help interpret words. Have younger children point to pictures. Use assisted technologies such as a picture board or drawings or gestures if necessary. This is especially helpful for communicating feelings of pain and hunger during hospitalization. If the child signs or fingerspells, make sure that you understand the signs for important functions. Give older children a pad of paper and pencil to write requests. People other than parents should be able to understand what the child is trying to communicate. Have an interpreter available if the child uses American Sign Language. Learn some common signs yourself in order to communicate simple words or phrases.

Help Parents to Meet Child's Educational Needs

Public laws apply to the education of children who are hearing impaired (see Chap. 1). After diagnosis, the parents and professionals together agree on an Individualized Education Plan (see discussion in Chap. 5). Day care and preschool are recommended for children with hearing problems.

- Provide parents with information about adjustments that may have to be made for the hearing-impaired child who attends public school. By sitting at the front of the classroom, the child can hear and see more clearly. The teacher should always face the child when speaking, and background noise should be reduced.

- Tell parents that children who are hearing impaired have the same intelligence quotient (IQ) distribution as children without hearing impairment. However, communication and learning can be difficult, and extra support is needed.

- Children with hearing impairment should reach their intellectual potential, although development in certain areas may take place more slowly than it does in non-hearing-impaired children.

Provide Emotional Support

By recognizing the effects of the diagnosis on the family, the nurse can help the family deal with their reaction to the child's hearing loss. Supporting healthy coping is an important intervention to help the parents carry on with their lives.

- Help the parents understand the child's disability and its effect on speech and language development. Provide accurate information about their concerns. Work jointly with other health care professionals and social service workers if necessary.
- Tell the family about the community services available for medical, nursing, psychologic, and financial assistance. Refer to Appendix F for a list of resources for families of children with hearing disorders.

17-13   Emergency Treatment of Ear Injuries

Injury	Treatment
Pinna	
Minor cuts or abrasions	Wash thoroughly with soap and water and rinse well; leave exposed to air if possible or apply adhesive bandage; monitor for infection.
Hematomas	Needle aspiration should be performed and pressure dressing applied; undrained hematomas may become fibrotic; "cauliflower ear" deformity may develop.
Cellulitis or abscesses	Apply moist heat intermittently; make sure that prescribed antibiotic is taken; minor surgery may be performed for an abscess.
Deep lacerations	Apply pressure to stop bleeding; transport to physician's office or emergency department for suturing.
Ear Canal	
Foreign bodies	Have child lie on back and turn head over edge of bed, with affected side down; wiggle earlobe and have child shake head; foreign object may fall out as result of gravity; if object remains in ear, call physician; do not try to remove foreign body with tweezers since this may push the object further into the ear.
Insects	Shine flashlights into ear to try to attract insect; instilling a few drops of mineral oil, olive oil, or alcohol kills insect, and irrigating ear canal gently may remove dead insect (see *Quick Reference to Pediatric Clinical Skills* accompanying this text).
Tympanic Membrane	
Ruptures	Call physician if child has persistent ear pain after blow, blast injury, or insertion of foreign object; cover external ear loosely with piece of sterile cotton or gauze; if tympanic membrane has been ruptured, systemic antibiotics are prescribed.

NURSING ALERT

If an alkaline button battery (like those found in many toys or watches) is inserted in a child's ear, it can rapidly destroy tissue, causing perforation of the tympanic membrane, destruction of the ossicles, and local tissue ulceration. Removal should be performed with the child under sedation or general anesthesia.

SAFETY PRECAUTIONS

Both parents and children should be instructed never to put any object in the child's ear. Some parents believe that the ear canal should be cleaned with a cotton-tipped swab. If the cleaning is too vigorous or the child moves unexpectedly, a ruptured tympanic membrane could result.

INJURIES OF THE EAR

Ear injuries of many types commonly occur in children. Lacerations, infections, and hematomas may occur in the external ear structures, especially the pinna. Children may place foreign objects in the ear, and insects may enter the ear canal. Rupture of the tympanic membrane may result from head injuries, blows to the ear, or insertion of objects into the ear canal.

Table 17–13 presents information on the emergency treatment of ear injuries. Any injury resulting in earache, decreased hearing, persistent bleeding, or other discharge should be seen by a physician.

► DISORDERS OF THE NOSE AND THROAT

EPISTAXIS

Epistaxis, or nosebleed, is common in school-age children, especially boys. Kiesselbach's plexus, an area of plentiful veins located in the anterior nares, is the most common source of bleeding. The most common cause is irritation from nosepicking, foreign bodies, or low humidity. Other causes include forceful coughing, allergies, or infections resulting in congestion of the nasal mucosa. Bleeding from the posterior septum is more serious and may be life threatening. Hospitalization may be necessary. Posterior nosebleeds have a variety of causes, some of which may indicate systemic disease (ie, bleeding disorder) or injury.

Children with nosebleeds are sometimes brought to the emergency department by a parent who has been unable to stop the flow of blood within a few minutes. Both parent and child may be frightened. Ask the parent briefly about any history of nosebleeds and other contributing factors, including medications. Take the child's pulse and blood pressure to assess for excessive blood loss. Carefully examine the nasal mucosa by asking the child to blow any clots out gently, if possible. Suctioning may be necessary.

Observing the flow may help determine whether the blood is coming from an anterior or a posterior location. A nosebleed confined to one side of the nose is almost always anterior, but posterior bleeding can flow on one or both sides. If blood cannot be seen, the child may be swallowing it and may become nauseated. Suspect posterior bleeding in children who have sustained blunt trauma or in other children at high risk.

The child with anterior bleeding should sit upright quietly. The head should be tilted forward to prevent blood from trickling down the throat, which can lead to vomiting. The nares should be squeezed just below the nasal bone and held for 10–15 minutes while the child breathes through the mouth. If the bleeding does not stop, a cotton ball or swab soaked with Neo-Synephrine, epinephrine, thrombin, or lidocaine may be inserted into the affected nostril to promote topical vasoconstriction or anesthesia. Once the bleeding has stopped, the nostril may have to be cauterized with silver nitrate or electrocautery. If the bleeding cannot be stopped, absorbable packing may be used.

Posterior bleeding must also be stopped by packing, and the child must be monitored carefully. Arterial ligation is occasionally needed.[25]

17-14	Discharge Teaching: Prevention and Home Management of Epistaxis

Prevention
- Humidify the child's room, especially during the winter.
- Discourage the child from picking or rubbing the nose or inserting foreign objects in the nose.
- Instruct the child to blow the nose gently and release sneezes through the mouth.
- Apply a thin layer of petroleum jelly twice a day to the septum to relieve dryness and irritation.

Home Management
- Keep the child calm.
- Sit the child upright with head tilted slightly forward so blood does not run down the throat.
- Press a roll of cotton under the upper lip to compress the labial artery.
- Apply steady pressure to both nostrils just below the nasal bone with the thumb and forefinger for 10–15 minutes. Time by the clock.
- Apply an ice pack or cold compress to the bridge of the nose or the back of the neck.
- Call health care provider if the bleeding does not stop.

Modified from Wolff, R. (1982). Nurse Practitioner, 7(10), 16. Reprinted with permission of Elsevier Science Publishing. Copyright © 1982.

Nursing Management

Assess the child's hematocrit or hemoglobin if significant bleeding has occurred. Children with frequent epistaxis should have a complete history taken and physical examination performed to rule out systemic disease.

After the nosebleed has stopped, the child is more vulnerable to rebleeding and should avoid bending over, stooping, strenuous exercise, hot drinks, and hot baths or showers for the next 3–4 days. Sleeping with the head elevated on two or three pillows and humidifying the air with a vaporizer may also prevent a recurrence. Provide parents with suggestions for prevention and home management of epistaxis (Table 17–14).

NASOPHARYNGITIS

Nasopharyngitis, also known as the "common cold," causes inflammation and infection of the nose and throat and is probably the most common illness of infancy and childhood. More than 200 viruses and numerous bacteria can cause this condition. The most common viruses include rhinovirus and coronavirus, and the most frequently occurring bacterium is group A *Streptococcus*. The organisms incubate in 1–3 days, and the infection is communicable several hours before symptoms develop and for 1–2 days after they begin.[25] Symptoms may last 4–10 days or longer. The pathogens are believed to spread when the infected person touches the hand of an uninfected person, who then touches his or her mouth or nose, resulting in self-inoculation.

A red nasal mucosa with clear nasal discharge and an infected throat with enlarged tonsils may be apparent in children with nasopharyngitis.

17-15	Clinical Manifestations of Nasopharyngitis

Infants Younger Than 3 Months of Age
Lethargy
Irritability
Feeding poorly
Fever (may be absent)

Infants 3 Months of Age or Older
Fever
Vomiting
Diarrhea
Sneezing
Anorexia
Irritability
Restlessness

Older Children
Dry, irritated nose and throat
Chills, fever
Generalized muscle aches
Headache
Malaise
Anorexia
Thin nasal discharge, which may later become thick and purulent
Possible sneezing

Vesicles may be present on the soft palate and in the pharynx. Clinical manifestations may vary, depending on the child's age (Table 17–15).

Between episodes of nasopharyngitis, the child should be asymptomatic. If a child continues to have upper respiratory infections, the presence of an underlying condition such as allergy, asthma, or polyps should be ruled out.

Nursing Management

For infants who cannot breathe through the mouth, normal saline nose drops can be administered every 3–4 hours, especially before feeding. (Refer to the *Quick Reference to Pediatric Clinical Skills* accompanying this text for instructions on how to administer nose drops.) For infants over 9 months of age, nasal stuffiness can be treated with either normal saline nose drops or a decongestant such as phenylephrine (0.125–0.25%, depending on the child's age). Older children can use nasal sprays.

Although nose drops and sprays are more effective than systemic decongestants, they should not be used for more than 4 or 5 days or more often than recommended. Antihistamines may be helpful for children with allergic rhinitis or profuse nasal drainage. Long-acting nasal sprays and medications with several ingredients are not recommended.

Room humidification may help prevent drying of nasal secretions. Antipyretics such as acetaminophen reduce fever and make the child more comfortable. Aspirin is not recommended because of its association with Reye syndrome (refer to Chap. 18).

Children should avoid strenuous physical activity and engage in quiet play such as reading, listening to music or stories, or watching television or videotapes. Children should not be forced to eat, but the intake of favorite fluids to liquify secretions should be encouraged. Parents should be told that no medicine or vaccine can prevent the common cold, but eliminating contact with infected persons can reduce the spread of infection. Proper hand-washing and disposal of tissues helps to decrease the spread of the infection.

SINUSITIS

Sinusitis is an inflammation of one or more of the paranasal sinuses. These sinuses, which have respiratory epithelium and are continuous with the respiratory tract, include the maxillary, ethmoid, frontal, and sphenoid sinuses. The sinuses may become infected with bacteria following a viral upper respiratory infection. In most cases, the child's history reveals a cold for several days, followed by improvement in the cold symptoms, but an increase in purulent nasal drainage. There is accompanying facial pain, headache, and fever.[26, 27] Chronic sinusitis may occur in children with uncontrolled allergies and asthma.

Although most physicians treat suspected sinusitis with antibiotics, many cases will clear spontaneously without treatment. Amoxicillin is the first choice for therapy; trimethoprim–sulfamethoxazole and cephalosporins are also sometimes used.[27] Chronic sinusitis may be treated with a prophylactic antibiotic (amoxicillin–clavulanate).

Parents whose child has persistent and purulent nasal drainage should be told to have the child seen by a health care provider, particularly if the drainage is accompanied by facial pain, headache, and fever. Teach parents the correct administration of antibiotics (ie, to take for the full course) if prescribed, and the use of saline nose drops if needed for comfort. Infants may need to have the nose cleared with nose drops and a bulb syringe prior to feedings. (Refer to the *Quick Reference to Pediatric Clinical Skills* accompanying this text for correct use of a bulb syringe.) Antipyretics can be given for fever and to relieve pain.

PHARYNGITIS

Acute pharyngitis is an infection that primarily affects the pharynx, including the tonsils (Fig. 17–11). It is seen most frequently in children 4–7 years of age and is rare in children less than 1 year of age.[28] Approximately 80% of these infections are caused by viruses; the rest are caused by bacteria. Bacterial pharyngitis is commonly known as "strep throat," since it is most often caused by group A beta-hemolytic *Streptococcus* (GABHS). Viral pharyngitis is caused by a large number of enteroviruses.

The major complaint is a sore throat. Table 17–16 contrasts clinical manifestations of viral pharyngitis and strep throat. Children with symptoms of strep throat who have minimal throat redness and pain, exudate, mild lymphadenopathy, and a low-grade fever, and who have been exposed to someone who has pharyngitis should have a throat culture. The classic signs of purulent drainage and white patches are not present in all cases of strep throat. A child who finds swallowing difficult or extremely painful, who drools, or who exhibits

CULTURAL CONSIDERATIONS

Many Hispanic and Asian cultural groups believe in the "hot and cold theory" of disease, in which health problems are viewed as the result of imbalance. For example, Mexican-Americans traditionally treat a "cold disease" such as an earache or common cold with "hot" substances. Ask families if they prefer to eat certain foods during an illness. Incorporating such preferences can help the child to get better and increase the confidence of the family in health care providers.

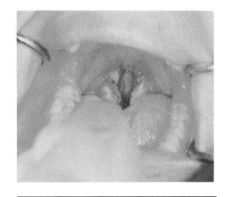

FIGURE 17–11. Acute pharyngitis primarily affects the pharynx but often involves the tonsils, as in this child.
From Malasanos, L., Barkauskas, V., & Stoltenberg-Allen, K. (1990). Health assessment (4th ed., Plate 2). St. Louis: Mosby–Year Book. Courtesy of Edward L. Applebaum, M.D., Chicago, IL.

17-16	Clinical Manifestations of Viral Pharyngitis and Strep Throat (Group A Beta-Hemolytic *Streptococcus* [GABHS])[a]
Viral Pharyngitis	**Strep Throat**
Nasal congestion	Tonsillar exudate[b]
Mild sore throat	Painful cervical lymphadenopathy[b]
Conjunctivitis	Abdominal pain
Cough	Vomiting
Hoarseness	Severe sore throat
Mild pharyngeal redness	Headache
Minimal tonsillar exudate	Fever >38.3°C (101°F)
Mildly tender anterior cervical lymphadenopathy	Petechial mottling of soft palate
Fever <38.3°C (101°F)	

[a]Children 6 months to 3 years of age may have streptococcus with symptoms that resemble those of viral pharyngitis. Children with scarlet fever have the symptoms of strep throat plus a sandpaper-textured erythematous generalized rash and pallor around the lips.
[b]Classic signs of strep throat.

CLINICAL TIP

Throat cultures must be properly performed for accurate diagnosis. A sterile cotton-tip applicator is swabbed across the tonsils, posterior edge of the soft palate, and uvula. Cooperative children can be asked to put their hands under their buttocks, open their mouth, and laugh or pant like a dog. The throat is quickly swabbed. Uncooperative and young children are placed on their back with their hands next to their head and held by a parent or an assistant. The tongue is gently depressed with a tongue blade and the throat is swabbed.

CLINICAL TIP

Children may be more willing to gargle with salt water if the mixture is placed in a spray bottle and sprayed gently toward the throat. Do you know why? The salt water bypasses the salt sensation on the outer part of the tongue and is not as distasteful. The gentle spray does not stimulate a gag reflex; it delivers the salt solution directly to the throat area where it can be gargled and then spit out.

signs of dehydration or respiratory distress should be seen by a physician immediately. These signs could be indicators of serious conditions such as epiglottitis, peritonsillar or retropharyngeal abscess, or diphtheria.

The diagnosis of strep throat is made by throat culture, using the rapid or traditional strep tests. Results of the rapid strep test may be available within minutes; those for the traditional test are available in 24–48 hours. Early signs of strep throat should be treated with oral penicillin for 10 days or by long-acting penicillin given in one injection immediately, even before the result of the culture is available. If the child is allergic to penicillin, erythromycin is given. Acute symptoms should resolve within 24 hours of therapy, at which time the child is no longer contagious.[28] For pharyngitis that is caused by a virus, symptomatic treatment alone is used.

Nursing Management

Nursing care focuses on symptomatic relief. Acetaminophen reduces throat pain and generalized fever. Cool, nonacidic fluids and soft foods, ice chips, or frozen juice pops given frequently in small amounts facilitate swallowing and prevent dehydration. Humidification, chewing gum, and gargling with warm salt water (1 teaspoon [5 g] salt to 8 oz. [250 mL] water) soothe an irritated throat. Commercial throat sprays or throat lozenges are not generally more effective than these home remedies. Encourage the child to rest, to conserve energy and promote recovery.

Teach parents the importance of completing the 10–day course of antibiotics if prescribed for bacterial pharyngitis. Reinforce to parents the importance of treating streptococcal infections, as untreated infections may lead to rheumatic fever, cervical adenitis, sinusitis, glomerulonephritis, or meningitis.

TONSILLITIS

Tonsillitis is an infection or inflammation (hypertrophy) of the palatine tonsils. Although most children with pharyngitis may have infected tonsils, they do not necessarily have tonsillitis.

Clinical Manifestations

Symptoms suggestive of tonsillitis include frequent throat infections with breathing and swallowing difficulties; persistent redness of the anterior pillars; and enlargement of the cervical lymph nodes. If children breathe through their mouths continuously, the mucous membranes may become dry and irritated.

Etiology and Pathophysiology

Like pharyngitis, tonsillitis may be caused by a virus or bacterium. The primary site of infection is the tonsils.

Diagnostic Tests and Medical Management

Diagnosis is made on the basis of visual inspection and clinical manifestations. Symptomatic treatment for tonsillitis is the same as for pharyngitis. Surgical removal of tonsils (tonsillectomy) is often recommended when children have recurrent throat infections (about three per year for 3 years), chronic tonsillitis, obstructive sleep apnea, or malformations causing nasal speech or a facial growth abnormality.[29] If the child is under 3 years of age, the surgery is postponed if possible because it may stimulate growth of other lymphoid tissue in the nasopharynx. If the pharyngeal tonsils (adenoids) are enlarged, as suggested by mouth breathing, cough, impaired taste and smell, a muffled quality to the voice, and chronic otitis media, they may be removed at the same time.

Nursing Assessment

Assess the throat carefully during each physical examination. Observe for tonsils that are simply large (a common finding in childhood) and those that are inflamed. Look for the degree of redness and presence of any exudate. Ask if the child has pain or difficulty swallowing. Ask about the history of past tonsillar infections and the length of time of the present discomfort.

   If surgery is indicated, take a complete history of the child preoperatively. Monitor vital signs and observe for respiratory distress, hemorrhage, and dehydration postoperatively.

Nursing Diagnosis

Several nursing diagnoses may apply to the child with tonsillitis. They include:

- Pain related to inflammation of the pharynx
- Pain related to surgical procedure
- Risk for Fluid Volume Deficit related to throat pain and reluctance to swallow
- Risk for Ineffective Breathing Pattern related to obstruction by enlarged tonsils
- Risk for Injury related to postoperative complications

- Impaired Swallowing related to inflammation and pain
- Knowledge Deficit (Parents) related to home care following discharge

Nursing Management

The nurse provides general supportive care and, if medication is prescribed, encourages completion of the full course of treatment. The nursing management of children with tonsillitis is similar to that of children with pharyngitis (see earlier discussion).

If surgery is indicated, the parents are helped to prepare their child for a short-term surgical procedure with a possible overnight stay in the hospital. Children should be free of sore throat, fever, or upper respiratory infection for at least 1 week before surgery. They should not be given aspirin or ibuprofen for 2 weeks before surgery, since these medications can increase bleeding.

Discharge Planning and Home Care Teaching

Discharge planning includes teaching parents about pain management, fluid and nutrition intake, activity restrictions, and possible complications in the postoperative period. Most children will have a sore throat for 7–10 days after tonsillectomy. Advise parents that to relieve the child's throat pain, they should:

- Have the child drink adequate cool fluids or chew gum, as this reduces spasms in the muscles surrounding the throat.
- Give acetaminophen elixir, as ordered.
- Apply an ice collar around the child's neck.
- Have the child gargle with a solution of ½ teaspoon (2.5 g) each of baking soda and salt in a glass of water.
- Have the child rinse the mouth well with viscous lidocaine and then swallow the solution.

17-17   Discharge Teaching: Complications of Tonsillectomy and Adenoidectomy

Bleeding
- To prevent bleeding, aspirin or ibuprofen should not be given for pain for the first postoperative week. Use acetaminophen instead.
- Bleeding is most likely to occur within the first 24 hours or 7–10 days after the tonsillectomy, when the scar is forming. Report any trickle of bright red blood to the physician immediately.

Infection
- The back of the throat will look white and have an odor for the first 7–8 days after the surgery. The child may also have a low-grade fever. These are not signs of infection.
- For temperatures over 38.3°C (101°F), acetaminophen may be used.
- Call the physician if the child develops a fever above 38.8°C (102°F).

Pain
- Administer acetaminophen as ordered.
- Offer frequent small amounts of cool liquids. Avoid citrus juice.
- Provide for rest and quiet activities for several days.

Children may experience ear pain, especially when swallowing, between 4 and 8 days after tonsillectomy. Advise parents that this is the result of pain referred from the tonsillar area and does not indicate an ear infection.

Emphasize to parents the importance of adequate fluid intake. Children should be given any liquid they prefer for the first week, except citrus juices, which may produce a burning sensation in the throat. Soft foods such as gelatin, applesauce, frozen juice pops, and mashed potatoes can be added as tolerated.

Children do not need to be confined to bed, but vigorous exercise should be avoided for the first week after surgery. Advise parents that the child may return to school approximately 10 days after tonsillectomy.

Any surgery carries with it the risk of postoperative complications. Teach parents the normal signs of healing in the postoperative period, as well as signs of complications (Table 17–17).

REFERENCES

1. Scheiner, A.P. (1996). Vision problems: Impairment to blindness. In A.M. Rudolph, J.I.E. Hoffman, & C.D. Rudolph (Eds.), *Rudolph's pediatrics* (20th ed., p. 167). Stamford, CT: Appleton & Lange.

2. O'Hara, M.A. (1993). Ophthalmia neonatorum. *Pediatric Clinics of North America, 40*(4), 715–726.

3. Apt, L., & Miller, K. (1996). The eyes. In A.M. Rudolph, J.I.E. Hoffman, & C.D. Rudolph (Eds.), *Rudolph's pediatrics* (20th ed., pp. 2063–2066). Stamford, CT: Appleton & Lange.

4. Wagner, R.S. (1997). Eye infections and abnormalities: Issues for the pediatrician. *Contemporary Pediatrics, 14*(6), 137–153.

5. Phelps, D.L. (1993). Retinopathy of prematurity. *Pediatric Clinics of North America, 40*(4), 705–714.

6. Nelson, L. (1996). Disorders of the eye. In R.E. Behrman, R.M. Kliegman, & A.M. Arvin (Eds.), *Nelson textbook of pediatrics* (15th ed., pp. 1764–1803). Philadelphia: Saunders.

7. Moller, M. (1993). Working with visually impaired children and their families. *Pediatric Clinics of North America, 40*(4), 881–890.

8. Menacker, S.J. (1993). Visual function in children with developmental disabilities. *Pediatric Clinics of North America, 40*(3), 659–674.

9. Espezel, H. (1994). The visually impaired child. *The Canadian Nurse, 90*(5), 23–25.

10. Catalano, R. (1992). Special considerations in the pediatric patient. In *Ocular emergencies* (pp. 91–105). Philadelphia: Saunders.

11. Coody, D., Banks, J.M., Yetman, R.J., & Musgrove, K. (1997). Eye trauma in children: Epidemiology, management, and prevention. *Journal of Pediatric Health Care, 11*(4), 182–188.

12. Catalano, R.A. (1993). Eye injuries and prevention. *Pediatric Clinics of North America, 40*(4). 827–840.

13. Novak, J.C., & Novak, R.E. (1993). Impact of otitis media on hearing and communication. *Small Talk, 5*(2), 1, 3–7.

14. Facione, N. (1990). Otitis media: An overview of acute and chronic disease. *Nurse Practitioner, 15*(10), 11–19.

15. Rosenfeld, R.M. (1996). An evidence-based approach to treating otitis media. *Pediatric Clinics of North America, 43*(6), 1165–1182.

16. Arnold, J.E. (1996). The ear. In R.E. Behrman, R.M. Kliegman, & A.M. Arvin (Eds.), *Nelson textbook of pediatrics* (15th ed., pp. 1804–1826). Philadelphia: Saunders.

17. Barnett, E.D., & Klein, J.O. (1995). The problem of resistant bacteria for the management of acute otitis media. *Pediatric Clinics of North America, 42*(3), 509–518.

18. Otitis Media Guideline Panel. (1994). *Otitis media with effusion in young children.* Rockville, MD: U.S. Department of Health and Human Services.

19. Brookhauser, P.E. (1996). Sensorineural hearing loss in children. *Pediatric Clinics of North America, 43*(6), 1195–1216.

20. Kelly, D.P. (1996). Hearing problems: Impairment to deafness. In A.M. Rudolph, J.I.E. Hoffman, & C.D. Rudolph (Eds.), *Rudolph's pediatrics* (20th ed., pp. 162–168). Stamford, CT: Appleton & Lange.

21. Letko, M.D. (1992). Detecting and preventing infant hearing loss. *Neonatal Network, 11*(5) 33-37.

22. Joint Committee on Infant Hearing. (1994). Position statement. *ASHA, 36,* 38–41.

23. Schilling, L.S., & DeJesus, E. (1993). Developmental issues in deaf children. *Journal of Pediatric Health Care, 7*(4), 161–166.

24. Nash, D.D.B., Schochat, E., Rozycki, A.A., & Musiek, F.E. (1997). When loud noises hurt. *Contemporary Pediatrics, 14*(6), 97–109.

25. Handler, S.D., & Myer, C.M. (1996). The nose and paranasal sinuses. In A.M. Rudolph, J.I.E. Hoffman, & C.D. Rudolph (Eds.), *Rudolph's pediatrics* (20th ed., pp. 953–958). Stamford, CT: Appleton & Lange.

26. Abbasi, S., & Cunningham, A.S. (1996). Are we overtreating sinusitis? *Contemporary Pediatrics, 13*(10), 49–62.

27. Isaacson, G. (1996). Sinusitis in childhood. *Pediatric Clinics of North America, 43*(6), 1297–1318.

28. Kenna, M.A. (1990). Sore throat in children. In C.D. Bluestone, & S. Stool (Eds.), *Pediatric otolaryngology* (2nd ed., Vol. II, pp. 837–842). Philadelphia: Saunders.

29. Deutsch, E.S. (1996). Tonsillectomy and adenoidectomy. *Pediatric Clinics of North America, 43*(6), 1319–1338.

ADDITIONAL RESOURCES

Denny, F.W. (1994). Tonsillopharyngitis 1994. *Pediatrics in Review, 15,* 185–191.

Dowd, T.R., & Stewart, F.M. (1994). Primary care approach to lymphadenopathy. *Nurse Practitioner, 19*(12), 36–44.

Friendly, D.S. (1993). Development of vision in infants and young children. *Pediatric Clinics of North America, 40*(4), 693–704.

Gardner, S.L., & Hagedorn, M.I. (1990). Physiologic sequelae of prematurity: The nurse practitioner's role. Part II. Retinopathy of prematurity. *Journal of Pediatric Health Care, 4*(2), 72–76.

George, D., Stephens, S., Fellows, R.R., & Bremer, D.L. (1988). The latest on retinopathy of prematurity. *American Journal of Maternal–Child Nursing, 32*(4), 254–258.

Harbeck, R.J., Teague, J., Crossen, G.R., Maul, D.M., & Childres, P.L (1993). Novel, rapid optical immunoassay technique for detection of group A streptococci from pharyngeal specimens: Comparison with standard culture methods. *Journal of Clinical Microbiology, 31,* 839–844.

Harrison, C.J., & Belhorn, T.H. (1992). Acute otitis media. *Clinical Reviews, 2*(4), 53–65.

Isaacson, G., & Rosenfeld, R.M. (1996). Care of the child with tympanotomy tubes. *Pediatric Clinics of North America, 43*(6), 1183–1194.

Jackson, C.B. (1990). Primary health care for deaf children. Part II. *Journal of Pediatric Health Care, 4*(1), 39–40.

Jackson, C.B. (1989). Primary health care for deaf children. Part I. *Journal of Pediatric Health Care, 3*(6), 316-318.

Kaye, B. (1990). The cure for lazy eye. *Journal of Ophthalmic Nursing and Technology, 9*(3), 90–93.

Kempthorne, J., & Giebink, G.S. (1991). Pediatric approach to diagnosis and management of otitis media. *Otolaryngologic Clinics of North America, 24*(2), 905–929.

Lanphear, B.P., Byrd, R.S., Auinger, P. & Hall, C.B. (1997). Increasing prevalence of recurrent otitis media among children in the United States. *Pediatrics, 99*(3), el. [http://www.pediatrics.org/cgi/content/full/99/3/el]

Lavrich, J.B., & Nelson, L.B. (1993). Diagnosis and treatment of strabismus disorders. *Pediatric Clinics of North America, 40*(4), 737–752.

Long, C.A. (1989). Cryotherapy: A new treatment for retinopathy of prematurity. *Pediatric Nursing, 15*(3), 269–272.

Neumann, E., Friedman, Z., & Able-Peleg, B. (1987). Prevention of strabismic amblyopia of early onset. *Journal of Ophthalmic Nursing and Technology, 6*(6), 242–237.

Orlin, M.N., Effgen, S.K., & Handler, S.D. (1997). Effect of otitis media with effusion on gross motor ability in preschool-aged children: Preliminary findings. *Pediatrics, 99*(3), 334–337.

Paradise, M.D., Rockette, H.E., & Colburn, K. (1997) Otitis media in 2,253 Pittsburgh-area infants: Prevalence and risk factors during the first two years of life. *Pediatrics, 99*(3), 318–333.

Riley, M.A. (1987). *Nursing care of clients with ear, nose and throat disorders* (pp. 179–184). New York: Springer.

Rubin, S.E., & Nelson, L.B. (1993). Amblyopia: Diagnosis and management. *Pediatric Clinics of North America, 40*(4), 727–736.

U.S. Public Health Service. (1994). Put prevention into practice: Screening for hearing loss. *Journal of the American Academy of Nurse Practitioners, 6*(9), 439–442.

Wetmore, R.F., & Willging, J.P. (1996). The oral cavity and oropharynx. In A.M. Rudolph, J.I.E. Hoffman, & C.D. Rudolph (Eds.), *Rudolph's pediatrics* (20th ed., pp. 959–969). Stamford, CT: Appleton & Lange.

Wheeler, L.C., Griffin, H.C., Taylor, J.R., & Taylor, S. (1997). Educational intervention strategies for children with visual impairments with emphasis on retinopathy of prematurity. *Journal of Pediatric Health Care, 11*(6), 275–279.

White, G.L., Liss, R.P., & Crandall, A.S. (1991). Congenital glaucoma. *Physician Assistant, 15*(1), 45–46, 48–49, 69–71.

Wurst, J., & Stern, P.N. (1990). Childhood otitis media: The family's endless quest for relief. *Issues in Comprehensive Pediatric Nursing, 13*(1), 25–39.

Yetman, R.J., & Coody, D.K. (1997). Conjunctivitis: A practical guideline. *Journal of Pediatric Health Care, 11*(5), 238–241.

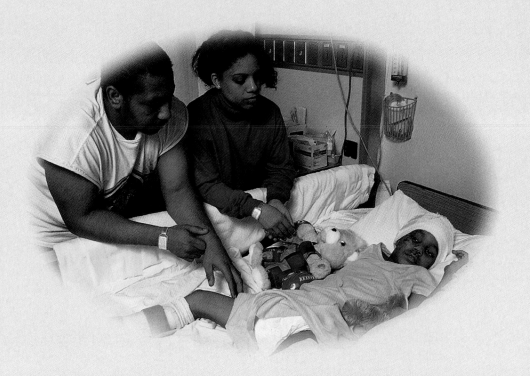

Antwan, 7 years old, was injured when he was struck by a car and thrown several feet into the air. He was unconscious upon admission to the emergency department and showed some signs of increased intracranial pressure (dilated and fixed pupils). He was treated for shock, and his neurologic status and vital signs were frequently assessed. The initial evaluation revealed that Antwan had sustained several contusions of the brain, but no skull fracture. He was intubated and medicated to manage the increased intracranial pressure.

Antwan's intracranial pressure has now stabilized, but he still has not totally regained consciousness. He is restless and agitated, and unable to follow directions. His parents stay at his bedside and provide auditory and tactile stimulation, hoping he will eventually respond. Physical therapy has been initiated to prevent contractures and to maintain function. Long-term rehabilitation will be needed to help Antwan and his family achieve the best outcome possible after this injury.

What is the role of the nurse in acute care of the brain-injured child? What support does the family need to contribute to the child's care? How does the nurse work with other health care professionals to plan the long-term care of a child such as Antwan?

ALTERATIONS IN NEUROLOGIC FUNCTION 18

"It's so hard to watch your child experience an injury like this. All we can do is be here every day for Antwan and hope that he will fully recover."

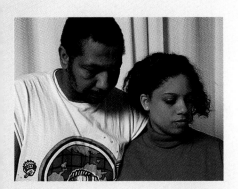

TERMINOLOGY

- **areflexia** No reflex response to verbal, sensory, or pain stimulation.
- **aura** Subjective sensation, often olfactory or visual in nature, that is an early sign of a seizure.
- **cerebral edema** Increase in intracellular and extracellular fluid in the brain that results from anoxia, vasodilation, or vascular stasis.
- **cerebral perfusion pressure** Amount of pressure needed to ensure that adequate oxygen and nutrients will be delivered to the brain.
- **clonic** Alternating muscular contraction and relaxation; often used to describe seizure activity.
- **coma** State of unconsciousness in which the child cannot be aroused, even with powerful stimuli.
- **confusion** Disorientation to time, place, or person.
- **Cushing's triad** Reflex response associated with increased intracranial pressure or compromised blood flow to the brainstem; characterized by hypertension, increased systolic pressure with wide pulse pressure, bradycardia, and irregular respirations.
- **delirium** State characterized by confusion, fear, agitation, hyperactivity, or anxiety.

- **encephalopathy** Cerebral dysfunction resulting from an insult (toxin, injury, inflammation, or anoxic event) of limited duration; the tissue damage is often permanent, but the dysfunction may improve over time.
- **focal** Specific area of the brain; often used to describe seizures or neurologic deficits.
- **intracranial pressure** Force exerted by brain tissue, cerebrospinal fluid, and blood within the cranial vault.
- **level of consciousness** General description of cognitive, sensory, and motor response to stimuli.
- **obtunded** Diminished level of consciousness with limited response to the environment; the child falls asleep unless given verbal or tactile stimulation.
- **postictal period** Period after seizure activity during which the level of consciousness is decreased.
- **posturing** Abnormal position assumed after injury or damage to the brain that may be seen as extreme flexion or extension of the limbs.
- **stupor** Diminished level of consciousness with response only to vigorous stimulation.
- **tonic** Continuous muscular contraction; often used to describe seizure activity.

Why do certain neurologic disorders occur more often in children than in adults? What effect do these disorders have on a child's growth and development? Why are some neurologic injuries more likely to be seen in children and why do children recover from these injuries more completely than adults? What role do nurses play in ensuring early diagnosis and treatment of neurologic disorders? This chapter will enable you to answer these questions by examining some of the more common disorders of neurologic function in children.

▶ ANATOMY AND PHYSIOLOGY OF PEDIATRIC DIFFERENCES

Knowledge of the anatomy of the nervous system makes neurologic symptoms easier to understand. The brain, spinal cord, and nerves are the major structures of the nervous system (Fig. 18–1). The spinal cord transmits impulses to and from the brain, conveying sensory information and relaying impulses that stimulate motor responses. Because the nervous system helps to control and coordinate many body functions, alterations in neurologic function can have widespread effects on the body's metabolism.

The brain and spinal cord are formed early in gestation from the neural tube. Any insult or critical event (teratogen, infection, substance abuse, or trauma) during this period can result in a central nervous system malformation. Such defects account for approximately one third of all apparent congenital malformations.[1]

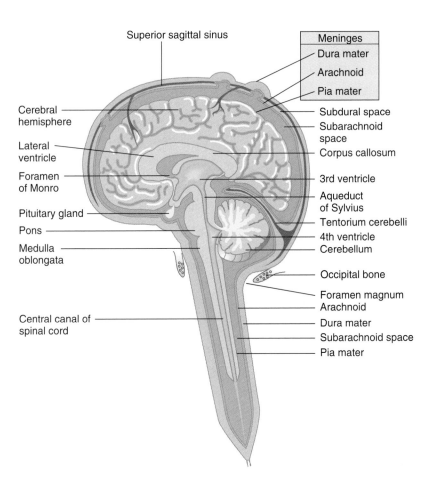

FIGURE 18–1. Transverse section of the brain and spinal cord. Knowledge of the anatomy of the brain is helpful in understanding the symptoms of neurologic dysfunction.

18-1	Summary of Anatomic and Physiologic Differences Between Children and Adults	

Difference in Children	Significance
Top heavy; head is large in proportion to body; neck muscles not well developed	Prone to head injuries with falls; neck may not be able to support large head
Thin cranial bones that are not well developed; unfused sutures	Prone to fracture
Highly vascular brain; subarachnoid space small; dura firmly attached but can strip away from pericranium	Brain prone to hemorrhage; there is less cerebrospinal fluid to cushion the brain
Excessive spinal mobility; muscles, joint capsules, and ligaments of cervical spine immature	Greater risk for high cervical spine injury at C1–C2 level
Wedge-shaped, cartilaginous vertebral bodies; ossification of vertebral bodies incomplete	Greater risk for compression fractures of vertebrae with falls

At birth, the nervous system is complete but immature. The infant is born with all of the nerve cells that will exist throughout life. However, the number of glial cells and dendrites, which enable receipt of nerve impulses, continues to increase until approximately 4 years of age. Myelination, which increases the speed and accuracy of nerve impulses, is also incomplete at birth. This process continues throughout childhood, proceeding in a cephalocaudal direction.

The anatomic and physiologic differences between the nervous systems of children and adults help explain why children and adults have different neurologic problems (Table 18–1). For example, the brain and spinal cord are protected by the skeletal structures of the skull and vertebrae. In infants, however, the cranial bones and vertebrae are not completely ossified. The infant's brain and spinal cord are thus at greater risk for injury resulting from trauma.

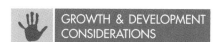

GROWTH & DEVELOPMENT CONSIDERATIONS

The myelination process accounts for the progressive acquisition of fine and gross motor skills and coordination during early childhood.

▶ ALTERED STATES OF CONSCIOUSNESS

Level of consciousness (LOC) is perhaps the most important indicator of neurologic dysfunction. Consciousness, the responsiveness of the mind to sensory stimuli, has two components: *alertness,* or the ability to react to stimuli, and *cognitive power,* or the ability to process the data and respond either verbally or physically. Unconsciousness, on the other hand, is depressed cerebral function, or the inability of the brain to respond to stimuli.

Levels of deterioration can be further categorized as:

- **Confusion:** disorientation to time, place, or person. The child may seem alert. Answers to simple questions may be correct, but responses to complex ones may be inaccurate.

- **Delirium:** state characterized by confusion, fear, agitation, hyperactivity, or anxiety.

- **Obtunded:** limited response to the environment; the child falls asleep unless given verbal or tactile stimulation.

- **Stupor:** response to vigorous stimulation only; the child returns to the unresponsive state when the stimulus is removed. For example, the child may react to a needle stick but not respond to a milder stimulus such as touching the skin.
- **Coma:** state characterized by severely diminished response; the child cannot be aroused even by painful stimuli.

Clinical Manifestations

Decline in a child's level of consciousness often follows a sequential pattern of deterioration. A child may first appear awake and alert, and may respond appropriately. Initial changes may be subtle: a slight disorientation to time, place, and person. The child may become restless or fussy, and actions that normally calm or soothe the child only increase irritability. As responsiveness decreases, the child may become drowsy but still respond to loud verbal commands and withdraw from painful stimuli. Keeping the child awake is sometimes difficult. Then response to pain progresses from purposeful to nonpurposeful. Decorticate or decerebrate **posturing,** the abnormal positions assumed after injury or damage to the brain, may occur (Fig. 18–2).

Etiology and Pathophysiology

Trauma, infection, poisoning, seizures, or any other process that affects the central nervous system may alter the level of consciousness (Table 18–2). Discovering the cause of the decreased level of consciousness is essential so that immediate treatment can begin, to prevent possible secondary effects of the illness or injury.

Diagnostic Tests and Medical Management

Medical management focuses on early diagnosis, intervention, and prevention of complications.

A thorough history is taken to assess whether the child had a recent head trauma, has an infection, or has ingested toxins. It is also important to

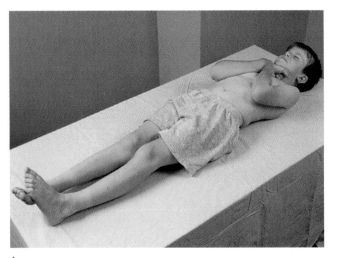

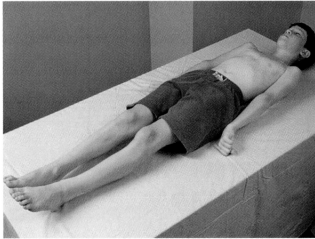

A   B

FIGURE 18–2. **A,** Decorticate posturing, characterized by rigid flexion, is associated with lesions above the brain stem in the corticospinal tracts. **B,** Decerebrate posturing, distinguished by rigid extension, is associated with lesions of the brain stem.

18-2   Causes of Decreased Level of Consciousness

Hypoxia

Trauma

Infection

Poisoning

Seizures

Endocrine or metabolic disturbances (eg, hypoglycemia)

Electrolyte or biochemical imbalance

Acid–base imbalances

Cerebrovascular pathology (eg, neoplasms or degenerative disorders)

Congenital structural defect

---

determine if the child has a shunt, a tumor, or a condition that could affect his or her level of consciousness.

Laboratory tests include a complete blood cell count, blood chemistry, clotting factors, and blood culture; toxicology assessments of both blood and urine; and urinalysis with culture.

A lumbar puncture may be performed to assess the cerebrospinal fluid for protein, glucose, or blood cells. An electroencephalogram (EEG) identifies damaged or nonfunctioning areas of the brain.

Radiologic examination is an essential part of the diagnostic workup. Computed tomography (CT) or magnetic resonance imaging (MRI) is used to detect any lesions, structural abnormalities, vascular malformations, or edema. Skull x-ray studies are used to detect fractures or bony malformations.

The Glasgow Coma Scale is used to quantify the level of consciousness, thus enabling future comparison of improvement or deterioration in the child's condition. Pediatric criteria, which take into account the child's developmental age for each category of the test, have been established to assess responses (Table 18–3).

- Eye opening. Note whether eye opening is spontaneous or occurs in response to a command.

- Verbal response. Crying in an infant is a positive response. The 2-year-old child who says "no" to each command is also responding in an age-appropriate way.

- Motor response. Motor score is probably the most critical aspect of this test, since the child cannot control reflexes. A fearful toddler may refuse to open his or her eyes or talk to strangers, but the child's reflexes should automatically respond to appropriate stimuli.

Increased **intracranial pressure** (force exerted by brain tissue, cerebrospinal fluid, and blood within the cranial vault) may be noted in the comatose child. If this increased pressure level is marked and results from the accumulation of cerebrospinal fluid because of obstruction, a ventricular tap can be performed to decrease the pressure, thus relieving a life-threatening condition that can lead to coma.

Depending upon the cause of altered level of consciousness, the child may recover after an acute illness or injury, or acquire a disability.

18-3	Glasgow Coma Scale for Assessment of Coma in Infants and Children		
Category	**Score**	**Infant and Young Child Criteria**	**Older Child and Adult Criteria**
Eye opening	4	Spontaneous opening	Spontaneous
	3	To loud noise	To verbal stimuli
	2	To pain	To pain
	1	No response	No response
Verbal response	5	Smiles, coos, cries to appropriate stimuli	Oriented to time, place, and person; uses appropriate words and phrases
	4	Irritable; cries	Confused
	3	Inappropriate crying	Inappropriate words or verbal response
	2	Grunts, moans	Incomprehensible words
	1	No response	No response
Motor response	6	Spontaneous movement	Obeys commands
	5	Withdraws to touch	Localizes pain
	4	Withdraws to pain	Withdraws to pain
	3	Abnormal flexion (decorticate)	Flexion to pain (decorticate)
	2	Abnormal extension (decerebrate)	Extention to pain (decerebrate)
	1	No response	No response

Add the score from each category to get the total. The maximum score is 15, indicating the best level of neurologic functioning. The minimum is 3, indicating total neurologic unresponsiveness.
From Teasdale, G., & Jennett, B. (1974). Assessment of coma and impaired consciousness. Lancet 2, 81–84; and James, H.E. (1986). Neurologic evaluation and support in the child with acute brain insult. Pediatric Annals, 15(1), 17.

18-4	Guidelines for Initial Physiologic Assessment
Assessment Area	**Questions**
Responsiveness	How does the child respond to verbal or tactile stimuli or the environment?
Airway	Is the child's airway patent?
	Is it maintainable (eg, with a jaw thrust) or is intubation necessary?
Breathing	Is the child's color normal? Does the child appear pale or cyanotic?
	What are the heart and respiratory rates?
	Is the child's breathing more labored? Does the child have nasal flaring, retractions, or grunting?
	What are the breath sounds?
	What is the pulse oximetry or arterial blood gas measurement?
Circulation	What are the heart rate and blood pressure?
	Is the capillary refill time greater than or less than 2 seconds?
Disability	What is the level of consciousness?
	What is the pediatric Glasgow Coma Scale score?
Exposure	Is the body temperature normal or above or below normal? Are there any signs of injury or trauma?

Nursing Assessment

Initially assess the child's physiologic status, using the guidelines described in Table 18–4. Assess the child's level of consciousness, vital signs, and breathing patterns frequently, as they can be indicators of neurologic deterioration.

A child's responses may differ significantly when stress and anxiety are reduced. Encourage the parents to take part in the examination to reduce the child's anxiety.

Assess the child's cranial nerves (see Table 3–24). This is not difficult to perform in the conscious child, but the inability of an unconscious child to cooperate makes assessment difficult (Table 18–5).

Assess the child's respiratory effort and color. Monitor pulse oximetry or arterial blood gas measurements. The child must be able to maintain adequate air exchange to keep oxygen and carbon dioxide levels within normal ranges; otherwise there is a risk of increased intracranial pressure. If the child cannot maintain an adequate tidal volume, mechanical ventilation will be necessary.

Nursing Diagnosis

Among the nursing diagnoses that might be appropriate for the child with an altered level of consciousness are:

- Ineffective Breathing Pattern related to decreased level of consciousness or increased intracranial pressure
- Risk for Aspiration related to decreased level of consciousness
- Risk for Impaired Skin Integrity related to decreased level of consciousness and impaired mobility
- Impaired Social Interaction related to diminished response to environment
- Altered Family Processes related to care of a child with an acquired disability

CLINICAL TIP

When assessing the motor skills of a toddler, ask the child to reach for a finger puppet or doll rather than your hand. This makes the child feel less threatened. The toy is a reward.

| 18-5 | Assessment of Cranial Nerves in the Unconsious Child |

Cranial Nerves	Reflex	Assessment Procedure and Normal Findings[a]
II, III	Pupillary	Shine a light source in eye. *Rapid, concentrically constricting pupils indicate intact cranial nerves II, III.*
II, IV, VI	Oculocephalic	Should be performed with eyes held open (doll's eyes) and head turned from side to side. *Eyes gazing straight up or lagging slightly behind head motion indicate intact cranial nerves.* Precaution: Cervical spine injury must be ruled out before this assessment is performed.
III, VIII	Oculovestibular	Place the head in a midline and slightly elevated position. Inject ice water into ear canal. *Eyes deviating toward the irrigated ear indicate intact cranial nerves III, VIII.* Precautions: Cervical spine injury must be ruled out before this assessment is performed. Tympanic membrane must be intact; otherwise brain may be filled with bacteria-laden fluid. Note: This assessment is usually performed by a physician.
V, VII	Corneal	Cornea is gently swabbed with sterile cotton swab. *A blink indicates intact cranial nerves V, VII.*
IX, X	Gag	Pharynx is irritated with tongue depressor or cotton swab. *Gagging response indicates intact cranial nerves IX, X.*

[a]Italic indicates normal findings.

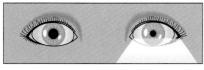

A

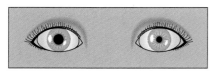

B

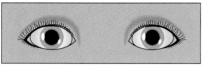

C

FIGURE 18–3. Pupil findings in various neurologic conditions with altered consciousness. **A,** A unilateral dilated and reactive pupil is associated with an intracranial mass. **B,** A fixed and dilated pupil may be a sign of impending brainstem herniation. **C,** Bilateral fixed and dilated pupils are associated with brainstem herniation from increased intracranial pressure.

Nursing Management

Nursing care focuses on maintaining airway patency, monitoring neurologic status, performing routine care, providing sensory stimulation, and providing emotional support to parents.

Maintain Airway Patency

Make sure the child's airway is clear at all times. Pulse oximetry or arterial blood gas analysis is performed at regular intervals to ensure that gas exchange is adequate. Mechanical ventilation may be required. If the child is having difficulty swallowing secretions or does not have a gag reflex, intubation or a tracheostomy is performed. Frequent suctioning may be required. Keep suction apparatus with catheters, oxygen, resuscitation bag and mask, and extra tracheostomy tubes (if applicable) at the bedside.

Monitor Neurologic Status

Perform routine neurologic checks. Evaluate pupil size and reactivity, eye movements, and motor function (Fig. 18–3). Monitor vital signs. Increased systolic blood pressure, a wide pulse pressure, and bradycardia indicate increased intracranial pressure. Watch for other signs of increased intracranial pressure listed in Table 18–6.

Be sure that adequate **cerebral perfusion pressure** (the amount of pressure needed to ensure that adequate oxygen and nutrients will be delivered to the brain) is maintained. Fluids are given if the child is hypovolemic (see Chap. 8). If the child shows signs of poor perfusion and fluid overload, dopamine or dobutamine may be administered.

If seizures occur, the side rails should be padded to protect the child from injury.

18-6	Signs of Increased Intracranial Pressure

Early Signs
Headache
Visual disturbances, diplopia
Nausea and vomiting
Dizziness or vertigo
Slight change in vital signs
Pupils not as reactive or equal
Sunsetting eyes
Seizures
Slight change in level of consciousness

Infant has above signs plus:
Bulging fontanel
Wide sutures, increased head circumference
Dilated scalp veins
High-pitched, catlike cry

Late Signs
Significant decrease in level of consciousness
Cushing's triad
  • Increased systolic blood pressure and widened pulse pressure
  • Brachycardia
  • Irregular respirations
Fixed and dilated pupils

18-7   Care of the Immobile Child

- Help keep body in proper alignment with splints or rolls made of towels or blankets.
- Perform passive or gentle range-of-motion exercises three or four times per day according to physician's orders.
- Maintain skin integrity:
  - Change position every 2 hours.
  - Place child on foam or egg-crate mattress or sheepskin covering.
  - Massage child gently using lotion.

Perform Routine Care

If the corneal reflex is absent, artificial tears are placed in the eyes, and they are covered with gauze that is taped in place so they remain closed. Perform routine mouth care by brushing the teeth and using glycerine swabs.

Provide adequate nutrition. Initially nutrients may be supplied intravenously. A gastrostomy tube may be inserted if the child remains unconscious or is not alert enough to take food by mouth.

Prevent complications associated with immobility (muscle atrophy, contractures, and skin breakdown) as described in Table 18–7.

Provide Sensory Stimulation

Explain all procedures and actions. Because the child with a severely altered level of consciousness may still be able to hear, talking to him or her may be beneficial.

When the child becomes more alert, orient the child to time, place, and person, depending on his or her age and level of understanding. Encourage parents to bring objects or toys from home to make the environment more familiar and promote a feeling of security.

Provide Emotional Support

Explain the child's condition in simple terms. Encourage parents to take part in the child's care and therapy as much as possible. If the child's normal functioning has been permanently impaired, refer the family to the appropriate psychologic and social services for emotional support. (See Chapter 6 for more information about helping families cope with a child's life-threatening illness.) Provide family members with opportunities to express their feelings.

Discharge Planning and Home Care Teaching

The child's transition from the hospital to home, a long-term care facility, or inpatient rehabilitation center must be planned well in advance of discharge. A case manager or social worker who can help plan the child's long-term care needs, including home health nursing, adaptation of the home, and the purchase of special equipment, should be identified.

Care in the Community

Home care nurses play a vital role in the care of the child with an acquired neurologic dysfunction. They coordinate care and services for the child and teach family members how to care for the child. For the child with severe neurologic dysfunction, the family needs to learn to perform routine procedures such as maintaining the airway, skin care, feeding, positioning, exercises, and stimulation. Regular follow-up visits are needed to assess the child's progress and to modify the treatment plan.

 CLINICAL TIP

Listening to music or tapes of family members talking or reading can soothe a child who has an altered level of consciousness.

The child also needs to be linked with community rehabilitation services through an early intervention program or school-based program. The home health nurse or case manager should assist the family to have an Individualized Education Plan developed for the child (see Chap. 5).

► SEIZURE DISORDERS

Seizures are periods of sudden disturbance of brain function that cause involuntary muscle activity, change in level of consciousness, or altered behavioral and sensory manifestations. They are a common neurologic disorder in children. Approximately 5% of children have seizures during childhood, most often during infancy. Epilepsy is a chronic disorder characterized by recurrent seizures. It is secondary to underlying brain dysfunction and is often a sign of a central nervous system disorder.[2,3]

Clinical Manifestations

The symptoms of a seizure depend on the type and duration of the seizure. Seizures are classified into two types: *partial (focal) seizures* and *generalized seizures* of nonfocal origin. The specific characteristics of the various types of partial and generalized seizures are presented in Table 18–8. The initial manifestations of the **tonic** phase of a generalized seizure are unconsciousness and continuous muscular contraction. The tonic phase is followed by the **clonic** phase, characterized by alternating muscular contraction and relaxation. In the **postictal period,** following seizure activity, the level of consciousness is decreased. The length of the postictal period varies among children.

Febrile seizures—generalized seizures that usually occur in children as the result of rapid temperature rise above 39°C (102°F)—involve generalized tonic–clonic movements that last less than 15 minutes.

Etiology and Pathophysiology

Seizures are believed to be the result of a spontaneous electrical discharge of hyperexcited cells in the brain. These cells can be triggered by either environmental or physiologic stimuli such as emotional stress, anxiety, fatigue, infection, or metabolic disturbances.

Some seizures are idiopathic. Genetic factors may lower the seizure threshold by making brain cells more vulnerable to abnormal electrical discharges. Acquired seizures may be caused by underlying pathologic conditions such as trauma, infection, hypoglycemia, endocrine dysfunction, toxins, tumors, or lesions that may be manifested at any time. Table 18–9 lists some of the causes of the different types of seizures.

Partial, or **focal,** seizures are caused by abnormal electrical activity in a specific area of the cerebral cortex, most often the temporal, frontal, or parietal lobes. The symptoms that are displayed depend on the region of the cortex affected.

In contrast, generalized seizures are the result of diffuse electrical activity that begins in one area of the brain and spreads throughout the cortex into the brainstem. Movements and spasms displayed by the child are bilateral and symmetric, since both hemispheres are affected.

The length of a seizure, especially that of a generalized seizure, is important because the airway may be compromised during the tonic phase. The basal metabolic rate rises during the peak of seizure activity. This

SAFETY CONSIDERATIONS

During the postictal period, monitor the child's vital signs, perform neurologic checks, and keep the environment safe.

18-8 Clinical Manifestations of Seizures

Type of Seizure	Clinical Manifestations
Partial Seizures	
Complex partial seizures (psychomotor seizures) *Onset:* 3 years of age to adolescence	Consciousness not completely lost, although level of consciousness decreases Aura frequently present Feelings of anxiety, fear, or déjà vu (sensation that an event has occurred before) Abdominal pain Unusual taste or odor Staring into space Mental confusion Posturing Performing repeated purposeless activities (automatisms) Lip smacking, lip chewing, or sucking
Simple partial seizures (focal seizures) *Onset:* any age	Consciousness generally not lost unless the seizure becomes generalized No aura Motor responses may involve one extremity, part of that extremity, or ipsilateral extremities with eyes and head turning in opposite direction Sensory responses involve paresthesias (decreased sensation or tingling) as well as auditory or visual sensations Motor and sensory involvement may be combined Jacksonian march (rare in young children): Tonic contractions of either fingers of one hand, toes of one foot, or one side of the face become clonic or tonic–clonic movements; activity then "marches" up to adjacent muscles of either affected extremity or same side of body (such as face)
Generalized Seizures	

Tonic–clonic seizures (grand mal seizures) *Onset:* any age	Abrupt onset seizure in which there may not be aura
	Tonic phase of seizure lasts 10–30 seconds; clonic phase may persist from 30 seconds to 30 minutes
	Falling to ground during initial tonic phase when loss of consciousness occurs
	Intense muscular contractions
	Eyes rolling upward or deviating to one side with pupils dilated
	Abdominal and chest muscle rigidity with leg, head, and neck extended and arms flexed or contracted
	Pallor or cyanosis
	Cry or grunt as air is forced through rigid diaphragm
	Urinary or bowel incontinence
	Postictal phase of variable duration (few minutes to several hours)
	Characterized by:
	  Sleepiness, difficulty in arousal
	  Hypertension
	  Diaphoresis
	  Headache, nausea, vomiting
	  Poor coordination, decreased muscle tone
	  Confusion, amnesia
	  Slurred speech
	  Visual disturbances
	  Combativeness

Absence seizures (petit mal, or lapse seizures) *Onset:* age 4 years with remission in adolescence More prevalent in females	Brief loss of consciousness; usually last 5–10 seconds, rarely exceeding 30 seconds Attacks occur frequently (as often as 20 or more times daily) No aura Abrupt cessation of current activity Rolling of eyes Ptosis or fluttering of eyelids Staring Slight loss in muscle tone (head may droop, hand-held objects may be dropped) Amnesia Episodes may often be confused with inattentiveness or daydreaming

Continued . . .

18-8   Clinical Manifestations of Seizures (continued)

Type of Seizure	Clinical Manifestations
Myoclonic seizures *Onset:* as early as 2 years, but more prevalent in school-age child and adolescent	No loss of consciousness; child recovers in seconds Attacks occur most often upon falling asleep or awakening Head, extremity, or body contractions No postictal period
Infantile spasms (myoclonic epilepsy of infancy, salaam seizures) *Onset:* begin at age 3 months and resolve by 2 years	Possible loss of consciousness Episodes usually occur when infant is sleepy or drowsy Several seizures can occur throughout day Dropping of head, flexion of neck, extension of arms, and flexion of legs Rolling of eyes either upward or downward Crying, pallor, or cyanosis Children who display these seizures with positive history of gestational difficulties, developmental delays, or other neurologic abnormalities most likely have mental retardation and other types of seizures
Akinetic or atonic seizures (drop attacks) *Onset:* first seen at age 2 years and disappear by age 6 years	Momentary loss of consciousness Loss of muscle tone after which child falls to ground Inability to break fall

change, in turn, increases the demand for oxygen and glucose. During a seizure the child may become pale or cyanotic as a result of hypoxia or hypoglycemia.

Febrile seizures occur in connection with an acute, febrile illness. They are most common in children from 6–18 months of age, but may be seen from 3 months to 5 years.[4] There is often a family history of febrile seizures. In addition, children who have one febrile seizure have a 30% greater chance of having future seizures. The lower convulsive threshold of infants may explain this type of seizure.

Diagnostic Tests and Medical Management

After the child's first seizure, it is essential that a thorough history be taken from the parent, primary caretaker, or witnesses to the event. Table 18–10 lists the questions that should be asked. Details such as the description and length of the seizure, presence or absence of an **aura** (an early sign or warning of an impending seizure, most often olfactory or visual in nature), and whether or not the child lost consciousness should be noted.

A complete physical and neurologic examination is performed. Based on the physical findings and history, diagnostic tests are ordered. Laboratory tests include a complete blood cell count and blood chemistry. If the child is taking any anticonvulsants, blood levels of the medication should be monitored. Lumbar puncture and EEG may be performed. Radiologic tests include CT scanning or MRI and angiography.

Children with febrile seizures may be treated with an anticonvulsant for the remainder of the presenting febrile illness. However, long-term anticonvulsants are not generally used. Instead, parents are taught to lower fevers by use of antipyretics and environmental control (keeping the child cool with sponge bathing and light clothing).

18-9   Common Causes of Seizures

Type of Seizure	Cause
Partial	
Complex partial seizure	Lesions, cysts, or tumors
	Perinatal trauma
	Prolonged febrile seizures that may cause scarring of mediotemporal lobe
	Hamartomatous lesions
	Arteriovenous malformations
	Trauma
Simple partial seizure	Focal damage (eg, with cerebral palsy)
	Tumors or lesions
	Arteriovenous malformation
	Brain abscesses
Generalized	
Tonic–clonic seizure	Cerebral damage from birth injury, trauma, tumors, lesions, and metabolic and neuromuscular degenerative disorders; many are idiopathic
Absence seizure	Possible genetic link
Infantile spasm	Prenatal and perinatal encephalopathy
	Tuberous sclerosis
	Microcephaly
Akinetic–myoclonic seizures	Gray matter degenerative diseases and subacute sclerosing panencephalitis; many are idiopathic
Febrile seizure	Rapid rise in temperature, reaching 39°C (102°F)
	Associated with infections:
	Upper respiratory
	Urinary tract
	Otitis media
	Pharyngitis
	Roseola

Many convulsions are self-limiting and require no emergency intervention; however, status epilepticus is considered a medical emergency. Status epilepticus is a continuous seizure that lasts more than 30 minutes or a series of seizures during which consciousness is not regained. The postictal period ranges from 30 minutes to 2 hours. Management of the child in status epilepticus is described in Table 18–11.

Most seizure disorders are treated with anticonvulsants (Table 18–12). Serum drug levels are monitored to maintain therapeutic levels. Maintaining a balance between seizure control and medication toxicity is difficult because as the child grows, the medication dosage may need to be increased.

A ketogenic diet is occasionally used for children with myoclonic and absence seizures. This diet involves a high intake of fat and low intake of carbohydrates and protein (Fig. 18–4). Family motivation must be high to maintain the diet and to frequently monitor the child's urine ketone values.[4]

Surgery may occasionally be performed to remove a tumor, lesion, or portion of the brain that has been identified as causing the seizures.[5]

CLINICAL TIP

Children under the age of 8 years with specific types of seizures may be put on a ketogenic diet, which consists of a ratio of 3–5 grams of fat to 1 gram of protein plus carbohydrates.[1] This high-fat diet causes a mild state of starvation, resulting in ketosis as the body uses fat for metabolism. A mild state of dehydration is maintained so the level of ketones in the circulation is not diluted. Ketosis is believed to slow the electrical impulses that cause seizures. Medium-chain triglycerides may be given as a supplement to increase the acidosis.

18-10   Questions to Ask About Seizures

- Did the child complain of not feeling well or feeling "funny" just before the seizure?
- Did the child complain of headache, nausea, muscle pain? Did the child vomit?
- Did the child suffer any trauma before the seizure?
- Did the child get into any medications or poisons before the seizure?
- Was the child sick or feverish before the seizure?
- Were the child's movements tonic–clonic (periods of muscle rigidity followed by relaxation)?
- Was the child's vision normal?
- Were the pupils dilated or the eyes deviated to one side?
- Was the child incontinent of urine or stool?
- How long did the episode last?
- When did the child begin to wake up?
- Was the child lethargic, weak, or uncoordinated upon arousal?
- Did the child's movements involve one side of the body or one arm or leg?
- Did the child injure himself or herself during the convulsion?
- Did the child become pale or did the skin change color (eg, red or blue)?
- Did the child lose consciousness?

18-11   Management of Status Epilepticus

- Maintain a patent airway. Muscle rigidity may compromise the airway.
- Perform a jaw thrust maneuver if the airway is obstructed.
- Keep suction equipment at the bedside in case secretions are excessive.
- Give oxygen by mask, as increased metabolic demands deplete oxygen stores.
- Monitor vital signs and circulation with pulse oximeter and cardiorespiratory monitor.
- Assess neurologic level.
- Establish an intravenous line to administer any necessary fluids or medications.
- Administer glucose if the child is hypoglycemic; the physical stress of the seizure may result in declining glucose levels.
- Insert a nasogastric tube.
- Protect the child from injury.
- Manage thermoregulation.
- Administer benzodiazepines such as diazepam, lorazepam, or midazolam. If there is no response, the dose may be repeated. Phenytoin or phenobarbital may be necessary if seizure activity continues.

18-12   Anticonvulsants Used to Treat Seizure Disorders

Carbamazepine	Lamotrigine
Clonazepam	Phenobarbital
Ethosuximide	Phenytoin
Felbamate	Primidone
Gabapentin	Valproic acid

Nursing Assessment

Assess the child's physiologic status (see Table 18–4). Once the child is stable, a more definitive assessment can be made. Level of consciousness is one of the most important indicators of neurologic function. Remember that the child's lack of response may be the result of the postictal state.

Nursing Diagnosis

Common nursing diagnoses for the child with a seizure disorder include:

- Ineffective Breathing Pattern related to decreased respiratory effort during the tonic phase of a seizure
- Ineffective Airway Clearance related to seizure activity and inability to control secretions
- Risk for Aspiration related to decreased level of consciousness and possible vomiting
- Risk for Injury related to seizure activity
- Body Image Disturbance related to loss of bowel and bladder control during seizure activity
- Risk for Anxiety related to distressing aspects of seizure disorder
- Knowledge Deficit (Parent) related to care during seizures
- Knowledge Deficit (Parent) related to pharmacologic management of seizures
- Altered Family Processes related to care of a child with a chronic disorder

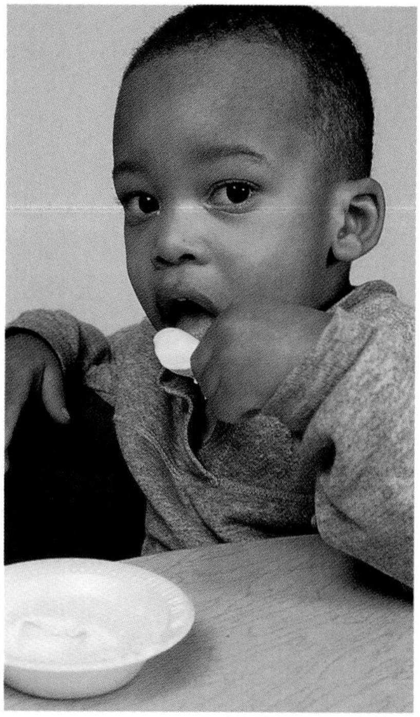

FIGURE 18–4. The family must make an effort to make the high-fat diet appealing to the child on a ketogenic diet, despite their personal feelings about eating large amounts of foods such as mayonnaise as this child is doing.

Nursing Management

Nursing care focuses on maintaining airway patency, ensuring safety, administering medications, and providing emotional support. Both acute care and long-term management are involved.

Maintain Airway Patency

Be sure that nothing is placed in the child's mouth during a seizure. Monitor the child to ensure adequate oxygenation: the child's color should be pink, the heart rate at a normal or slightly above normal rate for age, and the pulse oximetry reading greater than 95%. Oxygen is usually given at levels below 95%.

Ensure Safety

Protect the child from self-harm during violent seizures (Fig 18–5). If the child is in bed, the side rails should be padded to prevent injury.

Administer Medications

Take special precautions when administering intravenous medications for the acute management of seizures. These medications should be given very slowly to minimize the risk of respiratory or circulatory collapse.

Medications for the management of chronic seizures are given orally. Crushing pills and mixing them in a teaspoonful of applesauce, pudding, or other soft food make them more palatable and easier for the child to swallow.

 SAFETY PRECAUTIONS

Do not force a bite block between the teeth of a child during a seizure. Loose teeth may be knocked out and aspirated.

 SAFETY PRECAUTIONS

Children who have frequent, recurrent seizures should wear helmets to protect their heads in case they fall. All children with seizure disorders should wear some form of medical identification (eg, a Medic-Alert bracelet).

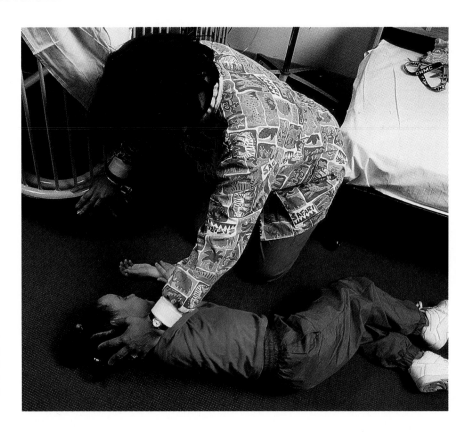

FIGURE 18–5. A child who has a seizure when standing should be gently assisted to the floor and placed in a side-lying position. Clear the area of any objects that might cause harm to the child.

Provide Emotional Support

The loss of control of body movements and possible loss of consciousness make seizures frightening and difficult to accept for the child, parents, and other family members.

Parents often feel guilty about the child's seizure disorder and compensate by not disciplining or restricting the child appropriately. Stress the need to treat the child as normally as possible. Refer the child and family to support groups and counseling services if indicated.

Discharge Planning and Home Care Teaching

Encourage parents to express their fears and anxieties. Answer their questions honestly, and refer them to organizations such as the Epilepsy Foundation of America, where they can obtain more information about the child's disorder (Appendix F). Be sure parents know how to administer medications and provide for the child's safety. Discuss with them whom to call with questions and when to return for follow-up.

Care in the Community

Educate the child and parents about medication regimens. Explain the purpose of each drug, its schedule for administration, and the importance of giving all doses. Teaching the older child to take medications without parental intervention gives the child a feeling of control. Provide information about the side effects of medications ordered, and alert parents to the signs of toxic reactions or undermedication. Regular dental care is important because of the effect of certain anticonvulsants on the gingiva. Explain the importance of follow-up visits to health care providers so the effectiveness of the child's medications can be monitored. Often blood levels will be measured to identify whether serum levels are being maintained within therapeutic ranges.

Assist the family to develop an Individual School Health Plan so the child can receive medications during school hours, if necessary. Teachers and school administrators should know what actions to take if the child has a seizure and what information to report about the seizure. They should also be aware that contact sports are not recommended, and swimming should be permitted only with close supervision.

The child may be afraid of having a seizure in front of friends. Reassure the child and family that taking medications regularly should control seizures. Children need to be able to explain to peers what a seizure is and what to do if they are present when one occurs. Summer camps for children with seizures can be a safe and comfortable place for the child to enjoy outdoor activities. Tell parents to boost the child's self-image by emphasizing what the child can do, rather than focusing on contraindicated activities. Depending on state laws, most adolescents can drive after they have been seizure free for at least 2 years.

Parents of children with recurrent febrile seizures should be taught how to give antipyretics and the proper dose. Antipyretic doses will need to be updated as the child grows. Parents can be reassured that complications for these children are rare.

► INFECTIOUS DISEASES

BACTERIAL MENINGITIS

Meningitis, an inflammation of the meninges, can be caused by either bacterial or viral agents. Bacterial meningitis is more virulent than viral meningitis and is sometimes fatal.[4] The child who is less than 1 year of age is at greatest risk for acquiring bacterial meningitis. Seventy percent of all cases appear before 5 years of age.[1]

Clinical Manifestations

Symptoms are variable and depend on the child's age, the pathogen, and the length of the illness before diagnosis. Onset may be sudden or the illness may develop over about a 1–week period. Symptoms in the young infant may include fever, change in feeding pattern, vomiting, or diarrhea. The anterior fontanel may be bulging or flat. The infant may be alert, restless, lethargic, or irritable. Rocking or cuddling, which normally calms a fussy infant, only irritates the infant with meningitis.

Older children are usually febrile, can be irritable, lethargic, or confused, have vomiting, and complain of muscle or joint pain. A hemorrhagic rash, first appearing as petechiae and changing to purpura or large necrotic patches, may be seen in meningococcal meningitis. The child displays other symptoms consistent with meningeal irritation: headache (most often frontal), photophobia, and nuchal (resistance to neck flexion) rigidity. The child is comfortable only in an opisthotonic position (hyperextension of the head and neck to relieve discomfort; Fig. 18–6). The child may have a positive Kernig or Brudzinski sign, or both, on examination (Figs. 18–7 and 18–8).

Symptoms can progress to include seizures, apnea, cerebral edema, subdural effusion, hydrocephalus, disseminated intravascular coagulation (DIC), shock, and increased intracranial pressure. The bacteria may also colonize within a joint, causing septic arthritis.

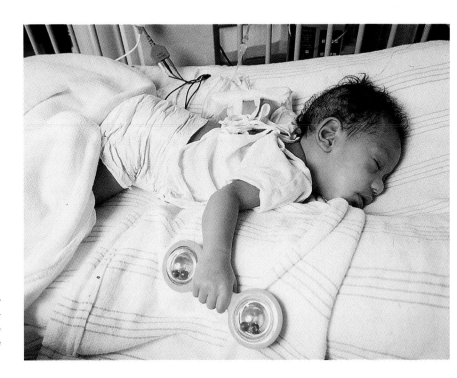

FIGURE 18-6. The child with bacterial meningitis assumes an opisthotonic position, with the neck and the head hyperextended, to relieve discomfort.

Etiology and Pathophysiology

Meningitis may occur secondary to other infections such as otitis media, sinusitis, pharyngitis, cellulitis, pneumonia, or septic arthritis; head trauma; or a neurosurgical procedure. The most common causal agents in children are listed in Table 18-13. Previously, *Haemophilus influenzae* type b was the most common causative organism, but its incidence has decreased markedly in recent years because most infants are now immunized against it. Pneumococcal meningitis has the highest morbidity and mortality.[6]

In many cases bacteremia spreads the infectious agent to the central nervous system (Fig. 18-9). An inflammatory response follows. White blood cells accumulate, covering the surface of the brain with a thick, white, purulent exudate. The brain then becomes hyperemic and edematous. If the

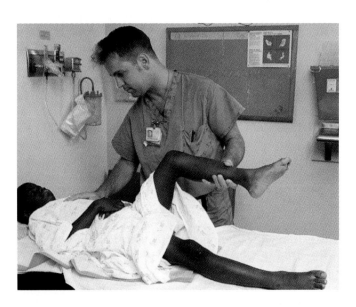

FIGURE 18-7. To test for Kernig sign, raise the child's leg with the knee flexed. Then extend the child's leg at the knee. If any resistance is noted or pain is felt, the result is a positive Kernig sign. This is a common finding in meningitis.

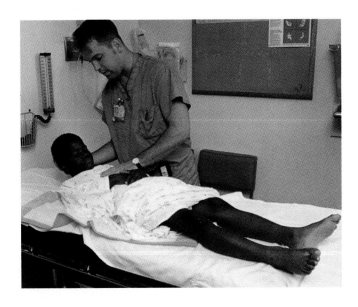

FIGURE 18–8. To test Brudzinski sign, flex the child's head while in a supine position. If this action makes the knees or hips flex involuntarily, a positive Brudzinski sign is present. This is a common finding in meningitis.

infection spreads to the ventricles, they can become obstructed and impede the flow of cerebrospinal fluid, causing hydrocephalus.

Diagnostic Tests and Medical Management

Diagnosis is based on the history, clinical presentation, and laboratory findings. A thorough history should be taken and a physical examination performed.

Laboratory tests include a complete blood count, blood cultures, serum electrolytes and osmolality, and clotting factors. A lumbar puncture is performed to evaluate the cerebrospinal fluid for number of white blood cells and protein and glucose levels. A Gram stain and culture are done on the cerebrospinal fluid.

18-13	Common Organisms That Cause Bacterial and Viral Meningitis	
Age	**Bacterial Agents**	**Viral Agents**
Neonates (age: less than 1–2 months)	*Escherichia coli*; group B *Streptococcus*; *Listeria monocytogenes*; *Haemophilus influenzae* type b; *Neisseria meningitidis*; *Streptococcus pneumoniae*	Herpes
Beyond neonatal period to early adolescence (age: 2 months to 12 years)	*Haemophilus influenzae* type b (in those not immunized); *Neisseria meningitidis*; *Streptococcus pneumoniae*	Enterovirus, mumps, adenovirus
Adolescence (age: more than 12 years)	*Neisseria meningitidis*; *Streptococcus pneumoniae*	Herpes, arbovirus, adenovirus

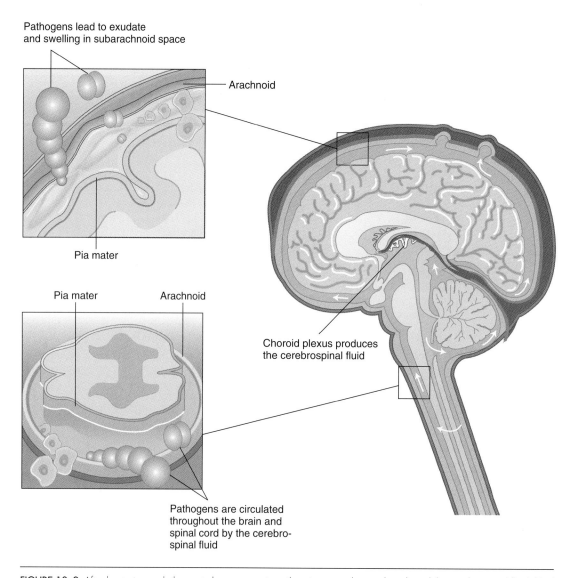

Pathogens lead to exudate and swelling in subarachnoid space

Arachnoid

Pia mater

Pia mater   Arachnoid

Choroid plexus produces the cerebrospinal fluid

Pathogens are circulated throughout the brain and spinal cord by the cerebrospinal fluid

FIGURE 18–9. After bacteria reach the central nervous system, the pia mater, the arachnoid, and the cerebrospinal fluid–filled subarachnoid space become infected. The cerebrospinal fluid then circulates the pathogens throughout the brain and spinal cord.

NURSING ALERT

Remember that gastrointestinal bleeding is a potential complication of corticosteroid use. Monitor the child receiving these drugs for signs of intestinal discomfort and for blood in the stools.

Medical management consists primarily of treating the child with appropriate antibiotics. Antibiotics are administered as soon as diagnostic tests are obtained (Table 18–14). These drugs are administered intravenously for 7–21 days, depending on the organism and the child's clinical response. Depending on the causative organism, the disease may need to be reported to the local health department, and contacts may need to take prophylactic antibiotics, such as rifampin. Corticosteroids are given as an adjunct to children over 6 weeks of age because these drugs result in less severe neurologic sequelae (eg, sensorineural hearing loss is reduced).[6,7] An adrenocortico-steroid (dexamethasone is the drug of choice) is given with or before the first dose of antibiotics and continued over several days.[6, 8] Anticonvulsants and antipyretics may be given.

Some infants and children who have had bacterial meningitis suffer neurologic damage despite early, aggressive management. The most common sequelae involve cranial nerves, especially the eighth, resulting in hearing loss. In addition, attention deficits, seizures, developmental delay, septic arthritis, or other focal signs may occur (Table 18–15). Another potential complication

18-14	Antibiotics Used in the Treatment of Bacterial Meningitis
Age Group	**Antibiotic**
Neonates	Ampicillin
	Aminoglycosides
	Cefotaxime
Infants	Ampicillin
	Cefotaxime
	Ceftriaxone
Children >6 years old	Penicillin G
	Ceftriaxone

From Tureen, J. (1996). Meningitis. In A.M. Rudolph, J.I.E. Hoffman, & C.D. Rudolph (Eds.), Rudolph's pediatrics (20th ed., p. 547). Stamford, CT: Appleton & Lange.

is meningococcal septicemia, which is characterized by high fever, hypotension, disseminated intravascular coagulation, and multisystem organ failure.[9]

Nursing Assessment

Assess the child's physiologic status, including vital signs and level of consciousness. Measure head circumference frequently in infants because of the potential for hydrocephalus to develop. Be alert to any signs of a change in the child's condition and response to treatment. Monitor the child's ability to control secretions and to drink sufficient fluids. Monitor intake and output. Assess for any sensory deficits. Identify parents' concerns related to this potentially life-threatening condition.

Nursing Diagnosis

Several nursing diagnoses that may apply to the child with bacterial meningitis are given in the accompanying Nursing Care Plan. Additional nursing diagnoses might include the following:

- Ineffective Airway Clearance related to altered level of consciousness
- Risk for Fluid Volume Deficit related to poor oral fluid intake
- Anticipatory Grieving (Parent) related to the child's potentially life-threatening condition
- Caregiver Role Strain related to a hospitalized child and other family responsibilities

18-15	Complications of Bacterial Meningitis

Syndrome of inappropriate antidiuretic hormone secretion (SIADH)
Disseminated intravascular coagulation (DIC)
Subdural effusion
Septicemia
Septic arthritis
Seizures
Hearing Loss
Hydrocephalus

NURSING CARE PLAN
THE CHILD WITH BACTERIAL MENINGITIS

GOAL	INTERVENTION	RATIONALE	EXPECTED OUTCOME

1. Inability to Sustain Spontaneous Ventilation related to decreased level of consciousness

GOAL	INTERVENTION	RATIONALE	EXPECTED OUTCOME
The child will not have respiratory arrest from apneic spells.	• Place the child on either an apnea monitor or respiratory monitor with a 20-second alarm.	• The alarm on the monitor alerts staff that the child is having an apneic spell.	The child's respiratory failure is easily managed with prompt assessment and treatment.
	• Have resuscitation equipment, including oxygen, resuscitation bag with mask, and suction apparatus at the bedside.	• Equipment should be at the bedside in case of respiratory arrest. Month-to-mouth resuscitation is not advised because the child's respiratory secretions include bacteria.	
	• Stimulate the child if apneic; if no response, begin manual ventilations and call for emergency resuscitation.	• Stimulation may encourage spontaneous respirations; if not, ventilation is necessary. Calling for emergency resuscitation ensures help in managing the child in a timely manner.	
	• Monitor heart rate and perform compressions if necessary.	• The apneic child may have bradycardia resulting from cardiac hypoxia.	

2. Risk for Infection related to pathogens in cerebrospinal fluid

GOAL	INTERVENTION	RATIONALE	EXPECTED OUTCOME
The child will be free of infection as quickly as possible.	• Administer prescribed antibiotics and corticosteroids as scheduled.	• Antibiotics and corticosteroids help eradicate the pathogen and prevent cerebral edema.	The child responds to the medication within 72 hours.
	• Monitor vital signs, assess for signs of increased intracranial pressure, check head circumference for swelling, note changes in level of consciousness.	• Watching for common sequelae such as subdural effusions or septic arthritis ensures prompt treatment.	
Caretakers or family members will have no apparent evidence of infection.	• Explain rationale and dose and schedule for taking rifampin.	• Rifampin provides prophylaxis for many bacterial pathogens responsible for meningitis.	Family members and other close contacts verbalize schedule of rifampin therapy.

NURSING CARE PLAN

THE CHILD WITH BACTERIAL MENINGITIS— *Continued*

GOAL	INTERVENTION	RATIONALE	EXPECTED OUTCOME

3. Risk for Ineffective Thermoregulation related to infection

GOAL	INTERVENTION	RATIONALE	EXPECTED OUTCOME
The child's thermoregulation will return to normal.	• Administer antipyretics such as acetaminophen as ordered (aspirin is not advised because of risk of Reye syndrome). May give tepid bath. May use hypothermia blanket.	• Administration of antipyretics and use of other techniques safely reduce fever.	Body temperature decreases or returns to normal.

4. Risk for Injury related to infection of cerebrospinal fluid and potential sequelae

GOAL	INTERVENTION	RATIONALE	EXPECTED OUTCOME
The child will suffer minimal central nervous system injury secondary to infection.	• Give antibiotics and corticosteroids as soon as possible. Note return of fever, nuchal rigidity, or irritability. Be alert for signs and symptoms of effusion, cerebrospinal fluid obstruction, or cerebral edema, and notify the physician immediately if they occur. • Measure head circumference once or twice daily.	• Prompt administration of antibiotics enhances eradication of the pathogen. Administration of corticosteroids diminishes inflammatory response and reduces the chance of neurologic sequelae. • Increasing head circumference may indicate subdural effusion or hydrocephalus.	The child's condition significantly improves within 48–72 hours (fever decreases, photophobia becomes less severe).
The child will not develop cerebral edema as result of water retention.	• Monitor for syndrome of inappropriate antidiuretic hormone secretion (SIADH) and watch for signs of increased intracranial pressure (ICP). • Perform strict intake and output measurements. Determine urine specific gravity. Check electrolytes and osmolality of both serum and urine. Weigh the child daily. Administer fluids at two thirds of maintenance requirements.	• SIADH can be either avoided or quickly managed if early recognition is achieved. • Low urine output with a high specific gravity is a sign of fluid retention and SIADH. The child is maintained with lower fluids to reduced the possibility for cerebral edema.	Cerebral edema does not develop. If SIADH or increased ICP occurs, the condition is treated promptly so effects on the child are minimal.
The child will be free of injury resulting from disseminated intravascular coagulation (DIC).	• Be aware of needle sticks that continue to bleed and lesions that continue to ooze. Monitor clotting times.	• Prompt recognition leads to management of the coagulopathy.	The child does not sustain injury from DIC.

Continued . . .

NURSING CARE PLAN
THE CHILD WITH BACTERIAL MENINGITIS– *Continued*

GOAL	INTERVENTION	RATIONALE	EXPECTED OUTCOME

4. Risk for Injury related to infection of cerebrospinal fluid and potential sequelae (continued)

GOAL	INTERVENTION	RATIONALE	EXPECTED OUTCOME
The child will be free of injury secondary to shock.	• Administer blood products, vitamin K, or heparin as ordered.	• Prompt recognition allows for early initial treatment of DIC. The child may bleed to death if treatment is delayed.	The child recovers from shock quickly with no complications. Prompt management of shock can enhance the child's recovery, since it prevents complications associated with poor perfusion (tissue acidosis and ischemia).
	• Maintain a safe environment. Protect the child from injury.	• Additional injury can be prevented.	
	• Monitor vital signs including pulse, respirations, and blood pressure. Note perfusion (capillary refill, central versus proximal pulses). Check level of consciousness. Note urine output.	• Monitoring allows for prompt diagnosis of shock based on clinical signs.	
	• Begin fluid resuscitation as ordered.	• Intravenous fluid bolus may improve perfusion.	
	• Administer inotropes if ordered.	• Inotropes enhance perfusion when response to fluid challenge is minimal.	
The child with any degree of hearing loss will be identified.	• Arrange for hearing assessment prior to discharge.	• Hearing loss is a common complication. Early intervention is needed to promote growth and development.	The child with identified hearing loss is referred to appropriate specialist or program for intervention.

5. Impaired Social Interaction related to decreased level of consciousness, hospitalization, and isolation

GOAL	INTERVENTION	RATIONALE	EXPECTED OUTCOME
The child's social interactions will be near normal despite isolation.	• Educate parents and other visitors to use proper infection control techniques.	• Family members help fulfill the emotional and social needs of the ill and contagious child.	The child's social and developmental needs are met by family members despite the child's illness and hospitalization.
	• Encourage parents to help with daily activities such as feeding and bathing.	• Parental involvement in the child's care provides the child with a sense of security and emotional well-being. Parents have a sense of control and a feeling that they are doing something to enhance the child's recovery.	

NURSING CARE PLAN
THE CHILD WITH BACTERIAL MENINGITIS— *Continued*

GOAL	INTERVENTION	RATIONALE	EXPECTED OUTCOME

5. Impaired Social Interaction related to decreased level of consciousness, hospitalization, and isolation (continued)

GOAL	INTERVENTION	RATIONALE	EXPECTED OUTCOME
	• Have age-appropriate games and toys in the room. Play with the child. When the child is feeling better, encourage watching television or a videotape or listening to the radio or an audio tape.	• Providing the child with toys and games as well as sensory stimulation helps the child achieve a sense of well-being.	The child engages in age-appropriate play.

6. Pain related to meningeal irritation

GOAL	INTERVENTION	RATIONALE	EXPECTED OUTCOME
The child will be as comfortable as possible.	• Minimize tactile stimulation	• Sensory stimulation increases discomfort.	The child is calm and expresses increased comfort.
	• Allow the child to assume a position of comfort.	• The child determines the most comfortable position. Opisthotonic position, with the head and neck hyperextended, may be the most comfortable.	
	• Keep the lights dim.	• Dim lights reduce the discomfort from photophobia.	
	• Maintain a quiet environment. Keep doors closed.	• Noise can disturb the child.	

Nursing Management

The preceding Nursing Care Plan summarizes care for the child with bacterial meningitis. Nursing care begins with emergency treatment and continues as the child's condition stabilizes. Monitor respiratory and neurologic status, maintain hydration, administer medications, and prevent complications. Promote the child's comfort with reduced stimulation (dim lights, quiet room) and by placing in a side-lying position. Monitor the child's response to antibiotic therapy. Isolate the child and use standard and droplet precautions until the causative organism is identified and effective treatment is underway.

Respond to parents' concerns about their child's condition, explaining all measures to reduce the child's discomfort and provide adequate treatment. Identify ways parents can participate in meeting the child's comfort needs. Parents may also need assistance in identifying the best strategies for meeting the needs of other children at home while spending time with the hospitalized child.

NURSING ALERT

Maintenance and replacement fluids are usually given to children with bacterial meningitis. However, it is important to monitor the serum sodium concentration and urine specific gravity because these children are at risk for developing the syndrome of insufficient antidiuretic hormone (SIADH; see Chap. 16). In addition, the degree of hyponatremia has been found to correlate with the presence of neurologic abnormalities, seizures, and subdural effusions.[10]

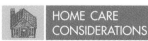

Discharge Planning and Home Care Teaching

Home care needs should be identified and addressed well in advance of discharge. Follow-up visits are important to monitor for complications and sequelae. Help parents deal with any physical requirements resulting from the child's illness and any emotional, social, and financial repercussions of the child's condition. Teach parents what to do if the child has a seizure.

Infants and toddlers with neurologic sequelae should be referred to an early intervention program. If the child has had a hearing loss, referral to an otolaryngologist and speech and language specialist should be made. Early identification of other neurologic sequelae, such as learning problems, should be encouraged.

VIRAL (ASEPTIC) MENINGITIS

Viral meningitis is an inflammatory response of the meninges characterized by an increased number of blood cells and protein in the cerebrospinal fluid. In the United States, an enterovirus is often the cause of aseptic meningitis.[11]

Generally, the child with aseptic meningitis does not appear to be as ill as the child with bacterial meningitis. The child may be irritable or lethargic and usually has a fever. Other symptoms include general malaise, headache, photophobia, gastrointestinal distress, upper respiratory symptoms, and a maculopapular rash. The child may also show signs of meningeal irritation such as stiff neck, back pain, and positive Kernig and Brudzinski signs (see Figs. 18–7 and 18–8). The infant may have a tense anterior fontanel. Seizures are rare. Symptoms usually resolve spontaneously within 3–10 days.

The child with fever and meningeal signs is hospitalized. Blood, urine, and cerebrospinal fluid analyses are performed. Until the diagnosis of aseptic meningitis is confirmed, the child is treated aggressively, as if he or she has bacterial meningitis.

Nursing Management

Initial nursing care focuses on providing supportive care as described for the child with bacterial meningitis. Give acetaminophen as ordered to reduce fever, headache, and muscle or joint pain. Keep the room dark and quiet (to decrease stimuli and meningeal irritation), give fluids either intravenously or orally, and promote comfort with proper positioning.

The child and family need information about the disease. Explain medical and nursing procedures in terms that the child and family can understand. Keep parents informed about the child's progress. Once the diagnosis of viral meningitis is made, discharge planning and teaching for home care must begin immediately. Explain that recovery may take several weeks but that complete recovery is expected.[11]

ENCEPHALITIS

Encephalitis is an inflammation of the brain usually caused by a viral infection. Inflammation of the meninges and the brain is also common.[12]

Signs and symptoms depend on the causative organism and the location of the infection within the brain. An acute onset of a febrile illness with neurologic signs is the classic manifestation of encephalitis. Initially the child may have a severe headache, signs of an upper respiratory infection, and nausea or vomiting. There may be signs of meningeal irritation such as nuchal rigidity, photophobia, and positive Kernig and Brudzinski signs (see Figs. 18–7 and 18–8). Other neurologic signs vary. The child may be disoriented or confused, with behavioral or personality changes. Speech disturbances; motor dysfunction such as hemiparesis, ataxia, or weakness; cranial nerve deficits; or alterations in reflex response may be present. Focal or generalized seizures may occur, alternating with periods of screaming, hallucinating, and moving in a bizarre fashion. The child's level of consciousness may deteriorate from stupor to coma.

Viruses are believed to cause most cases of encephalitis (Table 18–16). Herpes simplex type I is the most common cause after the newborn period.

Diagnosis is based on history and laboratory findings. Information about recent immunizations, insect bites, or travel to areas where vectors are present should be obtained. Cerebrospinal fluid analysis, blood serologic tests, and nasopharyngeal and stool specimens are evaluated to identify viral pathogens. A CT scan, MRI, and EEG may also be performed. The nucleic acid detection test is used to assay for herpes DNA in the spinal fluid. Brain biopsy is rarely performed to diagnose herpes simplex and parasitic infections.

The child with encephalitis is at risk for seizures, respiratory failure, and increased intracranial pressure and should be cared for in an intensive care unit. Treatment is both pharmacologic and supportive. The child with a suspected bacterial infection should be treated with antibiotics until bacterial pathogens have been ruled out. A child with herpesvirus infection should receive acyclovir or other antiviral agents.[13]

Children with encephalitis have many neurologic sequelae. Although some children recover completely, many more are left with intellectual, motor, visual, or auditory deficits. The cardiovascular system, lungs, or liver may also be affected. Generally, the younger the child, the more serious the illness and the more severe the residual effects.

Nursing Management

Nursing care focuses on monitoring cardiorespiratory function, preventing complications resulting from immobility, reorienting the child, and teaching the parents about the child's condition.

Monitor the child's cardiorespiratory function. Check the child's airway and ability to handle secretions. Monitor respiratory status by observing color, pulse oximetry readings, and arterial blood gas values. Observe cardiopulmonary status by monitoring heart rate, blood pressure, capillary refill time, and urine output. Provide seizure precautions, and have appropriate equipment for managing seizures at the bedside.

Prevent complications resulting from immobility as described in Table 18–7. Maintain skin integrity. Proper positioning with frequent turning is important. When indicated by the physician, perform chest physiotherapy to prevent pneumonia.

The child whose level of consciousness begins to improve may at first be confused and disoriented and may have residual effects of the disease. Orient the child to the hospital environment. Have the family help to reorient the child by bringing favorite stuffed animals or music from home. Engage in therapeutic play (refer to Chapter 4 for techniques). Give the child age-appropriate toys to encourage a return to normal behavior.

Provide the parents with information about their child's condition and prognosis. If the child receives physical, occupational, or speech therapy, explain the treatment regimen to the parents.

18-16 Causative Viruses of Encephalitis

Enteroviruses
- Poliovirus
- Echovirus
- Coxsackievirus

Adenoviruses and herpesviruses
Arboviruses
Measles
Mumps
Rubella
Rabies
Hepatitis B

Discharge Planning and Home Care Teaching

Encourage parents to take an active role in the child's physical and emotional care in the hospital, and give them written instructions concerning care for their child at home. Encourage the parents to learn specific physical, occupational, and speech therapies so they can work with their child at home between home care visits. Refer parents to home care, social services, family counseling, and support groups. Plan follow-up visits so the child can be evaluated for neurologic sequelae.

REYE SYNDROME

Reye syndrome is an acute metabolic encephalopathy of childhood that also affects the liver, causing hepatic dysfunction. It is characterized by cerebral edema and an enlarged, fatty, poorly functioning liver.

The clinical manifestations of Reye syndrome have been divided into five stages, as described in Table 18–17. The condition is most severe in younger children.[14]

The etiology of Reye syndrome is unclear. The disorder usually develops after a mild viral illness, such as varicella, an upper respiratory infection, or gastroenteritis. It has also been associated with aspirin use.[14] Since more and more parents have begun giving children acetaminophen rather than aspirin for flu-like symptoms and varicella, the incidence of Reye syndrome has declined. Only 25 cases were reported to the National Reye Syndrome Surveillance System in 1990.[1] About 70% of children who develop Reye syndrome survive.

The diagnosis of Reye syndrome is based on an abrupt change in the child's level of consciousness and diagnostic laboratory tests. The child has often progressed to coma or stage III by the time of diagnosis. Liver enzyme levels (aspartate aminotransferase [AST] or alanine aminotransferase [ALT]) are elevated to twice their normal levels, ammonia levels are elevated, blood glucose levels are below normal, and prothrombin time is prolonged. A liver biopsy is sometimes performed to confirm the diagnosis (by showing small droplet fat deposits).

> **CLINICAL TIP**
>
> Make sure all parents understand the link between aspirin and Reye syndrome. Instruct them to check all over-the-counter medicines for the presence of aspirin compounds. Emphasize the importance of obtaining health care whenever a child's condition worsens at the end of a viral illness.

18-17 Stages of Reye Syndrome

Stage	Clinical Manifestations
I	Vomiting; lethargy; appropriate responses to verbal commands; purposeful responses to pain; brisk pupillary reaction
II	Combativeness; stupor; inappropriate language; confusion; anxiety, fear; purposeful and nonpurposeful responses to pain; sluggish pupillary reaction; conjugate deviation with oculocephalic reflex; hyperactive reflexes; progresses to coma but interrupted by periods of screaming and ranting
III	Coma; decorticate rigidity; conjugate deviation with diminished oculocephalic reflex; sluggish pupillary reaction; decorticate posturing
IV	Coma with brainstem dysfunction; decerebrate rigidity; inconsistent or absent oculocephalic reflex; loss of corneal reflex; sluggish pupillary reaction; decerebrate posturing
V	Coma with seizures; flaccidity; loss of deep tendon reflexes; respiratory arrest

The child with Reye syndrome should be placed in a pediatric intensive care unit because of the potential for rapid deterioration in his or her condition. The goal of medical management is to provide supportive treatment and to prevent the secondary effects of cerebral edema and metabolic injury. Assisted ventilation is often needed once the child is comatose. The child is monitored for signs of increased intracranial pressure, which can be secondary to cerebral edema. Hypoglycemia is treated with intravenous glucose, and electrolytes, blood chemistry, and blood pH are monitored.

Nursing Management

Nursing care focuses on monitoring the child's physical status, providing emotional support, and teaching parents about disease prevention.

Check the child's respiratory and neurologic status frequently, and note any signs of improvement or deterioration. Orient the child who awakens from coma. Refer to the discussion of nursing management of altered states of consciousness at the beginning of this chapter for specific nursing interventions. Look for changes in laboratory values that indicate acidosis, an elevation of ammonia levels, or hypoglycemia. Monitor the child's intake and output. Correct imbalances by administering fluids, electrolytes, or medications as ordered. Prevent complications associated with immobility (see Table 18–7).

Provide emotional support to the parents, who may feel guilty because they did not seek medical attention sooner. Keep them informed about the child's condition, and prepare them for potential deterioration in the course of the disease. Explanations of treatments can help reduce anxiety. Encourage the parents to participate in the child's care whenever possible.

Once the child is discharged, monitoring is needed to observe for sequelae of the illness. Developmental and neurologic deficits may occur and are more severe in children under 2 years of age. Be sure the parents are informed about resources in the community that can assist them in dealing with the child's recovery.

GUILLAIN-BARRÉ SYNDROME (POSTINFECTIOUS POLYNEURITIS)

Guillain-Barré syndrome is an acute demyelinating disease of the nervous system. This condition may lead to deteriorating motor function and paralysis that progresses in an ascending pattern. It affects persons of all ages but is most commonly seen in children between the ages of 4 and 9 years.

Pain or paresthesia initially develops in the lower extremities and is followed by symmetric weakness or hypotonia. This weakness spreads to the upper extremities, trunk, chest, neck, face, and head. Deep tendon reflexes are absent. Respiratory effort may be inadequate to ensure proper ventilation. Facial paresis and difficulty swallowing follow. Cranial nerves may be affected. A dysfunctional autonomic nervous system may cause such symptoms as hypertension, postural hypotension, sinus tachycardia or bradycardia, excessive diaphoresis, urinary and bowel incontinence, and facial flushing.[12]

The etiology of Guillain-Barré syndrome is unknown. The disorder has been associated with viral illnesses (1–4 weeks before the onset) and noninfectious factors such as surgery, trauma, drugs, immunizations, and heredity.

Two tests are used to diagnose Guillain-Barré syndrome. Lumbar puncture is performed to obtain cerebrospinal fluid; increased protein levels with fewer than 10 lymphocytes per cubic millimeter are a positive indicator of the condition.[15] Electroconduction tests such as electromyography are also used. An abnormal pattern of nerve conduction is indicative of Guillain-Barré syndrome.

Treatment for Guillain-Barré syndrome is supportive. Intravenous immune globulin may be given. In most cases the progression of weakness and paralysis ceases in 2 to 4 weeks, and children usually recover completely with aggressive rehabilitation.

Nursing Management

Nursing care focuses on monitoring respiratory status, meeting nutritional needs, managing autonomic nervous system dysfunction, preventing complications associated with immobility, providing emotional support, and teaching the parents how to care for the child after discharge.

Monitor Respiratory Status

Monitor the child's respiratory status closely, especially in the early phase of illness. Look for such signs as fatigue, inadequate effort, color changes, and PaO_2 less than 70 mm Hg, which indicate the need for endotracheal intubation and mechanical ventilation.[15]

Meet Nutritional Needs

Assess whether the child is having difficulty swallowing. If the child has no gag reflex, nutritional needs are maintained with intravenous supplements or nasogastric tube feedings.

Manage Autonomic Nervous System Dysfunction

Monitor the child's vital signs closely for alterations such as hypotension and arrhythmias. Observe frequently for decreased level of consciousness. Intervene promptly if these or other signs of autonomic nervous system dysfunction are noted.

Prevent Complications

Prevent complications associated with immobility (see Table 18–7). Ensure good postural alignment, and turn the child every 2 hours. Maintaining skin integrity is also important.

Evaluate the child's muscle tone, strength, and symmetry. When the child's condition begins to improve, recovery of lost strength is the priority. Active exercise is emphasized in physical therapy. Encourage family members to participate in the child's care, especially during the recovery phase. They can help with the activities of daily living and reinforce what the child has learned in physical therapy.

Provide Emotional Support

Explain the progression of Guillain-Barré syndrome to the parents during the initial stages. Witnessing a rapid deterioration in their child's physical status can be frightening; therefore, preparation is essential to reduce their anxieties. Be honest when discussing recovery and prognosis for the child.

Have parents bring in favorite toys, dolls, or books to make the child feel more secure. Playing with or reading to the child can be comforting.

Discharge Planning and Home Care Teaching

Home care needs should be identified and addressed well in advance of discharge. Support the parents as they prepare for the child's return home.

Provide referral to home care nurses who can manage all aspects of treatment, rehabilitation, and follow-up. Refer the parents to social workers, who can help with financial arrangements and school considerations.

Care in the Community

Help the child to adjust to any residual effects of Guillain-Barré syndrome. Help the child practice exercises learned in physical therapy sessions, and encourage the child to perform activities of daily living, such as brushing the teeth or combing the hair.

To promote a positive self-image, praise any effort the child makes to be self-sufficient. The child may have feelings of frustration and anger. Allow the child to express these feelings in an appropriate way, either during play or in conversation.

▶ STRUCTURAL DEFECTS

HYDROCEPHALUS

Hydrocephalus is the body's response to an imbalance between the production and absorption of cerebrospinal fluid. The condition is often congenital, but may be related to prematurity. The incidence is 3–4 per 1000 births. An X-linked hydrocephalus is the most common inherited form, accounting for 2–7% of cases.[16] Hydrocephalus can develop in older children as a complication of illness or trauma.

Clinical Manifestations

The signs and symptoms of hydrocephalus, which vary depending on the age of the child, are listed in Table 18–18. The predominant manifestation of the condition in infants is rapid head growth (Fig. 18–10). Older children show signs of increased intracranial pressure (see Table 18–6).

Etiology and Pathophysiology

Hydrocephalus may be either communicating or obstructive. Communicating hydrocephalus involves reduced absorption of cerebrospinal fluid in the subarachnoid space at the arachnoid villi. It can be acquired, such as from postinfectious meningitis or subarachnoid hemorrhage; congenital; or of unknown etiology.

Obstructive hydrocephalus, which is responsible for 99% of all occurrences in children,[17] results from a blockage in the ventricular system that prevents cerebrospinal fluid from entering the subarachnoid space (Fig. 18–11). This obstruction can be caused by infection, hemorrhage, tumor, or structural deformity. Congenital structural defects such as the Arnold-Chiari II malformation (found in most children with myelomeningocele) and the Dandy-Walker syndrome have obstructions that block the flow of cerebrospinal fluid.[18]

Diagnostic Tests and Medical Management

The diagnosis of hydrocephalus in infants is based on clinical manifestations. In the hospital setting, daily measurements of the infant's head circumference are critical. In older children, signs of increased intracranial pressure are noted.

| 18-18 | Clinical Manifestations of Hydrocephalus |

Congenital Hydrocephalus in Infant
Rapid head growth (cranial sutures may separate)
Bossing (protrusion) of frontal area
Prominent scalp veins
Translucent skin
Sunsetting eyes (sclera visible above iris)
Tense or bulging anterior fontanel
Macewen's or "cracked pot" sign
Irritability or lethargy
Decline in level of consciousness
Late stages:
• Shrill, high-pitched cry
• Difficulty swallowing or feeding
• Cardiopulmonary depression (severe cases)

Acquired Hydrocephalus in Older Child
No head enlargement
Headache upon arising with nausea or vomiting
Fussiness, sleepiness, confusion, or apathy
Personality change
Poor judgment or verbal incoherence
Ataxia, spasticity, or other alterations in motor development
Visual defects secondary to pressure on optic nerve
Signs of increased intracranial pressure

CT scanning and MRI definitively identify hydrocephalus, and in some cases reveal the anatomic cause. In the infant whose fontanel is still open, ultrasonography or echoencephalography may be used to confirm the diagnosis.

Medical management of hydrocephalus involves treating the cause (which may involve surgical removal of a lesion), and diverting the excess

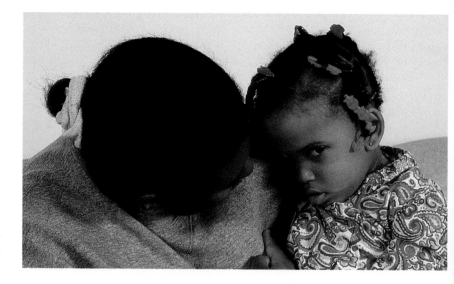

FIGURE 18–10. In communicating hydrocephalus, an excessive amount of cerebrospinal fluid accumulates in the subarachnoid space, producing the characteristic head enlargement seen here. Note the downward deviation of the eyes so that the lower half of the iris is hidden by the lower eyelid. This finding occurs in severe hydrocephalus.

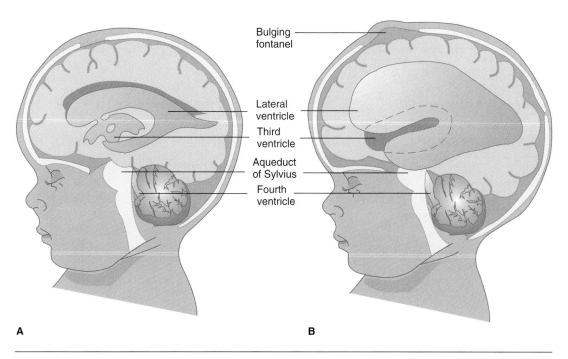

Bulging fontanel
Lateral ventricle
Third ventricle
Aqueduct of Sylvius
Fourth ventricle

A   B

FIGURE 18–11. A, Normal size of ventricle. B, Enlarged ventricles, characteristic of hydrocephalus.

cerebrospinal fluid by placement of a shunting device. Ventriculoperitoneal shunts (Fig. 18–12) are commonly used. Shunt systems consist of four parts: a ventricular catheter, a pumping chamber or reservoir, a unidirectional pressure valve, and a distal catheter. Initial shunt placement usually occurs at 3–4 months of age, with replacement two to four times as the child grows.

Mechanical complications may include blockage at either the proximal or the distal end of the catheter, kinking of the tubing, or valve breakdown. Infants or children with shunt failure show signs and symptoms of recurrent hydrocephalus and increased intracranial pressure. Shunt failure and ventricular size is confirmed by CT scanning or MRI.

The most serious complication is shunt infection, which may occur at any time but is most prevalent in the first 2 months after placement. Symptoms include ventriculitis, low-grade fever, malaise, headache, and nausea. Antibiotics are usually prescribed, but if the infection is overwhelming, the shunt is removed and an external drainage device is placed. A new shunt is inserted when the infection resolves.

Some children are placed on the same prophylactic antibiotic treatment regimen used for children with cardiac anomalies to reduce the risk of shunt infections (refer to Chap. 12).

Nursing Assessment

It is important for nurses to become familiar with the clinical manifestations of hydrocephalus to ensure prompt identification and treatment of children with this condition. Head circumference of all infants is measured at each well-child visit to detect the condition at an early stage.

Assess the child with a ventriculoperitoneal shunt for signs and symptoms of shunt failure and infection. Report any abnormalities to the physician immediately.

RESEARCH CONSIDERATIONS

Researchers in neuroendoscopy are developing techniques to create a new pathway for cerebrospinal fluid to flow between the ventricles and spinal cord in individuals with obstructive hydrocephalus. The new endoscopy procedure may be used in some patients in the future to avoid shunt placement.[18]

CLINICAL TIP

The most important signs of shunt infection are changes in responsiveness and irritability after fever is controlled.[18]

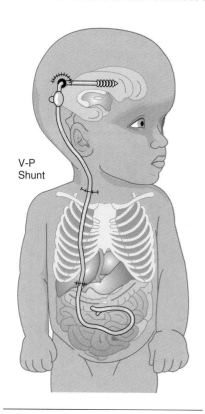

FIGURE 18–12. A ventriculoperitoneal shunt, commonly used to treat children with hydrocephalus, is usually placed at 3–4 months of age.

Nursing Diagnosis

Nursing diagnoses that might be appropriate for the child with hydrocephalus include:

- Risk for Infection related to presence of shunt
- Impaired Physical Mobility related to increased weight of head
- Risk for Caregiver Role Strain related to care of a child with a chronic condition or life-threatening illness
- Anxiety (Parent) related to repeated surgeries and life-threatening illness
- Risk for Injury related to shunt blockage

Nursing Management

Nursing care in the hospital setting focuses on providing preoperative and postoperative care and providing emotional support.

Provide Preoperative Care

Measure the child's head circumference daily and watch for signs of increased intracranial pressure (see Table 18–6).

Measure fluid intake and output as ordered. Carefully assess respiratory status. Provide good skin care.

Position the child carefully; do not stretch or strain the neck muscles, since they must support the large head. Holding the child may be difficult because of the additional weight of the head. Reduce the chances for skin breakdown by placing sheepskin or a lamb's wool blanket under the head. Prevent any other complications associated with immobility (see Table 18–7).

Attend to the child's special nutritional needs. Because the infant is prone to vomiting, frequent small feedings with frequent burping are beneficial.

Provide Postoperative Care

The child is usually placed in a flat position to prevent rapid cerebrospinal fluid drainage. The head of the bed is elevated gradually.

Take vital signs every 2–4 hours. Monitor the child carefully for any signs of shunt malfunction, increased intracranial pressure (see Table 18–6), or infection.

Provide Emotional Support

Provide parents with explanations about the child's condition and all procedures to be performed. Encourage parents and family to help with the child's care in the hospital when appropriate. Be sympathetic and understanding, and allow parents to express their concerns. If hydrocephalus occurs during early infancy, the parents will be anxious about the impact of the chronic condition and subsequent surgical procedures. If hydrocephalus is secondary to neoplasm, however, the parents' anxieties are compounded by their child's life-threatening illness.

Assure parents that most children with shunts lead normal lives, attending school and interacting with others no differently than their peers.

Discharge Planning and Home Care Teaching

Home care needs should be identified and addressed well in advance of discharge. Parents need to be taught how to care for a child with a shunt. Parents and other family members should be made aware of the signs and symptoms of both shunt failure (signs of increased intracranial pressure) and infection. Give them the telephone numbers of the pediatrician and the neurosurgeon, and make sure that they understand that they should contact a physician immediately if they suspect a problem. Inform them that the shunt may need to be replaced one or more times in childhood as the child grows. Appropriate home care referrals should be arranged. Refer families to the appropriate psychologic and social services, such as the Hydrocephalus Association (see Appendix F).

Care in the Community

Infants and children need frequent monitoring to ensure proper functioning of the shunt. Head circumference is measured at each visit to monitor growth. Assess the child for cognitive, speech, and motor developmental delays. Children with hydrocephalus often have better verbal skills than fine motor skills. The child and family should be referred to an early intervention program to promote developmental progress. School-age children may need to have an Individualized Education Plan developed (see Chap. 5). Impaired cognitive functioning is usually the result of additional complications rather than hydrocephalus alone.

Parents seeking child care for their infant should be encouraged to use a setting with fewer children to decrease exposure to infection. Review the signs of shunt failure and infection with parents at each visit and make sure they have a plan to manage the emergency of a shunt failure.

Encourage parents not to be overprotective and to allow the child to develop normally. Participation in contact sports should be discouraged.

SPINA BIFIDA

Spina bifida, a congenital neural tube defect that affects the head and spinal column, is the most common developmental disorder of the central nervous system. It is a malformation of the neural tube that can occur anywhere along the spine. The condition occurs in 0.4–1 per 1000 births in the United States each year but varies by region of the country.[19] Because the diagnosis can be made prenatally, delivery by cesarean section is usually performed to reduce trauma to the open spine.

There are several different types of spina bifida (Table 18–19). A saclike protrusion on the infant's back indicates meningocele or myelomeningocele (Fig. 18–13). The clinical manifestations seen depend on the location of the defect: the higher the defect, the greater the neurologic dysfunction. The lower extremities may be completely paralyzed or there may be varying degrees of immobility with orthopedic problems. Bowel and bladder sphincters may be affected. Renal involvement may occur secondary to neurologic impairment and urinary retention. Hydrocephalus is usually present in children with myelomeningocele because of the Arnold-Chiari II malformation. The range of potential problems for the child with spina bifida is listed in Table 18–20.

The cause of spina bifida is unknown, although environmental factors such as chemicals, medications, and poor maternal nutrition (especially low levels of folic acid) have been implicated. The increased incidence of the condition in families indicates a possible genetic influence.

Diagnosis is made by examination of the lesion and evaluation of the child's neurologic status. Radiologic imaging by CT scan, MRI, and flat films of the spinal column can pinpoint the bony defect. Surgery to close and repair the lesion usually occurs within days of the infant's birth.

 SAFETY CONSIDERATIONS

Infants with poor head control due to an enlarged head should not be placed in forward-facing car safety seats, regardless of their age. This position increases the risk of cervical spine injury and death to these children in the event of a car crash.

ARNOLD-CHIARI II MALFORMATION

In this malformation, there is downward displacement of the cerebellum, brainstem, and fourth ventricle. Because these structures control respiration and the protective reflexes, as well as house the cranial nerves, the displacement can have varying effects such as sudden death, the need for assisted ventilation, or swallowing difficulties. Signs and symptoms may occur at any time.

18-19   Types of Spina Bifida

Spina bifida occulta	Failure of posterior vertebral arches to fuse, most commonly at fifth lumbar or first sacral vertebrae; no herniation of spinal cord or meninges; condition usually not visible externally; tuft of hair, a dermoid cyst, or hemangioma may be found over the site
Spina bifida cystica	Defect in closure of posterior vertebral arch with protrusion through bony spine
Meningocele	Saclike protrusion through bony defect containing meninges and cerebrospinal fluid; sac covering defect may be translucent or membranous
Myelomeningocele	Saclike herniation through bony defect holding meninges, cerebrospinal fluid, as well as a portion of spinal cord or nerve roots; fluid leakage may also occur; lesion poorly covered with imperfect tissue

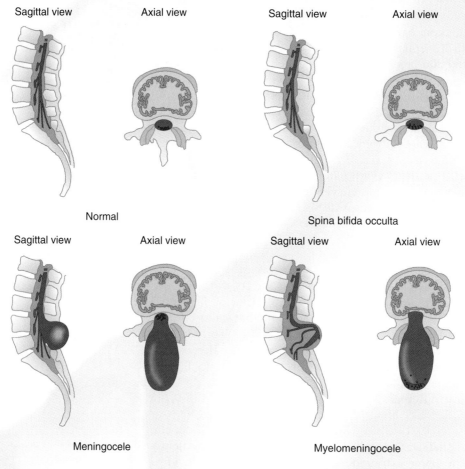

Prognosis depends on the type of defect, the level of the lesion, and the presence of other complicating factors. A team of physicians, nurses, and therapists from the neurosurgery, orthopedic, urology, and physical medicine departments should work with the child and family to form a comprehensive care plan.

Nursing Management

Nursing care in the hospital focuses on providing preoperative and postoperative care, promoting mobility, and providing emotional support.

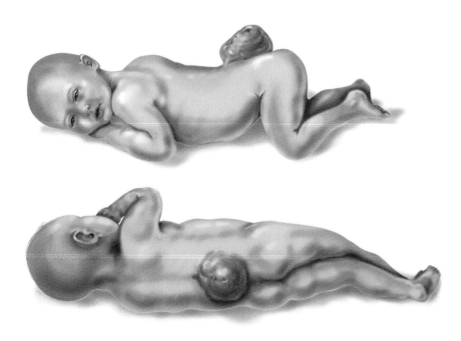

FIGURE 18-13. Lumbosacral myelomeningocele is caused by a neural tube defect that results in incomplete closure of the vertebral column. As shown here, the meninges (and sometimes the spinal cord) protrude as a saclike structure.

Provide Preoperative Care

Cover the sac with a sterile saline dressing to protect its integrity. Place the infant in a prone position with hips slightly flexed and legs abducted to minimize tension on the sac. Maintain this position using towel rolls placed between the knees. Assess the infant regularly for motor deficits as well as bladder and bowel involvement.

The infant is difficult to handle before surgery. Feed the infant with the head turned to one side until surgery has been performed. Comfort the infant before surgery with tactile stimulation such as touching, patting, and cuddling.

18-20	Common Health Problems of Children With Spina Bifida
System	**Health Problem**
Musculoskeletal	Clubfoot Dislocated hip Poor musculoskeletal alignment Scoliosis, kyphosis
Genitourinary	Neurogenic bladder Hydronephrosis, renal damage Urinary reflux and urinary tract infection Incontinence
Gastrointestinal	Constipation, impaction Incontinence
Neurologic	Cognitive deficit, learning disability Visual perceptual problems Sensory dysfunction Paralysis, muscle weakness Feeding difficulties, swallowing problems Sleep apnea

GROWTH & DEVELOPMENT CONSIDERATIONS

Older children should be treated according to their intellectual level, not their motor development. Encourage them to take responsibility for self-care, and recognize their need to control their bodily functions. Promote interaction with peers in the hospital and participation in activities. If children are hospitalized for an extended time, schooling should be arranged.

Provide Postoperative Care

Monitor the infant's vital signs carefully. Watch closely for symptoms of infection, especially meningitis. If a ventriculoperitoneal shunt was placed, watch for hydrocephalus, increased intracranial pressure, or infection. Inspect the surgical site for cerebrospinal fluid leakage. The infant should be placed in the prone or side-lying position, or in some cases may be held upright.

Promote Mobility

Begin gentle range-of-motion exercises as soon as possible to prevent muscle contractures and atrophy. Extreme caution should be used because these children have brittle bones and are subject to idiopathic fractures.

Provide Emotional Support

Keep parents informed about their child's status. Allow them to express their frustrations and anger. As soon as parents are able to cope with the child's condition, encourage them to become involved in the child's care in the hospital.

Discharge Planning and Home Care Teaching

Home care needs should be identified and addressed well in advance of discharge. Make sure family members understand how to care for the child at home. Help them obtain special devices such as splints, wedges, and rolls, if indicated, to prevent complications. Instruct parents how to position, handle, feed, and perform range-of-motion exercises. Teach parents the signs and symptoms of increased intracranial pressure, hydrocephalus, shunt infection or malfunction, and urinary tract infection. Home care nursing should be arranged, if necessary. The home care nurse will reinforce the skills learned in the hospital setting and coordinate the numerous health care professionals who will be working with the child and family.

Refer parents to resource groups such as the Spina Bifida Association of America (see Appendix F).

Care in the Community

To reduce complications and promote optimal development, children with spina bifida need comprehensive care planned and coordinated by a knowledgeable team of health care professionals. This care may be provided in partnership with the primary care physician.

Promote safety and independent mobility with proper use of braces, walkers, crutches, canes, and in some cases custom-designed wheelchairs (Fig. 18–14). Because the child has poor sensation in the lower extremities and does not feel scratches, rubbing by braces, or burns, it is important to teach parents to conduct a daily assessment of the skin for signs of irritation or pressure sores (see Chap. 21). Gel-filled cushions and frequent shifting of position are used by the child in a wheelchair to prevent pressure sores. Do not place in a car seat children whose bare skin is exposed without first checking to see how hot the seat is. Check water temperature for baths. The family will need to make sure that all health care providers, including dentists, are aware of the child's latex sensitivity.

Parents may need to learn how to catheterize the child and then at an appropriate age teach the child intermittent self-catheterization to prevent urinary tract infections and other renal complications (see Table 16–6). Good nutrition planning is important to prevent obesity and to reduce constipation and complications such as fecal impaction. Children need to be taught to assume greater responsibility for self-care as they get older.

SAFETY PRECAUTIONS

Between 18% and 40% of children with spina bifida have a latex allergy (see Chap. 9). Cases in which latex exposure has caused anaphylaxis in a child have been reported. All children with latex allergy need to carry a kit with premeasured adrenaline for emergency treatment of anaphylaxis. Use nonlatex materials when providing care to the child in the hospital, in the outpatient setting, or at home. The Spina Bifida Association can provide an updated list of products containing latex and potential substitutes (Table 9–9).

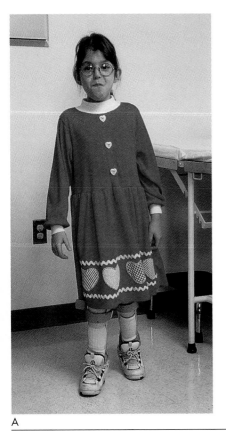 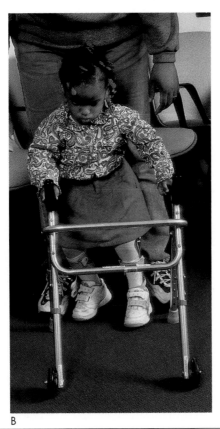 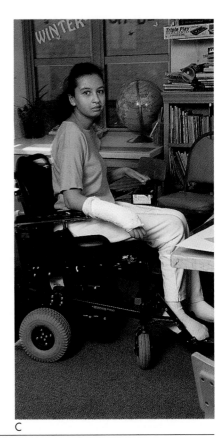

A   B   C

FIGURE 18–14. Help determine the best assistive device for the child to gain the most independence for mobilizing and to promote development. The child may change devices in different settings to promote optimal independence. **A and B,** Braces and walkers may be best for young children to promote an upright posture that encourages a normal interaction with the environment. **C,** A motorized wheelchair can assist the child with a significant neurologic impairment to achieve independence and mobility.

Parents are faced with the long-term financial issues of caring for the child who needs regular new adaptive equipment to match growth, as well as other medical supplies. Parents thus need to learn how to act as the child's case manager, or to work effectively with another individual in this role.

CRANIOSYNOSTOSIS

Craniosynostosis is the premature closing of the cranial sutures. This condition occurs in up to 1 in 2000 births. Most children have no family history of the condition, although 10–20% have other inherited syndromes.[20] More than 50 syndromes with craniosynostosis have been documented.[21]

Closure of the sutures usually takes place at predetermined times during the child's development. Problems arise if one or more sutures close early. Bone growth continues in a direction parallel to the suture line, which leads to compensatory overgrowth at normal suture lines and the classic skull deformities associated with craniosynostosis (Fig. 18–15).

The cause of craniosynostosis is unknown. Diagnosis is made by clinical appearance. Palpation of the skull reveals a bony ridge along a suture. Skull x-ray films, CT scan, and MRI confirm the diagnosis. The hands and feet should be carefully examined to detect any skeletal defect that could be associated with a syndrome.[20]

Reconstructive surgery is the most common form of treatment. After surgery, it is important for the incision to remain dry and intact. The nurse

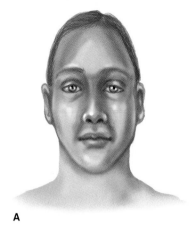
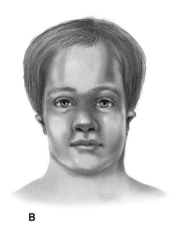

FIGURE 18–15. In craniosynostosis, the head shape is dependent upon which sutures are involved. Examples of different head shapes include those shown in **A** and **B**.

A   **B**

should also observe the child for symptoms of increased intracranial pressure (see Table 18–6).

Explain to parents that surgery will improve the child's appearance. Assure them that most children with craniosynostosis are healthy, and that their brains develop normally.

CLINICAL TIP

Illicit substances that may cause neonatal abstinence syndrome when used by the mother during pregnancy include: heroin, cocaine, meperidine, methadone, propoxyphene, amphetamines, alcohol, and marijuana.

CLINICAL TIP

Crying accompanied by poor feeding constitutes clinical signs that should increase the nurse's suspicion of neonatal abstinence syndrome.

► NEONATAL ABSTINENCE SYNDROME (DRUG-ADDICTED INFANT)

Repeated use of narcotics and other substances leads to tolerance and physical dependence. All narcotics, regardless of their mode of administration, readily cross the placenta, enter the fetal circulation, and have the same effects on the fetus that they do in the mother. When the mother stops taking drugs during pregnancy, both she and the fetus have withdrawal symptoms. If the infant is born to a mother who is still actively using drugs, the neonate goes into withdrawal shortly after birth.

In the newborn, irritability and jitteriness are the most common symptoms of drug withdrawal. These infants may have excoriated skin, especially on the heels, toes, hands, elbows, nose, or chin, as a result of their continuous movements on the crib sheets. They may also have a high-pitched, shrill cry; hyperreflexia; poor temperature control; episodes of tachypnea; abnormal sleep–wake patterns; flushing of the skin; and excessive diaphoresis. Additional symptoms may include poor feeding and poor coordination between sucking and swallowing, which can lead to aspiration and inadequate nutritional intake. Anemia may be present. Vomiting and diarrhea may occur as a result of a hyperactive bowel. These infants also have an increased risk of seizures.

Between 50% and 90% of infants of drug-addicted mothers suffer withdrawal. Withdrawal symptoms usually appear 12–28 hours after birth. However, it is not uncommon for these symptoms to appear between 7 and 14 days after birth if the mother was taking heroin or methadone. The onset of symptoms may be attributed to the type and amount of drug taken by the mother and how soon before birth it was taken. Signs of narcotic withdrawal in neonates are given in Table 18–21. Long-term exposure to these substances can result in intrauterine growth retardation, prematurity, small head circumference, shorter length, and low Apgar scores.

Diagnosis is based on the history of maternal substance abuse and physical signs in the infant. EEG abnormalities may be noted.[22] Identifica-

18-21	Signs of Narcotic Withdrawal in Neonates

W = wakefulness
I = irritability
T = tremulousness, temperature variation, tachypnea
H = hyperactivity, high-pitched cry, hyperacusis, hyperreflexia, hypertonia, hiccups
D = diarrhea, diaphoresis, disorganized suck
R = rub marks (excoriations on knees and face), regurgitation (vomiting)
A = apneic spells, autonomic dysfunction
W = weight loss (or failure to gain weight)
A = alkalosis (respiratory)
L = lacrimation
S = stuffy nose, sneezing, seizures

From Rudolph, A.M., Hoffman, J.I.E., & Rudolph, C.D. (Eds.). (1996). Rudolph's pediatrics (20th ed., p. 840). Stamford, CT: Appleton & Lange.

tion of the drug may be determined in some cases from maternal and infant urine. Meconium and hair of the infant may also be tested.

Treatment is generally supportive. Medications such as phenobarbitol, chlorpromazine, and paregoric may be prescribed to alleviate symptoms. The most serious and prevalent complication with drug abuse is acquired immunodeficiency syndrome (AIDS), since the human immunodeficiency virus (HIV) readily crosses the placenta and is transmitted to the fetus. Hepatitis B is likewise a risk. If the mother tests positive for hepatitis B, the infant should be given the hepatitis B vaccine, as well as hepatitis B immune globulin.

Nursing Management

Nursing care focuses on monitoring withdrawal symptoms, administering prescribed medications, and meeting the infant's emotional needs.

The drug-addicted infant should be observed closely for poor sucking, seizures, vomiting and diarrhea, dehydration, and an increased metabolic rate. Many of the symptoms of withdrawal are identical to those seen in other conditions such as infection, bowel obstruction, hydrocephalus, and intracranial anomaly. The infant could potentially have neonatal abstinence syndrome along with another condition.

Administer prescribed medications, if ordered; however, many infants are managed without drugs. Provide frequent, small, high-calorie feedings, which are more readily tolerated by these infants. Special attention is given to dietary intake during hospitalization and at home for several months, as the infant may not eat well. Keep the infant in a quiet environment with subdued lighting and minimal stimulation.

Satisfy the emotional needs of the neonate by swaddling, rocking, holding, and cuddling. Volunteers or hospital-based foster grandparents, if available, may help fulfill these needs. Such positive interaction with adults promotes comfort and supplies necessary emotional support for the infant. The infant should be held with the spine flexed to decrease extensor tone.[23]

Care in the Community

Long-term follow-up care of the child should be planned to ensure regular developmental testing and assessment for catch-up growth, neurobehavioral

HOME CARE CONSIDERATIONS

Infants with neonatal abstinence syndrome are at a significantly higher risk (5–10:1) for sudden infant death syndrome when their mother used heroin or cocaine. Home apnea monitoring should be implemented for these children.[24]

ETHICAL CONSIDERATIONS

As the health care of women in labor and newborns has improved, new health issues have emerged. Fetal monitoring has led to the early diagnosis of fetal distress and improved the mortality rate of newborns. However, as more premature infants survive, more anoxic episodes also occur. Thus the incidence of cerebral palsy has not decreased, and indeed the incidence of spastic diplegia has increased with technology improvements.[26] How should health care practitioners weigh the benefits and risks of certain procedures or interventions? Are parents always well informed about the benefits and risks of procedures involving their newborns? How can nurses deal with their feelings about these issues?

problems, and fetal alcohol syndrome. Interventions for any identified problem will need to be initiated. The mother will also need follow-up to determine whether her drug problem has been overcome and whether the infant is safe from neglect or other harmful situations. Care of the infant with neonatal abstinence syndrome and the substance-abusing mother can be a difficult health care challenge for the pediatric nurse, and support from social services is often needed. The infant is at risk for neurobehavioral problems that a substance-abusing parent has difficulty meeting. Family resources and foster care may need to be considered if the infant does not have adequate growth. The long-term effects of this condition on cognitive function are not known at this time.

► CEREBRAL PALSY

Cerebral palsy is a nonprogressive motor and posture dysfunction that occurs secondary to anoxic damage in the motor centers of the brain during the prenatal, perinatal, or postnatal (up to 2 years) periods. The categories of this dysfunction are presented in Table 18–22. Cerebral palsy is the most common chronic disorder of childhood, occurring in an estimated 2.7 in 1000 children.[25]

Clinical Manifestations

Cerebral palsy is characterized by abnormal muscle tone and lack of coordination (Fig. 18–16). Children have a variety of symptoms depending on their ages, as listed in Table 18–23. There is wide variability in symptoms depending on the area of the brain involved and the degree of anoxia. Children with cerebral palsy usually are delayed in meeting developmental milestones. They frequently have other problems, including visual defects such as strabismus, nystagmus, or refractory errors; hearing

18-22	Categories of Cerebral Palsy
Categories	**Characteristics**
Physiologic	
Hypotonia	Floppiness, increased range of motion of joints, diminished reflex response
Hypertonia	
Rigidity	Tense, tight muscles
Spasticity	Uncoordinated, awkward, stiff movements; scissoring or crossing of the legs; exaggerated reflex reactions
Athetosis	Constant involuntary writhing motions that are more severe distally
Ataxia	Irregularity in muscle coordination or action
Topographic	
Hemiplegia	Involvement of one side of the body with the upper extremities being more dysfunctional than the lower extremities
Diplegia	Involvement of the lower extremities, usually spastic
Quadriplegia	Involvement of all extremities with the arms in flexion and legs in extension

loss; speech or language delay; speech impediment; seizures; or mental retardation.

Etiology and Pathophysiology

Cerebral palsy may be due to prenatal, antenatal, or postnatal trauma or to an infection or a lesion. During gestation, insufficient nutrients and oxygen can cause damage to the developing brain of the fetus. Premature infants are at high risk because of their immature central nervous systems and the measures taken at birth to promote their survival. Injury at birth may be due to direct trauma to the brain or to asphyxia resulting from cord collapse or strangulation. In older children, head trauma is the major source of acquired brain injury and subsequent motor dysfunction.

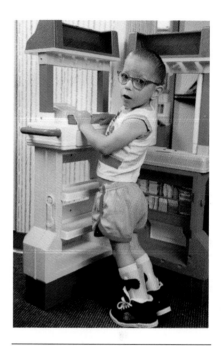

FIGURE 18–16. A child with cerebral palsy has abnormal muscle tone and lack of physical coordination.

18-23 | Characteristic Signs of Cerebral Palsy in Infancy

Birth to 1 Month
Weak or absent sucking or swallowing
Episodes of bradycardia or apnea
High-pitched cry
Jitteriness
Hypotonia
Seizures
Difficulty in eliciting primitive reflex responses

3 Months
Feeding difficulties
Tongue thrust
Irritability
Hypotonia but with advanced head control while prone
One or both hands fisted
Brisk tendon reflexes
Strabismus
Persistence of primitive reflexes

6 Months
Delayed developmental milestones
Handedness (one hand dominant); continued fisting
Hypertonia; difficult to dress
Little spontaneous movement
Arching; tendency to stand
Persistence of primitive reflexes

9 Months
Delayed motor milestones
    Abnormal crawl: may be asymmetric, using only arms for movement
    Abnormal reach: splaying of fingers with wrist extended; tremor
Abnormal movements
Keeping arms flexed

12 Months
Scissoring
Toe walking
Athetoid (writhing) motions
Handedness

Neonatal infections such as meningitis and kernicterus or infantile bilirubin **encephalopathy** (cerebral dysfunction after an insult of limited duration, in this case bilirubin, in which the lesion will not change or improve over time) may also lead to the development of cerebral palsy.

Diagnostic Tests and Medical Management

Diagnosis is usually based on clinical findings. Generally cerebral palsy is difficult to diagnose in the early months of life. Suspicious findings include an infant who is small for age, has a history of prematurity or other anoxic event, and demonstrates abnormal positions and developmental delays.[27] It is not uncommon for children who are delayed in meeting developmental milestones or have neuromuscular abnormalities at 1 year of age to show gradual improvement in function. In some cases, signs of dysfunction disappear entirely with physical maturation.

Medical management focuses on helping the child develop to his or her maximum potential. Referrals are made for physical, occupational, and speech therapy, as well as special education. Surgical interventions may be required to improve function as spasticity leads to progressive deformities. The Achilles tendon may be lengthened to increase range of motion in the ankle, which allows the heel to touch the floor and thus improves ambulation. The hamstrings may be released to correct knee flexion contractures. Other procedures may be performed to improve hip adduction or correct the natural position of the foot.

The prognosis for infants and children with cerebral palsy depends on the level of physical involvement and on the presence of intellectual, visual, or hearing deficits. Many children with hemiplegia or ataxia show some improvement with maturation and are able to ambulate. Others will need assistance with mobility and activities of daily living. They are usually cared for in their homes, but in some cases receive care in long-term care facilities.

Nursing Assessment

Be alert for children whose histories indicate an increased risk for cerebral palsy. Assess all children at each health care visit for developmental delays. Any orthopedic, visual, auditory, or intellectual deficits should be noted. Assess for the presence of newborn reflexes, which may persist beyond the normal age in a child with cerebral palsy. Record dietary intake as well as height and weight percentiles for children suspected to have or diagnosed with the condition.[28]

Nursing Diagnosis

Nursing diagnoses for the child with cerebral palsy vary, depending on the type of cerebral palsy, the particular child's symptoms and age, and the family situation. The accompanying Nursing Care Plan includes several diagnoses that might be appropriate for the child with cerebral palsy. Additional nursing diagnoses might include:

- Constipation related to low intake of fiber and fluids and effects of immobility on the gastrointestinal tract
- Bowel Incontinence related to central nervous system damage
- Risk for Injury related to seizures and impaired mobility and adaptive devices
- Impaired Tissue Integrity related to decreased mobility and limited self-care

CLINICAL TIP

All infants who show symptoms of developmental delays, feeding difficulties caused by poor sucking, or abnormalities of muscle tone should be evaluated. Two simple screening assessments are:

- Place a clean diaper on the infant's face. The normal child will use two hands to remove it, but the infant with cerebral palsy will either use one hand or not remove the cloth at all.
- Turn the infant's head to one side. A persistent asymmetric tonic neck reflex (beyond 6 months of age) is an indicator of a pathologic condition. Cerebral palsy should be suspected in any infant who has persistent primitive reflexes.

- Impaired Verbal Communication related to hearing and/or speech impairment
- Social Isolation related to mobility limitation
- Impaired Home Maintenance Management related to child's physical immobility, medications, nutritional needs, and other required care
- Self-Care Deficit (feeding, bathing/hygiene, dressing/grooming, toileting) related to physical abilities
- Altered Growth and Development related to lack of muscle strength or limited social interaction
- Body Image Disturbance related to spastic, athetoid movements or neuromuscular limitations
- Chronic Low Self-Esteem related to dependence on others

Nursing Management

The accompanying Nursing Care Plan summarizes care for the child with cerebral palsy. Nursing care focuses on providing adequate nutrition, maintaining skin integrity, promoting physical mobility, promoting safety, promoting growth and development, teaching parents how to care for the child, and providing emotional support.

Provide Adequate Nutrition

Children with cerebral palsy require high-calorie diets or supplements to the diet because of feeding difficulties associated with spasticity. Many children have difficulty chewing and swallowing. Give the child small amounts of soft foods at a time. Feeding utensils with large, padded handles may be easier for the child to use.

Maintain Skin Integrity

Take special care to protect the bony prominences from skin breakdown. See Table 18–7 for specific nursing interventions.

Proper body alignment should be maintained at all times. Support the child with pillows, towels, and bolsters whether the child is in bed or in a chair. Support the head and body of a floppy infant. A spastic child with scissored, extended legs or an athetoid child who writhes constantly is difficult to carry and transport.

Promote Physical Mobility

Range-of-motion exercises are essential to maintain joint flexibility and prevent contractures. Consult with the physical therapists who work with the child and assist with recommended exercises. Teach parents to position the child to foster flexion rather than extension so that interaction with the environment can be enhanced (eg, the child can bring objects closer to the face). Encourage parents to bring the child's adaptive appliances (customized wheelchairs, braces) to the hospital to prevent deterioration during hospitalizations. Refer parents to the appropriate resources for help with the acquisition of adaptive devices.

Promote Safety

Teach parents the importance of using safety belts with children in strollers and wheelchairs. A helmet should be worn by the child with chronic seizures to protect the child from further injury during seizures.

NURSING CARE PLAN
THE CHILD WITH CEREBRAL PALSY

GOAL	INTERVENTION	RATIONALE	EXPECTED OUTCOME

1. Impaired Physical Mobility related to disruption of neuromuscular development

The child will attain maximum physical abilities possible.	• Perform development assessment and record age of achievement of milestones (eg, reaching for objects, sitting, etc).	• Delayed developmental milestones are common with cerebral palsy. Once one milestone is achieved, interventions are revised to assist in the next skill necessary.	The child reaches maximum physical mobility and all developmental milestones possible.
	• Plan activities to use gross and fine motor skills (eg, holding pen or eating utensils, toys positioned to encourage reaching and rolling over, etc).	• Many activities of daily living and play activities promote physical development.	
	• Allow time for the child to complete activities.	• The child may perform tasks more slowly than most children.	
	• Perform range-of-motion exercises every 4 hours for the child unable to move body parts. Position the child to promote tendon stretching (eg, foot plantar flexion instead of dorsiflexion, legs extended instead of flexed at knees and hips).	• Promotes mobility and increased circulation, and decreases the risk of contractures.	
	• Arrange for and encourage parents to keep appointments with a rehabilitation therapist.	• A regular and frequently reevaluated rehabilitation program assists in promoting development.	
	• Teach the family to maintain appropriate brace wear.	• Adaptive devices are often necessary to maximize physical mobility.	

2. Sensory/Perceptual Alteration: Visual, Auditory, or Kinesthetic related to cerebral damage

The child will receive and benefit from varied forms of sensory and perceptual input.	• Facilitate eye and auditory examinations by specialists. Promote the use of adaptive devices (glasses, contact lenses, hearing aids), and encourage recommended return visits to specialists.	• Adaptive devices often enhance sensory input. These devices need frequent changes as the child grows.	The child receives adequate sensory/perceptual input to maximize developmental outcome.

NURSING CARE PLAN
THE CHILD WITH CEREBRAL PALSY— *Continued*

GOAL	INTERVENTION	RATIONALE	EXPECTED OUTCOME

2. Sensory/Perceptual Alteration: Visual, Auditory, or Kinesthetic related to cerebral damage (continued)

	INTERVENTION	RATIONALE	
	• Maximize the use of intact senses (ie, describe verbally the surroundings to a child with poor vision, allow touching of objects, provide visual materials to enhance learning in the child with impaired hearing, use computers to promote communication).	• Other senses can compensate for those that are impaired.	

3. Altered Nutrition: Less Than Body Requirements related to impaired chewing and swallowing, high metabolic rate

GOAL	INTERVENTION	RATIONALE	EXPECTED OUTCOME

The child will receive nutrients needed for normal growth.	• Monitor height and weight and plot on a growth grid. Perform hydration status assessment.
	• Teach the family techniques to promote caloric and nutrient intake:
	  • Position the child upright for feedings.
	  • Place foods far back in mouth to overcome tongue thrust.
	  • Use soft and blended foods.
	  • Allow extra time and quiet environment for meals.
		• Insufficient intake can lead to impaired growth and dehydration.
		
		• Special techniques can facilitate food intake.
			The child shows normal growth patterns for height, weight, and other physical parameters.

	• Perform frequent respiratory assessment. Teach the family to avoid aspiration pneumonia. Teach care of gastrostomy and tube feeding technique as appropriate.	• Aspiration pneumonia is a risk for the child with poor swallowing. Special feeding techniques may be needed.	The child does not develop aspiration pneumonia.

Continued . . .

NURSING CARE PLAN
THE CHILD WITH CEREBRAL PALSY— *Continued*

GOAL	INTERVENTION	RATIONALE	EXPECTED OUTCOME

4. Altered Family Processes related to ongoing, complex child care needs

GOAL	INTERVENTION	RATIONALE	EXPECTED OUTCOME
The family will adapt to growth and development needs of the child with cerebral palsy.	• Allow opportunities for parents to verbalize the impact of cerebral palsy on the family. Provide referral to other parents and support groups.	• The family needs an opportunity to explore the emotional and social impact of the child's care in order to integrate and grow from the experience.	The family continues its development and provides support for all of its members.
	• Explore community services for rehabilitation, respite care, child care, and other needs and refer family as appropriate.	• Diverse services are available and will be needed due to the multiple impacts of cerebral palsy on the child.	
	• During home and office visits review the child's achievements and praise the family for care provided.	• The child's achievements are positive reinforcement of the family's efforts.	
	• Teach the family skills needed to manage the child's care (eg, medication administration, physical rehabilitation, seizure management, etc). Teach case management techniques.	• The child requires care by many specialists. Many parents become case managers to plan the complex care required.	
	• Involve siblings in care for the child with cerebral palsy. Review for parents the needs of all children in the family.	• Siblings of the child with cerebral palsy may feel left out because of the care required. Special efforts contribute to meeting the developmental needs of all family members.	

5. Diversional Activity Deficit (Child and Parent) related to lack of mobility

GOAL	INTERVENTION	RATIONALE	EXPECTED OUTCOME
The child will engage in adequate diversional activity to maximize potential growth and development.	• Refer the family to early childhood stimulation programs. Encourage contact with other children. When hospitalized, place the child in a room with other children whenever possible.	• The child needs a variety of activities and contact with other children and adults to maximize development.	The child engages in activities that maximize development.

NURSING CARE PLAN
THE CHILD WITH CEREBRAL PALSY– *Continued*

GOAL	INTERVENTION	RATIONALE	EXPECTED OUTCOME

5. Diversional Activity Deficit (Child and Parent) related to lack of mobility (continued)

GOAL	INTERVENTION	RATIONALE	EXPECTED OUTCOME
Parents will meet their own diversional activity needs.	• Work with the local school to develop an Individualized Education Plan that allows the child contact with other children and a variety of activities. • Assist parents in locating appropriate child care and encourage them to engage in meaningful activities for themselves.	• Public schools must provide an Individualized Education Plan. Parents may need assistance to interact effectively with the school system. • Parents need to obtain respite care, and engage in diversional or work activities to meet their own developmental needs.	Parents meet their own diversional activity needs.

Promote Growth and Development

Remember that many children with cerebral palsy are physically but not intellectually disabled. Use terminology appropriate for the child's developmental level. Help the child develop a positive self-image to ensure emotional health and social growth. Children with a hearing impairment may need referral to learn American Sign Language or other communication methods.

Foster Parental Knowledge

Teach parents about the disorder and arrange sessions to teach them about all of the child's special needs. Teach administration, desired effects, and side effects of medications prescribed for seizures. Make sure parents are aware of the need for dental care when anticonvulsants are prescribed.

Provide Emotional Support

Refer parents to individual and family counseling if appropriate. Listen to the parents' concerns and encourage them to express their feelings and ask questions. Explain what they can expect regarding future treatment. Work with other health care professionals to help families adjust to this chronic disease.

Care in the Community

Children with cerebral palsy need continuous support in the community. A case manager such as the parent or nurse will likely be needed to coordinate care. As they grow, these children will need new adaptive devices, ongoing developmental assessment and care planning, and possibly surgery. Although the brain lesion does not change, it manifests itself in different ways as the child grows. For example, once the child begins to

 CLINICAL TIP

Provide audio and visual activities for the child who is quadriplegic. Television, videotapes, and music are good diversions. Encourage the child who is paraplegic to use his or her arms and hands in interactive games. Children can use special hand controls or pointers to play video games or other adaptive devices to manipulate the television or radio.

walk, the extensor tone may cause Achilles cord tightening. Braces may be used to decrease deformities, but surgery may eventually be needed. Later, surgery may be needed to loosen tight tendons in the knees or hips.[29] Speech therapy may be needed, as well as new glasses and eye examinations as the child grows. The child may need an Individualized Education Plan to maximize learning potential (see Chap. 5). Other parents of children with cerebral palsy can provide needed support.

Early intervention programs can help parents learn how to meet their child's special needs, including physical, occupational, and speech therapy, as well as educational needs. Parents may need financial assistance to provide the care that the child needs and to obtain appliances such as braces, wheelchairs, or adaptive utensils. Technology offers many new strategies to promote communication and self-care by these children. The nurse can be instrumental in helping parents meet the needs of the child with cerebral palsy in preschools, schools, offices, clinics, and other settings. In addition, the nurse makes referrals as appropriate to early intervention programs, support groups, and organizations such as the United Cerebral Palsy Association and Shriners Hospitals. Recreational activities may be identified through the National Association of Sports for Cerebral Palsy (see Appendix F).

► INJURIES OF THE NEUROLOGIC SYSTEM

HEAD INJURY

A head injury can be defined as any trauma involving the scalp, cranial bones, or structures within the skull resulting from force or penetration. Head injuries are the most common injuries in childhood, with an incidence of 200 per 100,000 children per year. About 5% of all head injuries are fatal. Approximately 20% of head injury survivors acquire a significant disability, such as mental retardation, physical disability, seizures, sensory deficits, and attention deficit disorders.[30, 31]

Children are prone to skull fractures, often resulting in hematomas and brain injury. They may suffer from the secondary effects of trauma, such as diffuse cerebral edema, malignant brain edema, and increased intracranial pressure.

Children under the age of 10 years have the best chance of recovering from head injuries. Because of their anatomic immaturity (as described in Table 18–1) and compensatory abilities, many of these children continue to improve and recuperate for up to 5 years after their injury.

Clinical Manifestations

The signs and symptoms of head injuries in children depend on the pathologic features and severity of the injury. The child with a mild head injury may remain conscious or lose consciousness for less than 5 minutes. The child with a moderate head injury loses consciousness for 5–10 minutes. Following mild and moderate head injuries, children may have amnesia about the event, headache, nausea, and vomiting. A child with a severe head injury is usually unconscious for more than 10 minutes and may show signs of increased intracranial pressure. This was the case with Antwan, in the opening scenario.

GROWTH & DEVELOPMENT CONSIDERATIONS

The younger the child, the greater the risk of head injuries. Fatalities from head injuries occur in children less than 1 year of age twice as often as they do in children aged 1–6 years, and three times as often as in children aged 6–12 years.[32]

Unconsciousness may result from increased intracranial pressure, edema, hemorrhage, or parenchymal damage to both cerebral cortices or the brainstem.

Vital signs are important indicators of head injury. Changes in respiratory effort or periods of apnea can occur secondary to shock, injury to the spinal cord above C4, or damage to or pressure on the medulla. Heart rate and blood pressure are indices of brainstem function. Tachycardia can be a sign of blood loss, shock, hypoxia, anxiety, or pain. **Cushing's triad,** associated with increased intracranial pressure or compromised blood flow to the brainstem, is characterized by hypertension, increased systolic pressure with wide pulse pressure, bradycardia, and irregular respirations. Refer to the discussion of altered states of consciousness earlier in this chapter for more information about increased intracranial pressure.

Reflexes may be hyporesponsive, hyperresponsive, or nonexistent. The child may assume a decorticate, decerebrate, **areflexic,** or flaccid posture (see Fig. 18–2).

Etiology and Pathophysiology

Falls are a major cause of unintentional head injuries in young children. Infants fall from dressing tables, beds, and sofas and also tumble down stairs, especially in walkers. Child abuse accounts for a large number of head injuries in the child less than 1 year old. Toddlers and preschool-age children lack good judgment, and they may run out into the street without looking where they are going or may lean out of windows and fall. School-age children may be injured in motor vehicle crashes, either as passengers or as pedestrians, and they may also be injured in bicycle, roller-blading, or skateboard mishaps. Adolescents are frequently the drivers in motor vehicle crashes; often alcohol or drugs are involved. Teenagers may also be injured in sports-related accidents.

Head injuries can be categorized as either primary or secondary. Primary injuries occur at the time of the insult when the initial cellular damage takes place. These injuries result from either a direct blow to the head (coup injury) or from acceleration-deceleration movement of the brain within the skull (contrecoup injury; Fig. 18–17). At the time of impact, arterial and intracranial pressures increase, and apnea and loss of consciousness occur.

The secondary phase of head trauma, which involves both the brain and the body's response to the initial injury, can be manifested immediately or several hours, days, or weeks later. Damage usually results from destruction of brain tissue secondary to hypoxia, hypotension, edema, change in the blood–brain barrier, or hemorrhage.[33] Whatever the underlying cause, however, the result is increased intracranial pressure. Irreversible brain damage may result if the condition is left untreated.

Diagnostic Tests and Medical Management

Identifying the pathologic results of a head injury involves history, observation, examination, and diagnostic testing. The questions in Table 18–24 can be used to determine what happened.

Neurologic evaluation with the pediatric Glasgow Coma Scale is performed frequently to detect changes in the child's condition (see Table 18–3). Cranial nerves are assessed (see Table 18–5). See Chapter 3 and the discussion of altered states of consciousness at the beginning of this chapter for further details.

NURSING ALERT

Any infant who arrives in the emergency department with seizures, failure to thrive, vomiting, lethargy, respiratory irregularities, or coma should be evaluated for child abuse, particularly "shaken child" syndrome.

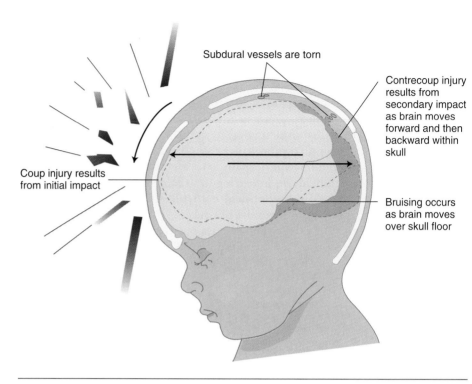

Subdural vessels are torn

Contrecoup injury results from secondary impact as brain moves forward and then backward within skull

Coup injury results from initial impact

Bruising occurs as brain moves over skull floor

FIGURE 18–17. Head trauma can result from a direct blow to the head (coup injury) or the acceleration–deceleration movement of the brain (contrecoup injury).

NURSING ALERT

Most children with head injuries are the victims of multiple trauma, and even though cervical spine injuries are rare, all children should be suspected of having a cervical spine injury until this possibility has been ruled out by radiologic examination.

Laboratory tests include a complete blood cell count, blood chemistry, toxicology screening, and urinalysis.

Radiologic examination is performed to identify the specific injury. Skull films are used to detect fractures. A CT scan is used to detect fractures, hematomas, lacerations, or contusions. An MRI scan may be performed in order to visualize subtle damage or injury.

The initial medical management of a child with a head injury is based on findings from the assessment of the child's physiologic status (see Table 18–4). The airway must be clear and stable. If indicated, the child is intubated, sedated, and chemically paralyzed.

Perfusion must be maintained to ensure that the brain gets adequate oxygen and nutrients. Shock is treated aggressively with fluid boluses. Until adequate cerebral perfusion pressure is ensured, the head of the bed should be kept flat.[34] Inotropes may be used to ensure perfusion if **cerebral edema** (the increase in intracellular and extracellular fluid in the brain that results from anoxia, vasodilation, or vascular stasis) is present.

18-24	Questions to Ask About Head Injuries in Children

- How did the injury occur?
- How did the child respond initially?
- How is the child different now?
- Did the child lose consciousness?
- Did the child have a seizure?
- What interventions were performed at the scene?
- Does the child remember the event?

Increased intracranial pressure must be controlled. Hypoxia and hypercapnia have disastrous effects on cerebral function, as they can cause vasodilation and increased intracranial pressure. Effective assisted ventilation with 100% oxygen at the child's normal respiratory rate is the initial treatment of choice.[35] If there is no cervical spine injury, the head of the bed is elevated to 30 degrees. The child's head is kept in the midline to promote venous (jugular) drainage. Hip flexion is avoided. Acetaminophen can be given for pain. The child's body temperature is kept within normal limits. The environment is kept as quiet as possible. Fluids may be restricted only after the child is hemodynamically stable. Diuretics such as mannitol or furosemide may be given to shrink brain volume. A urinary catheter is inserted to monitor output, and electrolytes should be checked frequently.

Invasive procedures may be necessary to reduce increased intracranial pressure. Burr holes may be made or more extensive surgery may be performed as a method of evacuating a lesion or hematoma. A ventricular catheter may be placed to drain cerebrospinal fluid and to monitor pressure.

Aggressive support continues until the child regains consciousness and rehabilitation can be initiated. Reliable predictions of outcome in the child who has suffered a severe head injury cannot be made until 6–12 months postinjury.

Nursing Assessment

Assess the child's neurologic status frequently. Evaluate the child's level of consciousness continually using the pediatric Glasgow Coma Scale (see Table 18–3). Monitor vital signs closely. Changes in these signs may indicate hypoxia, decreased perfusion, shock, or increased intracranial pressure. The child's neurologic status is compared to his or her previous state, with improvement, stability, or deterioration noted. The cause of any deterioration must be quickly determined and appropriate interventions taken.

CLINICAL TIP

A child who has a decreased level of consciousness shortly after a head injury may have had a posttraumatic seizure and may still be in the postictal state.

Nursing Diagnosis

Nursing diagnoses that might be appropriate for the child with a head injury include:

- Altered Cerebral Tissue Perfusion related to poor respiratory effort, hypovolemia, and/or increased intracranial pressure
- Impaired Gas Exchange related to poor respiratory effort
- Ineffective Airway Clearance related to decreased level of consciousness
- Risk for Caregiver Role Strain related to long-term care of a child with neurologic complications
- Risk for Altered Family Processes related to the child's acquired disability
- Altered Growth and Development related to motor, cognitive, and perceptual deficits

Nursing Management

Nursing care focuses on maintaining cardiopulmonary function, preventing complications, promoting recovery, and providing emotional support. Nursing management is based on prevention of secondary injury and return to an optimal level of function.

NURSING ALERT

In the child with moderate head injury, the oxygen saturation should remain over 95%. For the severely injured child who is intubated, monitor arterial blood gas results. The PaO_2 should be between 70 and 100 mm Hg.

Maintain Cardiopulmonary Function

In the moderately injured child, observe breathing patterns and check color and level of consciousness. Check the pulse oximeter. Report any sign of decreased oxygenation to the physician immediately.

Make sure that the side rails of the bed are padded to protect the child if a seizure occurs. Equipment for suction and ventilation should be at the bedside.

Prevent Complications

Position the child properly, maintain a quiet environment, and control body temperature. Administer medications as ordered. Check intracranial monitors or surgical sites if invasive measures have been taken. Report any signs and symptoms of increased intracranial pressure (see Table 18–6) to the physician immediately.

Promote Recovery

Prevent physical deformities. Physical, occupational, and speech therapy should begin in the hospital. Work with these therapists to reinforce exercises and help teach parents the techniques so they can work with the child in the hospital and at home. The nurse can reinforce what has been done during these sessions, noting positive changes. Using toys, books, music, or games, provide stimulation based on the child's age and ability. Encourage parents to bring in favorite toys, stuffed animals, and tape recordings of the child's favorite music or of family members talking.

Provide Emotional Support

Nurses, social workers, physicians, psychologists, rehabilitation therapists, and members of the clergy can support and help parents adjust to having a child with a new disability.

Discharge Planning and Home Care Teaching

Home care needs should be identified and addressed well in advance of discharge. Children with significant injuries will benefit from inpatient or outpatient rehabilitation to promote optimal achievement of function. A case manager may be needed to coordinate services and resources during rehabilitation.

Give parents information about caring for children with head injuries at home and possible behaviors to expect from the child. For children with disabilities, determine what adaptations are needed in the home to care for the child, such as a wheelchair, walker, braces, or special bed. Social work and home health agencies can often help the parents make special arrangements.

HOME CARE CONSIDERATIONS

Even though the child looks normal within days of a mild or moderate head injury, brain healing takes up to 6 weeks. Parents and teachers should be made aware that typical behavior during this period may include any of the following behaviors: tiring easily, memory loss or forgetfulness, easy distractibility, difficulty concentrating, difficulty following directions, irritability or short temper, and needing help starting and finishing tasks.

Care in the Community

Arrange for home care nursing and follow-up care, if necessary. The home care nurse can take over the case management for the disabled child and make sure the environment is safe. Many children with head injuries are disabled enough to qualify for Social Security Supplemental Security Income (SSI) benefits or the state program for children with special health care needs.

Parents of children with mild or moderate injuries need to be prepared for typical behavior after a head injury, until full recovery has occurred. If the child returns to school, help prepare the teachers, school administrators, and other children for how their classmate is "different." Such sensitivity training makes reintegrating the child into the classroom easier. The child or adolescent facing long-term rehabilitation needs support to adjust to the disability and to find the strength to maximize his or her abilities. The adolescent may need to gain vocational skills and learn to live independently. Refer parents to the Brain Injury Association for further information (see Appendix F).

Specific Head Injuries

Scalp Injuries

Injuries to the scalp, which can be caused by falls, blunt trauma, or penetration of a foreign body, are usually benign. Although bleeding may be extensive, hypovolemia or shock is uncommon unless the patient is an infant.

Lacerations should be irrigated with copious amounts of sterile normal saline solution and inspected for bony fragments or depressions, cerebrospinal fluid leakage with a dural tear, or debris. If the injury is simple, the laceration can be sutured and the child discharged from the emergency department. If not, a neurosurgeon should be consulted.

Concussion

A concussion can involve transient impairment of consciousness that usually results from blunt head trauma. It is secondary to stretching, compression, or shearing of nerve fibers.[33] There is usually no gross structural damage or focal injury. The child may have amnesia of the event, headache, nausea with or without vomiting, or dizziness. Concussions are categorized by three levels of severity (Table 18–25).

Treatment is supportive. Children are observed in the emergency department for several hours before being sent home with instructions to the parents to watch them closely. Any child who is unconscious for more than 5 minutes or has amnesia of the event may be admitted to the hospital or observed in a short-stay unit to rule out other injury.

Pediatric concussive syndrome, which is believed to be caused by an injury to the brainstem, is seen in children who are less than 3 years old. Toddlers seem stunned at the time of injury, but they do not lose consciousness. Later, however, these children become pale, clammy, and lethargic, and they may vomit. They are usually brought to the hospital for treatment when these symptoms appear. These children may be placed in a short-stay unit for observation and usually recover within 24 hours.

⚖️ **LEGAL & ETHICAL CONSIDERATIONS**

Public Law 104-166, the Traumatic Brain Injury Act, was enacted by Congress in 1996 to prevent head injuries and to minimize the severity of dysfunction as a result of head injury by providing funding to states to identify mechanisms to improve access to services.[36]

18-25 Levels of Concussion Severity

Grade 1
Transient confusion, no loss of consciousness, and a duration of mental status abnormalities of less than 15 minutes.

Grade 2
Transient confusion, no loss of consciousness, and a duration of mental status abnormalities of 15 minutes or longer.

Grade 3
Loss of consciousness, either brief (seconds) or prolonged (minutes or longer).

Adapted from the Quality Standards Subcommittee, American Academy of Neurology. (1997). Practice parameters: The management of concussion in sports. Neurology, 48, 581–585.

Postconcussive syndrome, which is common in both children and adults, may occur anytime after the initial head injury. Signs and symptoms can include headache, dizziness or vertigo, photophobia, subtle changes in personality, poor concentration, and poor memory. Treatment is supportive. Symptoms usually disappear within several weeks. Parents and teachers should be informed to expect altered behavior in the child. They should be encouraged to help the child maintain self-esteem.

Young athletes suffering a second concussion before complete recovery from the first develop *"second impact" syndrome.* This syndrome results in acute brain swelling, neurologic or cognitive deficits, and sometimes death from the cumulative effect of these concussions. Recommendations now exist for the management of sports-related concussions to reduce the risk of disability and death. Removal from sports participation ranges from 1 week to the entire season, depending on the severity of concussion and neurologic symptoms.[37]

Skull Fractures

A fracture to any of the eight cranial bones is caused by a considerable force to the head. Any area of the skull with swelling or a hematoma should be evaluated for possible fracture. Diagnosis is made by visual inspection, palpation, radiologic study, or CT scan. Treatment should always include neurosurgical consultation.

Management of skull fractures depends on the type and extent of the injury (Table 18–26 and Fig. 18–18).

Cerebral Contusion

A cerebral contusion, or the bruising of brain tissue, is secondary to blunt trauma and can occur with either coup or contrecoup injuries (see Fig. 18–17). Such injuries are rare in children less than 1 year of age. The temporal or frontal sections of the skull are the most common sites of this injury, which involves damage to the parenchyma with tears in vessels or tissue, pulping, and subsequent areas of necrosis or infarction.

The child may have focal symptoms depending on the area of injury. Altered levels of consciousness range from confusion and disorientation to being obtunded. A CT scan is used for diagnosis.

Treatment involves hospitalization for observation and to rule out other injuries. Surgical treatment is rarely necessary.

Sequelae are focal and specific to the area of the brain that was injured. For example, an injury to the left temporal area may affect speech.

Intracranial Hematomas

Intracranial hematomas are space-occupying lesions that expand rapidly or slowly, depending on whether they are arterial or venous in origin. They must be located quickly. Some lesions require evacuation as soon as possible to minimize the secondary effects of the injury. Table 18–27 describes types of intracranial hematomas and their treatment.

Subarachnoid hemorrhages, associated with severe head injuries such as intracranial hematomas or contusions, result from laceration of arteries or veins in the subarachnoid space. Symptoms include decreased level of consciousness, ipsilateral pupil dilation, diplopia, hemiparesis, nausea and vomiting, nuchal rigidity, and headache.

Diagnosis is confirmed by CT scan. There is no specific treatment, and the clinical course depends on associated injuries.

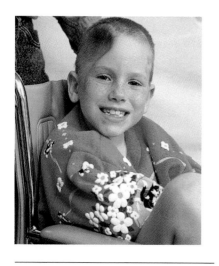

FIGURE 18–18. This child had a significant depressed skull fracture that required removal of bony fragments over a section of the skull.

18-26 | Skull Fractures

Injury	Diagnosis and Management
Linear Fracture Results from impact to large area of the skull; usually no symptoms unless fracture cuts across suture lines near middle meningeal artery, in which case epidural hematoma may form	On x-ray study, fracture appears as a thin, clear line; child is hospitalized overnight for observation; fracture heals within 6 months A growing skull fracture may appear if the dura mater has been torn; management is surgical
Depressed Fracture Break in skull itself, which usually shatters it into many fragments; pieces of broken bone can be depressed into brain tissue, with hematoma forming on top; most common sites for injury are frontal or parietal areas	Diagnosis confirmed by x-ray study or CT scan, although fracture usually palpable; any depressed area greater than thickness of skull or 5 mm must be elevated by surgery or possibly vacuum extraction to prevent damage to underlying brain tissue; brain contusion or laceration may be associated with the fracture; tetanus prophylaxis and antibiotics are given to prevent infection; seizures are common sequelae
Compound Fracture Combination of scalp laceration and depressed skull fracture	Diagnosis made visually, by x-ray study, or by CT scan; treatment involves surgical debridement and elevation of bony fragments, tetanus prophylaxis, and antibiotics
Basilar Fracture Occurs in the inferior, posterior portion of the skull; can involve frontal, ethmoid, sphenoid, temporal, or occipital bones; may have dural tear; classic signs are blood behind tympanic membrane with cerebrospinal fluid leaking from nose and ears; child also has periorbital ecchymosis (raccoon's eyes) and bruising of mastoid (Battle's sign)	Diagnosis confirmed by CT scan; treatment includes hospitalization with observation; often dural tear heals in 1 week; however, if cerebrospinal fluid leakage persists, leak should be surgically repaired; possible damage to cranial nerves I, II, III, VII, and VIII; antibiotic prophylaxis

Data from Semonin-Holleran, R. (1994). Head, neck, and spinal cord trauma. In Kelly, S. (Ed.). Pediatric emergency nursing (2nd ed., pp. 318–319). Stamford, CT: Appleton & Lange.

Penetrating Injuries

Gunshot wounds to the head can damage tissue, bone, and vessels. Low-velocity bullets enter but do not exit the skull; instead they ricochet within the cranial vault, destroying brain tissue and vessels. Although the child may be conscious just after the injury, the level of consciousness quickly deteriorates because of the edema surrounding the penetration tract. High-velocity bullets, on the other hand, cause immediate, severe damage on impact.

CT is used to evaluate gunshot trauma and to pinpoint the location of bullet and bone fragments as well as parenchymal damage. Treatment involves surgical debridement of the tract, evacuation of any hematomas, and removal of accessible bone or bullet particles.

Approximately 50% of children with gunshot wounds to the head die. Those who survive may suffer multiple focal deficits and seizures.

18-27 Intracranial Hematomas

Type of Hematoma	Diagnosis and Management

Subdural Hematoma

Result of severe head injuries such as falls, assaults, motor vehicle crashes, or shaken child syndrome

Occurs most frequently in children less than 1 year old

Caused by laceration of the bridging veins; clot forms and presses directly on brain, leading to damage from two sources: original contusion and hematoma

Symptoms (may not appear until 48–72 hours after the injury) include:

Change in level of consciousness (confusion, agitation, or lethargy)

Nausea or vomiting

Headache

Retinal hemorrhages in both eyes

Pupil on side of injury may be fixed and dilated

Seizures

Fever

Diagnosis confirmed by CT scan

Treatment is usually surgical; subdural taps may be necessary after surgery to give the brain room to expand

More than half of children with subdural hematomas die; those who survive have 75% chance of developing seizures

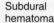
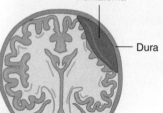

Bleeding occurs between dura and brain

Epidural Hematoma

Rare in children and almost never occurs in children less than 4 years of age

Results from blunt trauma (most often falls), motor vehicle crashes, or assaults

Temporal and parietal areas are most common sites

May be associated with linear skull fracture

May be fatal if bleeding is arterial

Symptoms include:

Sleepiness or lethargy

Headache

Full fontanel

Paresis of cranial nerves III and VI

Papilledema

Fixed and dilated pupil

Signs of increased intracranial pressure

Diagnosis confirmed by CT scan

Treatment involves immediate surgical intervention; craniotomy is performed followed by evacuation of the hematoma

Prognosis is good, although 25% of children have seizures

Bleeding occurs between dura and skull

Intracerebral Hematoma

Result of deep contusion or intracerebral laceration (secondary to foreign body or bony penetration or impalement)

Causes diffuse bleeding in parenchyma; there may be a hematoma with associated small areas of bleeding

Diagnosis confirmed by CT scan

Surgical treatment not indicated

Neurologic effects depend on size and location of lesion and whether bleeding can be controlled; hemiplegia or visual loss may result

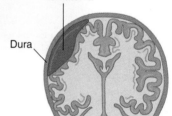

Bleeding occurs within cerebrum

Impalement injuries frequently occur in children in association with lawn darts or dog bites. All objects must be left in place and removed in the operating room by a neurosurgeon.

The child with an impalement injury is at high risk for focal injury and infection.

After surgery children with this type of injury are managed as with other postoperative head injuries, with attention focused on level of consciousness, increased intracranial pressure, and infection control.

SPINAL CORD INJURY

Less than 10% of spinal cord injuries occur in children.[38] Yet over half of the children with these injuries die within the first hour of trauma, and approximately 20% die during the first 3 months after trauma.[39]

Almost half of all spinal cord injuries are the result of motor vehicle crashes. In young children they are pedestrian–vehicular, bicycle–vehicular, or passenger related. By adolescence the incidence of passenger-related injuries increases significantly, with alcohol and drugs contributing to about 25% of crashes.[39] Other causes of spinal injuries, especially in toddlers and young children, include falls and child abuse. Recreation-related trauma accounts for more injuries as children grow older. Penetrating injuries such as stab and gunshot wounds are becoming more prevalent.

The mechanism of injury determines the type of lesion that occurs (Fig. 18–19). Hyperflexion injuries produce tears or avulsions and fractures of vertebral bodies, as well as subluxation and dislocation. Lateral flexion (rotation) may cause joint dislocations or unstable spinal fractures. Extension may result in the so-called hangman's fracture, ligament tears, avulsion fractures of vertebral bodies, as well as central or posterior spinal cord syndrome. Compression injuries cause anterior cord syndrome.

Spinal cord injuries are classified as complete or incomplete. Complete lesions are irreversible and involve a loss of sensory, motor, and autonomic function below the level of the injury. Incomplete lesions involve varying degrees of sensory, motor, and autonomic function below the level of injury.

Children are prone to specific kinds of spinal cord injuries because of the extreme mobility and flexibility of their spinal column. Table 18–28 describes the spinal cord injuries most common in children.

The higher the level of spinal cord injury, the more severe the neurologic damage. The child is often a victim of multiple trauma and may display signs of hypovolemic shock resulting from other injuries, increased intracranial pressure, or respiratory depression. Children can also experience neurogenic or spinal shock (see Chap. 12).

At the time of injury, the child is flaccid and areflexic below the lesion and responds only to stimuli above the level of the injury. Priapism may be present. Muscle spasticity below the lesion occurs later.

Diagnosis is made by observation, neurologic examination, and x-ray studies. X-ray studies include lateral cervical spine and anteroposterior and lateral views of the thoracic and lumbosacral spine. In addition, CT scanning, MRI, fluoroscopy, or myelography may be performed. Many children have spinal cord injury without radiographic abnormality (SCIWORA).[40]

Spinal injuries are managed aggressively. The child with a spinal cord injury may be placed in skeletal traction or a halo device. Further surgical management of the injury may be necessary. Debridement and decompression should be accomplished within the first 8 hours after penetrating injury. A fusion using bone from another part of the body may be performed to stabilize the spinal cord. If more drastic measures are necessary, an internal fixation device may be required.

SCIWORA

Spinal cord injury without radiographic abnormality (SCIWORA) accounts for 15–25% of all pediatric spinal cord trauma. SCIWORA occurs when initial films or CT scans show no bony deformity and the child is believed to be free of injury. Profound or progressive paralysis is found either immediately or within 48 hours. Children under 8 years of age are most at risk because of the elasticity of their spinal column. The young child's spinal column can withstand up to 2 inches of stretch without disruption, while the cord itself ruptures with an elongation of only ¼ inch. This incongruity may account for the normal radiograph despite cord injury.[40]

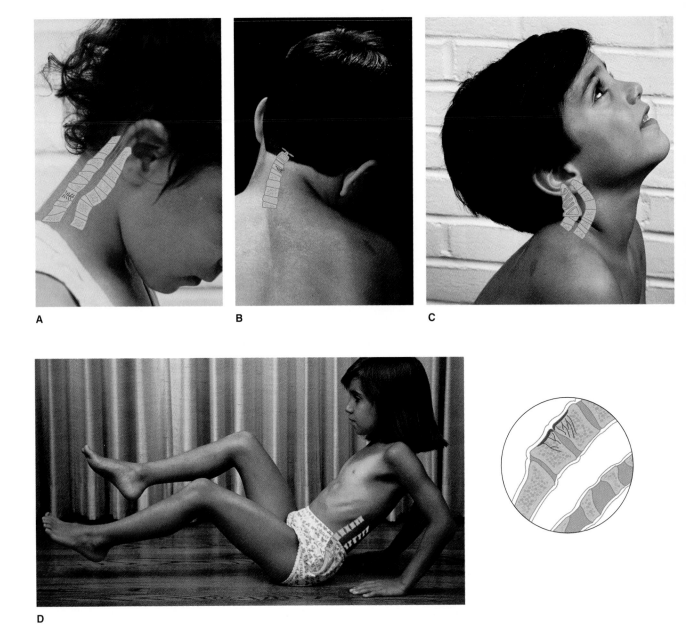

FIGURE 18-19. Mechanics of injury to the spinal cord. A, Hyperflexion. B, Lateral flexion. C, Extension. D, Compression.

To further decrease neurologic sequelae, methylprednisolone is administered in high doses to children with motor deficits. Administration must be started within 8 hours of the injury.

Nursing Management

Nursing care focuses on monitoring vital signs, meeting nutritional needs, maintaining skin integrity, promoting independent functioning, encouraging therapeutic play, providing emotional support, and promoting rehabilitation.

Monitor Vital Signs

Be alert for any changes in vital signs, especially those that may signify increased intracranial pressure (see Table 18-6). Monitor the child's respira-

18-28	Spinal Cord Injuries in Children

Cervical Region
- Site of 75% of spinal injuries in children through 8 years and 60% between 8 and 14 years
- Highest incidence above C3 segment
- Many of these injuries are fatal

Thoracolumbar Region
- Second most common area of injury; probably a result of improperly placed lap belts[a]

Thoracic Region
- Site of 20% of spinal injuries usually between 8 and 14 years

[a]Data from Luerssen, T. (1993). General characteristics of the neurological injury. In M. Eichelberger (Ed.), Pediatric trauma: Prevention, acute care, rehabilitation. St. Louis: Mosby–Year Book.

tory status. Some children with cervical lesions have tracheostomies performed to help maintain airway patency; others with very high lesions are dependent on ventilators. Proper emergency equipment should be at the bedside at all times.

Meet Nutritional Needs
Ensure adequate nutrition. A child with complete paralysis may require a gastrostomy tube.

Maintain Skin Integrity
Prevent skin breakdown (see Table 18–7). Observe surgical sites for signs of infection or inflammation. Good skin care should be performed at the insertion of the external fixation device (see Table 19–16).

Promote Independent Functioning
Reinforce the exercises and skills learned in physical and occupational therapy. Use supports, boots, footboards, splints, and braces as recommended by the therapists to prevent contractures (Fig. 18–20). Encourage the child to be as independent as possible in a wheelchair.

Bowel and bladder control may be hard to achieve. Intermittent catheterizations may be necessary (see Table 16–6). Bowel training involves a diet high in fiber and the use of stool softeners.

Encourage Therapeutic Play
Therapeutic play appropriate for the child's developmental level is an important part of the healing process. Provide as many normal activities for the child as possible, but do not give the child tasks that he or she will have difficulty completing. Child life teachers or tutors can help the child keep up with schoolwork.

Television, videotapes, and music can offer diversion for prolonged hospitalization. Paraplegic children can learn to use their arms and hands to play interactive games. Devices can also be adapted so that the child can play video games or manipulate the television or radio.

Provide Emotional Support
Support the child emotionally. Encourage the child to meet small, short-term goals, including those that involve self-care. Encourage the child to express fears and frustrations.

FIGURE 18–20. Splints are often used to prevent contractures, thus maintaining optimal functioning of the child's hands or feet.

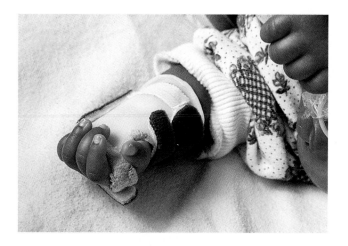

FIGURE 18–20. Splints are often used to prevent contractures, thus maintaining optimal functioning of the child's hands or feet.

Be compassionate and understanding. Encourage siblings to visit, answer their questions honestly, and help them to discuss their feelings. Involve the parents and siblings in the care of the child as much as possible. When appropriate, encourage them to help with activities of daily living.

Discharge Planning and Home Care Teaching

Many children are discharged to rehabilitation facilities. Assist with arrangements for the child's transfer from the hospital to the rehabilitation facility. Work closely with the child, parents, and other members of the health care team concerning placement. Home care needs and safety issues should be identified and addressed well in advance of discharge from the rehabilitation facility. Refer families to social services, family counseling, and support groups if indicated.

HYPOXIC–ISCHEMIC BRAIN INJURY (DROWNING AND NEAR-DROWNING)

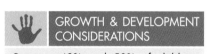

GROWTH & DEVELOPMENT CONSIDERATIONS

Between 40% and 50% of children who are injured in drowning incidents are under 4 years of age, with peak incidence between ages 1 and 2 years.

Drowning is defined as death within 24 hours of a submersion incident. Over 90% of drownings occur in fresh water. Fifty percent of these incidents occur in swimming pools, and 90% of these children drown in residential pools.[41]

Drowning is the third most common cause of injury-related deaths in children. The majority of pediatric victims are very young (under age 4 years) or in their teen years. Boys are five times more likely than girls to die from drowning.

There are two types of drowning. Wet drowning, which occurs more frequently, is the result of aspiration of fluid into the lungs. Dry drowning, which is seen in 10–15% of cases, is due to hypoxemia resulting from laryngospasm, with small or insignificant amounts of liquid aspirated.

The events preceding drowning follow a sequential pattern. The child trapped in water panics, struggles, attempts to move using swimming motions, and holds his or her breath. Then the child swallows a small amount of fluid, vomits, and aspirates the vomitus. This leads to a brief period of laryngospasm, which lasts no more than 2 minutes. Because of the increasing panic and hypoxia, the child swallows more liquid. Then either the child goes into profound laryngospasm, becomes severely hypoxic, has a seizure, and dies (dry drowning), or the child becomes unconscious, the laryngospasm relaxes as reflexes are lost, and the child passively aspirates even greater amounts of water into the airway and stomach (wet drowning).

Hypoxemia is the major insult associated with drowning. Aspiration leads to impaired gas exchange and ultimately affects pulmonary, cardiac, cerebral, and renal functions. See Chapter 11 for a brief discussion of the effects of drowning on the respiratory system.

Prognosis and outcome are highly individual. The length of time submerged and the immediacy of intervention and treatment, especially cardiopulmonary resuscitation, affect the child's chances for survival.[42,43]

The child who has been immersed exhibits a wide variety of signs and symptoms depending on the length of time underwater, the temperature of the water, the response to the episode, and the initial treatment performed at the scene. Children who are immersed for short periods have few symptoms and recover without complication. The child with a longer immersion can experience the following symptoms: decreased level of consciousness ranging from stupor to total unresponsiveness, cerebral edema, increased intracranial pressure, seizures, respiratory acidosis, irregular respirations, apnea, and gastric distention.

Medical intervention begins at the scene of the drowning with immediate ventilation and compressions, when indicated. The sooner the treatment is started, the better the child's prognosis.

Nursing Management

Nursing care of the child who survives a submersion incident focuses on monitoring the child's cardiopulmonary status and providing emotional support.

Monitor the child's respiratory status, cardiopulmonary function, and neurologic status. Administer prescribed medications and position the child properly. Other nursing interventions, especially for the obtunded child, are similar to those for any child in coma (see the earlier discussion of altered states of consciousness).

Provide emotional support to the family. Be nonjudgmental and provide a forum for parents to express their feelings. Reassure parents who exhibit guilt reactions that their child is receiving all possible medical treatment. Parents may be faced with an unknown prognosis. Encourage parents to seek assistance from social workers, members of the clergy, close friends, and relatives. Arrange for appropriate referrals.

Home care needs should be identified and addressed well in advance of discharge. Assist with arrangements for the child with minor deficits. Help the parents decide whether the comatose child will go home or to a long-term facility.

NURSING ALERT

All near-drowning victims should be admitted to the hospital for at least 24 hours or observed in a short-stay observation unit for several hours, even when asymptomatic. Many life-threatening complications, including respiratory distress and cerebral edema, may not become evident for at least 12 hours after the incident.

SAFETY PRECAUTIONS

Drowning can be prevented by education, legislation, and changes in the environment. Pool owners should erect unclimbable 5-foot fences around all four sides of the pool. Local ordinances may require such fences. Adolescents should learn the dangers of mixing alcohol and swimming. Five- and 10-gallon buckets should be kept empty when not in use. The nurse should emphasize the importance of closely supervising children when near or in the water, whether at pools, at the beach, or in the bathtub.

REFERENCES

1. Farley, J.A., Mooney, K.H., & Andrews, M.M. (1994). Alterations of neurologic function in children. In K.L. McCance & S.E. Huether (Eds.), *Pathophysiology: The biologic basis for disease in adults and children* (2nd ed., pp. 587–623). St. Louis: Mosby.

2. Nordli, D.R., Pedley, T.A., & De Vivo, D.C. (1996). Seizure disorders in infants and children. In A.M. Rudolph, J.I.E. Hoffman, & C.D. Rudolph (Eds.), *Rudolph's pediatrics* (20th ed., pp. 1941–1959). Stamford, CT: Appleton & Lange.

3. Kelley, S.J. (1994). *Pediatric emergency nursing* (2nd ed., pp. 509–517). Stamford, CT: Appleton & Lange.

4. Moe, P.G., & Seay, A.R. (1997). Neurologic and muscular disorders. In W.W. Hay, J.R. Groothius, A.R. Hayward, & M.J. Levin (Eds.), *Current pediatric diagnosis and treatment* (13th ed., pp. 644–656). Stamford, CT: Appleton & Lange.

5. Lannon, S.L. (1997). Epilepsy surgery for partial seizures. *Pediatric Nursing, 23*(5), 453–459.

6. Booy, R., & Kroll, S. (1994). Bacterial meningitis in children. *Current Opinion in Pediatrics, 6,* 29–35.

7. Jafari, H., & McCracken, G. (1993). Update on steroids for bacterial meningitis. *The Report on Pediatric Infectious Diseases, 3*(2), 1–2.

8. Tureen, J. (1996). Meningitis. In A.M. Rudolph, J.I.E. Hoffman, & C.D. Rudolph (Eds.), *Rudolph's pediatrics* (20th ed., pp. 544–548). Stamford, CT: Appleton & Lange.

9. Chiocca, E.M. (1995). Meningococcal meningitis. *American Journal of Nursing, 95*(12), 25.

10. Brown, L.W., & Feigin, R.D. (1994). Bacterial meningitis: Fluid balance and therapy. *Pediatric Annals, 23*(2), 93–98.

11. Rotbart, H.A. (1996). Enterviruses. In A.M. Rudolph, J.I.E. Hoffman, & C.D. Rudolph (Eds.), *Rudolph's pediatrics* (20th ed., pp. 633–638). Stamford, CT: Appleton & Lange.

12. Moe, P.G., & Seay, A.R. (1997). Neurologic and muscular disorders. In W.W. Hay, J.R. Groothius, A.R. Hayward, & M.J. Levin (Eds.), *Current pediatric diagnosis and treatment* (13th ed., pp. 686–689). Stamford, CT: Appleton & Lange.

13. Prober, C.G. (1996). Herpes simplex virus infections. In A.M. Rudolph, J.I.E. Hoffman, & C.D. Rudolph (Eds.), *Rudolph's pediatrics* (20th ed., p. 654). Stamford, CT: Appleton & Lange.

14. Sokol, R.J., & Narkewicz, M.R. (1997). Liver and pancreas. In W.W. Hay, J.R. Groothius, A.R. Hayward, & M.J. Levin (Eds.), *Current pediatric diagnosis and treatment* (13th ed., pp. 598–599). Stamford, CT: Appleton & Lange.

15. Glaze, D. (1992). Guillain-Barré syndrome. In R. Feigin, & J. Cherry (Eds.), *Textbook of pediatric infectious diseases* (3rd ed.). Philadelphia: Saunders.

16. Jouet, M., & Kenwrick, S. (1995). Gene analysis of L2 neural cell adhesion molecule in prenatal diagnosis of hydrocephalus. *The Lancet, 345*(Jan 21), 161–163.

17. Page, R. (1992). Hydrocephalus. In R. Hoekelman (Ed.-in-chief), *Primary pediatric care* (3rd ed.). St. Louis: Mosby–Year Book.

18. Jackson, P.L., & Harvey, J. (1996). Hydrocephalus. In P.L. Jackson, & J.A. Vessey (Eds.), *Primary care of the child with a chronic condition* (2nd ed.). St. Louis: Mosby.

19. Carey, C.M., Tullows, M.W., & Walker, M.L. (1994). Hydrocephalus: Etiology, pathologic effects, diagnosis, and natural history. In W.R. Check (Ed.), *Pediatric neurosurgery: Surgery of the developing nervous system* (3rd ed.). Philadephia: Saunders.

20. McIntyre, F.L. (1997). Craniosynostosis. *American Family Physician, 55*(3), 1173–1177.

21. Carey, J.C. (1996). Malformations and syndromes that involve the craniofacies. In A.M. Rudolph, J.I.E. Hoffman, & C.D. Rudolph (Eds.), *Rudolph's pediatrics* (20th ed., pp. 412–415). Stamford, CT: Appleton & Lange.

22. Forrest, D.C. (1994). The cocaine-exposed infant, part I: Identification and assessment. *Journal of Pediatric Health Care, 8*(1), 3–6.

23. Forrest, D.C. (1994). The cocaine-exposed infant, part II: Intervention and teaching. *Journal of Pediatric Health Care, 8*(1), 7–11.

24. Olson, K.R., & McGuigan, M.A. (1996). Toxicology and accidents. In A.M. Rudolph, J.I.E. Hoffman, & C.D. Rudolph (Eds.), *Rudolph's pediatrics* (20th ed., p. 841). Stamford, CT: Appleton & Lange.

25. Dzienkowski, R.C., Smith, K.K., Dillow, K.A., & Yucha, C.B. (1996). Cerebral palsy: A comprehensive review. *Nurse Practitioner, 21*(2), 45–59.

26. Wollack, J.B., & Nichter, C.A. (1996) Static encephalopathies. In A.M. Rudolph, J.I.E. Hoffman, & C.D. Rudolph (Eds.), *Rudolph's pediatrics* (20th ed., pp. 1892–1897). Stamford, CT: Appleton & Lange.

27. DeLuca, P.A. (1996). The musculoskeletal management of children with cerebral palsy. *Pediatric Clinics of North America, 43*(5), 1135–1150.

28. Zickler, C.F., & Dodge, N.N. (1994). Office management of the young child with cerebral palsy and difficulty in growing. *Journal of Pediatric Health Care, 8*(3), 111–120.

29. Eicher, P.S., & Batshaw, M.L. (1993). Cerebral palsy. *Pediatric Clinics of North America, 40*(3), 537–551.

30. Low, C. (1996). Head injury. In P.L. Jackson, & J.A. Vessey (Eds.), *Primary care of the child with a chronic condition* (2nd ed.). St. Louis: Mosby.

31. Michaud, L.J., Duhaime, A.C., & Batshaw, M.L. (1993). Traumatic brain injury in children. *Pediatric Clinics of North America, 40,* 553–565.

32. Reynolds, E. (1992). Controversies in caring for the child with a head injury. *Maternal Child Nursing, 17*(5), 246–251.

33. Bruce, D. (1993). Head trauma. In M. Eichelberger (Ed.), *Pediatric trauma: Prevention, acute care, rehabilitation.* St. Louis: Mosby–Year Book.

34. Pilmer, S., Duhaime, A., & Raphaely, R. (1993). Intracranial pressure control. In M. Eichelberger (Ed.), *Pediatric trauma: Prevention, acute care, rehabilitation.* St. Louis: Mosby–Year Book.

35. Brain Trauma Foundation and American Foundation for Neurologic Surgeons, the Joint Section on Neurotrauma and Critical Care. (1995). *Guidelines for the management of severe head injury.* New York: Brain Trauma Foundation.

36. United States Congress, (1996). Traumatic brain injury act of 1996. *Congressional Record, 142*(July 29, 1996), 110 STAT, 1445–1449.

37. Centers for Disease Control. (1997). Sports-related recurrent brain injuries—United States. *Morbidity and Mortality Weekly Report, 46*(10), 224–227.

38. Luerssen, T. (1993). General characteristics of neurological injury. In M. Eichelberger (Ed.), *Pediatric*

trauma: Prevention, acute care, rehabilitation. St. Louis: Mosby–Year Book.

39. Dickman, C., & Rekate, H. (1993). Spinal trauma. In M. Eichelberger (Ed.), *Pediatric trauma: Prevention, acute care, rehabilitation.* St. Louis: Mosby–Year Book.

40. Kriss, V.M., & Kriss, T.C. (1996). SCIWORA (spinal cord injury without radiographic abnormality in infants and children). *Clinical Pediatrics, 35*(3), 119–124.

41. Ochsenschlager, D. (1996). Drowning and near drowning. In R. Barkin (Ed.), *Pediatric emergency med-*

icine: Concepts and clinical practice (2nd ed.). St Louis: Mosby–Year Book.

42. Walsh, E.A., & Ioli, J.G. (1994). Child near drowning: Nursing care and primary prevention. *Pediatric Nursing, 20*(3), 265–269, 292.

43. Fields, A. (1993). Near-drowning. In M. Eichelberger (Ed.), *Pediatric trauma: Prevention, acute care, rehabilitation.* St. Louis: Mosby–Year Book.

ADDITIONAL RESOURCES

Batchelor, L., Nance, J., & Short, B. (1997). An interdisciplinary team approach to implementing the ketogenic diet for the treatment of seizures. *Pediatric Nursing, 23*(5), 465–471.

Bernes, S.M., & Kaplan, A.M. (1994). Evolution of neonatal seizures. *Pediatric Clinics of North America, 41*(5), 1069–1104.

Carter, J.R. (1994). The use of new antiepileptic medications in pediatric patients with epilepsy. *Journal of Pediatric Health Care, 8*(6), 277–282.

Chameides, L., & Hazinski, M.F. (Eds.). (1994). *Textbook of pediatric advanced life support.* Dallas: American Heart Association.

Farley, J.A., & Dunleavy, M.J. (1996). Myelodysplasia. In P.L. Jackson, & J.A. Vessey (Eds.), *Primary care of the child with a chronic condition* (2nd ed.). St. Louis: Mosby.

Ferrara, P.C., & Chan, L. (1997). Initial management of the patient with altered mental status. *American Family Physicians, 55*(4), 1773–1780.

George, J.E., Quattrone, M.S., & Goldstone, M. (1995). Triage protocols. *Journal of Emergency Nursing, 21*(1), 65–66.

Lollar, D.J. (Ed.). (1994). *Preventing secondary conditions associated with spina bifida and cerebral palsy: Proceedings and recommendations of a symposium.* Washington, DC: Spina Bifida Association of America.

McDonald, M.E. (1997). Use of the ketogenic diet in treating children with seizures. *Pediatric Nursing, 23*(5), 461–464.

Nichols, D., Yaster, M., Lappe, D., et al. (1995). *Golden hour: The handbook of advanced pediatric life support.* St. Louis: Mosby–Year Book.

Slater, J., Mostello, L., & Shaer, C. (1991). Rubber-specific IgE in children with spina bifida. *The Journal of Urology, 146*(578), 578–579.

Stegbauer, C.C. (1996). Parents' opinions concerning possible causes of cerebral palsy. *Nurse Practitioner, 21*(4), 116–118, 128.

Wald, E.R., Kaplan, S.L., Mason, E.O., Sabo, D., Ross, L., and others (1995). Dexamethosone therapy in children with bacterial meningitis. *Pediatrics, 95*(1), 21–28.

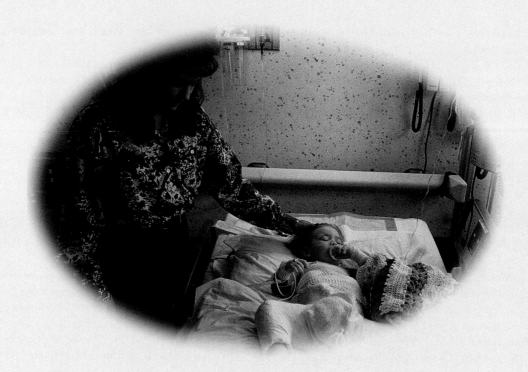

Zachary was born after a normal pregnancy of 39 weeks' gestation. He was healthy at birth but was noted to have syndactyly (fusion of fingers) of the third and fourth fingers of each hand. Syndactyly had occurred in other members of his family, so his parents were neither surprised nor alarmed by its presence. They knew that when he was about 2 years of age, the fused fingers could be surgically separated, resulting in nearly perfect function.

Zachary grew and developed normally. At about 2 years of age, his parents brought him to an outreach clinic in their small rural community for evaluation of his syndactyly. There, the examining nurse noted that Zachary limped when walking. Further examination revealed a dislocated left hip. He was immediately scheduled for surgery. The hip was repositioned within the joint and held in place with screws. A spica cast was applied to hold the hips in an adducted position during healing.

Early in Zachary's hospitalization, the nurses helped his mother to obtain a car seat that would accommodate his cast. Plans were made for follow-up visits. Zachary's cast will be removed in about 8 weeks, and he will be placed in a brace to facilitate hip adduction while he begins physical therapy. After treatment, Zachary will have a stable hip with nearly full range of motion.

ALTERATIONS IN MUSCULOSKELETAL FUNCTION 19

"When I first learned that Zachary had this condition, I wondered if he would be able to run and play like other children. I felt guilty that we had not noticed his limp. It is hard to see Zachary in this big cast, especially in these first days after surgery when he is in pain. But the doctor says that he is expected to recover and be able to walk and run normally."

TERMINOLOGY

- **chondrolysis** The breaking down and absorption of cartilage.
- **dislocation** Displacement of a bone from its normal articulation with a joint.
- **dysplasia** Abnormal development resulting in altered size, shape, and cell organization.
- **equinus** A condition that limits dorsiflexion to less than normal; usually associated with clubfoot.

- **ossification** Formation of bone from fibrous tissue or cartilage.
- **osteotomy** Surgical cutting of bone.
- **pseudohypertrophy** Enlargement of the muscles as a result of infiltration by fatty tissue.
- **subluxation** Partial or complete dislocation of a joint.
- **varus** A condition in which the hindfoot turns inward; usually associated with clubfoot.

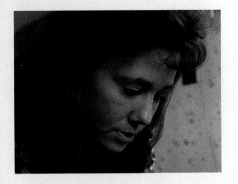

Varus

An abnormal position of a limb that involves bending inward toward the midline of the body

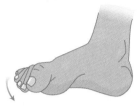

Valgus

An abnormal position of a limb that involves bending outward away from the midline of the body

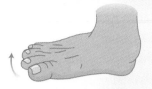

Adduction

Lateral movement of limbs toward the midline of the body

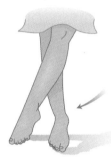

Abduction

Lateral movement of limbs away from the midline of the body

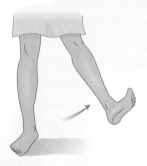

Inversion

Turning inward, usually more than normal

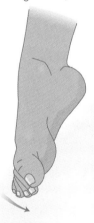

Eversion

Turning outward

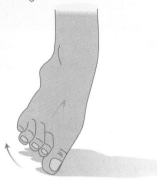

Supination

Lying on the back or placing the hand so the palm faces upward

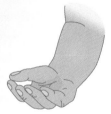

Pronation

Lying on the stomach or placing the hand so the palm faces downward

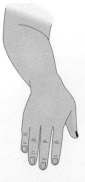

What causes developmental dysplasia of the hip? What are the consequences of uncorrected hip dysplasia? How can Zachary's parents and nurses meet his developmental needs during immobilization? The information in this chapter will enable you to answer these questions, and to provide effective care for children like Zachary who have musculoskeletal disorders.

The musculoskeletal system helps the body to protect its vital organs, support weight, control motion, store minerals, and supply red blood cells. Bones provide a rigid framework for the body, muscles provide for active movement, and tendons and ligaments hold the bones and muscles together. Alterations in musculoskeletal functioning thus can have a significant impact on a child's growth and development.

Musculoskeletal disorders may be congenital, such as clubfoot, or acquired, such as osteomyelitis. They may require short- or long-term management, and may be treated on an outpatient basis or require hospitalization. Many musculoskeletal disorders require surgical correction, casting, or braces.

Table 19–1 provides a review of several terms that will be used throughout this chapter in describing the positioning of a child's limbs.

► ANATOMY AND PHYSIOLOGY OF PEDIATRIC DIFFERENCES

BONES

Several differences exist between the bones of children and those of adults. Although primary centers of **ossification** (bone formation) are nearly complete at birth, a fibrous membrane still exists between the cranial bones (fontanels) (see Fig. 3–11). The posterior fontanel closes between 2 and 3 months of age. The anterior fontanel does not close until approximately 18 months of age, allowing for growth of the brain and skull. In addition, the ends of the long bones (epiphyses) remain cartilaginous (Fig. 19–1). Long bone growth continues until approximately age 20, when skeletal maturation is complete.

Secondary ossification occurs as the long bones grow. Cartilage cells at the epiphyses are replaced by osteoblasts (immature bone cells), resulting in the deposition of calcium. Calcium intake during childhood and adolescence is essential to provide adequate bone density that will prevent osteoporosis and fractures in adulthood. Because growth takes place at the epiphyseal plates, injuries to this portion of a long bone are of particular concern in young children.

The long bones of children are porous and less dense than those of adults. For this reason, children's bones can bend, buckle, or break as a result of a simple fall. In addition to the structural differences between the bones of children and adults, there are also functional differences in the skeletal system of children (see Fig. 3-1). Before birth, the thoracic and sacral regions of the spine are convex curves. As the infant learns to hold up its head, the cervical region becomes concave. When the child learns to stand, the lumbar region also becomes concave. Failure of the spine to assume these final curves results in an abnormal curvature of the spine (kyphosis or lordosis).

RESEARCH CONSIDERATIONS

Research that measures the intake and excretion of calcium has shown that the present Recommended Dietary Allowance (RDA) of calcium for adolescence of 1200 mg/day is not sufficient to saturate bones with calcium. Because calcium deposition at this age is critical for adequate bone density in later adulthood, the National Institutes of Health (NIH) now recommends that adolescents increase their consumption to between 1200 and 1500 mg/day.[1,2]

MUSCLES, TENDONS, AND LIGAMENTS

The muscular system, unlike the skeletal system, is almost completely formed at birth. As a child grows, muscles do not increase in number, but

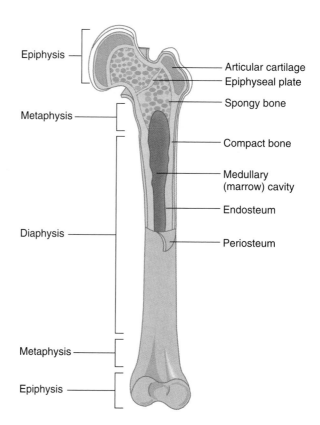

FIGURE 19–1. The parts of long bones.

rather in length and circumference.[3] Until puberty, both tendons and ligaments are stronger than bone. When these structural differences are not recognized, a childhood fracture is sometimes mistaken for a sprain.

► DISORDERS OF THE FEET AND LEGS

METATARSUS ADDUCTUS

Metatarsus adductus, the most common congenital foot deformity, is characterized by an inward turning of the forefoot at the tarsometatarsal joints (Fig. 19–2). Often referred to as "intoeing," metatarsus adductus affects male and female infants equally and occurs in approximately 2 in 1000 births. This condition is most likely caused by both intrauterine positioning and genetic factors.[3,4]

Treatment depends on the degree of foot flexibility. If the foot can be readily maneuvered past the neutral position, simple exercises may correct the problem. Most cases will resolve spontaneously by the time the infant is about 3 months of age. Serial casting is the treatment of choice. The infant's feet are placed in a position as close to neutral as possible and are held secure with casts. Casts are changed weekly until the desired correction is achieved. Braces and orthopedic shoes may also be used.[4]

Nursing Management

Reassure parents that the child's condition can be corrected. If the child's deformity is mild, teach parents simple stretching exercises that can be performed at each diaper change. If casting is necessary, provide cast care as outlined in Table 19–2 and teach parents how to care for the child in a cast

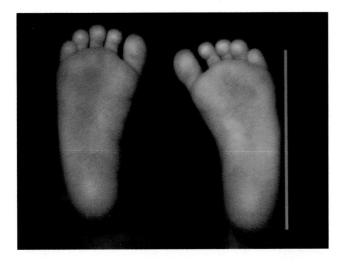

FIGURE 19–2. Metatarsus adductus is characterized by convexity (curvature) of the lateral border of the foot, as shown by the red line. *From Staheli, L.T. (1992). Fundamentals of pediatric orthopedics (p. 5.7). New York: Raven Press.*

19-2 Nursing Care of the Child in a Cast

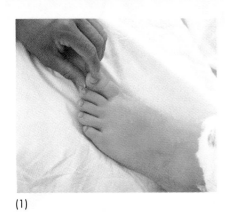

(1)

- A plaster cast takes anywhere from 24 to 48 hours to dry. When handling the cast, be gentle and use the palms of your hands, as fingertips can indent plaster and create pressure areas.
- After the cast is applied, elevate the extremity on a pillow above the level of the heart. Elevation helps to reduce swelling and increases venous return.
- If the cast is applied after surgery, there may be drainage or bleeding through the cast material. Circle the stain and note the date and time on the cast to provide a means of assessing the amount of fluid lost.
- Assess the distal pulses, and check the fingers and toes for color, warmth, capillary refill, and edema. Assess sensation as well as movement. Any deviation from normal may indicate nerve damage or decreased blood supply.
- During the first 24 hours, the casted extremity should be checked every 15–30 minutes for 2 hours, then every 1–2 hours thereafter. The skin should be warm. It should blanch when slight pressure is applied and then return to its normal color within 3 seconds (1). For the next 2 days, the casted extremity should be assessed at least every 4 hours.

- Check the edges of the cast for roughness or crumbling. If necessary, pull the inner stockinette over the edge of the cast and tape.
- The rough edges of the cast may also be alleviated by "petaling." This is done by securing adhesive tape to the inside of the cast and pulling it over the edge, covering the jagged or broken pieces of plaster, and securing it to the outer surface of the cast (2, 3, 4). Moleskin may be used on the cast as well.

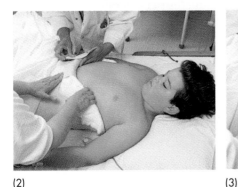

(2)

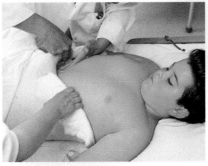

(3)

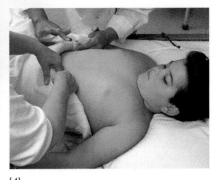

(4)

- Keep the cast as clean and dry as possible. Cover the cast with a plastic bag or plastic wrap when the child bathes or showers.
- The skin under the cast may itch; however, do not use powders or lotions near the edges or under the cast as they can cause skin irritation.
- Be sure that children do not put small objects between the casts and their extremities; these actions can cause skin irritation as well as neurovascular compromise.

19-3   Discharge Teaching: Home Care Instructions for Care of the Child With a Cast

Skin Care
- Check the skin around the cast edges for irritation, rubbing, or blistering. The skin should be clean and dry.
- You may cleanse the skin just under the cast edges and between the toes or fingers with a cotton-tipped applicator and rubbing alcohol. Avoid using lotions, oils, and powders near the cast as they may cause caking.
- Avoid poking sharp objects down inside the cast as this may result in sores.

Cast Care
- Keep the cast dry. Protect plaster with a cast shoe, thick sock, or sling.
- Allow a new, wet cast to air-dry for 24 hours.
- You may begin walking on a leg cast only if your physician has given you permission to do so.

Be Alert for Possible Complications
- Toes or fingers should be pink, not blue or white.
- Skin should be warm and the tips of the toes should blanch when pinched.
- Raise the casted arm or leg above heart level and rest it on pillows to prevent or reduce any swelling.

Notify Your Health Care Provider If Any of the Following Occur
- Unusual odor beneath the cast
- Tingling
- Burning or numbness in the casted arm or leg
- Drainage through the cast
- Swelling or inability to move the fingers or toes
- Slippage of the cast
- Cast cracked, soft, or loose
- Sudden unexplained fever
- Unusual fussiness or irritability in an infant or child
- Fingers or toes that are blue or white
- Pain that is not relieved by any comfort measures (ie, repositioning or pain medication)

Adapted from Shriners Hospital for Crippled Children, Spokane, WA, 1992, 1998.

CLINICAL TIP

To perform stretching exercises for metatarsus adductus:
1. Hold the infant's foot securely in the natural position.
2. Move the forefoot away from the body with the other hand.
3. Hold the foot in this position for 5 seconds.
4. Repeat five times at every diaper change.

CULTURAL CONSIDERATIONS

The incidence of talipes equinovarus (clubfoot) varies among ethnic groups. The condition is least common in Asian groups and Caucasians, with a higher incidence in groups from the Middle East, South Africa, and Mexico. It is most common in Polynesian groups.[6]

---

at home (Table 19–3). If metatarsus adductus persists into childhood without correction, the challenge is to find shoes that accommodate the unusual shape of the foot.

CLUBFOOT

Clubfoot is a congenital abnormality in which the foot is twisted out of its normal position. It occurs in approximately 1–2 in 1000 births and affects boys nearly twice as often as girls.[5]

Clinical Manifestations

A true clubfoot (talipes equinovarus) involves three areas of deformity: the midfoot is directed downward **(equinus),** the hindfoot turns inward **(varus),** and the forefoot curls toward the heel (adduction) and turns upward in partial supination.[7] Most children have this combination of findings. The foot is small with a shortened Achilles tendon. Muscles in the lower leg are atrophied, but leg lengths are generally normal. Clubfoot is bilateral in

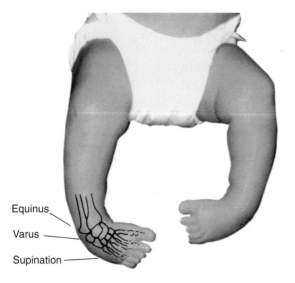

FIGURE 19–3. Bilateral clubfoot deformity. Parents of a child with a clubfoot will have many questions. Can the condition be treated? Will the child be able to walk normally after surgery? Will they need help caring for the infant? How much will surgery and other care cost? Will any subsequent children have a clubfoot?
Modified from Staheli, L.T. (1992). Fundamentals of pediatric orthopedics (p. 5.10). New York: Raven Press.

50% of cases (Fig. 19–3). Clubhand is a rare occurrence that has similar characteristics to the foot deformity (Fig 19–4).

Etiology and Pathophysiology

The exact cause of clubfoot is unknown; however, several possible etiologies have been proposed. Some authorities believe abnormal intrauterine positioning causes the deformity. Neuromuscular or vascular problems are suspected as causes by others. Yet other experts believe there is a genetic component, either at the chromosomal level or by the arrest of normal fetal development. A positive family history increases the chance of the deformity. [5-7]

Diagnostic Tests and Medical Management

Diagnosis is made at birth on the basis of visual inspection. Radiographs are used to confirm the severity of the condition.

Early treatment is essential to achieve successful correction and reduce the chance of complications. Serial casting is the treatment of choice. Casting should begin as soon as possible after birth. Timing is critical because the short bones of the foot, which are primarily cartilaginous at birth, begin to ossify shortly thereafter. The foot is manipulated to achieve maximum correction first of the varus deformity and then of the equinus deformity. A long leg cast is applied to hold the foot in the desired position (Fig. 19–5). The cast is changed every 1–2 weeks. This regimen of manipulation and casting continues for approximately 8–12 weeks until maximum correction is achieved. If the deformity has been corrected, the child may begin wearing reverse or corrective shoes to maintain the correction. If the deformity has not been corrected, surgical intervention is required. Casting is maintained to hold the foot in position until surgery is performed.

The age at which a child undergoes clubfoot surgery varies from surgeon to surgeon. However, most children have surgery between 4 and 12 months of age. The one-stage posteromedial release procedure, which involves realignment of the bones of the foot and release of the constricting soft tissue, is most commonly performed. The foot is held in the proper position by one or more stainless steel pins. A cast is then applied with the knee flexed to prevent damage to the pin and to discourage weight bearing.

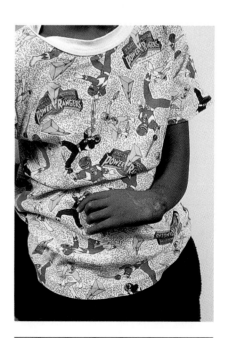

FIGURE 19–4. A clubhand deformity is a less common condition than clubfoot.

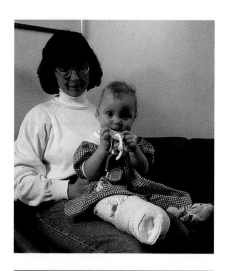

FIGURE 19–5. This girl has a long leg cast, which was applied after surgery to correct her clubfoot deformity.

Casting continues for 6–12 weeks. The child may then need to wear a brace or corrective shoes, depending on the severity of the deformity and the surgeon's preference.

More severe cases or those not corrected in infancy may require more than one surgery to correct the foot.

Nursing Assessment

Nursing assessment, which begins at birth and continues throughout the child's subsequent outpatient casting visits and hospitalization for surgery, includes taking a genetic and birth history, performing a physical examination (including position and appearance of the foot), and assessing the child's motor development and family's coping mechanisms. Because parents will need to bring the child for frequent cast changes, ask about transportation and other arrangements that are necessary to facilitate these visits.

Nursing Diagnosis

Among the nursing diagnoses that might apply to the child with a clubfoot deformity are the following:

- Impaired Physical Mobility related to cast wear
- Risk for Impaired Skin Integrity related to cast wear
- Altered Parenting related to emotional reaction following birth of a child with a physical defect
- Knowledge Deficit (Parent) related to deformity, treatment, and home care

Nursing Management

Nursing management involves providing emotional support, educating the family about home care of the child in a cast and the importance of keeping appointments at the outpatient facility for cast changes, preparation of the family for the child's hospitalization if surgery is to occur, and providing postsurgical care.

Provide Emotional Support

Clubfoot is a condition that affects both the child and the family. The child's foot deformity is upsetting to parents, and they need emotional support to allay their fears. Helping parents understand the condition and its treatment is essential.

Encourage parents to hold and cuddle the child and to take an active role in the child's care to help promote bonding. Explain that, with treatment, the child will grow and develop normally.

Provide Cast and Brace Care

Routine cast care is outlined in Table 19–2. After serial casting is complete, or following surgery, the child may progress to wearing a brace or special shoe for 6–12 months. Braces should fit snugly but should not interfere with neurovascular function. Before the child begins to wear a brace, check the skin for any areas of redness or breakdown. Provide parents with guidelines for brace wear (Table 19–4). Emphasize that proper skin care is essential. If skin redness develops, arrange to have the fit of the brace evaluated and modified if necessary.

19-4   Guidelines for Brace Wear

- Braces should be as comfortable as possible and the child should have adequate mobility while wearing the brace.
- Begin wearing the brace for periods of 1–2 hours and then progress to 2–4 hours.
- Check the skin at 1–2-hour intervals initially, then lengthening to every 4 hours once skin has been clear for several days. If redness is apparent, leave the brace off and allow the skin to clear. If breakdown has occurred, the brace cannot be replaced until healing is complete. (See Chapter 21 for a discussion of pressure ulcers.)
- Always have the child wear a clean white sock, T-shirt, or other thin white liner beneath the brace. Be sure the liner is wrinkle-free under the brace. Avoid using powders or lotions that can cause skin to break down. Toughen any sensitive areas using alcohol wipes.
- Reapply the brace when the skin returns to its normal color.
- Return to the physician or orthotic specialist if discomfort or red areas persist or if the brace needs adjustment or repair or is outgrown.
- Check the brace daily for rough edges.

Provide Postsurgical Care
Routine postoperative care after surgical correction includes neurovascular status checks every 2 hours for the first 24 hours and observing for any swelling around the cast edges (see Table 19–2). Apply ice bags to the foot, and keep the ankle and foot elevated on a pillow for 24 hours. This promotes healing and helps with venous return. Check for drainage or bleeding. Administer pain medication routinely for 24–48 hours.

Discharge Planning and Home Care Teaching
Parents should be given written instructions for care of the child with a cast (see Table 19–3). In addition, assist them in the following ways:

- Demonstrate the use of a sponge bath to protect the cast.
- Discuss several options for clothing that accommodates a cast, for example, one-piece snap suits or sweatpants.
- Discuss potential safety hazards that may result from awkward positioning.
- Suggest that parents make an effort to place toys within the child's reach, since the movements of a child in a cast may be slowed.

 SAFETY PRECAUTIONS

Advise parents that umbrella strollers may not be sturdy enough to support an infant's casted leg. Some infant swings do not provide a foot rest; its absence can contribute to cast slippage or breakdown.

GENU VARUM AND GENU VALGUM

Genu varum (bowlegs) is a deformity in which the knees are widely separated and the lower legs are turned inward (varus). In genu valgum (knock-knees), the knees are close together and the lower legs are directed outward (valgus).

At certain stages of a child's development, the appearance of bowlegs or knock-knees is normal. However, the appearance of knock-knees beyond the age of 2–4 years necessitates further evaluation. Chapter 3 discusses the assessment of bowlegs and knock-knees in children.

Braces are often used to correct mild deformities that could worsen as the child grows. Braces for bowlegs are worn at night; those for knock-knees both day and night. Duration of brace wear is determined by the severity of the deformity, which is usually evaluated by radiographs. If the deformity continues to worsen, surgical intervention is necessary. An **osteotomy** (cutting of the bone) is performed and the tibiofemoral angle surgically corrected. The child is then placed in a cast for approximately 6–10 weeks, or until full healing has occurred.

Nursing Management

Reassure parents that bowlegs and knock-knees are usually a normal part of a child's growth and development. These conditions often resolve on their own and require no treatment other than continued observation.

Nursing care focuses on educating the parents and child about the condition and its treatment. Provide the child and family with guidelines for brace wear and maintenance (see Table 19–4).

▶ DISORDERS OF THE HIP

DEVELOPMENTAL DYSPLASIA OF THE HIP

Developmental dysplasia of the hip (DDH) refers to a variety of conditions in which the femoral head and the acetabulum are improperly aligned. These conditions include **dislocation** (displacement of the bone from its normal articulation with the joint), **subluxation** (in this instance, a partial dislocation), and acetabular **dysplasia** (abnormal cellular or structural development). In the past, DDH was referred to as congenital dislocated hip (CDH). The revised name of the disorder emphasizes that many cases of dislocation, subluxation, and dysplasia occur well after the neonatal period and involve more than a simple dislocation. Zachary, described in the opening scenario, is an example of a child who presented with DDH after the newborn period.

DDH occurs in 1–2 in 1000 births, and the condition affects girls four times as often as boys.[8] It is unilateral in 80% of affected children, and the left hip is affected three times as often as the right.[8]

Clinical Manifestations

Common signs and symptoms of DDH include limited abduction of the affected hip, asymmetry of the gluteal and thigh fat folds, and telescoping or pistoning of the thigh (Fig. 19–6). The older child with untreated DDH walks with a significant limp, which results from telescoping of the femoral head into the pelvis. The longer the disorder goes untreated, the more pronounced the clinical manifestations become, and the worse the prognosis.

Etiology and Pathophysiology

Although the exact cause of DDH is unknown, genetic factors appear to play a role. DDH is 20–50 times more common in first-degree relatives of an infant with the condition than in the general population. If one child of a set of identical twins has DDH, the other twin is affected 30–40% of the time.

Prenatal conditions may affect the development of DDH. The left hip is involved more often than the right hip as a result of intrauterine positioning of the left side of the fetus against the mother's sacrum. Maternal estrogen may cause laxity of the hip joint and capsule, leading to joint instability. DDH is more common in infants born in the breech position. Cultural factors may also be associated with DDH.

CULTURAL CONSIDERATIONS

Infants who are positioned on cradle boards or traditionally swaddled, as in some Native American cultures, have a high incidence of developmental dysplasia of the hip (DDH). Among cultures in which mothers carry infants on their hips or backs with the infants' legs abducted—as in Korean, Chinese, and some African groups—the incidence of DDH is low.[8]

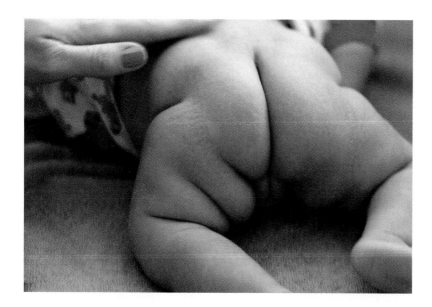

FIGURE 19–6. The asymmetry of the gluteal and thigh fat folds is easy to see in this child with developmental dysplasia of the hip.

Diagnostic Tests and Medical Management

Physical examination reveals Allis' sign (one knee lower than the other when the knees are flexed) and a positive Ortolani-Barlow maneuver. Refer to Chapter 3 for a discussion of the assessment of hip dysplasia in newborns and infants. Radiographs are generally not reliable until approximately 4 months of age because the pelvis in a newborn is still primarily cartilaginous. Before 4 months of age, ultrasonography may be useful for diagnosis. After that age, radiographs are used for diagnosis.

Treatment plans vary according to the child's age. For infants younger than 3 months of age, the Pavlik harness is the most commonly used method for hip reduction (Fig. 19–7). The Pavlik harness is a dynamic splint, that is, a splint that allows movement. It ensures hip flexion and abduction and does

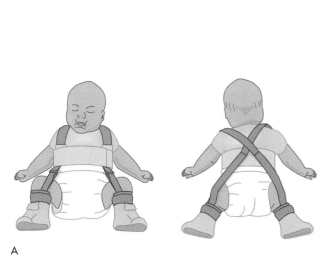

A

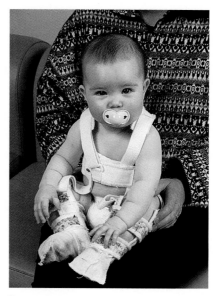

B

FIGURE 19–7. The most common treatment for DDH in a child under 3 months of age is a Pavlik harness. A shirt should be worn under the harness to prevent skin irritation. (It was omitted for clarity in this photograph.)

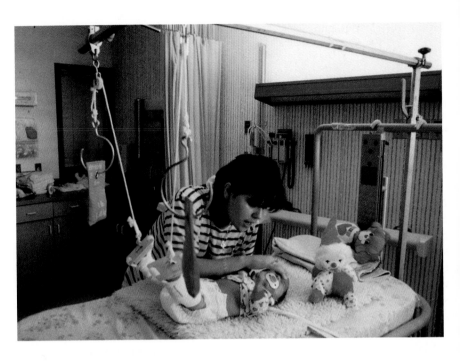

FIGURE 19–8. For infants older than 3 months of age, skin traction is commonly used for treatment of DDH.

not allow hip extension or adduction. For infants older than 3 months of age, skin traction is used (Fig. 19–8). Correct positioning, which involves relocating the femoral head into the acetabulum while gently stretching the restrictive soft tissue, is essential. Surgery and the application of a spica cast may be necessary. In children over 18 months of age, surgery and casting are usually necessary and bracing may also be required. In the opening scenario, Zachary had surgery to correct his dislocated hip and was placed in a hip spica cast to maintain correct position of the hip during healing.

Early screening, detection, and treatment enable the majority of affected children to attain normal hip function.

Nursing Assessment

Assessment for DDH begins at delivery and continues through all well-child checkups. The specific family history or birth data may indicate a high-risk infant. Instructions for performing the physical examination to assess the infant for DDH are given in Chapter 3.

Nursing Diagnosis

Several nursing diagnoses may apply to the child with DDH. They include:

- Impaired Physical Mobility related to treatment (Pavlik harness, traction, spica cast, brace)
- Risk for Impaired Skin Integrity related to irritation from harness straps or skin traction
- Risk for Altered Urinary Elimination or Constipation related to immobility caused by treatment
- Risk for Altered Nutrition related to immobility and decreased appetite
- Risk for Altered Growth and Development related to limited mobility and potential decreased exposure to stimulation
- Knowledge Deficit (Parent) related to disease process and treatment
- Knowledge Deficit (Parent) related to home care of a child in a Pavlik harness or spica cast

Nursing Management

The infant with DDH may be hospitalized only briefly for diagnosis and initial management. Nursing care varies according to the medical treatment and the child's age. Management includes maintaining traction, if ordered; providing cast care; preventing complications resulting from immobility; promoting normal growth and development; and teaching parents how to care for a child in a cast, traction, or a Pavlik harness at home. Because treatment interferes with the child's normal movement, the treatment plan should take into consideration the age and developmental stage of the child.

Maintain Traction

Bryant skin traction is the most common form of traction used in the treatment of DDH. (Types of traction are discussed later in the chapter and presented in Table 19–15.) Check the traction apparatus frequently to ensure that proper alignment and healing occur. Increasingly traction is being used as a treatment in the home. The family needs to be given careful instruction in how to care for the child in traction. In addition, arrangements should be made for a nurse to make several home visits to set up the traction apparatus and monitor the child's progress after discharge[9,10] (see Table 19–16).

Provide Cast Care

The principles of routine cast care presented in Table 19–2 apply to the care of spica casts. Special techniques should be used to help keep the cast clean and dry in children who are not toilet trained. Female and male urinals can be used for older children. Use a plastic lining to protect the cast edges and use a small disposable diaper to cover the perineum, tucking edges beneath the cast. Be sure to change the diaper frequently to prevent soiling of the cast.

Prevent Complications Resulting From Immobility

Immobilization from traction or a cast can cause alterations in physiologic functioning. Take the following actions to prevent complications:

- Assess breathing patterns and lung sounds frequently for congestion or respiratory compromise.
- Perform skin and neurovascular assessments approximately every 2 hours.
- Use adequate padding and skin wrapping to avoid placing pressure on the popliteal space. Such pressure could lead to nerve palsy.
- For the child in a cast, change the child's position every 2–3 hours while awake to help avoid areas of pressure and promote increased circulation. The child can be placed either prone or supine on a spica board or positioned on the floor and supported with pillows.
- Help prevent skin irritation and breakdown in the child with a cast. Use moleskin to provide protection from rough edges. Place tape around the perineal opening of the cast to prevent soiling.
- Increase fluids and fiber in the child's diet, as a change in bowel or bladder status is commonly associated with immobility.
- Permit limited mobility, if ordered by the physician, and release the child from traction for meals and daily care. The time out of traction should not exceed 1 hour per day. Encourage parents to hold and cuddle the child at this time to promote comfort and bonding.

CLINICAL TIP

Inspect the traction apparatus. Make sure that:
- Nuts and bolts are tight.
- Knots are well tied and secured with tape.
- Weight amounts are correct and weights are hanging free.
- Ropes are unfrayed.
- The line of pull is straight.

SAFETY PRECAUTIONS

Use caution in selecting toys appropriate for the child's developmental age. If the child is in a cast, be sure that toys or parts cannot be swallowed or stuck inside the cast.

Promote Normal Growth and Development

Engage the child in activities that stimulate the upper extremities and all five senses. Provide stimulating toys such as stacking blocks, brightly colored mobiles, Koosh balls, or musical toys. Position toys within the child's reach and interact with the child as much as possible.

Discharge Planning and Home Care Teaching

Parents need to be taught how to care for a child in a spica cast at home. The active participation of family members in the daily care of the child while hospitalized gradually increases their confidence in their ability to provide care once home. Home care needs should be identified and addressed well in advance of discharge. Before discharge, be sure the parents have:

- Information about general cast care (see Table 19–3), positioning, bathing, toileting, and age-appropriate diversional activities.
- Appropriate referrals for periodic assessment by a visiting nurse or home health nurse.
- Family resources to care for the child.

19-5	Resources for Transportation of Children in Casts and Orthopedic Devices

Manufacturers of Special Car Seats[a]

Columbia Medical Manufacturing
Pacific Palisades, CA
310–454–6612

Cosco
Columbus, IN
800–457–5276

E-Z-On Products, Inc.
Jupiter, FL
800–323–6598

Little Cargo Vest
St. Louis, MO
800–933–8580

Ortho-Kinetics, Inc.
Waukesha, WI
800–558–7786

J.A. Preston Corp.
Jackson, MI
800–631–7277

Renolux F.B.S., Inc.
Greer, SC
803–244–5273

Quickie Designs
Fresno, CA
800–456–8156

Shinn and Associates
Okemos, MI
800–955–8870

Snug Seat, Inc.
Matthews, NC
704–847–0772 or 800–336–SNUG

Teaching Materials for Parents of Children in Casts

Safely Home (16-minute video)
Available from:
Riley Children's Hospital
Room S-139
702 Barnhill Drive
Indianapolis, IN 46202

Slide show and script, available from:
Massachusetts Passenger Safety Program
150 Tremont Street, 3rd floor
Boston, MA 02111

Special Kids Are Riding Safe
Educational program development information, available from:
Regional Manager, Affiliate Service
National Easter Seal Society
70 East Lake Street
Chicago, IL 60601-5907

[a]Be sure that any car seat selected meets federal safety standards.
From Stout, J.D., Bandy, P., Feller, N., Stroup, K.B., & Bull, M.J. (1992). Transportation resources for pediatric orthopaedic clients. Orthopaedic Nursing, 9(2), 18–27.

19-6   Guidelines for Pavlik Harness Application

1. Position the chest halter at nipple line and fasten with Velcro.
2. Position the legs and feet in the stirrups, being sure the hips are flexed and abducted. Fasten with Velcro.
3. Connect the chest halter and leg straps in front.
4. Connect the chest halter and leg straps in back.

Mark all the straps at the first fitting with indelible ink so they can be reattached easily after the harness is rinsed and dried.

Before discharge, have parents demonstrate how to dress and feed a child in a spica cast. Ensure that safe travel arrangements have been made for the day of discharge. Help parents to obtain an appropriate car seat in advance of discharge (Table 19–5).[11] Encourage parents to let the child interact with other children at home, and to provide the child in a cast with similar opportunities for play and social activities.

Care in the Community

Have parents of an infant in a Pavlik harness demonstrate proper application of the harness (Table 19–6) and care of the infant in the harness. Teach family members about daily care (bathing, dressing, and feeding) of the infant. Ideally, the harness is worn 23 hours per day and is removed only for skin checks and bathing. The hips and buttocks should be supported carefully when the infant is out of the harness. Demonstrate how to feed the infant in an upright position to maintain abduction and how to change a diaper without removing the harness. Double diapering may be recommended to provide support for the hips.

Instruct the parents of an infant with a harness or a child in a cast to look for any reddened or irritated areas near the harness or cast edges and to check toes frequently for proper circulation. Frequent repositioning reduces the risk of pressure sores or circulatory compromise. The infant should wear an undershirt and socks under the harness to prevent rubbing of the skin.

Safety precautions are important as the child will not have normal mobility. Parents will need to use a specially designed car seat that accommodates the child with abducted hips (see Table 19–5). Strollers and cribs should provide sufficient room to protect the legs from injury and to prevent hip adduction.

CLINICAL TIP

A stroller can be built for the child in a spica cast from a golf club cart. This allows the child to have some mobility and to eat and play in a sitting position. Be sure to give clear instructions to the parents to ensure that the child is securely held in place.

LEGG-CALVÉ-PERTHES DISEASE

Legg-Calvé-Perthes disease is a self-limiting condition in which there is avascular necrosis of the femoral head. The disease occurs in approximately 1 in 12,000 children and affects boys four times more often than girls. It usually occurs between the ages of 2 and 12 years, with a peak incidence between 5 and 7 years. The disease is bilateral in 10–15% of cases.[12,13]

Clinical Manifestations

Early symptoms of Legg-Calvé-Perthes disease include a mild pain in the hip or anterior thigh and a limp, which are aggravated by increased activity and relieved by rest. The child favors the affected hip and limits hip movement to avoid discomfort.

As the disease progresses, range of motion becomes limited and weakness and muscle wasting develop. The affected thigh is 2–3 cm smaller than the unaffected thigh. Over time, prolonged hip irritability may produce muscle spasms.

Etiology and Pathophysiology

The necrosis associated with Legg-Calvé-Perthes disease results from an interruption of the blood supply to the femoral epiphysis. How and why this occurs is not completely understood, but several predisposing factors have been identified. The incidence of Legg-Calvé-Perthes disease is up to 20% higher in families with a history of the disease than in the general population, which suggests that genetic factors may play a role. In one quarter of the cases, onset of the disease is preceded by a mild traumatic injury. Trauma may cause a subchondral fracture and resultant synovitis, which in turn causes pressure that occludes the blood supply. Children with Legg-Calvé-Perthes disease often have delayed skeletal maturation and may have abnormal thyroid levels.[13]

Legg-Calvé-Perthes disease progresses through four distinct stages after the original insult (usually unknown) occurs, over a period of 1–4 years (Table 19–7).

Diagnostic Tests and Medical Management

Because the child's initial symptoms are so mild, parents often do not seek medical attention until symptoms have been present for several months. Diagnosis is made using standard anteroposterior and frog-leg radiographs. As noted in Table 19–7, radiographs taken early in the course of the disease may be normal or show vague widening of the cartilage space. Bone scans and magnetic resonance imaging (MRI) may show the disease process earlier than radiographs.

Medical management and prognosis depend on the degree of femoral involvement. Early detection is important. The desired outcome is a pain-

19-7	Stages of Legg-Calvé-Perthes Disease

Stage	Description
Prenecrosis	An insult causes loss of blood supply to the femoral head.
I—Necrosis	Avascular stage (3–6 months); the child is asymptomatic, bone radiographs are normal, and the head of the femur is structurally intact but avascular.
II—Revascularization	Period of 1–4 years characterized by pain and limitation of movement. Bone radiographs show new bone deposition and dead bone resorption. Fracture and deformity of the head of the femur can occur.
III—Bone healing	Reossification takes place.
IV—Remodeling	The disease process is over, and improvement in joint function occurs.

free hip that functions properly. To promote healing and prevent deformity, the femoral head must be contained within the hip socket until ossification is complete. Adequate containment will be achieved only if the hips remain in an abducted position. At the beginning of treatment, traction is often used to maintain the hips in an abducted and internally rotated position. Once abduction is accomplished, treatment consists of Petrie casting, or surgical soft tissue releases such as adductor tenotomy, followed by bracing. Toronto (Fig. 19–9) and Scottish-Rite braces are most commonly used. Prognosis is good if the femoral head can be contained long enough for proper healing to occur. Children with untreated disease or those diagnosed late in the disease process can develop osteoarthritis and hip dysfunction later in life. Prognosis is better for younger children and those with less severe involvement of the epiphysis.

Nursing Assessment

Legg-Calvé-Perthes disease should be suspected in any child, especially a boy aged 2–12 years, who complains of hip discomfort accompanied by a limp. The school nurse may be the first person to observe the child with symptoms of Legg-Calvé-Perthes disease. The child may complain of pain and have to rest during physical education classes. Referral should be made to the health care provider immediately. Question the child who has an apparent limp about pain, and assess the child's range of motion. Ask if the child injured the hip at some time in the past.

Nursing Diagnosis

Nursing diagnoses, which center on altered activities and compliance, might include the following:

- Impaired Physical Mobility related to brace or cast
- Knowledge Deficit related to potential complications resulting from noncompliance with the treatment regimen
- Risk for Noncompliance related to prolonged treatment period
- Diversional Activity Deficit related to impaired mobility
- Potential Body Image Disturbance related to brace

Nursing Management

Children with Legg-Calvé-Perthes disease often receive all of their treatment at home. Helping the child and family comply with the prescribed treatment plan may be challenging, because children develop the disease at an age when they are usually very active. The child, who may have little pain, often finds immobilization difficult.

Promote Normal Growth and Development
Parents should be given suggestions to help redirect the child's energy within the limitations in mobility imposed by treatment. A return to school promotes a feeling of normalcy. Activities that involve peers also help the child achieve developmental milestones. Help the child adjust to wearing a brace.

Care in the Community
Both the child and the family should be aware that treatment generally takes more than 2 years. Emphasize the importance of following the treatment

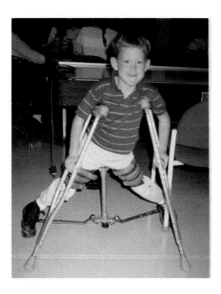

FIGURE 19–9. Although the Toronto brace may seem formidable for a child to wear, you can see by this photograph that, as usual, children adapt quite well to it.

 GROWTH & DEVELOPMENT CONSIDERATIONS

Legg-Calvé-Perthes disease primarily affects boys with an average age of 6 years. These school-age children are industrious and independent. Offer suggestions for activities that redirect energy and promote normal development. These may include horseback riding, which promotes hip abduction; swimming to increase mobility; handcrafts to promote fine motor skills; and computer activities to stimulate cognitive development.

plan to ensure adequate hip containment and proper healing. Teach the family how to care for a child in traction and how to check the child's skin for breakdown (see Table 19–16). Follow-up visits should be arranged at regular intervals, in addition to home care visits during the period of traction.

SLIPPED CAPITAL FEMORAL EPIPHYSIS

Slipped capital femoral epiphysis (SCFE) occurs when the femoral head is displaced from the femoral neck. This condition is commonly seen during the adolescent growth spurt, between ages 11 and 14 in girls and ages 13 and 16 in boys. Boys are affected twice as often as girls.[14]

Clinical Manifestations

Symptoms include limp, pain, and loss of hip motion. The condition is categorized as acute (sudden onset with less than 3 weeks' duration), chronic (longer than 3 weeks' duration), or acute-on-chronic (an additional slippage in a child with a chronic condition), depending on the onset and severity of symptoms. The child with an acute slip has sudden, severe pain and cannot bear weight. An acute slip may be associated with traumatic injury.

A chronic slip presents with persistent hip pain, which is generally aching or mild and can be referred to the thigh, knee, or both. A limp and decreased range of motion may also occur.

When the child has had a chronic slip and then sustains a traumatic incident that causes further slippage of the femoral head, an acute-on-chronic slip is said to have occurred. The child experiences sudden, severe pain.

Etiology and Pathophysiology

The cause of SCFE is unknown. Predisposing factors include obesity, a growth spurt resulting in a tall and thin stature, and endocrine disorders such as hypothyroidism and hypogonadism.[13,14] There may be a genetic predisposition to the development of the disorder.

Slippage of the femoral head occurs at the proximal epiphyseal plate, and the femur displaces from the epiphysis (Fig. 19–10). Slippage is usually

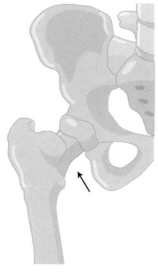
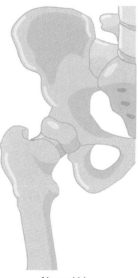

Slipped epiphysis   Normal hip

FIGURE 19–10. In slipped capital femoral epiphysis, the femoral head is displaced from the femoral neck at the proximal epiphyseal plate.

gradual (chronic), but may also result from an accident or other trauma (acute). The synovial membrane becomes inflamed, edematous, and painful. If untreated, callous formation occurs, resulting in a deformed hip with limited range of motion.

Diagnostic Tests and Medical Management

A complete history provides information about risk factors and the development of the condition. Radiographs are used to confirm the diagnosis. A bone scan may also be performed.

The goal of medical management is to stabilize the femoral head while keeping displacement to a minimum and retaining as much hip function as possible. Surgical treatment is usually necessary; this involves fixation of the epiphysis with screws or pins. Medical treatment, which is occasionally used, includes a regimen of no weight bearing, bedrest, a spica cast, and Buck or Russell traction (see Table 19–15).

Prognosis is related to the severity of the deformity and the occurrence of complications, such as avascular necrosis of the femoral head or **chondrolysis** (the breaking down and absorption of cartilage).[15]

Nursing Assessment

The child usually presents with hip pain or referred pain to the groin, thigh, or knee, and limited mobility. A thorough history is needed to assess for injury or trauma as a cause. Assess the child's range of motion, pain, and limp, if apparent. Refer the child for treatment immediately if SCFE is suspected. This condition is considered to be an emergency, and it is essential that the child be treated immediately to keep weight off the affected joint.

Nursing Diagnosis

Among the nursing diagnoses that may apply to the child with SCFE are:

- Impaired Physical Mobility related to non-weight-bearing treatment regimen
- Pain related to displacement of the femoral head or surgery
- Risk for Body Image Disturbance related to treatment regimen or surgery
- Risk for Altered Growth and Development related to mobility restrictions of treatment regimen
- Risk for Altered Nutrition: More than Body Requirements related to immobility
- Risk for Infection related to surgery
- Altered Tissue Perfusion: Peripheral related to traction, casting, and other treatments
- Knowledge Deficit (Child and Parent) related to disease process and treatment

Nursing Management

Nursing management involves caring for the child in traction or after surgery, administering medications and other pain-control interventions, maintaining mobility within the limits imposed by treatment, providing adequate nutrition, educating the child and family about the disorder, providing emotional support, and promoting compliance with the treatment plan.

Encourage Appropriate Nutritional Intake

A growing adolescent needs increased amounts of proteins, carbohydrates, and calcium to promote skeletal healing. Provide written instructions about nutritional requirements necessary to promote bone healing and maintain an ideal body weight. If a child is overweight, encourage weight loss, which decreases pressure on the femoral epiphysis and also leads to a more positive self-image.

Provide Emotional Support

Because the onset of SCFE is usually unexpected, the child and family may find themselves facing surgery with little warning. Explain the treatment plan simply and thoroughly. Reassure the child and family that with proper compliance, treatment should be successful.

Discharge Planning and Home Care Teaching

Follow-up visits are necessary until the child's epiphyseal plates close. It is not uncommon for SCFE to occur in the other hip. Make sure the child and family are aware of symptoms such as decreased range of motion or pain that could indicate onset of the disorder in the other hip. Tell parents to contact their health care provider immediately if these symptoms occur.

▶ DISORDERS OF THE SPINE

SCOLIOSIS

Scoliosis is a lateral S- or C-shaped curvature of the spine that is often associated with a rotational deformity of the spine and ribs. Many individuals exhibit some degree of spinal curvature, with curvatures of more than 10 degrees considered abnormal. Curves are either structural or compensatory, as the spine curves to compensate for a structural deformity along its length. Idiopathic scoliosis occurs most often in girls, especially during the growth spurt between the ages of 10 and 13 years.[16]

Clinical Manifestations

The classic signs of scoliosis include truncal asymmetry, uneven shoulders and hips, a one-sided rib hump, and a prominent scapula. The child does not complain of pain or discomfort.

Etiology and Pathophysiology

The cause of scoliosis is complex. Structural scoliosis may be congenital, idiopathic, or acquired (associated with neuromuscular disorders such as muscular dystrophy or myelodysplasia, or secondary to spinal cord injuries).

In idiopathic structural scoliosis (the most common type), the spine for unknown reasons begins to curve laterally, with vertebral rotation. The most common curve is a right thoracic and left lumbar deformity. As the curve progresses, structural changes occur. The ribs on the concave side (inside of the curve) are forced closer together, while the ribs on the convex side separate widely, causing narrowing of the thoracic cage and formation of the rib hump. The lateral curvature affects the vertebral structure. Disk spaces are narrowed on the concave side and spread wider on the convex side, resulting in an asymmetric vertebral canal (Fig. 19–11).

Scoliosis can also occur in congenital diseases involving the spinal structure and in the musculoskeletal changes seen in conditions such as myelomeningocele. It can also be acquired after injury to the spinal cord. (The child in Figure 19–13 acquired scoliosis after chemotherapy and radiation to the chest during treatment for cancer.)

Diagnostic Tests and Medical Management

Generally, observation and radiographic examination are used to diagnose scoliosis. Additional diagnostic studies include magnetic resonance imaging, computed tomography, and bone scanning, which are used occasionally to assess the degree of curvature. Moiré photography using a special screen and a point light source documents asymmetry of the spine and other bony landmarks (Fig. 19–12).

The goal of medical management is to limit or stop progression of the curvature. Early detection is essential to successful treatment. Adequate treatment and follow-up maximize the child's chances for proper spinal alignment. The treatment regimen chosen depends on the degree and progression of the curvature and the reaction of the child and family to medical management.

Treatment of children with mild scoliosis (curvatures of 10–20 degrees) consists of exercises to improve posture and muscle tone and to maintain, or possibly increase, flexibility of the spine. Emphasis is placed on bending strength toward the outside of the curve while stretching the inside of the curve. These exercises are not a cure, however, and the child should be evaluated by a physician at 3–month intervals, with radiographic evaluation every 6 months.

Medical management of moderate scoliosis (curvatures of 20–40 degrees) includes bracing with either a Boston or Milwaukee brace. The goal of wearing a brace is to maintain the existing spinal curvature with no increase. Brace wear begins immediately after diagnosis. To achieve maximum effectiveness, the brace should be worn 23 hours per day. Brace treatment is lengthy and requires a high degree of compliance, which can be difficult for adolescents, for whom body image or sports involvement is often important.

Electrical stimulation is used occasionally as an alternative treatment. An electric current stimulates the back muscles to contract, thus helping to correct the spinal curvature. This treatment, which is performed at night, eliminates the need for bracing. There is controversy about the usefulness of this therapy.

Children with severe scoliosis (curvatures of 40 degrees or more) require surgery, which involves spinal fusion. The majority of spinal fusions are performed using instrumentation. The Harrington rod, Luque wire, or Coutrel-Dubosset (CD) instrumentation may be used. The Harrington rod has the fewest complications but is less stable than the Luque wire or CD instrumentation and requires prolonged immobilization in a cast or halo brace. Following surgery with wires or instrumentation, the child will be on bedrest during a recovery period and then will be fitted with anteroposterior plastic shells that must be worn for several months to provide stability for the spine. Occasionally in severe cases, halo traction is used postoperatively to provide support for the unstable spine (Fig. 19–13).

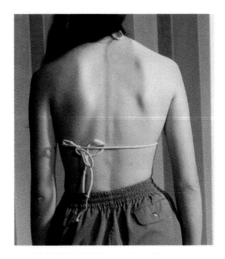

FIGURE 19–11. A child may have varying degrees of scoliosis. For mild forms, treatment will focus on strengthening and stretching. Moderate forms will require bracing. Severe forms may necessitate surgery and fusion. Clothes that fit at an angle, such as this teenage girl's shorts, and anatomic asymmetry of the back provide clues for early detection.

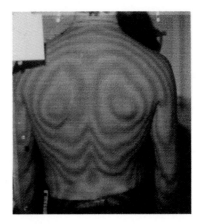

FIGURE 19–12. Moiré photography is sometimes used to document the degree of spinal asymmetry.
From Staheli, L.T. (1992). Fundamentals of pediatric orthopedics (p. 8.12). New York: Raven Press.

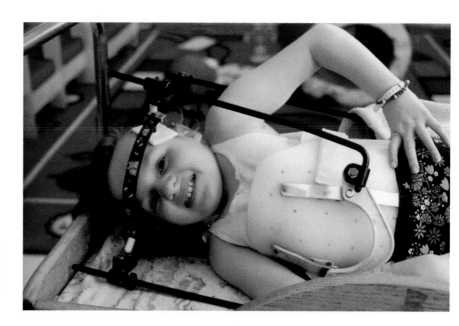

FIGURE 19–13. In moderate to severe forms of scoliosis, the child may need to wear a halo brace, shown here, to hold the body in position after surgery.

Nursing Assessment

School nurses often screen children for scoliosis, generally in the fifth and seventh grades. This screening is mandated by law in several states. When abnormalities are noted, the child is referred to an orthopedic center for further evaluation. Children should be examined every 6–9 months thereafter. If scoliosis is detected, the child's brothers and sisters should be examined and observed closely. Chapter 3 discusses screening children for scoliosis.

Once scoliosis has been identified, the nurse's focus becomes education and follow-up. Any child with scoliosis should have a comprehensive neurologic, cardiac, and respiratory examination, since the rib cage deformity can influence the functioning of these systems.

Nursing Diagnosis

The following nursing diagnoses may apply to the child with scoliosis who is not undergoing surgery:

- Risk for Noncompliance with exercise program related to lack of knowledge about the condition and its complications
- Activity Intolerance related to brace wear
- Impaired Physical Mobility related to brace wear
- Risk for Impaired Skin Integrity related to brace wear, or electrodes from electrical stimulation therapy
- Risk for Knowledge Deficit (Child and Parent) related to disease process

Common nursing diagnoses for the child who is having surgery can be found in the accompanying Nursing Care Plan.

Nursing Management

An important aspect of nursing care is patient education. Patient compliance is critical to the success of treatment. Children and their families need

Text continues on page 842.

NURSING CARE PLAN
THE CHILD UNDERGOING SURGERY FOR SCOLIOSIS

GOAL	INTERVENTION	RATIONALE	EXPECTED OUTCOME

1. Knowledge Deficit (Child and Parents) related to disease process and surgical procedure

GOAL	INTERVENTION	RATIONALE	EXPECTED OUTCOME
The child and parents will verbalize understanding of the disease, its treatment, and the surgical procedure.	• Teach the child and family about the course of the disease, its signs and symptoms, and treatment. Provide appropriate handouts. Encourage the child and parents to ask questions. • Begin preoperative teaching at the time of admission. Orient the child to hospital and postoperative procedures. Before surgery, have the child demonstrate log-rolling, range-of-motion exercises, and the use of an incentive spirometer. Discuss pain management.	• Understanding and involvement increase motivation and compliance while reducing fear. • Preoperative teaching and familiarity with hospital procedures reduces the stress related to surgery and postoperative complications.	The child and family accurately verbalize knowledge about the disease and its treatment. The child and family ask appropriate questions about postoperative care.

2. Ineffective Breathing Pattern related to administration of analgesics and operative procedure

GOAL	INTERVENTION	RATIONALE	EXPECTED OUTCOME
The child will show no signs of respiratory compromise.	• Monitor respiratory status, especially after the administration of analgesics. • Administer oxygen if ordered. • Have the child use an incentive spirometer. • Monitor intake and output. • Reposition the child at least every two hours.	• Evaluation of the child's respiratory condition anticipates and avoids complications. Analgesics such as morphine may increase or potentiate respiratory compromise. • Oxygen increases peripheral oxygen saturation to 95–100%. • Spirometry increases lung expansion and aeration of the alveoli. • Good hydration promotes loose secretions and helps prevent infection. • Repositioning ensures inflation of the lung fields.	The child has no respiratory complications.

Continued . . .

NURSING CARE PLAN
THE CHILD UNDERGOING SURGERY FOR SCOLIOSIS– *Continued*

GOAL	INTERVENTION	RATIONALE	EXPECTED OUTCOME

3. Risk for Injury related to neurovascular deficit secondary to instrumentation

GOAL	INTERVENTION	RATIONALE	EXPECTED OUTCOME
The child's neurovascular system will remain intact as evidenced by circulation, sensation, and motor checks. The child will feel no numbness or tingling.	• Monitor the child's color, circulation, capillary refill, warmth, sensation, and motion in all extremities. Perform neurovascular checks every 2 hours for the first 24 hours and then every 4 hours for the next 48 hours. Record presence of pedal and distal tibial pulses every hour for 48 hours. • Have the child wear antiembolism stockings until ambulatory. The stockings may be removed for 1 hour per shift. • Check for any pain, swelling, or a positive Homans' sign in the legs. Record any evidence of edema. • Monitor input and output. • Encourage and assist the child with range-of-motion exercises, both passive and active.	• When the spinal column is manipulated during surgery, altered neurovascular status, thrombus formation, and paralysis are possible complications. Postoperative risks include loss of bowel or bladder control, weakness or paralysis, and impaired vision or sensation. • Antiembolism stockings prevent blood clots and promote venous return. Thrombus formation is a postoperative risk. • Swelling may indicate a tight dressing and tissue damage. A positive Homans' sign and pain may indicate thrombus formation. • Abnormalities may indicate a fluid shift problem. • Activity promotes mobility and reduces risk of thrombus formation.	The child exhibits only temporary alteration (pale skin, faint pulse, and edema occur but then resolve within the initial postoperative phase). The child returns to the preoperative baseline state by discharge.

4. Pain related to spinal fusion with instrumentation

GOAL	INTERVENTION	RATIONALE	EXPECTED OUTCOME
The child will verbalize an adequate level of comfort or show absence of pain behavior within 1 hour of a specific nursing intervention.	• Assess the level of pain and initiate pain management strategies as soon as possible. Use patient-controlled analgesia if ordered. • Administer pain medication around-the-clock to help ensure pain relief, especially during the first 48 hours.	• Adequate pain management allows for faster healing and a more cooperative patient. Patient-controlled analgesics may be effective. • Medicating around-the-clock helps to maintain comfort.	The child experiences pain relief early in the postoperative period.

NURSING CARE PLAN

THE CHILD UNDERGOING SURGERY
FOR SCOLIOSIS– *Continued*

GOAL	INTERVENTION	RATIONALE	EXPECTED OUTCOME

4. Pain related to spinal fusion with instrumentation (continued)

GOAL	INTERVENTION	RATIONALE	EXPECTED OUTCOME
	• Use nonpharmacologic pain management techniques, such as imagery, relaxation, touch, music, application of heat and cold, and reduced environmental stimulation to supplement medications (see Chap. 7).	• Alternative treatments also interrupt the pain stimulus and provide relief. Non-pharmacologic methods can be an effective adjunct to pain management.	
	• Document pain assessment, interventions, and the child's reactions.	• Proper documentation guides the selection of the most effective means of pain control.	
	• Reassure the child that some discomfort is expected and that a variety of measures can be tried to reduce discomfort.	• Realistic expectations decrease anxiety and give the child a sense of control.	

5. Impaired Physical Mobility related to surgical procedure, pain management, or muscle spasms

GOAL	INTERVENTION	RATIONALE	EXPECTED OUTCOME
The child will maintain proper body alignment and progress with activity as ordered by the physician. If no anteroposterior shell bracing is required, the child will have active mobility by the third to fifth postoperative day.	• Reposition the child every 2 hours using the log-roll technique. Support the back, feet, and knees with pillows. • Have the child do passive and active range-of-motion exercises every 2 hours for 48 hours and then every 4 hours while awake. Have the child dangle his or her legs at the bedside by the second to fourth postoperative day. Begin ambulation by the third to fifth postoperative day. Note any complaints of dizziness, pallor, etc. Proceed slowly.	• Proper positioning prevents twisting or turning the spine. • Exercises help maintain strength, circulation, and muscle tone. If the spine is stable and the physician has ordered no external support, the child may progress to full ambulation as tolerated. If the spine is not stable, great care must be taken until external supportive devices are used.	The child is as mobile as appropriate for condition with 3–5 days after surgery.

Continued . . .

NURSING CARE PLAN
THE CHILD UNDERGOING SURGERY
FOR SCOLIOSIS– *Continued*

GOAL	INTERVENTION	RATIONALE	EXPECTED OUTCOME

6. Risk for Body Image Disturbance related to brace or cast wear or surgery

The child will verbalize feelings about body image and self-esteem in relation to the disease and its treatment. The child will be informed about available support services and use them as needed.	• Encourage independence in daily activities within allowable limits. Use positive reinforcements. Encourage the child to participate in community activities, if possible. Involve the child in scoliosis support groups.	• Involvement in activities demonstrates that a "normal" life is realistic.	The child has a positive self-image and is involved in community activities or support groups.
	• Provide contact with a peer resource person who has undergone treatment for scoliosis.	• Peers are an effective means of support.	

7. Risk for Knowledge Deficit (Child and Parent) related to discharge planning and home care

The child and family will verbalize reduced anxiety about home care. The child will demonstrate knowledge of self-care and permitted activities.	• Teach cast or brace care as appropriate (see Tables 19–3 and 19–4). Provide oral and written instructions and a list of activity limitations (see Table 19–8). Have the child and family demonstrate adequate knowledge.	• Providing education decreases anxiety and increases compliance with treatment plan. Demonstration reinforces the learning process.	The child and family demonstrate home care and implementation of discharge teaching.
	• Arrange for follow-up appointments as ordered by the physician. Encourage the child and family to notify the nurse or physician if they have any questions or concerns.	• Follow-up visits help the nurse and physician evaluate the effectiveness of the treatment plan and patient compliance.	

to understand the condition and the stages of treatment. This is particularly true for adolescents undergoing treatment for scoliosis. Children or adolescents facing surgery require education, reassurance, and support. The accompanying Nursing Care Plan summarizes nursing care for the child undergoing surgery for scoliosis.

Promote Compliance with the Treatment Plan
Provide instructions about exercises that will help to decrease the severity of the spinal curvature. Demonstrate the exercises, and explain their purpose (ie, to strengthen back muscles). Help the child adjust to wearing a brace.

Adolescents, in particular, may be reluctant to wear an external device such as a brace. To promote a sense of control, allow the adolescent to choose when to exercise and when to be out of the brace, within the treatment guidelines. Provide reassurance and encouragement and promote interaction with peers. Suggesting that the adolescent work with a peer support person who is being treated for scoliosis or has had the condition in the past may be beneficial. Provide information about fashionable clothing that can be worn with the brace.

Discharge Planning and Home Care Teaching

Home care needs should be identified and addressed well in advance of discharge. The child will need to learn to adapt to a new set of body mechanics. Show the child how to do simple tasks *without bending or twisting the torso*. Have the child demonstrate the ability to perform daily activities before discharge from the hospital.

Activities for the child who has had spinal surgery are limited (Table 19–8). Restrictions usually should be followed for 6–8 months, depending on the type of surgery and the surgeon. Emphasize to both the child and the family the importance of compliance. Give written discharge instructions to the child and family. The child and parent may be encouraged to sign a written contract to promote compliance. Follow-up visits are important. The child should be examined 4–6 weeks after discharge, then every 3–4 months for 1 year, and every 1–2 years thereafter.

Several organizations provide information and assistance to families of children with scoliosis (see Appendix F). The National Scoliosis Foundation is concerned with the early detection and prevention of spinal curvature; the Scoliosis Association is a self-help group. The Scoliosis Research Society, a group of physicians and scientists, has published an informative book, *Scoliosis: A Handbook for Patients*.

KYPHOSIS AND LORDOSIS

Kyphosis (hunchback) and lordosis (swayback) are two other types of spinal curvature that may occur in children (Table 19–9). Medical management

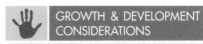

GROWTH & DEVELOPMENT CONSIDERATIONS

Postural lordosis is a characteristic finding in toddlers but should disappear by the school-age years.

19-8	Discharge Teaching: Postoperative Activities After Spinal Surgery

Recommended
Lying
Sitting
Standing
Walking (including normal stair climbing)
Swimming, gentle (not with a cast); diving is *not* permitted

Not Recommended
Bending or twisting at the waist
Lifting more than 10 pounds
Household chores such as vacuuming, unloading groceries, mowing the lawn, taking out the garbage
Sports such as bicycle riding, horseback riding, skiing, roller blading, skating
Physical education classes

19-9 Kyphosis and Lordosis: Clinical Manifestations and Treatment

Condition	Diagnostic Tests and Medical Management	Nursing Management
Kyphosis Excessive convex curvature of the cervical thoracic spine *Clinical manifestations:* Visible hunchback or rounded shoulders; shortness of breath or fatigue; abdominal creases and tight hamstrings in severe cases	*Diagnostic tests:* Spinal curvature is assessed by having the child bend 90 degrees at the waist and looking at the scapular area from side. Diagnosis is confirmed by radiograph. *Medical management:* Exercises are prescribed for mild condition; bracing is commonly used; surgery is performed in severe cases.	*Nursing management:* Provide support. Encourage exercises and diligent brace wear. Help the child to deal with the psychologic stress of altered body image.
Lordosis Excessive concave curvature of the lumbar spine with an angle of more than 60 degrees; most common in prepubescent girls and African-Americans *Clinical manifestations:* Presence of sway-back; prominent buttocks; hip flexion contractures; tight hamstrings	*Diagnostic tests:* Spinal curvature is assessed by looking at the standing child from the side. Lumbar lordosis is confirmed by visualizing the spine on standing, lateral radiograph. *Medical management:* Treatment focuses on exercises and postural awareness. Bracing and surgery are rarely prescribed.	*Nursing management:* Provide support. Reassure the child and family that the condition is often outgrown as the child matures. Encourage physical conditioning exercises and follow-up examinations on a yearly basis.

depends on the cause and degree of the curvature, and the age of the child at onset. Nurses can perform thorough musculoskeletal assessments of children (see Chap. 3) and refer any children with abnormalities for further evaluation.

► DISORDERS OF THE BONES AND JOINTS

OSTEOMYELITIS

Osteomyelitis is an infection of the bone, most often one of the long bones of the lower extremity. It may be acute or chronic and may spread into surrounding tissues. Although osteomyelitis may occur at any age, it is most common in children between the ages of 1 and 12 years. Boys are affected two to three times as often as girls, primarily because they have a greater incidence of trauma.[17,18]

Clinical Manifestations

Symptoms include pain and tenderness with swelling, decreased mobility of the infected joint, and fever. Redness over the area may occur. The onset of acute osteomyelitis is generally rapid.

Etiology and Pathophysiology

Osteomyelitis is caused by a microorganism, which is usually bacterial but can be viral or fungal. *Staphylococcus aureus* is the most common causative pathogen, followed by *Escherichia coli,* group B streptococci, *Streptococcus aureus, Streptococcus pyogenes,* and *Haemophilus influenzae.* A common source of infection is an upper respiratory infection. Trauma to the bone or surgical interventions are other common causes of infection.

The infecting organism spreads through the bloodstream or via a penetrating injury to the bone, where it becomes established. Most infections in children begin in the metaphysis (see Fig. 19–1), which has a sluggish blood supply. Eventually the infection may penetrate the bone cortex and periosteum.[19] Inflammation and abscess formation can lead to interruption of the blood supply to the underlying bone, involvement of the surrounding soft tissue, and, if the infection is left untreated, to necrosis.

Diagnostic Tests and Medical Management

A history suggestive of osteomyelitis includes an upper respiratory infection or blunt trauma followed by pain at the area of a growth plate. Laboratory evaluation shows leukocytosis and an elevated erythrocyte sedimentation rate (ESR). The degree of ESR elevation is directly related to the severity of the infection. Radiographs and bone scans may identify the area of involvement. A needle aspiration of the site can confirm the diagnosis and provide a culture of the causative organism.

Medical management begins with the intravenous administration of a broad-spectrum antibiotic, even before culture results are available. Once the culture results are obtained, the antibiotic may be altered. Oral antibiotics are given once an adequate response has occurred. However, extended intravenous home therapy may be used. Antibiotic therapy continues for about 6 weeks. When an adequate response is not obtained within 2–3 days, the area may be aspirated again, or surgical drainage may be carried out. Intravenous fluids may be administered to ensure adequate hydration.

Prompt diagnosis and treatment usually result in complete resolution of the infection. The prognosis is related to the initiation of therapy—the earlier treatment begins, the better the outcome. Long-term unfavorable outcomes include disruption of the growth plate, which can interrupt growth and damage the joints from septic arthritis.

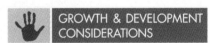

GROWTH & DEVELOPMENT CONSIDERATIONS

Osteomyelitis in a newborn is of great concern, as before 18 months of age the blood vessels cross the growth plates. This creates a higher risk of epiphyseal involvement with resultant limb length discrepancy.

Nursing Assessment

A thorough history, including information about the onset of symptoms and a history of recent infections or puncture wounds, is essential. Assess the affected area for signs of redness, swelling, pain, and decreased range of motion.

Nursing Diagnosis

Among the nursing diagnoses that may apply to the child with osteomyelitis are:

- Pain related to disease process or surgical drainage of abscess
- Impaired Physical Mobility related to disease process, destruction of bone, or joint tenderness

- Risk for Infection related to spread of infecting organism to other body sites
- Risk for Fluid Volume Deficit related to infection
- Risk for Altered Nutrition: Less Than Body Requirements related to disease process
- Risk for Noncompliance related to long course of antibiotic therapy
- Knowledge Deficit (Child and Parent) related to disease process

Nursing Management

Nursing management focuses on administering antibiotics, protecting the child from spread of the infection, and encouraging a well-balanced diet. Standard precautions should be used, with transmission-based precautions for any drainage from the site of infection.

Administer Fluids and Medications

Administer intravenous fluids as ordered to maintain the hydration status of the child. Antibiotics are administered intravenously, at first, then orally. Monitor the intravenous site and provide care for the central line, if one is used. (Refer to the *Quick Reference to Pediatric Clinical Skills* accompanying this text.) In the early stages of the infection, analgesics are prescribed to relieve the associated pain and joint tenderness.

Protect From the Spread of Infection

Strict aseptic technique and transmission-based precautions should be used during all dressing changes. Children and family members should avoid direct contact with any dressings or drainage. Teach good hygiene practices, including handwashing, to maintain infection control. Take vital signs and evaluate the child frequently for symptoms indicating the spread of infection (eg, increasing pain, difficulty breathing, increased pulse rate, fever).

Encourage a Well-Balanced Diet

Educate both the child and the parents about healthy dietary choices that promote the healing process. Providing a high-protein diet and extra vitamin C will contribute to this process. Encourage increased fluid intake to provide adequate hydration and circulation.

Discharge Planning and Home Care Teaching

Emphasize the importance of completing the full course of antibiotic therapy, especially for children who have undergone surgical drainage of an abscess or lesion. Failure to follow the prescribed antibiotic therapy may result in chronic infection. Provide suggestions for the family if the child will be immobilized at home. They may need to contact the school to obtain schoolwork or tutoring for the child. Help them plan activities that foster development during the child's immobilization. Parents may need the assistance of social services to plan care for the child if they must return to work.

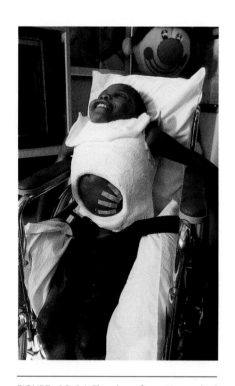

FIGURE 19–14. This boy from Kenya had surgery to correct severe kyphosis and scoliosis, caused by tuberculosis of the spine. A Risser cast has been applied to maintain stability of the spine and thoracic cage during healing. Notice the area cut out of the cast to allow for auscultation of the abdomen, as well as to facilitate the child's comfort and adequate intake of food.

SKELETAL TUBERCULOSIS AND SEPTIC ARTHRITIS

Skeletal tuberculosis (Fig. 19–14) and septic arthritis are two infections that, although infrequent, may affect children and adolescents. Table 19–10 summarizes the clinical manifestations, diagnostic tests, and medical and nursing management for these infections.

19-10 Skeletal Tuberculosis and Septic Arthritis: Clinical Manifestations and Management

Condition	Diagnostic Tests and Medical Management	Nursing Management
Skeletal Tuberculosis Rare microbacterial infection that can be very destructive. The spine is the most frequent site of infection (Pott's disease), with joints and other sites sometimes affected. *Clinical manifestations:* Depending on the site, pain, limp, severe muscle spasms, kyphosis, muscle atrophy, "doughy" swelling of joints, decreased joint motion, changes in reflexes, low-grade fever	*Diagnostic tests:* Diagnostic studies include tuberculosis skin test, complete blood count, synovial fluid analysis, and radiographs of affected limb or joint. *Medical management:* Antibiotic therapy (using a combination of drugs) for 6–9 months is the treatment of choice. The affected site is immobilized. Disease may become resistant to these drugs, and additional drug therapy may be necessary.	*Nursing management:* Educate the child and family about the disorder and stress the importance of complying with long-term antibiotic therapy. Test all members of the family for tuberculosis. Report the disease to the local health department. Facilitate the immobilization and physical therapy of the child at home.
Septic Arthritis Joint infection of the synovial space most often caused by *Haemophilus influenzae, Staphylococcus,* and *Streptococcus.* The most common site of infection is the knee, followed by the hip, ankle, and elbow. *Clinical manifestations:* Fever, pain and local inflammation, joint tenderness, swelling, loss of spontaneous movement	*Diagnostic tests:* Diagnosis is made based on joint aspiration findings. Radiographic changes may not be evident until later in the disease process. *Medical management:* This is a medical emergency requiring prompt treatment to avoid permanent disability. Treatment involves joint aspiration, open drainage, and irrigation, followed by intravenous antibiotic therapy for 3–4 weeks and then oral antibiotics. If the full course of antibiotic treatment is not completed, the child risks recurrent infection and further degeneration of the infected joint.	*Nursing management:* Educate the child and family about the disorder and emphasize the importance of proper antibiotic therapy. Carefully position the painful joint.

OSTEOGENESIS IMPERFECTA

Osteogenesis imperfecta, also known as brittle bone disease, is a connective tissue disorder that primarily affects the bones. Children with this condition have fragile bones that are more likely to fracture. The major type of osteogenesis imperfecta occurs in 1 in 30,000 live births and affects boys and girls equally.[20]

Clinical manifestations include multiple and frequent fractures; blue sclerae; thin, soft skin; increased joint flexibility; enlargement of the anterior fontanel; weak muscles; soft, pliable, brittle bones; and short stature. Conductive hearing loss can occur by adolescence or young adulthood.

The underlying disorder is a biochemical defect in the production of collagen. The disease is genetically transmitted, generally in an autosomal dominant inheritance pattern, although some types are now known to be transmitted in a recessive pattern.

The disease is classified into four types. In type I disease, the most common form, children have fragile bones, blue sclerae, weakened tooth dentin, and hearing loss that manifests in adolescence. In type II disease, the ribs and skeleton are extensively involved; most children with this form of the disease die in utero or shortly after birth. Type III disease is identified in the newborn period or in infancy when the child sustains numerous fractures and manifests blue sclera. Severe bone fragility and kyphoscoliosis are observed. Most children with type III disease die in childhood as a result of cardiorespiratory failure. Type IV disease is characterized by fractures without other symptoms of the disease. Bowing of the legs and other structural deformities can occur; however, the incidence of fractures decreases beginning in puberty.

Improved knowledge about the genetic transmission of this disease means that some cases of osteogenesis imperfecta can be identified before birth using ultrasound or collagen analysis of chorionic villus cells. In many cases, however, diagnosis of osteogenesis imperfecta is made only when the child has a delay in walking or sustains a fracture. Radiographic evaluation may detect old as well as new fractures. This may lead to an erroneous diagnosis of child abuse.

There is no cure for osteogenesis imperfecta. Medical management consists primarily of fracture care and prevention of deformities. The goal is to maximize the child's independence and mobility while minimizing the risk of fractures. Treatment includes physical therapy; casting, bracing, or splinting; and surgical stabilization.

SAFETY PRECAUTIONS

Handle infants with osteogenesis imperfecta gently and use a blanket for additional support when lifting and moving them. Never pull the legs upward when changing a diaper as this can cause a fracture. Instead, gently slip a hand under the hips to raise them, sliding the diaper carefully in, and then bringing it up as the legs are slightly abducted.

Nursing Management

Nursing care is primarily supportive and focuses on educating the parents and child about the disease and its treatment. The family may have been suspected of child abuse before the disease was diagnosed, and they should be given an explanation about the similar presenting symptoms of these cases.

To prevent fractures, children with osteogenesis imperfecta must be handled gently. The trunk and extremities should be supported whenever the child is moved. Such tasks as bathing and diapering may cause fractures and should be performed carefully.

Emphasize the importance of maintaining normal patterns of growth and development. Toddlers should be helped to explore and interact safely in their environment. Socialization is essential during the school-age and adolescent years. Encourage exercise, such as swimming, to improve muscle tone and prevent obesity. Independent functioning is promoted by the use of adaptive equipment and motorized wheelchairs. Maintenance of function can depend on proper rehabilitation services. The nurse can arrange and manage such services for the family.

The Osteogenesis Imperfecta Foundation provides information about the disease and can put families in touch with others who have the disease (see Appendix F). Parents should receive genetic counseling.

► MUSCULAR DYSTROPHIES

The muscular dystrophies are a group of inherited diseases characterized by muscle fiber degeneration and muscle wasting. These disorders can begin early or late in life, and onset can be at birth or gradual.

Many kinds of muscular dystrophies affect children and adults (Table 19–11 and Fig. 19–15). The most common form of childhood muscular dystrophy is Duchenne's muscular dystrophy (pseudohypertrophic), which occurs in 1 in 3500 live male births.[21] **Pseudohypertrophy** refers to enlargement of the muscles as a result of their infiltration with fatty tissue.

Diagnosis and classification are most often based on clinical signs and the pattern of muscle involvement. Children with muscular dystrophy have

RESEARCH CONSIDERATIONS

Researchers have found that the gene in the Xp21.2 region shows evidence of deletion or mutation in children with Duchenne's muscular dystrophy. This finding makes genetic screening and prenatal diagnosis possible.

19-11   Muscular Dystrophies of Childhood

Type of Dystrophy	Clinical Manifestations	Treatment and Prognosis
Duchenne's Muscular Dystrophy X-linked recessive disorder seen in boys (on Xp21 gene); however, 30–50% of affected children have no family history Onset: within the first 3–4 years of life	Delayed walking; frequent falls; easily tired when walking, running, or climbing stairs; toe walking, hypertrophied calves; waddling gait; lordosis; positive Gower's maneuver; mental retardation frequently seen	Supportive care; physical therapy and braces to help maintain mobility and prevent contractures Most children are wheelchair bound by 12 years of age; death usually occurs during adolescence from respiratory or cardiac failure
Becker's Muscular Dystrophy X-linked recessive disorder Onset: usually after 5 years	Symptoms are similar to those of Duchenne's muscular dystrophy, but milder and delayed; child is mobile until late teens; normal intelligence; congestive heart failure; contractures	Supportive care, same as for Duchenne's muscular dystrophy Slow progression (same as for Duchenne's muscular dystrophy); death usually occurs from the third to the fifth decade of life
Fascioscapulohumeral Muscular Dystrophy Autosomal dominant disorder (on 4q35 chromosome) Onset: later childhood and adolescence	Face, shoulder girdle, lower limbs affected; unable to raise arms over head; lordosis; cannot close eyes, whistle, smile, or drink from a straw because of inability to move face; characteristic appearance includes facial weakness, winging of the scapula, thin arms, well-developed forearms	Physical therapy Slow progression; confined to wheelchair as older adult, but usually attains normal life span
Emery-Dreyfuss Muscular Dystrophy X-linked recessive disorder (on Xq28 gene) Onset: childhood	Early onset of contractures followed by weakness; Achilles tendon, elbow, and spine affected; muscle weakness in upper body follows, with lower body weakness occurring later; cardiac conduction defect may occur	Physical therapy Surgery Pacemaker insertion
Congenital Muscular Dystrophies Autosomal recessive group of disorders Onset: present at birth	Muscle weaknesses present at birth; motor development delay; contractures and joint deformities; hypotonia	Correction of skeletal deformity (orthosis or surgery) Usually nonprogressive

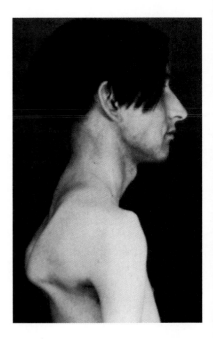

FIGURE 19–15. Scapulohumeral muscular dystrophy is characterized by atrophy of the upper limb muscles and winged scapulae.
From Walton, J. (1981). Disorders of voluntary muscle (4th ed., p. 449). Essex, England: Longman Group UK Ltd. By permission of Churchill Livingstone, London, England.

generalized muscle weakness. They compensate for weak lower extremities by using the upper extremity muscles to raise themselves to a standing position (Gower's maneuver) (Fig. 19–16). Biochemical examinations such as serum enzyme assay, muscle biopsy, and electromyography confirm the diagnosis. Serum creatine kinase (CK) is elevated early in the disease. Dystrophin, the muscle protein that is deficient in muscular dystrophy, can be measured by muscle biopsy.[22]

There is no effective treatment for childhood muscular dystrophy. Progressive weakness and muscle deformity result in chronic disability (Fig. 19–17). The goal of medical management is to provide support and prevent complications such as infection or spinal deformities. The team approach to managing the child with muscular dystrophy ensures a comprehensive management plan. Team members should include physicians (pediatrician, orthopedic surgeon, neurologist), nurses, physical and occupational therapists, a nutritionist, and a social worker.

Nursing Management

Nursing care focuses on promoting independence and mobility and providing psychosocial support that helps the child and family deal with this progressive, incapacitating disease.

Monitor cardiac and respiratory functioning frequently. Perform periodic developmental assessments, and provide parents with suggestions for encouraging the child's development. Meet with teachers to evaluate the child's learning needs and functioning in the classroom.

Encourage the child to be independent for as long as possible. Concentrate on what the child can accomplish and do not ask the child to complete tasks that may prove frustrating. Reading books to the child, listening to tapes, and watching television offer the child stimulation during hospitalization. Exercise as tolerated contributes to muscle strength. Physical therapy helps the child ambulate and prevents joint contractures. It is important to provide good back support and posture by keeping the child's body in alignment when confined to a wheelchair.

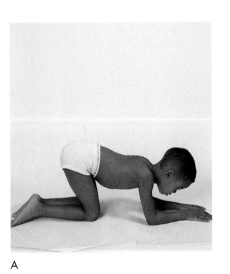
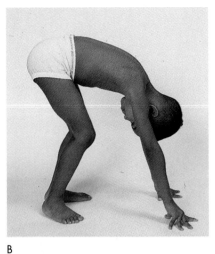
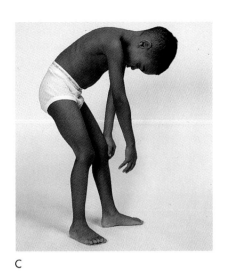

A   B   C

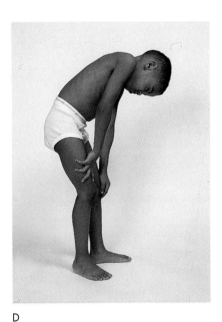
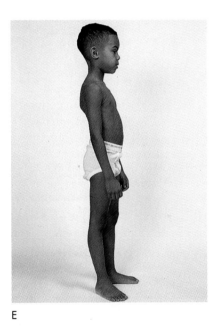

D   E

FIGURE 19–16. Since the leg muscles of children with muscular dystrophy are weak, these children must perform the Gower's maneuver to raise themselves to a standing position. **A and B,** The child first maneuvers to a position supported by arms and legs. **C,** The child next pushes off the floor and rests one hand on the knee. **D and E,** The child then pushes himself upright.

Parents may exhibit feelings of guilt and hopelessness. Encourage parents to express their feelings. Genetic counseling is recommended for the entire family, and it is especially important to identify women who are carriers of one of X-linked disorders. Siblings may feel neglected because their brother or sister is receiving so much attention. They may be concerned that they will develop the disease. Encourage the parents to involve siblings in the child's care to reassure them of their importance.

Refer family members to resource and support groups such as the Muscular Dystrophy Association (see Appendix F).

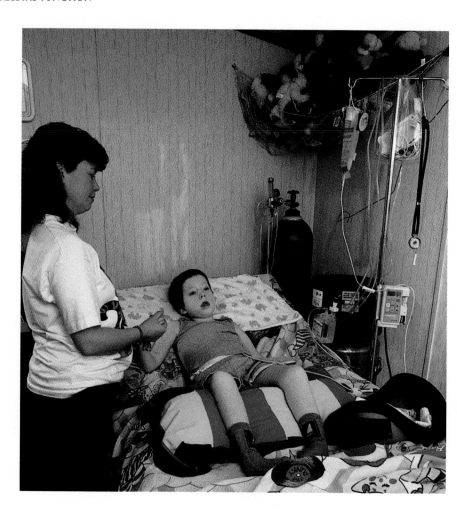

FIGURE 19–17. This young boy with muscular dystrophy needs to receive tube feedings and home nursing care. He attends school when possible and is able to use an adapted computer.

NURSING ALERT

When in doubt about the nature of an injury, apply a splint. Splinting immobilizes the site, prevents further damage, and decreases pain. Be sure to immobilize both the joints above and below the injury.

▶ INJURIES TO THE MUSCULOSKELETAL SYSTEM

Musculoskeletal injuries are classified according to the mechanism, the location, and the force of the injury. Strains, sprains, dislocations, and fractures are the most common musculoskeletal injuries in children. Distinguishing among these injuries is often difficult. Table 19–12 summarizes management of strains, sprains, and dislocations. A detailed discussion of fractures follows.

FRACTURES

A fracture is a break in a bone that occurs when more stress is placed on the bone than the bone can withstand. Fractures, which may occur at any age, occur frequently in children because their bones are less dense and more porous than those of adults.[23] Table 19–13 outlines several types of fractures.

Clinical Manifestations

Signs and symptoms of fractures vary depending on the location, type, and nature of the causative injury. Fractures are generally characterized by pain, abnormal positioning, edema, immobility or decreased range of motion, ec-

19-12   Strains, Sprains, and Dislocations

Strain

- Stretching or tearing of either a muscle or a tendon, usually from overuse (example: back strain resulting from improper or overly heavy lifting).
- Clinical manifestations vary according to the type and severity of the strain. Pain can be acute or chronic.
- Management involves rest and support of the injured part until the muscle or tendon heals and normal activity can occur.

Sprain

- Stretching or tearing of a ligament, usually caused by falls, sports injuries, or motor vehicle crashes.
- Clinical manifestations include edema, joint immobility, and pain.
- Management (generally continued for 24–36 hours) includes
  Rest
  Ice
  Compression, and
  Elevation

Dislocation

- Complete displacement of an articular joint surface, usually associated with falls, sports injuries, or motor vehicle crashes. Although almost any joint may be dislocated, most dislocations occur in the shoulder, knee, and hip.
- Clinical manifestations include pain and tenderness, swelling and obvious deformity, and instability of the joint.
- Management varies according to the site and severity of the injury, and consists of:
  Shoulder: Open or closed reduction followed by the application of a sling.
  Knee: Closed reduction with gentle traction, then immobilization with a splint.
  Hip (posterior): Immediate closed reduction or possibly open reduction, traction, or hip spica cast.
  Hip (anterior): Immediate closed reduction, extension traction, and hip spica cast.

---

chymosis, guarding, and crepitus. Childhood fractures most often involve the clavicle, tibia, ulna, and femur, with distal forearm fractures the most common type. Epiphyseal (growth plate) injuries are also common in children. These injuries are described using the Salter-Harris classification system (Fig. 19–18).

Etiology and Pathophysiology

Fractures in children may result from direct trauma to a bone (falls, sports injuries, abuse, motor vehicle crashes) or bone diseases (osteogenesis imperfecta) that result in weakening of the bone.

Diagnostic Tests and Medical Management

Radiographs are useful for determining the exact location and type of the fracture. Medical management consists of two basic steps: (1) reduction to realign displaced or fragmented bones, and (2) immobilization so that healing can take place.

A closed reduction aligns the bone by manual manipulation or traction. An open reduction requires surgical alignment of the bone, often

GROWTH & DEVELOPMENT CONSIDERATIONS

Stress fractures are becoming more common in adolescents who limit their intake of calories and calcium in an attempt to remain lean for sports such as distance running or gymnastics. These fractures may present with chronic pain that changes in intensity. Be alert to this possibility when teenagers' diets and athletic activities place them at risk.

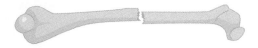

19-13   Classification and Types of Fractures

Classification

Complete (transverse) fracture

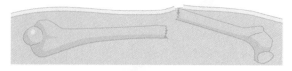

Break across entire section of a bone at a right angle to the bone shaft, resulting in two or more fragments

Open fracture

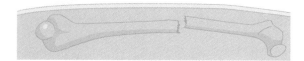

Broken bone protrudes through the skin, leaving a path to the fracture site; high risk of infection exists

Closed fracture

Broken bone does not protrude through the skin

Type

Spiral fracture

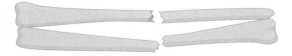

Associated with twisting force; fracture coils around the bone

Greenstick fracture

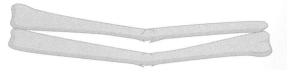

Caused by compression force; often seen in young children

Comminuted fracture

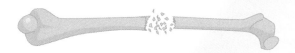

Associated with high impact forces; bone breaks into three or more segments

Additional types of fractures include: *incomplete,* in which the break occurs in only one side of the cortex; *oblique,* in which the fracture slants across the long axis of the bone; *compression,* in which two bones are jammed together (usually occurs in spinal area); and *compacted,* in which one bone fragment is wedged into another.

NURSING ALERT

Fractures involving the epiphyseal plate disrupt the growth process in children. If not treated properly, such injuries can cause limb length discrepancy, joint incongruity, and angular deformities.

using pins, plates, wires, or screws. Casting is the most common external method of immobilization. Other external methods include traction and splinting.

Healing of fractures is influenced by factors including age, size of the involved bone, and fracture site. Fractures heal in less time in children than in adults. Immobilization is essential for the bone healing process to take place. If a fracture is properly reduced, complications should be minimal (Table 19–14).

Nursing Assessment

When dealing with an injured child, be alert to the signs and symptoms of fractures before moving the child. Try to identify the cause of the injury by asking the child, parents, or other family members what happened. Evaluate pain, swelling, and any abnormal positioning of the injured area. When a child is admitted to the emergency department or hospital, nursing assessment includes the extent of the injury, the degree of pain, and the child's vital signs (respiratory status, pulse, blood pressure).

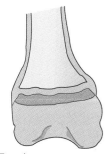

Type I
Common
Growth plate undisturbed
Growth disturbances rare

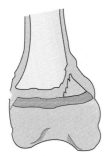

Type II
Most common
Growth disturbances rare

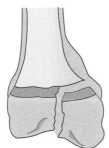

Type III
Less common
Serious threat to growth
    and joint

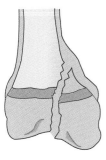

Type IV
Serious threat to growth

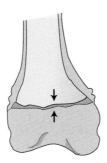

Type V
Rare
Crush injury causes cell death in growth plate,
    resulting in arrested growth and limited
    bone length
If growth plate is partially destroyed, angular
    deformities may result

FIGURE 19–18. The Salter-Harris classification system is based on the angle of the fracture in relation to the epiphysis.

19-14	Complications of Fracture Reduction
Complication	**Medical Management**

Infection
  Acute (may occur with open fractures)
  Chronic (osteomyelitis)
	Debridement, drainage, culture, and treatment with antibiotics

Neurovascular injury resulting from physical nerve damage	Nerve repair
Vascular injury	Vascular repair, amputation, tendon lengthening
Malunion (undesired healed alignment of bone) or delayed union	Corrective osteotomy; prolonged immobilization
Nonunion	Surgical intervention; internal fixation
Leg length discrepancy	Shoe lift

Nursing Diagnosis

Several nursing diagnoses may apply to the child with a fracture. They include:

- Pain related to fracture, trauma, or muscle spasm
- Risk for Impaired Skin Integrity related to trauma, traction, cast, or splint
- Risk for Infection related to open fracture or trauma
- Impaired Physical Mobility related to cast, splint, or traction
- Knowledge Deficit with increased anxiety related to unknown course of treatment

Nursing Management

Nursing care focuses on care of the child before and after fracture reduction, encouraging mobility as ordered, maintaining skin integrity, preventing infection, and teaching the parents and child how to care for the fracture. If conscious sedation is used, nursing care for this procedure is needed. When caring for a child who has undergone fracture reduction, it is important to be aware of the signs of complications. Notify the physician immediately if these signs occur.

Maintain Proper Alignment

Immobilization is used to maintain proper alignment of the fracture. Casts and traction are methods used for immobilizing an injured child. Cast care guidelines are included in Table 19–2, earlier in this chapter.

Different types of traction are used, depending on the location and type of fracture (Table 19–15). Nursing care for the child in traction is described in Table 19–16.

Monitor Neurovascular Status

Monitor the child's sensation to touch, temperature, movement, strength of the pulse, and capillary refill time in the extremity distal to the injury. Monitor every 15 minutes after the cast is applied for at least 2 hours and then every 1–2 hours, depending on your facility's policy and the child's condition. Keep the cast elevated above heart level to minimize edema.

Promote Mobility

The amount of mobility the child is allowed is ordered by the physician and restrictions depend on the extent and site of the fracture. Fractures of the hip or pelvis may involve body casts, and providing wheeled carts makes mobility possible. Children with leg fractures can move around with crutches, walkers, or wheelchairs.

Discharge Planning and Home Care Teaching

Most fractures can be easily managed at home. Activities are generally limited for approximately 8 weeks. Teach the parents and child cast care, activity restrictions, and how to identify problems that should be reported (see Table 19–3). Help parents to identify any modifications that may be needed at home and school. The child who has to manage steps at home or school may need special training with crutches or a temporary ramp. Refer parents to home health nurses or home teaching services if indicated.

NURSING ALERT

Compartment syndrome may occur with a crush injury or when a fracture is reduced. Swelling associated with inflammation reduces blood flow to the affected area, and casting causes further constriction of blood flow. Deep pain unrelieved by analgesics is an important sign of compartment syndrome. This syndrome is a medical emergency. Notify the physician immediately so that constricting dressings or casts can be removed to prevent progressive neurologic damage.

19-15   Types of Traction

Type

Skin Traction

Pull is applied to the skin surface, which puts traction directly on the bones and muscles. Traction is attached to the skin with adhesive materials or straps, or foam boots, belts, or halters.

Dunlop Traction (can be either skeletal or skin)

Used for fracture of the humerus. The arm, which is flexed, is suspended horizontally with straps placed on both the upper and lower portions for pull from both sides.

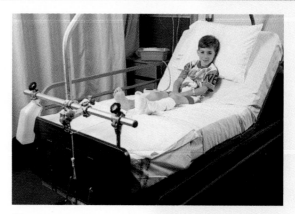

(2)

Buck Traction (2)

Used for knee immobilization; to correct contractures or deformities; or for short-term immobilization of a fracture. It keeps the leg in an extended position, without hip flexion. Traction is applied to the extremity in one direction (straight line) with a single pulley system.

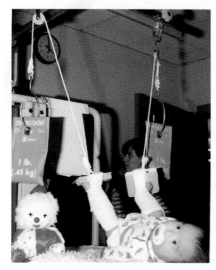

(1)

Bryant Traction (1)

Used specifically for the child under 3 years of age and weighing less than 35 pounds (17.5 kg), who has developmental dysplasia of the hip or a fractured femur. This bilateral traction is applied to the child's legs and kept in place by wrapping the legs from foot to thigh with elastic bandages. The hips are flexed at a 90-degree angle, with knees extended. This position is maintained by attaching the traction appliance to weights and pulleys, which are suspended above the crib. The buttocks do not rest on the mattress, but are slightly elevated off the bed.

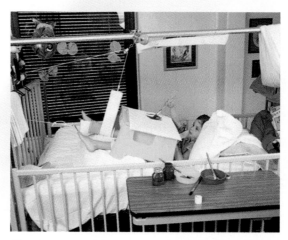

(3)

Russell Traction (3)

Used for fractures of the femur and lower leg. Traction is placed on the lower leg while the knee is suspended in a padded sling. The hips and knees, which are slightly flexed, are immobilized. One force is applied by a double pulley to the foot and another force is applied upward using a sling under the knee and an overhead pulley.

Continued . . .

19-15   Types of Traction (continued)

Type

Skeletal Traction
Pull is directly applied to the bone by pins, wires, tongs, or other apparatus that have been surgically placed through the distal end of the bone.

Skeletal Cervical Traction
Used for cervical spine injuries to reduce fractures and dislocations, Crutchfield Gardner-Wells, or Vinke tongs are placed in the skull with burr holes. Weights are attached to the apparatus with a rope and pulley system to the hyperextended head.

Halo Traction
Used to immobilize the head and neck after cervical injury or dislocation. Also used for positioning and immobilization after cervical injury.

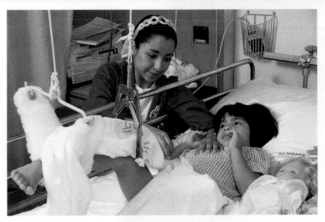

(4)

90–90 Traction (4)
Used for fractures of the femur or tibia. A skeletal pin or wire is surgically placed through the distal part of the femur, while the lower part of the extremity is in a boot cast. Traction ropes and pulleys are applied at the pin site and on the boot cast to maintain the flexion of both the hip and knee at 90 degrees. This traction can also be used for treatment of an upper extremity fracture.

External Fixators (5)
These devices can be used in the treatment of simple fractures, both open and closed; complex fractures with extensive soft tissue involvement; correction of bony or soft tissue deformities; pseudoarthroses; and limb length discrepancy. They are attached to the extremity by percutaneous transfixing of pins or wires to the bone.

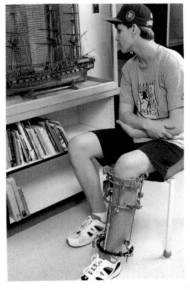

(5)

AMPUTATIONS

Amputation—the complete absence of a body extremity—can be either congenital or acquired. Approximately two thirds of amputations in children are congenital and one third are acquired. Congenital amputations can be caused by constrictive amniotic bands, drugs, or irradiation. Acquired amputations are generally associated with trauma or the result of a disease or disorder.

The child with an absent limb should be fitted with a prosthesis as soon as feasible. This fosters a positive body image, independence, and self-confidence and also ensures that motor skills develop as normally as possible. The prosthetic device should be reevaluated as the child progresses physically and developmentally. Frequent stump reconstructions are often necessary in children with traumatic amputations because as children grow, so do their bones, and the skin tends to adhere to the bone. Bone may need

19-16   Care of the Child in Traction

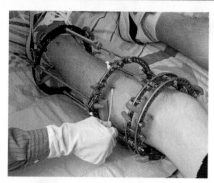

Providing pin care

1. Assess the child in traction by first checking the equipment. Make sure that the equipment is in the proper position. Observe both the body appliance and the attached weights and pulleys. Make certain that the child's body is in proper alignment.
2. Assess the skin under the straps and pin insertion sites for any signs of redness, edema, or skin breakdown.
3. Assess the extremity by checking neurovascular status frequently (check warmth, color, distal pulses, capillary refill time, movement, sensation).
4. Provide pin care when ordered using sterile technique. Clean the area surrounding the pin with cotton-tipped applicators saturated with normal saline or half-strength hydrogen peroxide. Clean the area again with sterile water or more saline. Apply an antibacterial ointment, if ordered, using another cotton-tipped applicator.
5. When the traction equipment can be removed, skin care should be performed every 4 hours.
6. Place a sheepskin pad under the child's extremity if orders permit.

to be cut and soft tissue added to keep the stump rounded. Joint fusions or stump lengthenings may also be needed to allow for the effective use of a prosthesis.

Nursing Management

Nursing care focuses on providing emotional support regarding altered body image, maintaining skin integrity, and encouraging maximal independent functioning.

Provide Emotional Support
Recovering from the loss of a limb is one of the most difficult challenges facing a child. Emphasize what the child can do rather than what he or she cannot do. Good listening skills are important.

Maintain Skin Integrity
The child usually begins wearing the prosthetic device for 1–2-hour intervals. Check the skin for any redness or breakdown. If redness or breakdown develops, leave the prosthesis off and allow the skin to clear before reapplying. Have the prosthesis adjusted if necessary, and increase wearing time as tolerated by the child.

Maximize Independent Functioning
Children with amputated limbs quickly learn how to accommodate to the prosthetic device. Make use of physical therapy programs that are specifically designed to help the child perform activities of daily living.

Discharge Planning and Home Care Teaching
Answer any questions the family has about how to care for the prosthetic device and how to perform skin checks. Encourage parents to allow the child to participate in peer activities that are physically and emotionally challenging. Sporting activities that enable the child to participate using modified equipment are a good way to build self-confidence and motivation. Several ski resorts offer programs that teach children with physical disabilities how to ski. Assess the need for counseling and offer referrals as appropriate.

REFERENCES

1. Matkovic, V., & Heaney, R.P. (1992). Calcium balance during human growth: Evidence for threshold behavior. *American Journal of Clinical Nutrition, 55,* 992–996.

2. National Institute of Health. (1994). Optimal calcium intake. *Journal of the American Medical Association, 272,* 1942–1948.

3. Skinner, S.R. (1996). Orthopedic problems in childhood. In A.M. Rudolph, J.I.E. Hoffman, & C.D. Rudolph (Eds.), *Rudolph's pediatrics* (20th ed., pp. 2129–2158). Stamford, CT: Appleton & Lange.

4. Hoffinger, S.A. (1996). Evaluation and management of pediatric foot deformities. *Pediatric Clinics of North America, 43*(5), 1091–1112.

5. Craig, C. (1995). Congenital talipes equinovarus. *Professional Nurse, 11*(1), 30–32.

6. Blakeslee, T.J. (1997). Congenital idiopathic talipes equinovarus (clubfoot). *Clinics on Podiatric Medicine and Surgery, 14*(1), 9–55.

7. Kyzer, S.P., & Stark, S.L. (1995). Congenital idiopathic clubfoot deformities. *Association of Operating Room Nurses, 61*(3), 492–503.

8. Novacheck, T.F. (1996). Developmental dysplasia of the hip. *Pediatric Clinics of North America, 43*(4), 829–848.

9. Hayes, M.A.B. (1995). Traction at home for infants with developmental dysplasia of the hip. *Orthopaedic Nursing, 14*(1), 33–40.

10. Stevens, B., Stockwell, M., Browne, G., Dent, P., Gafni, A., Martin, R., & Anderson, M. (1995). Evaluation of a home-based traction program for children with congenital dislocated hips and Legg Perthes disease. *Canadian Journal of Nursing Research, 27*(4), 133–150.

11. Stout, J.D., Bandy, P., Feller, N., Stroup, K.B., & Bull, M.J. (1992). Transportation resources for pediatric orthopaedic clients. *Orthopaedic Nursing, 11*(4), 26–30.

12. Dunst, R.M. (1990). Legg-Calvé-Perthes disease. *Orthopaedic Nursing, 9*(2), 18–27.

13. Koop, S., & Quanbeck, D. (1996). Three common causes of childhood hip pain. *Pediatric Clinics of North America, 43*(5), 1053–1066.

14. Benchot, R. (1996). The adolescent with slipped capital femoral epiphysis. *Journal of Pediatric Nursing, 11*(3), 175–182.

15. Gerberg, L., & Micheli, L.J. (1996). Nontraumatic hip pain in active children. *The Physician and Sportsmedicine, 24*(1), 69–74.

16. Boachie-Adjei, O., & Lonner, B. (1996). Spinal deformity. *Pediatric Clinics of North America, 43*(4), 883–898.

17. Nelson, J.D. (1996). Osteomyelitis. In A.M. Rudolph, J.I.E. Hoffman, & C.D. Rudolph (Eds.), *Rudolph's pediatrics* (20th ed., pp. 548–551). Stamford, CT: Appleton & Lange.

18. Sonnen, G.M., & Henry, N.K. (1996). Pediatric bone and joint infections: Diagnosis and antimicrobial management. *Pediatric Clinics of North America, 43*(4), 933–948.

19. Almekinders, L.C. (1994). Osteomyelitis: Essentials of diagnosis and treatment. *Journal of Musculoskeletal Medicine, 11*(11), 31–32, 34–36, 38, 40.

20. Sillence, D.O. (1996). Genetic skeletal dysplasias. In A.M. Rudolph, J.I.E. Hoffman, & C.D. Rudolph (Eds.), *Rudolph's pediatrics* (20th ed., pp. 377–392). Stamford, CT: Appleton & Lange.

21. Janas, J. (1996). Muscular dystrophy. *Nurse Practitioner Forum, 7*(4), 167–173.

22. DiMauro, S., Hays, A.P., & Bonilla, E. (1996). Myopathies. In A.M. Rudolph, J.I.E. Hoffman, & C.D. Rudolph (Eds.), *Rudolph's pediatrics* (20th ed., pp. 1977–1989). Stamford, CT: Appleton & Lange.

23. Urbanski, L.F., & Hanlon, D.P. (1996). Pediatric orthopedics. *Topics in Emergency Medicine, 18*(2), 73–90.

ADDITIONAL RESOURCES

Binder, H., Conway, A., & Gerber, L.H. (1993). Rehabilitation approaches to children with osteogenesis imperfecta: A ten-year experience. *Archives in Physical Medicine Rehabilitation, 74,* 386–390.

Brand, P.W. (1997). A personal revolution in the development of clubfoot correction. *Clinics in Podiatric Medicine and Surgery, 14*(1), 1–7.

Chestnut, M.A. (1998). *Pediatric home care manual.* Philadelphia: Lippincott.

Corbett, D. (1988). Information needs of parents of a child in a Pavlik harness. *Orthopaedic Nursing, 7*(2), 20–23.

Dicke, T.E., & Nunley, J.A. (1993). Distal forearm fractures in children. *Orthopedic Clinics of North America, 24*(2), 333–340.

Folcik, M.A., Carini-Garcia, G., & Birmingham, J.J. (1994). *Traction: Assessment and management.* St. Louis: Mosby–Year Book.

Gallo, A.M. (1996). Building strong bones in childhood and adolescence: Reducing the risk of fractures in later life. *Pediatric Nursing, 22*(5), 369–374, 422.

Grossman, M. (1996). Tuberculosis. In A.M. Rudolph, J.I.E. Hoffman, & C.D. Rudolph (Eds.), *Rudolph's pediatrics* (20th ed., pp 614–623). Stamford, CT: Appleton & Lange.

Harrigan, J. (1996). Muscular dystrophy. *Journal of School Nursing, 12*(2), 38, 40.

Jonides, L. (1995). Congenital scoliosis: A case presentation. *Journal of Pediatric Health Care, 9*(3), 139–140.

Killam, P.E. (1989). Orthopedic assessment of young children: Developmental variations. *Nurse Practitioner, 14*(7), 27–32.

Maitra, R.S., & Johnson, D.L. (1997). Stress fractures. *Clinics in Sports Medicine, 16*(2), 259–274.

McDonald, C.M., Abresch, R.T., Carter, G.T., Fowler, W.M., Johnson, R., Kilmer, D.D., & Sigford, B. J. (1995). Profiles of neuromuscular diseases: Duchenne muscular dystrophy. *American Journal of Physical Medicine and Rehabilitation, 74*(5), S70–S92.

Osebold, W.R., & King, H.A. (1994). Kyphoscoliosis in Williams syndrome. *Spine, 19*(3), 367–371.

Smith, M.D. (1994). Congenital scoliosis of the cervical or cervicothoracic spine. *Orthopedic Clinics of North America, 25*(2), 301–310.

Waters, E. (1995). Toxic synovitis of the hip in children. *Nurse Practitioner, 20*(4), 44–48.

Williamson, M. (1994). Pediatric forearm fractures. *Orthopaedic Nursing, 13*(3), 65–68.

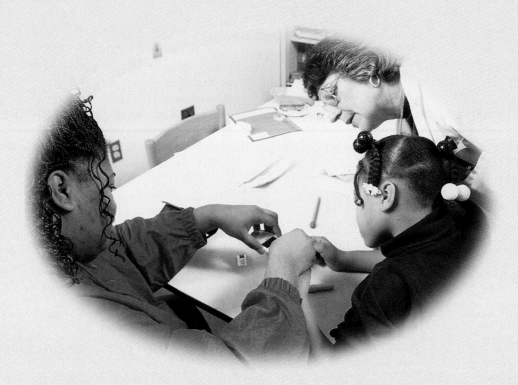

*S*hawnda, 6 years old, has just been diagnosed with diabetes mellitus. Her parents have brought her to their family physician after Shawnda complained of being constantly thirsty and hungry for over a week. Despite this she lost 5 pounds. They note that she had a viral illness about 1 month ago but seemed to recover from it. Her mother says that Shawnda has seemed lethargic for the past 3 days.

Shawnda and her family must now learn to manage her diabetes using a combination of diet, exercise, and insulin therapy. Monitoring her blood glucose level is important in determining how much insulin she will need in the first weeks of treatment, until her system stabilizes. Shawnda's mother will need to learn to schedule her daughter's meals and provide specific amounts of protein, fat, and carbohydrates at each meal. Shawnda's meals and activity will need to be coordinated with the insulin doses. Her parents will need to monitor Shawnda closely for signs of hypoglycemia.

What causes diabetes? What potential problems need prompt treatment? What are the long-term implications of the diagnosis? During Shawnda's short hospitalization and follow-up sessions, the nurse answers these questions and addresses other concerns raised by Shawnda's parents. As she begins to teach Shawnda and her family about the condition, the nurse also reassures them that Shawnda can live a normal life despite her disease.

ALTERATIONS IN ENDOCRINE FUNCTION 20

"Families are really challenged when a child develops diabetes. It is amazing how well they learn all the things they need to do to help keep their child's condition under control."

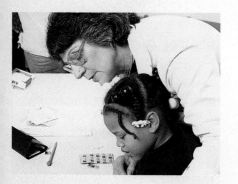

TERMINOLOGY

- **glucagon** A hormone produced by the pancreas that helps release stored glucose from the liver.
- **glycosuria** Abnormal amount of glucose in the urine.
- **goiter** Enlargement of the thyroid gland.
- **hormone** A chemical substance produced by a gland or organ and carried in the bloodstream to another part of the body where it has a regulatory effect on particular cells.
- **inborn errors of metabolism** Inherited biochemical abnormalities of the urea cycle and amino acid and organic acid metabolism.
- **karyotype** A microscopic display of the 46 chromosomes in the human body lined up from the largest to the smallest. The human female is 46,XX and the human male is 46,XY.
- **polydipsia** Excessive thirst.
- **polyphagia** Excessive or voracious eating.
- **polyuria** Passage of a large volume of urine in a given period.
- **pseudohermaphroditism** Ambiguous development of the external genitalia.
- **puberty** Period of life when the ability to reproduce sexually begins; characterized by maturation of the genital organs, development of the secondary sex characteristics, and (in females) the onset of menstruation.

The endocrine system controls the cellular activity that regulates growth and body metabolism through the release of hormones. **Hormones** are chemical messengers secreted by various glands that exert controlling effects on the cells of the body. Overlapping with all body systems, the general functions of the endocrine system include the following:

- Differentiation of the reproductive and central nervous systems in the fetus
- Regulation of the pace of growth and development in concert with the central nervous system throughout childhood and adolescence
- Coordination of the male and female reproductive systems, enabling sexual reproduction
- Maintenance of an optimal level of hormones for body functioning
- Maintenance of homeostasis, a healthy internal environment, in the presence of a constantly changing external environment

Endocrine disturbances result in alterations in metabolism, growth and development, and behavior that may have significant implications for children.

Inborn errors of metabolism—inherited biochemical abnormalities of the urea cycle and amino acid and organic acid metabolism—often have a significant impact on the endocrine system's ability to support growth and development. Some chromosomal abnormalities also result in disturbances in growth and sexual development. For these reasons inborn errors of metabolism and some chromosome disorders are included in this chapter.

Most endocrine malfunctions are present at birth. They are often observed at birth or during the routine newborn assessment or detected by health care providers within the first year of life. If not diagnosed and treated early, these conditions can result in delays in growth and development, mental retardation, and, occasionally, death. However, treatment, which usually consists of supplementation of missing hormones, adjustment of hormone levels, or dietary measures, allows most children to live a normal life.

Most children with endocrine and metabolic disorders are treated on an outpatient basis. Children may be admitted to the hospital in cases of an acute metabolic disturbance that occurs before diagnosis or when treatment is inadequate. Children may also be admitted to the hospital for other acute problems even though their endocrine disorder is well controlled.

▶ ANATOMY AND PHYSIOLOGY OF PEDIATRIC DIFFERENCES

The endocrine glands include the hypothalamus, pituitary gland, thyroid gland, parathyroid glands, adrenal glands, ovaries, testes, and islets of Langerhans in the pancreas (Fig. 20–1). These glands secrete hormones into the bloodstream that are carried to target organs or tissues. Most hormones exert their influence through interaction with receptors in the target cells of specific tissues (Table 20–1).

The regulation of hormone secretion occurs through a negative feedback mechanism that functions to maintain an optimal internal environment in the body. Negative feedback occurs when an endocrine gland or secretory tissue receives a message that an adequate amount of hormone has been received by the target cells. In response further secretion is inhibited. Secretion is resumed only when the secretory tissue receives another message indicating that levels of the hormone are low.

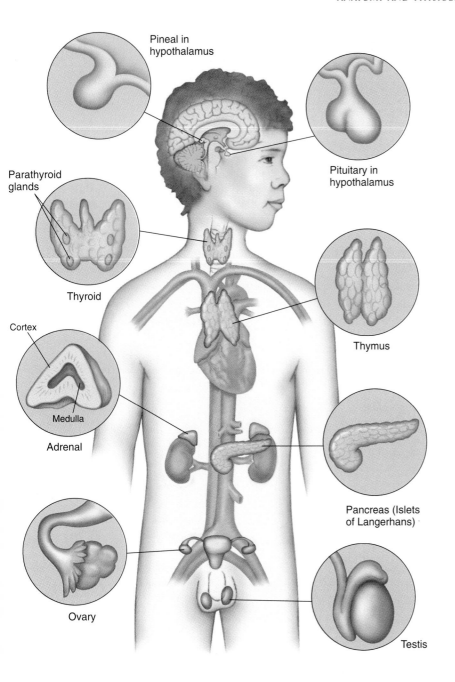

Pineal in
hypothalamus

Pituitary in
hypothalamus

Parathyroid
glands

Thyroid

Thymus

Cortex

Medulla

Adrenal

Pancreas (Islets
of Langerhans)

Ovary

Testis

FIGURE 20–1. Major organs and glands of the
endocrine system.

The endocrine system is responsible for sexual differentiation during
fetal development (Fig. 20–2) and for stimulating growth and development
during childhood and adolescence. This includes stimulating development
of the reproductive system in both sexes.

Puberty (sexual maturation, lasting 2–3 years) occurs when the gonads
secrete increased amounts of the sex hormones estrogen and testosterone.
At the average age of 10 years in girls and 11 years in boys, the hypothalamus produces increased amounts of gonadotropin-releasing hormone. This
hormone stimulates the anterior pituitary gland to increase the production
of luteinizing hormone (LH) and follicle-stimulating hormone (FSH).
These hormones in turn stimulate the gonads to secrete more sex hormones (Fig. 20–3), resulting in the development of primary and secondary
sex characteristics.

20-1   Endocrine Glands and Their Functions

Gland/Hormone	Function
Pituitary	
Growth hormone	Stimulates growth of all body tissues
Thyroid-stimulating hormone (TSH)	Stimulates thyroid hormone secretion
Adrenocorticotropic hormone (ACTH)	Stimulates secretion of glucocorticoids and androgens
Follicle-stimulating hormone (FSH)	Stimulates secretion of estrogen; supports follicle development in ovaries
Luteinizing hormone (LH)	Stimulates secretion of androgens in males and progesterone in females
Prolactin	Stimulates secretion of milk during lactation
Melanocyte-stimulating hormone (MSH)	Stimulates skin pigmentation
Antidiuretic hormone (ADH)	Stimulates permeability of renal tubules
Oxytocin	Stimulates uterine contractions and let-down reflex
Thyroid	
Thyroxine (T_4) and triiodothyronine (T_3)	Stimulate cellular growth rate
Thyrocalcitonin	Stimulates bone ossification and development
Parathyroid	
Parathyroid hormone	Stimulates reabsorption of calcium and excretion of phosphorus
Adrenal	
Aldosterone	Stimulates reabsorption of sodium and excretion of potassium
Androgens	Stimulates bone development and secondary sexual characteristics
Cortisol	Stimulates antiinflammatory reactions, among many other functions
Epinephrine	Activates sympathetic nervous system; stimulates increase in blood pressure and blood glucose levels
Pancreas (Islets of Langerhans)	
Insulin	Stimulates cellular glucose utilization
Glucagon	Stimulates hyperglycemia
Somatostatin	Stimulates inhibition of insulin and glucagon secretion; inhibits growth hormone; inhibits gastric acid secretion
Ovaries	
Estrogen	Stimulates development of breasts and ova
Progesterone	Stimulates breast glandular development; acts to maintain pregnancy
Testes	
Testosterone	Stimulates production of sperm, development of secondary sexual characteristics, and closure of epiphysis

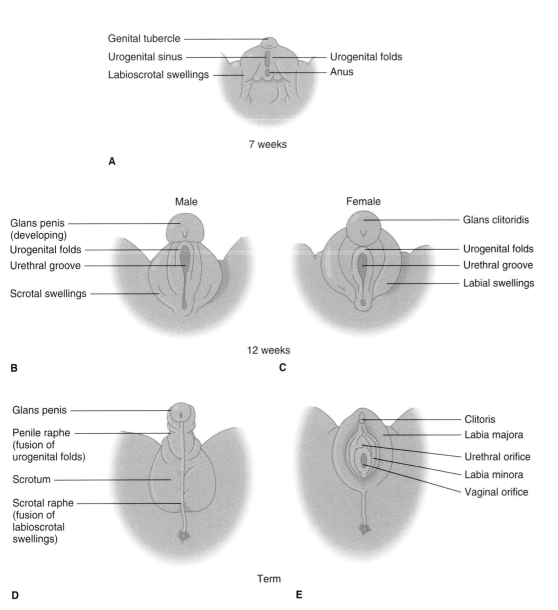

Undifferentiated

Genital tubercle
Urogenital sinus
Labioscrotal swellings
Urogenital folds
Anus

7 weeks

A

Male

Glans penis (developing)
Urogenital folds
Urethral groove
Scrotal swellings

Female

Glans clitoridis
Urogenital folds
Urethral groove
Labial swellings

12 weeks

B   **C**

Glans penis
Penile raphe (fusion of urogenital folds)
Scrotum
Scrotal raphe (fusion of labioscrotal swellings)

Clitoris
Labia majora
Urethral orifice
Labia minora
Vaginal orifice

Term

D   **E**

FIGURE 20–2. Sexual differentiation. **A,** At 7 weeks' gestation, male and female genitalia are identical (undifferentiated). **B** and **C,** By 12 weeks' gestation, noticeable differentiation begins to occur. **D** and **E,** Differentiation continues until birth but is almost complete at term.

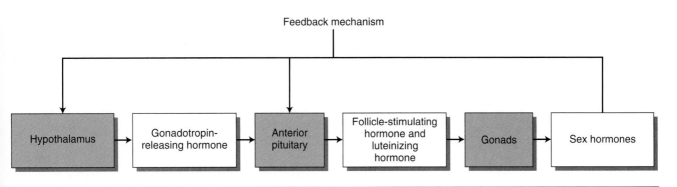

Feedback mechanism

Hypothalamus → Gonadotropin-releasing hormone → Anterior pituitary → Follicle-stimulating hormone and luteinizing hormone → Gonads → Sex hormones

FIGURE 20–3. Feedback mechanism in hormonal stimulation of the gonads during puberty.

▶ DISORDERS OF PITUITARY FUNCTION

HYPOPITUITARISM (GROWTH HORMONE DEFICIENCY)

Hypopituitarism is a disorder caused by decreased activity of the pituitary gland. Because most children with this disorder secrete inadequate amounts of growth hormone, the term *hypopituitarism* is often used interchangeably with *growth hormone deficiency*. An estimated 1 in 4000 school-age children has growth hormone deficiency.[1]

Children with hypopituitarism are of normal weight and length when born. By the age of 1 year, however, they are below the third percentile on the growth chart. They characteristically grow at a rate of less than 5 cm (2 in.) per year. Other characteristic findings in infants include hypoglycemic seizures, neonatal jaundice, pale optic discs, micropenis, and undescended testicles. Children with hypopituitarism tend to be overweight and to have youthful facial features, higher pitched voices, delayed dentition, "ripply" abdominal fat, delayed skeletal maturation, delayed sexual maturation, and hypoglycemia.

The release of growth hormone from the anterior pituitary gland is controlled by the hypothalamus, which secretes releasing and inhibitory factors. Growth hormone stimulates the growth of all body tissues. It also stimulates the synthesis of proteins in the liver, among them the somatomedins or insulinlike growth factors (IGFs), which promote glucose utilization by the cells and cell proliferation.

Infection, infarction of the pituitary gland (related to sickle cell disease), central nervous system disease, tumors of the pituitary gland or hypothalamus (primarily craniopharyngiomas and gliomas), and psychosocial deprivation may cause hypopituitarism or growth hormone deficiency by interfering with the production or release of growth hormone. In some cases, the disorder is caused by dominant or recessive inheritance or by a chromosomal mutation.[2] It is also suspected that the pituitary gland or hypothalamus either has developmental defects or may become damaged or malformed during fetal development or at birth.[1]

Any child whose height is 2–3 standard deviations below the mean height for age or whose measurement is falling off the normal growth chart should be evaluated for short stature (Table 20–2). A child whose screening tests reveal low levels of IGF-1 requires further evaluation by a pediatric endocrinologist. A careful history, physical examination, and radiologic studies are necessary to rule out familial short stature, constitutional growth delay, skeletal dysplasias, or psychosocial dwarfism. Provocative growth hormone testing, in which various medications (arginine, clonidine, glucagon, insulin, L-dopa) are administered to stimulate release of growth hormone, is the definitive diagnostic test in most children.

Treatment depends on the cause of the deficiency. In most cases it consists of replacement of the missing growth hormone and outpatient follow-up to monitor the child's growth. The development of a synthetic form of growth hormone has greatly increased the supply of this medication. Most children receive subcutaneous injections three times a week. Replacement therapy is continued until the child achieves an acceptable height or fails to respond to treatment. Early diagnosis and treatment are important to ensure attainment of maximum adult height potential. Testosterone injections are needed by some boys and estrogen by some girls to stimulate puberty.

PSYCHOSOCIAL DWARFISM

Psychosocial dwarfism is a syndrome of emotional deprivation that causes suppression of production of pituitary hormones resulting in adrenocorticotropic hormone (ACTH) and growth hormone deficiencies. The child is often withdrawn, with bizarre eating habits and polydipsia, and may also gorge and vomit.[1] Treatment involves removing the child from the stressful environment and providing for normal dietary intake. Pituitary secretion is usually restored, and dramatic catchup growth in height is observed.

LEGAL & ETHICAL CONSIDERATIONS

The increased availability of synthetic growth hormone has led to questions about the use of this medication for children who are below average for height but not growth hormone deficient. The medication is expensive (up to $20,000 per year), and its long-term effects, such as actually increasing adult height, are still being investigated.

20-2	Diagnostic Tests for Short Stature	
Test	**Purpose Related to Short Stature**	
IGF-1 and IGFBP-3	Excludes growth hormone deficiency if normal	
Radiographic views of the sella turcica (site of the pituitary gland)	Demonstrates size of the sella turcica or a tumor	
Karotype (girls)	Detects Turner's syndrome (see pages 899–900)	
Serum thyroxine level	Detects hypothyroidism (see pages 873–875)	
Urine creatinine, pH, specific gravity, urea nitrogen, electrolytes	Detects chronic renal failure (see Chap. 16)	
Bone age	Identifies other potential causes of delayed growth	
Complete blood count and erythrocyte sedimentation rate	Screens for inflammatory bowel disease with anemia	

Modified from D'Ercole, A.J., & Underwood, L. (1996). Anterior pituitary gland and hypothalamus. In A.M. Rudolph, J.I.E. Hoffman, & C.D. Rudolph (Eds.), Rudolph's pediatrics (20th ed., p. 1692). Stamford, CT: Appleton & Lange.

Nursing Management

Nursing care consists of monitoring growth, teaching the child and family about the disorder and its treatment, and providing emotional support. The child's height and weight are carefully measured (refer to the *Quick Reference to Pediatric Clinical Skills* accompanying this text) and plotted on a growth chart (see Appendix A).

Teach the parents and child about the growth hormone replacement therapy and provide the parents with educational resources (Table 20–3). Since replacement therapy is expensive and usually is not covered by insurance, parents may need help with finances. National organizations such as the Human Growth Foundation and the Short Stature Foundation (see Appendix F) are sources of additional information. The best results occur when treatment is initiated at an early age, before psychologic effects of short stature become apparent.

Children with growth hormone deficiency may have academic problems resulting from learning disabilities and below-average intelligence.[3]

20-3	Resources for Children With a Growth Disorder

Short and OK: A Guide for Parents of Short Children, by Patricia Rieser and Heino F.L. Meyer-Bahlburg; available from the Human Growth Foundation (see Appendix F); for parents

Tall and Small: A Book About Height, by Kate Phifer; New York: Walker & Co., 1987; for adolescents

Why Is Everybody Always Picking on Me?, by Terence Webster-Doyle; Middlebury, VT: Atrium Publications, 1991; for school-age children and adolescents

Before the child enters school, a comprehensive evaluation should be performed to identify potential problems.

People often treat short children on the basis of their size rather than their age, and such children experience social prejudice related to height.[3] Teasing is a common problem. The teenage years may be particularly stressful because of the preoccupation with body image characteristic of adolescence.

Encourage parents and teachers to treat the child in an age-appropriate manner. The child should dress in clothing that reflects chronologic age. Emphasize the child's strengths, support independence, and encourage participation in age-appropriate activities to aid in the development of a positive self-image. Suggest that the child take part in sports in which ability does not depend on size (eg, swimming, gymnastics, wrestling, ice skating, and martial arts). Identifying positive role models, short individuals who are successful in accomplishing their goals, is another approach that promotes a positive image. Refer the child for counseling if appropriate.

HYPERPITUITARISM

Hyperpituitarism, a disorder in which excessive secretion of growth hormone increases the growth rate, is rare in children. Oversecretion of growth hormone is usually caused by a pituitary adenoma. Another possible cause is a tumor of the hypothalamus. Affected children can grow to 7 or 8 feet in height when oversecretion occurs before closure of the epiphyseal plates.

Because tall stature is valued in our society, assessment of children (particularly boys) with accelerated growth is often delayed.[4] Any child whose predicted height exceeds that consistent with parental height should be evaluated for possible growth problems and underlying pathologic conditions.

A complete history is obtained, and physical examination and laboratory testing are performed. Increased levels of IGF-1 establish the diagnosis of hyperpituitarism. A bone scan is usually obtained to determine whether the epiphyseal plates have begun to fuse. Radiologic studies are used to detect a tumor. Thorough evaluation is required to differentiate hyperpituitarism from familial tall stature.

Treatment depends on the cause of the excessive growth and may involve surgical removal of a tumor, radiation therapy, or oral administration of bromocriptine, which suppresses secretion of growth hormone.

Nursing Management

Tall stature, like short stature, can be stressful for children. Tall children are often treated as if they are older than their chronologic age. Tall adolescents may have problems with self-image, and girls in particular may worry about their appearance.

Nursing care focuses on teaching the parents and child about the disorder and its treatment, providing emotional support, and, if surgery is required, providing preoperative and postoperative teaching and care (see Chap. 4).

DIABETES INSIPIDUS

Diabetes insipidus, a rare disorder of the posterior pituitary gland, is characterized by a deficiency of antidiuretic hormone (ADH), or vasopressin. ADH facilitates concentration of the urine by stimulating reabsorption of water from the distal tubule of the kidney. When ADH is inadequate, the tubules do not resorb, leading to **polyuria** (passage of a large volume of urine in a given period). Two forms of diabetes insipidus occur in children: true (or central) ADH deficiency and familial nephrogenic diabetes insipidus, in which the kidneys are unable to respond to the ADH that is present.

Polyuria and **polydipsia** (excessive thirst) are the cardinal signs of diabetes insipidus. The child is constantly thirsty even at night and becomes irritable when fluid is withheld. Nocturia and enuresis may occur in the previously toilet-trained child. Constipation, fever, and dehydration also may occur because body fluid is depleted or thirst is not satisfied. Although the onset of symptoms is usually sudden, diagnosis is often delayed. Children who are able to quench their thirst may not complain to parents about symptoms. With X-linked familial nephrogenic diabetes insipidus, symptoms of dehydration, fever, vomiting, mental status changes, and hypernatremia occur early in the neonatal period.

True ADH deficiency in children is usually familial or idiopathic. Secondary causes include damage to the neurohypophyseal system such as tumors of the hypothalamus, infections such as encephalitis or meningitis, and trauma. The result is a deficiency in secretion of the antidiuretic hormone, arginine vasopressin (AVP). Most cases of nephrogenic diabetes insipidus are familial, with either an X-linked or an autosomal recessive form. It may also result from drug toxicity or recurrent infection. In nephrogenic diabetes insipidus, the renal collecting tubules or the medulla, which are directly involved in the concentration of urine, are abnormal.[5]

In all forms of diabetes insipidus, the urine cannot be concentrated, no matter how dehydrated the child becomes. Dehydration usually precipitates diagnosis. Serum sodium concentration and osmolality increase rapidly to pathologic levels. Often an unconscious child is admitted to the emergency department with dehydration accompanied by hypernatremia.

Serum electrolytes and both serum and urine osmolalities are tested. Diagnosis is confirmed by measuring the plasma AVP level before and during a standard fluid deprivation test, which is usually conducted in the hospital or in a carefully controlled outpatient setting for 7 hours. Urine osmolality, urine specific gravity, serum sodium, and serum osmolality are monitored hourly. The child's output will exceed intake, and urine will not be excessively concentrated. The specific gravity will remain less than 1.010 even after dehydration.

Treatment of true ADH deficiency consists of the intramuscular administration of desmopressin acetate (DDAVP) or intranasal DDAVP, a synthetic analog of vasopressin with an effect lasting 8–12 hours. DDAVP reduces urinary output, enabling the child to live a more normal life with a decrease in thirst, urinary output, and nocturia. The dose of DDAVP must be titered so the child receives adequate caloric intake for growth and development. DDAVP is not effective in controlling nephrogenic diabetes insipidus. Children with nephrogenic diabetes insipidus are treated with diuretics, a high fluid intake, and a salt- and protein-restricted diet. The child's sodium and potassium levels must be carefully monitored to prevent hypernatremia and hypokalemia (see Chap. 8).

Nursing Management

Nursing care centers on administering medications and teaching parents how to manage the condition and recognize signs of altered fluid status. Parent education is of primary importance. Infants usually need fluid in-

 CLINICAL TIP

During the fluid deprivation test, advise parents that the child will be frustrated and irritable from thirst. No one should drink in front of the child during the testing period. Monitor the child's vital signs and intake and output carefully. The test is stopped if the child loses 3–5% of body weight and develops a fever and hypotension.[6]

take even during the night. Many infants have coexisting brain damage and decreased thirst and require nasogastric or gastrostomy feeding to maintain adequate hydration and nutrition.

Help parents monitor fluid intake after DDAVP treatment is initiated. When the child has compensated for the condition with an excessive fluid intake, the diminished need for fluids must be learned. The child will not have the ability to excrete the excess water load with DDAVP treatment.

Teach parents to recognize signs of inadequate fluid intake (see Chap. 8) and to adjust the child's fluid intake to prevent dehydration. When an acute illness occurs, the child's physician should be notified immediately because the increase in metabolic activity will necessitate the administration of additional fluids to prevent dehydration.

Parents may need assistance to manage the child's care. Arrangements for a visiting nurse, a home health nurse, or respite care may be needed.

PRECOCIOUS PUBERTY

Puberty normally occurs between 8 and 13 years of age in girls and between 9½ and 14 years of age in boys. Precocious puberty is defined as the appearance of any secondary sexual characteristics before 8 years of age in girls and 9 years of age in boys. Early puberty is inherited in 5–10% of boys.[8]

Early secretion of the normal hormones responsible for pubertal changes usually is not associated with abnormalities. However, a benign hypothalamic tumor may be present. Other causes include cerebral trauma, central nervous system disorder, infection, chronic adrenal insufficiency, hydrocephalus, neoplasms, and irradiation.[9] Children with precocious puberty have premature skeletal maturation and may appear unusually tall for their age. Their growth ceases prematurely, however, as the hormones stimulate closure of the epiphyseal plates, resulting in short stature.

Because the cause of the condition usually cannot be treated, the child's development may be monitored for 6–12 months to see how quickly pubertal changes are occurring. If development is stalled or slow, no treatment is initiated. If pubertal changes are occurring rapidly, management sometimes focuses on altering hormonal balance.[10] A synthetic form of luteinizing hormone–releasing factor (Lupron Depot) is used to slow or arrest the progression of puberty. The medication is administered either monthly by intramuscular injection or daily by subcutaneous injection. Treatment is continued until the child reaches a more appropriate age for puberty. Hormone levels are monitored to ensure maintenance of prepubertal levels, which results in regression or cessation of accelerated physical development.

Nursing Management

Nursing care centers on teaching the child and parents about the condition and its treatment and providing emotional support. The child should be informed in age-appropriate terms that physiologic changes are normal but occurring at an earlier than usual age. Reassure the child that friends will go through the same stages of development eventually. Remember that the child's social, cognitive, and emotional development matches his or her age, even though the physical development is advanced.

Children with precocious puberty become self-conscious as body changes occur. Parents should be advised to dress the child in a manner appropriate to his or her chronologic age, even though the child may look older. Looser clothing may help hide some of the body changes that are oc-curring. Provide privacy during examinations. Encourage the child to ex-press his or her feelings about the changes. The child may need to practice role playing as a coping mechanism to manage teasing by other children.

Boys may become more aggressive and develop a sex drive as a result of hormonal changes. Parents should be advised that they may need to dis-cuss issues of sexuality with the child at an earlier age than normal. Refer the child for counseling if appropriate.

▶ DISORDERS OF THYROID FUNCTION

HYPOTHYROIDISM

Hypothyroidism is a disorder in which levels of active thyroid hormones are decreased. It may be congenital or acquired. Congenital hypothyroidism oc-curs in approximately 1 in 4000 live births and is twice as common in girls as in boys. It is less prevalent in African-American infants but more frequent in Hispanic infants (1 in 2000 births).[11] It also occurs more commonly in children with Down syndrome. Acquired hypothyroidism occurs after the child is 2 years old and is more common in girls than in boys.

Clinical Manifestations

Infants with congenital hypothyroidism have few clinical signs of the disor-der in the first weeks of life. The characteristic cretinoid features (thick-ened protuberant tongue, thick lips, dull appearance) appear during the first few months of life in untreated infants. These signs are rarely seen today because routine screening within a few days of birth identifies most infants with the disorder, allowing early treatment. Other signs of congeni-tal hypothyroidism include prolonged neonatal jaundice, hypotonia, brady-cardia, decreased pulse pressure, cool extremities, mottling, umbilical her-nia, a posterior fontanel larger than 1 cm in diameter, difficulty feeding, lethargy, constipation, and a hoarse cry.

Children with acquired hypothyroidism have many of the same signs as adults: decreased appetite, dry skin, coarse hair or hair loss, depressed deep tendon reflexes, bradycardia, constipation, sensitivity to cold temperatures, and an enlarged thyroid gland or a **goiter.** Manifestations unique to chil-dren include change in past normal growth patterns with a weight increase and weight-for-age greater than height-for-age, delayed bone age, muscle hypertrophy with muscle weakness, and delayed or precocious puberty.

Etiology and Pathophysiology

Thyroid hormones are important for growth and development and for the metabolism of nutrients and energy. When these hormones are not avail-able for stimulation of other hormones or specific target cells, growth is de-layed and mental retardation develops.

Congenital hypothyroidism is usually caused by a spontaneous gene mutation, an autosomal recessive genetic transmission of an enzyme defi-ciency, failure of the central nervous system–thyroid feedback mechanism to develop, or iodine deficiency. Mental retardation is irreversible if the dis-order is not treated.

Acquired hypothyroidism can result from autoimmune thyroiditis (Hashimoto's thyroiditis), late-onset thyroid dysfunction, isolated thyroid-stimulating hormone (TSH) deficiency, an inborn error of thyroid hormone synthesis, or exposure to drugs or substances such as lithium that interfere with thyroid hormone synthesis. The family history is positive for thyroid disease in 30–40% of cases of autoimmune thyroiditis.[11]

Diagnostic Tests and Medical Management

Congenital hypothyroidism is usually detected during newborn screening of thyroxine (T_4) and TSH levels, which is mandatory in all 50 states. An elevated TSH level indicates that the disease originated in the thyroid, not the pituitary. If the T_4 level is below normal and the TSH level is increased, the synthetic thyroid hormone levothyroxine (Synthroid) is prescribed. The dose is increased gradually as the child grows to ensure a euthyroid (normal thyroid) state. Treatment is monitored by a pediatric endocrinologist. Periodic evaluation of T_4 and TSH serum levels, bone age, and growth parameters is necessary to assess for signs of excess or inadequate thyroid hormone. Antithyroid antibodies are measured in children with a goiter and suspected Hashimoto's thyroiditis, as increased titers of antithyroglobin are often found.[11]

To ensure an adequate growth rate and prevent mental retardation, the hormone must be taken throughout life. Children with congenital hypothyroidism that is diagnosed before 3 months of age have the best prognosis for optimal mental development. Children with acquired hypothyroidism usually have normal growth following a period of catch-up growth. Up to 30% of adolescents with Hashimoto's thyroiditis have a spontaneous remission.[11]

Nursing Assessment

Routine neonatal screening is usually performed before discharge from the hospital to evaluate levels of circulating thyroid hormones. However, many newborns are currently discharged before 24 hours of life. Nurses frequently make home visits a few days later to assess the health of the mother and infant. Neonatal screening may be performed at that visit (Table 20–4). Alternatively, T_4 and TSH screenings may be performed in a health care facility soon after birth.

Serial measurement and recording of height and weight are performed at each follow-up visit. The child is assessed for signs of inadequate growth to determine if the dose of thyroid hormone needs to be adjusted and to monitor compliance with medication.

Nursing Diagnosis

Among the nursing diagnoses that might be appropriate for the child with hypothyroidism are the following:

- Altered Nutrition: Less Than Body Requirements related to poor appetite or inability to utilize nutrients fully
- Hypothermia related to lowered metabolic rate
- Constipation related to decreased bowel motility
- Fatigue related to an imbalance in energy production
- Risk for Altered Health Maintenance related to lack of understanding about the treatment regimen

Nursing Management

Nursing care focuses on teaching the parents and child about the disorder and its treatment and monitoring the child's growth rate. When the cause is genetic, a referral for genetic counseling should be made. Explain how to

20-4 Blood Collection Tips for Neonatal Screening

To reduce errors in collection of blood for neonatal screening:
1. Collect blood before 72 hours of age. If blood is collected before 24 hours of age, repeat screening before 14 days of age.
2. Perform a heel stick and collect one large drop on the infant's heel. A capillary tube may be used.
3. Fill the entire circle on a clean filter paper. Apply blood to only one side of the filter paper.
4. Allow the paper to air dry at room temperature in a horizontal position.
5. Make sure all patient information is provided on the screening form to ensure that the infant can be found if the result is abnormal.
6. Mail the specimen to the laboratory within 24 hours of collection.

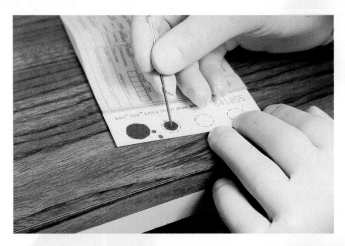

Collecting a blood sample from the newborn for neonatal metabolic screening. Blood from the capillary tube is placed in the circles of the filter paper, completely filling each circle.

administer thyroid hormone (eg, tablets can be crushed and mixed in a small amount of formula or applesauce). Advise parents that the child may experience temporary sleep disturbances or behavioral changes in response to therapy. Teach the parents how to assess for an increased pulse rate, which could indicate the presence of too much thyroid hormone, and advise them to report problems such as fatigue, which could indicate an improper drug dose that needs to be readjusted.

Caution parents to dress the child appropriately for the season to prevent hypothermia. Modify the child's diet by increasing the amount of fruits and bulk if constipation is a problem.

Reassure the family that the child will develop normally with hormone replacement therapy. Reinforce the importance of follow-up visits to assess growth rate and response to therapy and to regulate drug dosages as the child grows. Parents should be informed that therapy will be lifelong and is needed to promote the child's mental development.

HYPERTHYROIDISM

Hyperthyroidism occurs when thyroid hormone levels are increased (thyrotoxicosis). It is most common in adolescent girls and is almost always due to Graves' disease.

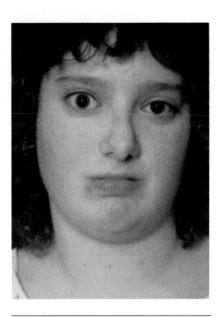

FIGURE 20–4. Exophthalmos and an enlarged thyroid in an adolescent with Graves' disease. *From Zitelli, B., & Davis, H. (Eds.) (1997). Atlas of pediatric physical diagnosis (3rd ed., p 271). St Louis: Mosby–Wolfe.*

NURSING ALERT

Propylthiouracil therapy can cause temporary side effects, including skin rashes, urticaria, and lymphadenopathy. If fever or sore throat develops, the child should be evaluated by a health care professional to rule out granulocytopenia.

Clinical Manifestations

Characteristic findings include an enlarged, nontender thyroid gland (goiter), prominent or bulging eyes (exophthalmos) (Fig. 20–4), tachycardia, nervousness, irritability, increased appetite, weight loss, emotional lability, heat intolerance, and muscle weakness. The thyroid gland may be slightly enlarged or grow to three to four times its normal size, feel warm, soft, and fleshy, and have an auditory bruit on auscultation. The disorder often presents in the preschool years, but with an increased incidence in adolescence. Onset is subtle, and the condition often goes unrecognized for 1–2 years. The condition is rare in children, with an incidence of 8 cases per million children per year.[12]

Children with Graves' disease usually manifest behavioral problems and declining performance in school. They become easily frustrated in the classroom and overheated and fatigued during physical education class. It is difficult for them to relax or sleep. These symptoms usually prompt parents to seek medical treatment for them. Other symptoms include an increased appetite with weight loss, tremors, and tachycardia. Exophthalmos is less common in children than in adults.

Etiology and Pathophysiology

Graves' disease is an autoimmune disorder in which the body produces antibodies that attack the cells of the thyroid gland. It has a high familial incidence. Immunoglobulins produced by the B lymphocytes stimulate oversecretion of thyroid hormones, resulting in the clinical symptoms. Signs and symptoms such as tachycardia, tremor, excessive perspiration, irritability, and emotional lability are caused by hyperactivity of the sympathetic nervous system. The remission rate is approximately 25% every 2 years.[12]

Other, more unusual forms of hyperthyroidism result from thyroiditis and thyroid hormone–producing tumors, including thyroid adenomas and carcinomas, and pituitary adenomas. Congenital hyperthyroidism can occur in infants of mothers with Graves' disease because of transplacental transfer of immunoglobulins.

Diagnostic Tests and Medical Management

Diagnostic studies include laboratory evaluation of serum TSH, T_3 (triiodothyronine) and T_4 levels, and a thyroid scan. Blood studies are also performed to detect autoantibodies specific for the various thyroid disorders.

The goal of medical management is to inhibit excessive secretion of thyroid hormones. Treatment may include antithyroid drug therapy, radiation therapy, or surgery. Drug therapy is most often used as the initial treatment modality, but compliance is often a problem because of drug side effects. Methimazole (Tapazole) and propylthiouracil (PTU) are given to inhibit thyroid hormone secretion. Treatment continues for 18 months to 2 years or until the thyroid decreases in size. Symptoms usually improve within weeks of starting treatment.

If drug therapy is ineffective, radiation therapy using radioactive iodine (^{131}I) is the next treatment choice. Thyroidectomy is the third alternative; however, destruction or removal of the thyroid gland often results in permanent hypothyroidism, necessitating hormone replacement therapy.

Nursing Assessment

Assess the child's vital signs, as blood pressure and pulse may be elevated. Keep a record of food intake. Accurate measurement and recording of height and weight are important to establish baselines and identify patterns of growth. Observe the child's behavior, activity, and level of fatigue.

Nursing Diagnosis

Common nursing diagnoses for the child with hyperthyroidism include the following:

- Ineffective Thermoregulation (Elevated) related to excessive activity of the sympathetic nervous system
- Altered Nutrition: Less Than Body Requirements related to increased metabolic rate
- Body Image Disturbance related to presence of prominent eyes, excessive perspiration, and tremors
- Fatigue related to imbalance in energy production, muscle weakness, and sleep disturbance
- Self-Esteem Disturbance related to declining school performance and behavior problems

Nursing Management

Nursing care focuses on teaching the child and parents about the disorder and its treatment, promoting rest, providing emotional support, and, if the child requires surgery, providing preoperative and postoperative teaching and care. Promote increased caloric intake by providing five or six moderate meals per day. Encourage the child and family to express their feelings and concerns about the disorder. Pointing out even slight improvements in the child's condition increases compliance with therapy.

Children with hyperthyroidism are easily fatigued. Rest periods should be scheduled at school and home and physical activities kept to a minimum until symptoms resolve. Encourage parents to provide a cool environment and allow the child to wear fewer clothes until symptoms subside.

Children who have partial or total removal of the thyroid gland receive antithyroid drugs, such as iodine, for approximately 2 weeks before surgery. Teach the child and parents about drug therapy and instruct parents to watch for side effects of antithyroid drugs, including fever, urticaria, and lymphadenopathy. Provide preoperative teaching (see Chap. 4). Young children, in particular, may be fearful about having their throat "cut." Postoperatively, observe for signs of severe thyrotoxicosis (thyroid "storm") and hypercalcemia, which can be life threatening. Treatment includes administration of antithyroid drugs and propranolol. Monitor the child's surgical site. Assess the child for bleeding, hoarseness, and difficulty breathing, which may be signs of inflammation.

Teach the family about the need for lifelong thyroid hormone replacement if radiation or surgery is performed. Make sure the child is monitored regularly to assure that the T_4 level is adequate to sustain growth.

NURSING ALERT

Thyroid storm may occur when thyroid hormone is suddenly released into the bloodstream during surgery. The child experiences fever, diaphoresis, and tachycardia, progressing to shock and, if untreated, death.

► DISORDERS OF ADRENAL FUNCTION

CUSHING'S SYNDROME

Cushing's syndrome, also called adrenocortical hyperfunction, is characterized by a group of symptoms resulting from excess levels of glucocorticoids (especially cortisol) in the bloodstream. It is uncommon in children and the true incidence is unknown. During infancy and childhood, most cases are due to malignant adrenal tumor. After 8 years of age more than half of the cases are due to secretion of adrenocorticotropic hormone (ACTH) by a pituitary adenoma.[13]

The initial sign in most children is gradual excessive weight gain and growth retardation. It generally takes up to 5 years for the child to develop the characteristic "cushingoid" appearance, which includes a moon face (chubby cheeks and a double chin) and fat pads over the shoulders and back (buffalo hump). Other signs and symptoms include hypertension, weight gain with distribution primarily on the trunk, striae on the abdomen, buttocks, and thighs, fatigue, muscle weakness and wasting, acne, bruising, osteoporosis, growth failure with delayed bone age, mental changes, and delayed puberty.

Causes of Cushing's syndrome include tumors of the pituitary gland that result in an overproduction of ACTH (which stimulates cortisol secretion), tumors of the adrenal glands, and hyperplasia of one or both adrenal glands. The increased secretion of cortisol alters metabolism, resulting in the following physiologic changes:

- Catabolism of protein, leading to capillary weakness and poor wound healing
- Decreased absorption of calcium from the intestines, leading to demineralization of the bone and osteoporosis
- An increased appetite, leading to the accumulation of fat
- Salt-retaining activity of cortisol, leading to an increase in blood volume and hypertension

Diagnosis is based on characteristic physical findings and laboratory values, including reduced serum levels of potassium and phosphorus; elevated serum calcium concentration; increased 24-hour urinary levels of free cortisol, and 17–hydroxycorticosteroid (17-OHCs); and loss of diurnal rhythm in serum cortisol (usually elevated at night).

The adrenal suppression test is used for the initial screening of children with suspected adrenocortical hyperfunction. If this test reveals that adrenal cortisol output is not suppressed overnight after a dose of dexamethasone, further diagnostic testing is necessary to determine the cause of hypercortisolism. Computed tomography (CT) and magnetic resonance imaging (MRI) are used to detect tumors in the adrenal and pituitary glands.

Surgical removal is the current treatment of choice for adrenal tumors or pituitary adenomas. Cortisol replacement is required when both adrenal glands are removed. The prognosis for children with malignant adrenal tumors is poor.

Nursing Management

The nurse usually encounters a child with Cushing's syndrome when the child is hospitalized for diagnostic evaluation or surgery. Nursing assessment includes monitoring the child's vital signs and fluid and nutritional status, and assessing muscle strength and endurance during hospital play activities.

Teach the child and family about the disorder and its treatment, and, for children undergoing surgery, provide preoperative and postoperative teaching and care. Answer any questions the child and family may have and explain all laboratory and diagnostic tests. Explain to parents that the child's cushingoid appearance is reversible with treatment. Provide nutritional guidance or refer the child and parents to a nutritionist to promote maintenance of an appropriate weight.

Preoperative and postoperative teaching and care are similar to those for the child undergoing surgery (see Chap. 4). Refer to Chapter 14 for general nursing care of the child with cancer.

For children who require cortisol replacement therapy, administering the drug early in the morning or every other day causes fewer symptoms than daily administration and mimics the normal diurnal pattern of cortisol secretion. Cortisol replacement in the postoperative period must be explained carefully to parents. Hydrocortisone (Cortef, Solu-Cortef, cortisone acetate) comes in liquid, tablet, or injectable form. Teach parents how and when to administer the injectable form, usually when the child is vomiting or has diarrhea, or cannot take the oral medication. The oral preparations of cortisone have a bitter taste and can cause gastric irritation. Giving the dose at mealtimes and using antacids between meals helps reduce these side effects.

Teach parents to be alert to signs of acute adrenal insufficiency during the withdrawal of corticosteroid therapy, and to inform all health care providers of the child's condition and medication. A medical alert bracelet should be worn at all times.

NURSING ALERT

Signs of acute adrenal insufficiency may include increased irritability, headache, confusion, restlessness, nausea and vomiting, diarrhea, abdominal pain, dehydration, fever, loss of appetite, and lethargy. If untreated, the child will go into shock. In newborns, the symptoms include failure to thrive, weakness, vomiting, and dehydration. Hyponatremia and hyperkalemia are key signs.

CONGENITAL ADRENAL HYPERPLASIA

Congenital adrenal hyperplasia, sometimes called adrenogenital syndrome, adrenocortical hyperplasia, or congenital adrenogenital hyperplasia, is an autosomal recessive disorder that causes a deficiency of one of the enzymes necessary for the synthesis of cortisol and aldosterone. The defective gene is located on the short arm of chromosome 6. It occurs in 1 in 5000–15,000 live births, and males and females are affected equally.[14] There are two classic forms of the disorder: salt-losing, caused by the blockage of aldosterone production, and non-salt-losing, or simple virilization.

More than 80% of children with congenital adrenal hyperplasia have partial or complete 21-hydroxylase enzyme deficiency. Another 10% have 11-hydroxylase deficiency. The remainder have deficiencies involving five other enzymes. In its most severe form the disorder can be life threatening.

Clinical Manifestations

Congenital adrenal hyperplasia is the most common cause of **pseudohermaphroditism** (ambiguous genitalia) in newborn girls. The female infant is born with an enlarged clitoris and labial fusions (Fig. 20–5). Severely virilized females may be mistaken for males with cryptorchidism, hypospadias, or micropenis. The male infant may look normal at birth or may have a slightly enlarged penis and hyperpigmented scrotum. The boy may have an adult-sized penis by school age, but the testes are appropriately sized for age. Partial enzyme deficiency produces less obvious symptoms. Precocious puberty and tall stature for age may be noted later. Recurrent vomiting, dehydration, metabolic acidosis, hypotension, and hypoglycemia are characteristic signs of the salt-wasting form of the disorder. Hypertension with hypokalemic alkalosis is alternately found in children with 11-hydroxylase deficiency.

Etiology and Pathophysiology

In all forms, increased secretion of ACTH occurs in response to diminished cortisol levels. In cases of 21-hydroxylase enzyme deficiency, there is usually

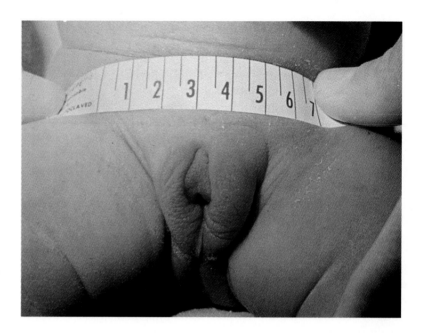

FIGURE 20–5. Newborn girl with ambiguous genitalia.
Courtesy of Patrick C. Walsh, M.D.

deficient aldosterone synthesis leading to excessive renal excretion of salt (salt losing).

During fetal development the lack of cortisol triggers the pituitary to continue secretion of ACTH. This in turn stimulates overproduction of the adrenal androgens. Female virilization of the external genitalia begins in week 10 of gestation. If untreated, the overproduction of androgens results in accelerated height, early closure of the epiphyseal plates, and premature sexual development with both pubic and axillary hair.

Acute adrenal insufficiency (see p. 000) can develop with any significant illness or injury because cortisol, which the child cannot produce, is an important hormone in the stress response.

Diagnostic Tests and Medical Management

Diagnosis in infants and children is usually confirmed by laboratory evaluation of serum 17-hydroxyprogesterone level. Routine newborn screening for congenital adrenal hyperplasia is performed in 14 states.[15] Prenatal screening is available. In instances of ambiguous genitalia, a **karyotype** (chromosome study) is obtained to determine the gender of the infant. Ultrasonography may be used to visualize pelvic structures. In the salt-wasting form of the disorder the child may have hyponatremia, hyperkalemia, a high urine sodium level, and low serum and urinary aldosterone levels.

The goal of treatment is to suppress adrenal secretion of androgens by replacing deficient hormones. This is accomplished by the oral administration of glucocorticoids (hydrocortisone). The glucocorticoid replacement leads to a reduction in secretion of ACTH which had overstimulated the adrenal cortex. As a result, excessive adrenal androgen production is suppressed. Growth parameters and sexual development are closely monitored to watch for return to a more normal rate. If the infant has the salt-wasting form of the disorder, salt is added to the infant's formula and a mineralocorticoid (Florinef) is given to replace the missing hormone. Hormone dosage must be doubled or tripled during acute illnesses or injury and for surgery. Injectable hydrocortisone is used for severe stress.

RESEARCH CONSIDERATIONS

Neonatal screening studies have revealed that the salt-losing form of congenital adrenal hyperplasia is more common than the non-salt-losing form by a 2- or 3-to-1 ratio. Early deaths in undiagnosed infants probably account for the lack of previous knowledge of the true incidence.[14]

Reconstructive surgery of the enlarged clitoris is often performed on girls during the first year of life. Vaginal reconstruction is performed in a later procedure.

Nursing Assessment

Assess the infant and child for signs of dehydration, electrolyte imbalance, and shock in the salt-wasting form of the disease. Monitor vital signs and assess peripheral perfusion (capillary refill, distal pulses, color and temperature of the extremities) frequently to detect early changes in condition.

Assess the parents' emotional response to a child with ambiguous genitalia and a chronic condition. Explore their values and beliefs regarding gender roles and sexuality while awaiting results of the karyotype.

Nursing Diagnosis

Nursing diagnoses for the child with congenital adrenal hyperplasia might include:

- Risk for Altered Parenting related to a child with undetermined gender identity
- Risk for Caregiver Role Strain related to care of a child with a chronic, potentially life-threatening condition
- Risk for Fluid Volume Deficit related to excess excretion of salt by the kidneys
- Altered Growth and Development related to premature development of secondary sex characteristics and accelerated growth

Nursing Management

Nursing care of the newborn with congenital adrenal hyperplasia focuses on teaching parents about the disorder and its treatment, providing emotional support, and preoperative and postoperative teaching for parents of infants undergoing reconstructive surgery. Because of the risk for adrenal insufficiency, the child will most likely be hospitalized for surgery rather than having outpatient surgery.

It is often difficult for parents to accept that their infant, whose genitalia look male, is really female. With medication and surgery the genitalia assume a female appearance and all organs necessary for future childbearing are usually functional. Several surgeries may be performed before 2 years of age and then during adolescence to dilate the vagina.

Nurses can assist parents in educating the child's siblings, grandparents, other family members, and day-care workers about the condition. In the newborn nursery the infant should be referred to as "your beautiful infant," not "your son" or "your daughter," until gender identity is confirmed.

Inform parents that genetic counseling should be provided for the child during adolescence. Parents considering a future pregnancy should also be informed that prenatal testing may detect congenital adrenal hyperplasia in the fetus. Refer the family for counseling if indicated.

Care in the Community

Teach parents about the special problems that develop in the salt-wasting form of the disease during acute illness. Explain the medication regimen and help the family develop an emergency care plan. Teach parents how to administer intramuscular injections of hydrocortisone. Make sure the parents have an emergency kit of injectable hydrocortisone at home to be used when the child is vomiting or has diarrhea. If injectable hydrocortisone is not available, the child needs urgent treatment in an emergency department. The child may become dehydrated quickly and need intravenous fluid and electrolyte replacement in addition to higher doses of hydrocortisone. The child should wear a medical alert bracelet.

ADRENAL INSUFFICIENCY (ADDISON'S DISEASE)

Adrenal insufficiency, also known as Addison's disease, is a rare disorder in childhood characterized by a deficiency of glucocorticoids (cortisone) and mineralocorticoids (aldosterone). It may be acquired after trauma; with tuberculosis, acquired immunodeficiency syndrome (AIDS), or fungal infections that cause destruction of the adrenal glands; or as the result of an autoimmune process.

Adrenal insufficiency usually develops slowly as the adrenal glands deteriorate. The early signs may not be noticed but include weakness with fatigue; anorexia and salt craving; poor weight gain or weight loss; hyperpigmentation at pressure points, lip borders and buccal mucosa, nipples, body creases, and scarred areas of the body; abdominal pain; nausea and vomiting; and diarrhea. Symptomatic hypoglycemia may also be present. If the child experiences a stressful period (illness, injury, or surgery), acute adrenal insufficiency may occur. Signs of an adrenal crisis include weakness, fever, abdominal pain, hypoglycemia with seizures, hypotension, dehydration, and shock.

Serum cortisol and urinary 17-hydroxycorticoid levels are measured in the early morning. Low levels are associated with adrenal insufficiency. The ACTH stimulation test is used to detect adrenal gland reserve. Electrolyte values generally reveal low serum sodium, elevated serum potassium, and low fasting blood glucose levels. CT may be used to visualize the adrenal glands.

Treatment involves replacement of the deficient hormones. Oral hydrocortisone is given in the lowest therapeutic dose to control symptoms and promote normal growth. Fludrocortisone acetate (Florinef) is administered to replace the missing mineralocorticoid in children with aldosterone deficiency. Adrenal crisis is treated by fluid and electrolyte resuscitation, treatment of the precipitating illness or injury, adequate doses of glucocorticoid, and maintenance doses of mineralocorticoid.

Nursing Management

Nursing management focuses on educating the child and parents about the disorder, providing emotional support, and caring for the child during acute episodes. See the earlier discussion of congenital adrenal hyperplasia for further detail.

PHEOCHROMOCYTOMA

Pheochromocytoma is a tumor that usually originates in the chromaffin cells of the adrenal medulla. In most cases these tumors are benign and curable. They can occur in a familial pattern (autosomal dominant trait) with a 3:2 male to female ratio.[16] Most tumors are diagnosed in children between the ages of 6 and 14 years.

Clinical manifestations include labile hypertension with a systolic reading that may reach 250 mm Hg, tachycardia, profuse sweating with cool extremities, headache, nausea and vomiting, weight loss, visual disturbances, polydipsia, and polyuria. The classic triad of signs includes new onset hypertension, new or worsening diabetes mellitus, and hypertensive crisis. Because release of catecholamines (norepinephrine and epinephrine) from the tumor is not continuous, these symptoms occur intermittently. Attacks may occur daily or monthly. In some cases the condition may be silent until a stressor such as surgery causes a hypertensive crisis.

Diagnosis is based on 24-hour urine studies to detect the presence of catecholamines and CT, MRI, and ultrasound studies to localize the tumor. The treatment of choice is surgical removal of the tumor; however, the procedure is dangerous and may result in pheochromocytoma crisis.[17] Alpha- and beta-adrenergic blocking agents to control hypertension are given for 10–14 days before surgery. Postoperatively, for several days, a 24–hour urine collection is measured for catecholamines to determine if all tumor sites were removed. With successful removal of all tumor sites, the prognosis is generally good. Follow-up is important to assess for recurrence.

NURSING ALERT

Pheochromocytoma crisis manifests with seizures, shock, altered level of consciousness, disseminated intravascular coagulation, rhabomyolysis (skeletal muscle destruction), and acute renal failure, which can result in death.

Nursing Management

Nursing care is mainly supportive. Provide preoperative and postoperative teaching and care (see Chap. 4). Preoperatively, monitor vital signs and observe for signs of complications associated with pheochromocytoma crisis. Administer antihypertensives and watch for any signs of hyperglycemia (see Table 20–5). Postoperatively, monitor blood pressure and observe for signs of shock. Lifelong follow-up care is required as symptoms have recurred more than 20 years after surgery.[17]

20-5	Comparison of the Signs and Symptoms of Hyperglycemia and Hypoglycemia	
Hyperglycemia	**Hypoglycemia**	
Gradual onset	Rapid onset	
Lethargy, sleepiness, slowed responses, or confusion	Irritability, nervousness, difficulty concentrating or speaking, behavior change	
Deep, rapid breathing	Shallow breathing	
Weak pulse	Tachycardia	
Flushed skin, dry skin	Pallor, sweating	
Dry mucous membranes, thirst, hunger, dehydration	Moist mucous membranes, hunger	
Weakness, fatigue	Tremors, shaky feeling	
Headache, abdominal pain, nausea, vomiting	Headache, dizziness	
Blurred vision	Blurred vision, double vision	
Shock	Numb lips or mouth	
	Confusion, repeating something over and over	
	Unconsciousness, seizure	
	Photophobia	

▶ DISORDERS OF PANCREATIC FUNCTION

DIABETES MELLITUS

Diabetes mellitus, the most common metabolic disease in children, is a disorder of carbohydrate, protein, and fat metabolism. There are two main types of diabetes.

The majority of children with diabetes have insulin-dependent diabetes mellitus (IDDM), or type I. Formerly this condition was known as juvenile diabetes. In the United States about 1–2 children per 1000 have IDDM. There are 12 new cases per 100,000 children per year.[18] The peak ages of occurrence are between 10 and 12 years of age in girls and 12 and 14 years of age in boys.[19]

Non-insulin-dependent diabetes mellitus (NIDDM), or type II, is usually contracted as an adult and is associated with being overweight. NIDDM that occurs in adolescents is referred to as maturity-onset diabetes of youth (MODY). Diet, exercise, and oral hypoglycemic drugs are used to treat non-insulin-dependent diabetes.

Because the majority of children with diabetes have IDDM, the remainder of the discussion focuses on this form of the disease.

Clinical Manifestations

The classic signs of IDDM are polyuria, polydipsia, and **polyphagia** (excessive appetite) with significant weight loss, as occurred with Shawnda in the opening scenario. Unexplained fatigue or lethargy, headaches, stomachaches, and occasional enuresis may also occur in a previously toilet-trained child. Adolescent girls may have vaginitis caused by *Candida,* which thrives in the hyperglycemic tissues. Symptoms develop gradually and insidiously but have usually been present less than a month. In severe cases diabetic ketoacidosis (DKA), a type of metabolic acidosis, may develop. This condition is discussed in more detail on p. 897.

Etiology and Pathophysiology

It is thought that IDDM is caused by a genetic component, environmental influences, and an autoimmune response. IDDM has strong familial tendencies but does not show any specific pattern of inheritance. The child inherits a susceptibility to the disease rather than the disease itself.

Environmental factors such as viruses or chemicals in the diet are believed to play an important role in damaging the beta cells in the islets of Langerhans (Fig. 20–6). These are the cells responsible for insulin production. The incidence of onset of IDDM is increased during winter when viral diseases are more prevalent. Often the child has a history of a viral infection 1–2 months before the onset of symptoms.

The presence of circulating antibodies in pancreatic islet cells indicates that the body is having an immunologic response to an inflammatory process. As the beta cells are destroyed, the level of circulating antibodies falls.

Insulin helps transport glucose into the cells so that this carbohydrate can be used as an energy source. It also prevents the outflow of glucose from the liver to the general circulation. In IDDM, over 90% of the beta cells in the islets of Langerhans are destroyed. The remaining beta cells are unable to produce sufficient insulin to maintain a normal blood glucose

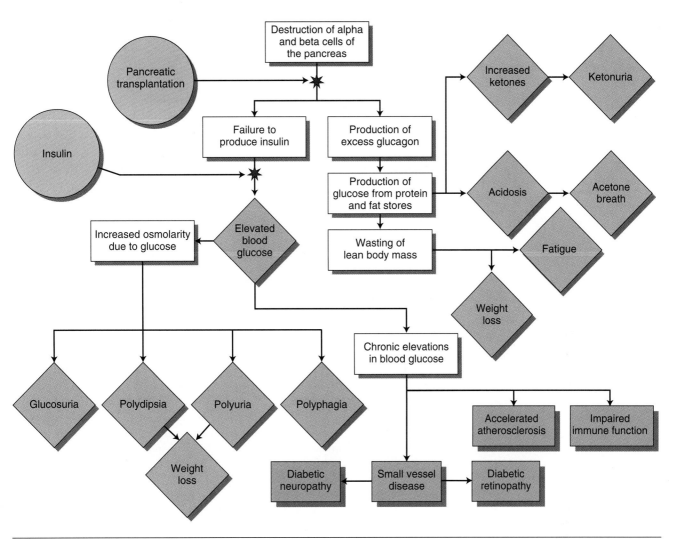

FIGURE 20–6. Pathophysiology of diabetes mellitus.
Adapted from Black, J.M., & Matassarian-Jacobs, E. (1997). Medical-surgical nursing: Clinical management for continuity of care (5th ed., p. 1958). Philadelphia: Saunders.

level, defined as 80–120 mg/dL. Lack of insulin results in a rise in blood glucose level and a decrease in the glucose level inside the cells. When the renal threshold for glucose (160 mg/dL) is exceeded, glycosuria occurs. Up to 1000 calories per day can be lost in the urine.

When glucose is unavailable to the cells for metabolism, an alternate source of energy is provided by free fatty acids. They are metabolized at an increased rate by the liver, producing acetyl coenzyme A (CoA). The by-products of acetyl CoA metabolism (ketone bodies) accumulate in the body, resulting in a state of metabolic acidosis, or ketoacidosis. (Refer to Chapter 8 for discussion of metabolic acidosis.)

Diagnostic Tests and Medical Management

Diagnosis is based on the presence of classic symptoms and a plasma glucose level above 200 mg/dL. A glucose tolerance test is not required when these findings are present. A careful history is necessary to rule out the presence of a stress-related illness, corticosteroid usage, fracture, acute infection, cystic fibrosis, pancreatitis, or liver disease.

IDDM DIAGNOSTIC CRITERIA

When classic signs are not present, diagnostic criteria include a fasting plasma glucose of 140 mg/dL on two occasions plus two oral glucose tolerance tests with 2-hour plasma glucose levels plus one intervening value >200 mg/dL.[21]

20-6	Insulin Action (Subcutaneous Route)		
Type	Onset	Peak	Duration
Rapid Acting			
Lispro/Humalog	5–15 min	1 hr	≤4 hr
Short Acting			
Regular	½–1 hr	2–4 hr	6–8 hr
Intermediate Acting			
NPH	1–2 hr	6–12 hr	18–26 hr
Lente	1–2 hr	6–12 hr	24–26 hr
Long Acting			
Ultralente	4–6 hr	14–24 hr	28–36 hr

Therapy for IDDM combines insulin, dietary management, an exercise regimen, and physiologic support. The goal of initial insulin therapy is to lower blood glucose levels to normal. Long-term insulin therapy is calculated to maintain a blood glucose level as close to the normal range as possible and to minimize episodes of hyperglycemia and hypoglycemia (see Table 20–5). Insulin therapy must be balanced by the child's dietary intake and exercise level. Stress, infection, and illness increase insulin needs. In addition, insulin doses must be adjusted for growth and at puberty.

Several forms of insulin are available (Table 20–6). The most common insulin regimen consists of daily administration of a combination of a short-acting (regular) insulin and an intermediate-acting (NPH or Lente) or long-acting insulin (Ultralente) before breakfast and before the evening meal (Fig. 20–7). However, other routines requiring more injections are preferred by some physicians; for example, short-acting and intermediate-acting insulin before breakfast, short-acting insulin at supper, and intermediate-acting insulin at bedtime. Rapid-acting insulin has recently become available and may be used by older children and adolescents to achieve tight glucose control. Insulin is usually provided in prepackaged doses of 100 units/mL. Diluted insulin prepared by a pharmacist may be used for infants and toddlers who require a small insulin dosage. Some highly motivated adolescents may choose to use an insulin

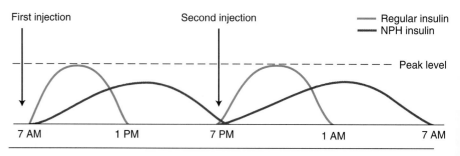

FIGURE 20–7. Insulin levels vary over a 24-hour period in relation to injections and mealtimes.

20-7	Advantages and Disadvantages of an External Insulin Infusion Pump	
Advantages	**Disadvantages**	

Advantages	Disadvantages
• Delivers a continuous infusion of insulin to match the basal rate needed plus an insulin bolus at mealtime • Helps maintain blood glucose control between meals • Improves growth in children • Reduces number of injections • Allows child to eat with less regard to a schedule	• Requires highly motivated child and supportive health care professionals • Requires willingness to live connected to a device (can be disconnected for short periods by removing or clamping the catheter) • Necessitates more time and energy to monitor blood glucose levels, dietary intake, and insulin bolus calculation • Involves changing syringe, catheter, and skin setup every 2–3 days

Based on information in Saudek, C.D. (1997). Novel forms of insulin delivery. Endocrinology and Metabolism Clinics of North America, 26(3), 599–610.

pump for diabetic management. Advantages and disadvantages of this approach are outlined in Table 20–7. A pen-shaped device that contains an insulin-filled cartridge may also be used by adolescents.

Daily blood glucose levels are tested and recorded before meals and at bedtime. Laboratory evaluation of glycosylated hemoglobin should be performed every 3 months.[19] Hemoglobin A_{1c} (HbA$_{1c}$) is considered the most precise measurement of glycosylated hemoglobin.[22] It provides an objective measurement of glycemic control because it represents the amount of glucose irreversibly attached to the hemoglobin molecule over an extended period (the life span of the red blood cell, approximately 120 days). The HbA$_{1c}$ level in persons without IDDM is 4–7%, and this level is higher in those with IDDM. The higher the level, the poorer has been the blood glucose control over the past 3 months.

Physical activity is associated with increased insulin sensitivity. Regular exercise and fitness improve metabolic control with a lower insulin dose. Blood lipid levels are also positively affected. However, the child must have an adequate caloric intake to prevent hypoglycemia.

Long-term complications of IDDM (retinopathy, heart disease, renal failure, and peripheral vascular disease) result from hyperglycemic effects on the blood vessels. Despite careful management, many diabetic children develop renal failure and loss of vision in adulthood. Careful management is important, however, to delay or lessen the severity of these complications.

Nursing Assessment

Physiologic Assessment
Children are generally admitted to the hospital at the time of diagnosis. Assess the child's physiologic status, focusing on vital signs and level of consciousness. Assess hydration by checking mucous membranes, skin turgor, and urine output. Blood initially is collected hourly to monitor blood gases, glucose, and electrolytes. Once the child is stable, assess dietary and caloric intake and the ability of the child or family to manage care.

 RESEARCH CONSIDERATIONS

The results of the Diabetes Control Complications Trial (DCCT) demonstrated that patients adhering to an intensive therapy regimen that focused on keeping both the blood glucose and HbA$_{1c}$ levels within the normal range were able to significantly decrease complications. Intensive therapy included:
• Monitoring blood glucose four times a day and once a week at 3 AM
• Monitoring dietary intake
• Varying the insulin dose to fit the carbohydrates eaten at each meal or snack if doing carbohydrate counting
• Anticipating exercise in the routine
As a result of the study findings, the American Diabetes Association recommends that all patients over 13 years of age strive for tight blood glucose control.[19]

 RESEARCH CONSIDERATIONS

An implantable insulin infusion pump with a glucose sensing device that can work for years without being accessed is now being used experimentally. FDA approval has not yet been sought.[21]

Psychosocial Assessment

Parents may feel guilty at the time of diagnosis if they waited to seek care until the child began to experience symptoms of DKA. Assess coping mechanisms, ability to manage the disease, and educational needs of both the child and parents.

Developmental Assessment

Assess the child's developmental level, particularly fine motor skills and cognitive level. The child will need to learn how to obtain and read a blood glucose sample and how to draw up and administer insulin. Children are usually able to perform some of these tasks with supervision by 6–8 years of age. Self-management is the eventual goal, and the child's responsibilities are gradually increased.

Adolescents perceive IDDM as a disability and often deny having the disease so they can be like their peers when eating and exercising. Talk with the adolescent to evaluate motivation to manage diet, the exercise regimen, blood glucose testing, and insulin therapy. Although the adolescent is cognitively able to manage self-care, the desire to be like peers often interferes with compliance.

Nursing Diagnosis

Several diagnoses that may apply to the child newly diagnosed with IDDM are provided in the accompanying Nursing Care Plans. Additional diagnoses that may be appropriate include the following:

- Risk for Fluid Volume Deficit related to hyperglycemia
- Ineffective Breathing Pattern related to effort to compensate for metabolic acidosis
- Powerlessness related to presence of a chronic illness requiring a rigorous dietary, exercise, and medication regimen
- Ineffective Management of Therapeutic Regimen related to denial of chronic condition

Nursing Management

Nursing care focuses on teaching the child and parents about the disease and its management, managing dietary intake, providing emotional support, and planning strategies for daily management in the community. Refer to the accompanying Nursing Care Plans, which summarize nursing care for the child who is hospitalized with newly diagnosed IDDM, and the child who is receiving care in the community.

Provide Education

The nurse is an important member of the management team (physician, nurse, nutritionist, and social worker) and is usually responsible for educating the child and family. Teaching often is performed in the home setting, since children may be hospitalized only briefly following diagnosis.

The timing and amount of information provided are especially important in the first days following diagnosis. Both the child and parents are often in a state of shock and disbelief; information presented during this period may need to be repeated. This time should be used to assess learning needs and to answer the family's questions. Initial teaching focuses on the skills necessary for home management (insulin administration, blood glucose testing, urine testing, record keeping, dietary management, and the recognition and treatment of both hypoglycemia and hyperglycemia).

Text continues on page 893.

NURSING CARE PLAN
THE CHILD HOSPITALIZED WITH NEWLY DIAGNOSED DIABETES MELLITUS

GOAL	INTERVENTION	RATIONALE	EXPECTED OUTCOME

1. Knowledge Deficit (Child and Parents) related to diabetic management in the newly diagnosed child

The child and parents will state diabetic home management regimen.	• Assess the child's developmental level and select an educational approach and self-care activities to match. Teach blood glucose monitoring, insulin administration, urine testing for ketones, and record keeping. • Use demonstration/return demonstration until the family and child are comfortable with procedures.	• Learning goals for the child must match knowledge and skill expectations appropriate for developmental stage. Diabetic management skills are needed for initial home management. • Evaluation permits positive reinforcement and guidance for modification of techniques.	The child and parents demonstrate proper technique for blood glucose monitoring, urine testing for ketones, insulin administration, and record keeping.

2. Risk for Injury related to periods of hypoglycemia and diabetic ketoacidosis

The child will experience few episodes of hypoglycemia and no episodes of diabetic ketoacidosis during hospitalization.	• Assess the child at least every 2 hours for signs of hypoglycemia (see Table 20–5). If hypoglycemia exists, check blood glucose to verify and administer source of quick sugar (sugar cube, hard candy). • When the child is NPO for a special procedure, withhold morning insulin and verify with physician when food, fluids, and insulin are to be given or if an intravenous infusion with dextrose is to be given. • Have glucose paste or 50% dextrose solution readily available.	• Hypoglycemia commonly occurs during hospitalization because of change in diet, lack of food intake, or illness. • Giving insulin without food intake can lead to hypoglycemia. Intravenous dextrose and insulin can be used when the child must be NPO. • Dextrose is used for emergency intravenous treatment of severe hypoglycemia. Glucose paste is used for oral treatment.	The child and staff manage episodes of hypoglycemia without a crisis developing.

Continued . . .

NURSING CARE PLAN
THE CHILD HOSPITALIZED WITH
NEWLY DIAGNOSED DIABETES MELLITUS– *Continued*

GOAL	INTERVENTION	RATIONALE	EXPECTED OUTCOME

2. Risk for Injury related to periods of hypoglycemia and diabetic ketoacidosis (continued)

GOAL	INTERVENTION	RATIONALE	EXPECTED OUTCOME
The child and parents will recognize signs and symptoms of poor glucose control.	• If signs of hyperglycemia are present, check blood glucose to confirm and administer insulin as ordered. Be prepared with intravenous equipment. • Check blood glucose three to four times daily, before each insulin dose. • Administer regular insulin doses on time and not more than 30 minutes before meals. • Have insulin doses checked by a second nurse. • Teach signs and symptoms of hypoglycemic and hyperglycemic reactions. • Teach child to test blood glucose when feeling different than usual, and record the reading and symptoms felt.	• If the child's condition is severe, insulin, fluid, and electrolyte therapy may be required. • Allows for consistent measurement and establishment of patterns. • Permits insulin peak action when food is available for digestion. • Doses are frequently small, and the possibility of error is great. • Recognition of and treatment of poor glucose control will prevent progression of symptoms. • Permits child to learn his/her specific symptoms of hyper- and hypoglycemia.	The child and family can describe symptoms of hypoglycemia and hyperglycemia.

3. Risk for Altered Nutrition: Less Than Body Requirements related to glycosuria

GOAL	INTERVENTION	RATIONALE	EXPECTED OUTCOME
The child will eat a well-balanced diet and maintain normal height and weight proportions. The child and parents will state understanding of dietary management of diabetes mellitus.	• Encourage and serve meals and snacks with consistent carbohydrates at the same time each day. • Make an appointment with a nutritionist who can assess the child's favorite foods and promote their utilization in the child's diet. Reinforce dietary information taught. • Provide sample menus and food exchanges, or teach the use of carbohydrate counting.	• Keeps blood glucose levels stable, thus reducing sequelae of disease. • The nutritionist can develop dietary recommendations that fit the specific needs of the child and include favorite foods, thereby increasing compliance with the diet. • Assists the family and adolescent in diet planning.	The child demonstrates normal growth without fluctuations in height, weight, and blood glucose level. The child and parents describe nutritional needs of the child and dietary management to meet those needs.

NURSING CARE PLAN
THE CHILD HOSPITALIZED WITH
NEWLY DIAGNOSED DIABETES MELLITUS– *Continued*

GOAL	INTERVENTION	RATIONALE	EXPECTED OUTCOME
4. Risk for Impaired Skin Integrity related to poor healing of injuries			
The child will maintain intact skin.	• Assess skin thoroughly each shift, especially extremities, mouth, and pressure areas.	• Diabetic patients may have decreased circulation and sensation, which can lead to skin breakdown.	The child's skin is free of any lesions.
	• Report and record any changes. • Keep lesions clean, keep them covered if draining, and check every 2 hours. • Take temperature at least every 4 hours. • Administer antibiotics if prescribed.	• Allows for close observation of changes. • Prevents infection or worsening of lesion. • Temperature elevation can indicate infection. • Diabetic patients may heal slowly because of circulatory changes and thus are more prone to infection. Antibiotics may be needed for treatment.	

NURSING CARE PLAN
THE CHILD WITH PREVIOUSLY DIAGNOSED
DIABETES MELLITUS BEING CARED FOR AT HOME

GOAL	INTERVENTION	RATIONALE	EXPECTED OUTCOME
1. Risk for Injury related to periods of hypoglycemia and diabetic ketoacidosis			
The child and parents will demonstrate emergency management of hypoglycemia.	• Identify sources of glucose to give in case of hypoglycemic reaction. Tell the child and parent to carry candy with them at all times.	• Access to sources of glucose and its rapid administration are important for emergency care.	The child and family can identify several glucose sources for emergencies. The child and family have candy or another source of glucose with them at each visit.
The child and parents will demonstrate management of sick days.	• Teach the child and family to test blood glucose and urine for ketones with acute symptoms and notify the physician.	• When the child is ill, hyperglycemia needs special management to prevent progression to ketoacidosis.	The child's hyperglycemic episodes do not progress to ketoacidosis.

Continued . . .

NURSING CARE PLAN
THE CHILD WITH PREVIOUSLY DIAGNOSED DIABETES MELLITUS BEING CARED FOR AT HOME– *Continued*

GOAL	INTERVENTION	RATIONALE	EXPECTED OUTCOME

2. Risk for Altered Nutrition: Less Than Body Requirements related to glycosuria

GOAL	INTERVENTION	RATIONALE	EXPECTED OUTCOME
The child will eat a well-balanced diet and maintain normal height and weight proportions.	• Assess height and weight regularly and plot on growth chart. • Make sure the child and family understand the importance of regularly spaced meals and snacks every day. Encourage them to keep a food diary.	• Inadequate insulin management can affect growth. • Nutritional intake should be balanced with insulin administration and exercise to prevent hypoglycemia.	Diet records indicate meals eaten at consistent times each day with appropriate distribution of carbohydrates, protein, and fats.

3. Altered Family Processes related to management of a chronic disease

GOAL	INTERVENTION	RATIONALE	EXPECTED OUTCOME
The child and family will manage medications, dietary modifications, and exercise regimen.	• Assess family's life-style. Attempt to fit the child's care needs to the family's schedule. • Discuss the family's routines for special occasions and vacations. Identify ways to modify the child's management for these occasions.	• Fitting the care to the family's life-style promotes compliance with regimen. • It is important for the child to participate in special events with the family and peers as a normal child to promote psychologic development.	The child and family make minimal changes in usual life-style while managing diabetes.

4. Body Image Disturbance related to perceived loss of health

GOAL	INTERVENTION	RATIONALE	EXPECTED OUTCOME
The child will demonstrate enhanced coping skills.	• Ask how the child has solved problems in the past. Review possible problems the child may encounter. Together evaluate the effectiveness of solutions. Suggest other solutions to consider.	• Children's success in mastering maturational conflicts and daily psychosocial problems will influence their pattern of coping.	The child demonstrates enhanced coping skills and expresses positive attitude toward self. The child displays warmth and affection toward family.
The child will develop positive self-esteem.	• Encourage the child to express feelings about disease to those he or she trusts. • Encourage the child to continue previous social activities and hobbies. Praise all endeavors. • Reassure the child that friends cannot see overt evidence of disease.	• Expressing feelings decreases anxiety. • Increased social interaction, especially in group sessions, improves self-esteem. • Self-esteem is closely linked to body image, especially during adolescence.	

NURSING CARE PLAN

THE CHILD WITH PREVIOUSLY DIAGNOSED DIABETES MELLITUS BEING CARED FOR AT HOME– *Continued*

GOAL	INTERVENTION	RATIONALE	EXPECTED OUTCOME
5. Altered Role Performance (Child) related to need to begin self-management of chronic disorder			
The child will develop independent ability to manage diabetes care.	• Allow the child to perform as many self-care procedures as possible at each developmental stage. • Encourage the child to make decisions regarding care. Review decisions and discuss possible alternative solutions. Role play possible scenarios. Provide 24-hour access to physician or diabetes nurse educator. Encourage the child to seek help early.	• Normal growth and development are ensured if the child is encouraged to participate in care from the beginning. • Feelings of trust are developed when children sense that their decisions are respected or at least considered by others.	The child is able to perform as many diabetic care techniques as possible for age.

Explain the goals of insulin therapy. Teach the child and parents how to administer insulin and test blood glucose (Fig. 20–8). Rotating the injection sites is important to decrease the chances of lipodystrophy (development of fibrotic tissue that interferes with absorption of insulin) (Fig. 20–9). An understanding of the different types of insulin and their actions is essential.

Once the child and parents demonstrate understanding of this information, guidelines for managing episodes of hyperglycemia during acute illness and using a sliding scale are taught. A sliding scale indicates specific insulin dosages appropriate for a particular blood glucose level. The family also needs to learn "sick day" care guidelines to prevent diabetic ketoacidosis.

Caution parents to check the blood glucose level of a toddler who is extremely sleepy or irritable, as these can be signs of either hypoglycemia or hyperglycemia.

Manage Dietary Intake

The preferred diet for children with IDDM is a low-saturated-fat, low-sodium diet that avoids concentrated sugars. The child needs adequate calories to reach or maintain a desirable body weight. Usually at the time of diagnosis the child needs to regain lost weight, so extra calories may be recommended.

Dietary intake should include three meals per day, eaten at consistent intervals, plus a midafternoon carbohydrate snack and a bedtime snack high in protein. A consistent intake of carbohydrates at each meal and

CLINICAL TIP

The recommended distribution of total calories by food group for children with IDDM is[23]:

Carbohydrates	55–60%
Protein	12–20%
Fat	<30%

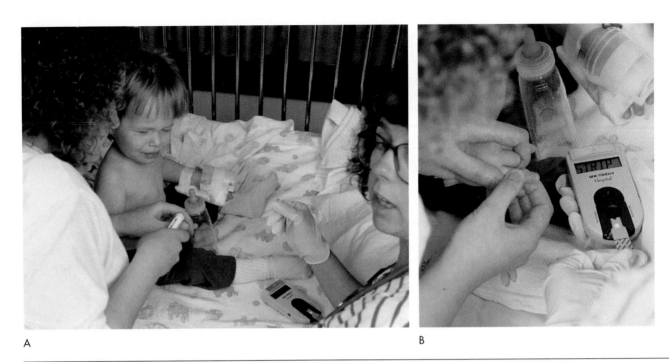

A   B

FIGURE 20–8. This mother is being taught how to test her child's blood glucose level.

snack is needed. The American Diabetes Association's exchange lists facilitate dietary management by suggesting portions and types of foods and noting allowed substitutions.

Many adolescents find that carbohydrate counting for dietary management gives them more flexibility in disease management. They learn the number of units of insulin needed to cover the grams of carbohydrates eaten.

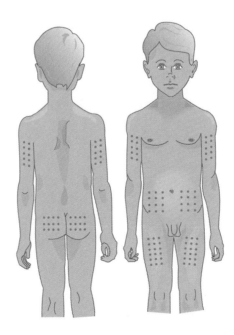

FIGURE 20–9. Insulin injection sites. Give all morning insulin in one site (eg, arms) and all evening insulin in another (eg, legs) because of different rates of absorption from these sites. Space injections about ½ inch (1.25 cm) apart.

Provide Emotional Support

The diagnosis of IDDM often comes as a shock to the family. If there is a familial history, parents may feel guilty about having caused the disease. The diagnosis of a chronic disease that requires daily management can be difficult to accept. Give parents information about diabetes education programs, put them in touch with other parents of diabetic children, and help them to learn the role they can play in managing the disease.

Support for the child depends on age and developmental stage. Encourage the child to express feelings about the disease and its management. The adolescent may benefit from contact with other adolescents who have IDDM.

Discharge Planning and Home Care Teaching

Home care needs should be identified and addressed before discharge. This is often difficult because of the short hospitalization of children with newly diagnosed diabetes. Home health or visiting nurses should be notified to visit the family within 24 hours of discharge. The goal of the teaching plan is to enable the child and family to assume the necessary responsibility for home care and to manage hyperglycemic episodes.

Make every effort to incorporate the diabetic regimen (insulin administration, diet, blood glucose monitoring, and exercise) into the family's present life-style. The fewer changes the family has to make, the greater the chance of compliance.

Provide written materials and refer parents to books and other materials they can use in teaching the child about diabetes (see Table 20–8). The American Diabetes Association is a good source of information (see Appendix F).

Care in the Community

During follow-up visits, ask the child or parents about signs indicating problems of diabetic control (Table 20–9). Record growth measurements and vital signs in the child's chart. Assess the child's sexual development using Tanner staging guidelines (see Chap. 3). Puberty may be delayed if diabetic control is inadequate. Review the child's typical dietary intake and exercise regimens.

20-8   Teaching Tools for Children With Diabetes Mellitus

Understanding Insulin Dependent Diabetes, by Peter Chase, M.D.; Pink Panther; for parents and adolescents

Kids, Food and Diabetes, by Gloria Loring; Chicago: Contemporary Books, 1986; for parents

The Truth About Stacy, by Ann M. Martin; one of The Babysitters Club books; excellent resource for girls age 9–12 years

Grilled Cheese at Four O'Clock in the Morning, an American Diabetes Association publication (see Appendix F); excellent for boys age 10–14 years

Several pamphlets and dolls are available that illustrate anatomy and physiology, provide step-by-step instructions on injecting insulin, and allow the child to practice injections.

20-9	Questions to Ask to Identify Problems in Diabetic Control

- Is the child hungry at meals? Between meals?
- How much fluid is the child drinking?
- Has the child been going to the bathroom frequently or had episodes of bedwetting?
- Does the child have dry skin?
- Are there sores on the feet? Do scratches or scrapes take a long time to heal?
- Has the child had any skin infections?
- Does the child have changes in mood (depression, unexplained sadness, irritability) or energy level from day to day or throughout the day?

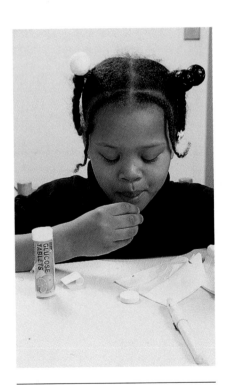

FIGURE 20-10. Shawnda is old enough to understand the need to take glucose tablets or another form of a rapidly absorbed sugar when her blood glucose level is low.

Continually work with the child to help him or her assume responsibility for self-care, and with parents to promote the child's self-care (Fig. 20–10). The child's developmental stage and cognitive level influence his or her readiness to take on responsibility for self-care. Summer camps and other programs for diabetic children are often helpful in providing support.

The preschool child's need for autonomy and control can be met by allowing the child to choose snacks or to pick which finger to stick for glucose testing and by helping parents to gather necessary supplies. School-age children can learn to test blood glucose, administer insulin, and keep records. They should be taught how to select foods appropriate for dietary management and how to plan an exercise program. School-age children need to learn to recognize the signs of hypoglycemia and hyperglycemia, and understand the importance of carrying a rapidly absorbed sugar product.[24]

Adolescents should take on total responsibility for self-care. Although they understand explanations about the potential complications of diabetes, they are present-time oriented and may rebel against the daily regimentation of insulin injections and dietary management. Successful self-care depends in part on the adolescent's adjustment to the chronic nature of the disease and feelings of being different from peers.

Children with IDDM often learn manipulative behaviors, using their disease to obtain something they want. Teach parents to be alert to signs of manipulation, such as helpless, demanding, or whining behaviors, and any evidence of poor coping. Food may become a battleground for toddlers who are picky eaters, but must have adequate intake for the insulin dose.[18] Referral for counseling may be appropriate for some families.

The child with IDDM may have circulatory and neurologic changes that make skin breakdown a greater risk than normal. If signs of infection occur, the parents should seek medical care. Emphasize the importance of good foot care, for example, wearing clean white cotton socks; changing socks and shoes when they are damp; washing, drying, and powdering feet; and keeping toenails short.

Explain to parents that the child should wear some type of medical alert identification. Assist them in having an Individual School Health Plan developed (see Chap. 5) to assure that school administrators and teachers can identify the signs of hypoglycemia or hyperglycemia and provide emergency management.

DIABETIC KETOACIDOSIS

Diabetic ketoacidosis (DKA) is the condition that results in children with IDDM when the body must burn fat for energy because no insulin is available to metabolize glucose. DKA is more likely to occur with stressors such as infections.

Characteristic signs of DKA include dehydration, weight loss, tachycardia, flushed ears and cheeks, Kussmaul respirations, acetone breath, depressed level of consciousness, and hypotension. The disorder may progress to electrolyte disturbances, arrhythmias, and shock. Children complain of abdominal or chest pain, begin to vomit, have labored breathing, and can slowly slip into a semiconscious state. Hyperglycemia, **glycosuria** (abnormal amount of glucose in the urine), and ketonuria are also present.

With decreased glucose metabolism and hyperglycemia, osmotic diuresis is triggered. This results in a hyperosmolar state with dehydration and hypotension. The hyperglycemia accounts for most of the osmolality. When lipids are used for an energy source, metabolic acidosis and ketone production result.

DKA is present when the following findings are present: blood glucose level greater than 300 mg/dL, ketones in the serum, acidosis (pH less than or equal to 7.30 and bicarbonate less than 15 mEq/L), glycosuria, and ketonuria. Electrolyte disorders also occur (hyperkalemia, hyperchloremia, hyponatremia, hypophosphatemia, hypocalcemia, and hypomagnesemia.) Diabetic coma occurs when the serum osmolality exceeds 350 mOsm/kg. Normal serum osmolality is 275–295 mOsm/kg. Cerebral edema is a life-threatening complication thought to be related to hyperosmolality.[25]

The child with ketoacidosis is usually hospitalized. Medical management includes insulin by continuous infusion pump to decrease the serum glucose level at a rate not to exceed 100 mg/dL/hr. Faster reduction of hyperglycemia and serum osmolality may be related to the development of cerebral edema.

Nursing Management

The child's vital signs, respiratory status, perfusion, and mental status are continuously monitored. Frequent tests are performed to assess the blood and urine for glucose levels and ketones. Intake and output are monitored.

Intravenous fluids are given in boluses of 20 mL/kg if the child is in shock. Adequate fluids are given to reverse the fluid deficit. Electrolytes are replaced as needed. The insulin infusion must be carefully maintained to control the gradual reduction in hyperglycemia.

The prevention of future episodes of DKA is important. The parents and child need to learn strategies to keep hyperglycemic episodes from progressing to DKA. For example, the child's urine should be tested for ketones if three or four consecutive blood glucose readings are higher than 200 mg/dL. If the child has a high blood glucose and moderate or large amounts of ketones, treatment with extra insulin and fluids can be initiated. This monitoring is especially important when the child has significant stressors such as an illness. Insulin is needed even when the child is not eating to counter the hormones secreted in response to the stressor.[20]

HYPOGLYCEMIA

Hypoglycemia can develop within minutes in children with diabetes mellitus. The symptoms outlined in Table 20–5 may occur when there is a sudden drop in blood glucose levels. Common causes include an error in insulin dosage, inadequate calories because of missed meals, or exercise without a corresponding increase in caloric intake.

Hypoglycemia can be diagnosed on the basis of the sudden onset of signs and symptoms. A blood glucose reading should be taken to confirm the diagnosis, since signs of hyperglycemia and hypoglycemia may be difficult to distinguish. Give glucose immediately in the form of a carbohydrate-containing snack or drink, cake frosting, glucose tablets, or glucose paste. In the hospital setting, administer an intravenous infusion of dextrose to prevent progression of symptoms. If the child becomes unconscious, cake frosting or glucose paste can be squeezed onto the gums. Retest the blood glucose level if the child is not better in 15–20 minutes. If the reading is still low, give more sugar. Give an extra snack if the next meal is not planned for more than 30 minutes or if activity is planned.

Nursing Management

Teach parents and children to recognize the signs of hypoglycemia and take appropriate action. Parents can be taught to give an intramuscular or subcutaneous dose of **glucagon** (a hormone produced by the pancreas that helps release stored glucose from the liver) for severe cases of hypoglycemia. Reinforce the importance of balancing dietary intake, insulin, and exercise every day.

▶ DISORDERS OF GONADAL FUNCTION

GYNECOMASTIA

Gynecomastia is the presence of unilateral or bilateral enlarged breast tissue in males. It is a common finding during adolescence and is sometimes confused with subcutaneous fat pads in obese boys. Gynecomastia occurs when the ratio of estrogen to testosterone is greater than the usual male ratio. The amount of breast tissue varies among boys. The condition usually disappears in 1–2 years.

Nursing care focuses on reassuring the boy and his parents that gynecomastia is a common and transient condition. Because of the concerns about body image that are common during adolescence, embarrassment is a frequent problem. Alerting the teen's teachers may be necessary if teasing becomes a problem.

AMENORRHEA

Amenorrhea, or lack of menstruation, may be primary or secondary. Primary amenorrhea is defined as the failure to have menstrual periods by 1 year beyond the average age of family members.[26] Primary amenorrhea is differentiated from delayed menarche, which is associated with well-developed secondary sexual characteristics and a strong family history of late menarche.[27] Secondary amenorrhea is the cessation of menstrual periods after menstruation has begun; it is characterized by an absence of spontaneous bleeding for at least 120 days. Pregnancy is the most common cause of secondary amenorrhea in adolescents.

Primary amenorrhea is most often caused by structural defects of the reproductive system; chromosomal abnormalities (such as Turner's syndrome); or hypothalamic (pituitary) tumors, thyroid dysfunction, or polycystic ovary disease. No underlying pathologic condition is found in some adolescents. Primary or secondary amenorrhea may be found in competitive athletes, particularly those who are pressured to be strong competitors, to maintain a perfect body type, and to have endurance. Excessive exercise can result in luteal phase deficiency, anovulation, and exercise-induced amenorrhea.[28]

A thorough history, physical examination, and laboratory evaluation are required to determine the cause of amenorrhea. The history focuses on asking questions about recent excessive weight loss or gain; excessive physical activity or sports training; chronic illness; use of illegal drugs, birth control pills, or phenothiazines; and emotional problems, all of which may result in the absence or cessation of menses.

The physical examination focuses on evaluating the adolescent's stage of sexual development (see Chap. 3). A bone scan is performed to determine bone age, and hormone levels are evaluated (estrogen, LH, FSH, and prolactin).

Treatment of amenorrhea depends on the specific cause. The most common approach is to give birth control pills containing both estrogen and progesterone. Athletic teenagers are encouraged to eat a well-balanced, high-calorie diet. Calcium supplements may be ordered. Estrogen with progesterone in low doses may be prescribed for athletes to reduce the risk for osteoporosis. Nursing management centers on patient education and emotional support. The goal is to maintain normal growth and development.

DYSMENORRHEA

Dysmenorrhea (menstrual pain or cramping) is a common complaint of adolescent girls. It is usually caused by an increased secretion of prostaglandins. Dysmenorrhea usually occurs following the beginning of ovulation and ends on the second day of the menstrual cycle. The pain can be mild or severe. Other symptoms may include nausea, vomiting, diarrhea, and urinary frequency.

Nonprescription analgesics, relaxation techniques, and application of a heating pad may relieve mild discomfort. Nursing care centers on providing patient education and emotional support.

▶ DISORDERS RELATED TO SEX CHROMOSOME ABNORMALITIES

TURNER'S SYNDROME

Turner's syndrome is a genetic condition that occurs in girls who have a missing or abnormal X chromosome. It occurs in approximately 1 in 2000–5000 live female births.[29] The cause of the chromosomal error is unknown.

Characteristic clinical findings include significant short stature; undeveloped ovaries; a short, webbed neck with a low posterior hairline; cubitus valgus (increased angle at the elbow); broad chest with widely spaced nipples; lymphedema; hyperconvex fingernails; dark, pigmented nevi; delayed puberty; amenorrhea; and infertility (Fig. 20–11). Few girls have all of these features.

Among the conditions that may be associated with Turner's syndrome are congenital heart disease; structural abnormalities of the kidney; con-

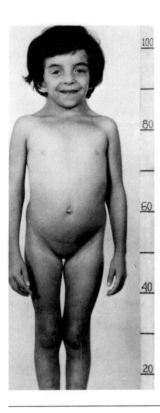

FIGURE 20–11. What characteristic physical manifestations of Turner's syndrome can you identify in this 8-year-old girl?
From Grumbach, M.M., & Barr, ML. (1958). Recent Progress in Hormone Research, 14, 255.

genital lymphedema; hypothyroidism or Hashimoto's thyroiditis; chronic or recurrent otitis media; ptosis, myopia, or amblyopia (lazy eye); inflammatory bowel disease; idiopathic hypertension; and scoliosis.[30] Kidney abnormalities are present in 25–30% of girls.

Growth usually proceeds at a normal rate for the first 2–3 years of life and then slows. Breast tissue, which begins to bud at about 10–12 years, fails to develop fully. Only in rare instances will a girl with Turner's syndrome menstruate spontaneously or be able to conceive. Final height is approximately 4 feet 8 inches.

The presence of characteristic physical findings may alert health care providers to suspect Turner's syndrome. Some infants, however, have few of these characteristics. In some instances diagnosis is made only when short stature and delayed puberty become apparent in the teenage years. The condition is diagnosed definitively by a karyotype, which reveals the classic 45,XO chromosome pattern or 46,XX pattern with one misshapen X chromosome.

Treatment involves carefully monitoring the child's growth. A growth chart made especially for girls with Turner's syndrome is available. Low-dose estrogen therapy is usually begun at about 15 years of age, with dosage increases over the next 2–3 years. Waiting until 15 years gives the girl the opportunity to achieve her maximum height before hormones cause the growth plates to close. This treatment produces pubertal changes such as breast development and pubic hair. Progesterone is added to the estrogen therapy to initiate menstrual periods. Approximately 20–30% of girls go through puberty spontaneously.[30]

Nursing Management

The lack of growth and sexual development associated with Turner's syndrome presents problems not only for physical growth but also for psychosocial development. Self-image, self-consciousness, and self-esteem are affected by the girl's perception of her body and how she differs from peers.

In the United States, cultural values place importance on attaining normal to tall stature. Short children tend to be treated according to their size rather than their age. Emphasis is also placed on sexual maturity. Television, advertisements, and movies encourage adolescents to dress and behave in a sexually mature manner. Girls with Turner's syndrome are often self-conscious and easily embarrassed and suffer from low self-esteem. Even though their intelligence is generally normal, they have a higher incidence of learning problems because of visual–spatial deficits that affect performance on mathematical and manual dexterity tasks.[3]

The nurse can be instrumental in helping the child adapt to the condition and gain self-esteem. Be an active listener and reinforce abilities and skills that the girl exhibits. Encourage parents to provide support. The Turner Syndrome Society (see Appendix F) can provide additional information about the disorder for parents and adolescents.

KLINEFELTER'S SYNDROME

Klinefelter's syndrome is a genetic condition that occurs in boys who have an extra X chromosome (usually 47,XXY). It occurs in approximately 1 in 1000 male births[31] and is the single most common cause of hypogonadism (decreased secretory activity of the gonad) and infertility in males.

Most infants appear normal at birth. The condition is usually diagnosed during the school-age years when the boy's behavior becomes a problem in the classroom. Boys with Klinefelter's syndrome may have emotional problems because of delayed language development and auditory processing problems that are frustrating to the child. Intelligence quotient (IQ) scores are often 10–15 points below those of unaffected siblings, and IQs below 80 are not uncommon. Boys with Klinefelter's syndrome are tall and thin, with overly long arms and legs. The arm span to height ratio is normal. The onset of puberty is often delayed, and testicular size is decreased at all ages. Development of the penis and pubic hair may be normal, but a full beard and mustache may not develop. Gynecomastia is a characteristic finding.

Diagnosis is confirmed by chromosomal analysis revealing one or more extra X chromosomes. The goal of treatment is to stimulate masculinization and the development of secondary sex characteristics when adolescence is delayed. Testosterone replacement is begun when the boy is 11 or 12 years of age. Depo-Testosterone is given by intramuscular injection every 3–4 weeks to maintain serum testosterone levels within the normal range. The dose is increased gradually until an adult dose is reached between 15 and 17 years of age; however, this does not improve fertility. Gynecomastia does not typically disappear with hormone treatment. Cosmetic surgery may be needed if breast size is distressing.

Nursing Management

Nursing care consists of educating the parents and child about the syndrome, evaluating the child's and family's coping mechanisms, assisting with school problems, and reinforcing the child's strengths. Encourage parents to channel their son's energy into areas that will provide opportunities for success and productive experiences. Emphasize the importance of rewarding the boy's successes in school, sports, or hobbies. Genetic counseling should be made available to adolescents, if indicated, because sexual functioning and fertility may be impaired.

▶ INBORN ERRORS OF METABOLISM

Inborn errors of metabolism are inherited biochemical abnormalities of the urea cycle, amino acid, and organic acid metabolism. Individually they are rare disorders; however, as a group they are a significant health problem in infancy.

Clinical manifestations usually occur within days or weeks of birth. Signs and symptoms may include lethargy and poor feeding, persistent vomiting, abnormal muscle tone and seizures, apnea and tachycardia, and an unusual urine or body odor (musty, sweet odor of maple syrup or burnt sugar, or cheesy or sweaty feet).

The biochemical defect usually causes an abnormal chemical by-product to accumulate in the blood, urine, or tissues or results in a decreased amount of normal enzymes. Most disorders are associated with a protein intolerance, with symptoms developing shortly after formula or breast milk feedings are begun.

In many states neonatal screening is used to detect several of these conditions before symptoms develop. However, most inborn errors of metabolism are not detected until signs and symptoms are present. Initial laboratory tests include measurement of serum glucose, electrolytes, blood gases, and serum ammonia. Results of these tests make it possible to classify the disorder by the presence of hypoglycemia, metabolic acidosis,

 LEGAL & ETHICAL CONSIDERATIONS

Neonatal screening for hypothyroidism and phenylketonuria is mandated by state law in all 50 states. When a state law exists, signed informed consent of the parents is not required. If parents refuse the test, obtain a signature of "informed dissent" to include in the child's medical record.[32]

hyperammonemia, or liver dysfunction. Further diagnostic laboratory tests are then performed.

Treatment, when available, focuses on replacing or reducing the amount of the substance causing the biochemical abnormality.

Two of the more common inborn errors of metabolism, phenylketonuria and galactosemia, are presented here. Congenital hypothyroidism and congenital adrenal hyperplasia, also considered inborn errors of metabolism, were discussed earlier in this chapter.

PHENYLKETONURIA

Phenylketonuria (PKU) is an inherited disorder of amino acid metabolism that affects the body's utilization of protein. Children with PKU have a deficiency of the liver enzyme phenylalanine hydroxylase, which breaks down the essential amino acid phenylalanine into tyrosine. As a result, phenylalanine accumulates in the blood, causing a musty body odor, musty urine odor, irritability, vomiting, hyperactivity, seizures, and an eczema-like rash. Persistence of elevated phenylalanine leads to disruption of cellular processes of myelination and protein synthesis and, after 2–3 years, results in a seizure disorder and mental retardation.

PKU is inherited as an autosomal recessive disorder or as a mutation. The incidence is 1 in 10,000–25,000 live births per year, with great ethnic variability.[33]

Infants appear normal at birth. Screening for PKU is required by state law in all 50 states. For best results the newborn should have begun formula or breast milk feeding before specimen collection. Early hospital discharge places newborns at risk for false negative screening tests if screened within 24 hours of birth. Screening needs to occur no sooner than 48 hours after birth, or the test should be repeated at 1–2 weeks of age.[33] If the test shows elevated levels of plasma phenylalanine, a repeat test is performed. If the second test is positive, the family is referred to a treatment center and treatment is begun on an outpatient basis.

PKU is treated using special formulas and a diet low in phenylalanine to keep plasma phenylalanine levels between 2 and 6 mg/dL. Mature breast milk, at least 10 days after birth, has a lower phenylalanine level and is a good source of protein for the infant with PKU. The diet must also meet the child's needs for optimal growth. High-protein foods (meats and dairy products) and aspartame are avoided because they contain large amounts of phenylalanine. Elemental medical foods (modified protein hydrosylates in which the phenylalanine has been removed) are used instead. The low-phenylalanine diet should be maintained until late school age or adolescence. If dietary control is lost before 8 years of age, there is a significant impact on IQ.[35] Affected adolescent girls and women who become pregnant should resume the low-phenylalanine diet before they conceive to prevent congenital defects (low birth weight, mental retardation, microcephaly) in the fetus.

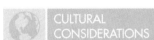

CULTURAL CONSIDERATIONS

Phenylketonuria is rare in African, Jewish, and Japanese populations. It is more commonly found in isolated communities with numerous intermarriages between families over several generations.

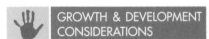

GROWTH & DEVELOPMENT CONSIDERATIONS

Infants with PKU who do not begin treatment as neonates lose 10 IQ points if their phenylalanine level is not stable by 1 month of age and 10 more points if it is not stable by 2 months of age. The IQ drops to 50 by 1 year of age and to 30 by 3 years of age.[34]

Nursing Management

Nursing care is mainly supportive and focuses on teaching parents about the disorder and its management. Serum levels of phenylalanine should be measured periodically throughout life. When the child begins to eat solid foods, parents need to watch the amount of phenylalanine consumed by the child daily and should not allow it to exceed the amount prescribed by the physician.

The low-phenylalanine diet is a rigid, strict diet that excludes many foods. Parents and children need a great deal of support to promote compliance. The formula and elemental medical food costs are relatively high. Usually only the formula is reimbursed by insurance. Like children with diabetes mellitus, children with PKU may rebel against the dietary limitations in an effort to be like their peers. For this reason the low-phenylalanine diet may be discontinued during the late school-age years or adolescence. If the child has problems concentrating or sitting still, resumption of the low-phenylalanine diet may be recommended. Some experts think lifelong dietary control may be needed. The long-term neurologic effects of this disorder are unknown.[34]

Parents of an affected child who are considering a future pregnancy and adolescents with the disorder should be referred for genetic counseling.

GALACTOSEMIA

Galactosemia is a disorder of carbohydrate metabolism that results from a deficiency of the liver enzyme galactose-1–phosphate uridyltransferase. This is one of three enzymes needed to convert galactose to glucose. Galactosemia has an autosomal recessive inheritance pattern and occurs in 1 in 60,000–80,000 live births.[36] Early signs include feeding problems, vomiting, weight loss, jaundice, and an enlarged liver. Later signs include mental retardation, sepsis, lethargy, hypotonia, cataracts, progressive hepatic cirrhosis, and coma. Death may occur within 1 month of birth without treatment, usually due to sepsis.[37]

Routine newborn screening for galactosemia is performed in 43 states.[14] Infants in other states are identified once they become symptomatic. Infants with galactosemia are placed on a lactose- or galactose-free formula (usually a soy formula), which remains the child's milk substitute for life. A galactose-free diet (no milk or cheese products) is prescribed when the infant is ready for solids. In spite of compliance with the diet, complications (learning disabilities, speech defects, ovarian failure, and neurologic syndromes) develop in many children.

Nursing management focuses on educating the parents and child about the disorder and required diet, assessing coping abilities, and providing emotional support. Refer the family to a nutritionist for diet counseling. Calcium supplementation may be needed. Advise parents that several galactose-free cheeses are sold commercially. Because the disorder is inherited, the family should be referred for genetic counseling.

REFERENCES

1. D'Ercole, A.J., & Underwood, L. (1996). Anterior pituitary gland and hypothalamus. In A.M. Rudolph, J.I.E. Hoffman, & C.D. Rudolph (Eds.), *Rudolph's pediatrics* (20th ed., pp. 1683–1695). Stamford, CT: Appleton & Lange.

2. Finegold, D. (1997). Endocrinology. In B.J. Zitelli, & H.W. Davis (Eds.), *Atlas of pediatric physical diagnosis* (3rd ed., p. 270). St. Louis: Mosby–Wolfe.

3. Rieser, P.A. (1992). Educational, psychologic, and social aspects of short stature. *Journal of Pediatric Health Care, 6*(5), 325–332.

4. Connaughty, M.S. (1992). Accelerated growth in children. *Journal of Pediatric Health Care, 6*(5), 316–324.

5. Robertson, G.L. (1995). Diabetes insipidus. *Endocrinology and Metabolism Clinics of North America, 24*(3), 549–572.

6. Segar, W.E., & Friedman, A.L. (1996). Primary disturbances of water homeostasis. In A.M. Rudolph, J.I.E. Hoffman, & C.D. Rudolph (Eds.), *Rudolph's pediatrics* (20th ed., pp. 1703–1710). Stamford, CT: Appleton & Lange.

7. Herman-Giddens, M.E., Slora, E.J., Wasserman, R.C., Bourdony, C.J., Bhapkar, M.V., Koch, G.G., & Hasemeier, C.M. (1997). Secondary sexual characteristics and menses in young girls seen in office practice: A study from the pediatric research in office settings network. *Pediatrics, 99*(4), 505–512.

8. Office of Research Reporting, National Institute of Child Health and Development (1989). *Facts about precocious puberty.* Washington, DC: National Institutes of Health.

9. Rosen, D., & Kelch, R.P. (1995). Precocious and delayed puberty. In K.L. Becker (Ed.), *Principles and practice of endocrinology and metabolism* (2nd. ed., pp. 830–842). Philadelphia: Lippincott.

10. Ball, J.B. (1998). *Mosby's pediatric patient teaching guides.* St. Louis: Mosby.

11. Fisher, D.A. (1996). The thyroid. In A.M. Rudolph, J.I.E. Hoffman, & C.D. Rudolph (Eds.), *Rudolph's pediatrics* (20th ed., pp. 1750–1773). Stamford, CT: Appleton & Lange.

12. Castiglia, P.T. (1997). Hyperthyroidism (Graves' disease). *Journal of Pediatric Health Care, 11*(5), 227–229.

13. Miller, W.L. (1996). The adrenal cortex. In A.M. Rudolph, J.I.E. Hoffman, & C.D. Rudolph (Eds.), *Rudolph's pediatrics* (20th ed., pp. 1711–1742). Stamford, CT: Appleton & Lange.

14. Ruble, J.A. (1996). Congenital adrenal hyperplasia. In P.L. Jackson, & J.A. Vessey (Eds.), *Primary care of the child with a chronic condition* (2nd ed., pp. 276–295). St. Louis: Mosby.

15. Elsas, L.J. (1996). Newborn screening. In A.M. Rudolph, J.I.E. Hoffman, & C.D. Rudolph (Eds.), *Rudolph's pediatrics* (20th ed., pp. 282–288). Stamford, CT: Appleton & Lange.

16. Voorhess, M.L. (1996). Adrenal medula, sympathetic nervous system, and multiple endocrine neoplasia syndromes. In A.M. Rudolph, J.I.E. Hoffman, & C.D. Rudolph (Eds.), *Rudolph's pediatrics* (20th ed., pp. 1742–1750). Stamford, CT: Appleton & Lange.

17. Werbel, S.S., & Ober, K.P. (1995). Pheochromocytoma: Update on diagnosis, localization, and management. *Medical Clinics of North America, 79*(1), 161–166.

18. Linder, B. (1997). Improving diabetic control with a new insulin analog. *Contemporary Pediatrics, 14*(10), 52–73.

19. Ahern, J.A., & Grey, M. (1996). New developments in treating children with insulin-dependent diabetes mellitus. *Journal of Pediatric Health Care, 10*(4), 161–166.

20. Grey, M., & Boland, E.A. (1996). Diabetes mellitus (Type 1). In P.L. Jackson, & J.A. Vessey (Eds.), *Primary care of the child with a chronic condition* (2nd ed., pp. 350–370). St. Louis: Mosby.

21. Saudek, C.D. (1997). Novel forms of insulin delivery. *Endocrinology and Metabolism Clinics of North America, 26*(3), 599–610.

22. White, N.H. (1996). Diabetes mellitus in children. In A.M. Rudolph, J.I.E. Hoffman, & C.D. Rudolph (Eds.), *Rudolph's pediatrics* (20th ed., pp. 1803–1827). Stamford, CT: Appleton & Lange.

23. Drash, A.L., & Becker, D.J. (1993). Nutritional considerations in the therapy of the child with diabetes mellitus. In R.M. Suskind, & L. Lewinter-Suskind (Eds.), *Textbook of pediatric nutrition* (2nd ed.). New York: Raven Press.

24. Giordano, B.P., Petrila, A., Banion, C.R., & Neuenkirchen, G. (1992). The challenge of transferring responsibility for diabetes management from parent to child. *Journal of Pediatric Health Care, 6*(5), 235–239.

25. Fagan, M.J. (1995). Nursing care of the child with DKA in the PICU. *Pediatric Nursing, 21*(4), 375–380.

26. Castiglia, P.T. (1996). Amenorrhea. *Journal of Pediatric Health Care, 10*(5), 226–227.

27. Tuttle, J.I. (1991). Menstrual disorders during adolescence. *Journal of Pediatric Health Care, 5*(4), 197–203.

28. Yurth, E.F. (1995). Female athlete triad. *Western Journal of Medicine, 162*(2), 149–151.

29. Committee on Genetics, American Academy of Pediatrics (1995). Health supervision for children with Turner syndrome. *Pediatrics, 96*(6), 1166–1173.

30. Sanger, P. (1996). Turner's syndrome. *Current Concepts, 335*(2), 1749–1754.

31. Grumbach, M.M. (1996). Abnormalities of sex determination and differentiation. In A.M. Rudolph, J.I.E. Hoffman, & C.D. Rudolph (Eds.), *Rudolph's pediatrics* (20th ed., pp. 1773–1389). Stamford, CT: Appleton & Lange.

32. Buist, N.R.M., & Tuerck, J.M. (1992). The practitioner's role in newborn screening. *Pediatric Clinics of North America, 39*(2), 199–211.

33. Sinai, L.N., Kim, S.C., Casey, R., & Pinto-Martin, J.A. (1995). Phenylketonuria screening: Effect of early newborn discharge. *Pediatrics, 96*(4), 605–608.

34. Bowe, K. (1995). Phenylketonuria: An update for pediatric community health nurses. *Pediatric Nursing, 21*(2), 191–194.

35. Yule, K.S. (1996). Phenylketonuria. In P.L. Jackson, & J.A. Vessey (Eds.), *Primary care of the child with a chronic condition* (2nd ed., pp. 623–649) St. Louis: Mosby.

36. Strobel, S.E., & Keller, C.S. (1993). Metabolic screening in the NICU population: A proposal for change. *Pediatric Nursing, 19*(2), 113–117.

37. Greene, C.L., & Goodman, S.I. (1997). Inborn errors of metabolism. In W.W. Hay, J.R. Groothuis, A.R. Hayward, & M.J. Levin (Eds.), *Current pediatric diagnosis & treatment* (13th ed., pp. 864–884). Stamford, CT: Appleton & Lange.

ADDITIONAL RESOURCES

Adam, P. (1997). Evaluation and management of diabetes insipidus. *American Family Physician, 55*(6), 2146–2152.

Brandt, P.A., & Magyary, D.L. (1993). The impact of a diabetes education program on children and mothers. *Journal of Pediatric Nursing, 8*(1), 31–40.

Davidson, A. (1992). Management and counseling of children with inherited metabolic disorders. *Journal of Pediatric Health Care, 6*(3), 146–152.

Donahoe, P.K, & Schnitzer, J.J. (1996). Evaluation of the infant who has ambiguous genitalia, and principles of operative management. *Seminars in Pediatric Surgery, 5*(1), 30–40.

Gidwani, G.P. (1997). Menstruation and the athlete. *Contemporary Pediatrics, 14*(1), 27–48.

Greve, L.C., Wheeler, M.D., Green-Burgeson, D.K., & Zorn, E.M. (1994). Breast-feeding in the management of the newborn with phenylketonuria: A practical approach to dietary therapy. *Journal of the American Dietetic Association, 94*(3), 305–310.

Henry, J., & Giordano, B. (1992). Assessment of growth in infants and children: Normal and abnormal patterns. *Journal of Pediatric Health Care, 5*(2), 289–334.

Heuther, S.E. (1994). Mechanisms of hormonal regulation. In K.L. McCance, & S.E. Huether (Eds.), *Pathophysiology: A biologic basis for disease in adults and children* (2nd ed., pp. 626–655). St. Louis: Mosby.

Kaufman, F.R. (1994). Outpatient management of children and adults with IDDM. *Clinical Diabetes, 12*(6), 146–151.

Magiakou, M.A., Mastorakos, G., Oldfield, E.H., Gomez, M.T., Doppman, J.L., Cutler, G.B., Nieman, L.K., & Chrousos, G.P. (1994). Cushing's syndrome in children and adolescents. *New England Journal of Medicine, 331*(10), 629–636.

Merke, D.P., & Cutler, G.B. (1997). New approaches to the treatment of congenital adrenal hyperplasia. *Journal of the American Medical Association, 277*(13), 1073–1076.

Rapone, K., & Brabston, L. (1997). A health care plan for the student with diabetes. *Journal of School Nursing, 13*(2), 30–34.

Saudek, C.D. (1992). Use of implanted insulin pumps to treat IDDM. *Journal of Pediatric Endocrinology, 5*(4), 217–227.

Seckl, J.R., & Miller, W.L. (1997). How safe is long-term prenatal glucocorticoid treatment? *Journal of the American Medical Association, 277*(13), 1077–1080.

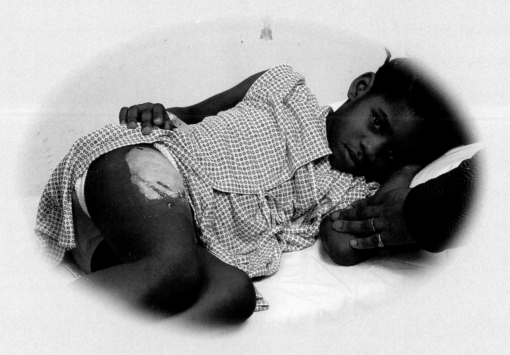

*S*herray, 6 years old, was admitted to the hospital with a deep partial-thickness burn after dropping a bowl of soup on her leg. By her second day in the hospital, it is clear that Sherray's burn is not full thickness and that no skin grafting is needed. The amount of scarring she will have cannot be anticipated at this time.

Sherray's treatment includes a bath with wound debridement and dressing changes twice a day. Although pain medication is provided, the debridement and dressing changes cause a lot of anxiety and pain. Sherray needs a high-protein, high-calorie diet to promote wound heeling. She has a hard time extending her leg and walking because movement stretches the burned skin, so she needs assistance to get out of bed and participate in child life activities.

Sherray's mother is rooming in, and remains at her side during the dressing changes. Her greatest concern right now is to help Sherray deal with the burn injury and to reduce the chance of infection. Over the next couple of days, Sherray's mother will take more responsibility for the dressing changes in anticipation of continuing her daughter's care at home.

ALTERATIONS IN SKIN INTEGRITY 21

"I didn't know that soup could cause such a bad injury. The hardest thing for me to deal with is all the pain Sherray has with each dressing change."

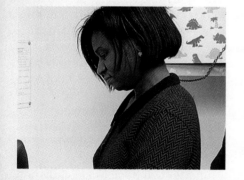

TERMINOLOGY

- **atopy** A hereditary allergic tendency.
- **debridement** Enzyme action to clean a lesion and dissolve fibrin clots or scabs; or removal of dead tissue to speed the healing process.
- **dermatophytoses** Fungal infections that affect primarily the skin but may affect the hair and nails.

- **eschar** Slough or layer of dead skin or tissue.
- **escharotomy** Incision into constricting dead tissue of a burn injury to restore peripheral circulation.
- **lichenification** Thickening of the skin.

What is the role of the nurse in providing care to the child with a burn injury? What nursing support may help the child deal with painful dressing changes and a disfiguring injury? What other health care team members are important in ensuring an optimal recovery for Sherray? What teaching must be provided to her mother to enable her to provide care at home? The information in this chapter will prepare you to answer these questions and to provide care to children such as Sherray with burn injuries or other alterations in skin integrity.

Skin disorders are seen frequently by nurses who work in outpatient clinics, schools, emergency departments, and pediatric units of hospitals. Many of these disorders are not unique to children, but children are at greater risk for some skin conditions for reasons that are discussed in this chapter.

The skin is the largest organ in the body. It performs several essential functions, among them perception, protection, temperature regulation, vitamin D synthesis, and excretion. The skin protects underlying tissues from invasion by microorganisms and from trauma. The nerves in the skin enable us to perceive pain, heat, and cold.

Temperature regulation of the body is achieved by dilation or constriction of blood vessels and sweat glands that act under the control of the central nervous system. The skin also supplements the body's intake of vitamin D by synthesizing this vitamin from ultraviolet light. Excretion is performed by the sweat glands, which secrete a solution of water, electrolytes, and urea, thus helping to rid the body of toxins.

► ANATOMY AND PHYSIOLOGY OF PEDIATRIC DIFFERENCES

The skin is made up of three distinct layers: the epidermis, the dermis, and the subcutaneous fatty layer that separates the skin from the underlying tissue (Fig. 21–1). Within the dermis are nerves, muscles, connective tissue, hair follicles, sebaceous and sweat glands, lymph channels, and blood vessels.

At birth the skin is thin, with little underlying subcutaneous fat. Because of this the infant loses heat more rapidly, has greater difficulty regulating body temperature, and becomes more easily chilled than an older child or an adult. The thinner skin also leads to increased absorption of harmful chemical substances. The newborn's skin contains more water than an adult's and has loosely attached cells. As the infant grows, the skin toughens and becomes less hydrated, making it less susceptible to bacteria.

The accessory structures of the skin (hair, sebaceous glands, eccrine glands, and apocrine glands) are present at birth. Like other body structures, however, they are still immature.

At birth the infant may have soft, downy hair, called lanugo, on the shoulders and back. Lanugo is usually shed by 2–3 weeks of age. The amount of hair on the head varies. Scalp hair usually is shed within a few months and replaced, sometimes with hair of a different color.

Sebaceous glands function at birth, although somewhat immaturely. They vary in size and appear all over the body except on the hands and soles of the feet. Sebum, a lipid substance produced and secreted into the hair follicle or directly onto the skin, provides lubrication to the skin and hair.

Eccrine glands, located in the dermis, open onto the skin surface. They secrete an odorless, watery fluid, primarily in response to emotional stress. They also respond to changes in body temperature. As body temperature increases, the glands increase production of sweat. The result is

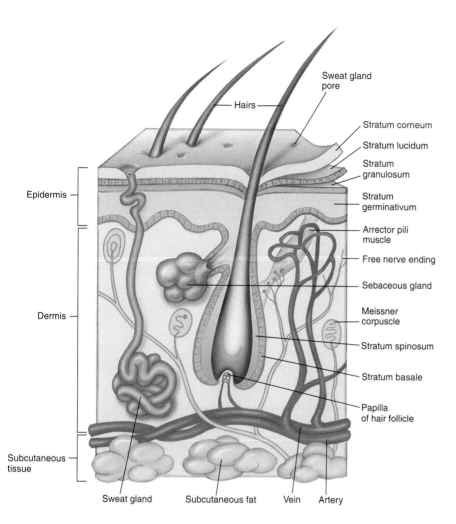

FIGURE 21-1. Layers of the skin with accessory structures.

decreased heat as the sweat evaporates. Because the eccrine sweat glands usually are not fully functional until middle childhood, infants and young children are unable to regulate temperature as effectively as older children and adults.

Apocrine glands, located mainly in the axillary and genital areas, do not function until puberty. Decomposition of the fluid secreted by these glands leads to body odor. Their biologic function, however, is unknown.

▶ SKIN LESIONS

Skin lesions vary in size, shape, color, and texture characteristics. The two major types of skin lesions are primary lesions and secondary lesions. Primary lesions arise from previously healthy skin and include macules, patches, papules, nodules, tumors, vesicles, pustules, bullae, and wheals (see Table 3–9). Secondary lesions result from changes in primary lesions. They include crusts, scales, **lichenification** (thickening of the skin), scars, keloids, excoriation, fissures, erosion, and ulcers (Table 21–1). It is important for the nurse to be able to identify and describe the primary and secondary skin lesions and understand their underlying cause and treatment.

21-1	Common Secondary Skin Lesions and Associated Conditions		
Lesion Name	**Description**		**Example**
Crust	Dried residue of serum, pus, or blood		Impetigo
Scale	Thin flake of exfoliated epidermis		Dandruff, psoriasis
Lichenification	Thickening of skin with increased visibility of normal skin furrows		Eczema (atopic dermatitis)
Scar	Replacement of destroyed tissue with fibrous tissue		Healed surgical incision
Keloid	Overdevelopment or hypertrophy of scar that extends beyond wound edges and above skin line due to excess collagen		Healed skin area following traumatic injury
Excoriation	Abrasion or scratch mark		Scratched insect bite
Fissure	Linear crack in skin		Tinea pedis (athlete's foot)
Erosion	Loss of superficial epidermis; moist but does not bleed		Ruptured chickenpox vesicle
Ulcer	Deeper loss of skin surface; bleeding or scarring may ensue		Chancre

► WOUND HEALING

Wound healing is a process that occurs in three overlapping phases: inflammation, reconstruction, and maturation (Table 21–2).[1,2]

Inflammation, the initial response at the injury site, lasts approximately 3–5 days. This phase prepares the injury site for the repair process. Coagulation occurs as platelets, red blood cells, and fibrin gather to form a clot. This seals the wound, preventing bacterial invasion and joining the wound edges. Vasodilation, which occurs shortly after injury, allows leukocytes to travel to the injury site, where they ingest bacteria and debris.

Reconstruction, the second phase, may last from 5 days to 4 weeks, depending on the extent of the injury. Capillary budding to reestablish the blood flow and natural **debridement** (enzyme action to clean the lesion and dissolve the clot or scab) occur. The wound contracts. Fibroblasts multiply, producing collagen and granulation tissue to fill the wound to skin level. A fine layer of epithelial cells forms over the site.

Maturation, the third phase, involves continued collagen production for scar production and remodeling. The scar gradually strengthens and devascularizes. Maturation can take months to years, depending on the extent of the injury.

► DERMATITIS

Many skin inflammations occur in early childhood. Most are easily treated and do not have long-term consequences. Dermatitis is a condition in which changes occur in the skin in response to external stimuli. The four most com-

21-2   Phases of Wound Healing

Inflammation (3–5 days)

Clot formation and wound sealing

Increased blood flow to area

Increased capillary permeability, causing swelling

Phagocytosis

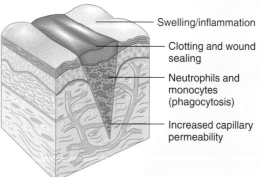

Inflammation

— Swelling/inflammation

— Clotting and wound sealing

— Neutrophils and monocytes (phagocytosis)

— Increased capillary permeability

Reconstruction (5 Days to 4 Weeks)

Debridement

Collagen production

Epithelialization with granulation tissue

Capillary budding

Wound contraction

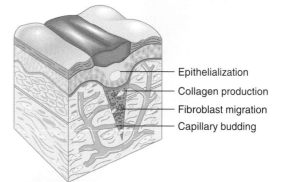

Reconstruction

— Epithelialization

— Collagen production

— Fibroblast migration

— Capillary budding

Maturation (Months to Years)

Remodeling

Scar formation and strengthening

Capillary disappearance

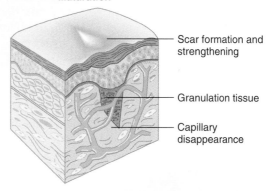

Maturation

— Scar formation and strengthening

— Granulation tissue

— Capillary disappearance

Based on information in O'Hanlon-Nichols, T. (1995). Commonly asked questions about wound healing. American Journal of Nursing, 95(4), 22–24; and Rote, N.S. (1994). Inflammation. In K.L. McCance & S.E. Huether (Eds.), Pathophysiology: The basis for disease in adults and children (2nd ed., pp 234–267). St. Louis: Mosby.

mon types of dermatitis that occur in infants, children, and adolescents are contact dermatitis, diaper dermatitis, seborrheic dermatitis, and eczema (atopic dermatitis). It is important for the nurse to understand that these skin disorders bring with them emotional problems for the family and child. Be sympathetic and remember that the family and child can see the skin condition and need to be reassured that the child is not infectious.

CONTACT DERMATITIS

Contact dermatitis is an inflammation of the skin that occurs in response to direct contact with an allergen or irritant. Common allergens include poison ivy, poison oak, rubber, shoe leather, and nickel. Common irritants include soaps, detergents, bleaches, lotions, urine, and stool. Reactions to latex, which can be found in many types of hospital equipment (gloves, intravenous equipment, airway equipment, plastic syringes, adhesive tape) as well as in products in the home and community, also have been reported (see Chap. 9).

The rash of allergic contact dermatitis is characterized by erythematous papules with oozing, crusting, and edema, and it is usually limited to the area of contact. Symptoms of allergic contact dermatitis can develop up to 18 hours after contact, peak between 48 and 72 hours, and can last up to 3 weeks. In contrast, irritant contact dermatitis usually develops within a few hours of contact, peaks within 24 hours, and quickly resolves.

Treatment involves removing the offending agent (eg, clothes, plant, soap). Calamine lotion or hydrocortisone cream or ointment can be applied to the affected skin. Sometimes reactions to poison ivy require treatment with corticosteroids.

Nursing Management

Patient education for home care management focuses on ways to avoid the offending agent and on care of the skin. Advise parents to wash all clothes before the first wearing and to rinse clothes an extra time to remove all the soap. Mild soap should be used to clean the skin. Familiarize parents with the symptoms of infection in the affected area (ie, increased redness, oozing, fever) and tell them when to return for follow-up care.

DIAPER DERMATITIS

Diaper dermatitis, the most common irritant contact dermatitis, occurs in approximately one third of young children, usually in a mild form.[3] It is most common in infants from 4–12 months of age.

The rash is characterized by erythema, edema, vesicles, papules, and scaling that appear in areas in direct contact with the diaper. Usually the perineum, genitals, and buttocks are affected, and the skin folds are spared. In severe cases, the infant develops a rash that is fiery red, raised, and confluent. Pustules with tenderness can also be present (Fig. 21–2).

Diaper dermatitis is a primary reaction to urine, feces, moisture, or friction. Urine and feces interact to cause dermatitis. The urine increases the hydration and pH of the skin, increasing its permeability to irritants, abrasion, and microbes. Fecal organisms provide more irritants.[4] *Candida albicans,* a secondary infection, is a common complication of diaper dermatitis or antibiotic therapy for another condition. It is frequently the underlying cause of severe diaper rash. Diaper candidiasis often occurs simultaneously with oral candidiasis (see later discussion).

Treatment for moderate or severe diaper dermatitis involves application of low potency (0.25% or 0.5%) hydrocortisone cream with each diaper change for 5 to 7 days and good basic hygiene. The cream must be applied before any protective sealant (eg, zinc oxide or Balmex) is used. Diaper candidiasis is treated with alternating applications of 1% hydrocortisone cream and antifungal creams (nystatin) applied to the affected areas at diaper change. Fluorinated topical corticosteroids should not be used because of the higher rate of absorption through damaged skin.

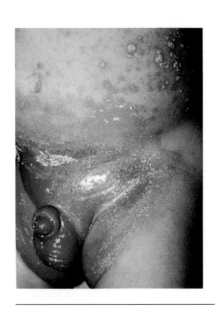

FIGURE 21–2. Diaper dermatitis.
Courtesy of the Centers for Disease Control, Atlanta, GA.

Nursing Management

Severe diaper dermatitis can be a major source of stress for parents who must deal with a child in constant discomfort. Instruct parents to change the diaper as soon as the infant is wet, or at least every 2 hours during the day and once during the night.

Encourage parents to use superabsorbent disposable diapers, which tend to reduce the frequency and severity of diaper dermatitis. When wet, these diapers form a gel that keeps the skin drier than cloth diapers. However, this should not be an excuse for waiting until the diaper is saturated to change it. Tell parents to avoid using tight diapers and waterproof pants. A & D ointment, zinc oxide, Desitin, and Balmex can be used to protect the skin from urine and stool.

Advise parents to wash the perianal area with warm water and a mild soap (such as Dove or Tone) or a cleanser not needing water (Acquanit HC lotion or Cetaphil) only after a bowel movement. Cornstarch or zeaSORB powder helps to decrease friction and moisture, but it is important to keep these powders away from the infant's face. Exposing the diaper area to air helps aid healing; for example, allowing the child to go without a diaper, while lying on an absorbable pad or cloth.

SEBORRHEIC DERMATITIS

Seborrheic dermatitis is a recurrent inflammatory skin condition thought to be caused by an overgrowth of *Pityrosporum* yeast, commonly found in areas of sebaceous gland activity.[4] The condition is also thought to be influenced by hormones and associated with an oily complexion. The rash is found over the areas of the body where the sebaceous glands are most plentiful: scalp (cradle cap), forehead, and postauricular and periorbital areas. It may also occur on the skin of the eyelids, inguinal area, or nasolabial folds. The condition is frequently seen in infants (beginning at 3–4 weeks of age) and adolescents.

Common symptoms are pruritus and an adherent waxy, scaling of the scalp (or "dandruff"). Yellow-red patches with greasy scaling may be present, typically on the scalp and nasolabial folds on the face, behind the ears, and on the upper chest (Fig. 21–3).

Treatment for seborrheic dermatitis consists of daily shampooing with a medicated shampoo (eg, Selsun or Head and Shoulders). The shampoo is left on the scalp for a few minutes to soften crusts. The hair is then rinsed thoroughly. Lesions on the body can be treated with shampoos containing selenium sulfide or salicylic acid.[5] Use baby shampoo to wash lesions on the eyelids and eyelashes. Treatments are continued for several days after the lesions disappear. Topical corticosteriods are used to treat seborrhea that is not on the scalp.

Nursing Management

Seborrheic dermatitis in newborns can often be prevented with proper scalp hygiene. Teach new parents that the infant's hair should be washed daily. Reassure parents that gentle cleansing will not harm the infant's "soft spot." Provide a bath demonstration to show them the proper technique, if necessary. Follow-up is seldom necessary, as the condition resolves with treatment. Advise adolescents that emotional distress may trigger future flare-ups and to initiate treatment promptly when symptoms begin.

NURSING ALERT

Instruct parents to avoid using such products as baby wipes on an infant with diaper dermatitis. The alcohol content in the wipes may exacerbate the condition.

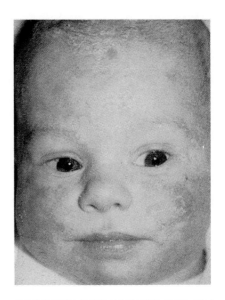

FIGURE 21–3. Seborrheic dermatitis.

DRUG REACTIONS

Adverse reactions to over-the-counter or prescription medications are relatively common. Children with drug allergies usually have reactions after ingestion (eg, aspirin, antibiotics, sedatives), injection (eg, penicillin), or direct skin contact with medications. Drug sensitivities may result from variations in an individual's ability to tolerate a particular drug or concentration of a drug or from allergic responses. (See Chapter 9 for a description of allergic reactions.)

Sensitivity reactions to a drug not previously administered may take up to 7 days to develop. If the child has been sensitized to a drug, the reaction is almost immediate. The most common reactions in children are the development of erythematous macules and papules or urticaria, which may be pruritic. See Table 21–3 for other signs of a serious systemic drug reaction. The nurse should be alert to the possibility of an anaphylactic reaction, which is a medical emergency.

The treatment of choice for most drug sensitivity reactions is discontinuation of the causative drug. In some cases, a drug may be continued when the child has a sensitivity reaction because it is the best treatment choice. Supportive measures should be taken to decrease the intensity of the reaction. An antihistamine may be used to block the release of histamine, which causes the rash. Topical corticosteroids, cool compresses, and baths may also be prescribed.

Nursing Management

Nurses can play an important role by teaching parents to be alert for the signs of drug sensitivity reactions. Obtain a careful history of the child's past reactions to medications before starting new therapies. If a reaction occurs, discontinue the medication until the physician is notified. Prominently mark the child's records so that all allergies are easily identified.

> **NURSING ALERT.**
>
> Children with a true drug allergy (having a past serious systemic reaction) should never be treated with that drug again. The child should wear a medical alert bracelet.

21-3	**Signs Indicating a Serious Systemic Drug Reaction**

Confluent erythema

Facial edema

Swelling of the tongue

Skin pain

Palpable purpura

Skin necrosis

Blisters

Urticaria

Fever higher than 40°C (104°F)

Enlarged lymph nodes

Arthalgias

Shortness of breath, wheezing

Hypotension

From Roujeau, J.C., & Stern, R.S. (1994). Severe adverse cutaneous reactions to drugs. New England Journal of Medicine, 331(19), 1272–1285. *Copyright © 1994. Massachusetts Medical Society: All rights reserved.*

ECZEMA (ATOPIC DERMATITIS)

Eczema, also called atopic dermatitis, is a chronic, superficial inflammatory skin disorder characterized by intense pruritus. The condition affects infants, children, and adolescents. It is a common skin condition, believed to affect 1 in 10 children.[6] The condition develops during the first year of life in 60% of affected children.[7]

Clinical Manifestations

Acute eczema is characterized by pruritus and erythematous patches with vesicles, exudate, and crusts (Fig. 21–4). Subacute eczema is characterized by scaling with erythema and excoriation. There are often postinflammatory pigment changes. Symptoms of chronic eczema are pruritus, dryness, scaling, and lichenification (thickening of the skin with increased visibility of normal skin furrows). Inflammation usually occurs on the face, upper arms, back, upper thighs, and back of the hands and feet.

Eczema occurs in three forms: infantile (ages 2 months to 2 years), childhood (ages 2 years to puberty), and adolescent (Table 21–4). In infantile eczema, lesions are exudative and crusted. Vesicles and erythema are common. Itching frequently interrupts the child's sleep patterns. In childhood eczema, lesions are drier, scaly, pruritic, well circumscribed, and rarely exudative. Lesions in adolescent eczema are similar to those in the childhood form; however, larger plaques and lichenification may also be present.

Etiology and Pathophysiology

The etiology of eczema is unknown, but the disorder tends to occur in children with hereditary allergic tendencies (**atopy**). If one parent has allergies (eg, hay fever, asthma, or contact dermatitis), the child has a 60% greater

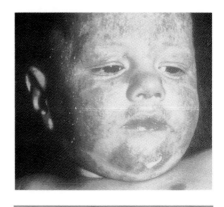

FIGURE 21–4. Chronic eczema.

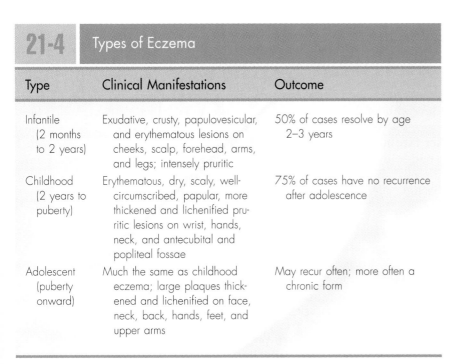

21-4	Types of Eczema	
Type	**Clinical Manifestations**	**Outcome**
Infantile (2 months to 2 years)	Exudative, crusty, papulovesicular, and erythematous lesions on cheeks, scalp, forehead, arms, and legs; intensely pruritic	50% of cases resolve by age 2–3 years
Childhood (2 years to puberty)	Erythematous, dry, scaly, well-circumscribed, papular, more thickened and lichenified pruritic lesions on wrist, hands, neck, and antecubital and popliteal fossae	75% of cases have no recurrence after adolescence
Adolescent (puberty onward)	Much the same as childhood eczema; large plaques thickened and lichenified on face, neck, back, hands, feet, and upper arms	May recur often; more often a chronic form

chance of having allergies. This increases to 80% if both parents have allergies. A family history of asthma or hay fever frequently predisposes a child to eczema. Infantile eczema is more likely to be food induced when the condition is severe.[8] Chronic eczema in older children and adults may be associated with allergies to house dust mites.[6] Eczema may be intensified by dry skin, irritating clothing, abrasive detergents, perspiration, emotional stress, cosmetics, and perfumed lotions and soaps.

Diagnostic Tests and Medical Management

Eczema is distinguished from other forms of dermatitis by its history and clinical manifestations. Eczema is more likely to have a generalized distribution with no known exposure to an allergen.

Goals of treatment are to hydrate and lubricate the skin, reduce pruritus, minimize inflammatory changes, and try to determine what triggers flare-ups. The cardinal principle of topical therapy for oozing or weeping is "wet on wet." If lesions are weeping, wet compresses (cotton cloths) soaked in aluminum acetate solution sometimes are used. Lubrication is achieved by applying lotion after bathing to trap moisture and prevent drying of the skin. Alphahydroxy acid can be applied to the skin twice a day to retain skin moisture and to decrease skin thickness in cases of chronic eczema. Noninflamed areas may also be treated with emollients such as Eucerin.

Topical corticosteroids are used to reduce inflammation. Ointments are preferred over creams because of their occlusive effect, which ensures a stronger barrier and absorption into the skin. Hydrocortisone 1% or triamcinolone 0.1% is usually the drug of choice. Corticosteroids are used two to three times daily for 2 weeks and must be applied before the skin moisturizer is used. Oral corticosteroids may be used for an acute exacerbation; however, there is often a rebound effect (ie, after the medication is discontinued, the rash returns). Systemic antibiotics are given only if the child has a superimposed infection.

Antihistamine agents such as hydroxyzine (Vistaril and Atarax) can be given to relieve itching. Methods to reduce pruritus include environmental controls, such as humidification in the winter and air conditioning in the summer. Use of a humidifier counteracts dryness of the surrounding air, minimizing loss of skin moisture. Air conditioning limits unnecessary sweating that can exacerbate inflamed areas.

Because of the high rate of food allergies in infants under 2 years of age, a food elimination test may be suggested for infants and young children with moderate to severe eczema needing daily treatment. Milk, wheat, eggs, soy products, citrus, and peanuts are the foods most often withheld for 2 or more weeks to determine if any change in skin condition occurs. Foods withheld are then introduced one at a time to determine which ones are the allergens. A RAST (radioallergosorbent) test is sometimes used to exclude allergens (see Chap. 9).

Nursing Assessment

A thorough history, including any family history of allergy, environmental or dietary factors, and past exacerbations, is necessary. Note distribution and type of lesions.

Nursing Diagnosis

Common nursing diagnoses that may be appropriate for the child with eczema include:

- Impaired Skin Integrity related to open vesicles and open lesions as a result of scratching
- Risk for Infection related to breaks in skin barrier
- Body Image Disturbance related to presence of noticeable skin lesions
- Self-Esteem Disturbance related to peer reaction to visible skin lesions
- Knowledge Deficit (Child and Parents) related to measures that will help keep the condition under control during and between flare-ups

Nursing Management

Nursing management focuses on education and emotional support. Although no "cure" has been found for eczema, the condition can be controlled. Advise parents that the lesions are not contagious and will not result in scarring. Help parents and adolescents deal with the frustration of the acute flare-ups of the condition by reinforcing that remissions do occur with good home care.

Instruct parents or adolescents to avoid using harsh or perfumed soaps. Use a mild soap (eg, Dove or Tone), but only where the skin is dirty. Washing clean skin with soap only dries it out. Use wet wraps for severely affected skin to give moisture back to the skin. Hot water can exacerbate the condition and increase itching. Recommend tepid baths and patting dry or air drying afterward. Moisturizers should be applied immediately after the bath to help retain moisture. Wool clothing should be avoided because it can increase skin irritation and pruritus. Encourage the wearing of loose cotton clothing.

Teach parents and adolescents appropriate application of topical ointments or creams. Instruct parents to place clean cotton gloves or socks over the infant or young child's hands and to keep the child's fingernails cut short to decrease scratching and reduce the chance of secondary infection.

Eczema produces visible changes that can affect a child's self-confidence and self-esteem. Children need to be educated about the disorder and its treatment. Emphasize the importance of following the treatment plan to promote healing of existing lesions and to reduce the risk of secondary infections.

Once the condition is under control, counsel the parents about the method for introducing a food that was previously eliminated when an allergen cause of eczema was suspected (see Chap. 9). Emphasize that increased itching within hours of eating a food may be associated with the eczema flare-up. Teach parents how to control the skin inflammation that results, as described above. Once a specific food allergy has been identified, refer the parents to a nutritionist for counseling related to alternative food options that will fulfill daily nutritional requirements. Refer the family to the Food Allergy Network (see Appendix F).

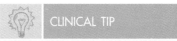

CLINICAL TIP

Children with acute exacerbations of eczema are often sleep deprived because of the discomfort and itching. Help parents recognize that this is often a cause of the child's irritability and offer strategies, such as scheduling the antihistamine medication just before naps and bedtime, to promote sleep.

▶ ACNE

Acne, an inflammatory disorder of the pilosebaceous unit (hair follicle and sebaceous gland), is the most common skin disorder in the pediatric population. It is believed to be triggered by the increased androgen production of puberty. The prevalence in adolescents aged 15–17 years is estimated to approach 85%. The condition is often more severe in the winter. Acne may also occur in neonates in response to maternal androgen hormones. This form of acne usually develops between 2 and 4 weeks of age and resolves by 4–6 months of age.

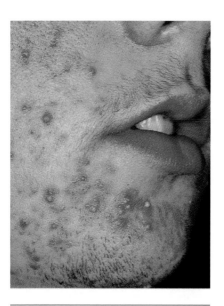

FIGURE 21–5. Pustular acne can have a signif-icant effect on an adolescent's self-esteem. *From Habif, T.P. (1990). Clinical dermatology: A color guide to diagnosis and therapy (2nd ed., p. 113). St. Louis: Mosby–Year Book.*

NURSING ALERT

Accutane is teratogenic. All females using Accutane must actively avoid pregnancy, through either abstinence or contraception. Some providers have adolescents sign a contract to emphasize the importance of this issue.

Clinical Manifestations

There are three main types of acne: comedomal (characterized by open and closed comedones), papulopustular (characterized by papules and pus-tules) (Fig. 21–5), and cystic (characterized by nodules and cysts). Lesions occur most often on the face, upper chest, shoulders, and back. In adoles-cents, the major complaint is an increase in the number of closed (black-head) or open (whitehead) comedones, pimples, and red papules that are tender to touch. Postinflammatory redness results. Cystic acne may result in permanent scarring and disfigurement.

Etiology and Pathophysiology

Keratin and sebum that usually flow to the skin surface are obstructed in the follicular canal, causing comedones (whiteheads and blackheads) and pimples. The closed comedones get larger and tend to rupture, sending sebum into the dermis. This sets off an inflammatory reaction. When the inflammatory reaction is close to the surface, a papule or pustule develops. If the inflammatory reaction is deeper, a larger papule or nodule develops. A bacterium, *Propionibacterium acnes,* resides on the skin and produces an enzyme that intensifies the inflammatory response.[9] The inflammatory re-action is not related to foods, and it is not caused by dirty skin. Although fa-milial trends are recognized, hard data to define the pattern of inheritance are not conclusive.

Diagnostic Tests and Medical Management

Treatment depends on the type of lesion. Most adolescent acne is treated with topical and oral medications, alone or in combination. Table 21–5 out-lines specific treatment protocols for comedomal, papulopustular, and cys-tic acne. The goal of treatment is to prevent infection and scarring and minimize psychologic distress.

Nursing Assessment

Physical assessment should include documentation regarding distribution, type, and severity of acne lesions. Assess the child's and parents' knowledge

21-5	Treatment Protocols for Acne	
Appearance	**Treatment**
Mild papular acne	2.5% benzoyl peroxide gel
Comedomal acne (comedones only)	Tretinoin (Retin-A) 0.025% cream daily, in the evening
Papulopustular acne (red papules, pus-tules)	Tretinoin (Retin-A) in evening and 10% ben-zoyl peroxide in morning
Cystic acne (red papules, many pustules, cysts)	Tretinoin (Retin-A) and benzoyl peroxide twice a day, with oral antibiotics (tetra-cycline or erythromycin)
Pustulocystic nodular (severe, resistant to other treatment)	Isotretinoin (Accutane)

Adapted from Hurwitz, S. (1995). Acne treatment for the '90s. Contemporary Pediatrics 12(8), 19–32.

about the cause and treatment of acne. Also explore the amount of emotional distress the acne is causing the adolescent.

Nursing Diagnosis

Common nursing diagnoses are presented in the Nursing Care Plan for the Adolescent With Acne.

Nursing Management

Nursing care for the adolescent with acne is summarized in the accompanying Nursing Care Plan. Nursing management focuses on educating the child and parents about acne and its treatment. Advise adolescents not to touch the affected areas and to avoid picking at lesions. Remind them that the inflammation occurs with the rupture of lesions below the skin surface, which picking and squeezing may cause. In addition, advise them to avoid using any cosmetics or cleansing products that have a greasy base, to shampoo hair regularly (to treat seborrhea that can accompany acne), to expect flare-ups despite treatment, and to eat a well-balanced diet.

Instruct adolescents to wash the face no more than two to three times a day with a mild soap, then wait about 20–30 minutes before applying tretinoin (Retin-A), if prescribed. Topical medications should be spread in a thin film over the skin, according to directions. Emphasize that treatment is often long term. Significant improvement may not be seen until at least 6–12 weeks after the start of treatment.

Correct misconceptions about dietary causes. (For example, there is no evidence that chocolate or other fatty foods cause acne.) Good nutrition is important. Teach parents and children that increased sweating, as well as heat and humidity, may exacerbate acne. Emotional stress may increase adrenal androgen production, resulting in increased sebum production and acne flare-ups.

Caution patients who are using tretinoin that this medication can make their skin sensitive to sunlight, resulting in sunburn with even minimal exposure. Applying tretinoin in the evening rather than in the morning can reduce this side effect. However, sunscreens should still be used whenever the skin is exposed to sunlight because of the increased skin sensitivity. Teach correct procedures for taking other prescribed drugs, such as tetracycline and isotretinoin (Accutane), and discuss possible side effects. Emphasize the importance of return visits to the adolescent's health care provider to monitor side effects of medications.

Psychologic support is an important aspect of care. Because adolescents are preoccupied with their body image and peer relationships, they often find having acne embarrassing. Encourage them to express their feelings and refer for counseling, if necessary.

▶ INFECTIOUS DISORDERS

IMPETIGO

Impetigo is a highly contagious, superficial infection caused by streptococci, staphylococci, or both. The most common sites are the face, around the mouth, the hands, the neck, and the extremities. It is the most common bacterial skin condition in children and accounts for nearly 10% of all skin problems.[10]

Clinical manifestations include pruritus, burning, and secondary lymph node involvement. The lesion begins as a vesicle or pustule that is surrounded by edema and redness, usually at a site that has been injured.

NURSING CARE PLAN
THE ADOLESCENT WITH ACNE

GOAL	INTERVENTION	RATIONALE	EXPECTED OUTCOME

1. Impaired Skin Integrity related to destruction of skin layers, multiple pustules, papules, and secretions

The adolescent will verbalize proper hygiene, nutrition, and treatment of acne[a].	• Teach good skin care:
	  • Wash skin with mild soap and water twice a day.
	  • Do not use astringents.
	  • Avoid vigorous scrubbing.
	• Praise good habits.
	• Advise the adolescent to wash hair with antiseborrheic shampoo, avoid oil-based cosmetics or lotions.
		• Good hygiene and appropriate skin care reduce surface oils and bacteria, which intensify inflammatory reactions.
		
		• Treats seborrhea, which frequently accompanies acne. Oil-based preparations can obstruct sebaceous glands, exacerbating acne.
			The adolescent exhibits habits of good hygiene.

	• Encourage a balanced diet, adequate fluids, exercise, and adequate rest. • Encourage the adolescent to keep a diary of health and diet habits.	• Adequate nutrients, water, and exercise promote healthy skin.	The adolescent keeps a diary for 1 week to support healthy habits.

2. Knowledge Deficit related to treatment of acne

The adolescent will verbalize understanding of treatment regimen.	• Educate the adolescent about medications (action, side effects, dosage, method of application). • Encourage application of tretinoin at night. Encourage use of non-oil sunscreens of at least SPF 15. • Educate the adolescent about time needed for response and importance of daily compliance.	• Proper application of medication enhances healing of lesions. • Helps reduce sensitivity to sun and avoid sunburn. • May take up to 3 months for significant improvement to occur. The adolescent needs a reason to continue with the care plan.	The adolescent states understanding of treatment regimen, resulting in a noticeable reduction in lesions.

[a]The care described for goal 1 also applies to goal 2.

This progresses to an exudative and crusting stage. The initially serous vesicular fluid becomes cloudy, and the vesicle ruptures, leaving a honey-colored crust covering an ulcerated base (Fig. 21–6). Less commonly bullous impetigo develops, sometimes in the skin folds. The vesicles enlarge

NURSING CARE PLAN
THE ADOLESCENT WITH ACNE— *Continued*

GOAL	INTERVENTION	RATIONALE	EXPECTED OUTCOME

3. Body Image Disturbance related to visible facial lesions as evidenced by decreased interest in self and self-degrading comments

GOAL	INTERVENTION	RATIONALE	EXPECTED OUTCOME
The adolescent will demonstrate increased self-confidence and self-esteem.	• Establish rapport with the adolescent.	• A trusting relationship promotes verbalization of concerns and fears.	The adolescent freely discusses concerns and fears.
	• Provide education about the condition and therapy modalities.	• Providing information better enables the adolescent to take control of the condition.	The adolescent demonstrates active involvement in own care.
	• Encourage the adolescent to be responsible for treatment and follow-up, and give positive reinforcement when compliance is noted.	• Responsibility reinforces sense of self-esteem.	
	• Encourage the adolescent to become involved with school activities and peers.	• Involvement in activities helps to enhance self-esteem and allows the adolescent to explore new experiences and friendships.	The adolescent shows increased confidence, as demonstrated by involvement in extracurricular activities.

into bullae with straw-colored fluid and then rupture, forming erosions with crusts. There is little erythema.

Infection occurs more commonly in children who are in close physical contact with one another. Children frequently pass the infection to one another in preschool or day-care settings.

Local treatment involves removal of the crusts and application of a topical antibiotic. Crusts are soaked in warm water and gently scrubbed with an antiseptic soap (pHisoHex). A topical bactericidal ointment (such as neosporin, bacitracin, or mupirocin) is applied for 5–7 days. If there is no response to topical antibiotics, a systemic antibiotic (eg, dicloxacillin or erythromycin) may be needed. The infection is communicable for 48 hours after antibiotic ointment treatment is begun.

Nursing Management

Advise parents that oral or topical medications must be continued for the full number of days prescribed. Tell the parents to observe all close contacts and family members for lesions. Caution parents that an infected child should not share towels or toiletries with others and that all linens and clothing used by the child should be washed separately with detergent in hot water. Fingernails should be kept short and clean to prevent the spread of infection from scratching.

 CLINICAL TIP

Inform the child's day care center about the infection, so toys and surfaces can be sanitized.

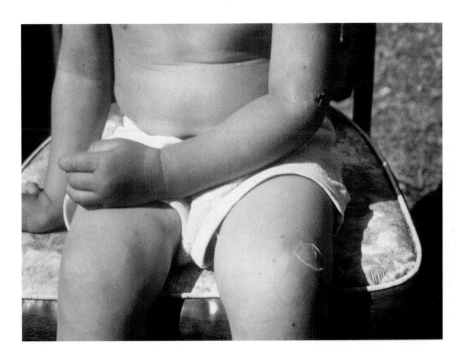

FIGURE 21–6. Characteristic lesions of impetigo.
Courtesy of the Centers for Disease Control, Atlanta, GA.

FOLLICULITIS

Folliculitis is a superficial inflammation of the pilosebaceous follicle caused by infection, trauma, or irritation. The condition is common in children and teenagers because of increased sweat production.

Symptoms include tenderness, localized swelling, and the formation of tiny dome-shaped, yellowish pustules and red papules at follicular openings with surrounding erythema. Individual lesions may become deeper and form an abscess. Lesions are usually seen in clusters on the face, scalp, and extremities. The causative organism is usually *Staphylococcus aureus*.

Treatment of inflamed follicles consists of washing the affected area with a topical antibiotic cleanser (eg, chlorhexidine or hexachlorophene) and water, followed by application of hot compresses for 20 minutes, four times a day. Complications are rare. If lesions do not resolve within a week, the child may need systemic antibiotics (eg, cephalexin or dicloxacillin) and, if the infection is deep, incision and drainage.

Nursing Management

Nursing management focuses on educating the parents and child about prevention. Advise children to shower daily and shortly after exercise, to cleanse with an antibacterial soap, and to wear loose cotton clothing.

CELLULITIS

Cellulitis is an acute inflammation of the dermis and underlying connective tissue characterized by red or lilac, tender, edematous skin that may have an ill-defined, nonelevated border.[11] The condition usually occurs on the face and extremities as a result of trauma or compromise of the skin barrier.

Clinical Manifestations

Children with cellulitis appear ill and are commonly febrile. Classic signs and symptoms include erythema, edema of the face or infected limb, warmth, and tenderness around the infected site (Fig. 21–7). Other symptoms include chills, malaise, and enlargement and tenderness of regional lymph nodes. In some cases, a rapidly progressive lesion may result in septicemia.

Etiology and Pathophysiology

Children with cellulitis often have a history of trauma, impetigo, folliculitis, or recent otitis media. Common causative organisms are *Staphylococcus aureus* and beta-hemolytic and group A *Streptococcus*. The condition may also result from a nearby abscess or sinusitis. Onset is usually rapid.

Diagnostic Tests and Medical Management

Blood studies may show an increase in white blood cells. Cultures are taken by needle aspiration, if possible, to identify the causative organisms. Blood cultures are taken if the child has a toxic (very ill) appearance. If the face is involved, antibiotic therapy is administered to avoid serious complications. (Periorbital cellulitis is discussed in Chapter 17.)

Children with cellulitis on the trunk, limbs, or perianal area may be treated on an outpatient basis with oral antibiotics. Recovery begins within 48 hours, but therapy should continue for at least 10 days.

Children with severe cases or a large affected surface area are hospitalized to prevent sepsis. Systemic antibiotics are administered. Untreated cellulitis or cellulitis that does not respond to treatment can lead to osteomyelitis or arthritis.

Nursing Assessment

Assessment centers on recognition of infection, documentation of location and related symptoms, and monitoring of vital signs.

Nursing Diagnosis

Among the nursing diagnoses that may be appropriate for the child with cellulitis are:

- Impaired Skin Integrity related to the inflammatory process and presence of infection
- Pain related to swelling and inflammation of the skin
- Knowledge Deficit (Parent or Child) related to care of the infected area

Nursing Management

Because of the risk of sepsis, cellulitis should be managed carefully. Administer prescribed antibiotics. Supportive care includes warm compresses to the affected area four times daily, elevation of the affected limb, and bed rest. Outpatient follow-up is crucial.

Advise parents about possible complications, such as abcess formation. Instruct parents of children who are treated at home to contact their health care provider if the child has any of the following signs: (1) spread of the infected area in the 24–48-hour period after the start of treatment, (2) temperature over 38.3°C (101°F), or (3) increased lethargy. Reinforce to parents the importance of compliance with the treatment regimen and the seriousness associated with complications.

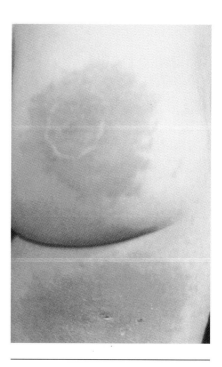

FIGURE 21–7. Characteristic appearance of cellulitis.
From Ben-Amitai, D., & Ashkenazi, S. (1993). Common bacterial skin infections in children. Pediatric Annals, 22(4), 226. Photograph courtesy of Dr. Aryeh Metzker.

PEDICULOSIS CAPITIS (LICE)

Pediculosis capitis is an infestation of the hair and scalp with lice. Head lice live and reproduce only on humans and are transmitted by direct or indirect contact such as sharing of brushes, hats, towels, and bedding. Lice do not fly or jump, but they can crawl quickly. The female louse lays her eggs (nits) on the hair shaft, close to the scalp (see Fig. 3–8). The incubation period is 8–10 days.

Clinical manifestations include intense pruritus and complaints of "dandruff" that sticks to the hair (actually the nits) and "bugs" in the hair. Nits look like silvery white 1-mm teardrops adhering to the hair shaft. Secondary effects of scratching include inflammation, pustules, and bacterial infection. Nits are found most commonly behind the ears and at the crown and back of the head. Lice move quickly away from light and are not commonly seen. Occipital nodes are frequently palpable.

Infestation occurs among children of all socioeconomic levels. The presence of lice may be noted by parents or teachers, or by health care providers during routine examination of the child (see Chap. 3). Outbreaks occur periodically among preschool and school-age children, particularly those in day care and elementary school.

Treatment involves the use of a pediculicide shampoo, such as pyrethrum with an enzymatic lice egg remover, or an ovicidal rinse, such as permethrin (Nix). Lindane shampoo is a treatment of last resort because of its toxicity.[12] The hair is towel dried, and the nits are removed with a fine-toothed comb. The treatment is repeated in 7 days.

Permethrin cream rinse is applied to washed and towel-dried hair. The preparation is applied, left in place for 10 minutes, and then rinsed. The hair is towel dried, and the nits are removed with a fine-toothed comb. Vinegar compresses (50% vinegar and 50% water) help loosen the nit's bond to the hair shaft. One-time treatment is effective in only 70–80% of cases, however, and a second treatment is usually needed in 7 days.

Nursing Management

Carefully assess children who have been exposed to head lice (see Chap. 3). To avoid potential reinfestation of other children, change gloves frequently when assessing several children in a classroom setting.

Infestation with lice can be upsetting for both the child and family. Emphasize to the family that anyone can get lice. Thorough interventions and education are essential for effective treatment.

Explain to parents that the shampoo and rinses prescribed are pesticides and must be used as directed. Keep these products out of the eyes and mouth of the child during their use. When combing the hair to remove nits, a creme rinse or oil may make combing easier. Comb 1–inch sections and pin these out of the way when done.

Although lice can survive for only about 48 hours away from a human host, nits that are shed are capable of hatching 8–10 days later. For this reason, bedding and clothing used by the child should be changed daily, laundered in hot water with detergent, and dried in a hot dryer for 20 minutes. Nonessential bedding and clothing can be stored in a tightly sealed bag for 10 days to 2 weeks and then washed. Hairbrushes and combs should be discarded or soaked in hot water (54.4°C [130°F]) for 10–15 minutes or washed with pediculicide shampoo. Furniture and carpets should be vacuumed and treated with a hot iron when possible. Seal toys that cannot be washed or dry cleaned in a plastic bag for 2 weeks.

CLINICAL TIP

Instruct parents that children infested with lice should not return to day care or school until after the first pediculicide treatment is completed. Parents of other children exposed to the infected child should be notified so they can watch for signs of infestation.

NURSING ALERT

Use of an insecticide in the home to kill the lice on carpets, furniture, and other items with which young children and pets come into contact is not recommended.

All contacts of the child should be examined for infestation and should be treated as necessary. Teach the child not to share clothing, headwear, or combs.

SCABIES

Scabies is a highly contagious infestation caused by the mite *Sarcoptes scabiei.* Symptoms include a rash with various types of lesions, severe pruritus that worsens at night, and restlessness. Lesions are usually located in the webs of the fingers, in the intergluteal folds, around the axillae, or on the palms, wrists, head, neck, legs, buttocks, chest, abdomen, and waist (Fig. 21–8). In infants the palms, soles, head, and neck can be affected. Lesions appear as linear, threadlike, grayish burrows 1–10 cm in length, which may end in a pinpoint vesicle. The lesion may have been obliterated by the child's scratching.

Children of all ages and both sexes can be affected. The female mite burrows into the outer layer of the epidermis (stratum corneum) to lay her eggs. The larvae hatch in approximately 2–4 days and proceed toward the surface of the skin. The cycle is repeated 14–17 days later. The intense pruritus is caused by sensitization to the ova and mite feces, which occurs approximately 1 month after infestation. Nodules, which can persist for weeks after effective treatment, develop as a granulomatous response to the dead mite antigens and feces. Because the mite usually takes at least 45 minutes to burrow into the skin, transient contact is unlikely to cause infestation.

Diagnosis is confirmed by examination under the microscope of scrapings from a burrow, which reveals eggs or nits. Treatment involves application of a scabicide, such as 5% permethrin lotion, over the entire body from the chin down. Lindane is no longer recommended for full-body application in infants and young children because seizures have been reported.[12]

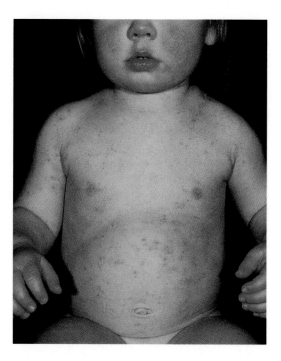

FIGURE 21–8. Diffuse scabies in an infant. The lesions are most numerous around the axillae, chest, and abdomen.
From Habif, T.P. (1990). Clinical dermatology: A color guide to diagnosis and therapy (2nd ed., p. 298). St. Louis: Mosby–Year Book.

Apply scabicide only to the scalp and forehead of infants. The lotion can be applied to the face of older children if lesions are present.

Application of 5% permethrin lotion is preceded by a warm soap and water bath. Skin must be cool and dry before the lotion is applied. The lotion is left in place for 8–12 hours before washing it off. Usually only one application is necessary; however, 2- or 3-day treatment cycles are sometimes recommended. All members of the household should be treated at the same time. An oral antihistamine (eg, Benadryl, Atarax) may be prescribed to help relieve itching.

Nursing Management

Advise parents that scabies is transmitted by close contact and is very contagious. All clothing, bedding, and pillowcases used by the child should be changed daily, washed with boiling water, and ironed before reuse. Nonwashable toys and other items should be sealed in plastic bags for 4 days.

Family members who are not infected should avoid touching the affected child until after treatment is completed. If contact is made, hands should be washed well. Inform the parents about signs of secondary infections and that itching and nodules may persist for weeks after effective treatment.

Scabies, like pediculosis, can be embarrassing or upsetting for the child and family. Educate the child and parents about the condition, its spread, and treatment measures to prevent recurrence.

FUNGAL INFECTIONS

Oral Candidiasis (Thrush)

Oral candidiasis (moniliasis or thrush) is a fungal infection that occurs as an acute condition in newborns (usually acquired during birth from the vaginal canal of an infected mother) and a chronic condition in young children who:

- Have an immune disorder
- Regularly use a corticosteroid inhaler
- Are receiving antibiotics, which have disturbed the normal flora, allowing the growth of the fungus

Thrush is characterized by white patches that look like coagulated milk on the oral mucosa and may bleed when removed (Fig. 21–9). The infant may refuse to nurse or feed because of discomfort and pain. The infant may also have diaper dermatitis superinfection with candidiasis. Fever is usually not present.

Treatment involves oral nystatin suspension, which is applied to the mouth and tongue after feedings. For infants, parents should use a swab to apply the suspension to the buccal mucosa and tongue surfaces, allowing the infant to swallow the remaining suspension. Older children are instructed to swish the solution around in the mouth before swallowing it.

If infection is severe, occurs in the esophagus, or invades other body systems, oral fluconazole or intravenous amphotericin B may be prescribed.

Nursing Management

To prevent a reinfection, educate parents about the appropriate sterilization technique for bottle nipples and pacifiers the infant puts in the mouth. A commercial antiseptic spray may be used on toys that cannot be auto-

CLINICAL TIP

The white patches of candidiasis are easily differentiated from coagulated milk. Milk residue can be removed from the oral mucosa with gentle swabbing. With candidiasis, however, attempts at gentle removal are unsuccessful. (Avoid scraping the patches, as this will result in bleeding.)

claved, but follow directions carefully so the child does not ingest any harmful residue. Teach parents and older children with asthma to rinse the mouth well with water after using a corticosteroid inhaler to prevent candidiasis.

Dermatophytoses (Ringworm)

Dermatophytoses are fungal infections that affect the skin, hair, or nails. Children of all ages may be affected. Dermatophytoses may be spread from person to person or from animal to person. The most common infections are tinea capitis, tinea corporis, tinea cruris, and tinea pedis. Table 21–6 compares and contrasts these infections.

Diagnosis is confirmed through microscopic examination of the scrapings using a potassium hydroxide (KOH) wet mount to reveal hyphae (threadlike fungal bodies). A Wood's lamp is also useful in identifying some forms of tinea that fluoresce under ultraviolet light. However, *Trichophyton tonsurans*, the most common cause of tinea capitis, does not fluoresce with a Wood's lamp.[13] Treatment involves application of an antifungal lotion, cream, or shampoo. An oral antifungal agent (eg, griseofulvin) is usually prescribed for tinea capitis (see Table 21–6).

Nursing Management

Advise parents to give oral griseofulvin with fatty foods such as whole milk to enhance absorption. Lotions, creams, and shampoos should be applied to the entire lesion, as well as to approximately 1 cm surrounding the lesion. The oral and topical medications must be used for the entire prescribed period, even if the lesions are gone, to prevent recurrence of the infection. Teach parents and older children or teenagers that fungi are found in soil and animals and are transmitted through direct contact. Household pets should be examined for signs of infection.

Since person-to-person transmission is common, personal contact with hair and the sharing of hair care products should be avoided. For children with tinea cruris, encourage the use of loose-fitting undergarments to promote dryness. With tinea pedis, feet should be kept clean and dry and nails clipped short. Discourage the wearing of occlusive footwear or nylon socks, which trap moisture.

Parents of children with tinea capitis should be told that hair regrowth is slow and may take 6–12 months. In some cases hair loss is permanent, which can be particularly stressful for older children or adolescents. Provide emotional support.

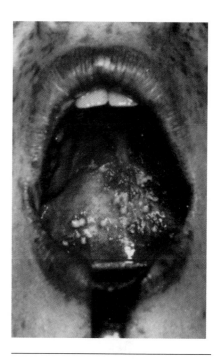

FIGURE 21–9. Thrush, an acute pseudomembranous form of oral candidiasis, is a common fungal infection in infants and young children. *From Orkin, M., Maibach, H.I., & Dahl, M.V. (1991). Dermatology (p. 575). Norwalk, CT: Appleton & Lange.*

► INJURIES TO THE SKIN

PRESSURE ULCERS

An increasing number of children with disabilities are cared for in hospital, community, and home care settings. Many of these children are at risk for skin breakdown and pressure ulcer formation. Soft tissues can be compressed for a prolonged period of time between a bony prominence and another surface in each of the following circumstances:

- Braces used for body alignment or mobility
- Wheelchairs used for mobility
- Confinement to bed

21-6	Types of Tinea Infection		
Site	**Clinical Manifestations**	**Incidence**	**Treatment**
Tinea capitis[13] (scalp)	Hair loss (one or several patches which slowly increase in size); broken hairs; black, dotted stubbed appearance where weakened hair has broken off; folliculitis; thickened, white scales; fine scaling; mild itching	Usually prepubertal children between 3 and 9 years of age	Griseofulvin orally for 8 weeks; selenium sulfide shampoo for up to 8 weeks, leave on 10 minutes before rinsing
Tinea corporis (trunk)	One or several circular erythematous patches; may be scaly or erythematous throughout; slightly raised borders with a clearing center	Children or adolescents	Topical cream (eg, clotrimazole, miconazole, tolnaftate) twice a day for 4 weeks
Tinea cruris ("jock itch") (inner thighs, inguinal creases)	Scaly, erythematous eruption symmetric bilaterally; possibly elevated lesions; possible papules or vesicles	Rare before adolescence	Same as for tinea corporis
Tinea pedis ("athlete's foot", (feet and toes)	Vesicles or erosions on instep or between toes (fissures, red scaly); itching	Usually postpubertal adolescents	Same as for tinea corporis and cruris

Tinea capitis

Tinea corporis

Photographs of tinea capitis and tinea corporis courtesy of the Centers for Disease Control and Prevention, Atlanta, GA.
Based on information in Givens, T.G., Murray M.M., & Baker, R.C. (1995). Comparison of 1% and 2.5% selenium sulfide in the treatment of tinea capitis. Archives of Pediatrics and Adolescent Medicine, 149(7), 808–812.

Children at greatest risk are those with limited mobility, sensory deficits, or the inability to change positions (Table 21–7).

Clinical Manifestations

The earliest sign of skin damage is an area of redness that does not go away within 30 minutes of removing the pressure or skin irritant. In the next stage the skin looks rubbed or raw (superficial or partial thickness injury), similar to an abrasion or blister. If intervention does not occur, the skin damage extends through the epidermis and dermis (full-thickness injury) and an ulcer forms. Damage to underlying tissue (muscles, bone, or connective tissue) occurs if the skin damage progresses.[14, 15] (Fig 21–10).

21-7	Sites and Potential Causes of Pressure Ulcers

Sites	Potential Causes
Occipital region of scalp	Inability to lift head
Sacrum and buttocks	Confinement to bed or wheelchair
Legs and feet	Leg braces
Spine and neck	Scoliosis brace
Knees and elbows	Rubbing against bed sheet

Etiology and Pathophysiology

Tissue ischemia occurs as the cells are deprived of oxygen and nutrients, and metabolic waste products accumulate, resulting in soft tissue injury. Without appropriate intervention, the injury becomes rapidly progressive and a pressure ulcer forms. Tissue ischemia occurs when high pressure is maintained over a short period of time or low pressure is maintained over a prolonged time.

Medical Management

Initial treatment for early stages of skin damage involves removing pressure from the affected site until the skin has healed. Children who use leg braces for alignment and mobility are often put in wheelchairs. Children who use wheelchairs are often put on bed rest on a pressure-reducing surface. Frequent repositioning is needed. A transparent film may be applied to affected red skin to minimize friction. Pressure ulcers are treated with various dressings, such as hydrocolloids, gels or hydrogels, and calcium alginates.[14]

Nursing Assessment

Carefully inspect the dependent skin surfaces of all infants and children confined to bed at least three times in each 24–hour period. Evaluate the risk for skin damage by considering factors that can contribute to skin breakdown, such as the following:[16]

- Ability to change and control body position
- Degree of physical activity
- Ability to respond to pressure-related discomfort
- Ability to perceive normal sensation
- Degree to which the skin is exposed to moisture
- Extent to which the skin rubs against support surfaces
- Nutritional status of the child
- Child's tissue perfusion and oxygenation

Identify the size (diameter and depth) and character of the skin lesion. Note any signs of infection, the appearance of wound edges, and the type of tissue at the wound base. Describe drainage amount, color, and type.

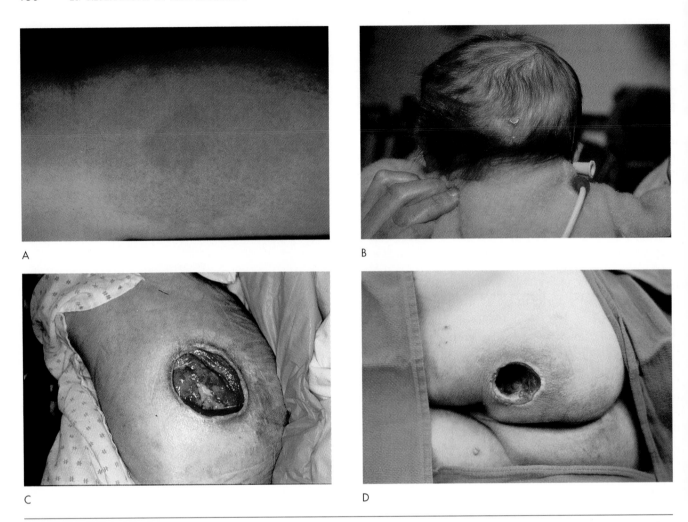

FIGURE 21–10. The four stages of pressure ulcer formation. **A,** Stage 1, abrasion or blister appearance; nonblanchable erythema of intact skin. **B,** Stage 2, damage through the epidermis, dermis, or both. **C,** Stage 3, damage and necrosis of subcutaneous tissue; deep crater with or without undermining of adjacent tissue. **D,** Stage 4, extensive destruction to muscle, bone, or supporting tissues.
Courtesy Sandra Quigley, Children's Hospital, Boston, MA.

Nursing Diagnosis

The following nursing diagnoses may be appropriate for the child at risk for pressure sores:

- Risk for Impaired Skin Integrity related to infant's inability to shift position
- Impaired Skin Integrity related to irritation from leg brace that is too small
- Impaired Physical Mobility related to pressure sores
- Risk for Infection related to breaks in the skin

Nursing Management

Develop protocols for pressure ulcer prevention so that children at high risk are identified and appropriate interventions are initiated. Such interventions may include increased ambulation, frequent position changes, use of pressure-reducing surfaces, and use of moisture barriers.

Provide wound care and dressing changes according to agency guidelines. These guidelines may include irrigating the site with saline, debridement, and the application of a dressing appropriate for the wound condition. Avoid the use of tape to hold dressings in place unless a protective skin barrier is used.

Care in the Community

Teach parents of children with impaired mobility and diminished pain sensation to inspect the braces and skin under the braces every day for signs of irritation (redness or blisters). Take the braces off and help the child to use a mirror with a long handle to inspect skin on the bottom and sides of the feet, behind the knees, and lower legs. Check all edges of the braces for roughness or breakage that can pinch or scrape the skin. If any sign of skin irritation is seen and redness does not go away within 30 minutes, do not put the brace back on until the skin heals. Inform the child's physician so that an appropriate treatment regimen can be started immediately. To prevent braces from rubbing on bare skin, have the child wear cotton socks under the braces. To avoid irritation of the foot, shoes should be purchased that are large enough to accommodate the brace and the foot in the shoe. Advise parents to return to a prosthetist regularly for refitting as the child grows.

Children who are confined to a wheelchair are at risk for skin breakdown on the buttocks and lower back because of the pressure from sitting for hours. A wheelchair cushion can distribute and shift the child's weight when sitting in the chair. Frequent position changes need to be made to relieve the pressure on the skin. Teach the child to do wheelchair push-ups or to shift the weight by leaning to the side or forward for several minutes every 10–15 minutes. Make sure the child wears a safety belt when sitting in the wheelchair. Teach school personnel about the child's recommended protocol so they can provide opportunities in school to change positions and reinforce the routine.

BURNS

Burns are the second leading cause of injury deaths (after motor vehicle crashes) in children between 1 and 9 years of age.[17] Boys between the ages of 1 and 4 years are twice as likely as girls to be burned. However, the national average age of pediatric burn patients is 32 months. Each year in the United States alone there are over 2 million injuries and thousands of deaths related to burns.

There are four main types of burns: thermal, chemical, electrical, and radioactive. Thermal burns, the most common burns in children, may occur through exposure to flames or scalds (such as coffee or grease), or contact with a hot object (such as a wood stove or curling iron). Sherray, described in the opening vignette, sustained a scald burn when a bowl of hot soup fell onto her leg. Chemical burns occur when children touch or ingest caustic agents. Electrical burns occur from exposure to direct or alternating current in electrical wires, appliances, or high-voltage wires. Radiation burns result from exposure to radioactive substances or sunlight.

Etiology

Children at different developmental stages are at risk for different types of burns (Table 21–8):

- Infants are most often injured by thermal burns (scalding liquids, house fires) (Fig. 21–11).
- Toddlers are at risk for thermal burns (pulling hot liquids or grease onto themselves), electrical burns (biting electrical cords) (Fig. 21–12),

CLINICAL TIP

A full-thickness burn can occur in adults after only 2 seconds' immersion in water with a temperature of 65°C (149°F). The amount of time for a burn to occur increases to 10 minutes when water temperature is 50°C (122°F). Because infants and children have more sensitive skin, less time is needed for them to receive a serious burn.[18]

21-8	Distribution of Children by Age and Burn Type Treated in a Burn Center Between 1991 and 1993		
Burn Type	0–2 Years	2–5 Years	5–20 Years
Scald	69.7%	62.5%	26.8%
Flame	7.5%	20.4%	60.7%
Contact	19.3%	13.9%	5.3%
Electrical	0.7%	1.7%	4.5%
All others	2.8%	1.5%	2.7%

Adapted from Saffle, J.R., Davis, B., Williams, P., & the American Burn Association Registry Participant Group. (1995). Recent outcomes in the treatment of burn injury in the United States: A report of the American Burn Patient Registry. Journal of Burn Care Rehabilitation, 16(3), 219–232.

contact burns, and chemical burns (ingesting cleaning agents and other substances) associated with exploring the environment.

- Preschool-age children are most often injured by scalding or contact with hot appliances (curling irons, ovens).
- School-age children are at risk for thermal burns (playing with matches), electrical burns (climbing high-voltage towers, climbing trees, and contact with electrical wires), and chemical burns (combustion experiments) associated with their curiosity and interest in experimentation (Fig. 21–13).
- Adolescents also experience thermal, chemical, and electrical burns.

Medical Management

Assessment of Burn Severity

Burn severity is determined by the depth of the burn injury, percentage of body surface area (BSA) affected, and involvement of specific body parts.

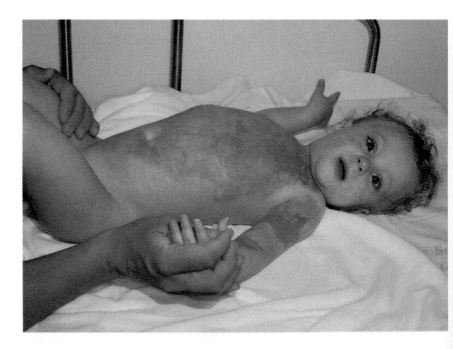

FIGURE 21–11. Thermal (scald) burns are the most common burn injury in infancy.

Burn depth may be defined as partial thickness or full thickness. Partial-thickness burns, in which the injured tissue can regenerate and heal, encompass first- and second-degree burns. Full-thickness burns, in which the injured tissue cannot regenerate, are also known as third-degree burns (Table 21–9).

A Lund and Browder chart with BSA distributions for various body parts at different ages is used to calculate the area affected by the burn injury (Fig. 21–14). Once the affected BSA is calculated, the burn can be classified as minor (less than 10% BSA partial thickness or 2% BSA full thickness), moderate (10–20% BSA partial thickness or 3–10% BSA full thickness), or major (greater than 20% BSA partial thickness or 10% BSA full thickness).[18] Children with moderate and major burns require hospitalization.

The involvement of specific body parts or specific burn distributions increases the burn severity, regardless of the percentage of BSA affected. Burns to the face, hands, feet, or perineal area are treated as major injuries because of the potential for functional impairment. Circumferential burns (injury completely surrounding the thorax or an extremity), anterior chest burns, and smoke inhalation are also classified as major burns.

Initial Treatment

The first step is to stop the burning process by removing any jewelry and all clothing. Emergency treatment of major burns is based on the ABCs of basic life support (*a*irway patency, *b*reathing, and *c*irculation). Assessment and treatment are necessary to ensure airway patency, especially when signs

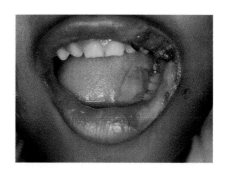

FIGURE 21–12. Electrical burn caused by biting an electrical cord.
Courtesy Dr. Lezley McIlveen, Department of Dentistry, Children's National Medical Center, Washington, DC.

 CLINICAL TIP

The palm of a child's hand is 1% of his or her body surface area and can be used to make a quick estimate of the burn size.

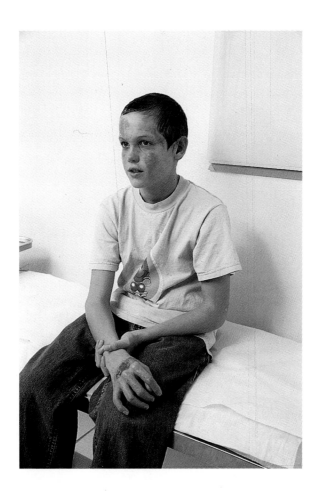

FIGURE 21–13. The burns on the face and hands of this school-age boy were the result of a flash burn caused by igniting gasoline.

21-9   Classification of Burns

Superficial Partial Thickness (first degree)	Partial Thickness (second degree)	Full Thickness (third degree)

Skin red, dry

Blisters; skin moist, pink or red

Charring: skin black, brown, red

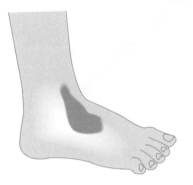

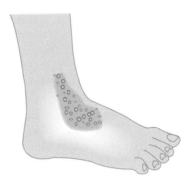

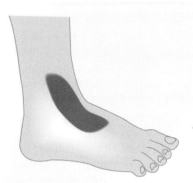

Damages only outer layer of skin; burn is painful and red; heals in a few days (example: sunburn)

Involves epidermis and upper layers of dermis; painful (partial thickness) and sensitive to cold air; results in blisters that blanch with pressure; heals in 10–14 days

Involves all of epidermis and dermis; may also involve underlying tissue; skin brown, black, or deep cherry red; usually no pain because nerve endings have been destroyed; injured area may appear sunken; requires skin grafting

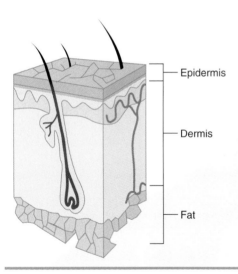

- Epidermis
- Dermis
- Fat

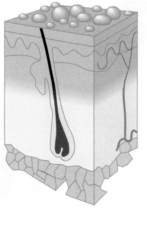

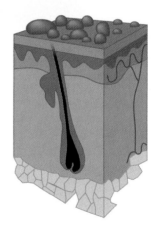

of smoke inhalation or burns to the face and neck are present. The child is assessed for other potential injuries when the mechanism of injury also includes a fall or explosion. Identify signs of respiratory distress and any potential bleeding source. If acid is the burning agent, neutralization in the emergency department is often required.

A weak, thready pulse, tachycardia, and pallor are important signs of early shock that may provide clues to an internal injury. Fluid replacement is necessary to prevent hypovolemic shock in cases of major burn injury. Fluid shifts from the vasculature to the interstitial spaces (third spacing) occur soon after the burn. Vascular integrity is usually restored after the first 24 hours.

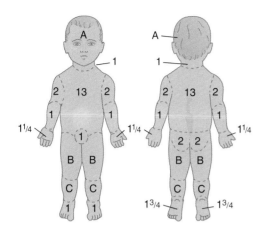

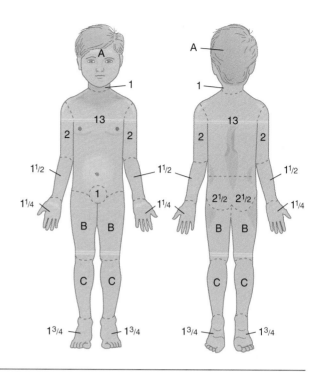

Relative Percentages of Areas Affected by Growth

Area	Age in years					
	0	1	5	10	11	Adult
A = 1/2 of head	9 1/2	8 1/2	6 1/2	5 1/2	4 1/2	3 1/2
B = 1/2 of one thigh	2 3/4	3 1/4	4	4 1/2	4 1/2	4 3/4
C = 1/2 of one lower leg	2 1/2	2 1/2	2 3/4	3	3 1/4	3 1/2

FIGURE 21–14. Lund and Browder chart for determining percentage of body surface area in pediatric burn injuries. *Adapted from Artz, C.P., & Moncrief, J.A. (1969). The treatment of burns (2nd ed.). Philadelphia: Saunders.*

Fluid replacement for the first 24 hours after the injury is based on a fluid volume formula calculated from the child's body weight, affected BSA, and normal maintenance needs. Several formulas exist for this calculation. Lactated Ringer's solution is the preferred fluid. Half of the total volume calculated for the 24-hour period is infused over the first 8 hours, and the remainder is distributed evenly over the next 16 hours. Resuscitation efforts are also focused on maintaining the child's temperature because heat is lost rapidly through burned skin.

Treatment of Major Burns

Children with major burns are monitored closely for fever and usually require more aggressive wound management. Intravenous narcotics are often necessary to alleviate pain, especially during treatment. Intake and output must be monitored closely. Intravenous fluids are administered to replace fluid lost through the skin. A urinary catheter may be inserted to enable close monitoring of urine output.

Fever is a normal, expected outcome of any significant thermal injury. Infection of the burned area is a frequent complication. Frequent checks of vital signs are necessary. Treatment may include analgesics, ice packs, cooling blankets, or cool hydrotherapy sessions. Enteral feedings are initiated within 24 hours of the burn injury to support the child's increased nutritional requirements, which result from the increased metabolic rate needed to support healing and the body's stress response to injury.

Special consideration is needed when burns involve certain areas of the body:

- Dependent edema is common with burn injuries. Elevation of the burned extremity helps to minimize edema. Check the pulse every hour in the burned extremity (distal to the circumferential or nearly circumferential burn). Any decrease, change, or absence of pulse requires immediate notification of the physician, since an **escharotomy** (incision into the constricting tissue) may be necessary to restore peripheral circulation.

- Facial burns usually cause significant edema. Care must be taken to ensure airway patency. For burns to the eye, an ophthalmologist should be consulted to assess damage. If damage has occurred, the affected eye should be covered with a dressing saturated with sterile saline solution. If the lips are burned, an infant may be unable to suck.

- Burns of the hands require careful management to maintain function. Special splinting and physical therapy are usually necessary.

- Perineal burns are at higher risk for infection because of frequent contamination with urine and stool. Perineal burns are treated with bacitracin on the urethral meatus and Silvadene (silver sulfadiazine) on the rest of the burn. The area is then wrapped with a burn pack and secured with a diaper. Frequent dressing changes are required. A urinary catheter is usually inserted but is removed once hydration status is stable to minimize the risk of urinary tract infection.

Treatment of Burn Wounds

Wound management is the most important aspect of caring for the burned child. Burn wound care has three main goals: (1) to speed wound debridement, (2) to protect granulation tissue and new grafts, and (3) to conserve body heat and fluids. Several treatment regimens are used to achieve these goals.

The entire body is bathed to initiate debridement. Conscious sedation may be ordered for pain management during debridement. Be sure to follow all agency guidelines for patient assessment and monitoring of conscious sedation during the debridement process (see Chap. 7). Anesthesiology support may be needed for the conscious sedation process, especially when patients are not fully stabilized. Hair can harbor bacteria and should be shaved or cut away from burned areas. Intact blisters provide a natural, pain-free, sterile dressing. If blisters break open, the tissue should be carefully cut away. After initial cleansing, antibacterial agents, such as Silvadene, are applied to prevent bacterial infection and dressings are added to cover the burned area (Table 21–10).

Dressing changes are performed at least twice daily, although once-a-day dressing changes are being evaluated for certain burn types.[20] These changes are often very painful. When an old dressing is removed, a layer of **eschar** (the tough leathery scab that forms over severely burned areas) is also removed, resulting in debridement (removal of necrotic tissue from a burned area). Children should be given analgesics 30–60 minutes before debridement procedures.

Hydrotherapy (whirlpool) baths are given before debridement to loosen eschar. Hydrotherapy is performed twice daily to increase vasodilation and circulation and to speed healing (Fig. 21–15). As a rule, tap water is used for debridement. Gentle washing is necessary to protect new epithelial cells. Granulation tissue forms as a result of daily debridement.

Skin grafting is necessary with any deep second- or third-degree burn that (1) has an impenetrable leathery layer of eschar that is preventing spontaneous regeneration of skin or (2) is so deep that not enough skin structures are left to permit spontaneous growth. The graft is placed only after the area is excised to reveal healthy, bleeding tissue. Wet-to-dry dressings may be used for a few days preoperatively to prepare an area for the

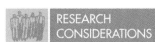

RESEARCH CONSIDERATIONS

Mepetel, an experimental mesh dressing, was shown to reduce eschar formation, the pain associated with dressing changes, and the amount of time needed for dressing changes for partial-thickness scald burns. In addition, healing time was also reduced.[19]

21-10   Burn Wound Care

Preparation

1. Check the physician's orders. Since burn care is often a painful procedure, check for pain medication orders and administer medication at least 30–60 minutes before starting burn care. Conscious sedation may be used for some debridement procedures.
2. Wash your hands. Gather supplies, including gloves (clean and sterile), a basin, sterile normal saline solution, a large supply of 4 × 4 gauze pads, forceps, scissors, a sterile tongue blade, the prescribed topical medication, tape, and an absorbent pad.
3. You may need an assistant to hold the child and the burned extremity during care.

Procedure

1. Place the absorbent pad under the area to be cleaned. Put on clean gloves. Soak the wound for about 10 minutes in normal saline solution, or apply a wet dressing to the area. This will soften the wound. Remove the gloves.
2. After approximately 10 minutes, put on sterile gloves and wash the burn with the gauze pads using a *firm*, circular motion, moving from the inside to the outer edges. As you do this, be sure to remove any medication or crusting. Bleeding may occur, but this is a sign of healing, healthy tissue. Rinse with more normal saline solution. Pat dry with sterile gauze.
3. Remove (per physician's orders) any loose or dead skin around the edges of the burn by gently lifting it with the forceps and snipping it. This is not painful to the child. You may rinse and dry again.
4. Place a thin layer of prescribed medication (about ⅛-inch thick) on the burn or gauze with fingers or a tongue blade. Place the medicated gauze on the burn and cover with a dry, sterile dressing.

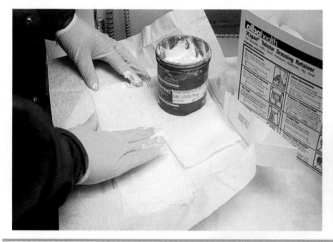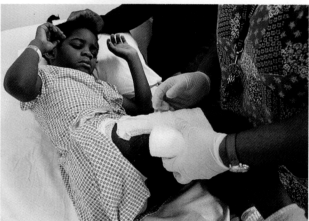

Burn wound care written by Marcia Wellington, R.N., M.S.

graft. However, these dressings are very painful, and the child will need analgesics and emotional support.

Four types of grafts are available: autografts, allografts, xenografts, and synthetic grafts. In an autograft, healthy skin is taken from a nonburned area of the child's body and placed on the burned area. This type of graft is permanent. The donor site (where the autograft was harvested) is a new wound, causing pain and requiring close monitoring for signs of infection.

Temporary grafts include allografts (use of skin of the same species, for example, cadaver), xenografts (use of skin from another species, such as pig skin), and synthetic grafts (artificial skin substitutes). Temporary grafts are used to promote epithelial stimulation in partial-thickness burns and to cover healing granulation tissue. They usually slough off in 4–5 weeks as a result of tissue rejection. These grafts provide for the functions of the skin that were lost in the burn (temperature regulation, pain control, fluid loss, infection barrier). Often they are used as a test to determine whether an autograft is likely to succeed in a burned area. The potential risk of HIV infection associated with the use of allografts needs to be taken into consideration.

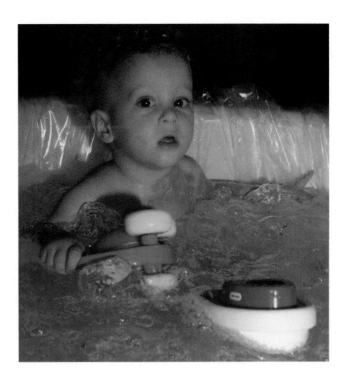

FIGURE 21–15. A whirlpool bath is being used to increase this child's circulation and speed the healing of his burns.

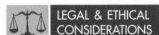

LEGAL & ETHICAL CONSIDERATIONS

When taking a burn history, carefully document the following:

- Type of injury
- Time of injury
- People present at the time of the injury
- First aid administered
- History of other unusual injuries or emergency department visits

Nursing Assessment

Obtain information about the type of burn (eg, thermal, electrical, chemical), as well as a complete history. Thorough documentation is essential to rule out child abuse. Be alert to signs of abuse (eg, glove and stocking burns, contact burns from cigarettes or irons, zebra burn lines from contact with a hot grate [Fig 21–16]). If a burn injury was preventable, parents may be emotionally stressed by feelings of guilt. Caution is needed to avoid sounding accusatory when questioning parents about the injury.

Physical assessment should be thorough, including frequent monitoring of vital signs and daily weight measurement. A head-to-toe assessment is performed at the beginning of every shift followed by system-specific assessments, depending on clinical findings and changes in the child's status.

Assess the child's concerns over appearance and the stress of hospitalization. Determine if the child has memories or nightmares about the burn so psychologic support can be provided as needed.

Nursing Diagnosis

Common nursing diagnoses for the child with a major burn injury are included in the accompanying Nursing Care Plan. Additional nursing diagnoses for the child with a major burn might include:

- Impaired Physical Mobility related to limb immobilization, contractures, and pain
- Body Image Disturbance related to possible disfigurement
- Anxiety related to crisis, memory of trauma experience, and threat of death or disfigurement

Nursing Management

Nursing care focuses on performing burn care, preventing complications, and providing emotional support. Care of the burned child involves various

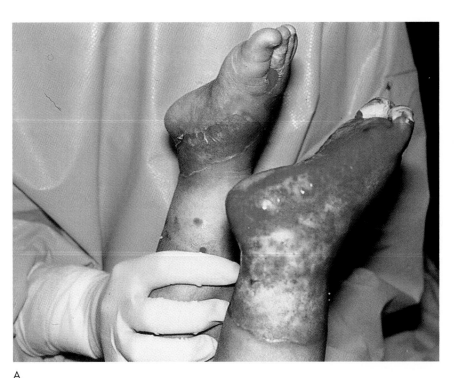

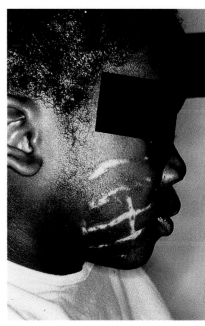

B

A

FIGURE 21–16. Burn injuries associated with child abuse. **A,** Burns of the hands or feet that are distributed like gloves or stockings. **B,** Zebra burns from a grate.
Courtesy American Academy of Pediatrics, Elk Grove Village, IL, and the C. Henry Kempe National Center on Child Abuse and Neglect, Denver, CO.

treatments designed to promote healing and prevent complications. These include dressing changes, hydrotherapy, antibiotic therapy, analgesic support, physical therapy, play therapy, and possibly skin grafting.

The accompanying Nursing Care Plan summarizes nursing care of the child with a major burn. Severe morbidity is likely with major burns. Severe scarring may occur regardless of autografting. Contractures and loss of function are also possible. If fluid replacement is inadequate, irreversible renal damage or cardiac damage may ensue, necessitating close follow-up unrelated to the actual burn injury. Children with major burns require comprehensive follow-up, sometimes involving repeated hospitalizations for surgery to release burn contractures, perform new grafting, or provide scar revision.

Prevent Complications

Severe complications of burns include infections, pneumonia, and renal failure, as well as possible irreversible loss of function of the burned area. The goal of the health care team is to prevent complications. Parents need to be involved in their child's care and to learn how to change dressings, assess for infection and dehydration (see Chap. 8), and perform range-of-motion exercises to aid in the child's recovery.

Play therapy is encouraged for children, even if they can only observe initially. Play therapy serves several purposes for the child with a major burn:

- It provides an outlet for frustration, independence, and creativity.
- It promotes activities that challenge range of motion.
- It normalizes the child's daily routine.
- It encourages the child, who sees the progress that other children make day by day.

NURSING CARE PLAN
THE CHILD WITH A MAJOR BURN INJURY

GOAL	INTERVENTION	RATIONALE	EXPECTED OUTCOME

1. Pain related to destruction of tissues and edema

GOAL	INTERVENTION	RATIONALE	EXPECTED OUTCOME
The child will verbalize adequate relief from pain and will be able to perform activities of daily living (ADLs).	• Assess level of pain frequently using pain scales (see Chap. 7).	• Pain scale provides objective measurement. Pain is always present, but changes in location and intensity may indicate complications.	The child verbalizes adequate relief from pain and is able to perform ADLs.
	• Cover burns as much as possible.	• Temperature changes or movement of air causes pain.	
	• Change the child's position frequently. Perform range-of-motion exercises.	• Reduces joint stiffness and prevents contractures.	
	• Elevate burned extremities.	• Helps reduce swelling and pain by promoting venous return.	
	• Encourage verbalization about pain.	• Provides an outlet for emotions and helps the child cope.	
	• Provide diversional activities.	• Helps to lessen focus on pain.	
	• Promote uninterrupted sleep with use of medications.	• Sleep deprivation can increase pain perception.	
	• Use analgesics before all dressing changes and burn care.	• Helps to reduce pain and decreases anxiety for subsequent dressing changes.	

2. Risk for Infection related to destruction of skin barrier, traumatized tissue, multiple indwelling catheters

GOAL	INTERVENTION	RATIONALE	EXPECTED OUTCOME
The child will be free of infection during healing process.	• Take vital signs frequently.	• Increased temperature is an early sign of infection.	The child is free of secondary infection.
	• Use standard precautions (gown, gloves, mask) when wounds of a major burn are exposed. Change dressings 1 or 2 times daily using sterile technique. Limit visitors (no one with an upper respiratory infection or other contagious disease).	• Reduces risk of contamination.	
	• Shave or clip hair around burns.	• Hair harbors bacteria.	

NURSING CARE PLAN
THE CHILD WITH A MAJOR BURN INJURY– *Continued*

GOAL	INTERVENTION	RATIONALE	EXPECTED OUTCOME

2. *Risk for Infection related to destruction of skin barrier, traumatized tissue, multiple indwelling catheters (continued)*

	• Debride necrotic tissue.	• Promotes formation of granulation tissue, which aids healing.	
	• Apply topical antibacterial agents.	• Helps to reduce the number of bacteria present on the burn.	

3. *Risk for Fluid Volume Excess or Deficit related to loss of fluid through wounds, hemorrhagic losses*

GOAL	INTERVENTION	RATIONALE	EXPECTED OUTCOME
The child will maintain normal vital signs and urine output.	• Monitor vital signs, central venous pressure, capillary refill time, pulses.	• The child is at risk initially for hypovolemic shock and needs fluid resuscitation (see Chap. 8).	The child maintains normal vital signs and urine output.
	• Administer intravenous and oral fluids as ordered.	• Careful calculation of fluid needs and ensuring proper intake helps to keep child properly hydrated.	
	• Estimate insensible fluid losses.	• Losses are increased during the first 72 hours after burn injury; may need replacement. Plasma is lost through burn site because of capillary damage.	
	• Monitor intake and output carefully.	• The child is at risk for fluid overload during hydration, and for edema in the tissues at the burn site.	
	• Weigh the child daily.	• Significant weight loss or gain can help determine amount of fluid needed. Gain is normal during the first 72 hours.	
	• Insert a urinary catheter.	• Helps maintain accurate intake and output measurements.	
	• Monitor for hyponatremia and hyperkalemia (see Chap. 8).	• Sodium is lost with burn fluid and potassium is lost from damaged cells, causing electrolyte imbalances.	

Continued . . .

NURSING CARE PLAN
THE CHILD WITH A MAJOR BURN INJURY – *Continued*

GOAL	INTERVENTION	RATIONALE	EXPECTED OUTCOME

4. Altered Peripheral Tissue Perfusion related to edema of burned extremities or circumferential burns

GOAL	INTERVENTION	RATIONALE	EXPECTED OUTCOME
The child will maintain adequate perfusion in burned extremities.	• Elevate extremities. Perform hourly distal pulse checks. Notify the physician of decreased or absent pulses. • Check eschar.	• Elevation helps to reduce dependent edema by promoting venous return. Dependent edema can constrict peripheral circulation. • Eschar can constrict peripheral circulation in edematous extremity.	The child has no episodes of poor perfusion in the burned extremity.

5. Risk for Ineffective Breathing Pattern related to hypervolemia, smoke inhalation, airway edema

GOAL	INTERVENTION	RATIONALE	EXPECTED OUTCOME
The child will maintain or demonstrate improvement in breathing pattern.	• Closely monitor quality of respirations, breath sounds, mucus secretions, pulse oximetry. • Provide thorough pulmonary care. • Elevate head of bed. Keep intubation tray at bedside. • Administer corticosteroids, as prescribed.	• Excess fluid replacement can cause pulmonary edema; toxins from burning products can cause airway inflammation. • Pulmonary care assists in removal of secretions to prevent infection. • Dyspnea, nasal flaring, air hunger (respiratory distress) may develop. • Reduces airway edema.	The child has regular and unlabored breathing pattern.

6. Impaired Physical Mobility related to burns involving joints

GOAL	INTERVENTION	RATIONALE	EXPECTED OUTCOME
The child will maintain maximum range of motion.	• Arrange physical and occupational therapy twice daily for stretching and range-of-motion exercises. Splint as ordered. Encourage independent ADLs.	• Good positioning, range-of-motion exercises, and alignment prevent contractures.	The child maintains maximum range of motion without contractures.

NURSING CARE PLAN
THE CHILD WITH A MAJOR BURN INJURY— *Continued*

GOAL	INTERVENTION	RATIONALE	EXPECTED OUTCOME

7. Altered Nutrition: Less Than Body Requirements related to hypermetabolic burn wound state

GOAL	INTERVENTION	RATIONALE	EXPECTED OUTCOME
The child will maintain weight and demonstrate adequate serum albumin and hydration.	• Provide an opportunity to choose meals. Offer a variety of foods. Provide snacks. • Encourage the child to have meals with other children. • Substitute milk and juices for water. • Provide a multivitamin supplement. • Provide nasogastric feedings as ordered. • Weigh the child daily.	• Encourages intake. General malaise and anorexia lead to poor healing. • Socialization improves intake • Provides additional calories. • Vitamin C aids zinc absorption; zinc aids in healing. • A child with a burn greater than 10% of BSA cannot usually meet nutrition requirements without assistance. • Provides objective evaluation.	The child maintains weight, adequate hydration, normal serum albumin.

8. Anxiety (Child) related to hospitalization and painful interventions

GOAL	INTERVENTION	RATIONALE	EXPECTED OUTCOME
The child will verbalize reduced anxiety.	• Provide continuity of care providers. • Encourage parents to stay with the child; calls from home; pictures from classmates. • Group tasks and activities.	• Helps to build a trusting relationship. • Familiar surroundings, people, and items encourage relaxation. • Reduces overstimulation and encourages rest.	The child expresses and shows signs of reduced anxiety.

9. Anxiety (Parent) related to child's hospitalization and fear

GOAL	INTERVENTION	RATIONALE	EXPECTED OUTCOME
Parents will verbalize decreased anxiety.	• Provide educational materials about healing, grafting, dressing changes, and course of care. • Be flexible when teaching parents about wound care. • Provide referral to social services or parent support group.	• Knowledge reduces anxiety. • Adults learn in many different ways. • Allows for venting of fears and guilt feelings, and provides exchange of ideas on dealing with hospitalization and long-term care.	Parents state decreased anxiety.

Provide Emotional Support

Burned children have received a profound insult to their body and their self-image. Fear and anxiety related to disfigurement and scarring are common responses, especially among adolescents. Increased stress occurs as a result of the shock and pain of the injury, as well as the unfamiliar surroundings and presence of health care providers.

An attitude of genuine interest and concern on the part of the nurse is essential. The child should be oriented to his or her surroundings frequently and given ample preparation for procedures, when possible. Continuity of care providers is important in developing a trusting relationship with the child. Encourage the child to voice concerns, and show understanding and support.

Families are at risk for emotional stress. They should be forewarned about the expected edema and the resulting gross changes in the child's body. Parents often feel guilty and responsible for the child's injury. It is important to help parents focus on recovery rather than past actions. Fear usually results from lack of knowledge about the severity of the burn and the child's status, especially in the early stages of burn care and admission to the hospital ICU. Include the family in the child's care whenever possible. The family needs to be given information and frequent updates. This promotes the development of trust between the family and the health care team.

Autografting procedures enable the child to recover from major burns, but the operation leaves visible scarring. Psychologic support is therefore essential to the child's recovery. Social workers, chaplains, art therapists, child life specialists, and play therapists are all trained to help the child and family deal with the stressors of recovery. Appropriate referrals should be made to ensure that the child and family receive necessary services.

Discharge Planning and Home Care Teaching

Home care needs should be identified and addressed well in advance of discharge. Thorough assessment is necessary to identify the family's needs related to the child's discharge home or to a rehabilitation facility. Discharge planning may include instructing parents in nutrition and diet needs, safety in the home, burn wound care, and range-of-motion exercises to prevent contractures.

Provide support and encouragement to parents when they are learning how to care for the burned child. Many parents find it difficult to perform procedures they know will inflict pain to their child. Outline specific guidelines so that parents and health care team members will have the same focus. Parents should first observe care being performed and then provide repeat demonstrations until competent.

Care in the Community

Care of the child with a burn requires long-term therapy and rehabilitation. Nurses in clinic and home care settings continue the care provided during hospitalization. Long-term care commonly occurs in the home, with frequent visits to health care professionals. In some cases, children return to the hospital clinic for dressing changes on a regular basis. Children with extensive burns or with burns in locations that have the potential to cause functional limitations related to scarring must often wear an elasticized (Jobst) garment, and sometimes a face mask if the face was burned. The Jobst garment may present a threat to the child's body image, but it is an important means of decreasing scarring. Scar management may also be handled through drug injections or surgery (ie, revision, grafting, or Z-plasty). Help families understand the need for the special garments and masks and how to clean and care for them.

Continued physical therapy and occupational therapy are often needed to increase strength and dexterity in performing activities of daily living (ADLs) and to prevent contractures. Emphasis is placed on returning to normal ADLs as soon as possible. This includes returning to school as soon as health permits. Some children have home tutors for a while to decrease their risk of exposure to infection.

School reentry is often a traumatic experience, especially for older children and adolescents, because of the fear of rejection, decreased self-esteem, and impaired body image. The child's primary nurse, social worker, and child life specialist may visit the school of a child with a burn injury before the child returns to school—bringing photographs of the child, pressure garments, or other items—to desensitize the class and allow them to explore their emotions relating to the child's burn injury. Several communities offer support groups for families and children with burn injuries. Referral to these groups may be beneficial.

Management of Minor Burns

Many children with minor burns are cared for at home after an initial visit to the emergency department or urgent care clinic. Any open blisters are debrided, and a thin layer of silver sulfadiazine is applied over the burn. The burn is then covered with one or two layers of gauze. Burn dressings should be changed twice daily. This involves cleaning the burn and reapplying antibiotic cream.

Instruct parents to increase the child's fluid intake to compensate for loss of fluid through damaged skin. A high-calorie, high-protein diet is necessary to meet the increased nutritional requirements of healing. Acetaminophen (Tylenol) with codeine is often given, especially before dressing changes. Infection is a common complication. The child should be seen within 48 hours of treatment to monitor progress. Reinforce to parents the importance of follow-up appointments.

SUNBURN

Sunburn is a burn injury to the outer layer of skin caused by ultraviolet rays. It occurs more often in fair-skinned children, who have less melanin (skin pigment) to protect their skin against these harmful rays.

Erythema and skin tenderness usually develop between 30 minutes and 4 hours after exposure to sunlight. Increased vasodilation and vascular permeability result in the extravasation of fluid to the tissues and white blood cell migration to the damaged skin. The erythema peaks at 24 hours. Prolonged exposure can result in edema, vesiculation, bullae, or ulceration. Systemic complaints include malaise, insomnia (because of skin tenderness), fatigue, headaches, and chilling (because of rapid heat loss).

Treatment is generally supportive. Pain can be relieved by cool compresses followed by the application of a topical corticosteroid to relieve discomfort. Children with severe sunburn may require antiinflammatory drugs, such as ibuprofen.

Nursing Management

Educate parents and children about ways to prevent sunburn (Table 21–11). Advise that repeated sunburns may lead to permanent skin damage and skin cancer. Recommend to parents that children use sunscreens of at least SPF 15, reapplied several times daily, wear protective clothing, and limit the amount of time they spend in the sun. Children should also wear sunglasses with 99% ultraviolet blockage.

CLINICAL TIP

Most minor burns can be handled at home by parents. For minor burns, exposure to cool, running water is the best treatment. This stops the burning process and helps to alleviate pain. Ice is contraindicated because it may add more damage to already injured skin. All jewelry and clothing are removed, and the burn area is placed under running water. A topical antibiotic (Neosporin) may then be applied, if desired.

NURSING ALERT

Caution parents to avoid placing WATERPROOF sunscreen near the eyes. Waterproof sunscreen in the eyes causes severe pain and a chemical burn that can damage the child's vision. Flushing the eyes with water does not stop the burning! Call the poison control center immediately and take the child to the emergency department. Special chemicals will be needed to flush the sunscreen out of the eyes and preserve vision.

CLINICAL TIP

It is estimated that 80% of a person's lifetime exposure to sunburns occurs before 21 years of age. This occurs at a time when the epidermis is relatively thin. Melanin is also present in low levels during infancy and childhood.[21] For these reasons, it is recommended that children use a sunscreen with an SPF of 15 or higher during outdoor activities.

| 21-11 | Parent Teaching: Preventing Sunburn |

- Keep children out of direct sunlight as much as possible.
- When outdoors, minimize exposed areas by wearing hats and long-sleeved, closely woven clothing and pants: wear T-shirts while swimming. Special sun protection clothing is now available from some manufacturers.
- Be aware that water, concrete, and sand reflect sunlight and increase exposure up to 90% by reflecting up to 85% of the ultraviolet rays.
- Avoid scheduling outdoor activities during the hours of maximum exposure (10 AM to 2 PM).
- Use sunscreen (preferably 15 SPF [sun protection factor]). For optimal protection, apply as thickly as directed to all exposed areas 30–45 minutes before sun exposure. Reapply every 2 hours as needed, or sooner if swimming, toweling off, or perspiring heavily.
- Use a waterproof sunscreen when swimming; this provides protection in water for approximately 60–80 minutes. Then reapply.
- Avoid using sunscreens in infants less than 6 months of age because of the possibility of absorption of the chemicals through their skin.
- Avoid the use of para-aminobenzoic acid (PABA) sunscreens as these can induce photosensitivity.
- Remember that a child can be burned even on a cloudy day. Up to 80% of ultraviolet rays can penetrate the cloud cover.
- If the child is taking any medications, check with your health care practitioner before exposure (some medications [tretinoin, tetracycline, nonsteroidal antiinflammatory drugs, and oral contraceptives] cause hypersensitivity to sunlight).

HYPOTHERMIA

Hypothermia is a condition in which the core body temperature falls below 35°C (95°F). This occurs when the heat produced by the body is less than the heat lost. Hypothermia is a life-threatening emergency.

Hypothermia is associated with near-drowning episodes because body heat is lost quickly in water, as compared with air. Children are at greater risk for hypothermia because of their thinner skin, limited subcutaneous fat, and high surface area to body mass ratio. As the body temperature falls, the body tries to conserve the core temperature at the expense of the extremities. Increased muscle tone and an increased metabolic rate occur. Shivering occurs to try to rewarm the blood before it returns to the core of the body.

Symptoms of mild hypothermia include slurred speech, incoordination, poor judgment, and shivering. Symptoms of moderate hypothermia include depressed respirations, slow pulse, low blood pressure, pale or cyanotic color, shivering, dilated pupils, and confusion. Profound hypothermia (body temperature below 29°C [84°F]) may result in absence of respirations and pulse, ventricular arrhythmia, dilated pupils, and loss of consciousness.

Treatment focuses on resuscitation, if necessary, and gradual rewarming of the body. The child who has been immersed in cold water for a long time (up to 30–45 minutes) should receive CPR until the body temperature returns to normal because the diving reflex may preserve vital organs. Body temperature is assessed with a rectal thermometer. For mild hypothermia (temperature above 35°C [95°F]), external heat lamps, immersion in warm water, and an electric blanket may be all that are necessary. More aggressive techniques are required for profound hypothermia. These may include use of humidified, warm oxygen; warmed intra-

CAUSES OF HYPOTHERMIA[18]

- Exposure
- Ingestion of alcohol or barbiturates
- Trauma or a brain disorder that interferes with temperature regulation
- Overwhelming sepsis

DIVING REFLEX

The diving reflex is a series of changes in the cardiovascular system that occurs when the face and nose are immersed. Heart rate decreases and blood flow is decreased to all body areas except the brain, thus conserving oxygen.

venous fluids; hemodialysis; or application of warmth to core circulation areas (axilla, groin, and posterior neck).

If a child becomes hypothermic during an outing such as a camping trip, a warm person should get into a sleeping bag (or under the blankets) next to the child. This action will warm the child and prevent further heat loss.

Nursing Management

Monitor vital signs and urine output during rewarming. Prevention is geared toward educating parents to layer children's clothing in cold climates, recognize signs of hypothermia, decrease time of exposure to cold, and be aware of actions to take for mild hypothermia. Teach school-age children and adolescents who go on camping and hunting trips how to recognize and manage hypothermia in themselves and others.

FROSTBITE

Frostbite is an extreme form of hypothermia that results from overexposure to extremely low temperatures. Areas of the body at high risk for frostbite include the hands, feet, cheeks, nose, and ears. Skin cells have a high concentration of water. Ice crystallizes in the tissues, resulting in cellular dehydration and ischemic damage.

Clinical manifestations depend on the severity of the cellular damage. The skin at first appears pale and is numb. Rapid rewarming causes a flush. The erythema and mild swelling develop into bullae. The extent of injury usually is not initially apparent.

If frostbite is suspected, loosen all constricting clothing and remove any wet clothes. Obtain health care as soon as possible. Rewarming is done slowly to decrease the chance of cellular damage. Immerse the affected part for 10–15 minutes in water warmed to between 38° and 40°C (100.4° and 104°F). Analgesics may be given to manage pain. Elevate the affected part, if possible, to improve venous return. Encourage the child to drink warm fluids. This will help to warm the child slowly. Because the frostbitten area is numb, extreme caution is needed to protect it from any trauma.

The child may complain of tingling, burning, or prickling in the affected area during rewarming. These are signs that sensation is returning.

Lengthy treatment and amputation are sometimes necessary when tissues are permanently damaged.

Nursing Management

As with hypothermia, the goal of management is prevention. Teach parents to layer children's clothing for warmth and to pack extra blankets and clothing if cold temperatures are expected during outdoor activities. Teach adolescents how to avoid frostbite during hunting and other cold weather expeditions. Wet clothing should be changed quickly. Early care is instrumental in minimizing permanent injury. Severe frostbite will require hospitalization, with fluid management, dressing changes, antibiotic therapy, and careful attention to diet.

BITES

Animal Bites

Each year 5 million people are bitten by animals in the United States. About 1 million dog bites occur each year and half of those require medical attention.[22] Children, especially in the 5–9-year-old age range, are at higher risk for animal bites, and boys are bitten twice as often as girls.[23]

FIRST AID FOR HYPOTHERMIA

If mild hypothermia occurs at home, move the child to a dry area and remove any wet clothing. Replace with warm, dry clothing, and encourage the child to drink a warm, high-calorie liquid, if able.

 NURSING ALERT

Do not rub a frostbitten extremity or body part. Do not use direct heat to rewarm the body part. The child will not be able to feel any trauma caused by these actions, and this could result in greater injury.

LEGAL & ETHICAL CONSIDERATIONS

If a child sustains an animal bite, a complete and accurate history is essential. Include:
- Extent of the injury
- Circumstances surrounding the attack
- Present location of the animal
- Attempts to assess the animal's health

RABIES PROPHYLAXIS

Rabies immune globulin (RIG) or human diploid cell rabies (HDVC) vaccine should be given to all children bitten by wild animals in which rabies cannot be excluded, as well as to children bitten by domestic animals (cats and dogs) suspected or proven to be rabid.

Assessment includes noting location and number of bites, breaks in the skin, redness or swelling at entry sites, redness extending out from site (possible cellulitis), and any drainage related to the bite. Check for nerve, muscle, tendon, or vascular damage. Findings should be carefully documented. Head and neck bites require radiographic examination to rule out any associated injury, such as trauma to the airway or breathing structures or a depressed skull fracture.

To decrease infection, initial treatment involves high-pressure wound irrigation with large quantities of sterile saline or lactated Ringer's solution rather than scrubbing. A 19-gauge needle on a 60-cc syringe may be used. Any devitalized tissue is debrided. Conscious sedation may be needed for some children. A clean pressure dressing is applied, and the affected part is elevated to reduce bleeding. Small wounds may be closed with adhesive strips rather than suturing because of the potential for infection. Severe bites sometimes require surgical closure or reconstruction. Wounds over joints should be immobilized and elevated. Puncture wounds should not be irrigated or sutured.

Dog bites tend to be crushing, rather than clean, sharp lacerations. The major complication of dog bites is infection. Antibiotics and early treatment of the wound can greatly decrease this sequela. Dog bites should be reported to the police, and the dog should be observed for 10 days for signs of rabies. Cat bites are also dangerous because they tend to be puncture wounds and are therefore associated with a higher rate of infection, cellulitis, and abscesses. Check the child's immunization record to determine whether a tetanus booster is necessary. (Refer to the immunization schedule in Chapter 10.) Instruct parents about how to care for the wound.

Human Bites

Human bites are more common than most people realize. They usually occur in toddlers and young children. Because the mouth harbors many bacteria, infection is fairly common. Assess the risk for hepatitis B and HIV infection. Antibiotics may be prescribed to prevent systemic complications. Initial treatment includes irrigating with sterile saline and debridement. Instruct parents about how to care for the wound. Follow-up is important to watch for infection.

Nursing Management

Educate parents about ways to prevent animal and human bites and the importance of teaching children appropriate behavior around other children and animals (Table 21–12). When these bites occur in a day-care or school setting, inform parents about the human bite so they can discuss potential risks and follow up with a health care provider.

As these children are often cared for at home, teach the parents about the normal healing process, proper wound care, and the signs and symptoms of infection.

Children who receive traumatic animal bites often experience significant psychologic trauma. They may develop a fear of strange animals and a decreased capacity to enjoy the presence of household pets. Counseling and follow-up may be necessary to evaluate such concerns.

INSECT BITES AND STINGS

Insect bites and stings occur frequently in children and usually are not a cause for concern. Exceptions include bites or stings by insects that carry parasites or communicable diseases (ticks, mosquitos), those of venomous

21-12 | Parent Teaching: Preventing Animal Bites

- Teach children the following rules:
  - —Avoid all unfamiliar animals.
  - —Avoid contact with all wild animals.
  - —Do not touch an animal when it is eating or sleeping.
  - —Never overexcite an animal, even in play.
  - —Never tease an animal.
  - —Never put your face close to an animal.
- If an animal is sick or acting strangely, notify the health department.
- Never leave a young child alone with an animal.
- Do not buy a pet unless you are confident of your child's ability to respect it.

insects (spiders), and those that produce an allergic reaction. (For a discussion of Lyme disease and Rocky Mountain spotted fever, see Chapter 10.)

Reactions to insect bites can be localized or systemic. Local reactions include discrete, red papules and edema at the bite site, as well as itching and pain. Local inflammation results from injected foreign protein or chemicals. Most bites produce minimal discomfort. Systemic reactions can include wheezing, urticaria, laryngeal edema, and shock.

Treatment is usually supportive and focuses on relieving itching and reducing inflammation. Pruritus is treated with cold compresses or ice applied to the site and an antihistamine. In children who are sensitized to insect bites, pruritic wheals and bullae tend to develop with repeat exposure. In rare cases exposure can lead to an anaphylactic reaction. If large wheals, swelling of extremities, or respiratory difficulty occurs, emergency medical treatment is needed.

Bees and fire ants (Hymenoptera) inject a hemolytic, neurotoxic venom that causes a histaminelike response. Fire ant bites have a black center at the point of the bite and cause vesicles with local swelling. Reactions to either bee stings or fire ant bites may be local inflammation or a systemic allergic response (wheezing, urticaria, diarrhea, vomiting, and dizziness). In some cases an anaphylactic response occurs. Treatment of local reactions includes antihistamines. For systemic reactions, treat with intravenous or subcutaneous 1:1000 epinephrine solution. Desensitization for the Hymenoptera group should also be considered when the child has a systemic reaction.

Black widow spider bites are characterized by a stinging sensation at the time of the bite followed by swelling, redness, and pain at the site. Red fang marks can be seen. Systemic symptoms can occur 15 minutes to 2 hours after the bite and include dizziness, fever, severe abdominal pain (abdominal muscle rigidity), and weakness. Muscle cramps begin near the bite and can involve all skeletal muscles. If large doses of venom are absorbed, the bite may lead to paralysis and death. A neurotoxin produced by the spider is responsible for the symptoms. The black widow spider can be recognized by the red and orange hourglass-shaped markings on its underside. It usually bites in self-defense and avoids light areas. Treatment involves cleansing the wound and immediately applying ice packs. Sedatives, antivenom, analgesics, or muscle relaxants may be prescribed. Hydrocortisone may decrease the inflammatory response. Symptoms can progress for 24 hours and then gradually decrease over 2–3 days.

The brown recluse spider bite is characterized by a sharp pain resembling a sting. Most bites are mild and cause only minimal edema and mild erythema. Severe bites can become necrotic within 4 hours. The child experiences mild to

CLINICAL TIP

A dash of meat tenderizer (papain powder) and a drop of water massaged into the skin for 5 minutes quickly relieves the pain of most insect bites and stings. Ice is also effective.

CLINICAL TIP

When removing a bee stinger, do not use tweezers or squeeze the venom sack. Use a straight edge, such as a piece of cardboard, to pull the stinger out in a scraping motion.

severe pain and tenderness. Within 3–4 days a purple, star-shaped area forms at the site. This is followed by necrotic ulceration in 7–14 days. Severe progressive reactions may include associated fever, restlessness, malaise, joint pain, and nausea and vomiting. The wound usually heals with scar formation in 6–8 weeks. The brown recluse spider is recognized by the fiddle-shaped marking on its head. It is usually unaggressive and bites only when provoked. Treatment involves antibiotics, analgesics, application of cool compresses to the site, and corticosteroids for inflammation. In some cases a skin graft is needed.

Nursing Management

The goal of nursing care is prevention. Children should be taught to avoid spiders and other biting or stinging insects. Many commercial repellents (OFF, Cutter's, Deep Woods OFF) are available. Most products contain DEET (diethyltoluamide) and are effective against many insects including mosquitos, fleas, ticks, and chiggers. DEET does not repel stinging insects. Warn parents against using heavily perfumed shampoos, powders, soaps, or lotions, or dressing children in bright clothing when outdoors, as these may attract insects. Household pets may be a source of fleas or ticks. Encourage frequent inspection of pets and preventive treatments against fleas and ticks before pets are allowed prolonged contact with children. When a known allergy to Hymenoptera has occurred, the child should wear a medical alert identification and carry an emergency kit with epinephrine. Teach parents and school personnel how to administer epinephrine.

CONTUSIONS

Contusions are soft tissue injuries that result from a variety of causes. Often it is difficult to assess whether an injury has caused underlying tissue damage. An injury does not have to break the skin to result in internal damage. Radiographic examination may be necessary to rule out broken bones or further tissue damage. Signs and symptoms that indicate a need for treatment include swelling that does not subside within 72 hours, intense pain, inability to move the injured part, and infection.

Elevate the injured extremity and apply ice as soon as possible after injury. This can reduce inflammation and swelling in the area.

FOREIGN BODIES

Many skin injuries result from penetration of foreign particles. Common substances include gravel from abrasions, bee stingers, and splinters. Treatment of superficial foreign bodies involves irrigating the wound to try to forcibly dislodge the debris. A deeply embedded foreign body is best removed under medical supervision to avoid permanent injury or scarring.

> **NURSING ALERT**
>
> Caution parents to avoid overuse of products containing DEET (diethyltoluamide), especially with infants and small children. Cases of toxic encephalopathy have been reported following repeated use on children's bedding and clothing.[24]

REFERENCES

1. O'Hanlon-Nichols, T. (1995). Commonly asked questions about wound healing. *American Journal of Nursing, 95*(4), 22–24.
2. Rote, N.S. (1994). Inflammation. In K.L. McCance, & S.E. Huether (Eds.), *Pathophysiology: The biologic basis for disease in adults and children* (2nd ed., pp. 234–267). St. Louis: Mosby.
3. Farrington, E. (1992). Diaper dermatitis. *Pediatric Nursing, 18*(1), 81–82.
4. Armsmeier, S.L., & Paller, A.S. (1997). Getting to the bottom of diaper dermatitis. *Contemporary Pediatrics, 14*(11), 115–129.

5. Hebert, A.A., & Goller, M.M. (1996). Papulosquamous disorders in the pediatric patient. *Contemporary Pediatrics, 13*(2), 69–88.

6. Tan, B.B., Weald, D., Strickland, I., & Friedman, P.S. (1996). Double-blind controlled trials of effect of housedust-mite allergen avoidance on atopic dermatitis. *Lancet, 347* (January 6), 15–19.

7. Kay, J., Gawrodger, D.J., Mortimer, M.J., & Jaron, A.G. (1994). The prevalence of childhood atopic eczema in a general population. *Journal of the American Academy of Dermatology, 30*(1), 35–39.

8. Hebert, P.W., Rakes, G.P., Loach, T.C., & Murphy, D.D. (1997). Recognizing the young atopic child. *Contemporary Pediatrics, 14*(4), 131–139.

9. Hurwitz, S. (1995). Acne treatment for the '90s. *Contemporary Pediatrics, 12*(8), 19–32.

10. Darmstadt, G.L. (1997). A guide to superficial strep and staph skin infections. *Contemporary Pediatrics, 14*(5), 95–116.

11. Ben-Amitai, D., & Ashkenazi, S. (1993). Common bacterial skin infections in childhood. *Pediatric Annals, 22*(4), 226–227.

12. Wittner, M. (1996). Diseases caused by arthropods. In A.M. Rudolph, J.I.E. Hoffman, & C.D. Rudolph (Eds.), *Rudolph's pediatrics* (20th ed., pp. 779–783). Stamford, CT: Appleton & Lange.

13. Givens, T.G., Murray, M.M., & Baker, R.C. (1995). Comparison of 1% and 2.5% selenium sulfide in the treatment of tinea capitis. *Archives of Pediatrics and Adolescent Medicine, 149*(7), 808–812.

14. Quigley, S.M., & Curley, M.A.Q. (1996). Skin integrity in the pediatric population: Preventing and managing pressure ulcers. *Journal of the Society of Pediatric Nurses, 1*(1), 7–18.

15. Ball, J.W. (1998). *Mosby's pediatric patient teaching guides.* St. Louis: Mosby.

16. Braden, B., & Bergstrom, N. (1989). Clinical utility of the Braden scale for predicting pressure sore risk. *Decubitus, 2*(3), 44–51.

17. National Center for Health Statistics (1995). National Vital Statistics System. Unpublished data.

18. Eichelberger, M.R., Ball, J.W., Pratsch, G.L., & Clark, J.R. (1998). *Pediatric emergencies* (2nd ed., p. 182). Upper Saddle River, CT: Prentice-Hall.

19. Gotschall, C.S., Morrison, M.I.S., & Eichelberger, M.R. (1998). Prospective randomized study of the efficacy of Mepetel on children with partial-thickness scalds. *Journal of Burn Care Rehabilitation,* in press.

20. Sheridan, R.L., Petras, L., Lydon, M., & Salvo, P.M. (1997). Once-daily wound cleansing and dressing change: Efficacy and cost. *Journal of Burn Care Rehabilitation, 18*(2), 139–140.

21. Kim, H.J., Ghali, F.E., & Tunnessen, W.W. (1997). Here comes the sun. *Contemporary Pediatrics, 14*(7), 41–69.

22. Peter, G. (Ed.) (1997). *1997 Red book: Report of the committee on infectious diseases* (24th ed.). Elk Grove Village, IL: American Academy of Pediatrics.

23. Connelly, K.P. (1997). Advising families about pets. *Contemporary Pediatrics, 14*(2), 71–86.

24. Rustad, O.J. (1992). Outdoors and active: Relieving summer's siege on skin. *Physician and Sportsmedicine, 20*(5), 162–168, 171–176, 178.

ADDITIONAL RESOURCES

Arendt, D.L., & Arendt, D.B. (1992). Rescue operations for snakebites. *American Journal of Nursing, 92*(7), 26–32.

Children's National Medical Center, Burn Unit Staff. (1996). *Burn wound care.* Washington, DC: Children's National Medical Center.

Dinman, S., & Jarosz, D.A (1996). Managing serious dog bite injuries in children. *Pediatric Nursing, 22*(5), 413–416.

Frey, C. (1992). Frostbitten feet: Steps to treatment and prevention. *Physician and Sportsmedicine, 20*(1), 67–72, 76.

Herndon, D.N. (1997). Perspectives in the use of allograft. *Journal of Burn Care Rehabilitation, 18*(1, part 2), S6.

Kealey, G.P. (1997). Disease transmission by means of allograft. *Journal of Burn Care Rehabilitation, 18*(1, part 2), S10–11.

Kizer, K.W. (1991). Treating insect stings. *Physician and Sportsmedicine, 19*(8), 33–34, 36.

Koo, J.Y.M., & Smith L.L. (1991). Psychologic aspects of acne. *Pediatric Dermatology, 8*(3), 185–188.

Ritchie, S.R. (1992). Primary bacterial skin infections. *Dermatology Nursing, 4*(4), 261–268.

Romeo, S.P. (1995). Atopic dermatitis: The itch that rashes. *Pediatric Nursing, 21*(2), 157–163.

Roujeau, J.C., & Stern, R.S. (1994). Severe adverse cutaneous reactions to drugs. *New England Journal of Medicine, 331*(19), 1272–1285.

Saffle, J.R., Davis, B., Williams, P., & the American Burn Association Registry Participant Group. (1995). Recent outcomes in the treatment of burn injury in the United States: A report of the American Burn Patient Registry. *Journal of Burn Care Rehabilitation, 16*(3), 219–232.

Schmitt, B.D. (1996). When your child has ringworm of the scalp. *Contemporary Pediatrics, 13*(1), 62–63.

Sokolof, F. (1994). Identification and management of pediculosis. *Nurse Practitioner, 19*(8), 62–63.

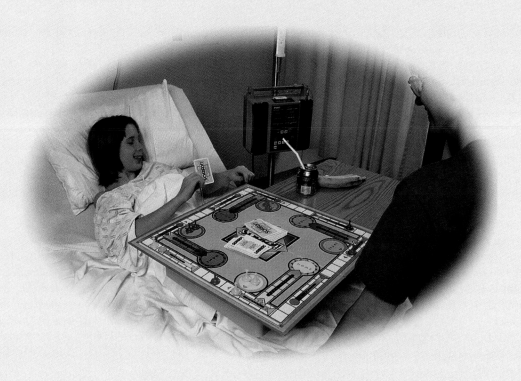

Ten-year-old Clara has attention deficit hyperactivity disorder (ADHD). She has been hospitalized to treat a dog bite to her lower leg. Although her hospitalization will be short, it offers particular challenges to the nurses who will be caring for her on the pediatric unit.

During admission, Clara pulled over a large pile of folders near the computer in the admission area. She ran into and around the emergency department in the next hallway. It was difficult for her mother to complete the admission history and supervise Clara at the same time. Clara's mother reports that her daughter has always been an active and impulsive child. In fact, she sustained her present injury when she ran into a neighbor's yard, despite her mother's instructions not to do so.

Clara was cared for at home until kindergarten. At that time, her teacher recommended that she be evaluated by a clinical psychologist, who diagnosed ADHD. Since the age of 7 years, Clara has been taking methylphenidate (Ritalin) to help control her behavior. Her mother reports that the medication has helped Clara to control her behavior and to perform better at school. However, at this time she is off Ritalin for a trial during summer vacation. In addition, Clara's parents have learned behavioral management techniques to assist them in setting clear limits for her.

ALTERATIONS IN PSYCHOSOCIAL FUNCTION 22

"Clara has always been such a challenge. Sometimes I feel exhausted by the amount of energy it takes to do anything with her. Going to the store, getting ready for school . . . these things seem so much simpler with our other children. She has so many talents, though, and is really smart. We want to help her learn to control her behavior and do well in school as she grows up."

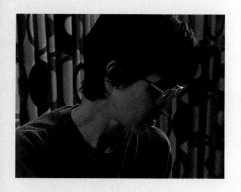

TERMINOLOGY

- **adaptive functioning** The ability of an individual to meet the standards expected for his or her age by his or her cultural group.
- **affect** Outward manifestation of feeling or emotion; the tone of a person's reaction or response to people or events.
- **behavior modification** A technique used to reinforce desirable behaviors, helping the child to replace maladaptive behaviors with more appropriate ones.
- **child sexual abuse** The exploitation of a child for the sexual gratification of an adult.
- **cognitive therapy** A therapeutic approach that attempts to help the person recognize automatic thought patterns that lead to unpleasant feelings.
- **emotional abuse** Shaming, ridiculing, embarrassing, or insulting a child.

- **emotional neglect** A caretaker's unavailability to meet the psychosocial needs of a child.
- **physical abuse** The deliberate maltreatment of another individual that inflicts pain or injury and may result in permanent or temporary disfigurement or even death.
- **physical neglect** The deliberate withholding of or failure to provide the necessary and available resources to a child.
- **play therapy** A therapeutic intervention often used with preschool and school-aged children. The child reveals conflicts, wishes, and fears on an unconscious level while playing with dolls, toys, clay, and other objects.
- **stereotypy** Repetitive, obsessive, machine-like movements, commonly seen in autistic or schizophrenic children.

As one of the nurses caring for Clara, how will you ensure her safety during her stay on the unit while still meeting her developmental needs? What special care will she require, in addition to that provided for her injury?

The purpose of this chapter is to give you the knowledge and tools that can help you provide appropriate care for children like Clara with alterations in psychosocial functioning. Because much of this care will be provided by psychiatric–mental health specialists, the nurse's role often centers on identification, support of the therapy, teaching, and referral.

Some psychosocial conditions in children originate from a genetic or physiologic cause. Examples include mental retardation and childhood schizophrenia. Others, such as child abuse, occur because of the environment in which the child lives. Still others, such as substance abuse, may be a result of both genetic and environmental influences.

Most psychosocial conditions are treated in community settings, and nurses in these settings play an active role in the treatment and support of the child and family. Nurses may function as case managers, assisting a family to deal with all areas of the child's care. Occasionally a child is hospitalized with a psychosocial condition, either for treatment of that condition or for treatment of another health problem.

► PSYCHOTHERAPEUTIC MANAGEMENT OF CHILDREN AND ADOLESCENTS

The primary treatment goal in the management of children and adolescents with psychosocial disorders is to assist the child and family to achieve and maintain an optimal level of functioning through interventions designed to reduce the impact of stressors. Therapeutic interventions and communications are based on the principle that one must look at the feelings motivating the behaviors. Parents and others close to the child often fall into the habit of reacting to the child's behaviors rather than trying to find out what feelings may be precipitating the undesirable actions.

TREATMENT MODES

Three basic treatment modes are used: individual, family, and group therapy.[1] The choice of treatment mode must take into account the child's age and developmental stage. Various strategies may be used within these modes, as discussed below. Most therapists incorporate several strategies simultaneously. Different strategies are more or less effective and appropriate for children and adolescents in various stages of development. A thorough understanding of developmental needs, expectations, and abilities is therefore essential.

Individual Therapy

Individual therapy involves only the child and the therapist. Treatment of specific emotional problems or disorders may involve various techniques such as play therapy, psychodrama, art therapy, and **cognitive therapy** (a technique used to help a person recognize automatic negative thinking). Individual therapy may be short term (four to six sessions) or long term (lasting for several years).

Family Therapy

Family therapy involves the exploration of a particular emotional problem and its manifestations among the family members. Family therapy is based on the idea that the emotional symptoms or problems of an individual are an expression of emotional symptoms or problems in the family. The focus is on the relationships among the family members, not the psychologic conflict within each individual member.

Group Therapy

Group therapy involves an ongoing or limited number of sessions in which several patients participate. The emphasis is on the interpersonal styles of relating to one another in the group. Group therapy is particularly effective with adolescents because of the importance of the peer group at this age. An advantage of group therapy is that stimuli and feedback come from multiple sources (the group members) instead of just one person (the therapist).

THERAPEUTIC STRATEGIES

Play Therapy

Play is often called the language or work of the child. From a developmental perspective, children progressively learn to express feelings and needs through action, fantasy, and finally language. The special quality of play buffers children against the pressures and demands of daily life. Play facilitates mastery of developmental stages by strengthening physical and neurologic processes. Play also assists in cognitive learning, setting the stage for problem solving and creativity.

Play therapy is a technique that reveals problems on a fantasy level through the use of toys, dolls, clay, art, and other creative objects. It is often used with preschool and school-age children who are experiencing anxiety, stress, and other specific nonpsychotic mental disorders. Play therapy encourages the child to act out feelings, such as anger, hostility, sadness, and fear. It also provides the opportunity for the therapist to help the child understand, on a conscious or unconscious level, his or her own responses and behavior in a safe, supportive environment.

Art Therapy

Children who may be apprehensive about playing can sometimes be encouraged to participate in art therapy, using brief drawing exercises. This technique is appropriate for children of all ages, including adolescents. The drawings can help the therapist gain information about the child, the family, and the interactions between the child and family. However, children's drawings should never be used solely to form a definitive diagnosis.

When used in conjunction with a thorough history and appropriate psychologic testing information, art therapy can guide the child's treatment. These drawing exercises provide an opportunity to help in the healing process. The therapist can assist the child to release feelings of anger, pain, or fear onto paper, where they can be examined objectively. (Figures 22–1 to 22–4 present several examples of this technique.)

Behavior Therapy

Behavior modification is a therapeutic technique that uses stimulus and response conditioning to alter inappropriate behaviors. It is used to reinforce

PLAY THERAPY

Play therapy, a technique used with children who have psychosocial disorders, is different from *therapeutic play,* which may be used with many hospitalized children (see Chap. 4). Although some techniques overlap, only a specialist is qualified to provide play therapy.

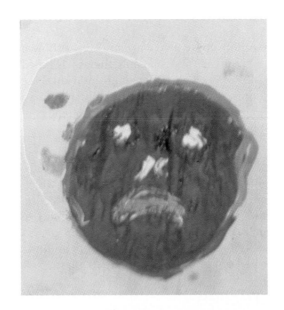

FIGURE 22-1. "Me." Drawn by a 14-year-old girl with major depression, anxiety, and school phobia who had experienced multiple losses over several years. Her mother had severe chronic lung problems and diabetes, and the girl had stopped attending school for fear that something would happen to her mother. This drawing represents the girl's obvious feelings of sadness and depression but also indicates a glimmer of hope (represented by yellow mask coming from behind dark mask of depression).

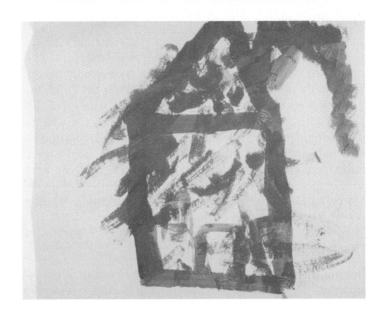

FIGURE 22-2. "Self-Portrait." Drawn by a 15-year-old boy who was admitted through the emergency department after a failed suicide attempt by hanging. He had a psychiatric diagnosis of depression and polysubstance abuse (including inhalants and alcohol) and insisted that he was a member of a satanic cult in his hometown. Most of his drawings depicted a preoccupation with violence and suicide. The boy said that he always felt a "darkness" like a shadow that followed him around and wanted him dead. His family history was significant for depression and suicide on both his mother's and his father's side. His father also had a lengthy history of polysubstance abuse and alcoholism. The boy was discharged to a long-term residential treatment facility for adolescents.

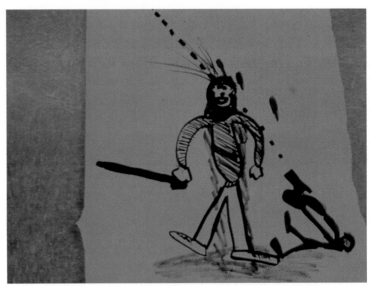

FIGURE 22-3. "An Activity." Drawn by an 8-year-old boy who was initially admitted to the medical-surgical floor of a pediatric hospital for dehydration resulting from vomiting and diarrhea. Psychiatric evaluation was ordered for extreme anxiety. These drawings, completed during the initial interview, led to further investigation, which revealed that the child had started a house fire in which his grandmother (his primary caretaker at the time) was killed. The family's home and all their belongings were lost. No one had known that the child had set the fire. Further sessions indicated that he had been setting neighborhood garage fires frequently and watching them burn from a distance.

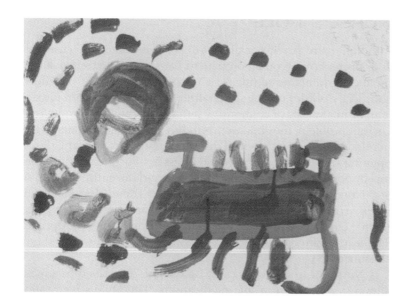

FIGURE 22–4. "A Family Activity." By the same boy who drew Figure 22–3. This drawing depicts a recurring incident of physical and emotional abuse by his mother's live-in boyfriend. It shows the family bathtub with feces and blood smeared on the floors and walls. The boy reported that when either he or his 3-year-old brother had a toileting accident, the boyfriend would make them go into the bathroom and stand in the bathtub while he smeared the feces on the walls. He would then hit the children and make them clean up the mess. The boy had been removed from the mother's custody previously for neglect. He was transferred from the medical-surgical area to the inpatient children's psychiatric unit, where he received a diagnosis of depression, overanxious disorder, and child abuse (physical and emotional). Charges were filed against the mother's boyfriend, and custody of both children was temporarily revoked.

desirable behaviors, helping the child to replace maladaptive behaviors with more appropriate ones. This technique is based on the assumption that any learned behavior can be unlearned. Thus, if parents, nurses, teachers, and other adults consistently reinforce desirable behaviors, the child will eventually alter or discontinue undesirable behaviors.

Behavior modification may include (1) removing the child from the home to a more structured environment, such as a hospital, for a brief time, and (2) teaching the parents, teachers, and other appropriate adults to be agents of behavioral change.[1] Several ongoing sessions may be required with the adults involved, using role play and other techniques. Consistency is the most important principle in the successful use of behavior modification.

Visualization and Guided Imagery

The techniques of visualization and guided imagery begin with specific directions for progressive relaxation according to the child's ability. This form of therapy uses the child's own imagination and positive thinking to reduce stress and anxiety, decrease the experience of pain or discomfort, and promote healing. The techniques are especially useful in the management of anxiety disorders and chronic pain. It is not easy for every child to use his or her imagination in this way, so the technique may not work or be appropriate for everyone.

Hypnosis

Hypnosis involves varying degrees of suggestibility and deep relaxation effects. This technique is useful for children and adolescents because they can usually be hypnotized more easily than adults. Hypnosis is especially helpful in treating physical symptoms with a psychologic component, anxiety, and phobias and in managing severe physical symptoms or discomfort (pain or nausea) associated with a physiologic disorder or its treatment (eg, cancer or juvenile rheumatoid arthritis).

NURSE'S ROLE

Although many psychosocial disorders are managed effectively with therapy and/or medication on an outpatient basis, some necessitate admission to an inpatient psychiatric setting. The nurse may encounter the child with a psychosocial disorder during hospitalization for a concurrent physiologic problem, or in a variety of community settings. If a child is hospitalized for a concurrent problem, the child's current level of functioning needs to be assessed in relation to the psychosocial disorder. In the case of Clara, described in the opening vignette, the nurse would assess her current attention deficit behaviors by observing Clara during admission and the entire hospital stay.

Nursing assessment also focuses on identifying medications being taken, common abnormal behaviors (what triggers them, what reduces them), family interactions, and routines to maintain appropriate behaviors. The nurse then considers how to support the child within the hospital environment.

Nursing care includes carrying out the prescribed treatment plan and administering psychotropic medications. The child's medication regimen should be evaluated for administration schedule, dosage, side effects, and effectiveness. Inform the therapist of the child's hospitalization if the child has been hospitalized for a concurrent condition, and consult with the therapist regarding appropriate approaches for the child. Provide supportive care for the child and family. Continuation of family involvement is critical. The nurse frequently is the liaison between the family and the therapist in making follow-up arrangements at the time of discharge.

The nurse in the community assesses how a child with a psychosocial disorder is functioning in each microsystem (see Chap. 2), such as home, day care, school, and with friends. Involvement in therapy sessions and ability to manage prescribed pharmacologic interventions are evaluated.

► AUTISTIC DISORDER

Autistic disorder is a complex childhood disorder that involves abnormalities in behavior, social interactions, and communication. It is the most common of the pervasive developmental disorders, of which Rett syndrome and Asperger's syndrome are two other examples. The essential features of autistic disorder typically become apparent by the time a child is 3 years of age. For every 10,000 births, 2–5 children are found to have autistic disorder. The disorder occurs four times more often in boys than in girls.[2]

Clinical Manifestations

Autistic children may manifest disturbances in the rate or sequence of development. Characteristically these children engage in repetitive behaviors, including head banging, twirling in circles, biting themselves, and flapping their hands or arms. Frequently a child's behavior is self-stimulating or self-destructive. Responses to sensory stimuli are frequently abnormal and include an extreme aversion to touch, loud noises, and bright lights.

Difficulties or delays in speech, language, and cognitive abilities are common and may correspond to intellectual deficits. Abnormal communication patterns include both verbal and nonverbal communication. Autistic children may eventually learn to talk, in some cases well, but their speech is likely to show certain abnormalities: use of "you" in place of "I"; echolalia (a compulsive parroting of what is heard); repeating questions rather than answering them; and fascination with rhythmic, repetitive songs and verses.

RETT SYNDROME

Rett syndrome is a pervasive developmental disorder similar in some ways to autistic disorder. Rett syndrome, however, occurs only in girls. The child usually appears normal until 6–18 months of age. Symptoms of increasing ataxia, hand-wringing, intermittent hyperventilation, dementia, and growth retardation then progress until the child requires total care.

ASPERGER SYNDROME

Asperger syndrome is manifested by impaired social interaction and repetitive behavior. However, cognition and language skills are usually normal for age.

Autistic children are unable to relate to people or to respond to social and emotional cues.[3] Emotional lability is common.

Etiology and Pathophysiology

The cause of autistic disorder is unknown. Brain dysfunction is thought to be a likely cause. Genetic transmission and biochemical imbalances may also be involved. Autistic children are frequently cognitively impaired but can demonstrate a wide range of intellectual ability and functioning. Only about 25% have an intelligence quotient (IQ) that measures within the normal range.[4]

Diagnostic Tests and Medical Management

Diagnosis is based on the presence of specific criteria, as described in the American Psychiatric Association's *Diagnostic and Statistical Manual of Mental Disorders*, 4th edition *(DSM-IV)*, outlined in Table 22–1.

22-1 | *DSM-IV* Diagnostic Criteria for Autistic Disorder

A. A total of six or more items from 1, 2, and 3, with at least two from 1, and one each from 2 and 3:
 1. Qualitative impairment in social interaction, as manifested by at least two of the following:
    a. Marked impairment in the use of multiple nonverbal behaviors such as eye-to-eye gaze, facial expression, body posture and gestures to regulate social interaction
    b. Failure to develop peer relationships appropriate to developmental level
    c. A lack of spontaneous seeking to share enjoyment, interests, or achievements with other people
    d. Lack of social or emotional reciprocity
 2. Qualitative impairments in communication as manifested by at least one of the following:
    a. Delay in, or total lack of, the development of spoken language (not accompanied by an attempt to compensate through alternative modes of communication such as gesture or mime)
    b. In individuals with adequate speech, marked impairment in the ability to initiate or sustain a conversation with others
    c. Stereotyped and repetitive use of language or idiosyncratic language
    d. Lack of varied, spontaneous make-believe play or social imitative play appropriate to developmental level
 3. Restricted repetitive and stereotyped patterns of behavior, interests, and activities, as manifested by at least one of the following:
    a. Encompassing preoccupation with one or more stereotyped and restricted patterns of interest that is abnormal either in intensity or in focus
    b. Apparently inflexible adherence to specific, nonfunctional routines or rituals
    c. Stereotyped and repetitive motor mannerisms (eg, hand or finger flapping or twisting, or complex whole-body movements)
    d. Persistent preoccupation with parts of objects
B. Delays or abnormal functioning in at least one of the following areas, with onset prior to age 3 years: (1) social interaction, (2) language as used in social communication, or (3) symbolic or imaginative play.
C. The disturbance is not better accounted for by Rett Syndrome or Childhood Disintegrative Disorder.

From American Psychiatric Association. (1994). Diagnostic and statistical manual of mental disorders (4th ed.). Washington DC: Author. Copyright © 1994 American Psychiatric Association.

Treatment focuses on behavior modification to reward appropriate behaviors, foster positive or adaptive coping skills, and facilitate effective communication. The goals of treatment are to reduce rigidity or **stereotypy** (repetitive, obsessive, machine-like movements) and decrease maladaptive behaviors. Often the child must be physically restrained from aggressive or self-destructive behaviors.

The overall prognosis for autistic children to become functioning members of society is guarded. The extent to which adequate adjustment is achieved varies greatly. Successful adjustment is more likely for children with higher IQs, adequate speech, and access to specialized programs.

Nursing Assessment

The nurse may encounter the autistic child when parents seek care for a suspected hearing impairment or developmental delay. Parents may report abnormal interaction such as lack of eye contact, disinterest in cuddling, minimal facial responsiveness, and failure to talk. Initial assessment focuses on language development, response to others, and hearing acuity (see Chaps. 3 and 17).

When a child with a diagnosis of autistic disorder is hospitalized for a concurrent problem, obtain a history from the parents regarding the child's routines, rituals, and likes and dislikes, as well as ways to promote interaction and cooperation. Ask about the child's behaviors as well as observing them on admission. Obtain a history of acute and chronic illnesses and injuries.

Autistic children may carry a special toy or object that they play with during times of stress. Ask parents about these objects and their use.

Nursing Diagnosis

Nursing diagnoses must be tailored to fit the individual needs of the child. Examples of nursing diagnoses that might be appropriate for autistic children include the following:

- Impaired Verbal Communication related to poor language skills
- Impaired Social Interaction related to slow developmental maturation
- Impaired Adjustment related to disruption of daily routine
- Altered Thought Processes related to abnormal response to environmental cues
- Sleep Pattern Disturbance related to hyperactivity and hypermobility
- Risk for Injury related to cognitive impairment
- Risk for Caregiver Role Strain related to child's delayed development, need for constant care, and inability to relate to caregivers
- Ineffective Family Coping: Compromised or Disabling related to child who does not become integrated into family

Nursing Management

Nursing care focuses on decreasing environmental stimuli, providing supportive care, maintaining a safe environment, giving the parents anticipatory guidance, and providing emotional support.

Decrease Environmental Stimuli

Autistic children interpret and respond to the environment differently from other individuals. Sounds that are not distressing to the average person may be interpreted by autistic children as louder, more frightening, and over-whelming. The child needs to be oriented to the hospital room and may adjust best to a room with only one other child. Encourage parents to bring the child's favorite objects from home, and try to keep these objects in the same places, because the child does not cope well with changes in the environment.

Provide Supportive Care

Developing a trusting relationship with the autistic child is often difficult. Adjust communication techniques and teaching to the child's developmental level. Ask parents about the child's usual home routines, and maintain these routines as much as possible. Because self-care abilities are often limited, the child may need assistance to meet basic needs. When possible, schedule daily care and routine procedures at consistent times to maintain predictability. Encourage parents to remain with the child and to participate in daily care planning. Identify rituals for naptime and bedtime, and maintain them to promote rest and sleep.

Maintain a Safe Environment

Monitor autistic children at all times, including bath time and bedtime. Close supervision is needed to ensure that the child does not obtain any harmful objects or engage in dangerous behaviors.

Provide Anticipatory Guidance

Approximately half of all children with autistic disorder require lifelong supervision and support. This is especially true if the disorder is accompanied by mental retardation. Some children may grow up to lead independent lives, although they will be socially inept and their social and interpersonal relationships will be limited. Encourage parents to promote the child's development through behavior modification and specialized educational programs. The overall goal is to provide the child with the guidance, education, and support necessary for optimal functioning.

Care in the Community

Families of autistic children need a great deal of support to cope with the challenges of caring for the autistic child. Help the family to identify resources for child care, such as special toddler programs and preschools. The child will need an Individualized Education Plan when old enough. The parent or primary caretaker often has difficulty obtaining respite care and may need assistance to find suitable resources. Siblings of the autistic child may need help to explain the disorder to their friends or teachers. Family support programs are available in some states to provide assistance to parents.

Local support groups for parents of autistic children are available in most areas. Parents can also be referred to the Autism Society of America (see Appendix F) for information.

 SAFETY PRECAUTIONS

If the autistic child or adolescent is particularly aggressive or self-abusive, bike helmets and mitts can be the least restrictive method used for the safety of the child, other patients, and staff. This may enable the child to participate in activities and engage in the social environment (to the degree capable) with specially trained professionals.

▶ ATTENTION DEFICIT DISORDER AND ATTENTION DEFICIT HYPERACTIVITY DISORDER

Attention deficit disorder (ADD) is characterized by developmentally inappropriate behaviors involving inattention. When hyperactivity accompanies inattention, the disorder is called attention deficit hyperactivity disorder

(ADHD). Since ADHD is the more common condition, the discussion below focuses on this disorder. ADHD affects approximately 3% of all children and is approximately six to nine times more common in boys than in girls.[5]

Clinical Manifestations

Children with ADD and ADHD have problems related to decreased attention span, impulsiveness, or increased motor activity. Symptoms can range from mild to severe. The disorders often coexist with various developmental learning disabilities. The child has difficulty completing tasks, fidgets constantly, is frequently loud, and interrupts others. Because of these behaviors, the child often has difficulty developing and maintaining social relationships and may be shunned or teased by other children. This only increases the anxiety of the already compromised child, whose behavior is set on a downward-spiraling course.

Typically, girls with ADHD show less aggression and impulsiveness than boys, but far more anxiety, mood swings, social withdrawal, rejection, and cognitive and language problems. Girls tend to be older at the time of diagnosis. However, like Clara in the opening vignette, children are frequently diagnosed with the disorder soon after beginning school, with its challenges for attentive behavior.

Etiology and Pathophysiology

The results of research have dramatically changed the thinking about ADHD in the past 40 years. Although a variety of physical and neurologic disorders are associated with ADHD, children with identifiable causes represent a small proportion of this population. Examples of known associations include exposure to high levels of lead in childhood and prenatal exposure to alcohol. There may be a deficit in the catecholamines dopamine and norepinephrine in some children, lowering the threshold for stimuli input. Probably there are many types of attention deficit, resulting from several different mechanisms. Genetic factors may be important, as well as family dynamics. Although ADHD occurs more commonly within families, a single gene has not been located and a specific mechanism of genetic transmission is not known. An interaction between the genetic and environmental factors is often an important part of the disorder.[2]

Diagnostic Tests and Medical Management

Children are usually brought for evaluation when behaviors escalate to the point of interfering with the daily functioning of teachers or parents. When children have learning disabilities or anxiety disorders, the problem is commonly misdiagnosed as ADHD without further evaluation of the child's symptoms. Therefore obtaining an accurate diagnosis by a pediatric mental health specialist is important.

Specific diagnostic criteria (Table 22–2) vary among children. Treatment depends on the severity of the disorder and may include one or more of the following approaches: environmental changes, behavior modification, or pharmacotherapy.

Children with milder cases of ADHD often benefit from environmental changes. Decreasing stimulation, for example, by turning off television, keeping the environment quiet, and maintaining an orderly and clutter-free desk or study area without distraction, may help the child to stay focused on the task at hand. Another relatively simple change is appropriate classroom placement, preferably in a small class with a teacher who can provide close

22-2 *DSM-IV Diagnostic Criteria for Attention Deficit Hyperactivity Disorder*

A. Either 1 or 2:
1. **Inattention:** Six (or more) of the following symptoms of inattention have persisted for at least 6 months to a degree that is maladaptive and inconsistent with developmental level:
   a. Often fails to give close attention to details or makes careless mistakes in schoolwork, work, and other activities
   b. Often has difficulty sustaining attention in tasks or play activities
   c. Often does not seem to listen when spoken to directly
   d. Often does not follow through on instructions and fails to finish schoolwork, chores, or duties in the workplace (not due to oppositional behavior or failure to understand instructions)
   e. Often has difficulty organizing tasks and activities
   f. Often avoids, dislikes, or is reluctant to engage in tasks that require sustained mental effort (such as schoolwork or homework)
   g. Often loses things necessary for tasks or activities (eg, toys, school assignments, pencils, books, or tools)
   h. Is often easily distracted by extraneous stimuli
   i. Is often forgetful in daily activities
2. **Hyperactivity-impulsivity:** Six (or more) of the following symptoms of hyperactivity-impulsivity have persisted for at least 6 months to a degree that is maladaptive and inconsistent with developmental level:

   Hyperactivity
   a. Often fidgets with hands or feet or squirms in seat
   b. Often leaves seat in classroom or in other situations in which remaining seated is expected
   c. Often runs about or climbs excessively in situations in which it is inappropriate (in adolescents or adults, may be limited to subjective feelings of restlessness)
   d. Often has difficulty playing or engaging in leisure activities quietly
   e. Is often "on the go" or often acts as if "driven by a motor"
   f. Often talks excessively

   Impulsivity
   g. Often blurts out answers before questions have been completed
   h. Often has difficulty awaiting turn
   i. Often interrupts or intrudes on others (eg, butts into conversations or games)
B. Some hyperactive-impulsive or inattentive symptoms that caused impairment were present before age 7 years.
C. Some impairment from the symptoms is present in two or more settings (eg, at school [or work] and at home).
D. There must be clear evidence of clinically significant impairment in social, academic, or occupational functioning.
E. The symptoms do not occur exclusively during the course of a Pervasive Developmental Disorder, Schizophrenia, or other Psychotic Disorder and are not better accounted for by another mental disorder (eg, Mood Disorder, Anxiety Disorder, Dissociative Disorder, or a Personality Disorder).

From American Psychiatric Association. (1994). Diagnostic and statistical manual of mental disorders (4th ed.). Washington DC: Author. Copyright © 1994 American Psychiatric Association.

supervision and a structured daily routine. Consistent limits and expectations should be set for the child.

Children with moderate to severe ADHD are treated with pharmacotherapy. Methylphenidate (Ritalin) is most often prescribed, as was true for Clara in the chapter opener. This drug acts mainly on the central nervous system, enhancing catecholamine effects to inhibit impulsiveness and hyperactivity while generally improving attention span and task performance.[6] Usually a favorable response (a decrease in impulsive behaviors and an increase in the ability to sit still and attend to an activity for at least 15 minutes) is seen in the first 10 days of treatment and frequently within the first few doses.

Approximately 20% of children do not respond to stimulants such as methylphenidate. Other medications that have been shown to be effective include antidepressants such as desipramine (Norpramin) and bupropion (Wellbutrin); carbamazepine (Tegretol), an anticonvulsant; magnesium pemoline (Cylert), a dopamine agonist; and lithium, an antimanic drug that is used occasionally in children with a coexisting conduct disorder.[7]

Although ADHD was once thought to be a disorder of childhood that gradually improved with age, it is now believed that symptoms continue into adulthood and that careful management in childhood assists in lessening problems of social functioning later in life.

Nursing Assessment

The nurse may encounter the child with ADHD in the hospital when parents bring the child for treatment of an injury (eg, fracture) or other problem. This was illustrated in the opening scenario. Explore the parent's report of the child's attention span in detail. Usually within a few minutes in an unstructured setting or waiting area, the child with ADHD becomes restless and searches for distraction. Remember the disruptive activities of Clara when she was admitted to the hospital. Gather information about the child's activity level and impulsiveness. Be alert for information that reveals a serious problem, such as hurting animals or other children. Obtain information about distractibility, attention deficit in activities of daily living, characteristic ways of reacting, and the extent of impulsiveness when the child is receiving medication. Find out how the family manages at home. Ask about a family history of the disorder, as that is a common finding among children with ADHD.[8]

Nursing Diagnosis

Examples of nursing diagnoses that might be appropriate for a child with ADHD include the following:

- Impaired Verbal Communication related to inattention
- Impaired Social Interaction related to chronic episodes of impulsive behavior
- Chronic Low Self-Esteem related to lack of positive feedback and lack of success in social interactions
- Anxiety related to mood swings and concern about ability to behave in a socially appropriate manner
- Risk for Injury related to high level of impulsiveness and excitability, and low impulse control
- Risk for Caregiver Role Strain related to unpredictable nature of child's moods and difficulty in managing a high-energy child

Nursing Management

Nursing care of the hospitalized child with ADHD focuses on administering medications, managing the child's environment, implementing behavioral

NURSING ALERT

Children receiving magnesium pemoline (Cylert) should continue to receive the drug during hospitalization. If the medication is stopped during hospitalization, the child may have behavioral problems for weeks after discharge.

management plans, providing emotional support to the child and family, and promoting self-esteem.

Administer Medications

Methylphenidate and other medications increase the child's attention span and decrease distractibility. Be alert for the common side effects of these medications, including anorexia, insomnia, and tachycardia. Administering medication early in the day helps to alleviate insomnia. Anorexia can be managed by giving medication at mealtimes. Careful monitoring of weight, height, and blood pressure is necessary.

Minimize Environmental Distractions

The child may need to be placed in an environment with minimal distractions. When hospitalized, this may mean a room with only one other child. Potentially harmful equipment should be kept out of reach. Television and video game time needs to be monitored and limited. Use shades to darken the room at nap- or bedtime, and minimize noise. Teach parents to minimize distractions at home during periods when the child needs to concentrate; for example, when doing schoolwork. Visits to areas such as shopping malls and playgrounds may need to be limited.

Implement Behavioral Management Plans

Behavior modification programs can help to reduce specific impulsive behaviors. An example is setting up a reward program for the child who has taken medication as ordered or completed a homework assignment. The rewards may be daily as well as weekly or monthly, depending on the child's age. (For example, one completed homework assignment might be rewarded with 30 minutes of basketball or a bike ride; assignments completed for a week might be rewarded with participation in an activity of the child's choice on the weekend.)

If punishment is necessary, the behavior should be corrected while simultaneously supporting the child as a person. Punishment should follow the offense quickly as the child may not otherwise connect the punishment with the behavior.

Provide Emotional Support

Children with ADHD offer a special challenge to parents, teachers, and health care providers. Parents must cope simultaneously with managing the difficult needs and demands of a hard-to-handle child, obtaining appropriate evaluation and treatment, and understanding and accepting the diagnosis, even when the child exhibits different behaviors with different people.[9] Family support is essential. Educate both the parents and the child about the importance of appropriate expectations and consequences of behaviors.

Promote Self-Esteem

Help the child to understand the disorder at an appropriate developmental level, and facilitate a trusting relationship with health care providers. Assist the child with social skills through the use of role-play, playing in small groups, and modeling. Promote the child's self-esteem by pointing out the positive aspects of behavior and treating instances of negative behavior as learning opportunities. Help the child to develop ego strengths (the consciousness to be able to screen outside stimuli and control internal demands), which will result in better impulse control and thus increase self-esteem over time.

Care in the Community

Most children with ADHD are not hospitalized. Only occasionally will a child be hospitalized when needing care for another condition. Parents need support to understand the diagnosis and to learn how to manage the child. Emphasize the importance of a stable environment, at home as well as at school. At home the child may have difficulty staying on task. Parents need to consider age and developmental appropriateness of tasks, give clear and simple instructions, and provide frequent reminders to ensure completion.

The nurse can serve as a liaison to teachers and school personnel. Special classrooms or periods of instruction free from the distractions of the entire class may enable the child to improve school performance. Parents may have difficulty understanding the need for these approaches because the child often tests with above-average intelligence. Reinforce the importance of providing a structured environment free from unnecessary external stimuli. Be sure that parents understand behavioral approaches that will help the child, how to administer prescribed medications, and the importance of returning for health care visits to monitor for side effects.

As the child grows older, provide explanations about the disorder and information about techniques that will assist in dealing with problems. Emphasize the importance of doing homework or other tasks requiring concentration in a quiet environment without background noise from a television or radio. Encourage children with ADHD to write down instructions from teachers and to use checklists to help them accomplish specific tasks.

▶ MENTAL RETARDATION

Mental retardation is defined as significantly subaverage general intellectual functioning (IQ below 70–75), as well as impairments in **adaptive functioning** (the ability of an individual to meet the standards expected for his or her age by his or her cultural group). The mentally retarded child has adaptive deficits in at least two areas such as communication, self-care, home living, social/interpersonal skills, use of community resources, self-direction, functional academic skills, work, leisure, health, or safety. A low IQ score by itself does not necessarily correlate with impairment in the ability to carry out adaptive skills. The IQ score and the level of adaptive skills together determine the degree of severity of mental retardation (see Table 22–3).

22-3	Severity of Mental Retardation	
Severity		**IQ**
Mild retardation		50–55 to approximately 70
Moderate retardation		35–40 to 50–55
Severe retardation		20–25 to 35–40
Profound retardation		below 20–25

Clinical Manifestations

Children who are mentally retarded manifest delays in all areas of development, including motor movement, language, and adaptive behavior. They usually achieve developmental milestones more slowly than the average child. These developmental delays may be the first indication to parents and care providers of the child's condition.

Mental retardation is sometimes accompanied by sensory impairment, speech problems, motor and orthopedic disabilities, and seizure disorders. Of children with mental retardation, 10–30% manifest one of these other disorders.[10] Table 22–4 lists several physical characteristics associated with three of the most common disorders that result in mental

---

22-4 | **Characteristics Associated With Three Common Types of Mental Retardation**

Down Syndrome (see Fig. 3–14)
Small head (microcephaly)
Flattened forehead
Wide, short neck
Epicanthal eye folds
White spots on eye iris (Brushfield spots)
Congenital cataracts
Flat nose
Small, low-set ears
Protruding tongue
Short broad hands
Simian line on palm
Wide space between first and second toes
Hearing loss
Increased incidence of diabetes, congenital heart defect, and leukemia
Hypotonia

Fragile X Syndrome
Long face
Prominent jaw
Large ears
Frequent otitis media
Large testicles
Epicanthal eye folds
Strabismus
High arched palate
Scoliosis
Pliable joints

Fetal Alcohol Syndrome (see Fig. 2–5)
Flat midface
Low nasal bridge
Long philtrum with narrow upper lip
Short upturned nose
Poor coordination
Failure to thrive
Skeletal and joint abnormalities
Hearing loss

Adapted from Ross, LJ. (1994). Developmental disabilities: Genetic implications. Journal of Obstetric and Neonatal Nursing, 23(6), 502–504.

22-5	Common Causes of Mental Retardation

Prenatal Conditions
Down syndrome
Fragile X syndrome
Fetal alcohol syndrome
Maternal infection (eg, rubella, cytomegalovirus)

Biologic Environment
Errors of metabolism (eg, phenylketonuria, hypothyroidism)

External Forces
Trauma (eg, accident)
Poison ingestion (acute or chronic)
Hypoxia
Infection (eg, meningitis)
Environmental deprivation

NURSING ALERT

Prematurity places the child at risk of displaying below-normal cognitive development. The premature infant needs frequent, thorough neurologic and developmental examinations, particularly in the first year of life.

retardation: Down syndrome, fragile X syndrome, and fetal alcohol syndrome.

Etiology and Pathophysiology

Mild retardation occurs in 3.7–5.9 per 1000 people, and the more severe types of retardation affect an additional 3–4 per 1000 population.[11] The causes of mental retardation can be grouped into three general categories: prenatal errors in the development of the central nervous system, prenatal or postnatal changes in the biologic environment of the person, and external forces leading to central nervous system damage. In each instance, the precipitating factor causes a change in the form, function, and adaptation of the central nervous system. Table 22–5 provides examples of common causes of mental retardation for each category.

Diagnostic Tests and Medical Management

Mental retardation is diagnosed on the basis of a comprehensive history and evaluation of the child's physical characteristics, developmental level, and intellectual and adaptive functioning. Table 22–6 presents the *DSM-IV* criteria for mental retardation. Laboratory tests such as chromosome analysis, blood enzyme levels, lead levels, or cranial imaging provide valuable information in some circumstances.

Developmental screening using a test such as the Denver II can help to identify at-risk children. Tests of intellectual and adaptive functioning are performed when mental retardation is suspected. A neurologic examination may indicate asymmetry of movement or strength, irritability or lethargy, or abnormal pitch to an infant's cry. Because mental retardation may be accompanied by physical abnormalities, it is important to observe the child for facial symmetry, distance between the eyes, level of the ears, hair growth, and palmar creases. These abnormalities may be cues to other health problems.

Medical management focuses on early intervention to improve the degree of adaptive functioning. Simultaneous treatment of associated physical, emotional, and behavioral problems is provided. Depending on the severity of the child's condition, special education programs and physical or

22-6	*DSM-IV* Diagnostic Criteria for Mental Retardation

A. Significantly subaverage intellectual functioning: an IQ of approximately 70 or below on an individually administered IQ test (for infants, a clinical judgment of significantly subaverage intellectual functioning)
B. Concurrent deficits or impairments in present adaptive functioning (ie, the person's effectiveness in meeting the standards expected for his or her age by his or her cultural group) in at least two of the following areas: communication, self-care, home living, social/interpersonal skills, use of community resources, self-direction, functional academic skills, work, leisure, health, and safety
C. The onset is before age 18 years

From American Psychiatric Association. (1994). Diagnostic and statistical manual of mental disorders (4th ed.). Washington DC: Author. Copyright © 1994 American Psychiatric Association.

occupational therapy may be necessary (Fig. 22–5). The child may require supportive care and assistance with activities of daily living.

Nursing Assessment

Nurses can help to identify mentally retarded children through history taking, observation, and developmental screening during early childhood. The history should provide information about the mental and adaptive functioning of birth parents and other family members, as mental retardation clusters in families and some conditions such as fragile X syndrome are genetic in origin. The pregnancy and birth history can provide important information relating to alcohol and drug use by the mother during preg-

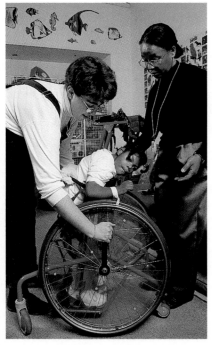

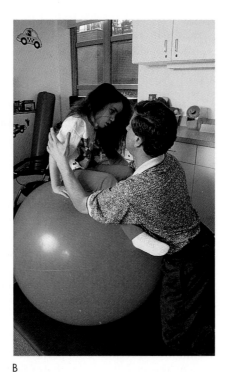

A   B

FIGURE 22–5. Physical therapy is an important component of medical management for many children who are mentally retarded. **A,** This severely retarded girl, who is wheelchair bound, is being positioned in a mobile prone stander, which enables her to interact in a different manner with her therapists and the environment. **B,** Physical therapists also provide outpatient care in the community to children with varying degrees of disability.

nancy. Be alert for a history of difficult pregnancy and problems during delivery. When genetic conditions in the family predispose family members to mental retardation, careful assessment of the child is needed. Children from deprived environments or those at risk because of environmental factors such as lead poisoning are more likely to manifest mental retardation.

Many mentally retarded children are not diagnosed with the condition until they reach school age, particularly if the condition is mild or moderate. Early intervention, however, can help to enhance the child's functioning later. During home visits, clinic appointments, in child care centers, and during hospitalization, be alert for signs such as developmental delays, multiple (more than three) physical anomalies (see Table 22–4), or neurologic alterations. Developmental assessment should be part of each health care visit.

Once the diagnosis of mental retardation has been made, assess the adaptive functioning of the child and family. A functional assessment of the child should be performed, including toileting, dressing, and feeding skills. Assess the child's language, sensory, and psychomotor functioning. Assess the home and community for safety hazards. Observe how the family is managing with the child. Assess the availability of services such as support groups for parents and special education opportunities for children. Evaluate the coping skills of family members.

Nursing Diagnosis

Several nursing diagnoses may be appropriate for the mentally retarded child, depending on the degree, cause, and outcome of the child's condition. Some of these diagnoses relate to impairments in adaptive functioning; others relate to the impact on the family. Examples include:

- Altered Growth and Development related to anoxia at birth
- Altered Nutrition: Less Than Body Requirements related to difficulty with self-feeding
- Toileting Self-Care Deficit related to delayed development
- Impaired Verbal Communication related to inability to understand and speak at age level
- Risk for Injury related to lack of understanding of environmental hazards
- Ineffective Family Coping: Compromised related to a child with significant intellectual and adaptive impairment
- Anticipatory Grieving (Parents) related to the loss of "perfect" child

Nursing Management

Nearly all children who are mentally retarded are cared for in the community. However, they may have conditions that require periodic hospitalization or frequent health care visits. Wherever nursing care occurs, it focuses on providing emotional support and information to family members, assisting the child with adaptive functioning, and fostering parental management of the child's activities. Whenever possible, the nurse uses preventive teaching to lower the risk of mental retardation.

Provide Emotional Support and Information

Family members need empathy and support both at the time of diagnosis and in the ensuing years. Parents may be in an acute or chronic state of grief over the loss of the perfect child. Encourage them to verbalize their feelings. Introducing them to parents of other mentally retarded children may provide assistance and support as they learn how to manage the child's needs. Discuss the availability of respite care to provide parents with a break from caretaking. Other family members such as grandparents and siblings may also be experiencing grief or guilt and should be given an opportunity to talk about their feelings.

Parents need honest information and answers to their questions about the child's condition. Reinforce information provided by genetic counselors and other health care professionals. Parents need to be informed about community resources designed to assist mentally retarded children. These may include the Zero to Three project early intervention programs, special education preschools and schools, county health services, and respite care, among others. See Appendix F for resources on mental retardation.

Maintain a Safe Environment

The mentally retarded child requires close supervision because he or she may lack an understanding of common hazards. Ensure safety in the hospital environment. Assist parents to provide safety at home, and teach the child necessary skills such as pedestrian safety. Consider both physical and emotional safety. The mentally retarded child may be trusting of others and sometimes is at risk for physical or sexual abuse.

Provide Assistance With Adaptive Functioning

Encourage parents' efforts to maximize the child's areas of strength and identify needs related to adaptive behaviors. Refer them to resources to assist in the areas of adaptive functioning in which the child has impairment, such as communication, self-care activities, or social skills. During hospitalization, support parents' efforts to maintain the child's skills in toileting, dressing, and self-care by planning interventions to use the skills being taught at home.

Care in the Community

Parents often act as case managers for the child's care. Assist parents as necessary to acquire the skills required to coordinate the child's plan of care. Evaluate the child's needs regularly and assist parents with the treatment plan as necessary. Assist with plans for education and for services such as physical or speech therapy. Most mentally retarded children will have an Individualized Education Plan designed to meet their specific learning needs. Parents, nurses, and others such as teachers and language therapists are part of the team that plans the child's Individualized Education Plan. Promote optimal development and socialization. As the child reaches adolescence, education is directed toward a vocation, issues of sexuality, and the goal of independent living, when appropriate.

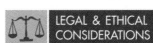

LEGAL & ETHICAL CONSIDERATIONS

The Education for All Handicapped Children Act, P.L. 94–142, provides free appropriate education to all handicapped children between 2 and 21 years of age. Amendments to this act in 1986 (P.L. 99–457) encouraged states to provide early intervention services for handicapped infants and toddlers by providing federal funding.

▶ EATING AND ELIMINATION DISORDERS

A number of eating and elimination disorders affect children and adolescents. Because food is intricately connected with emotional health, these disorders are often associated with both physiologic and psychologic problems. They can create increasing difficulty in family and social relationships for the child or adolescent and can be worsened by disturbed social relationships. The results are depression, isolation and withdrawal, and other self-destructive behaviors.

Eating symbolizes many things. On a basic level, eating represents parental nurturing. The act of being fed or cared for by a parent is the model for all future intimate relationships. For some individuals, however, eating creates anxiety related to a negative association with unpleasant or unsatisfactory parent–child interactions. Elimination, as the outcome of eating, can reflect the same anxieties connected with food intake.

A multidisciplinary team, including a pediatrician, pediatric mental health specialist (psychiatrist, child psychologist, clinical nurse specialist, or social worker), family therapist, and nutritionist, assesses the child's physical, developmental, mental health, familial, and nutritional status. Because nutritional deficiencies often accompany eating and elimination disorders, physical assessment focuses on identifying possible associated problems (eg, anemia). The overall strengths and weaknesses of the child and family must be evaluated to identify the various factors contributing to the child's inadequate or excessive caloric intake and caloric expenditure. Treatment is then designed to address these factors.

FEEDING DISORDER OF INFANCY OR EARLY CHILDHOOD (FAILURE TO THRIVE)

Failure to thrive (FTT) describes a syndrome in which infants or young children fail to eat enough food to be adequately nourished. This disorder accounts for 1–5% of pediatric hospitalizations in children under 1 year of age, and many more children are managed on an outpatient or home care basis.[12]

The cause of FTT can be organic, as in congenital acquired immunodeficiency syndrome (AIDS) (see Chap. 9), inborn errors of metabolism (see Chap. 20), neurologic disease, and esophageal reflux (see Chap. 15). Most cases of FTT, however, are nonorganic in origin. FTT resulting from nonorganic causes is now called feeding disorder of infancy or early childhood.

The characteristics of this feeding disorder are persistent failure to eat adequately or to gain weight in a child under 6 years of age, which is not associated with other medical conditions or mental disorders, and is not caused by lack of or unavailability of food[13] (Fig. 22–6). Infants with feed-

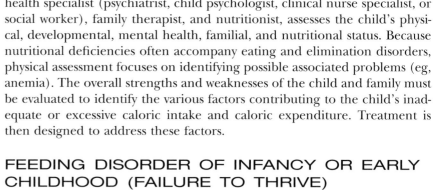

CULTURAL CONSIDERATIONS

Each child should maintain a height and weight growth curve similar to the population standard. Asian-American children may normally be below the fifth percentile on standard growth charts and not have FTT. Suspect FTT when the infant or child falls 1 standard deviation below *his or her own* curve as established by several prior measurements.

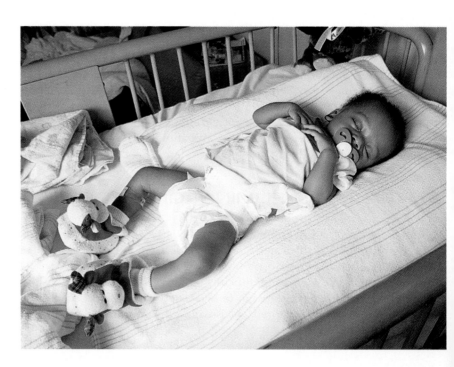

FIGURE 22–6. Infants with failure to thrive may not look severely malnourished, but they fall well below the expected weight and height norms for their age. This infant, who appears to be about 4 months old, is actually 8 months old. He has been hospitalized for evaluation of failure to thrive.

ing disorder refuse food, may have erratic sleep patterns, are irritable and difficult to soothe, and are often developmentally delayed.

Infants and children whose parents or caretakers suffer from depression, substance abuse, mental retardation, or psychosis are at risk for this disorder. Parents may be socially and emotionally isolated. A reciprocal interaction pattern may exist whereby the parent does not offer enough food or is not responsive to the infant's hunger cues, and the infant is irritable, not soothed, and does not give clear cues about hunger.

A thorough history and physical examination are needed to rule out any chronic physical illness. The infant or child may be hospitalized so that health care providers can establish a routine for feeding and sleeping. The goals of treatment are to provide adequate caloric and nutritional intake, promote normal growth and development, and assist parents in developing feeding routines and responding to the infant's cues of physical and psychologic hunger.

Nursing Management

Nursing care centers on observing parent–child interactions during feeding times and providing necessary teaching to enable parents to respond appropriately to their child's needs. Nurses weigh and measure infants and plot changes on grids to monitor growth. Often nurses feed the child to determine if he or she is eating, how much food is eaten, and the amount of time it takes to eat. Parents need to be taught how to feed the infant and provide other basic infant care in a warm, loving, and attentive environment. Referrals to home health care nurses are necessary after hospitalization so the child and family can be assisted over time with feeding and so that the child can be carefully evaluated for continued growth and developmental skills.

RECURRENT ABDOMINAL PAIN

Recurrent abdominal pain is a frequent problem among young children and adolescents, particularly girls of school age. The pain is generally located in the periumbilical area and occurs on a regular basis. Although there may be organic causes such as motility problems, constipation, or inflammatory bowel disease, in most cases an organic cause cannot be found. However, parents and health care professionals should not dismiss the child's pain just because the cause is unknown or unidentified.

A thorough history and physical examination are necessary to rule out organic causes. Children with recurrent abdominal pain often have little independence and feel controlled by their parents.[14] The history should explore the pressures and stresses in the child's life, the child's temperament or methods of coping, bowel elimination patterns, and history of sexual abuse.[15]

Laboratory studies such as a complete blood count may be ordered to rule out other illness. Gastrointestinal studies may be performed in an outpatient setting. Children are occasionally hospitalized when their condition is severe and not treatable at home.

When no organic cause can be identified, treatment of recurrent abdominal pain focuses on providing outlets for the release of stress within the family and in other settings in the child's life, enhancing the child's coping methods, and promoting dietary changes that encourage regular bowel movements.

CLINICAL TIP

Children commonly hold their feelings in their "tummies." When interviewing children to find out how they are feeling inside, you only need to ask, "What's your tummy feel like today? Right now? Yesterday when that happened?"

Nursing Management

Nursing care includes supporting the child during assessment and diagnostic testing. The child can be taught relaxation techniques and methods for coping with stress. Identify what life events are stressors for the child or what he or she worries about. Methods for giving more independence to the child in the family are explored. The importance of eating a high-fiber diet and maintaining a regular elimination pattern is taught. The child and family may need explanations to understand the pain, which can be compared to neck pain or a headache as an outcome of stress. Children with continuing or recurrent abdominal pain should be referred to a mental health professional.

ENCOPRESIS

Encopresis is an abnormal elimination pattern characterized by the recurrent soiling or passage of stool at inappropriate times by a child who should have achieved bowel continence. It occurs in approximately 1% of school-age children.[16] Children with primary encopresis have never achieved bowel control. Children with secondary encopresis have been continent of stool for several months.

Encopresis is usually associated with voluntary or involuntary retention of stool in the lower bowel and rectum, leading to constipation, dilation of the lower bowel, and incompetence of the inner sphincter. Loose stool leaks around the hard feces, and the child is unaware of a need to eliminate. Soiling may occur during the day or night. Bowel movements are irregular, painful, small, and hard. The child may be ridiculed by peers because of his or her offensive body odor. This rejection leads to withdrawal and behavioral problems, often resulting in altered school performance and attendance. Parents commonly seek health care, believing that the child has diarrhea or constipation.

The underlying constipation that leads to encopresis may be caused by the stress of environmental changes (birth of a sibling, moving to a new house, attending a new school), issues of anger and control related to bowel training, diet, or a genetic predisposition.

A thorough history, physical examination, and diagnostic studies (possibly including barium enema) are necessary to rule out organic causes and anatomic abnormalities. Examination of mental health and cognitive functioning may be indicated. Information about the child's toilet-training habits and parents' attitudes concerning those habits is obtained. A dietary history, including eating habits and types of foods eaten, is often helpful. Physical examination sometimes reveals a nontender mass in the lower abdomen.

Treatment may include behavior modification techniques, dietary changes, use of lubricants to clear the bowel of impacted stool and encourage normal defecation, and psychotherapy. Behavior modification programs that reward and reinforce appropriate toileting habits can be successful. Dietary changes include incorporating high-fiber foods such as fruits, vegetables, and whole-grain cereals into the diet. Limiting intake of refined and highly processed foods and dairy products also may be helpful. Drugs such as mineral oil, bulk-forming laxatives, and stool softeners are used temporarily to empty the bowel. The child should sit on the toilet for several minutes after morning and evening meals. It takes several months for the bowel to be retrained to respond to sphincter stimulation. Psychotherapy involving the child and family may be indicated in instances of dysfunctional parent–child relationships.

Nursing Management

Prevention of encopresis is a nursing goal. Teach toilet training techniques to parents, emphasizing the child's developmental readiness (see Chap. 2).

Parents should praise the child for successes and avoid punishment and power struggles. Encourage high-fiber diets and regular times for elimination. Nursing care when a child has encopresis centers on educating the child and parents about the disorder and its treatment and providing emotional support. Explain the treatment plan, including dietary changes and use of laxatives or stool softeners. Reassure the child that he or she has a healthy body and, with treatment, will achieve normal functioning. The child should be followed by the nurse for at least 6 months to be certain new patterns have been established.

ANOREXIA NERVOSA

Anorexia nervosa is a potentially life-threatening eating disorder that occurs primarily in teenage girls and young women, affecting an estimated 1% of young women in the United States.[17] The typical patient is white and from a middle- to upper middle-class family. Age at onset varies, and incidence peaks at 12–13 years and again at 17–18 years.[18]

Clinical Manifestations

Anorectic adolescents are characterized by extreme weight loss accompanied by a preoccupation with weight and food, excessive compulsive exercising, peculiar patterns of eating and handling food, and distorted body image. They may prepare elaborate meals for others but eat only low-calorie foods.[19] Characteristically the fear of becoming fat does not decrease with continued weight loss. Accompanying signs and symptoms of depression, crying spells, feelings of isolation and loneliness, and suicidal thoughts and feelings are common.

Physical findings include cold intolerance, dizziness, constipation, abdominal discomfort, bloating, cessation of menses, and malnutrition (Fig. 22–7). Lanugo (fine, downy body hair) may be present. Fluid and electrolyte imbalances, especially potassium imbalances, are common. The child or adolescent is usually energetic despite significant weight loss. Extreme weight loss often leads to cardiac arrhythmias (bradycardia).

Etiology and Pathophysiology

Many causes are now thought to contribute to the onset of anorexia. Cultural overemphasis on thinness may contribute to the overconcern with dieting, body image, and fear of becoming fat experienced by many adolescents. Chemical changes have been found in the brain and blood of anorectic patients, leading to theories about a biologic cause. However, it is not clear whether these changes are a cause or an effect of the disorder. Often a significant life stress, loss, or change precedes the onset of anorexia.

Many authorities view anorexia as a family problem. Intrafamilial conflicts and dysfunctional family patterns may occur when parents are overcontrolling and perfectionistic. The adolescent's eating behaviors may be an attempt to exercise independence and resolve internal psychologic conflicts.[18]

The adolescent may engage in lengthy and vigorous exercise (up to 4 hours daily) to prevent weight gain. Laxatives or diuretics may be used to induce weight loss. As the disorder progresses, the adolescent perceives the ever-thinner body as becoming more beautiful. The body responds to the abnormal eating behaviors as if starvation were occurring. Leukopenia, electrolyte imbalance, and hypoglycemia develop as a result of protein–calorie malnutrition.[19] Once the body mass decreases below a critical level, menstruation ceases.

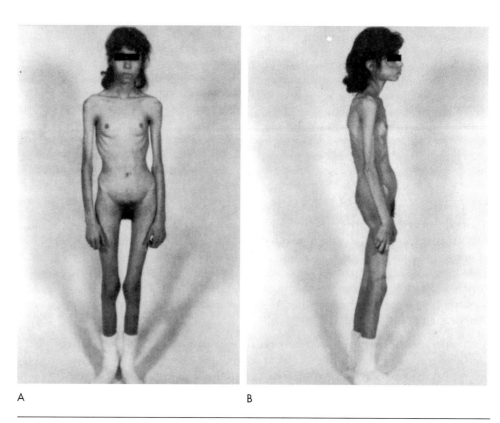

A   B

FIGURE 22–7. Characteristic physical appearance of an adolescent girl with anorexia nervosa.
From Rawlings, R.P., Williams, S.R., & Beck, C.K. (1992). Mental-health psychiatric nursing (3rd ed.). St. Louis: Mosby–Year Book.

Diagnostic Tests and Medical Management

Diagnosis is based on a comprehensive history, physical examination revealing characteristic clinical manifestations, and the *DSM-IV* criteria included in Table 22–7.

The goal of treatment is to address the physiologic problems associated with malnutrition, as well as the behavioral and cognitive components of the disorder. A firm focus is placed on reaching a targeted weight with a gradual weight gain of 0.1–0.2 kg/day (0.25–0.5 lb/day). Enteral feedings or total parenteral nutrition (TPN) may be necessary to replace lost fluid, protein, and nutrients. However, the adolescent often perceives these feedings as a punitive measure.

Individual treatment and family therapy are used to address dysfunctional family patterns and assist the family to accept and deal with the adolescent as an independent and less than perfect individual. Family involvement is crucial to effect a lasting change in the adolescent.

Long-term outpatient treatment, in either an individual or a group setting, is frequently necessary. Counseling may be continued for 2–3 years to ensure that weight gain and self-image are maintained. Antidepressant drugs such as imipramine (Tofranil) or desipramine (Norpramin) may be prescribed for coexisting conditions such as depression, anxiety, or obsessive-compulsive disorders.

Indications for hospitalization include loss of 25–30% of body weight, fluid and electrolyte imbalances or arrhythmias, or the need to provide a more intense period of therapy if outpatient treatment fails to produce improvement. Behavior modification techniques are used extensively in com-

22-7	*DSM-IV* Diagnostic Criteria for Anorexia Nervosa

A. Refusal to maintain body weight at or above a minimally normal weight for age and height (eg, weight loss leading to maintenance of body weight less than 85% of that expected; or failure to make expected weight gain during period of growth, leading to body weight less than 85% of that expected).

B. Intense fear of gaining weight or becoming fat, even though underweight.

C. Disturbance in the way in which one's weight or shape is experienced, undue influence of body weight or shape on self-evaluation, or denial of the seriousness of the current body weight.

D. In postmenarcheal females, amenorrhea, ie, the absence of at least three consecutive menstrual cycles. (A woman is considered to have amenorrhea if her periods occur only following hormone, eg, estrogen administration).

From American Psychiatric Association. (1994). Diagnostic and statistical manual of mental disorders (4th ed.). Washington, DC: Author. Copyright © 1994 American Psychiatric Association.

bination with counseling and other methods in care of the hospitalized anorectic adolescent.

Nursing Assessment

Obtain a thorough individual and family history. Ask about usual eating patterns, daily caloric intake, exercise patterns, and menstrual history. Is there a family history of eating disorders? Assess for signs of malnutrition. Obtain height and weight measurements, and compare with norms for the general population. Because the anorectic patient often wears layers of clothes when being weighed, attention is needed to obtain an accurate measurement.

Nursing Diagnosis

Nursing diagnoses for the adolescent with anorexia nervosa might include the following:

- Altered Nutrition: Less Than Body Requirements related to distorted beliefs about food requirements, inadequate food intake, or refusal to eat
- Risk for Fluid Volume Deficit related to inadequate fluid intake or overuse of laxatives and diuretics
- Risk for Altered Body Temperature related to excessive weight loss and absence of subcutaneous fat
- Constipation related to inadequate food intake and overuse of laxatives
- Body Image Disturbance related to distorted perception of body size and shape
- Self-Esteem Disturbance related to dysfunctional family dynamics
- Ineffective Family Coping: Compromised or Disabling related to parental tendency to be overcontrolling and perfectionistic

Nursing Management

Nursing care centers on meeting nutritional and fluid needs, preventing complications, administering medications, and providing referral to appropriate resources. Specific treatment measures vary depending on physical complications, length and degree of illness, emotional symptoms accompanying the disorder, and family dynamics. Resistance to treatment is common, and nurses who care for anorectic adolescents must deal with their own feelings of frustration and anger.

Meet Nutritional and Fluid Needs

Monitor nutritional and fluid intake, encourage consumption of food, and observe eating behaviors at mealtime. Elimination patterns may be altered as a result of increased intake during hospitalization. Monitor for possible problems, including abdominal distention, constipation, or diarrhea. Daily monitoring of serum electrolytes is necessary.

If TPN is administered, watch for complications such as circulatory overload, hyperglycemia, or hypoglycemia. Use strict aseptic technique when changing tubing or dressings.

Administer Medications

Monitor vital signs if the adolescent is receiving antidepressants. Watch for signs of hypertension and tachycardia. Administering medications after meals helps to prevent gastric irritation.

Provide Referral to Appropriate Resources

Refer parents and other family members to the American Anorexia and Bulimia Association, National Anorectic Aid Society, and National Association of Anorexia Nervosa & Associated Disorders for further information about the disorder and a list of support groups in their area (see Appendix F).

BULIMIA NERVOSA

Bulimia nervosa is an eating disorder characterized by binge eating (a compulsion to consume large quantities of food in a short period of time). Usually the episodes of bingeing are followed by various methods of weight control (purging), such as self-induced vomiting, large doses of laxatives or diuretics, or a combination of methods. Like anorexia, bulimia affects mainly adolescent girls and young women who are white and in the higher socioeconomic classes. It affects 5% or more of young women. The disorder usually begins in middle to late adolescence, frequently emerging during college.[20]

Clinical Manifestations

Bulimic adolescents, like anorectic ones, are preoccupied with body shape, size, and weight. They may appear overweight or thin and usually report a wide range of average body weight over the years. Physical findings depend on the degree of purging, starvation, dehydration, and electrolyte disturbance. Erosion of tooth enamel, increased dental caries, and gum recession, which result from vomiting of gastric acids, are common findings. The back of a hand can have callouses from inducing vomiting. Abdominal distention is often seen. Esophageal tears and esophagitis may also occur.

Etiology and Pathophysiology

Causes of bulimia nervosa are similar to those of anorexia nervosa: sensitivity to social pressure for thinness, body image difficulties, and long-standing dysfunctional family patterns. Families may be chaotic and distant from the girl, rather than overinvolved as with the anorectic. Many bulimic individuals experience depression. It is not clear whether the depression is a cause or a result of the bulimic individual's inability to control the bingeing and purging cycles. A bulimic adolescent often binges after any stressful event.[21]

Bingeing usually occurs in secret for several hours until the individual is stopped by abdominal discomfort, by another person, or by vomiting. At first the episodes of binge eating are pleasurable. Immediately following the binge episode, however, feelings of guilt, shame, anger, depression, and fear of loss of control and weight gain arise. As these feelings intensify, the bulimic adolescent becomes increasingly anxious. This usually initiates the purge behaviors.

Purging eliminates the discomfort from bloating and also prevents weight gain. This relieves the feelings of depression and guilt, but only temporarily. Adolescents with bulimia commonly practice the binge–purge cycle many times a day, losing their ability to respond to normal cues of hunger and satiety.

Diagnostic Tests and Medical Management

A comprehensive history is necessary because most bulimic adolescents appear normal in weight or only slightly underweight. Laboratory evaluation may identify signs of altered electrolyte and hematologic status. The diagnosis is confirmed by the presence of specific *DSM-IV* criteria (Table 22–8).

Treatment includes management of physiologic problems, behavior modification, and psychotherapy. Behavior modification focuses on modifying the dysfunctional eating patterns and restoring a normal pattern. Until the episodes of bingeing and purging are under control, feelings of discouragement and hopelessness prevail. Thus, the focus early in treatment is on initiating an immediate behavioral change. Once initial interventions have been successful, group therapy sessions work well for persons with anorexia or bulimia.[21, 22] Specific treatment measures may include the following:

- Educating the adolescent about good nutrition (including food choice and caloric content)

22-8	*DSM-IV Criteria for Bulimia Nervosa*

A. Recurrent episodes of binge eating. An episode of binge eating is characterized by both of the following:
   1. Eating, in a discrete period of time (eg, within any 2-hour period), an amount of food that is definitely larger than most people would eat during a similar period of time and under similar circumstances
   2. A sense of lack of control over eating during the episode (eg, a feeling that one cannot stop eating or control what or how much one is eating)
B. Recurrent inappropriate compensatory behavior in order to prevent weight gain, such as self-induced vomiting; misuse of laxatives, diuretics, enemas, or other medications; fasting; or excessive exercise.
C. The binge eating and inappropriate compensatory behaviors both occur, on average, at least twice a week for 3 months.
D. Self-evaluation is unduly influenced by body weight and shape.
E. The disturbance does not occur exclusively during episodes of Anorexia Nervosa.

- Encouraging the adolescent to keep a log or food journal and assisting the adolescent to make connections between emotional states and stress and the impulse to binge or purge
- Setting up a daily dietary routine of three meals and three snacks a day (using the same foods for each meal and snack every day to change misconceptions about the weight-gaining potential of certain foods and to decrease anxiety about what food must be eaten at the next meal)

Once these initial measures have been taken, the underlying psychosocial issues are explored. The goals of therapy are to provide the bulimic adolescent with adaptive coping skills and to improve self-esteem.

Most bulimic adolescents do not require hospitalization. Serious abnormalities in fluid and electrolyte levels caused by uncontrollable cycles of bingeing and vomiting, accompanied by depression or suicidal activity, are indications of the need for hospitalization. The prognosis is good with long-term therapy.

Nursing Assessment

Obtain a thorough individual and family history, including daily dietary intake and weight fluctuations. Inquire about problems such as abdominal pain or distention, which may indicate an abnormal eating or elimination pattern. Assess the oral mucosa for signs of damage to tooth enamel caused by purging; examine hands for evidence of vomiting-inducing calluses.

Nursing Diagnosis

Among the nursing diagnoses that might be appropriate for the adolescent with bulimia nervosa are the following:

- Altered Nutrition: Less Than or More Than Body Requirements related to binge–purge behaviors, vomiting, or laxative use
- Risk for Fluid Volume Deficit related to excess vomiting or laxative use
- Altered Oral Mucous Membrane related to damaging effects of vomited gastric acids
- Knowledge Deficit (Child) related to health risks of excessive use of laxatives and diuretics
- Anxiety related to weight gain and loss of control over eating behavior
- Self-Esteem Disturbance related to dysfunctional family dynamics
- Ineffective Individual Coping related to life stressors

Nursing Management

Nursing care includes monitoring nutritional intake and elimination patterns, preventing complications, and providing appropriate referrals.

During hospitalization a food diary is kept by the patient. Be alert to the adolescent who hides, gives away, or discards food from the tray or who exits to use the bathroom after meals. Withdrawal from laxatives and diuretics is managed with careful observation for alterations in fluid and electrolyte status. Cardiac monitoring may be necessary if potassium levels are seriously altered. Esophageal tearing or esophagitis is treated to promote mucosal healing. Medications such as antidepressants may be administered. Encourage continuation of group and other therapy sessions.

Bulimic adolescents and their families can be referred to various organizations for assistance and information about the disorder (see Appendix F).

CLINICAL TIP

Monitor bulimic adolescents for at least a half hour after each meal to ensure that they do not attempt purging behaviors. These patients should not be allowed to go into their rooms alone. One technique is to contract with the adolescent to sit at the nurse's station during this period.

COMPULSIVE OVEREATING AND OBESITY

Obesity is usually defined as an excessive accumulation of body fat. Whether obesity should be classified as an eating disorder is a matter of considerable discussion and disagreement, because many obese individuals appear to be well adjusted. However, a number of these persons have low self-esteem, poor body image, difficulty in relationships, and recurring bouts of anxiety and depression. The obese child is also at risk for a number of problems stemming from elevated blood lipid levels, hypertension, and minimal exercise. (See Chapter 12 for a discussion of risk factors for cardiovascular disease.)

Abnormal eating patterns may begin in childhood or adolescence. Obese children and adolescents may use compulsive overeating to make up for a lack of parental love and nurturance or in an attempt to relieve stress.[23] Treatment usually combines behavioral modification with dietary modifications and an exercise program. Family involvement in the treatment plan is essential.

Nursing Management

Obesity alone rarely necessitates hospitalization. Most often the nurse encounters the obese child when he or she is hospitalized for an orthopedic problem or recurrent abdominal pain. Nursing care focuses on meeting the child's nutritional needs, managing related problems, and promoting self-esteem. Exercise is encouraged; assist the child in choosing activities that are fun and will not be embarrassing. Nurses can use mealtimes to educate the child and family about nutritionally sound food choices. Referral to a nutritionist is usually appropriate. Caloric count and portion control need to be emphasized.

The child and family can be referred to local organizations that are devoted to nutrition education and support.

▶ SUBSTANCE ABUSE

Substance abuse occurs in children and adolescents of all socioeconomic levels and is a growing health problem. It is important to keep in mind that the use of any drug can pose a serious psychologic and physical risk to children and adolescents.

Although a decline in the daily use of marijuana by adolescents has been reported, abuse of other substances, particularly alcohol, cocaine, crack, and heroin, remains high.[24] A 1992 survey of high school seniors reported the following alarming statistics: 34% engaged in binge drinking of alcohol, and the average age for beginning alcohol and cigarette use was 12 years.[19] Synthetic drugs such as phencyclidine (PCP) (commonly referred to as "designer" drugs) mimic other narcotics, stimulants, and hallucinogens and are also dangerous.

Over-the-counter medications are legal substances that are frequently abused. Easily obtainable at grocery stores and drugstores, these drugs include antihistamines, atropine, bromides, caffeine, ephedrine, pseudoephedrine, phenylpropanolamine, and amphetamine-like substitutes. Volatile inhalants, such as glues, are dangerous substances of abuse, and their use appears to be rising among school-age children and adolescents. Anabolic steroids are the drugs of abuse most commonly used by athletes.

CLINICAL TIP

Adolescents who have some or all of the following symptoms may be experiencing alcohol withdrawal: anxiety, headache, tremors, nausea and vomiting, malaise or weakness, tachycardia, hypertension, insomnia, depressed mood or irritability, hallucinations.

Clinical Manifestations

Substance abuse in children and adolescents is commonly overlooked and underdiagnosed by health care providers.[25] This is due in part to the wide range of clinical presentations, which vary according to type of drug abused, amount, frequency, time of last use, and severity of drug dependence (Table 22–9).

22-9   Commonly Abused Drugs and Their Effects

Drug	Potential for Dependence	Effects of Intoxication
Depressants Alcohol, barbiturates (amobarbital, pentobarbital, secobarbital)	*Physical and psychologic:* High; varies somewhat among drugs	*Physical:* Decreased muscle tone and coordination, tremors *Psychologic:* Impaired speech, memory, and judgment; confusion; decreased attention span; emotional lability
Stimulants Amphetamines (eg, Benzedrine), caffeine, cocaine	*Physical:* Low to moderate *Psychologic:* High; withdrawal from amphetamines and cocaine can lead to severe depression	*Physical:* Dilated pupils, increased pulse and blood pressure, flushing, nausea, loss of appetite, tremors *Psychologic:* Euphoria; increased alertness, agitation, or irritability; hallucinations; insomnia
Opiates Codeine, heroin, meperidine (Demerol), methadone, morphine, opium, oxycodone (Percodan)	*Physical and psychologic:* High; varies somewhat among drugs; withdrawal effects are uncomfortable but rarely life threatening	*Physical:* Analgesia, depressed respirations and muscle tone (may lead to coma or death), nausea, constricted pupils *Psychologic:* Changes in mood (usually euphoria), drowsiness, impaired attention or memory, sense of tranquility
Hallucinogens Lysergic acid diethylamide (LSD), mescaline, phencyclidine (PCP)	*Physical:* None *Psychologic:* Unknown	*Physical:* Lack of coordination, dilated pupils, hypertension, elevated temperature; severe PCP intoxication can result in seizures, respiratory depression, coma, and death *Psychologic:* Visual illusions and hallucinations, altered perceptions of time and space, emotional lability, psychosis
Volatile Inhalants Glues, typing correction fluid, acrylic paints, spot removers, lighter fluid, gasoline, butane	*Physical and psychologic:* Varies with drug used	*Physical:* Impaired coordination, liver damage (in some cases) *Psychologic:* Impaired judgment, delirium
Marijuana	*Physical:* Low *Psychologic:* Usually low; occasionally moderate to high	*Physical:* Tachycardia, reddened conjunctiva, dry mouth, increased appetite *Psychologic:* Initial anxiety followed by euphoria; giddiness; impaired attention, judgment, and memory

Based on information in Finke, L. (1992). Nursing interventions with children and adolescents experiencing substance abuse. In P. West, & C.L. Sieloff Evans (Eds.), Psychiatric and mental health with children and adolescents (pp. 244–246). Gaithersburg, MD: Aspen Publications, Exhibit 17–1; and Lahmeyer, H.W., Channon, R.A., & Francis Schlemmer, R., Jr. (1993). Psychoactive substance abuse. In J.A. Flaherty, J.M. Davis, & P.G. Janicak (Eds.), Psychiatry: Diagnosis & therapy (2nd ed., pp. 268–283). Norwalk, CT: Appleton & Lange.

Common physical manifestations include alterations in vital signs, weight loss, chronic fatigue, chronic cough, respiratory congestion, red eyes, and general apathy and malaise. The mental status examination may reveal alterations in level of consciousness, impaired attention and concentration, impaired thought processes, delusions, and hallucinations. Low self-esteem, feelings of guilt or worthlessness, and suicidal or homicidal thoughts are also common.

Poor school performance and changes in mood, sleep habits, appetite, dress, and social relationships are nonspecific characteristics of the substance-abusing child.

Etiology and Pathophysiology

In most cases substance abuse represents a maladaptive coping response to the stressors of childhood and adolescence. A child may begin using drugs or alcohol to deal with stress because family members or peers do so. Children in families with a history of substance abuse are at higher risk of abusing drugs and alcohol. Other risk factors include rebelliousness, aggressiveness, low self-esteem, dysfunctional parental relationships, lack of adequate support systems, academic underachievement, poor judgment, and poor impulse control.

Initial experimentation with alcohol or drugs may be unpleasant. With continued use, however, the adolescent learns to "achieve the high," an illusion of power and well-being. The adolescent wants the high more frequently and actively seeks alcohol or drugs. Tolerance to the substance occurs with continued use, and ever-increasing amounts are required to achieve a pleasurable high. Physical and psychologic dependence ensues as the body's tissues require the substance to function properly. Withdrawal symptoms occur when the child or adolescent is deprived of the substance.

Diagnostic Tests and Medical Management

Multiple psychiatric diagnostic criteria exist for each drug class. Children and adolescents who have other psychosocial disorders commonly use or abuse drugs or alcohol. Treatment should therefore focus not only on the substance use or abuse, but also on the issues underlying the problem. Intervention includes the family as well as the substance-abusing child or adolescent.

The primary goal of treatment is to teach the child and other family members to develop and sustain positive coping patterns, and to support them during this process. Most treatment programs offer inpatient and outpatient services, as well as after-care programs. These programs usually consist of peer support focusing on the development of a life-style free of drugs or alcohol, healthy family relationships, and positive coping skills. Family involvement is strongly encouraged. Hospitalization is required if the physical dependence is significant and withdrawal places the child at risk for complications such as seizures, depression, or suicidal behavior.

Nursing Assessment

Nurses may encounter the substance-abusing child or adolescent in the emergency department or outpatient clinic or during hospitalization for an injury or other acute problem. Nursing assessment includes taking a thorough history from the parents and child, observing the child's behavior, and performing a physical examination. The history should include the age

CLINICAL TIP

Children who abuse drugs, alcohol, or other substances are at greater risk for injuries requiring hospitalization. Assess all children or adolescents involved in motor vehicle crashes (as driver), falls, near-drownings, or shootings for evidence of substance abuse.

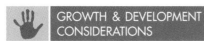

GROWTH & DEVELOPMENT CONSIDERATIONS

Nurses may need to interview older school-age children and adolescents privately to elicit information about drug use. The child or adolescent may provide this information only if trust in the nurse is established.

at which drug use began, pattern of use, length of time the drug has been used, amount of drug used, and psychologic state while on drugs. A history of parental drug use puts the child at higher risk for substance abuse, reflecting the combined effects of genetic and environmental influences.

Physiologic Assessment

Look for physical signs and symptoms of substance abuse, including bloodshot eyes, dilated pupils, slurred speech, and weight loss. The adolescent may appear sleepy or restless, or may show signs of clumsiness or inconsistent behavior. Consider all types of substance abuse, including model glue, gasoline, and other sources.

Psychologic Assessment

Changes in social habits may indicate substance abuse. Parents may report a drop in the school-age child's or adolescent's grades or decreased interest in school activities. New friends are not introduced to parents, and the adolescent has less contact with parents, teachers, and other adults who were previously important. The child's current drug use, potential for violence, and motivation to make changes are noted. Assess the degree of family support available.

Nursing Diagnosis

Nursing diagnoses for children and adolescents who abuse drugs or alcohol might include the following:

- Impaired Social Interaction related to substance abuse behaviors and effects of harmful materials
- Self-Esteem Disturbance related to dysfunctional family and social relationships
- Risk for Injury related to altered perceptions and sensorium
- Risk for Violence: Self-Directed or Directed at Others related to physiologic dependence on drugs, alcohol, and other substances and lack of concern about behaviors or actions necessary to obtain the next dose

Nursing Management

Care of children and adolescents who abuse drugs, alcohol, and other substances is challenging and often frustrating. Long-term mental health counseling may be necessary to resolve underlying issues and foster life-style and behavioral changes.

Prevention is the most desirable intervention. The nurse can play a major role in teaching children and their families about substance abuse. Education should begin in primary school. Nurses also can play a major role in community education. Various prevention programs have been developed by federal and private organizations. Referral to support organizations may be beneficial for the child, parents, and other family members (see Appendix F). Self-help groups, which are available in most communities, include Alcoholics Anonymous, Narcotics Anonymous, Al-Anon, Nar-Anon, and Ala-Teen.

► DEPRESSION AND ANXIETY

Both depression and anxiety can be seen as symptoms or disease states. *Symptoms* include both subjective feelings and physiologic manifestations of distress. A *disease state* is diagnosed when a pattern of symptoms exists as a result of an identified cause.

DEPRESSION

Only in recent years has depression in children been recognized as a clinical condition. Many children referred to child guidance centers and mental health professionals because of behavioral difficulties or poor achievement actually suffer from depression. The incidence of major depression is estimated to be about 2% in prepubertal children and about 5% in adolescents.[26] Before puberty, depression is more common in boys than girls. Depressive symptoms and disorders increase with age, as does the female:male ratio.[27]

Clinical Manifestations

Characteristic findings of major depression in children and adolescents include declining school performance; withdrawal from social activities; sleep disturbance (either too much or too little); appetite disturbance (too much or too little); multiple somatic complaints, especially headaches and stomachaches; decreased energy; difficulty concentrating and making decisions; low self-esteem; and feelings of hopelessness.

Etiology and Pathophysiology

Many theories have been proposed to explain the cause of depression in children and adolescents. Depression may be biologic in origin or a result of learned helplessness, cognitive distortion, social skills deficit, or family dysfunction.[27] Childhood depression sometimes occurs secondary to parental depression because the parental depression deprives the child of effective parenting. Abuse and neglect predispose children to depression, especially very young children. In about half of all children with depression, at least one other psychiatric diagnosis is made; these include conditions such as attention deficit hyperactivity disorder, anxiety disorder, or another personality disorder.[27]

Diagnostic Tests and Medical Management

Initial assessment is performed by a child psychologist or child psychiatrist. A variety of scales and techniques are used; however, very little guidance is available relating to evaluation of children under 6 years of age.[27]

Treatment may include psychotherapy in combination with psychotropic medication. Often a combination of individual, family, and group therapy provides the greatest benefits for young children and adolescents. Involving parents and other family members in the treatment plan is essential. Group therapy is an effective treatment measure for adolescents because of the importance of peer group relationships during the teenage years. Cognitive therapy may be used with adolescents, and play therapy with younger children (see discussion earlier in this chapter).

Antidepressant medications, most commonly imipramine (Tofranil), desipramine (Norpramin), and amitriptyline (Elavil), may be prescribed.

Nursing Assessment

A thorough history and physical examination, including observation of behavior, are obtained at the time of admission. Assess the child for common risk factors for depression and anxiety (Table 22–10).

| 22-10 | Risk Factors for Depression and Anxiety in Children and Adolescents |

Parental neglect, abuse, or loss
Stressful social relationships
Academic pressures and underachievement
Dysfunctional family relationships
Family history of depression, suicide, substance abuse, alcoholism, or other psychopathology
Chronic illness and frequent hospitalization

Nursing Diagnosis

Several nursing diagnoses that might be appropriate for the child or adolescent hospitalized with depression are included in the accompanying Nursing Care Plan. Other diagnoses might include the following:

- Altered Health Maintenance related to inability to perform or lack of interest in activities of daily living (ADLs)
- Altered Nutrition: More Than Body Requirements related to coping mechanism of compulsive eating
- Powerlessness related to overwhelming sense of doom or inability to cope
- Self-Esteem Disturbance related to dysfunctional family dynamics

Nursing Management

Nursing care of the child hospitalized for depression includes administering medications and providing supportive care. Monitor vital signs of children receiving antidepressant medications. Watch for common side effects, including hypertension and tachycardia. Refer to the Nursing Care Plan for specific nursing interventions for the child or adolescent hospitalized with depression.

Discharge Planning and Home Care Teaching

When the child has been hospitalized and is returning home, teach parents to recognize signs and symptoms of worsening anxiety and depression. Parents should also be taught dosages and side effects of any prescribed medications. Refer the family to appropriate health care professionals and to support groups for family members dealing with depression.

Care in the Community

Most children with depression are cared for in the community. Maintain regular contact with the family through their health care visits to outpatient agencies and by making home visits. School teachers and counselors often are aware of the child's ability to perform in the school setting. Have the family schedule after-school care so young children are not left at home alone for extended periods. Assist the family in finding support for financial and emotional needs related to managing the child's depression.

NURSING CARE PLAN
THE CHILD OR ADOLESCENT HOSPITALIZED WITH DEPRESSION

GOAL	INTERVENTION	RATIONALE	EXPECTED OUTCOME

1. Hopelessness related to fear and anxiety

The child or adolescent will discuss feelings of hopelessness.	• Encourage open expression of feelings. Explore hopeless, sad, or lonely feelings. Point out the connection between feelings and behavior. Assess the child or adolescent to identify the precipitating event when feelings of sadness arose.	• Expressing feelings may help to relieve sadness, loneliness, despair, and hopelessness. An accepting and nonjudgmental attitude must be maintained regarding any feelings expressed by the child.	By discharge, the child or adolescent expresses an interest in the future.
	• Encourage the child or adolescent to take part in self-care and unit activities. Use routines to establish feelings of control.	• An active role in self-care and treatment helps the child or adolescent to feel more in control.	
	• Medicate as ordered and document results.	• Antidepressants modify mood to a more hopeful outlook.	

2. Ineffective Individual Coping related to dysfunctional family system

The child or adolescent will use effective coping skills.	• Teach positive, effective coping strategies such as guided imagery and relaxation. Assist the child or adolescent to focus on strengths rather than weaknesses.	• Therapeutic techniques can help the child or adolescent to replace negative thoughts and images with more positive and effective beliefs and images.	The child or adolescent verbalizes and demonstrates ability to cope appropriately for his or her age.
	• Assist the child or adolescent to identify friends, family members, and others who are positive and supportive.	• Helps the child or adolescent to become aware that people can be caring and supportive (thus validating self-esteem).	

Continued . . .

NURSING CARE PLAN
THE CHILD OR ADOLESCENT HOSPITALIZED WITH DEPRESSION– *Continued*

GOAL	INTERVENTION	RATIONALE	EXPECTED OUTCOME

3. Impaired Social Interaction related to low self-esteem and negative body image

The child or adolescent will participate in and initiate activities and conversation.	• Assist the child or adolescent to identify topics and activities of interest.	• The more the child or adolescent focuses on areas of interest, the less he or she will focus on internal anxiety and depression.	By discharge, the child or adolescent initiates conversation and activities with staff and peers.
	• Encourage interaction with peers and staff.	• Each positive interaction reinforces feelings of success. Each success reinforces the desire for future social interaction.	
	• Facilitate visits from family and friends.	• Reinforces positive and rewarding relationships.	
	• Provide guidance to family regarding interaction that promotes self-esteem.	• The family's existing interaction style is often negative.	

4. Altered Nutrition: Less Than Body Requirements related to loss of appetite secondary to depression

The child or adolescent's daily intake will be adequate to maintain optimal nutritional status.	• Offer nutritious finger foods, sandwiches, and high-calorie liquid supplements frequently throughout the day.	• Convenient easy-to-eat foods encourage the child or adolescent to eat and maintain nutritional status.	The child or adolescent's daily intake will be adequate to maintain optimal nutritional status by discharge.
	• Offer easy-to-carry drinks that are high in vitamins, minerals, and calories.	• These are a convenient method for meeting hydration and electrolyte needs.	

SUICIDE

Suicide is the third leading cause of death in adolescents between 15 and 19 years of age.[28] Over the past 30 years, teenage suicide has increased by more than 250%. Suicide rates among children under age 14 have doubled since 1979, and in 1995, were the fifth most common cause of death in this age group.[28]

Boys die as a result of suicide four times more often than girls. This statistic is reversed for suicide attempts, perhaps because boys use lethal methods such as guns, hanging, and jumping more often than girls, who use drug overdose and wrist cutting. It is not unusual for health care professionals and parents to label suicide attempts by children and adolescents "accidents." Adults may have difficulty believing that young children, in particular, would have any reason to want to end their lives. Because of this, many children who are brought to the emergency department with indications of a suicide attempt are classified as unintentional injury victims and released without arrangements for appropriate follow-up care.

Many risk factors for suicide exist in children and adolescents (Table 22–11). The most common precursor to adolescent suicide is depression. Common signs or symptoms of an underlying depression that could lead to suicide include boredom, restlessness, problems with concentration, irritability, lethargy, intentional misbehavior, preoccupation with one's own body or health, and excessive dependence on or isolation from others (especially adults or caregivers).

The child or adolescent found to be at high risk for suicide may be admitted to a psychiatric unit for care or cared for in a community mental health facility. Treatment may include individual, group, or family therapy. Negotiating a "no suicide" contract is one method that may be used with a suicidal youth. In the contract, the child agrees not to attempt suicide during a specified time period. When a suicide attempt is made, the child or adolescent is generally hospitalized for at least 24 hours to ensure adequate assessment and monitoring.

Nursing Management

Be alert for children and adolescents at risk for suicide in any setting. Report threats of suicide and depressive behavior. Recognize that when one suicide has occurred, there may be an increased risk for friends of the victim. Provide supportive services to family and friends whenever suicide occurs.

Nursing care centers on taking appropriate precautions to ensure the child's safety. Both the child and the hospital environment are monitored for any object that could be used for self-harm. All potentially harmful objects, such as shoestrings, belts, pantyhose, and hair ribbons, are removed. All personal care items (including toothbrush and shampoo) are kept locked at the nursing station and monitored constantly when used by the child.

Children or adolescents who are considered at high risk for suicidal behaviors are attended by a nursing staff member at all times, including while using the bathroom and sleeping. It may be necessary for the child to dress in a plain hospital gown, be kept in a visually monitored seclusion room, or (if seriously impaired and self-abusive) be medicated or physically restrained for a period of time. Restraints are used only when ordered by the physician and interdisciplinary team caring for the child.

22-11	Risk Factors for Suicide in Children and Adolescents

School problems
Pregnancy
Drug use or abuse
Problems with a romantic relationship
Feelings of anxiety
History of chronic family problems
Chronic illness
Physical, emotional, or sexual abuse
History of suicide in a family member
History of depression
Chronic low self-esteem

 RESEARCH CONSIDERATIONS

Research has demonstrated that there may be different triggers for suicide in female and male adolescents. Female adolescents consider suicide more frequently when their situations are unstable, and it is often an impulsive act. Male adolescents think of suicide when they are depressed and when their social environment is unsatisfactory.[29]

 NURSING ALERT

If an adolescent or child persists in threatening suicide after the health care provider attempts to negotiate a "no suicide" contract, hospitalization is necessary to ensure the child's safety. *All suicide threats must be taken seriously.*

Hospitalization continues as long as the child's behavior is self-destructive. Children are referred for intensive individual and family therapy. Encourage parents to keep follow-up clinic appointments, to watch for self-destructive behaviors, and to administer any prescribed medications according to the treatment schedule.

SEPARATION ANXIETY AND SCHOOL PHOBIA

Anxiety is a subjective feeling of uncertainty and helplessness, usually accompanied by central nervous system signs, including restlessness, trembling, perspiration, and rapid pulse.[30]

Separation anxiety disorder is characterized by an extreme state of uneasiness when in unfamiliar surroundings and often by refusal to visit friends' homes or attend school for at least 2 weeks. This disorder occurs in approximately 3% of children and in twice as many girls as boys.[31]

Children with separation anxiety disorder tend to be perfectionistic, overly compliant, and eager to please. They appear to cling to the parent or caretaker. They may use physical complaints such as headaches, abdominal pain, nausea, and vomiting in an attempt to avoid being away from the parent. Depression frequently accompanies separation anxiety disorder. The resulting avoidant behaviors can interfere with personal growth and development, academic achievement, and social functioning.

School phobia (also called school avoidance or school refusal) is a persistent, irrational, or excessive fear of attending school. The child may fear being harmed or losing control. School phobia is common in children between 5 and 12 years of age but can occur in children up to age 16.[31] The child's avoidance of school is often a manifestation of his or her fear of leaving the parent or primary caretaker (usually the mother). Children commonly report that teachers and peers "pick on them." Somatic complaints are similar to those seen in children who have separation anxiety disorder. Characteristically symptoms are present only on school days and not on weekends or holidays.

Treatment of children with separation anxiety disorder or school phobia must include the family as well as the child. Establish firm limits defining the behavioral expectations and consequences for the child. Antidepressant medications (such as imipramine [Tofranil]) or antianxiety medications (such as lorazepam [Ativan] or clonazepam [Klonopin]) are often helpful in decreasing the child's overwhelming sense of anxiety.

Prompt intervention is needed in cases of school absenteeism. The longer the child is out of school, the greater the likelihood that a chronic, treatment-resistant condition will result. Referral for psychiatric evaluation is indicated if symptoms persist.

Nursing Management

Nursing care centers on educating parents about the disorder and management techniques. Children with separation anxiety disorder benefit from a predictable routine and environment. Advise children in advance of any expected changes in routine. Help parents to plan consistent and reassuring contacts for the child after school and during activities.

► SCHIZOPHRENIA

Schizophrenia is a psychotic disorder that is relatively rare in young children and adolescents, although it can occur in children as young as 5 years of age. The prevalence of schizophrenia increases after puberty and reaches adult levels by late adolescence (approximately 1% of the population).[32] Previously, autistic disorder was sometimes labeled as childhood schizophrenia. However, separate criteria have been developed for that disorder[2] (see the discussion earlier in this chapter).

The clinical manifestations of schizophrenia are the same in children as in adults. Characteristic behaviors of the schizophrenic individual include social withdrawal, impaired social relationships, flat **affect** (outward appearance of feeling or emotion), regression, loose associations (thought characterized by speech in which ideas shift from one subject to another that is unrelated), delusions, and hallucinations.

The cause of schizophrenia is unknown, but genetic predisposition may play a role in its occurrence. The disorder most often manifests between 15 and 20 years of age. Onset may be sudden or insidious. Most often the child demonstrates restlessness, poor appetite, and social withdrawal over a period of several weeks to months. Some children, however, become psychotic without any warning over a few days.

During adolescence, acute schizophrenia can occur while the teenager is making plans to leave home and family in order to attend college, marry, or work in another area. Onset of symptoms may be triggered by an important loss (death of a significant other, parent, child, or friend).

Treatment of childhood schizophrenia is multifaceted, including individual psychotherapy, family therapy, and various psychotropic medications (antipsychotics such as haloperidol [Haldol], antianxiety agents such as lorazepam [Ativan], and antidepressants such as imipramine [Tofranil]). Drugs are only moderately effective at controlling hallucinations and delusions, and responses vary considerably among individuals. Side effects will determine what drugs are used and for how long. Antipsychotic medication often must be continued for several months or years after recovery from an acute schizophrenic episode.

Most episodes of acute schizophrenia require several weeks to months of inpatient hospitalization on a psychiatric unit. Treatment may include an intensive school-based program in a structured, supervised setting with specially trained professionals. The goal of treatment initially is to reduce or control psychotic episodes and provide a safe, structured environment for the child or adolescent, enabling the child to live each day at an optimal level of functioning.

Most children require long-term treatment, including intermittent periods of hospitalization. Children or adolescents whose symptoms are difficult to control and who present a safety risk to themselves or others may require long-term residential treatment.

Nursing Management

The nurse may encounter the child or adolescent with schizophrenia during hospitalization for an acute episode, for treatment of another problem, or while working with the individual in the community. Nursing care centers on providing education and supportive care to the child and parents.

Educating the child and parents about the risk of recurrence and methods to alleviate side effects of prescribed medications may increase compliance with the treatment plan. Because most schizophrenic children return home after hospitalization for an acute episode, family education and involvement in the treatment plan are essential. The nurse may also need to communicate with school personnel in order to ensure understanding of the child's condition.

► CONVERSION REACTION

Conversion reaction is a disorder in which a disturbance or loss of sensory, motor, or other physical functions suggests neurologic or other somatic disease. The disturbance or loss cannot be explained by any known pathophysiologic mechanism. Instead, psychologic factors are involved.

Clinical manifestations include altered sensations, such as blindness or deafness; paralysis or ataxia, including inability to stand or walk and loss of ability to speak (aphonia); involuntary movements, such as pseudoepileptic convulsions; and constant complaints of pain with no physical basis (psychogenic pain). The onset of conversion symptoms is usually dramatic and sudden. Symptoms often appear to be neurologic, but on careful examination obvious discrepancies are found. Often the child or family members appear indifferent or unconcerned over what health care providers consider an overwhelming physical disability.

Children suspected of having a conversion reaction require a complete physical and neurologic evaluation to rule out any possible physiologic basis for the symptoms. Individual and family therapy is usually necessary to identify the source of the psychologic conflict, pain, or need resulting in the conversion symptoms.

► CHILD ABUSE

VIOLENCE AND CHILDREN

Violence is a major threat to the life of children in American society. One in every 680 U.S. children is killed by gunfire before the age of 20.[33]

Violence against children can take many forms; one of the most common types is child abuse, which is discussed in this section. Awareness of the problem of child abuse is increasing. More cases are being reported; however, these are probably only a small percentage of the total. Approximately 4% of children between the ages of 3 and 17 years—about 2 million children—are physically abused each year.[34]

Physical abuse is only one part of a larger problem. The definition of child abuse has expanded over the past 10 years to include physical neglect, emotional abuse and neglect, verbal abuse, and sexual abuse, as well as physical abuse. Many children who are sexually abused are under the age of 5 years, some as young as 3 months of age. The average age for sexual molestation is 4 years.[35]

An abused child is one whose parent or another person legally responsible for his or her care:

• Inflicts or allows another to inflict physical or emotional pain or injury, or

• Creates or allows another to create a significant risk of serious physical or emotional pain or injury, or

• Commits or allows another to commit an act of sexual abuse, as defined by law, against the child.

Abuse generally involves an act of commission, that is, actively doing something to a child physically, emotionally, or sexually, such as hitting, belittling, or molesting. Neglect more often involves an act of omission, such as not providing adequate nutrition, emotional contact, or necessary physical care. Because the evidence is often not visible, emotional abuse and neglect are more difficult to identify and prove than physical abuse or neglect. Risk factors for abuse and neglect are listed in Table 22–12.

22-12   Risk Factors for Child Abuse and Neglect

Factors Increasing Risk for Physical Abuse
Poverty
Violence in the family
Prematurity
Unrelated male primary caretaker
Parents who were abused as children
Age less than 3 years
Handicap or condition that requires a great deal of care (eg, mental retardation, attention deficit hyperactivity disorder)
Parental substance abuse or social isolation

Factors Increasing Risk for Sexual Abuse
Absence of natural father or having a stepfather
Being female
Mother's employment outside the home
Poor relationship with parent
Parental relationship characterized by conflict
Parental substance abuse or social isolation

Types of Abuse

Physical Abuse

Physical abuse is the deliberate maltreatment of another individual that inflicts pain or injury and may result in permanent or temporary disfigurement or even death. Common methods of physical abuse in children are listed in Table 22–13.

Physical Neglect

Physical neglect is the deliberate withholding of or failure to provide the necessary and available resources to the child. Behaviors constituting physical neglect include failure to provide for the following basic needs: adequate nutrition and hydration, hygiene (eg, clean diapers and clothes, bathing and toileting facilities), shelter (eg, warmth in winter), and appropriate health care (eg, immunizations, dental care, medications, eyeglasses).

Emotional Abuse

Emotional abuse usually involves shaming, ridiculing, embarrassing, or insulting the child. It can also include the destruction of a child's personal property, such as tearing up the child's favorite family photographs or letters or harming, killing, or giving away the child's pet. These actions are frequently used as a means of frightening or controlling the child.

Verbal abuse is a common method of emotional abuse. Words can be a violent and volatile weapon against a child, eroding the child's fragile sense of self and destroying self-esteem. Common examples of verbal abuse include yelling obscenities at the child, calling the child names, threatening to "put the child away" or to give away or kill the child's pet, telling the child "I wish you were never born" or "You're worthless," and using words to humiliate, shame, or degrade the child.

22-13 Methods of Physical Abuse in Children

Hitting, slapping, kicking, or punching

Whipping with belts, shoes, or electrical cords **(1)**

Inflicting burns with a lit cigarette or lighter **(2)**

Immersing child or body part in scalding water (commonly legs, perineal area, hands, or feet; see Fig. 21–16A)

Shaking the child violently ("shaken child" syndrome)

Tying the child to a fence, bed, tree, or other object

Throwing the child against a wall, down stairs, or against a window

Choking or gagging the child

Fracturing the legs, arms, ribs, or skull

Deliberately administering excessive doses of prescribed or nonprescribed drugs

Deliberately withholding prescribed medication

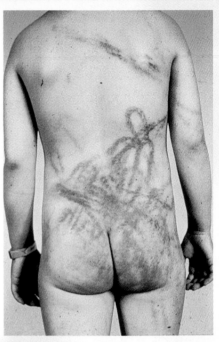

(1)

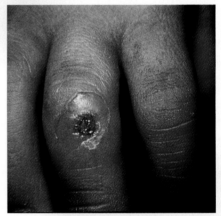

(2)

Photographs copyright © AAP/Kempe. Used with permission.

COMMON FORMS OF SEXUAL ABUSE

- Oral–genital contact
- Fondling and caressing the genitals
- Anal intercourse
- Sexual intercourse
- Rape
- Sodomy
- Prostitution

Emotional Neglect

Emotional neglect is characterized by the caretaker's emotional unavailability to the child. The usual style of interaction is cold and lacking in sensitive personal attention. The child suffers from a lack of nurturance and failure of the parent or caretaker to meet basic dependency needs.

Sexual Abuse

Child sexual abuse is the exploitation of a child for the sexual gratification of an adult. Between 100,000 and 500,000 children in the United States are sexually abused each year.[35] Approximately 75–80% of child sexual abusers are immediate family members, other relatives, friends, or neighbors. Male perpetrators make up 92–98% of all abusers.[35] Abusers often threaten to harm or kill the child or another family member if the child discloses the abuse.

Clinical Manifestations

Manifestations of physical abuse include but are not limited to:

- Multiple bruises in various stages of healing
- Scald burns with clear lines of demarcation and in a glove or stocking distribution (see Fig. 21–16A)
- Rope, belt, or cord marks, usually seen on the mouth, buttocks, back, legs, and arms [see Fig. 22–13(1)]
- Burn scars in various stages of healing
- Multiple fractures in various stages of healing
- Shortness of breath and distress upon being moved, indicating chest contusions and possible rib fractures
- Sedation from overmedication
- Exacerbation of chronic illness (such as diabetes or asthma) because of withholding of medication

Behaviors inconsistent with developmental stage may also be apparent. For example, the toddler or preschool child may be indiscriminately friendly with unfamiliar adults, including health care providers, rather than demonstrating shyness or anxiety.

Manifestations of physical neglect include undernourishment (evidenced by constantly feeling hungry, hoarding or stealing food, and being underweight), unclean clothes and body, poor dental health (extensive cavities or generally poor condition of teeth), and inappropriate clothing for the season.

Manifestations of emotional abuse, verbal abuse, and emotional neglect include fear, poor physical growth, and failure to meet appropriate developmental milestones. The child may have difficulty relating to adults, impaired communication skills, and developmental delays.

Children who have been sexually abused may exhibit a variety of physical and behavioral signs and symptoms (Table 22–14). However, sexual abuse does not always result in apparent injury. Among the many long-term consequences of child sexual abuse are ongoing feelings of shame, guilt, anger, and hostility; decreased self-esteem, which leads to increased self-destructive behavior and risk of suicide; recurrence of victimization experiences; substance abuse; and eating disorders. Factors associated with greater psychologic harm to the child include (1) a long period of abuse, (2) use of violent force or threat of violence, (3) abuse involving penetration (intercourse or oral–genital sex), and (4) abuse involving family members, especially the father or stepfather.

Etiology and Pathophysiology

Regardless of the type of abuse, the most common abuser is the child's parent or guardian or the boyfriend of the child's mother. Risk factors associated with abusive behavior in adults include the following:

- Psychopathology, such as drug addiction or alcoholism, low self-esteem, poor impulse control, and other personality disorders

RESEARCH CONSIDERATIONS

The impact of childhood sexual abuse is long lasting. Persons experiencing such abuse may experience posttraumatic stress syndrome. There is also a high rate of addictive behavior among those with a history of childhood sexual abuse.[36]

22-14	Physical and Behavioral Manifestations of Sexual Abuse in Children and Adolescents

Vaginal discharge

Bloodstained underpants or diaper

Genital redness, pain, itching, or bruising

Difficulty walking or sitting

Urinary tract infection

Sexually transmitted disease

Somatic complaints, such as headaches or stomachaches

Sleeping problems, such as nightmares or night terrors

Bedwetting

Unwillingness to go to babysitter, family member, neighbor, or other person

Fear of strangers

New or excessive sexual curiosity or play

Constant masturbation

Curling into fetal position

Excessively seductive behavior

Phobias about particular places, people, or things

Abrupt changes in school performance and attendance

Changes in eating habits

Abrupt changes in behavior (especially withdrawal)

Child or adolescent female acts like a wife or mother

- Poor parenting experiences, such as abuse in the abuser's own childhood, rejection by the abuser's own parent(s), lack of knowledge of alternative methods of discipline, strong belief in or family tradition of harsh discipline, and lack of parental affection
- Marital stressors and problems with partners, such as hostile-dependent, abusive, or nonsupportive relationships, and one-sided decision making
- Environmental stressors, such as legal, financial, medical, or housing problems
- Social isolation, such as few friends and limited use of sitters, family, or other resources
- Inappropriate expectations for the developmental level of the child

Diagnostic Tests and Medical Management

Diagnosis of abuse is made on the basis of a careful history and thorough physical examination. X-ray studies may be ordered to identify signs of recurrent abuse (eg, healed fractures). Some children are admitted directly to the hospital with the diagnosis of suspected abuse or neglect. Less obvious as a victim of abuse is the child admitted with a skull fracture who "fell off a chair."

Neglect, which is more difficult to define and identify, frequently requires hospitalization with a comprehensive medical, social, and psychiatric evaluation. Five basic categories must be considered when attempting to diagnose neglect: (1) medical care neglect (lack of necessary medical care), (2) gross safety neglect (lack of appropriate supervision), (3) physical neglect (lack of food and shelter), (4) emotional neglect, and (5) educational neglect.

All 50 states have extensive and complex statutes regarding reporting of child abuse and neglect. A specialist must be consulted, especially if the child's testimony will be used in court.

Children do not routinely make false allegations of abuse. If indeed there is reason to believe the allegations are false, a child and adolescent therapist (psychiatrist, psychologist, psychiatric clinical nurse specialist, or social worker) with special expertise should be consulted to determine the truth. Keep in mind that children who withdraw their accusations have often been threatened or coerced into doing so. Because children who have been physically, emotionally, or sexually abused are at risk for major depression, they require skilled care by mental health professionals who are specially trained in this area. Initially the treatment goals include prevention of self-destructive or other dangerous acts. Children must be encouraged to express their fears and feelings in a safe and supportive environment. Equally important is the child's need to build coping skills and self-esteem. The child must be reassured and convinced that he or she is in no way responsible or to blame for what happened.

Individual treatment with art therapy is used initially because it is the least threatening method in the early stages of treatment, it can easily be tailored to meet the child's individual needs, and it prepares the child for other forms of treatment such as family and group therapy. Family or group therapy may be of benefit in exploring the child's concerns and feelings. Anger is common, especially in children who were abused by a trusted adult such as the father or stepfather.

Nursing Assessment

Nursing assessment in instances of suspected child abuse or neglect requires a comprehensive history and physical examination, with documentation of findings. Consultation with social service agencies in the community is important if the family is receiving services.

Obtaining the history can be stressful for both the nurse and the parent. Use of therapeutic communication techniques and a quiet, unhurried environment are helpful. Maintaining a nonjudgmental attitude at all times is essential. It is important to differentiate true child abuse from cultural variations that might inaccurately be assumed to indicate abuse (Figs. 22–8A and 22–8B). Obtaining information about abusive and neglectful behaviors requires the nurse to establish a trusting relationship with parents, who are often afraid to trust any professional.

The health history sequence should include (1) parental concerns, (2) general family history, and (3) specific child history. This sequence begins with nonthreatening topics and allows the nurse to demonstrate concern before asking about abuse-related concerns. Obtain details about how injuries occurred. The parents' and child's own words should be documented verbatim using quotation marks. Compare reports obtained from each family member for lack of consistency and details that change over time.

It is desirable to interview the parent and child separately as well as together. Parent–child interaction during an intensive history-taking session provides an opportunity to observe the child's behavior and the parent's method of handling and responding to the child.

Data gathered during history-taking are particularly important in light of physical findings. Are there discrepancies between the history and physical assessment data? Do the parents give a history of an uncontrollable,

LEGAL & ETHICAL CONSIDERATIONS

Every state has a child abuse law specifying the particular behaviors that define every type of abuse. Any professional who works with children and reasonably suspects that a child has been abused is required to report his or her suspicions to the local agency for child protective services. Reports made in good faith are not liable to countersuits. However, professionals who suspect abuse and do not report it may be held responsible by the courts.

COMMUNICATION STRATEGIES

The nurse should communicate in an open manner. A clear statement of purpose is needed, for example, "Hello, Mr. S. My name is Joan T. I'm Jonathan's nurse. I will be talking with you and asking you some questions about his overall health."

CULTURAL CONSIDERATIONS

Traditional treatment practices are sometimes mistaken for signs of physical abuse. The Chinese practice of cupping, which involves heating a bamboo cup and placing it on the skin, is a traditional treatment for headaches or abdominal pain. The Vietnamese practice of *caogio* (rubbing out the wind), in which a coin or the fingers are forcefully rubbed on the chest, back, or neck, is used to treat minor ailments.

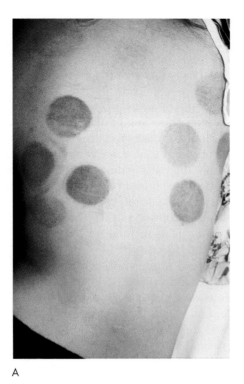
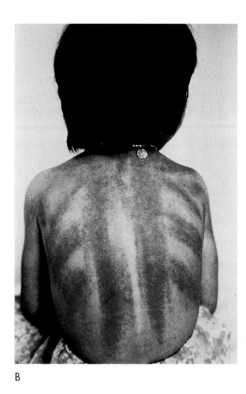

A   B

FIGURE 22–8. It is important to differentiate cultural practices such as cupping **(A)** and coining **(B)** from signs of child abuse.
Photographs copyright © AAP/Kempe. Used with permission.

 LEGAL & ETHICAL CONSIDERATIONS

Each person who handles a laboratory specimen or other item (eg, clothing soiled with semen) in cases of suspected child abuse, must be identified in the patient's record, and the specimen must never be left unattended. This documented chain of possession is necessary to ensure the admissibility of the evidence in court.

inattentive toddler when the nurse observes a child who is attentive throughout a 15–minute examination? Assess the child's general appearance, including dress and behavior during the assessment. How do the child's affect, behavior, and development compare with those of other children the same age?

Documentation of findings is important in all situations but is essential in cases of suspected child abuse and neglect. Physical findings should be recorded as observed. Figure diagrams should be used to document skin injuries. Photographs are taken to document the location, nature, and extent of injuries.[37]

Nursing Diagnosis

Among the nursing diagnoses that might be appropriate for the physically abused or neglected child are the following:

- Pain related to inflicted injuries
- Impaired Skin Integrity related to inflicted injuries
- Altered Growth and Development related to lack of supportive parenting and environment
- Altered Nutrition: Less Than Body Requirements related to inadequate caloric intake
- Altered Health Maintenance related to lack of parental provision of child's essential needs
- Fear related to actual physical harm or repeated risk of injury
- Risk for Injury related to physical abuse

- Risk for Violence (Parent) related to inability to manage anger

Additional diagnoses that might apply to the emotionally abused or neglected child include the following:

- Defensive Coping related to belittling or verbal threats by parents
- Chronic Low Self-Esteem related to lack of appropriate emotional support from parents
- Ineffective Family Coping: Disabling related to dysfunctional family dynamics and pattern of physical abuse

Diagnoses that might apply to the sexually abused child include the following:

- Anxiety related to potential separation from parent
- Rape-Trauma Syndrome related to sexual exploitation of the child
- Altered Role Performance related to expectation of meeting adults' sexual gratification needs
- Personal Identity Disturbance related to disturbance of usual activities of childhood and decreased self-esteem

Nursing Management

Nursing care focuses on helping to remove the child from an abusive environment, preventing further injury, providing supportive care, and reinforcing the importance of follow-up care and counseling.

Prevent Further Injury
Work with social services and community agencies to assess the child's home environment, individuals living in the home, and the actions surrounding the abuse. Assist in removing the child from the home to temporary custody of the court or foster care of another relative, if indicated. Counsel family members about abuse and refer for appropriate therapy.

Provide Supportive Care
Protect and treat the child's injuries (eg, fractures, burns). Include parents in the child's treatment plan, and keep them informed about the child's progress. Even if suspected of inflicting injuries to the child, the parent is still the child's primary caretaker. Talk with the parent as you would with any parent. Be supportive of any guilt expressed. Encourage the parent to assist with the child's care. Observe parent–child interactions and document supportive behaviors and the child's response to the parent versus other care providers.

Interacting nonjudgmentally with a parent suspected of abusing his or her child can be difficult. Talk with a colleague about any anger you feel toward the parents or about the child's injuries or specific actions surrounding the abuse. Use team meetings to develop strategies that enable you to work with the parents and child.

Discharge Planning and Home Care Teaching
If there is any question about the child returning to a potentially dangerous situation, support the child's removal from the situation. After discharge the child may receive supervised care in the home by court order. Day care, home nursing, and social worker visits may be arranged. Parents should be

referred to parent effectiveness classes, family therapy, and support groups as necessary.

MUNCHAUSEN SYNDROME BY PROXY

Munchausen syndrome by proxy is a potentially deadly form of child abuse that involves the fabrication of signs and symptoms of a health condition in a child. Usually it is the mother who creates these fictitious signs in her child (the proxy). The victim is usually under 6 years of age. Frequently the child's symptoms of illness are used to gain entry into the medical system to meet the abuser's own needs.[38]

The issues of abuse are multidimensional. The child is a victim of the feigned illness, repeated hospitalizations, and invasive procedures. Equally disruptive is the deprivation of the child's daily routine caused by the periodic medical crises.

Munchausen syndrome by proxy should be suspected when unexplained, recurrent, or extremely rare conditions occur; illness is unresponsive to treatment; and the history and clinical findings are inconsistent. The most commonly reported signs and symptoms are central nervous system dysfunction, apnea, diarrhea, vomiting, fever, seizures, signs of bleeding (in urine or stool), and rashes. The parent may overdose the child on medications, such as nonprescription drugs and even syrup of ipecac, causing a variety of side effects.[39] The symptoms occur in the presence of the same caretaker and disappear when the child is separated from that caretaker.

The child often appears uncooperative, extremely anxious, fearful, and negative. The caretaker, who in contrast appears very cooperative, competent, and loving, often expresses a desire for the child to recover. The caretaker may even suggest diagnostic procedures to try to determine "what's wrong." Characteristically the caretaker thrives in the health care environment.

The cause of Munchausen syndrome by proxy is often complex and rooted in the caretaker's own abusive or neglectful childhood. The disorder occurs in all socioeconomic classes. Often the perpetrator has some type of health care background, such as nursing or another allied health profession.

A suspicion of Munchausen syndrome by proxy requires a coordinated evaluation by an interdisciplinary team. Members of the team must organize and communicate a strategic plan regarding collection of evidence, confrontation of the abuser, and management of the hospitalized child.[40] The child's safety is the ultimate concern. The case must also be reported to the appropriate child protective services.

Nursing Management

Special care should be taken to maintain a trusting relationship with the caretaker so that he or she does not become suspicious and leave the hospital. Often the best person on the team to function in the role of "trusted other" is a member of the psychiatric consultation team.

Careful documentation of parent–child interactions, presence or absence of symptoms, and other pertinent observations is essential. The child must be closely monitored. When enough evidence is collected to prove Munchausen syndrome by proxy, the caretaker is confronted by the physician or another member of the psychiatric team.

REFERENCES

1. Herrick, C.A., Goodykoontz, L., & Herrick, R.H. (1992). Selection of treatment modalities. In P. West, & C.L. Sieloff Evans (Eds.), *Psychiatric and mental health with children and adolescents* (pp. 98–115). Gaithersburg, MD: Aspen Publications.

2. Elliot, G.R. (1996). Autistic disorder and other pervasive mental disorders. In A.M. Rudolph, J.I.E. Hoffman, & C.D. Rudolph (Eds.), *Rudolph's pediatrics* (20th ed., pp. 168–170). Stamford, CT: Appleton & Lange.

3. Stanley, S. (1992). Nursing interventions in children and adolescents experiencing communication disabilities. In P. West, & C.L. Sieloff Evans (Eds.), *Psychiatric and mental health with children and adolescents* (pp. 199–211). Gaithersburg, MD: Aspen Publications.

4. Gabel, S., Dolgan, J.I., & Hea, R.A. (1997). Behavioral, psychosocial, & psychiatric pediatrics. In G.B. Merenstein, D.W. Kaplan, & A.A. Rosenberg (Eds.), *Handbook of pediatrics* (pp. 199–200). Stamford, CT: Appleton & Lange.

5. Johnson, B.S. (1997). Children. In B.S. Johnson (Ed.). *Psychiatric-mental health nursing* (4th ed., pp. 375–409). Philadelphia: Lippincott.

6. Bindler, R.M., & Howry, L.B. (1997). *Pediatric drugs and nursing implications* (2nd ed., pp. 370–371). Stamford, CT: Appleton & Lange.

7. Greenhill, L.L. (1997). Attention-deficit hyperactivity disorder. In J.M. Weiner (Ed.), *Textbook of child and adolescent psychiatry* (2nd ed., pp. 261–275). Washington, DC: American Psychiatric Press.

8. Townsend, M.C. (1997). *Psychiatric mental health nursing: Concepts of care* (2nd ed., pp. 309–337). Philadelphia: FA Davis.

9. Yearwood, E. (1992). Nursing interventions with children experiencing attention and motor difficulties. In P. West, & C.L. Seiloff Evans (Eds.), *Psychiatric and mental health with children and adolescents* (pp. 169–181). Gaithersburg, MD: Aspen Publications.

10. Symanski, L.S., & Kaplan, L.C. (1997). Mental retardation. In J.M. Weiner (Ed.), *Textbook of child and adolescent psychiatry* (2nd ed., pp. 143–168). Washington, DC: American Psychiatric Press.

11. Chitty, K. (1996). Eating disorders. In H.S. Wilson, & C.C. Kneisl (Eds.), *Psychiatric nursing* (5th ed., pp. 468–483). Redwood City, CA: Addison-Wesley.

12. Maggioni, A., & Lifchitz, F. (1995). Nutritional management of failure to thrive. *Pediatric Clinics of North America, 42*(4), 791–810.

13. American Psychiatric Association. (1994). *Diagnostic and statistical manual of mental disorders* (4th ed.). Washington, DC: Author.

14. Kaufman, K.L., Cromer, B., Deleiden, E.L., Zaron-Aqua, A., Aqua, K., Greeley, T., & Li, B.U. (1997). Recurrent adolescent pain in adolescents: Psychosocial correlates of organic and nonorganic pain. *Children's Health Care, 26*(1), 15–30.

15. Neff, E.J., & Dale, J. (1996). Worries of school age children. *Journal of the Society of Pediatric Nurses, 1*(1), 27–32.

16. Dalton, R. (1996). Vegetative disorders. In R.E. Behrman, R.M. Kliegman, & A. Arvin (Eds.), *Nelson textbook of pediatrics* (15th ed., pp. 79–81). Philadelphia: Saunders.

17. National Institute of Mental Health. (1993). *Eating disorders: Decade of the brain* (NIH Publication No. 93-3477). Washington, DC: U.S. Government Printing Office.

18. Potts, N.W. (1995). Eating disorders. In B.S. Johnson (Ed.), *Child, adolescent, and family psychiatric nursing* (pp. 301–314). Philadelphia: Lippincott.

19. Irwin, C.E., & Ryan, S.A. (1996). Health problems of adolescents. In A.M. Rudolph, J.I.E. Hoffman, & C.D. Rudolph (Eds.), *Rudolph's pediatrics* (20th ed., pp. 40–45). Stamford, CT: Appleton & Lange.

20. Kaplan, D.W., & Mammel, K.A. (1997). Adolescence. In W.W. Hay, J.R. Groothuis, A.R. Hayward, & M.J. Levin (Eds.), *Current pediatric diagnosis and treatment* (13th ed., pp. 129–131). Stamford, CT: Appleton & Lange.

21. Owen, S.V., & Fullerton, M.L. (1994). A discussion group in a behaviorally oriented inpatient eating disorder program. *Journal of Psychosocial Nursing, 33*(11), 35–40.

22. McGowen, A., & Whitbread, J. (1996). Out of control! The most effective way to help the binge-eating patient. *Journal of Psychosocial Nursing, 34*(1), 30–37.

23. Deering, C.G. (1992). Nursing interventions with children and adolescents experiencing eating difficulties. In P. West, & C.L. Sieloff Evans (Eds.), *Psychiatric and mental health with children and adolescents* (pp. 343–360). Gaithersburg, MD: Aspen Publications.

24. Finke, L. (1992). Nursing intervention with children and adolescents experiencing substance abuse. In P. West, & C.L. Sieloff Evans (Eds.), *Psychiatric and mental health with children and adolescents* (pp. 242–254). Gaithersburg, MD: Aspen Publications.

25. Pagliaro, A.M., & Pagliaro, L.A. (1996). *Substance abuse among children and adolescents.* New York: John Wiley & Sons.

26. Kashani, J.H., & Eppright, T.D. (1997). Mood disorders in adolescents. In J.M. Weiner (Ed.), *Textbook of child and adolescent psychiatry* (2nd ed., pp. 248–260). Washington, DC: American Psychiatric Press.

27. Brantly, D.K., & Takacs, D.J. (1991). Anxiety and depression in preschool and school-aged children. In P. Clunn (Ed.), *Child psychiatric nursing* (pp. 351–365). St. Louis: Mosby–Year Book.

28. Guyer, B., Strobino, D.M., Ventura, S.J., MacDorman, M., & Martin, J.A. (1996). Annual summary of vital statistics—1995. *Pediatrics, 98*(6), 1007–1019.

29. Rohde, P., Seeley, J.R., & Mace, D.E. (1997). Correlates of suicidal behavior in a juvenile detention center. *Suicide and Life Threatening Behavior, 27*(2), 164–175.

30. Flaherty, J.A., Davis, J.M., & Janicak, P.G. (Eds). (1993). *Psychiatry: Diagnosis and therapy* (2nd ed.). Stamford, CT: Appleton & Lange.

31. Keefer, C.H. (1996). Pervasive developmental disorders. In B.S. Johnson (Ed.), *Child, adolescent, and family psychiatric nursing* (pp. 270–285). Philadelphia: Lippincott.

32. Volkmar, F.R. (1996). Childhood schizophrenia. In A.M. Rudolph, J.I.E. Hoffman, & C.D. Rudolph (Eds.), *Rudolph's pediatrics* (20th ed., pp 177–178). Stamford, CT: Appleton & Lange.

33. Association for Care of Children's Health. (1998). *The state of America's children.* Washington, DC: Author.

34. U.S. Bureau of the Census. (1996). *Statistical abstract of the United States—1996* (116th ed.). Washington, DC: Author.

35. Fontaine, K. (1996). Intrafamily abuse. In H.S. Wilson, & C.R. Kneisl (Eds.), *Psychiatric nursing* (5th ed., pp. 555–584). Menlo Park, CA: Addison-Wesley.

36. Walker, G.C., Scott, P.S., & Koppersmith, G. (1998). The impact of child sexual abuse on addiction severity and analysis of trauma processing. *Journal of Psychosocial Nursing, 36*(3), 10–18.

37. Campbell, J., & Humphreys, J. (1993). *Nursing care of survivors of family violence.* St. Louis: Mosby–Year Book.

38. Klebes, C., & Fay, S. (1995). Munchausen syndrome by proxy: A review, case study, and nursing implications. *Journal of Pediatric Nursing, 10*(2), 93–98.

39. Schender, D.J., Perez, A., Knilans, T.E., Daniels, S.R., Bove, K.E., & Bonnell, H. (1996). Clinical and pathologic aspects of cardiomyopathy from ipecac administration in Munchausen's syndrome by proxy. *Pediatrics, 97*(6), 902–906.

40. Castiglia, P. (1995). Munchausen syndrome by proxy. *Journal of Pediatric Health Care, 9*(2), 79–80.

ADDITIONAL RESOURCES

American Academy of Pediatrics. (1996). *Diagnostic and statistical manual for primary care.* Elk Grove Village, IL: Author.

Bursch, B., Weinburg, H.D., & Shilkoff, S. (1996). Nurses' knowledge of and experience with Munchausen syndrome by proxy. *Issues in Comprehensive Pediatric Nursing, 19*(2), 93–102.

Castiglia, P. (1993). *The time-solution: A parent's guide for handling everyday behavior problems.* Chicago: Contemporary Books.

Center for the Future of Children. (1996). *Special education for students with disabilities.* Los Angeles: Author.

Church, C.C., & Coplan, J. (1995). The high-functioning autistic experience: Birth to preteen years. *Journal of Pediatric Health Care, 9*(1), 22–29.

Dreikurs, R., & Cassel, P. (1990). *Discipline without tears: A reassuring and practical guide to teaching your child positive behavior.* New York: Dutton.

Eminson, D.M., & Postlethwaite, R.J. (1992). Factitious illness: Recognition and management. *Archives of Disease in Childhood, 67,* 1510–1516.

Fiesta, J. (1992). Protecting children: A public duty to report. *Nursing Management, 23*(7), 14–15.

Heatherington, E.M., & Blechman, E.A. (1996). *Stress, coping, and resiliency in children and families.* Mahwah, NJ: Lawrence Erlbaum Associates.

Ireys, H.T., Grason, H.A., & Guyer, B. (1996). Assuring quality of care for children with special needs in managed care organization: Roles for pediatricians. *Pediatrics, 98*(2), 178–185.

Jackson, B., Finkler, D., & Robinson, C. (1995). A cost analysis of a case management system for infants with chronic illnesses and development disabilites. *Journal of Pediatric Nursing, 10*(5), 304–310.

Kelleher, K., & Wolraich, M.L. (1996). Diagnosing psychosocial problems. *Pediatrics, 97*(6), 899–901.

Monteleone, J.A. (1996). *Recognition of child abuse for the mandated reporter* (2nd ed.). St. Louis: G.W. Medical Publishing.

Nehring, W.M. (1994). The nurse whose specialty is developmental disabilities. *Pediatric Nursing, 20*(1), 78–81.

Schraeder, B.D. (1995). Children with disabilities. *Journal of Pediatric Nursing, 10*(3), 166–172.

Smith, K., Wheeler, B., Pilecki, P., & Parker, T. (1995). The role of the pediatric nurse practitioner in educating teens with mental retardation about sex. *Journal of Pediatric Health Care, 9*(2), 59–66.

Spitzer, A., & Cameron, C. (1995). School-age children's perceptions of mental illness. *Western Journal of Nursing Research, 17*(4), 398–415.

St. Dennis, C., & Synoground, G. (1996). Pharmacology update. Methylphenidate. *Journal of School Nursing, 12*(1), 5–8,10.

Stein, M.A., Blonids, T.A., Schnitzler, E.R., O'Brien, T., Fishkin, J., Blackwell, B., Szumowski, E., & Roizen, N.J. (1996). Methylphenidate dosing: Twice daily versus three times daily. *Pediatrics, 98*(4), 748–756.

BOYS: BIRTH TO 36 MONTHS
PHYSICAL GROWTH
NCHS PERCENTILES*

NAME _____ RECORD # _____

AGE (MONTHS)

LENGTH

WEIGHT

AGE (MONTHS)

MOTHER'S STATURE _____ GESTATIONAL
FATHER'S STATURE _____ AGE _____ WEEKS

DATE	AGE	LENGTH	WEIGHT	HEAD CIRC.	COMMENT
	BIRTH				

*Adapted from: Hamill PVV, Drizd TA, Johnson CL, Reed RB, Roche AF, Moore WM: Physical growth: National Center for Health Statistics percentiles. Am J Clin Nutr 32:607–629. Data from the Fels Longitudinal Study, Wright State University School of Medicine, Yellow Springs, Ohio.

FIGURE A–1. Physical growth percentiles for length and weight—boys: birth to 36 months.
From NCHS Growth Charts, copyright © 1982 Ross Laboratories. Reprinted with permission of Ross Laboratories, Columbus, OH.

Physical Growth Charts

BOYS: BIRTH TO 36 MONTHS
PHYSICAL GROWTH
NCHS PERCENTILES*   NAME _____   RECORD # _____

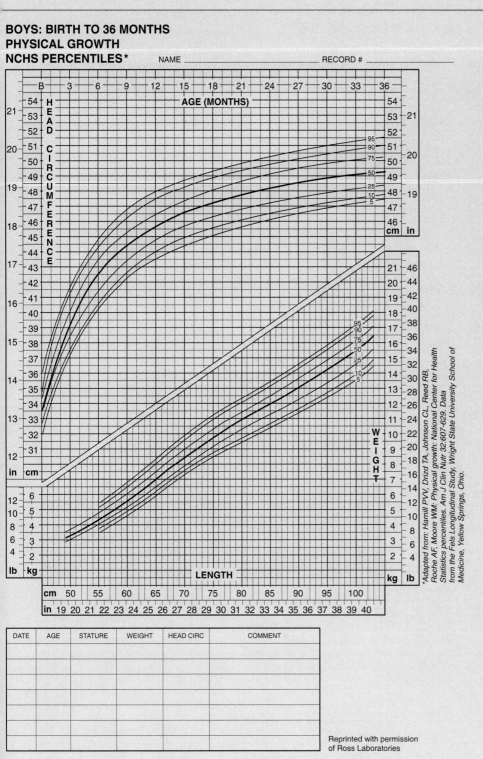

*Adapted from: Hamill PVV, Drizd TA, Johnson CL, Reed RB, Roche AF, Moore WM: Physical growth: National Center for Health Statistics percentiles. Am J Clin Nutr 32:607–629. Data from the Fels Longitudinal Study, Wright State University School of Medicine, Yellow Springs, Ohio.

DATE	AGE	STATURE	WEIGHT	HEAD CIRC	COMMENT

FIGURE A–2. Physical growth percentiles for head circumference, length, and weight—boys: birth to 36 months.

From NCHS Growth Charts, copyright © 1982 Ross Laboratories. Reprinted with permission of Ross Laboratories, Columbus, OH.

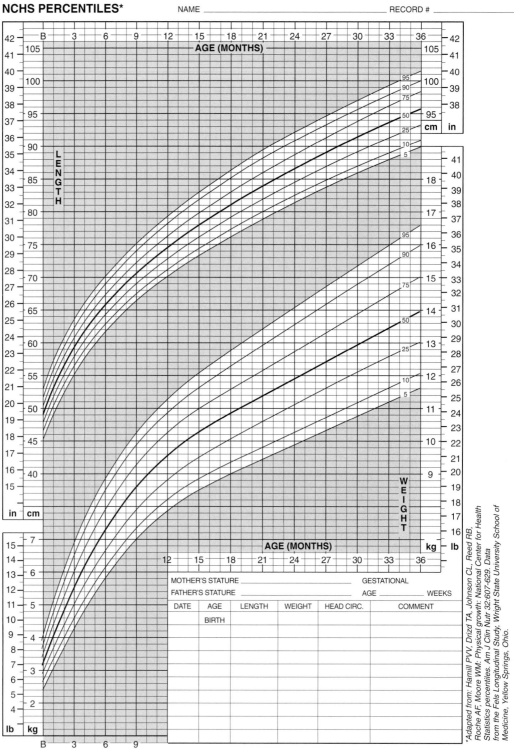

FIGURE A–3. Physical growth percentiles for length and weight—girls: birth to 36 months.
From NCHS Growth Charts, copyright © 1982 Ross Laboratories. Reprinted with permission of Ross Laboratories, Columbus, OH.

GIRLS: BIRTH TO 36 MONTHS
PHYSICAL GROWTH
NCHS PERCENTILES*

NAME _____   RECORD # _____

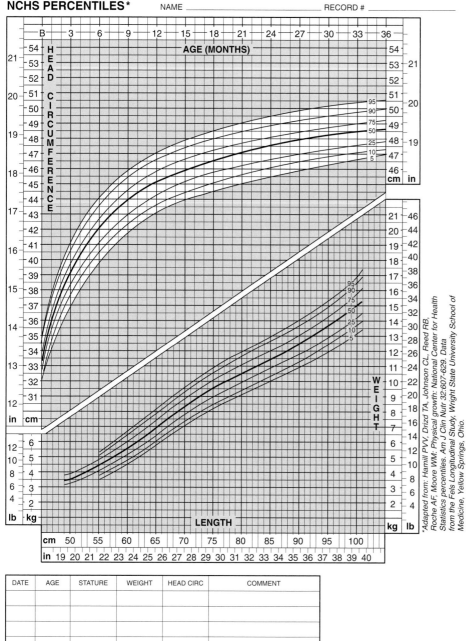

DATE	AGE	STATURE	WEIGHT	HEAD CIRC	COMMENT

FIGURE A–4. Physical growth percentiles for head circumference, length, and weight—girls: birth to 36 months.

From NCHS Growth Charts, copyright © 1982 Ross Laboratories. Reprinted with permission of Ross Laboratories, Columbus, OH.

BOYS: 2 TO 18 YEARS
PHYSICAL GROWTH ·
NCHS PERCENTILES*

FIGURE A–5. Physical growth percentiles for stature and weight according to age—boys: 2 to 18 years.
From NCHS Growth Charts, copyright © 1982 Ross Laboratories. Reprinted with permission of Ross Laboratories, Columbus, OH.

GIRLS: 2 TO 18 YEARS
PHYSICAL GROWTH
NCHS PERCENTILES*

NAME _____   RECORD # _____

FIGURE A–6. Physical growth percentiles for stature and weight according to age—girls: 2 to 18 years.
From NCHS Growth Charts, copyright © 1982 Ross Laboratories. Reprinted with permission of Ross Laboratories, Columbus, OH.

Food Guide Pyramid

The food guide pyramid shows the variety of foods that should be eaten each day to obtain the required nutrients and adequate energy. Foods in each of the five bottom groups are needed as no one group provides all of the nutrients required. Fats, oils, and sugars at the top of the food pyramid supply calories but little or no vitamins or minerals, so these should be used sparingly.

For toddlers and preschoolers, serving size can be based on 1 tablespoon of solid food for each year of age. Food serving sizes for older children and adolescents are about ½ cup or 2 to 3 ounces, depending upon the food category.

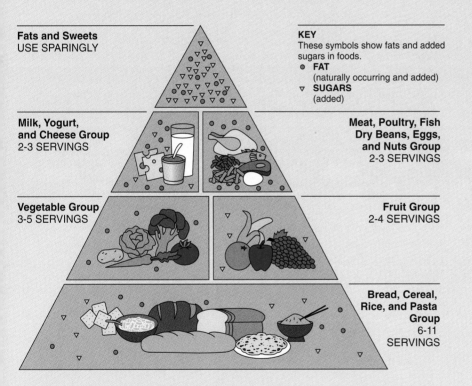

Fats and Sweets
USE SPARINGLY

KEY
These symbols show fats and added sugars in foods.
- ● **FAT**
  (naturally occurring and added)
- ▽ **SUGARS**
  (added)

Milk, Yogurt, and Cheese Group
2-3 SERVINGS

Meat, Poultry, Fish Dry Beans, Eggs, and Nuts Group
2-3 SERVINGS

Vegetable Group
3-5 SERVINGS

Fruit Group
2-4 SERVINGS

Bread, Cereal, Rice, and Pasta Group
6-11 SERVINGS

FIGURE B-1. Food Guide Pyramid: A Guide to Daily Food Choices.
U.S. Department of Agriculture and U.S. Department of Health and Human Services (1990). Nutrition and your health: Dietary guidelines for Americans (3rd ed.). Home and Garden Bulletin No. 232. Washington, DC: U.S. Government Printing Office.

Recommended Dietary Allowances[a] Designed for the Maintenance of Good Nutrition of Practically All Healthy People in the United States

Category	Age (yr) or condition	Weight[b] (kg)	Weight[b] (lb)	Height[b] (cm)	Height[b] (in.)	Protein (g)	Fat-Soluble Vitamins Vitamin A (μg RE)[c]	Vitamin D (μg)[d]	Vitamin E (mg/α-TE)[e]	Vitamin K (μg)
Infants	0.0–0.5	6	13	60	24	13	375	7.5	3	5
	0.5–1.0	9	20	71	28	14	375	10	4	10
Children	1–3	13	29	90	35	16	400	10	6	15
	4–6	20	44	112	44	24	500	10	7	20
	7–10	28	62	132	52	28	700	10	7	30
Males	11–14	45	99	157	62	45	1000	10	10	45
	15–18	66	145	176	69	59	1000	10	10	65
	19–24	72	160	177	70	58	1000	10	10	70
	25–50	79	174	176	70	63	1000	5	10	80
	51+	77	170	173	68	63	1000	5	10	80
Females	11–14	46	101	157	62	46	800	10	8	45
	15–18	55	120	163	64	44	800	10	8	55
	19–24	58	128	164	65	46	800	10	8	60
	25–50	63	138	163	64	50	800	5	8	65
	51+	65	143	160	63	50	800	5	8	65
Pregnant						60	800	10	10	65
Lactating	1st 6 months					65	1300	10	12	65
	2nd 6 months					62	1200	10	11	65

[a]The allowances, expressed as average daily intakes over time, are intended to provide for individual variations among most normal persons as they live in the United States under usual environmental stresses. Diets should be based on a variety of common foods in order to provide other nutrients for which human requirements have been less well defined.

[b]Weights and heights of reference adults are actual medians for the U.S. population of the designated age, as reported by National Health and Nutrition Examination Survey (NHANES) II. The median weights and heights of those under 19 years of age were taken from Hamill, P.V. et al. (1979). Physical growth: National Center for Health Statistics percentiles. *Am J Clin Nutr, 32*, 607–629. The use of these figures does not imply that the height-to-weight ratios are ideal.

Recommended Dietary Allowances

Water-Soluble Vitamins							Minerals						
Vitamin C (mg)	Thia-min (mg)	Ribo-flavin (mg)	Niacin (mg NE)[f]	Vitamin B_6 (mg)	Folate (µg)	Vitamin B_{12} (µg)	Cal-cium (mg)	Phos-phorus (mg)	Mag-nesium (mg)	Iron (mg)	Zinc (mg)	Iodine (µg)	Sele-nium (µg)
30	0.3	0.4	5	0.3	25	0.3	400	300	40	6	5	40	10
35	0.4	0.5	6	0.6	35	0.5	600	500	60	10	5	50	15
40	0.7	0.8	9	1.0	50	0.7	800	800	80	10	10	70	20
45	0.9	1.1	12	1.1	75	1.0	800	800	120	10	10	90	20
45	1.0	1.2	13	1.4	100	1.4	800	800	170	10	10	120	30
50	1.3	1.5	17	1.7	150	2.0	1200	1200	270	12	15	150	40
60	1.5	1.8	20	2.0	200	2.0	1200	1200	400	12	15	150	50
60	1.5	1.7	19	2.0	200	2.0	1200	1200	350	10	15	150	70
60	1.5	1.7	19	2.0	200	2.0	800	800	350	10	15	150	70
60	1.2	1.4	15	2.0	200	2.0	800	800	350	10	15	150	70
50	1.1	1.3	15	1.4	150	2.0	1200	1200	280	15	12	150	45
60	1.1	1.3	15	1.5	180	2.0	1200	1200	300	15	12	150	50
60	1.1	1.3	15	1.6	180	2.0	1200	1200	280	15	12	150	55
60	1.1	1.3	15	1.6	180	2.0	800	800	280	15	12	150	55
60	1.0	1.2	13	1.6	180	2.0	800	800	280	10	12	150	55
70	1.5	1.6	17	2.2	400	2.2	1200	1200	320	30	15	175	65
95	1.6	1.8	20	2.1	280	2.6	1200	1200	355	15	19	200	75
90	1.6	1.7	20	2.1	260	2.6	1200	1200	340	15	16	200	75

[c]Retinol equivalent. 1 retinol equivalent = 1 µg retinol or 6 µg β-carotene.
[d]As cholecalciferol. 10 µg cholecalciferol = 400 IU vitamin D.
[e]α-Tocopherol equivalents. 1 µg d-α-tocopherol = 1 α-TE.
[f]1 NE (niacin equivalent) is equal to 1 mg of niacin or 60 mg of dietary tryptophan.

From Food and Nutrition Board, National Research Council. (1989). Recommended dietary allowances (10th ed.). Washington, DC: National Academy of Sciences. Courtesy of the National Academy Press, Washington, DC.

All laboratory values listed are approximate. Consult your local laboratory for guidelines as to normal values for the specific testing procedures used.

NORMAL VALUES: BLOOD

Acid–Base Measurements (B)
pH: 7.38–7.42 from 14 minutes of age and older.

Pao_2: 65–76 mm Hg (8.66–10.13 kPa).

$Paco_2$: 36–38 mm Hg (4.8–5.07 kPa).

Base excess: 22–12 mEq/L, except in newborns (range, 24–20).

Albumin (S)
1–3 years: 3.4–4.2 g/dL.

4–6 years: 3.5–5.2 g/dL.

7–9 years: 3.7–5.6 g/dL.

10–19 years: 3.7–5.6 g/dL.

Aldolase (S)
Infants: 3.4–11.8 U/L.

Children: 1.2–8.8 U/L.

Adults: 1.7–4.9 U/L.

Aldosterone (S)
6–9 years: 1–24 ng/dL.

10–11 years: 2–15 ng/dL.

12–14 years: 1–22 ng/dL.

15–17 years: 1–32 ng/dL.

Alkaline Phosphatase (S)
Values in IU/L at 37°C (98.6°F) using p-nitrophenol phosphate buffered with AMP (kinetic).

Age	Males	Females
Newborns (1–3 days)	95–368	95–368
2–24 months	115–460	115–460
2–5 years	115–391	115–391
6–7 years	115–460	115–460
8–9 years	115–345	115–345
10–11 years	115–336	115–437
12–13 years	127–403	92–336
14–15 years	79–446	78–212
16–18 years	58–331	35–124
Adults	41–137	39–118

α_1-Antitrypsin (S)
1–3 months: 127–404 mg/dL.

3–12 months: 145–362 mg/dL.

1–2 years: 160–382 mg/dL.

2–15 years: 148–394 mg/dL.

Ammonia (P)
Newborns: 90–150 µg/dL (53–88 µmol/L); higher in premature and jaundiced infants.

Thereafter: 0–60 µg/dL (0–35 µmol/L) when blood is drawn with proper precautions.

Modified from Hathaway, W.E., Hay, W.W., Groothuis, J.R., & Paisley, J.W. (1997). *Current pediatric diagnosis and treatment* (13th ed.). Stamford, CT: Appleton & Lange; and Soldin, S.J., Brugnara, C., Gunter, K.C, & Hicks, J.M. (1997). *Pediatric reference ranges* (2nd ed.). Washington, DC: AACC Press.
Note: Values may vary with the procedure employed.
S, serum; B, whole blood; P, plasma; RBC, red blood cells.

Normal Laboratory Values

Bicarbonate, Actual (P)
Calculated from pH and Pa_{CO_2}.
Newborns: 17.2–23.6 mmol/L.
2 months–2 years: 19–24 mmol/L.
Children: 18–25 mmol/L.
Adult males: 20.1–28.9 mmol/L.
Adult females: 18.4–28.8 mmol/L.

Bilirubin (S)
Values in mg/dL (μmol/L).
Levels after 1 month are as follows:
Conjugated: 0–0.3 mg/dL (0–5 μmol/L).
Unconjugated:
    0.1–0.7 mg/dL (2–12 μmol/L).

Peak Newborn Level	Newborns (Birth Weight) Exceeding Peak Level (%)		
	<2001 g	2001–2500 g	>2500 g
20 (342)	8.2	2.6	0.8
18 (308)	13.5	4.6	1.5
16 (274)	20.3	7.6	2.6
14 (239)	33.0	12.0	4.4
11 (188)	53.8	23.0	9.3
8 (137)	77.0	45.4	26.1

Bleeding Time (Simplate)
2–9 min.

Blood Volume
Premature infants: 98 mL/kg.
At 1 year: 86 mL/kg (range, 69–112 mL/kg).
Older children: 70 mL/kg (range, 51–86 mL/kg).

Calcium (S)
Premature infants (first week): 3.5–4.5 mEq/L (1.7–2.3 mmol/L).
Full-term infants (first week): 4–5 mEq/L (2–2.5 mmol/L).
Thereafter: 4.4–5.3 mEq/L (2.2–2.7 mmol/L).

Carbon Dioxide, Total (S, P)
Cord blood: 15–20.2 mmol/L.
Children: 18–27 mmol/L.
Adults: 24–35 mmol/L.

Chloride (S, P)
Premature infants: 95–110 mmol/L.
Full-term infants: 96–116 mmol/L.
Children: 98–105 mmol/L.
Adults: 98–108 mmol/L.

Cholesterol, High-Density Lipoprotein (S)
1–9 years:
    35–82 mg/dL (0.91–2.12 mmol/L).
10–13 years:
    36–84 mg/dL (0.93–2.17 mmol/L).
14–19 years:
    35–65 mg/dL (0.91–1.68 mmol/L).

Cholesterol, Low-Density Lipoprotein (S)
Values in mg/dL (mmol/L).

Group	Males	Females
6–7 years	56–134 (1.44–3.46)	52–149 (1.34–3.85)
8–9 years	52–129 (1.34–3.33)	57–143 (1.47–3.69)
10–11 years	45–149 (1.16–3.85)	56–140 (1.44–3.61)
12–13 years	55–135 (1.42–3.48)	58–138 (1.49–3.56)
14–15 years	48–143 (1.24–3.69)	47–140 (1.21–3.61)
16–17 years	53–134 (1.36–3.36)	44–147 (1.13–3.79)

Cholesterol, Total (S, P)
Values in mg/dL (mmol/L).

Age	Males	Females
6–7 years	115–197 (2.97–5.09)	126–199 (3.25–5.14)
8–9 years	112–199 (2.89–5.14)	124–208 (3.20–5.37)
10–11 years	108–220 (2.79–5.68)	115–208 (2.97–5.37)
12–13 years	117–202 (3.02–5.21)	114–207 (2.94–5.34)
14–15 years	103–207 (2.66–5.34)	102–208 (2.68–5.37)
16–17 years	107–198 (2.76–5.11)	106–213 (2.73–5.50)

Complement (S)
C3: 96–195 mg/dL.
C4: 15–20 mg/dL.

Creatine (S, P)
0.2–0.8 mg/dL (15.2–61 µmol/L).

Creatine Kinase (S, P)
Newborns (1–3 days): 40–474 IU/L at 37°C (98.6°F).
Adult males: 30–210 IU/L at 37°C (98°F).
Adult females: 20–128 IU/L at 37°C (98.6°F).

Creatinine (S, P)
Values in mg/dL (µmol/L).

Age	Males	Females
Newborns (1–3 days)[a]	0.2–1.0 (17.7–88.4)	0.2–1.0 (17.7–88.4)
1 year	0.2–0.6 (17.7–53.0)	0.2–0.5 (17.7–44.2)
2–3 years	0.2–0.7 (17.7–61.9)	0.3–0.6 (26.5–53.0)
4–7 years	0.2–0.8 (17.7–70.7)	0.2–0.7 (17.7–61.9)
8–10 years	0.3–0.9 (26.5–79.6)	0.3–0.8 (26.5–70.7)
11–12 years	0.3–1.0 (26.5–88.4)	0.3–0.9 (26.5–79.6)
13–17 years	0.3–1.2 (26.5–106.1)	0.3–1.1 (26.5–97.2)
18–20 years	0.5–1.3 (44.2–115.0)	0.3–1.1 (26.5–97.2)

[a]Values may be higher in premature newborns.

Creatinine Clearance
Values show great variability and depend on specificity of analytical methods used.
Newborns (1 days): 5–50 mL/min/1.73 m^2 (mean, 18 mL/min/1.73 m^2).
Newborns (6 days): 15–90 mL/min/1.73 m^2 (mean, 36 mL/min/1.73 m^2).
Adult males: 85–125 mL/min/1.73 m^2.
Adult females: 75–115 mL/min/1.73 m^2.

Fibrinogen (P)
200–500 mg/dL (5.9–14.7 µmol/L).

Galactose (S, P)
1.1–2.1 mg/dL (0.06–0.12 mmol/L).

Galactose-1-Phosphate (RBC)
Normal: 1 mg/dL of packed erythrocyte lysate; slightly higher in cord blood.
Infants with congenital galactosemia on a milk-free diet: <2 mg/dL.
Infants with congenital galactosemia taking milk: 9–20 mg/dL.

Galactose-1-Phosphate Uridyl Transferase (RBC)
Normal: 308–475 mIU/g of hemoglobin.
Heterozygous for Duarte variant: 225–308 mIU/g of hemoglobin.
Homozygous for Duarte variant: 142–225 mIU/g of hemoglobin.
Heterozygous for congenital galactosemia: 142–225 mIU/g of hemoglobin.
Homozygous for congenital galactosemia: <8 mIU/g of hemoglobin.

Glucose (S,P)
Premature infants: 20–80 mg/dL (1.11–4.44 mmol/L).
Full-term infants: 30–100 mg/dL (1.67–5.56 mmol/L).
Children and adults (fasting): 60–105 mg/dL (3.33–5.88 mmol/L).

Glucose 6–Phosphate Dehydrogenase (RBC)
150–215 units/dL.

Glucose Tolerance Test Results in Serum[a]

Time	Glucose		Insulin	
	mg/dL	mmol/L	µU/mL	pmol/L
Fasting	59–96	3.11–5.33	5–40	36–287
30 min	91–185	5.05–10.27	36–110	258–789
60 min	66–164	3.66–9.10	22–124	158–890
90 min	68–148	3.77–8.22	17–105	122–753
2 hr	66–122	3.66–6.77	6–84	43–603
3 hr	47–99	2.61–5.49	2–46	14–330
4 hr	61–93	3.39–5.16	3–32	21–230
5 hr	63–86	3.50–4.77	5–37	36–265

[a]Normal levels based on results in 13 normal children given glucose, 1.75 g/kg orally in one dose, after 2 weeks on a high-carbohydrate diet.

Glycosylated Hemoglobin (Hemoglobin A$_1$)(B)
Normal: 4–7% of total hemoglobin.
Diabetic patients in good control of their condition: 8–10%.
Diabetic patients in poor control: >10%.
Values tend to vary with testing technique.

Growth Hormone (GH)(S)

After infancy (fasting specimen):
   0–5 ng/mL.
In response to natural and artificial provocation (eg, sleep, arginine, insulin, hypoglycemia): >8 ng/mL.
During the newborn period (fasting specimen):
   GH levels are high (15–40 ng/mL) and responses to provocation variable.

Hematocrit (B)

Values in %.

Age	Males	Females
Newborns	43.4–56.1	37.4–55.9
6 months–2 years	30.9–37.0	36.2–37.2
2–6 years	31.7–37.7	32.0–37.1
6–12 years	32.7–39.3	33.0–39.6
12–18 years	34.8–43.9	34.0–40.7
>18 years	33.4–46.2	33.0–41.0

Hemoglobin (B)

Values in g/dL.

Age	Males	Females
Newborns	14.7–18.6	12.7–18.3
6 months–2 years	10.3–12.4	10.4–12.4
2–6 years	10.5–12.7	10.7–12.7
6–12 years	11.0–13.3	10.9–13.3
12–18 years	11.5–14.8	11.2–13.6
>18 years	10.9–15.7	10.7–13.5

Hemoglobin A₁c

See Glycosylated Hemoglobin.

Hemoglobin Electrophoresis (B)

A_1 hemoglobin: 96–98.5% of total hemoglobin.
A_2 hemoglobin: 1.5–4% of total hemoglobin.

Hemoglobin, Fetal (B)

At birth: 50–85% of total hemoglobin.
At 1 year: <15% of total hemoglobin.
Up to 2 years: Up to 5% of total hemoglobin.
Thereafter: <2% of total hemoglobin.

Immunoglobulins (S)

Values in mg/dL.

Age	IgG	IgA	IgM
Cord blood	766–1693	0.04–9	4–26
2 weeks–3 months	299–852	3–66	15–149
3–6 months	142–988	4–90	18–118
6–12 months	418–1142	14–95	43–223
1–2 years	356–1204	13–118	37–239
2–3 years	492–1269	23–137	49–204
3–6 years	564–1381	35–209	51–214
6–9 years	658–1535	29–384	50–228
9–12 years	625–1598	60–294	64–278
12–16 years	660–1548	81–252	45–256

Iron (S, P)

Newborns:
   20–157 µg/dL (3.6–28.1 µmol/L).
6 weeks–3 years:
   20–115 µg/dL (3.6–20.6 µmol/L).
3–9 years:
   20–141 µg/dL (3.6–25.2 µmol/L).
9–14 years:
   21–151 µg/dL (3.8–27 µmol/L).
14–16 years:
   20–181 µg/dL (3.6–32.4 µmol/L).
Adults: 44–196 µg/dL (7.2–31.3 µmol/L).

Iron-binding Capacity (S, P)

Newborns: 59–175 µg/dL
   (10.6–31.3 µmol/L).
Children and adults: 275–458 µg/dL
   (45–72 µmol/L).

Lactate Dehydrogenase (LDH)(S, P)

Values using lactate substrate (kinetic).
Newborns (1–3 days): 40–348 IU/L at 37°C
   (98.6°F).
1 months–5 years: 150–360 IU/L at 37°C
   (98.6°F).
5–8 years: 150–300 IU/L at 37°C (98.6°F).
8–12 years: 130–300 IU/L at 37°C (98.6°F).
12–14 years: 130–280 IU/L at 37°C
   (98.6°F).
14–16 years: 130–230 IU/L at 37°C
   (98.6°F).
Adult males: 70–178 IU/L at 37°C
   (98.6°F).
Adult females: 42–166 IU/L at 37°C
   (98.6°F).

Lead (B)

<10 µg/dL (<0.48 µmol/L): Within normal range.

10–19 µg/dL (0.48–0.92 µmol/L): Prevention needed.

>20 µg/dL (>0.97 µmol/L): Evaluation, possible treatment, and environmental control.

>70 µg/dL (>3.38 µmol/L): Immediate treatment and environmental control.

Magnesium (P)

Values in mg/dL (mmol/L).

Age	Males	Females
1–30 days	1.7–2.4 (0.70–0.99)	1.7–2.5 (0.70–1.03)
31–365 days	1.6–2.5 (0.66–1.03)	1.9–2.4 (0.78–0.99)
1–3 years	1.7–2.4 (0.70–0.99)	1.7–2.4 (0.70–0.99)
4–6 years	1.7–2.4 (0.70–0.99)	1.7–2.2 (0.70–0.91)
7–9 years	1.7–2.3 (0.70–0.95)	1.6–2.3 (0.66–0.95)
10–12 years	1.6–2.2 (0.66–0.91)	1.6–2.2 (0.66–0.91)
13–15 years	1.6–2.3 (0.66–0.95)	1.6–2.3 (0.66–0.95)
16–18 years	1.5–2.2 (0.62–0.91)	1.5–2.2 (0.62–0.91)

Osmolality (S, P)

270–290 mOsm/kg.

Oxygen Saturation (B)

Newborns: 85–90%.

Thereafter: 95–99%.

Partial Thromboplastin Time (P)

Children: 42–54 sec.

Phenylalanine (S, P)

0.7–3.5 mg/dL (0.04–0.21 mmol/L).

Phosphorus, Inorganic (S,P)

Newborns: 5.0–9.0 mg/dL (1.81–3.78 mmol/L).

1 year: 3.8–6.2 mg/dL (1.23–2.0 mmol/L).

10 years: 3.6–5.6 mg/dL (1.16–1.81 mmol/L).

Adults: 3.1–5.1 mg/dL (1.0–1.65 mmol/L).

Platelet Count (RBC)

Value × 10^3/µL.

Age	Males	Females
Newborns	164–351	234–346
1–2 months	275–567	295–615
2–6 months	275–566	288–598
6 months–2 years	219–452	229–465
2–6 years	204–405	204–402
6–12 years	194–364	183–369
12–18 years	165–332	185–335
>18 years	143–320	171–326

Potassium (S, P)

Premature infants: 4.5–7.2 mmol/L.

Full-term infants: 3.7–5.2 mmol/L.

Children: 3.5–5.8 mmol/L.

Adults: 3.5–5.5 mmol/L.

Proteins in Serum[a]

Age	Total Protein	α_1-Globulin	α_2-Globulin
At birth	4.6–7.0	0.1–0.3	0.2–0.3
3 months	4.5–6.5	0.1–0.3	0.3–0.7
1 year	5.4–7.5	0.1–0.3	0.4–1.0
>4 years	5.9–8.0	0.1–0.3	0.4–0.8

Age	β-Globulin	λ-Globulin
At birth	0.3–0.6	0.6–1.2
3 months	0.3–0.7	0.2–0.7
1 year	0.4–1.0	0.2–0.9
>4 years	0.5–1.0	0.4–1.3

[a]Values are for cellulose acetate electrophoresis and are in g/dL. SI conversion factor: g/dL × 10 = g/L.

Prothrombin Time (P)

Children: 11–15 sec.

Protoporphyrin, "Free" (FEP, ZPP)(B)

Values for free erythrocyte protoporphyrin (FEP) and zinc protoporphyrin (ZPP) are 1.2–2.7 µg/g of hemoglobin.

Red Blood Cell Count (B)
Values $\times 10^6/\mu L$.

Age	Males	Females
Newborns	4.2–5.5	3.4–5.4
6 months–2 years	4.1–5.0	4.1–4.9
2–6 years	4.0–4.9	4.0–4.9
6–12 years	4.0–4.9	4.0–4.9
12–18 years	4.2–5.3	4.0–4.9
>18 years	3.8–5.4	3.8–4.8

Sedimentation Rate (Micro) (B)
<2 years: 1–5 mm/hr.
>2 years: 1–8 mm/hr.

Sodium (S, P)
Newborns: 133–146 mmol/L.
Children and adults: 135–148 mmol/L.

Thrombin Time (P)
Children: 12–16 sec.

Thyroid-stimulating Hormone (TSH) (P,S)
Values in $\mu U/mL$.

Age	Males	Females
1–30 days	0.52–16.00	0.72–13.10
1 month–5 years	0.55–7.10	0.46–8.10
6–18 years	0.37–6.00	0.36–5.80

Thyroxine (T_4) (S, P)
Values in $\mu g/dL$ (nmol/L).

Age	Males	Females
1–30 days	5.9–21.5 (76–276)	6.3–21.5 (81–276)
1–12 months	6.4–13.9 (82–179)	4.9–13.7 (63–176)
1–3 years	7.0–13.1 (90–169)	7.1–14.1 (91–180)
4–6 years	6.1–12.6 (79–162)	7.2–14.0 (93–180)
7–12 years	6.7–13.4 (86–172)	6.1–12.1 (79–156)
13–15 years	4.8–11.5 (62–148)	5.8–11.2 (75–144)
16–18 years	5.9–11.5 (76–148)	5.2–13.2 (67–170)

Throxine, "Free" (Free T_4)(S, P)
Newborns: 0.80–2.78 ng/dL (10–36 pmol/L).
1–12 months:
    0.76–2.00 ng/dL (10–26 pmol/L).
1–5 years: 0.90–1.72 ng/dL (12–22 pmol/L).
6–10 years: 0.81–1.68 ng/dL (10–22 pmol/L).
11–15 years:
    0.79–1.57 ng/dL (10–20 pmol/L).
16–18 years:
    0.83–1.53 ng/dL (11–20 pmol/L).

Throxine-binding Globulin (TBG) (P)
1–12 months: 16.2–32.9 mg/L.
1–3 years: 16.4–33.8 mg/L.
4–6 years: 16.6–30.8 mg/L.
7–12 years: 15.0–29.2 mg/L.
13–18 years: 13.4–28.7 mg/L.

Triglycerides (S)
Values in mg/dL (mmol/L).

Age	Males	Females
1–3 years	27–125 (0.31–1.41)	27–125 (0.31–1.41)
4–6 years	32–116 (0.36–1.31)	32–116 (0.36–1.31)
7–9 years	28–129 (0.32–1.46)	28–129 (0.32–1.46)
10–11 years	24–137 (0.27–1.55)	39–140 (0.44–1.58)
12–13 years	24–145 (0.27–1.64)	37–130 (0.42–1.47)
14–15 years	34–165 (0.38–1.86)	38–135 (0.43–1.52)
16–19 years	34–140 (0.38–1.58)	37–140 (0.42–1.58)

Triiodothyronine (T_3) (S)
1–3 days: 89–405 ng/dL.
1 week: 91–300 ng/dL.
1–12 months: 85–250 ng/dL.
Prepubertal children: 119–218 ng/dL.
Pubertal children and adults: 55–170 ng/dL.

Urea Clearance
Premature infants:
    3.5–17.3 mL/min/1.73 m².
Newborns: 8.7–33 mL/min/1.73 m².
2–12 months: 40–95 mL/min/1.73 m².
≥2 years: >52 mL/min/1.73 m².

Urea Nitrogen (S, P)
1–2 years: 5–15 mg/dL (1.8–5.4 mmol/L).
Thereafter: 10–20 mg/dL (3.5–7.1 mmol/L).

Uric Acid (S, P)
Males:
0–14 years: 2–7 mg/dL (119–416 µmol/L).
>14 years: 3–8 mg/dL (178–476 µmol/L).
Females:
All ages: 2–7 mg/dL (119–416 µmol/L).

White Blood Cell Count (B)
Values × 10^3/µL.

Age	Males	Females
Newborns	6.8–13.3	8.0–14.3
6 months–2 years	6.2–14.5	6.4–15.0
2–6 years	5.3–11.5	5.3–11.5
6–12 years	4.5–10.5	4.7–10.3
12–18 years	4.5–10.0	4.8–10.1
>18 years	4.4–10.2	4.9–10.0

NORMAL VALUES: URINE

Addis Count
Red cells (12-hr specimen): <1 million.
White cells (12-hr specimen): <2 million.
Casts (12-hr specimen): <10,000.
Protein (12-hr specimen): <55 mg.

Albumin
First month: 1–100 mg/L.
Second month: 0.2–34 mg/L.
2–12 months: 0.5–19 mg/L.

Ammonia
2–12 months: 4–20 µEq/min/m^2.
1–16 years: 6–16 µEq/min/m^2.

Calcium
4–12 years: 4–8 mEq/L (2–4 mmol/L).

Catecholamines (Norepinephrine, Epinephrine)
Values in µg/24 hr (nmol/24 hr).

Age	Total Cate-cholamines	Norepi-nephrine	Epinephrine
<1 year	20	5.4–15.9 (32–94)	0.1–4.3 (0.5–23.5)
1–5 years	40	8.1–30.8 (48–182)	0.8–9.1 (4.4–49.7)
6–15 years	80	19.0–71.1 (112–421)	1.3–10.5 (7.1–57.3)
>15 years	100	34.4–87.0 (203–514)	3.5–13.2 (19.1–72.1)

Chloride
Infants: 1.7–8.5 mmol/24 hr.
Children: 17–34 mmol/24 hr.
Adults: 140–240 mmol/24 hr.

Corticosteroids (17-Hydroxycorticosteroids)
0–2 years: 2–4 mg/24 hr (5.5–11 µmol).
2–6 years: 3–6 mg/24 hr (8.3–16.6 µmol).
6–10 years:
    6–8 mg/24 hr (16.6–22.1 µmol).
10–14 years: 8–10 mg/24 hr
    (22.1–27.6 mmol).

Creatine
18–58 mg/L (1.37–4.42 mmol/L).

Creatinine
Newborns: 7–10 mg/kg/24 hr.
Children: 20–30 mg/kg/24 hr.
Adult males: 21–26 mg/kg/24 hr.
Adult females: 16–22 mg/kg/24 hr.

Growth Hormone
2.2–13.3 years (Tanner 1): 0.4–6.3 ng/24 hr
    (0.9–12.3 ng/g creatinine).
10.3–14.6 years (Tanner 2): 0.8–12.0 ng/24 hr
    (1.0–14.1 ng/g creatinine).
11.5–15.3 years (Tanner 3): 1.7–20.4 ng/24 hr
    (1.9–17.0 ng/g creatinine).
12.7–17.1 years (Tanner 4): 1.5–18.2 ng/24 hr
    (1.3–14.4 ng/g creatinine).
13.5–19.9 years (Tanner 5): 1.2–14.5 ng/24 hr
    (0.8–11.0 ng/g creatinine).

Homovanillic Acid
Children: 3–16 µg/mg of creatinine.
Adults: 2–4 µg/mg of creatinine.

Mucopolysaccharides

Acid mucopolysaccharide screen should yield negative results. Positive results after dialysis of the urine should be followed up with a thin-layer chromatogram for evaluation of the acid mucopolysaccharide excretion pattern.

Osmolality

Infants: 50–600 mosm/L.
Older children: 50–1400 mosm/L.

Phosphorus, Tubular Reabsorption

78–97%.

Porphyrins

δ-Aminolevulinic acid: 0–7 mg/24 hr (0–53.4 μmol/24 hr).
Porphobilinogen: 0–2 mg/24 hr (0–8.8 μmol/24 hr).
Coproporphyrin: 0–160 μg/24 hr (0–244 nmol/24 hr).
Uroporphyrin: 0–26 μg/24 hr (0–31 nmol/24 hr).

Potassium

26–123 mmol/L.

Sodium

Infants: 0.3–3.5 mmol/24 hr (6–10 mmol/m^2).
Children and adults: 5.6–17 mmol/24 hr.
Specific Gravity 1.010–1.030

Urobilinogen

<3 mg/24 hr (<5.1 μmol/24 hr).

Vanillymandelic Acid (VMA)

Because of the difficulty in obtaining an accurately timed 24-hour collection, values based on microgram per milligram of creatinine are the most reliable indications of VMA excretion in young children.
1–12 months: 1–35 μg/mg of creatinine (31–135 μg/kg/24 hr).
1–2 years: 1–30 μg/mg of creatinine.
2–5 years: 1–15 μg/mg of creatinine.
5–10 years: 1–14 μg/mg of creatinine.
10–15 years: 1–10 μg/mg of creatinine (1–7 mg/24 hr; 5–35 μmol/24hr).
Adults: 1–7 μg/mg of creatinine (1–7 mg/24 hr; 5–35 μmol/24 hr).

NORMAL VALUES: FECES

Fat, Total

2–6 months: 0.3–1.3 g/d.
6 months–1 year: <4 g/d.
Children: <3 g/d.
Adolescents: <5 g/d.
Adults: <7 g/d.

NORMAL VALUES: SWEAT

Electrolytes

Normal: <40 mmol/L for both sodium and chloride.
Patients with cystic fibrosis: >60 mmol/L for both sodium and chloride.

NORMAL VALUES: CEREBROSPINAL FLUID

Protein

Newborns: 40–120 mg/dL.
<1 month: 20–80 mg/dL.
>1 month: 15–45 mg/dL.

Glucose

All ages: 60–80% of blood glucose.

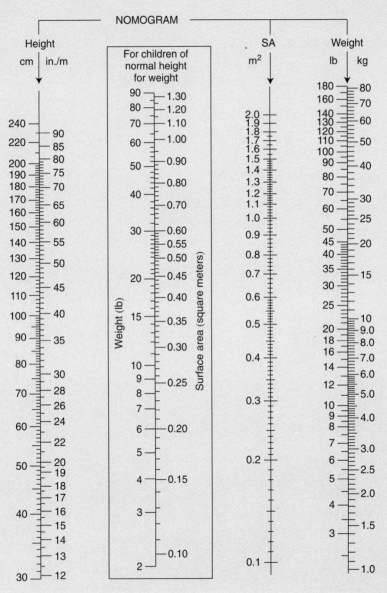

NOMOGRAM

Nomogram modified from data of E. Boyd by C.D. West; from Behrman, R.E., & Vaughan, V.C. (Eds.). (1992). Nelson's textbook of pediatrics (14th ed.). Philadelphia: W.B. Saunders.

West Nomogram for Calculation of Body Surface Area

EXAMPLE

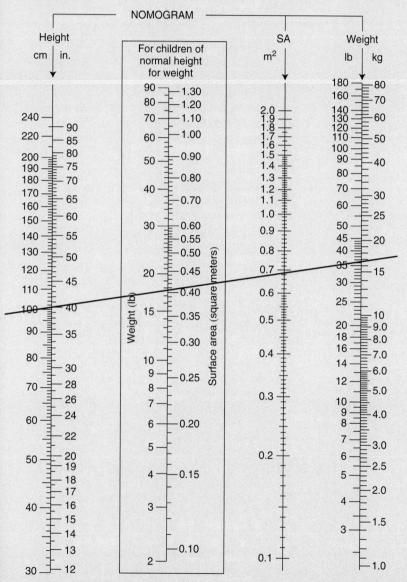

Pediatric doses of medications are generally based on body surface area (BSA) or weight. To calculate a child's BSA, draw a straight line from the height (in the left-hand column) to the weight (in the right-hand column). The point at which the line intersects the surface area (SA) column is the BSA (measured in square meters [m^2]). If the child is of roughly normal proportion, BSA can be calculated from the weight alone (in the enclosed area).

The following formula can then be used to estimate the pediatric drug dose:

$$\frac{\text{BSA of child}}{\text{Mean BSA of adult}} \times \text{Adult dose} = \text{Estimated pediatric dose}$$

►CHAPTER 4
Nursing Considerations for the
Hospitalized Child

Association for the Care of Children's
    Health (ACCH)
19 Mantua Road
Mount Royal, NJ 08061
(609) 224–1742; fax: (609) 423–3420
www.acch.org

Brain Injury Association
105 N. Alfred Street
Alexandria, VA 22314
(703) 236–6000; fax: (703) 236–6001
www.biausa.org

Institute for Family Centered Care
7900 Wisconsin Ave., Suite 405
Bethesda, MD 20814
(301) 652–0281; fax: (301) 652–0186
www.familycenteredcare.org
e-mail: *info@familycenteredcare.org*

►CHAPTER 5
Nursing Considerations for the Child
in the Community

American Academy of Pediatrics
(TIPP injury prevention program and guide-
    lines for primary care)
141 Northwest Point Blvd.
Elk Grove Village, IL 60007–1098
(847) 228–5005; fax: (847) 228–5097
www.aap.org

American Red Cross
(for child health and safety education
    programs)
430 17th Street, N.W.
Washington, DC 20006
(202) 737–8300
www.crossnet.org
e-mail: *usa.redcross.org*

Children's Safety Network
55 Chapel Street
Newton, MA 02160
(617) 969–7100; fax: (617) 244–3436

Emergency Medical Services for Children
    National Resource Center
111 Michigan Ave., N.W.
Washington, DC 20010
(202) 884–4927; fax: (301) 650–8045
www.ems-c.org
e-mail: *info@emscnrc.com*

Family Voices
(parent support for families with children
    with special health care needs)
P.O. Box 769
Algodones, NM 87001
(505) 867–2368; fax: (505) 867–6517
www.FamilyVoices.org
e-mail: *kidshealth@familyvoices.org*

Federation for Children with Special Needs
95 Berkeley Street, #104
Boston, MA 02116
(617) 482–2915; fax: (617) 695-2939
www.fcsn.org
e-mail: *kidinfo@fcsn.org*

National SAFE KIDS Campaign
1301 Pennsylvania Ave., N.W., Suite 1000
Washington, DC 20004–1707
(202) 662–0600; fax: (202) 393–2072
www.safekids.org

►CHAPTER 6
The Child with a Life-threatening
Illness or Injury

Candlelighter's Childhood Cancer
    Foundation
(for parents of children with cancer)
7910 Woodmont Ave., Suite 460
Bethesda, MD 20814
(800) 266–2223
(301) 657–8401; fax: (301) 718–2686
www.candlelighters.org
e-mail: *info@candlelighters.org*

Organizations and Resources

Children's Hospice International
(for care of the terminally ill)
2202 Mt. Vernon Ave., Suite 3C
Alexandria, VA 22301
(800) 242–4453; fax: (703) 684–0226
www.chionline.org
e-mail: *chiorg@aol.com*

The Compassionate Friends
(for bereaved parents)
P.O. Box 3696
Oak Brook, IL 60522–3696
(630) 990–0010; fax: (630) 990–0246
e-mail: *TCF_National@prodigy.com*

The Compassionate Friends
685 Williams Ave.
Winnipeg, Manitoba
Canada R3E 0Z2
e-mail: *TCFLAC@aol.com*

Ronald McDonald Children's Charities
One Kroc Drive
Oak Brook, IL 60523
(630) 623–7048; fax: (630) 623–7488

The Ronald McDonald House
405 E. 73rd Street
New York, NY 10021
(212) 639–0100;
fax (212) 396–2870 or (212) 472–0376
www.rmdh.org/ronald.htm

►CHAPTER 9
Alterations in Immune Function

The American Juvenile Arthritis Organization and The Arthritis Foundation
1330 West Peachtree Street
Atlanta, GA 30309
(800) 283–7800 or (404) 872–7100
www.arthritis.org

Arthritis Society
393 University Ave., Suite 1700
Toronto, Ontario
Canada M5G 1E6
(800) 321–1433
(416) 979–3760; fax: (416) 979–8366
www.arthritis.ca

Canadian Latex Allergy Association
96 Cavan Street
Port Hope, Ontario
Canada L1A 3B7
(905) 885–5270; fax: (905) 885–2839
www.interlog.com/~polar/latex/latex.html

Delaware Valley Latex Allergy Support
  Network, Inc.
P.O. Box 6010
Philadelphia, PA 19114
(800) 528–3966 (LATEX-NO)
(215) 637–6289; fax: (215) 637–2028
www.latex.org

Elizabeth Glaser Pediatric AIDS Foundation
1311 Colorado Ave.
Santa Monica, CA 90404
(310) 395–9051; fax: (310) 395–5149
www.pedaids.org
e-mail: *info@pedaids.org*

The Lupus Foundation of America, Inc.
1300 Piccard Drive, Suite 200
Rockville, MD 20850–4303
(800) 558–0121
(301) 670–9292; fax: (310) 670–9486
http://internet-plaza.net/lupus/

Lupus Foundation of America
17985 Sky Park Circle, Suite J
Irvine, CA 92614
(888) 532–2322
(714) 833–2121; fax: (714) 833–1183

National Institute of Allergy and Infectious
Diseases (NIAID)
(for information about AIDS, allergies, immunology)
NIAID Office of Communications
Bldg. 31, Room 7A–50
31 Center Drive MSC 2520
Bethesda, MD 20892–2520
(301) 496–5717; fax: (301) 402–0120
www.niaid.nih.gov
e-mail: *niaidoc@nih.gov*

National Institute of Arthritis and
Musculoskeletal and Skin Disorders
(NIAMS)
Information Clearinghouse
National Institutes of Health
1 AMS Circle
Bethesda, MD 20892–3675
(301) 495–4484; fax: (301) 587–4352
TTY: (301) 565–2966
www.nih.gov/niams/

National Pediatric and Family HIV Resource
Center
UMDNJ
30 Bergen Street, ADNC #4
Newark, NJ 07103
(800) 362–0071 or (973) 972–0399
www.pedhivaids.org

Pediatric AIDS Canada
269 Juniper Ave.
Burlington, Ontario
Canada L7L 2T5
(905) 631–8818; fax: (905) 631–8819
www.cgocable.net/~pac/
e-mail: *pac@cgocable.net*

►CHAPTER 10
Infectious and Communicable Diseases

American Lyme Disease Foundation, Inc.
Mill Pond Offices
293 Route 100
Somers, NY 10589
(914) 277–6970; fax: (914) 277–6974
www.aldf.com
e-mail: *inquire@aldf.com*

Hepatits B Foundation
700 East Butler Avenue
Doylestown, PA 18901
(215) 489–4900; fax: (215) 489–4920
www.hepb.org
e-mail: *info@hepb.org*

Immunization Action Coalition
1573 Selby Ave., Suite 229
St. Paul, MN 55104–6328
(612) 647–9009; fax: (612) 647–9131
www.immunize.org
e-mail: *mail@immunize.org*

National Immunization Program
Centers for Disease Control and Prevention
1600 Clifton Road
Atlanta, GA 30333
(800) CDC–SHOT
www.cdc.gov/nip/default.htm

National Institute of Allergy and Infectious
Diseases (NIAID)
(for information about AIDS, allergies, immunology)
NIAID Office of Communications
Bldg. 31, Room 7A–50
31 Center Drive MSC 2520
Bethesda, MD 20892–2520
(301) 496–5717; fax: (301) 402–0120
www.niaid.nih.gov
e-mail: *niaidoc@nih.gov*

►CHAPTER 11
Alterations in Respiratory Function

Allergy and Asthma Network/Mothers of
Asthmatics, Inc.
2751 Prosperity Ave., Suite 150
Fairfax, VA 22031
(800) 878–4403
(703) 573–7782; fax: 573–7794
www.nma.org
e-mail: *aanma@aol.com*

Asthma and Allergy Foundation of America
1125 15th Street, N.W., Suite 502
Washington, DC 20005
(800) 7–ASTHMA (US only)
(202) 466–7643; fax: (202) 466–8940
www.aafa.org

American Lung Association
1740 Broadway, 14th Floor
New York, NY 10019–4374
(800) LUNG–USA or (212) 315–8700
www.lungusa.org

Canadian Cystic Fibrosis Foundation
2221 Young Street, Suite 601
Toronto, Ontario
Canada M4S 2B4
(800) 378–2233 (Canada)
(416) 485–9149; fax: (416) 485–0960
www.ccff.ca/~cfwww/index.html
e-mail: *info@ccff.ca*

Canadian Lung Association
75 Albert Street, Suite 908
Ottawa, Ontario
Canada K1P 5E7
(613) 237–1208

Council of Guilds for Infant Survival
(has 12 guilds in 7 states)
2724 Scott Street
Davenport, IA 52803
(319) 322–4870; fax: (319) 322–4870

Cystic Fibrosis Foundation
6931 Arlington Road, Suite 200
Bethesda, MD 20814
(800) FIGHT–CF
(301) 951–4422; fax: (301) 951–6378
http://208.196.156.141/
e-mail: *info@cff.org*

Food Allergy Network
10400 Eaton Place, Suite 107
Fairfax, VA 22030–2208
(703) 691–3179; fax: (703) 691–2713
www.foodallergy.org
e-mail: *fan@worldweb.net*

The Lung Association
365 Bloor Street East, Suite 601
Toronto, Ontario
Canada M4W 3L4
(416) 922–9440; fax: (416) 922–9430

National Asthma Education & Prevention
    Program
P.O. Box 30105
Bethesda, MD 20824–0105
(301) 251–1222; fax: (301) 251–1223
www.nhlbi.nih.gov/nhlbi/nhlbi.htm

National SIDS Resource Center
2070 Chain Bridge Road, Suite 450
Vienna, VA 22181
(703) 821–8955; fax: (703) 821–2098
www.circsol.com/SIDS
e-mail: *info@circsol.com*

National SHARE (Source of Help in Airing
    and Resolving Experiences) Office
St. Joseph Health Center
300 First Capitol Drive
St. Charles, MO 63301–2893
(800) 821–6819
(314) 947–6164; fax: (314) 947–7486
www.NationalSHAREOffice.com

SIDS Alliance
1314 Bedford Ave., Suite 210
Baltimore, MD 21208
(800) 221–7437; fax: (410) 653–8709

SIDS Network
P.O. Box 520
Ledyard, CT 06339
http://sids-network.org

►CHAPTER 12
Alterations in Cardiovascular Function

American Heart Association
7272 Greenville Ave.
Dallas, TX 75231
(800) 242–8721
(214) 706–1179; fax: (214) 706–2139
www.americanheart.org

National Heart, Lung and Blood Institute
NHLBI Information Center
P.O. Box 30105
Bethesda, MD 20824–0105
(301) 251–1222; fax: (301) 251–1223
www.nhlbi.nih.gov/nhlbi/nhlbi.htm

►**CHAPTER 13**
Alterations in Hematologic Function

Aplastic Anemia Foundation of America
P.O. Box 613
Annapolis, MD 21404–0613
(800) 747–2820
(410) 867–0242; fax: (410) 867–0240
www.aplastic.org
e-mail: *aafacenter@aol.com*

Bone Marrow Transplant Family Support
    Network
P.O. Box 845
Avon, CT 06001
(800) 826–9376

Canadian Hemophilia Society
625 President Kennedy, Suite 1210
Montreal, Quebec
CANADA H3A 1K2
(800) 668–2686
(514) 848–0503; fax: (514) 848–9661
e-mail: *chs@odyssee.net*

Cooley's Anemia Foundation and
    Thalassemia Action Group
129–09 26th Ave., #203
Flushing, NY 11354
(800) 522–7222
(718) 321–2873; fax: (718) 321–3340
www.thalassemia.org
e-mail: *ncaf@aol.com*

Sickle Cell Disease Association of America
200 Corporate Point, Suite 495
Culver City, CA 90230–7633
(310) 216–6363; fax: (310) 215–3722
e-mail: *lascdaa@aol.com*

National Hemophilia Foundation
116 West 32nd Street, 11th Floor
New York, NY 10001
(212) 328–3700; fax: (212) 328–3777
www.infohf.org
e-mail: *info@hemophilia.org*

Sickle Cell Association of Ontario
3199 Bathurst Street, Suite 202
Toronto, Ontario
CANADA M6A 2B2
(416) 789–2855; fax: (416) 789–1903

Sickle Cell Information Center
P.O. Box 109
Grady Memorial Hospital
80 Butler Street
Atlanta, GA 30335
(404) 616–3572; fax: (404) 616–5998
www.emory.edu/PEDS/SICKLE/

►**CHAPTER 14**
Alterations in Cellular Growth

American Amputee Foundation
P.O. Box 250218
Hillcrest Station
Little Rock, AR 72225
(501) 666–2523; fax: (501) 666–8367

American Cancer Society
1599 Clifton Road, N.E.
Atlanta, GA 30329
(800) ACS–2345
www.cancer.org

American Red Cross
(for child health and safety education
    programs)
430 17th Street, N.W.
Washington, DC 20006
(202) 737–8300
www.crossnet.org
e-mail: *usa.redcross.org*

Brain Tumor Foundation for Children, Inc.
2231 Perimeter Park Drive, Suite 9
Atlanta, GA 39341
(770) 458–5554; fax: (770) 458–5467
e-mail: *eallman1@juno.com*

Candlelighter's Childhood Cancer Family
    Alliance
705 Balmoral Court
Friendswood, TX 77546
(218) 996–1174
http://candle.org
e-mail: *candle@cois.com*

Candlelighter's Childhood Cancer
    Foundation
(for parents of children with cancer)
7910 Woodmont Ave., Suite 460
Bethesda, MD 20814
(800) 266–2223
(301) 657–8401; fax: (301) 718–2686
www.candlelighters.org
e-mail: *info@candlelighters.org*

Children's Leukemia Research Association, Inc.
585 Stewart Ave., Suite 536
Garden City, NY 11530
(516) 222–1944; fax: (516) 222–0457

Make a Wish Foundation
100 West Clarendon, Suite 2200
Phoenix, AZ 85013
(800) 722–WISH; fax: (602) 279–0855
www.wish.org

National Cancer Institute of the NIH
Pediatric Oncology Branch
Bldg. 10, Room 13N240
Bethesda, MD 20892–1928
(301) 402–0696; fax: (301) 402–0575
cancernet.nci.nih.gov/pedpage/pedbrhome.html

National Childhood Cancer Foundation
440 E. Huntington Drive, Suite 300
P.O. Box 60012
Arcadia, CA 91066–6012
(800) 458–6223; fax: (800) 723–2822
www.nccf.org

National Kidney Cancer Association
1234 Sherman Ave.
Evanston, IL 60202
(847) 332–1051; fax: (847) 332–2978
www.nkca.org
e-mail: *office@nkca.org*

St. Jude's Children's Research Hospital
322 N. Lauderdale Street
Memphis, TN 38105
(901) 495–3300
www.stjude.org

►CHAPTER 15
Alterations in Gastrointestinal Function

American Celiac Society
58 Musano Court
West Orange, NJ 07052
(973) 325–8837; fax: (973) 669–8808

American Cleft Palate-Craniofacial
  Association (ACPA) and Cleft Palate
  Foundation (CPF)
1829 East Franklin Street, Suite 1022
Chapel Hill, NC 27514
(800) 242–5338 (hotline)
(919) 933–0944; fax: (919) 933–9604
www.cleft.com

American Liver Foundation
1425 Pompton Ave.
Cedar Grove, NJ 07009
(800) 465–4837
(888) 443–7222; fax: (973) 256–3214
www.liverfoundation.org

American Pseudo-obstruction &
  Hirschsprung's Disease
158 Pleasant Street
North Andover, MA 01845–2797
(978) 685–4477; fax: (978) 685–4488
e-mail: *aphs@mail.tiac.net*

Canadian Celiac Association, Inc.
Britannia Road East, Unit 11
Mississauga, Ontario
CANADA L4Z 1W6
(800) 363–7296
(905) 507–6208; fax: (905) 507–4673

Canadian Foundation for Ileitis and Colitis
21 St. Clair Ave. E., Suite 301
Toronto, Ontario
CANADA M4T 1L9
(800) 387–1479
(416) 920–5035; fax: (416) 929–0364
www.ccfc.ca

Celiac Disease Foundation
13251 Ventura Blvd., Suite 1
Studio City, CA 91604–1838
(818) 990–2354; fax: (818) 990–2379
www.celiac.org/cdf
e-mail: *cdf@primenet.com*

Celiac Sprue Association USA, Inc.
P.O. Box 31700
Omaha, NE 68131–0700
(402) 558–0600; fax: (402) 558–1347
www.csaceliacs.org
e-mail: *celiacs@csaceliacs.org*

Children's Memorial Hospital
2300 Children's Plaza
Chicago, IL 60614
(773) 880–4000

Crohn's and Colitis Foundation of
   America, Inc.
386 Park Ave. South, 17th Floor
New York, NY 10016–8804
(800) 932–2423
(212) 685–3440; fax: (212) 779–4098
www.ccfa.org
e-mail: *info@ccfa.org*

Food Allergy Network
10400 Eaton Place, Suite 107
Fairfax, VA 22030–2208
(703) 691–3179; fax: (703) 691–2713
www.foodallergy.org
e-mail: *fan@worldweb.net*

Gluten Intolerance Group of North America
P.O. Box 23053
Seattle, WA 98102–0353
(206) 325–6980; fax: (206) 320–1172
e-mail: *gig@accessone.com*

International Foundation for Functional
   GI Disorders
P.O. Box 17864
Milwaukee, WI 53217
(888) 964–2001
(414) 964–1799; fax: (414) 964–7176
www.execpc.com/iffgd
e-mail: *iffgd@execpc.com*

National SAFE KIDS Campaign
1301 Pennsylvania Ave., N.W., Suite 1000
Washington, DC 20004–1707
(202) 662–0600; fax: (202) 393–2072
www.safekids.org

Pediatric/Adolescent Gastroesophagel
   Reflux Association, Inc. (PAGER)
P.O. Box 1153
Germantown, MD 20875–1153
(301) 601–9541
www.reflux.org
e-mail: *GERGROUP@aol.com*

Pediatric Crohn's and Colitis Association,
   Inc.
P.O. Box 188
Newton, MA 02168
(617) 489–5854

TEF/VATER Support Network
15301 Grey Fox Road
Upper Marlboro, MD 20772
(301) 952–6837; fax: (301) 952–6837

United Ostomy Association, Inc.
19772 MacArthur Blvd., Suite 200
Irvine, CA 92612–2405
(800) 826–0826
(949) 660–8624; fax: (949) 660–9262
www.uoa.org

United Ostomy Association, Canada
4 Hamilton Ave.
Hamilton, Ontario
CANADA L8V 2S3

►CHAPTER 16
Alterations in Genitourinary Function

American Association of Kidney Patients
100 South Ashley Drive, Suite 280
Tampa, FL 33602
(800) 749–2257
(813) 223–7099; fax: (813) 223–0001
http://cybermart.com/aakpaz/aakp.html

Children's Organ Transplant Association
2501 Cota Drive
Bloomington, IN 47403
(800) 366–2682
(812) 336–8872; fax: (812) 336–8885

Hereditary Nephritis Foundation
P.O. Box 57294
Murray, UT 84107
(801) 581–7818

Kidney Foundation of Canada
5 Sherbrooke West, Suite 300
Montreal, Quebec
CANADA H4A 1T6
(800) 361–7494
(514) 369–4806; fax: (514) 369–2472

National Kidney Foundation
30 E. 33rd Street
New York, NY 10016
(800) 622–9010
(212) 889–2210; fax: (212) 689–9261
www.kidney.org

National Kidney & Urologic Diseases Information Clearinghouse
3 Information Way
Bethesda, MD 20892–3560
(301) 654–4415; fax:(301) 907–8906
www.niddk.nih.gov
e-mail: *nkudic@info.niddk.nih.gov*

Polycystic Kidney Research Fund
4901 Main Street, Suite 200
Kansas City, MO 64112–2634
(800) PKD–CURE
(816) 931–2600; fax: (816) 931–8655
www.kumc.edu/pkrf/

Transplant Foundation
8002 Discovery Drive, Suite 310
Richmond, VA 23229
(804) 285–5115; fax: (804) 288–2408

United Network for Organ Sharing (UNOS)
1100 Boulders Parkway, Suite 500
Richmond, VA 23225–8770
(800) 24–DONOR
(804) 330–8500; fax: (804) 330–8507
www.unos.org

►CHAPTER 17
Alterations in Eye, Ear, Nose, and Throat
Function

American Council of the Blind
1155 15th Street, N.W., Suite 720
Washington, DC 20005
(800) 424–8666
(202) 467–5081; fax: (202) 467–5085
www.acb.org

American Speech-Language-Hearing
    Association
10801 Rockville Pike
Rockville, MD 20852
(800) 498–2071 or (301) 897–5700;
(301) 571–0457 (TTY); fax: (301) 897–0157
www.asha.org

Canadian Hearing Society
271 Spadina Road
Toronto, Ontario
CANADA M5R 2V3
(416) 964–9595; fax: (416) 928–2506
www.chs.ca
e-mail: *inf@chs*

Canadian National Institute for the Blind
1931 Bayview Ave.
Toronto, Ontario
CANADA M4G 3E8
(416) 486–2500; fax: (416) 480–7503
www.cnib.ca

Institute for Families of Blind Children
P.O. Box 54700, Mailstop 111
Los Angeles, CA 90054–0700
(213) 669–4649; fax: (213) 665–7869

Low Vision Association of Canada
263 Russell Hill Road, Suite 101
Toronto, Ontario
CANADA M4V 2T4
(416) 921–6609; fax: (416) 921–6085

National Association of the Deaf
814 Thayer Ave.
Silver Spring, MD 20910–4500
(301) 587–1788
fax: (301) 587–1791 (TTY); (301) 587–1789
www.nad.org
e-mail: *NADH@juno.com*

National Association for Parents of the
    Visually Impaired
2011 Hardy Circle
Austin, TX 78757

National Federation of the Blind
1800 Johnson Street
Baltimore, MD 21230
(410) 659–9314
www.nfb.org

National Institute on Deafness and Other
    Communication Disorders (NIDCD)
NICDC Information Clearinghouse
1 Communication Ave.
Bethesda, MD 20892–3456
(800) 241–1044
fax: (301) 907–8830; TTY: (800) 241–1055
www.nih.gov/nidcd
e-mail: *nidcd@aerie.com*

National Society to Prevent Blindness
500 E. Remington Road
Schaumburg, IL 60173
(800) 331–2020
(847) 843–2020; fax: (847) 843–8458
www.preventblindess.org

►CHAPTER 18
Alterations in Neurologic Function

Brain Injury Association, Inc.
105 North Alfred Street
Alexandria, VA 23314
(703) 236–6000; fax: (703) 236–6001
www.biausa.org

Epilepsy Canada
1470 Peel Street, Suite 745
Montreal, Quebec
CANADA H3A 1T1
(514) 845–7855; fax: (514) 845–7866

Epilepsy Foundation of America
4351 Garden City Drive
Landover, MD 20785–2265
(800) 332–1000
(301) 459–3700; fax: (301) 577–2684
www.EFA.org

National Easter Seal Society
230 West Monroe Street, Suite 1800
Chicago, IL 60606
(800) 221–6827
(312) 726–6200; fax: (312) 726–1494
www.easter-seals.org

National Hydrocephalus Foundation
12413 Centralia
Lakewood, CA 90715
(562) 402–3523; fax: (562) 924–6666

Ontario Federation for Cerebral Palsy
1630 Lawrence Ave. West, Suite 104
Toronto, Ontario
CANADA M6L 1C5
(416) 244–9686; fax: (416) 244–6543

Spina Bifida Association of America
4590 MacArthur Blvd., N.W. Suite 250
Washington, DC 20007–4226
(800) 621–3141
(202) 944–3285; fax: (202) 944–3295
sbaa.org
e-mail: *spinabifda@aol.com*

United Cerebral Palsy Association, Inc.
1660 L Street, N.W., Suite 700
Washington, DC 20036
(800) 872–5827; fax: (800) 766–0414
www.UCPA.ORG
e-mail: *ucpnatl@ucpa.org*

U.S. Cerebral Palsy Athletic Association
200 Harrison Ave.
Newport, RI 02840
(401) 848–2460; fax: (401) 848–5280
www.wucpaa.org

►CHAPTER 19
Alterations in Musculoskeletal Function

International Federation of Spine Association
9908 Cape Scott Court
Raleigh, NC 27614–9025
(919) 846–2204
www.ifosa.org

Muscular Dystrophy Association of America
3300 East Sunrise Drive
Tucson, AZ 85718
(800) 572–1717
www.mdausa.org
e-mail: *mda@mdausa.org*

Muscular Dystrophy Association of Canada
2345 Yonge Street, Suite 900
Toronto, Ontario
Canada M4P 2E5
(800) 567–2873
(416) 488–0030; fax: (416) 488–7523

National Scoliosis Foundation
5 Cabot Place
Stoughton, MA 02072
(800) 673–6922
(781) 341–6333; fax: (781) 341–8333
e-mail: *scoliosis@aol.com*

Osteogenesis Imperfecta Foundation, Inc.
(OIF)
804 W. Diamond Ave., Suite 204
Gaithersburg, MD 20878
(800) 981–2663
(301) 947–0083; fax: (301) 947–0456
www.oif.org

Scoliosis Association, Inc.
P.O. Box 811705
Boca Raton, FL 33481–1705
(800) 800–0669; fax: (561) 914–2455

Scoliosis Research Society
6300 N. River Road, Suite 727
Rosemont, IL 60018–4226
(847) 698–1627; fax: (847) 923–0536
http://srs.org
e-mail: *goulding@aaos.org*

Shriners Hospitals
2900 Rocky Point Drive
Tampa, FL 33607–1435
(800) 237–5055 (USA)
(813) 281–0300; (800) 361–7256 (Canada)
www.shrinershq.org/Hospitals

►CHAPTER 20
Alterations in Endocrine Function

Alliance of Genetic Support Groups
4301 Connecticut Ave., N.W., Suite 404
Washington, DC 20008–2304
(800) 336–GENE or (301) 652–5553
http://medhelp.org/geneticalliance
e-mail: *info@geneticalliance.org*

American Diabetes Association, Inc.
1660 Duke St.
Alexandria, VA 22314
(800) 232–3472
(703) 549–1500; fax: (703) 549–6995
www.diabetes.org

American Dietetic Association
216 W. Jackson Blvd.
Chicago, IL 60606–6995
(800) 877–1600
(312) 899–0040; fax: (312) 899–1979
www.eatright.org

Canadian Diabetes Association
15 Toronto Street, Suite 800
Toronto, Ontario
Canada M5C 2E3
(800) 266–8464
(416) 363–3373; fax: (416) 214–1899

Children's PKU Network
1520 State Street, Suite 240
San Diego, CA 92101
(619) 233–3202; fax: (619) 233–0838

Human Growth Foundation
7777 Leesburg Pike, Suite 202 South
Falls Church, VA 22043
(800) 451–6434
(703) 883–1773; fax: (703) 883–1776
www.genetic.org/hgf
e-mail: *hgfound@erols.com*

Juvenile Diabetes Foundation and the
  Diabetes Research Foundation
120 Wall Street
New York, NY 10005–4001
(800) JDF–CURE
(212) 785–9500; fax: (212) 785–9595
www.jdfcure.org

Little People of America
P.O. Box 745
Lubbock, TX 79408
(888) LPA–2001; fax: (806) 829–2160
www-bfs.ucsd.edu/dwarfism

March of Dimes Birth Defects Foundation
1275 Mamaroneck Ave.
White Plains, NY 10605
(800) 663–4637; fax: (914) 997–4764
www.modimes.org

Metabolic Information Network
P.O. Box 670847
Dallas, TX 75367–0847
(800) 945–2188
(214) 696–2188; fax: (800) 955–3258
e-mail: *mizesg@ix.netcom.com*

National Diabetes Information Clearinghouse
1 Information Way
Bethesda, MD 20892–3560
(301) 654–3327; fax: (301) 907–8906
e-mail: *ndic@infor.niddk.nih.gov*

National Graves Disease Foundation
2 Tsitsi Court
Brevard, NC 28712
(704) 877–5251
www.ngdf.org

National Organization for Rare Disorders
P.O. Box 8923
New Fairfield, CT 06812–8923
(800) 999–6673
(203) 746–6518; fax: (203) 746–6481
www.NORD–RDB.com/~orphan/

National PKU News
6869 Woodlawn Ave., N.E., Suite 116
Seattle, WA 98115
(206) 525–8140; fax: (203) 525–5023
e-mail: *schuett@pkunews.org*

Short Stature Foundation
P.O. Box 5356
Huntington Beach, CA 92615
(800) 24–DWARF (help line)

Thyroid Foundation of America, Inc.
350 Ruth Sleeper Hall – RSL 350
Parkman Street
Boston, MA 02114–2690
(800) 832–8321
(617) 726–8500; fax: (617) 726–4136
www.clark.net/pub/tfa
e-mail: *tfa@clark.net*

Turner Syndrome Society
1313 Southeast 5th Street, Suite 327
Minneapolis, MN 55414
(800) 365–9944; fax: (612) 379–3619
www.turner-syndrome-us.org

Turner Syndrome Society of Canada
814 Glencairn Ave.
Toronto, Ontario
Canada M6B 2A3
(800) 465–6744
(416) 781–2086; fax: (416) 781–7245
e-mail: *tssincan@web.net*

▶CHAPTER 21
Alterations in Skin Integrity

American Burn Association
625 N. Michigan Ave., Suite 1530
Chicago, IL 60611
(800) 548–2876
(312) 642–9260; fax: (312) 642–9130

Skin Phototrauma Foundation
P.O. Box 6312
Parsippany, NJ 07054

▶CHAPTER 22
Alterations in Psychosocial Function

Al-Anon
Ala-Teen
Alcoholics Anonymous
(check Yellow Pages under Health Agencies or Social
    Services)

American Anorexia and Bulimia Association, Inc.
165 West 46th Street, Suite 1108
New York, NY 10036
(212) 575–6200; fax: (212) 278–0698
members.aol.com/amanbu
e-mail: *amanbu@aol.com*

The Arc of the United States
(formerly Association for Retarded Citizens)
500 E. Border Street, Suite 300
Arlington, TX 76010
(800) 433–5255 or (817) 261–6003;
fax: (817) 277–3491; TDD (817) 277–0553
www.thearc.org
e-mail: *thearc@metronet.com*

Autism Society of America
7910 Woodmont Ave., Suite 650
Bethesda, MD 20814–3015
(800) 3AUTISM
(301) 657–0881; fax: (301) 657–0869

Canadian Down Syndrome Society
811–14 Street, N.W.
Calgary, Alberta
Canada T2N 2A4
(800) 883–5608 Canada
(403) 270–8500; fax: (403) 270–8291
http://home.ican.net/~cdss
e-mail: *cdss@ican.net*

Children and Adults with Attention Deficit Disorders
499 Northwest 70th Ave., Suite 101
Plantation, FL 33317
(800) 233–4050
(954) 587–3700; fax: (954) 587–4599
www.chadd.org

Cyclic Vomiting Syndrome Association
13180 Caroline Court
Elm Grove, WI 53122
(414) 784–6842; fax: (414) 821–5494
www.breaker.iupui.edu/cvsa

Learning Disabilities Association of America
4156 Library Road
Pittsburgh, PA 15234–1349
(412) 341–1515; fax: (412) 344–0224
www.ldanatl.org
e-mail: *ldanatl@usaor.net*

Nar-Anon
Narcotics Anonymous
(check Yellow Pages under Health Agencies or Social
    Services)

National Anorectic Aid Society, Inc.
1925 E. Dublin-Granville Road
Columbus, OH 43229
(614) 436–1112

National Association of Anorexia Nervosa &
    Associated Disorders, Inc.
Box 7
Highland Park, IL 60035
(847) 831–3438; fax: (847) 433–4632
members.aol.com/anad20/index.html

National Attention Deficit Disorder Association
9930 Johnnycake Ridge Road, Suite 3E
Mentor, OH 44064
(800) 487–2282
(440) 350–9595; fax: (440) 350–0223
www.add.org
e-mail: *NatlADDA@aol.com*

National Clearinghouse for Alcohol and Drug
    Information
P.O. Box 2345
Rockville, MD 20847–2345
(800) 729–6686 or (301) 468–2600
(800) 487–4899 (Spanish); fax: (301) 468–6433
http://naswi.health.org/

National Clearinghouse on Child Abuse and Neglect
P.O. Box 1182
Washington, DC 20013–1182
(800) 394–3366
(703) 385–7565; fax: (703) 385–3206
www.calib.com/nccanch/
e-mail: *nccanch@calib.com*

National Committee to Prevent Child Abuse
200 S. Michigan Ave., 17th Floor
Chicago, IL 60604
(312) 663–3520; fax: (312) 939–8962
www.childabuse.org

National Down Syndrome Society
666 Broadway, 8th Floor
New York, NY 10012–2317
(800) 221–4602
(212) 460–9330; fax: (212) 979–2873
www.ndss.org
e-mail: *info@ndss.org*

Public Information Office
National Council on Alcoholism and Drug
    Dependence, Inc.
12 West 21st Street
New York, NY 10010
(800) 622–2255
(212) 206–6770; fax: (212) 645–1690
www.ncadd.org
e-mail: *national@ncadd.org*

accommodation The process of changing one's cognitive structures to include data from recent experiences.

acellular vaccine A vaccine that uses proteins from the microorganism rather than the whole cell to stimulate the process of active immunity.

acidemia Decreased blood pH.

acidosis Condition caused by excess acid in the blood.

active immunity Stimulation of antibody production without causing clinical disease.

acute pain Sudden pain of short duration, associated with a tissue-damaging stimulus.

adaptive functioning The ability of an individual to meet the standards expected for his or her age by his or her cultural group.

advance directives A patient's living will or appointed durable power of attorney for health care decisions.

adventitious Breath sounds that are not normally heard, such as crackles and rhonchi.

affect Outward manifestation of feeling or emotion; the tone of a person's reaction or response to people or events.

airway resistance The effort or force needed to move oxygen through the trachea to the lungs.

alkalemia Increased blood pH.

alkalosis Condition caused by too little acid in the blood.

allergen An antigen capable of inducing hypersensitivity.

alveolar hypoventilation The condition in which the volume of air entering the alveoli during gas exchange is inadequate to meet the body's metabolic needs.

anemia Reduction in the number of red blood cells, the quantity of hemoglobin, and the volume of packed red cells per 100 mL of blood to below-normal levels.

antibody A protein capable of reacting to a specific antigen.

anticipatory guidance The process of understanding upcoming developmental needs and then teaching caretakers to meet those needs.

antigen A foreign substance that triggers an immune system response.

anxiolysis Sedation by medication.

apnea Cessation of respiration lasting longer than 20 seconds.

areflexia No reflex response to verbal, sensory, or pain stimulation.

assent Voluntary agreement to participate in a research project or to accept treatment.

assessment The process of collecting information about a child and family to develop the nursing diagnoses. The assessment process includes the patient history, physical examination, and analysis of the collected data to identify relevant information.

assimilation The process of incorporating new experiences into one's cognitive awareness.

associative play A type of play that emerges in preschool years when children interact with one another, engaging in similar activities and participating in groups.

atopy A hereditary allergic tendency.

audiography A test used to assess hearing in which sounds of various pitches and intensity are presented to children through earphones.

aura Subjective sensation, often olfactory or visual in nature, that is an early sign of a seizure.

auscultation The technique of listening to sounds produced by the airway, lungs, stomach, heart, and blood vessels to identify their characteristics. Auscultation is usually performed with the stethoscope to enhance the sounds heard.

azotemia Accumulation of nitrogenous wastes in the blood.

behavior modification A technique used to reinforce desirable behaviors, helping the child to replace maladaptive behaviors with more appropriate ones.

benign A growth that does not endanger life or health.

binocularity Ability of the eyes to function together.

biotherapy Use of biologic response modifiers to treat cancer.

body fluid Body water that has substances (solutes) dissolved in it.

buffer Related acid–base pair that gives up or takes up hydrogen ions as needed to prevent large changes in the pH of a solution.

carcinogens Chemicals or processes that, when combined with genetic traits and in interaction with one another, cause cancer.

case manager Person who coordinates health care to prevent gaps or overlaps.

cephalocaudal development The process by which development proceeds from the head downward through the body and toward the feet.

cerebral edema Increase in intracellular and extracellular fluid in the brain that results from anoxia, vasodilation, or vascular stasis.

cerebral perfusion pressure Amount of pressure needed to ensure that adequate oxygen and nutrients will be delivered to the brain.

chemotherapy Treatment to combat cancer that involves drugs taken orally, intravenously, intrathecally, or by injection, which kill both normal and cancerous cells.

child life specialist Trained professional who plans therapeutic activities for hospitalized children.

child sexual abuse The exploitation of a child for the sexual gratification of an adult.

cholestasis Disruption of bile flow.

chondrolysis The breaking down and absorption of cartilage.

chronic condition A health condition that lasts or is expected to last 3 months or more.

chronic pain Persistent pain lasting longer than 6 months, generally associated with a prolonged disease process.

clinical judgment Analyzing and synthesizing data from the patient history, physical examination, screening tests, and laboratory studies to make decisions about the child's health problems. This is also called diagnostic reasoning.

clonic Alternating muscular contraction and relaxation; often used to describe seizure activity.

cognitive therapy A therapeutic approach that attempts to help the person recognize automatic thought patterns that lead to unpleasant feelings.

collective monologue A type of speech demonstrated when two people talk about separate subjects, wait for each other to speak, and do not respond to each other's topics; common during preschool years.

coma State of unconsciousness in which the child cannot be aroused, even with powerful stimuli.

communicable disease An illness that is transmitted directly or indirectly from one person to another.

compliance Amount of distention or expansion the ventricles can achieve to increase stroke volume.

conductive hearing loss Hearing loss caused by inadequate conduction of sound from the outer to the middle ear.

confusion Disorientation to time, place, or person.

conscious sedation Light sedation during which the child maintains airway reflexes and responds to verbal stimuli.

conservation The knowledge that matter is not changed when its form is altered.

constipation Difficult and infrequent defecation with passage of hard, dry stool.

continuity of care An interdisciplinary process of facilitating a patient's transition between and among settings based on changing needs and available resources.

continuum of care A system of care that includes each of the following elements: primary care, illness or injury prevention, acute care in the hospital, and restorative care in either the home or a rehabilitation center until the patient is reintegrated into family and community.

cooperative play A type of play that emerges in school years when children join into groups to achieve a goal or play a game.

critical pathways Comprehensive interdisciplinary care plans for a specific condition that describe the sequence and timing of interventions that should result in desired patient outcomes.

Cushing's triad Reflex response associated with increased intracranial pressure or compromised blood flow to the brainstem; characterized by hypertension, increased systolic pressure with wide pulse pressure, bradycardia, and irregular respirations.

deamination Removal of an amino group from an amino compound.

death anxiety A feeling of apprehension or fear of death.

death imagery Any reference to death or death-related topics, such as going away, separation, funerals, and dying, given in response to a picture or story that would not usually stimulate other children to discuss death-related topics.

debridement Enzyme action to clean a lesion and dissolve fibrin clots or scabs; or removal of dead tissue to speed the healing process.

decibels Units used to measure the loudness of sounds.

deep sedation A controlled state of depressed consciousness or unconsciousness in which the child may experience partial or complete loss of protective reflexes.

defense mechanisms Techniques used by the ego to unconsciously change reality, thereby protecting itself from excessive anxiety.

dehydration The state of body water deficit.

delirium State characterized by confusion, fear, agitation, hyperactivity, or anxiety.

dermatophytoses Fungal infections that affect primarily the skin but may affect the hair and nails.

desaturated blood Blood with a lower than normal oxygen level resulting when a heart defect causes oxygenated and unoxygenated blood to mix.

development An increase in capability or function.

developmental surveillance A continuous process of skilled observations of a child's fine and gross motor, language, and psychosocial behavior milestones throughout encounters during child health visits.

dialysate The solution used in dialysis.

diarrhea Frequent passage of abnormally watery stool.

digitalization Process of giving a higher than normal dose of digoxin initially to speed response to the drug.

direct transmission The passage of an infectious disease through physical contact between the source of the pathogen and a new host.

disability Impairment in one or more of five categories of function—cognition, communication, motor abilities, social abilities, or patterns of interactions.

dislocation Displacement of a bone from its normal articulation with a joint.

distraction The ability to focus attention on something other than pain, such as an activity, music, or a story.

dramatic play A type of play in which a child acts out the drama of daily life.

dysphonia Muffled, hoarse, or absent voice sounds.

dysplasia Abnormal development resulting in altered size, shape, and cell organization.

dyspnea Shortness of breath; difficulty in breathing.

ecchymosis A bruise.

effective communication Information exchanged among the nurse, parent, and child that is clearly understood by all persons involved in the conversation.

electroanalgesia A method of delivering electrical stimulation to the skin, to compete with pain stimuli for transmission to the spinal cord; also known as transcutaneous electrical nerve stimulation (TENS).

electrolytes Charged particles (ions) dissolved in body fluid.

emancipated minors Self-supporting adolescents under 18 years of age not subject to parental control.

emotional abuse Shaming, ridiculing, embarrassing, or insulting a child.

emotional neglect A caretaker's unavailability to meet the psychosocial needs of a child.

encephalopathy Cerebral dysfunction resulting from an insult (toxin, injury, inflammation, or anoxic event) of limited duration; the tissue damage is often permanent, but the dysfunction may improve over time.

end-stage renal disease Irreversible kidney failure.

enuresis Involuntary micturition by a child who has reached the age at which bladder control is expected.

equianalgesic dose The amount of a drug, whether administered orally or parenterally, needed to produce the same analgesic effect.

equinus A condition that limits dorsiflexion to less than normal; usually associated with clubfoot.

erythropoiesis Formation of red blood cells.

eschar Slough or layer of dead skin or tissue.

escharotomy Incision into constricting dead tissue of a burn injury to restore peripheral circulation.

expressive jargon Use of unintelligible words with normal speech intonations as if truly communicating in words; common in toddlerhood.

extracellular fluid The fluid in the body that is outside the cells.

extravasation Damage that occurs when a chemotherapeutic drug leaks into the soft tissue surrounding the infusion site.

family-centered care A philosophy of care that integrates the family's values and potential contributions in the plans for and provision of care to the child.

family crisis An event occurring when a family encounters problems that for a time seem insurmountable and with which the family is unable to cope in its usual ways.

filtration Movement into or out of capillaries as the net result of several opposing forces.

focal Specific area of the brain; often used to describe seizures or neurologic deficits.

glucagon A hormone produced by the pancreas that helps release stored glucose from the liver.

gluconeogenesis Formation of glycogen from noncarbohydrate sources such as protein or fat.

glycosuria Abnormal amount of glucose in the urine.

goiter Enlargement of the thyroid gland.

graft-versus-host disease A series of immunologic responses mounted by the host of a transplanted organ with the purpose of destroying the transplant cells.

growth An increase in physical size.

health supervision The process of health promotion services, growth and development monitoring, and disease and injury prevention throughout the child's life.

hemarthrosis Bleeding into joint spaces.

hematopoiesis Blood cell production.

hemodynamics Pressures generated by blood and passage of blood through the heart and pulmonary system.

hemoglobinopathy Disease characterized by abnormal hemoglobin.

hemosiderosis Increased storage of iron in body tissues; associated with diseases involving the destruction of red blood cells.

hernia Protrusion or projection of a body part or structure through the muscle wall of the cavity that normally contains it.

hormone A chemical substance produced by a gland or organ and carried in the bloodstream to another part of the body where it has a regulatory effect on particular cells.

hospice A philosophy of care that focuses on helping persons with short life expectancies to live their remaining lives to the fullest—without pain and with choices and dignity.

hydronephrosis Collection of urine in the renal pelvis as a result of obstructed outflow.

hypercapnia Greater than normal amounts of carbon dioxide in the blood.

hypersensitivity response An overreaction of the immune system, responsible for allergic reactions.

hypertonic fluid Fluid that is more concentrated than normal body fluid.

hypotonic fluid Fluid that is more dilute than normal body fluid.

hypoxemia Lower than normal amounts of oxygen in the blood.

hypoxia Lower than normal amounts of oxygen in the tissues.

immunodeficiency A state of the immune system in which it cannot cope effectively with foreign antigens.

immunoglobulin A protein that functions as an antibody. Immunoglobulins are responsible for humoral immunity.

inborn errors of metabolism Inherited biochemical abnormalities of the urea cycle and amino acid and organic acid metabolism.

indirect transmission The passage of an infectious disease involving survival of pathogens outside humans before they invade a new host.

Individualized Education Plan Formulation of a specific learning approach for a child with a physical or mental disability, following thorough assessment of the child's capabilities and areas of need.

infectious disease Illness, caused by a microorganism, that is commonly communicated from one host (human or otherwise) to another.

informed consent A formal preauthorization for an invasive procedure or participation in research.

inspection The technique of purposeful observation by carefully looking at the characteristics of the child's physical features and behaviors. Physical feature characteristics include size, shape, color, movement, position, and location.

interstitial fluid That portion of the extracellular fluid that is between the cells and outside the blood and lymphatic vessels.

intracellular fluid The fluid in the body that is inside the cells.

intracranial pressure Force exerted by brain tissue, cerebrospinal fluid, and blood within the cranial vault.

intravascular fluid That portion of the extracellular fluid that is in the blood vessels.

isotonic fluid Fluid that has the same osmolality as normal body fluid.

karyotype A microscopic display of the 46 chromosomes in the human body lined up from the largest to the smallest. The human female is 46,XX and the human male is 46,XY.

killed virus vaccine A vaccine that contains a killed microorganism that is still capable of inducing the human body to produce antibodies to the disease.

laryngospasm Spasmodic vibrations of the larynx, which create sudden, violent, unpredictable, involuntary contraction of airway muscles.

leukocytosis A higher than normal white cell count.

leukopenia A lower than normal white cell count.

level of consciousness General description of cognitive, sensory, and motor response to stimuli.

lichenification Thickening of the skin.

live virus vaccine A vaccine that contains the microorganism in a live but attenuated, or weakened, form.

malignant The progressive growth of a tumor that will, if not checked by treatment, result in death.

mature minors Adolescents of 14 and 15 years of age who are able to understand treatment risks and who in some states can consent to or refuse treatment.

medical home A primary care provider or regular source of health care.

medically fragile Children who need skilled nursing care with or without medical equipment to support vital functions.

menorrhagia Increased menstrual bleeding.

metastasis The spread of cancer cells to other sites in the body.

mixed hearing loss Hearing loss having a combination of conductive and sensorineural causes.

moral dilemma A conflict of social values and ethical principles that support different courses of action.

morbidity An illness or injury that limits activity, requires medical attention or hospitalization, or results in a chronic condition.

myelosuppression A decreased production of blood cells in the bone marrow.

myringotomy A procedure whereby an incision is made in the tympanic membrane to drain fluid.

nature The genetic or hereditary capability of an individual.

neoplasms Cancerous growths.

nonverbal behavior The use of facial expression, eye contact, touch, posture, gestures, and body movements that communicate feelings during a conversation.

nosocomial infection An infection acquired in a health care agency, not present at the time of entrance to the agency.

NSAIDs Nonsteroidal antiinflammatory drugs, used for the treatment of pain.

nurture The effects of environment on an individual's performance.

object permanence The knowledge that an object or person continues to exist when not seen, heard, or felt.

obtunded Diminished level of consciousness with limited response to the environment; the child falls asleep unless given verbal or tactile stimulation.

occult blood Blood that is present in minute quantities and can be seen only on microscopic examination or through chemical testing.

oliguria Diminished urine output (less than 0.5–1 mL/kg/hr).

oncogene A portion of the DNA that is altered and, when duplicated, causes uncontrolled cellular division.

oncotic pressure The part of the blood osmotic pressure that is due to plasma proteins; also called blood colloid osmotic pressure.

opioids Synthetic narcotic drugs used for the treatment of pain.

opportunistic infection An infection that is often caused by normally nonpathogenic organisms in persons who lack normal immunity.

osmolality The amount of concentration of a fluid; technically, the number of moles of particles per kilogram of water in the solution.

osmosis Movement of water across a semipermeable membrane into an area of higher particle concentration.

ossification Formation of bone from fibrous tissue or cartilage.

osteodystrophy Defective mineralization of bone caused by renal failure and chronic hyperphosphatemia.

osteotomy Surgical cutting of bone.

ostomy An artificial abdominal opening into the urinary or gastrointestinal canal that provides an outlet for the diversion of urine or fecal matter.

pain An unpleasant sensory and emotional experience associated with actual or potential tissue damage. Pain exists when the patient says it does.

palliative procedure Intervention used to preserve life in children with a potentially fatal or lethal condition.

palpation The technique of touch to identify characteristics of the skin, internal organs, and masses. Characteristics include texture, moistness, tenderness, temperature, position, shape, consistency, and mobility of masses and organs.

pancytopenia A decreased number of blood cell components.

paradoxical breathing Severe respiratory distress in which the chest falls and the abdomen rises on inspiration.

parallel play A type of play that emerges in toddlerhood when children play side by side with similar or different toys, demonstrating little or no social interaction.

passive immunity Immunity produced through introduction of specific antibodies to the disease, which are usually obtained from the blood or serum of immune persons and animals. *Does not confer lasting immunity.*

patient-controlled analgesia (PCA) A method for administering an intravenous analgesic, such as morphine, using a computerized pump that the patient controls.

percussion The technique of striking the surface of the body, either directly or indirectly, to set up vibrations that reveal the density of underlying tissues and borders of internal organs.

periodic breathing Pauses in respiration lasting less than 20 seconds; a normal breathing pattern in infancy and childhood.

peristalsis A progressive, wavelike muscular movement that occurs involuntarily throughout the gastrointestinal tract.

petechiae Pinpoint red lesions.

pH Negative logarithm of the hydrogen ion concentration; used to monitor the acidity of body fluid.

physical abuse The deliberate maltreatment of another individual that inflicts pain or injury and may result in permanent or temporary disfigurement or even death.

physical neglect The deliberate withholding of or failure to provide the necessary and available resources to a child.

physiologic anorexia A decrease in appetite manifested when the extremely high metabolic demands of infancy slow to keep pace with the more moderate growth rate of toddlerhood.

play therapy A therapeutic intervention often used with preschool and school-aged children. The child reveals conflicts, wishes, and fears on an unconscious level while playing with dolls, toys, clay, and other objects.

polycythemia Above-normal increase in the number of red cells in the blood to increase the amount of hemoglobin available to carry oxygen.

polydipsia Excessive thirst.

polyphagia Excessive or voracious eating.

polypharmacy The use of many drugs at one time to treat multiple health conditions.

polyuria Passage of a large volume of urine in a given period.

postictal period Period after seizure activity during which the level of consciousness is decreased.

posturing Abnormal position assumed after injury or damage to the brain that may be seen as extreme flexion or extension of the limbs.

preload Volume of blood in the ventricle at the end of diastole that stretches the heart muscle before contraction.

primary immune response The process in which B lymphocytes produce antibodies specific to a particular antigen on first exposure.

projectile vomiting Vomiting in which the stomach contents are ejected with great force.

protocol A plan of action for chemotherapy that is based on the type of cancer, its stage, and the particular cell type.

protooncogene A gene that regulates cellular growth and development but can become an oncogene, capable of causing cancerous growth.

proximodistal development The process by which development proceeds from the center of the body outward to the extremities.

pseudohermaphroditism Ambiguous development of the external genitalia.

pseudohypertrophy Enlargement of the muscles as a result of infiltration by fatty tissue.

puberty Period of life when the ability to reproduce sexually begins; characterized by maturation of the genital organs, development of the secondary sex characteristics, and (in females) the onset of menstruation.

pulmonary hypertension Condition resulting from a chronic blood volume overload through the pulmonary arteries. It is often irreversible and leads to a life-threatening increase in pulmonary vascular resistance.

purpura Bleeding into the tissues, particularly beneath the skin and mucous membranes, causing lesions that vary from red to purple.

quality assurance A process for monitoring the procedures and outcomes of care that uses indicators to measure compliance with standards of care.

quality improvement The continuous study and improvement of the processes and outcomes of providing health care services to meet the needs of patients by examining the system and processes of care and service delivery.

radiation Cancer treatment using unstable isotopes that release varying levels of energy to cause breaks in the DNA molecule and thereby destroy cells.

range of motion The direction and extent to which a particular joint is capable of moving, either independently or with assistance.

rehabilitation Assisting a child with physical or mental challenges to reach his or her fullest potential through therapy and education that considers the physiologic, psychologic, and environmental strengths and limitations of the child.

renal insufficiency Any degree of renal failure in which the kidneys' ability to conserve sodium and concentrate the urine decreases.

retractions A visible drawing in of the skin of the neck and chest, which occurs on inhalation in infants and young children in respiratory distress.

review of systems A comprehensive interview to identify and record the parent's or child's health concerns and health problems by body system; provides an overview of the child's health status.

risk management A process established by a health care institution to identify, evaluate, and reduce the risk of injury to patients, staff, and visitors and thereby reduce the institution's liability.

rooming in Practice in which parents stay in the child's hospital room and care for the child.

saline A mixture of salt and water; *normal saline* refers to the mixture of salt and water in equal concentration in body fluids.

screening tests Procedures used to detect the presence of a health condition before symptoms are apparent.

sensitive periods Times when an individual is especially responsive to certain environmental effects; sometimes called critical periods.

sensitivity Screening test value stated as the percentage of children testing positive for a condition who truly have that condition.

sensorineural hearing loss Hearing loss caused by damage to the inner ear structures or the auditory nerve.

separation anxiety Distress behaviors observed in young children separated from familiar caregivers.

shunt Movement of blood or body fluid through an abnormal anatomic or surgically created opening.

specificity Screening test value stated as the percentage of children testing negative for a condition who do not have that condition.

stent A device used to maintain patency of the urethral canal after surgery.

stereotypy Repetitive, obsessive, machinelike movements, commonly seen in autistic or schizophrenic children.

stranger anxiety Wariness of strange people and places, often shown by infants between 6 and 18 months of age.

stridor An abnormal, high-pitched musical respiratory sound caused when air moves through a narrowed larynx or trachea.

stupor Diminished level of consciousness with response only to vigorous stimulation.

subluxation Partial or complete dislocation of a joint.

support systems The extended network of family, friends, and religious and community contacts that provide nurturance, emotional support, and direct assistance to parents.

syncope Transient loss of consciousness and muscle tone.

tachypnea An abnormally rapid rate of respiration.

therapeutic play Planned play techniques that provide an opportunity for children to deal with their fears and concerns related to illness or hospitalization.

thrombocytopenia A lower than normal platelet count.

tolerance An altered state of response to an opioid or other pain agent in which increasing amounts of the drug are needed to produce or maintain the same level of pain relief.

tonic Continuous muscular contraction; often used to describe seizure activity.

toxoid A toxin that has been treated (by heat or chemical) to weaken its toxic effects but retain its antigenicity.

transplacental immunity Passive immunity that is transferred from mother to infant.

trigger A stimulus that initiates an asthmatic episode; a substance or condition, including exercise, infection, allergy, irritants, weather, or emotions.

tumor suppressor genes Genetic material that controls the growth of cells, decreasing the effects of oncogenes.

tympanogram A graph showing the ability of the middle ear to transmit sound energy; measured by inserting an airtight probe into the external ear entrance and emitting a tone.

tympanotomy tubes Small Teflon tubes inserted surgically into the tympanic membrane to equalize pressure, promote fluid drainage, and ventilate the middle ear.

uremia Toxicity resulting from the buildup of urea and nitrogenous waste in the blood.

varus A condition in which the hindfoot turns inward; usually associated with clubfoot.

vaso-occlusion Blockage of a blood vessel.

vesicoureteral reflux The backflow of urine from the bladder into the ureters during voiding.

vision A complex process of acquiring meaning from what is seen, involving the eye, brain, and related neurologic and physiologic structures.

visual acuity Measurement of the ability to discriminate a letter or other object used in testing sight.

INDEX

A

ABCs, in burn treatment, 933–934
Abdomen
    assessment of, 145–149, 608
    inspection of, 145–146
    movement during respiratory effort, 133, 146
    palpation of, 148–149
        cooperation of child during, 148
        deep, 148–149
        light, 148
        precautions for, with Wilms' tumors, 574
    percussion of, 147f, 147–148
    topographic landmarks of, 145, 146f
Abdominal mass, palpation of, 149, 574
Abdominal pain, recurrent, 973–974
Abdominal trauma, 651–652
    nursing management of, 652
Abducens nerve, assessment of, 166t
Abduction, 818f
Abuse
    child. See Child abuse
    definition of, 992
    diagnosis of, 996
    emotional, 953, 992–993, 1036
        clinical manifestations of, 995
        nursing diagnoses related to, 999
    and head injuries, 801
    physical, 953, 992–993, 994t, 1038
        clinical manifestations of, 995
        nursing diagnoses related to, 998–999
    sexual. See Sexual abuse
    substance. See Substance abuse
    verbal, 993
        clinical manifestations of, 995
Accident. See Injury(ies)
Accommodation, 27, 37, 1036
    pupillary response test for, 114
Accountability, 17
Acellular vaccine, 367, 1036
    pertussis, 370, 371t
Acetaminophen
    poisoning with, 653t
    recommended doses of, 278t
Acetyl coenzyme A, 885
Achilles reflex, assessment of, 170t
Acid-base balance, 324–327
    kidneys in, 327, 327f
    pediatric differences in, 290–293
    physiology of, 324–327
    respiratory system in, 326–327

Acid-base imbalances, 328–336
    mixed, 336
Acidemia, 289, 325, 1036
Acidosis, 289, 1036. See also Diabetic
        ketoacidosis; Metabolic acidosis;
        Respiratory acidosis
    definition of, 328
Acne, 917–919
    clinical manifestations of, 918, 918f
    comedonal, 918, 918t
    cystic, 918, 918t
    diagnosis of, 918
    epidemiology of, 917
    etiology of, 918
    medical management of, 918, 918t
    mild papular, 918t
    neonatal, 917
    nursing assessment for, 918–919
    nursing care plan for, 920t–921t
    nursing management of, 919
    papulopustular, 918, 918f, 918t
    pathophysiology of, 918
    pustulocystic, 918t
    types of, 918
Acoustic nerve, 165
    assessment of, 166t
Acquired immunity, 340
Acquired immunodeficiency syndrome
        (AIDS), 347–355
    clinical manifestations of, 347–348
    congenital, 48
    diagnosis of, 347–349
    discharge planning for, 354–355
    emotional support in, 354
    etiology of, 348
    home care teaching for, 354–355
    infection prevention in, 350, 351t
    medical management of, 346t, 348–349
    nursing assessment for, 349–350
    nursing care plan for, 351t–353t
    nursing diagnoses related to, 350,
        351t–353t
    nursing management of, 350–355
    nutritional support in, 354
    opportunistic infections in, 347–348
    pathophysiology of, 348
    pediatric
        deaths from, 347
        epidemiology of, 347
    viral agent of, 347, 347f. See also HIV
        (human immunodeficiency virus)
Activated charcoal, for poisoning, 654t

Active immunity, 367, 370, 1036
Activities. See also Play
    of adolescents, 85, 87, 87f
    for adolescents, during hospitalization,
        192–193, 193f
    of infants, 58t
    of preschool child, 76t
Acute lymphoblastic leukemia, 577f, 577–
        580. See also Leukemia(s)
    chemotherapy for, 578–579
Acute myelogenous leukemia, 577–580. See
        also Leukemia(s)
    chemotherapy for, 578–579
Acute pain, 265–266, 1036
Acute postinfectious glomerulonephritis,
        697–702
    clinical manifestations of, 698
    diagnosis of, 698–699
    discharge planning in, 702
    epidemiology of, 697–698
    etiology of, 698
    fluid balance in, 699–701
    home care teaching for, 702
    medical management of, 698–699
    nursing assessment for, 699
    nursing care plan for, 700t–701t
    nursing diagnoses related to, 700t–701t
    nursing management of, 699–702
    pathophysiology of, 698, 698f
    and streptococcal infection, 697–698
    urinalysis results in, 699
Acute renal failure, 680–686
    in adolescent, risk factors for, 680
    clinical manifestations of, 680–682, 681t
    complications of, drug therapy for, 683,
        683t
    diagnosis of, 682t, 683
    diet in, 686
    discharge planning for, 685–686
    drug-induced, 682
    electrolyte imbalances in, 680–682, 681t
    etiology of, 682
    home care teaching for, 685–686
    intrinsic, 682
    laboratory findings in, 682t
    medical management of, 683, 683t
    in newborn, risk factors for, 680
    nursing assessment for, 684
    nursing diagnoses related to, 684
    nursing management of, 685–686
    pathogenesis of, 680
    pathophysiology of, 682

F

G

O

► NANDA APPROVED NURSING DIAGNOSES

PATTERN 1: EXCHANGING

Altered Nutrition: More than Body Requirements
Altered Nutrition: Less than Body Requirements
Altered Nutrition: Risk for More than Body
  Requirements
Risk for Infection
Risk for Altered Body Temperature
Hypothermia
Hyperthermia
Ineffective Thermoregulation
Dysreflexia
Constipation
Perceived Constipation
Colonic Constipation
Diarrhea
Bowel Incontinence
Altered Urinary Elimination
Stress Incontinence
Reflex Incontinence
Urge Incontinence
Functional Incontinence
Total Incontinence
Urinary Retention
Altered (Specify Type) Tissue Perfusion (Renal,
  Cerebral, Cardiopulmonary, Gastrointestinal,
  Peripheral)
Fluid Volume Excess
Fluid Volume Deficit
Risk for Fluid Volume Deficit
Decreased Cardiac Output
Impaired Gas Exchange
Ineffective Airway Clearance
Ineffective Breathing Pattern
Inability to Sustain Spontaneous Ventilation
Dysfunctional Ventilatory Weaning Response (DVWR)
Risk for Injury
Risk for Suffocation
Risk for Poisoning
Risk for Trauma
Risk for Aspiration
Risk for Disuse Syndrome
Altered Protection
Impaired Tissue Integrity
Altered Oral Mucous Membrane
Impaired Skin Integrity
Risk for Impaired Skin Integrity
Decreased Adaptive Capacity: Intracranial
Energy Field Disturbance

PATTERN 2: COMMUNICATING

Impaired Verbal Communication

PATTERN 3: RELATING

Impaired Social Interaction
Social Isolation
Risk for Loneliness
Altered Role Performance
Altered Parenting
Risk for Altered Parent/Infant/Child Attachment
Sexual Dysfunction
Altered Family Processes
Caregiver Role Strain
Risk for Caregiver Role Strain
Altered Family Process: Alcoholism
Parental Role Conflict
Altered Sexuality Patterns

PATTERN 4: VALUING

Spiritual Distress (Distress of the Human Spirit)
Potential for Enhanced Spiritual Well-Being

PATTERN 5: CHOOSING

Ineffective Individual Coping
Impaired Adjustment
Defensive Coping
Ineffective Denial
Ineffective Family Coping: Disabling
Ineffective Family Coping: Compromised
Family Coping: Potential for Growth
Potential for Enhanced Community Coping
Ineffective Community Coping
Ineffective Management of Therapeutic Regimen
  (Individuals)
Noncompliance (Specify)
Ineffective Management of Therapeutic Regimen:
  Families
Ineffective Management of Therapeutic Regimen:
  Community
Effective Management of Therapeutic Regimen:
  Individual
Decisional Conflict (Specify)
Health-Seeking Behaviors (Specify)